HANDBOOK OF PEDIATRIC PSYCHOLOGY

The Society of Pediatric Psychology (Division 54 of the American Psychological Association) is pleased to sponsor the publication of this *Handbook*. Such sponsorship recognizes the scholarly significance of the volume and the care taken in the development of the chapters on scientific and professional issues. Topics were selected by experts in pediatric psychology, and recognized professionals in the field were solicited to contribute chapters. This was followed by an extensive peer review process for each chapter. This *Handbook* has not been considered by the Council of Representatives of the American Psychological Association, however, and does not represent official policy of the organization as a whole.

Handbook of Pediatric Psychology

FOURTH EDITION

Edited by

MICHAEL C. ROBERTS
RIC G. STEELE

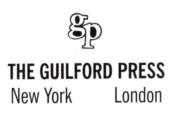

THE GUILFORD PRESS
New York   London

Library of Congress Cataloging-in-Publication Data

Handbook of pediatric psychology / edited by Michael C. Roberts.–4th ed. / Ric G. Steele.
   p. cm.
  Includes bibliographical references and index.
  ISBN 978-1-60623-328-3 (hardcover)
  1. Pediatrics—Psychological aspects. 2. Sick children—Psychology. I. Roberts,
Michael C.   II. Steele, Ric G.
  RJ47.5.H38 2009
  618.92—dc22

                                                          2009003750

*To the pioneers of pediatric psychology
and the founders of the Society of Pediatric Psychology—
those whose efforts and insights
propelled the field to where it is today*

About the Editors

Michael C. Roberts, PhD, ABPP, is Professor and Director of the Clinical Child Psychology Program at the University of Kansas. He holds academic appointments in the Departments of Psychology, Applied Behavioral Science, and Pediatrics. Dr. Roberts has published close to 200 journal articles and book chapters related to the application of psychology to understanding and influencing children's physical and mental health. He has authored or coedited 18 books. Currently the Editor of the American Psychological Association journal *Professional Psychology: Research and Practice*, Dr. Roberts has served as Editor for the *Journal of Pediatric Psychology*; *Children's Health Care*; and *Children's Services: Social Policy, Research, and Practice*. He has also served as Associate Editor for the *Journal of Consulting and Clinical Psychology*. Dr. Roberts is a recipient of the 2006 Award for Distinguished Contributions to Education and Training from the American Psychological Association and the 2008 Martin P. Levin Mentorship Award from the Society of Pediatric Psychology.

Ric G. Steele, PhD, ABPP, is Associate Professor in the Clinical Child Psychology Program at the University of Kansas. He is an Associate Editor for the *Journal of Child and Family Studies* and is on the editorial boards of the *Journal of Pediatric Psychology*, the *Journal of Clinical Child and Adolescent Psychology*, *Children's Health Care*, and *Professional Psychology: Research and Practice*. Dr. Steele has published more than 60 journal articles and book chapters and has coedited several handbooks related to health and mental health services for children and youth. His empirical research examines the promotion of physical and mental health across a continuum of health risk categories, with particular emphasis on the promotion of weight-related health.

Contributors

Natalie Walders Abramson, PhD, Division of Psychosocial Medicine, National Jewish Health, Denver, Colorado

F. Daniel Armstrong, PhD, Department of Pediatrics, Mailman Center for Child Development and Sylvester Comprehensive Cancer Center, University of Miami Miller School of Medicine, Miami, Florida; Holtz Children's Hospital at UM/Jackson Memorial Medical Center, Miami, Florida

Brandon S. Aylward, MA, Clinical Child Psychology Program, University of Kansas, Lawrence, Kansas

Glen P. Aylward, PhD, ABPP, Division of Developmental and Behavioral Pediatrics/Psychology, Southern Illinois University School of Medicine, Springfield, Illinois

Gerard A. Banez, PhD, Pediatric Pain Rehabilitation Program, Cleveland Clinic Children's Hospital, Cleveland, Ohio

Lamia P. Barakat, PhD, Department of Pediatrics, University of Pennsylvania School of Medicine and The Children's Hospital of Philadelphia, Philadelphia, Pennsylvania

David H. Barker, MS, Department of Psychology, University of Miami, Coral Gables, Florida

Amy E. Baughcum, PhD, Department of Pediatrics, The Ohio State University, and Department of Psychology, Nationwide Children's Hospital, Columbus, Ohio

Jade A. Bender, MA, Clinical Child Psychology Program, University of Kansas, Lawrence, Kansas

Ronald L. Blount, PhD, Department of Psychology, University of Georgia, Athens, Georgia

Barbara L. Bonner, PhD, Center on Child Abuse and Neglect and Child Study Center, Department of Pediatrics, University of Oklahoma Health Sciences Center, Oklahoma City, Oklahoma

Stephen M. Borowitz, MD, Department of Pediatrics, University of Virginia Health Sciences Center, Charlottesville, Virginia

Glendaliz Bosques, MD, Division of Physical Medicine and Rehabilitation, Department of Pediatrics, Cincinnati Children's Hospital Medical Center, University of Cincinnati College of Medicine, Cincinnati, Ohio

Ronald T. Brown, PhD, ABPP, Department of Public Health, Temple University, Philadelphia, Pennsylvania

Keri J. Brown Kirschman, PhD, Department of Psychology, University of Dayton, Dayton, Ohio

Donald Brunnquell, PhD, Office of Ethics, Children's Hospitals and Clinics of Minnesota, Minneapolis and St. Paul, Minnesota

Lisa M. Buckloh, PhD, Division of Psychology and Psychiatry, Nemours Children's Clinic, Jacksonville, Florida

Jonathan M. Campbell, PhD, Department of Educational Psychology, University of Georgia, Athens, Georgia

Laura K. Campbell, PhD, Department of Behavioral Medicine, University of Virginia Health Sciences Center, Charlottesville, Virginia

Johanna L. Carpenter, MA, Department of Psychology, Temple University, Philadelphia, Pennsylvania

Bryan D. Carter, PhD, Division of Child, Adolescent, and Family Psychiatry, Departments of Psychiatry and Pediatrics, University of Louisville School of Medicine, Kosair Children's Hospital, Louisville, Kentucky

Edward R. Christophersen, PhD, ABPP, Section of Developmental and Behavioral Sciences, Children's Mercy Hospitals and Clinics, Kansas City, Missouri

Daniel L. Clay, PhD, College of Education, Auburn University, Auburn, Alabama

Jeremy S. Cohen, MA, Department of Psychology, Temple University, Philadelphia, Pennsylvania

Lindsey L. Cohen, PhD, Department of Psychology, Georgia State University, Atlanta, Georgia

Daniel J. Cox, PhD, ABPP, Department of Behavioral Medicine, University of Virginia Health Sciences Center, Charlottesville, Virginia

Carin L. Cunningham, PhD, Department of Pediatrics, Case Western Reserve School of Medicine, Cleveland, Ohio

Lynnda M. Dahlquist, PhD, Department of Psychology, University of Maryland Baltimore County, Baltimore, Maryland

Brian P. Daly, PhD, Department of Public Health, Temple University, Philadelphia, Pennsylvania

Lauren C. Daniel, MS, Department of Psychology, Drexel University, Philadelphia, Pennsylvania

Kathleen K. M. Deidrick, PhD, Thompson Center for Autism and Neurodevelopmental Disorders, University of Missouri, Columbia, Missouri

Alan M. Delamater, PhD, ABPP, Department of Pediatrics, University of Miami Miller School of Medicine, Miami, Florida

Katie A. Devine, PhD, Department of Psychology, Loyola University Chicago, Chicago, Illinois

Aila K. Dommestrup, BA, Department of Educational Psychology, University of Georgia, Athens, Georgia

Angela Celio Doyle, PhD, Department of Psychiatry and Behavioral Neuroscience, University of Chicago, Chicago, Illinois

George J. DuPaul, PhD, Department of Education and Human Services, Lehigh University, Bethlehem, Pennsylvania

Michelle M. Ernst, PhD, Division of Behavioral Medicine and Clinical Psychology, Department of Pediatrics, Cincinnati Children's Hospital Medical Center, University of Cincinnati College of Medicine, Cincinnati, Ohio

Subhadra Evans, PhD, Pediatric Pain Program, University of California Los Angeles, Los Angeles, California

Janet E. Farmer, PhD, Thompson Center for Autism and Neurodevelopmental Disorders, University of Missouri, Columbia, Missouri

Bernard F. Fuemmeler, PhD, MPH, Department of Community and Family Medicine, Duke University Medical Center, Durham, North Carolina

Cynthia A. Gerhardt, PhD, Center for Biobehavioral Health, The Research Institute at Nationwide Children's Hospital, and Departments of Pediatrics and Psychology, The Ohio State University, Columbus, Ohio

Stephen R. Gillaspy, PhD, Department of Pediatrics, University of Oklahoma Health Sciences Center, Oklahoma City, Oklahoma

Montserrat M. Graves, PhD, Clinical Child Psychology Program, University of Kansas, Lawrence, Kansas

Peggy Greco, PhD, Division of Psychology and Psychiatry, Nemours Children's Clinic, Jacksonville, Florida

Mary E. Grimley, MS, Department of Psychology, University of Miami, Coral Gables, Florida

Maureen O. Grissom, PhD, Thompson Center for Autism and Neurodevelopmental Disorders, University of Missouri, Columbia, Missouri

Chantelle N. Hart, PhD, Department of Psychiatry and Human Behavior, Warren Alpert Medical School, Brown University, Providence, Rhode Island

Lauren Herlihy, BS, Yale Child Study Center, Yale University, New Haven, Connecticut

Grayson N. Holmbeck, PhD, Department of Psychology, Loyola University, Chicago, Illinois

Tiina Jaaniste, MPsychol, Department of Pain Medicine, Sydney Children's Hospital, Randwick, New South Wales, Australia

Elissa Jelalian, PhD, Department of Psychiatry and Human Behavior, Alpert Medical School, Brown University, Providence, Rhode Island

Jason F. Jent, PhD, Department of Pediatrics, University of Miami Miller School of Medicine, Miami, Florida

Cynthia Karlson, MA, Department of Pediatrics, University of Kansas Medical Center, Kansas City, Kansas

Nancy Kassam-Adams, PhD, Center for Injury Research and Prevention, The Children's Hospital of Philadelphia, Philadelphia, Pennsylvania

Anne E. Kazak, PhD, ABPP, The Children's Hospital of Philadelphia, Philadelphia, Pennsylvania

William G. Kronenberger, PhD, Division of Child and Adolescent Psychiatry, Department of Psychiatry, Riley Hospital for Children, Indiana University School of Medicine, Indianapolis, Indiana

Annette M. La Greca, PhD, ABPP, Departments of Psychology and Pediatrics, University of Miami, Coral Gables, Florida

Hannah G. Lawman, BS, Department of Psychology, Barnwell College, University of South Carolina, Columbia, South Carolina

Daniel le Grange, PhD, Department of Psychiatry and Behavioral Neuroscience, University of Chicago, Chicago, Illinois

Kathleen L. Lemanek, PhD, Department of Pediatrics, The Ohio State University College of Medicine and Department of Psychology, Nationwide Children's Hospital, Columbus, Ohio

Carol B. Lindsley, MD, Department of Pediatrics, University of Kansas Medical Center, Kansas City, Kansas

Eleanor Race Mackey, PhD, Department of Psychiatry, Children's National Medical Center, Washington, DC

Kristen K. Marciel, PhD, Departments of Psychology and Pediatrics, University of Miami, Coral Gables, Florida

Sunnye Mayes, PhD, Department of Pediatrics, University of Oklahoma Health Sciences Center, Oklahoma City, Oklahoma

Katie McGoron, BS, Department of Psychology, Loyola University, Chicago, Illinois

Elizabeth L. McQuaid, PhD, Department of Psychiatry and Human Behavior, Warren Alpert Medical School, Brown University, Providence, Rhode Island

Lisa J. Meltzer, PhD, Division of Pulmonary Medicine, The Children's Hospital of Philadelphia, University of Pennsylvania School of Medicine, Philadelphia, Pennsylvania

Jodi A. Mindell, PhD, Department of Psychology, Saint Joseph's University, Philadelphia, Pennsylvania

Lindsay Moriarty, BA, Department of Community and Family Medicine, Duke University Medical Center, Durham, North Carolina

Marni Switkin Nagel, PhD, Department of Pediatric Psychology, Children's Hospital of Orange County, Orange, California

Neha Navsaria, PhD, The Children's Hospital of Philadelphia, Philadelphia, Pennsylvania

Timothy D. Nelson, PhD, Department of Psychology, University of Nebraska, Lincoln, Nebraska

Robert B. Noll, PhD, Department of Pediatrics, Child Development Unit, University of Pittsburgh Medical Center, Pittsburgh, Pennsylvania

Lisa Opipari-Arrigan, PhD, Department of Pediatrics and Communicable Diseases, University of Michigan Medical School, Ann Arbor, Michigan

Tonya M. Palermo, PhD, Department of Anesthesiology and Peri-Operative Medicine, Oregon Health and Science University, Portland, Oregon

Jennifer Shroff Pendley, PhD, Department of Pediatrics, Division of Behavioral Health, A. I. duPont Hospital for Children, Wilmington, Delaware

Michael S. Perciful, BA, Department of Psychology, University of Dayton, Dayton, Ohio

Ellen C. Perrin, MD, Division of Developmental–Behavioral Pediatrics, The Floating Hospital for Children and Tufts Medical Center, Boston, Massachusetts

Thomas J. Power, PhD, Department of Pediatrics, The Children's Hospital of Philadelphia, University of Pennsylvania School of Medicine, Philadelphia, Pennsylvania

Elizabeth R. Pulgaron, MA, Department of Psychology, Drexel University, Philadelphia, Pennsylvania

Alexandra L. Quittner, PhD, Departments of Psychology and Pediatrics, University of Miami, Coral Gables, Florida

William A. Rae, PhD, Department of Educational Psychology, Texas A&M University, College Station, Texas

Lisa Ramirez, MA, Department of Psychology, Case Western Reserve University, Cleveland, Ohio

Mark Ranalli, MD, Department of Pediatrics, The Ohio State University College of Medicine and Division of Hematology/Oncology/BMT, Nationwide Children's Hospital, Columbus, Ohio

Michael A. Rapoff, PhD, Department of Pediatrics, University of Kansas Medical Center, Kansas City, Kansas

Jennifer Reiter-Purtill, PhD, Division of Behavioral Medicine and Clinical Psychology, Cincinnati Children's Hospital Medical Center, Cincinnati, Ohio

Michael C. Roberts, PhD, ABPP, Clinical Child Psychology Program, University of Kansas, Lawrence, Kansas

James R. Rodrigue, PhD, The Transplant Institute, Beth Israel Deaconess Medical Center, and Department of Psychiatry, Harvard Medical School, Boston, Massachusetts

Susan L. Rosenthal, PhD, Department of Pediatrics, Children's Hospital South and Departments of Pediatrics and Psychology, Columbia University, New York, New York

Mary T. Rourke, PhD, The Children's Hospital of Philadelphia, Philadelphia, Pennsylvania

Kimberlee M. Roy, PhD, Department of Pediatrics, Primary Children's Medical Center, University of Utah School of Medicine, Salt Lake City, Utah

Christina G. Salley, MA, Center for Biobehavioral Health, The Research Institute at Nationwide Children's Hospital, and Department of Psychology, The Ohio State University, Columbus, Ohio

Stephanie Schneider, MS, The Children's Hospital of Philadelphia, Philadelphia, Pennsylvania

Eric Scott, PhD, Division of Child and Adolescent Psychiatry, Department of Psychiatry, Riley Hospital for Children, Indiana University School of Medicine, Indianapolis, Indiana

Matthew J. Segall, MA, Department of Educational Psychology, University of Georgia, Athens, Georgia

Michael Seid, PhD, Divisions of Pulmonary Medicine and Health Policy and Clinical Effectiveness, Cincinnati Children's Hospital Medical Center, Cincinnati, Ohio

Edward S. Shapiro, PhD, Department of Education and Human Services, Lehigh University, Bethlehem, Pennsylvania

Mary B. Short, PhD, Department of Psychology, University of Houston–Clear Lake, Houston, Texas

Alan H. Silverman, PhD, Department of Pediatric Gastroenterology and Nutrition, Medical College of Wisconsin, Milwaukee, Wisconsin

Elisa J. Sobo, PhD, Department of Anthropology, San Diego State University, San Diego, California

Mikle South, PhD, Department of Psychology, Brigham Young University, Provo, Utah

Terry Stancin, PhD, Division of Pediatric Psychology, MetroHealth Medical Center, Case Western Reserve University, Cleveland, Ohio

Ric G. Steele, PhD, ABPP, Clinical Child Psychology Program, University of Kansas, Lawrence, Kansas

Meredith Lutz Stehl, PhD, Department of Pediatrics, Division of Behavioral Health, A. I. duPont Hospital for Children, Wilmington, Delaware

Lynne Sturm, PhD, Department of Pediatrics, Riley Child Development Center, Indiana University School of Medicine, Indianapolis, Indiana

Jeremy R. Sullivan, PhD, Department of Educational Psychology, University of Texas at San Antonio, San Antonio, Texas

Sally Tarbell, PhD, Pediatric Gastroenterology and Nutrition, Medical College of Wisconsin, Milwaukee, Wisconsin

Kenneth J. Tarnowski, PhD, ABPP, Psychology Program, Florida Gulf Coast University, Fort Myers, Florida

Kenneth P. Tercyak, PhD, Lombardi Comprehensive Cancer Center, Georgetown University Medical Center, Washington, DC

William Douglas Tynan, PhD, ABPP, Center for Children's Health Innovation, Nemours Health and Prevention Services, Newark, Delaware

Kathryn Vannatta, PhD, Center for Biobehavioral Health, The Research Institute at Nationwide Children's Hospital, and Departments of Pediatrics and Psychology, The Ohio State University, Columbus, Ohio

Susan M. VanScoyoc, PhD, ABPP, College of Arts and Sciences, University of Phoenix, Phoenix, Arizona

Shari L. Wade, PhD, Division of Physical Medicine and Rehabilitation, Department of Pediatrics, Cincinnati Children's Hospital Medical Center, University of Cincinnati College of Medicine, Cincinnati, Ohio

Jennifer M. Waller, BA, Department of Psychology, University of Pittsburgh, Pittsburgh, Pennsylvania

Nicolay Chertkoff Walz, PhD, Division of Behavioral Medicine and Clinical Psychology, Department of Pediatrics, Cincinnati Children's Hospital Medical Center, University of Cincinnati College of Medicine, Cincinnati, Ohio

Anna C. Wilson, PhD, Department of Anesthesiology and Peri-Operative Medicine, Oregon Health and Science University, Portland, Oregon

Dawn K. Wilson, PhD, Department of Psychology, Barnwell College, University of South Carolina, Columbia, South Carolina

Julie Wolf, PhD, Child Study Center, Yale University School of Medicine, New Haven, Connecticut

Yelena P. Wu, MA, Clinical Child Psychology Program, University of Kansas, Lawrence, Kansas

Tim Wysocki, PhD, ABPP, Center for Pediatric Psychology Research, Nemours Children's Clinic, Jacksonville, Florida

Tammi Young-Saleme, PhD, Department of Psychology, Nationwide Children's Hospital, and Department of Pediatrics, The Ohio State University, Columbus, Ohio

Kathy Zebracki, PhD, Department of Psychology, Loyola University Chicago, Chicago, Illinois

Nataliya Zelikovsky, PhD, Department of Pediatrics, Division of Nephrology, The Children's Hospital of Philadelphia, University of Pennsylvania, Philadelphia, Pennsylvania

Lonnie K. Zeltzer, MD, Pediatric Pain Program, Mattel Children's Hospital, University of California Los Angeles, Los Angeles, California

William T. Zempsky, MD, Division of Pain Medicine, Department of Pediatrics, Connecticut Children's Medical Center, Hartford, Connecticut

Gregory D. Zimet, PhD, Department of Pediatrics, Section of Adolescent Medicine, Indiana University School of Medicine, Indianapolis, Indiana

Preface

Pediatric psychology as a single phrase is—at best—an incomplete label for a diversity of activities and interests at the intersection of pediatric medicine and applied child psychology, with unique contributions to understanding and clinical service of children, adolescents, and their families. In its American incarnation, pediatric psychology points to the developmental years of the 1960s and 1970s as critical to the formalization of concepts, research, and clinical applications of psychology to pediatric problems. With the more formal milestones of the formation of the Society of Pediatric Psychology in 1969 by the first committee of Dorothea Ross, Lee Salk, and Logan Wright, and a pivotal article in *American Psychologist* by Logan Wright in 1967, the foundations of today's field were laid. We offer this *Handbook* as evidence that the development of pediatric psychology as a field of research and practice has been dramatic and sustained.

The field did not just appear when we as individual pediatric psychologists became cognizant of it; past work by a number of brilliant predecessors laid the groundwork for clinical science and scientific applications at the interface of psychology and pediatrics. Although this volume is an indication of the advances in the field, the topics, to a large degree, are very similar to the primary issues in pediatric psychology at its founding and throughout its existence. Of course, pediatric psychology is not just an American invention, but an international idea of investigation and application of concepts.

As can be seen in these pages, the conceptualizations, research, and practice activities that were present at the founding of the field are here, as are the expansions built on the scientist-practitioner model that epitomized the years of progression to convey a vital and developing clinical profession built on clinical science. Notably, as a reflection of the field, this fourth edition builds on the foundations of the first three editions (Roberts, 1995, 2003; Routh, 1988), while adding some new concepts and topics (and a coeditor). The additions indicate the field is evolving while retaining many of its traditional elements (if a field that is 40 years old can be considered old enough to have traditions).

At the outset of this edition, we requested the assistance of an Advisory Panel of experts for their input on retention or deletion of topics, as well as questions about organization. Although the field continues to evolve with new topics of interest and activities, we find it intriguing that most of the issues remain ubiquitous as they were early in the field's development and in previous editions, even as the technologies and methodologies used to address the topics have changed over time. Once again, these panelists viewed the field from the perspectives of their particular interests, and often recommended changes to the *Handbook* that might have diminished other panelists' primary interests. These sometimes conflicting views of the field were not competitive recommendations, but more a reflection of each panel member's own activities and what he or she values about the field. As we developed the *Handbook*'s outline of topics, we attempted to be open-minded and inclusive of our pediatric psychology colleagues' range of activities and interests. Our task was to combine these various inputs to cover the full range of pediatric psychology, ever mindful of the page restrictions within a single volume for chapters on whose topics entire books have been published. Although we have tried to make it comprehensive, this *Handbook* cannot be exhaustive. Because of the space requirements, our authors could not include everything they would have liked to include (although several very clever authors did attempt to disguise overlength manuscripts by changing font size, spacing, and margins!). We asked the authors not to comment on the lack of space to cover their topic fully, because all authors had these restrictions, and the comment itself took up space. We greatly appreciate the diligence, insight, and scholarship of these chapter authors, as they represent those who have contributed to the development of the field and present significant information for science and practice.

This *Handbook* is a peer-reviewed publication of the Society of Pediatric Psychology. The reviewers are acknowledged in the list of the Board of Editors. All chapters were reviewed by professional-level psychologists who are experts on the topics, and by graduate students from the Clinical Child Psychology Program at the University of Kansas, in addition to our (the editors') own reviewing and editing. We acknowledge the contributions of these editorial consultants in improving the quality of the *Handbook* and making it worthy of the imprimatur of the Society of Pediatric Psychology. We also appreciate the contributions of Brandon S. Aylward and Yelena P. Wu as editorial assistants in the preparation of the volume, from conceptualization to final packaging.

The first edition of the *Handbook* was dedicated to Logan Wright, who passed away in 1999 and will be remembered for his contributions in founding the field of pediatric psychology and for early research and professional writings (Willis, 2000). The second edition was dedicated as a living memorial to Donald K. Routh, who edited the first edition and was an early editor of the *Journal of Pediatric Psychology*, in addition to his important work in developing the Society and the field. The third edition was dedicated to honor both Don Routh and Lizette Peterson-Homer, who died in 2002. Lizette made significant contributions to the scientific base of pediatric psychology through her theoretical conceptualizations and empirical research in a variety of topics (Roberts, 2002).

We dedicate this edition to the pioneers of pediatric psychology in research, scholarship, and clinical mentorship, and to the founders of the Society of Pediatric Psychology in its first 10–15 years. In doing so, we recognize that without their creative and organizational efforts and insights, the field of pediatric psychology and the Society would be very different or nonexistent. We hesitate to list specific pioneers at this point, lest we neglect one or more important professional. In presenting this volume, we recognize those who found ways to fund the development and maintenance of the Society in its early years despite financial troubles, and who often encountered resistance to the new contributions of pediatric psychologists in research and practice. We gratefully acknowledge those whose ideas and seminal work as psychological researchers and practitioners of pediatric psychology shaped the development of the vibrant field we can appreciate today.

MICHAEL C. ROBERTS
RIC G. STEELE

References

Roberts, M. C. (Ed.). (1995). *Handbook of pediatric psychology* (2nd ed.). New York: Guilford Press.

Roberts, M. C. (2002). The legacy of Lizette Peterson-Homer in pediatric psychology (1951–2002). *Journal of Pediatric Psychology, 27,* 765–769.

Roberts, M. C. (Ed.). (2003). *Handbook of pediatric psychology* (3rd ed.). New York: Guilford Press.

Routh, D. K. (Ed.). (1988). *Handbook of pediatric psychology.* New York: Guilford Press.

Willis, D. J. (2000). In memoriam: Logan Wright, Jr., PhD (1933–1999). *Journal of Pediatric Psychology, 25,* 359–361.

Contents

PART III. MEDICAL, DEVELOPMENTAL, BEHAVIORAL, AND COGNITIVE-AFFECTIVE CONDITIONS

PART IV. PUBLIC HEALTH ISSUES

PART V. SYSTEMS

PART VI. EMERGING ISSUES

PART I

Professional Issues

CHAPTER 1

Historical Developments and Trends in Pediatric Psychology

BRANDON S. AYLWARD
JADE A. BENDER
MONTSERRAT M. GRAVES
MICHAEL C. ROBERTS

As reflected in its official definition, pediatric psychology is a multifaceted and integrated field of both scientific research and clinical practice that focuses on addressing a wide range of physical and psychological issues related to promoting the health and development of children, adolescents, and their families, with an emphasis on evidence-based methods. These health-related issues are considered by pediatric psychologists within a developmental context and reflect a systems-oriented approach to examining the multitude of factors that can affect children and their families (see Steele & Aylward, Chapter 43, this volume). The dynamic field of pediatric psychology developed to address unmet needs for psychological services in the pediatric setting, and the field represents the confluence of development within several areas of psychology (Roberts, Maddux, Wurtele, & Wright, 1982). Although the mission of pediatric psychology has always been interdisciplinary, the field's official vision statement was amended in 2006 to include the following statement: "Founded in 1969, the field has broad interdisciplinary theoretical underpinnings and draws from clinical, developmental, social, cognitive, behavioral, counseling, community and school psychology" (Society of Pediatric Psychology, n.d.). This development did not occur overnight; it has emerged over time, and the field has had remarkable growth since its early conception (Roberts, 1986, 1993). Ultimately, the recurrent as well as emerging issues that help both define the field and shape the future of pediatric psychology are worth a "look in the mirror" (Kronenberger, 2006).

History of Pediatric Psychology

Conceptual Origins

The beginnings of pediatric psychology can be linked to the late 19th century, when Lightner Witmer established the first psychological clinic in the United States. Resembling some of the current work in the field, Witmer interacted with both pediatricians and schools to help children with general and pediatric-related problems, served on the editorial board of a pediatric journal, and published case studies describing interventions for pediatric-related cases (Routh, 1975, 1990). Early in the 20th century, several psychologists and pediatricians began to perceive the importance of recognizing the link between psychology and medicine. For example, Arnold Gesell bridged the fields of pediatrics and psychology by earning both a PhD in psychology and an MD, combining the two disciplines into a "single skull" (Routh, 1990). Gesell was also one of the first to discuss the need for clinical psychologists to address the psychological issues of children in medical settings (Gesell, 1919). For example, as the scope of practice in pediatrics broadened in the early to mid-1900s to include physical growth and child development, Gesell (1926) highlighted the need for psychological norms "to lay down for various ages of infancy and childhood certain concrete minimum essentials of normal health expressed in tangible behavior terms" (p. 48). The potential benefits of collaboration between clinical psychologists and pediatricians were reiterated by J. E. Anderson (1930) in an address to the American Medical Association. In particular, he noted the potential benefits of collaboration, particularly with regard to child assessments and advice for parents about child rearing.

However, little collaboration seems to have resulted from these presentations. Furthermore, although the early descriptions of potential collaborative efforts were written primarily by pediatricians, some pediatricians were not as open to collaboration with other professions. For example, Brennemann (1933) was wary of the emphasis on child development; he termed psychologists, as well as psychiatrists, "child guiders" who would cause unnecessary parental worry regarding their child's development and behavior.

Early Teaching and Training

In the early 1900s, there was a significant rise in the scientific standards of medical instruction in the United States. This development was associated with a 1910 report by Abraham Flexner, which was sponsored by the Carnegie Foundation to improve medical education and practice (Moll, 1968). This rise in scientific standards for medicine was presumably a factor in the establishment of the 1911 American Psychological Association (APA) Committee on the Relations between Psychology and Medical Education. This committee served as one of the earliest efforts in collaborative teaching (Fernberger, 1932; Routh, 1975). In addition, articles highlighting the need for psychological training in pediatrics to address patients with such issues as behavioral, speech, hearing, or developmental delays were published in the 1930s and 1940s (e.g., Caecae, 1936; Rubin-Rabson, 1948). Although a survey of medical students and faculty by the APA Committee revealed that many recognized the potential benefits of general psychology and clinical psychology, and recommended adding related courses to medical education, no formal action was taken for some time (Routh, 1975).

In the early 1940s, fewer than 12 medical schools had a psychologist as a faculty member (Mensh, 1953). However, after World War II, a significant increase occurred in the number of psychologists working in medical school departments. For example, Matarazzo and Daniel (1957) reported that in 1955, about four psychologists, on average, were listed on medical school faculties (for additional reviews, see Buck, 1961; Routh, 1970). Although some clinical psychologists had completed practica or internships in children's hospitals, none of these medical school positions had been formally identified as "pediatric psychology" (Routh, 1975).

Despite the early recognition of the benefits of a working relationship between pediatrics and psychology, progress toward more collaboration did not occur until the mid-1960s. At about this time, pediatricians were being faced with a large number of problems in development, behavior, education, and child management when treating patients in their clinics (McClelland, Staples, Weisberg, & Berger, 1973). For example, Duff, Rowe, and Anderson (1973) found that only 12% of all patients in a pediatric practice presented with purely physical problems, whereas 36% had primarily psychological issues, and 52% had issues that were both physical and psychological in nature. Thus, as pediatrician Richmond (1967) highlighted, pediatrics was in need of an expansion and application of knowledge in child development. Similarly, psychologists later discovered that clients and their families who had medically related problems continued not having their needs met by traditional office or outpatient psychology clinics (summarized by Roberts, Mitchell, & McNeal, 2003). Ultimately, both groups of professionals found that they could not meet the challenges of critical childhood problems within their traditional frameworks. Thus the growing need for collaboration between psychology and medicine was becoming apparent (Roberts, 1986).

In response to these ongoing needs, developmental psychologist and researcher Jerome Kagan (1965) called for a "new marriage" between psychology and pediatrics. Kagan specifically described the role a psychologist might play in a pediatric setting, and outlined areas in which collaboration would be most fruitful in the decade ahead. Some of his suggested benefits included early detection of severe psychopathology and psychosocial problems, as well as the study of the relationship between prenatal and perinatal factors to psychological problems (Kagan, 1965). Kagan's article was published in the *American Journal of Diseases of Children*, and unlike Anderson's (1930) more general treatise, it "struck a responsive chord among professional clinical psychologists" (Routh, 1975, p. 7). Kagan was bold in his assertions; he stated the benefits of direct observation of psychopathology and developmental issues for psychologists, and the opportunity to utilize research inquiry to examine the etiology of symptoms for pediatricians (Drotar, 1995). However, as Mesibov (1984) suggested, Kagan viewed the role of the psychologist in pediatrics as research-oriented, and he seems to have underestimated the applied, direct service role within medical settings that would be required of psychologists. Moreover, not everyone was in agreement with the proposed "marriage" between psychologists and pediatricians. For instance, Cushna (1968) suggested that such a union might produce "immature interspecies mules" (p. 288).

Despite these challenges, development in the field moved forward, and the term "pediatric psychology" was first coined by Logan Wright in 1967 in an article entitled "The Pediatric Psychologist: A Role Model." This work was pivotal in the early conceptualization and vitalization of the field (Roberts, 1993). Wright defined pediatric psychology as "dealing primarily with children in a medical setting which is nonpsychiatric in nature" (1967, p. 323). Central to optimal collaboration, Wright (1967) urged psychologists to understand the requirements of pediatric practice and, furthermore, to develop and utilize both assessment and prevention treatments that best fit with the setting. This description of the role of the pediatric psychologist was consistent with Kagan's marriage metaphor between the two disciplines (Drotar, 1995); however, Wright was the first to recognize the important clinical role of pediatric psychologists in the medical setting (Mesibov, 1984). To further ensure the future of pediatric psychology, Wright called for (1) a group identity for the field through a formal organization and distribution of a newsletter, (2) more specific training for future pediatric psychologists, and (3) an accumulation of a body of knowledge though applied research. Following these recommendations ultimately led to concrete developments within the field and the emergence of the field of pediatric psychology as a distinct area in psychology (Roberts, 1993).

Organizational Developments

One of Wright's perceived needs for the field of pediatric psychology was a group identity through a formal organization within the APA. This group identity was primarily formed through the Society of Pediatric Psychology (SPP), which began as an interest group within Section I (Clinical Child Psychology) of the APA Division of Clinical Psychology and focused on the delivery of psychological services to children in medical settings and research in child health psychology (Routh, 1994). In 1967, the president of the APA Division of Clinical Psychology, George Albee, suggested that the Section on Clinical Child Psychology evaluate the increasing role of psychologists in pediatric settings and the potential for the organization of a special interest group. The outgoing and incoming presidents of this section then assembled a committee on pediatric psychology consisting of Logan Wright (chair), Dorothea Ross, and Lee Salk. This committee sent letters to the chairs of pediatrics departments in all the medical schools in the United States asking for the names of psychologists on their staff. In response to this inquiry, over 250 names were identified of psychologists interested in a society for addressing the needs of pediatric psychologists. This group formed the basis for the interest group in pediatric psychology, out of which SPP was formed in August 1968, as an affiliate of the Section of Clinical Child Psychology. The majority of the initial members was recruited from university medical schools; however, as the society developed, individuals from such settings as community hospitals and pediatric group practices also became involved (Routh, 1994).

   At the Executive Committee meeting in December 1974, SPP was defined as a group whose purpose is "to exchange information on clinical procedures and research and to define training standards for the pediatric psychologist" (Kenny, 1975, p. 8). The early members of the SPP were mostly faculty members in pediatric departments. Given the research-based nature of these positions, the increase in research in the field was to be expected (Routh, 1982). The first newsletter of the society, *Pediatric Psychology*, was organized by Lee Salk in 1968 and edited by G. Gail Gardner. The first newsletter issue was distributed in March 1969, and later issues provided an outlet to distribute research and practice related to the field of pediatric psychology. Eventually this newsletter was transformed into the *Journal of Pediatric Psychology* (*JPP*) in 1976 by the founding editor, Diane J. Willis; this, according to Roberts and colleagues (1982), solidified SPP's foundation and established the field as "a truly scientific and professional enterprise" (p. 198).

On October 1, 1980, the SPP became a regular section within the APA Division of Clinical Psychology (Section 5). Due to the increasing identity of the field as a separate area within psychology, SPP formally assumed independent status as a separate division in 2000 as Division 54 of the APA. Today the society is vibrant and continues to be involved in such activities as forming important task forces on issues in the field, testifying before the U.S. Senate, developing liaisons with other academies and societies (e.g., the American Academy of Pediatrics [AAP] and the Society of Developmental and Behavioral Pediatrics [SDBP]), publishing professional texts, and sponsoring regional and national conferences, as well as programming events at the APA conventions (see also Roberts, 1993; Routh, 1994).

SPP originally consisted of 75 full members and 22 affiliate members. Today, these membership numbers have increased dramatically, with 1,818 members across all categories. The society faced some financial hardships in its early years (see Routh, 1994). Yet, in his presidential message early in SPP's existence, Mesibov (1984) highlighted the society's increased strength, noting the increase in memberships, financial stability, and respectability of the flagship journal, as well as acceptance of the field itself. These trends continue in the present day, and SPP serves as the formal organization by which the field of pediatric psychology continues to prosper. Furthermore, SPP maintains relationships with the AAP and SDBP, as well as other related organizations (see Armstrong, Chapter 52, this volume).

Research in Pediatric Psychology

In his seminal article, Wright (1967) asserted that an accumulation of research was crucial to the development of the field. Although there was no specific outlet for research in pediatric psychology in the late 1960s and early 1970s, various medical and psychological journals published early research in the field, which centered on examining the psychological impact of medical disorders and the outcomes of effective intervention (e.g., Cassell & Paul, 1967; Friedman, 1972; Salk, Hilgartner, & Granich, 1972; Wright & Jimmerson, 1971; Wright, Nunnery, Eichel, & Scott, 1968; Wright, Woodcock, & Scott, 1970).

In describing the early scientific research in the field of pediatric psychology, Routh and Mesibov (1979) defined it as including developmental disabilities (e.g., mental retardation, autism); infant development; noncompliance; toilet training; the development of self-help skills in preschool children; parental neglect and child abuse; failure to thrive; psychological aspects of physical illness in children; death and bereavement; hospitalization; and child neuropsychology. This list of research areas was representative of topics early in the field, and many of these topics still remain as continuing areas of research within pediatric psychology today, as indicated by their representation in this edition of the *Handbook*.

As noted previously, *Pediatric Psychology*, the original SPP newsletter, served as an initial outlet for the dissemination of research in the field of pediatric psychology. Also as noted earlier, this newsletter eventually changed its name and format, becoming *JPP* in 1976. According to Roberts and colleagues (2003), *JPP* is isomorphic with research

in the field, reflecting the breadth and depth of research activities, and is the most concentrated scientific representation of the field of pediatric psychology. Over time, *JPP*
has continued to show steady growth in such areas as the number of submissions, papers
published, issues published annually, and journal impact factor. A brief overview of the
history of *JPP* is provided below (see Kazak, 2000, for a more detailed history).

History of JPP

The first several volumes of *JPP* were published quarterly and focused on such issues
as training, reviews and treatment of child/medical issues (e.g., encopresis and enuresis,
child abuse and neglect), and professional issues. Today, much of the research published
in *JPP* has an interest in a range of chronic illnesses, primarily cancer, diabetes, and
sickle cell disease; however, other conditions (e.g., obesity, asthma, and pediatric sleep)
are now seen more frequently in the journal. As Brown (2007) discussed in his editorial
vale dictum, trends reflected in *JPP* highlight the evolution of scientific research in the
field and can highlight changes in the empirical basis of pediatric psychology. Previous
editors' perspectives on progress in the field similarly reflect growth in topics, methodology, theory, and applications (Kazak, 2002; La Greca, 1997; Roberts, 1992).
   In looking at influences on pediatric psychology in its early existence, Routh and
Mesibov (1979) examined data regarding the journals most frequently cited in the first
three issues of *JPP*, and selected 23 journals that were cited a minimum of 20 times over
the issues published in this time span. The researchers concluded that the authors in *JPP*
cited articles in pediatric and general medical literature, psychiatry, neurology, developmental disabilities, and (to a large extent) literature on child development, clinical psychology, and behavioral approaches to treatment. In a similar, more recent study, Kazak
(2000) examined articles published from 1997 to 1998, and found that "competitive
and respectable" pediatric, psychology, and psychiatry journals were highly cited in
the articles published. Most recently, in examining research articles citing *JPP* between
2000 and 2004, Steele, Graves, Roberts, and Steele (2007) found that *JPP* articles are
being cited both within and outside the field of pediatric psychology. Collectively, these
results indicate that the field of pediatric psychology is both influencing and being influenced by other fields. This influence is even long-standing from early works in the field.
Specifically, classic articles in *JPP* have recently been identified, and their continued
impact in such areas as developmental and behavioral pediatrics, clinical psychology,
child development, and specialty medicine has been highlighted (see Aylward, Roberts,
Colombo, & Steele, 2008).
   Since its early years, several content analyses have been conducted to examine trends
in such areas as the types of research and populations studied in the articles appearing
in *JPP*. The first comprehensive analysis was conducted by Elkins and Roberts (1988)
on the first 10 years of articles appearing in *JPP* (1976–1985). The results indicated that
over time there was an increase in the number of basic and applied research articles that
focused predominantly on medically ill children or children with developmental delays.
In addition, the age of children in theses studies often spanned two or more age groups.
Finally, in this 10-year span, the number of female authors increased (indeed, females
became the majority of authors), and more of the senior authors were affiliated with college or universities rather than medical centers. The past editors of *JPP* have conducted
similar analyses in their closing articles (i.e., Brown, 2007; Kazak, 2002; La Greca,

1997; Roberts, 1992). Many of these analyses revealed similar results to the Elkins and Roberts study; however, some of the findings indicated new changes in the field that are worth noting. For example, in the Roberts (1992) analysis, the majority of senior authors were affiliated with medical settings rather than colleges or universities. In addition, almost 75% of *JPP* articles were explicative research (i.e., examining the relationship between physical and psychological phenomena), whereas intervention, prevention, and assessment articles accounted for only about 25% of the articles. As a result, Roberts highlighted the need to translate explicative research into effective intervention work. At the end of La Greca's editorship (La Greca, 1997), many of the similar trends identified in the previous analyses were found; yet, La Greca noted a 45.8% increase in articles on assessment and a 52.9% increase on intervention articles from the previous analysis. However, there was also a subsequent increase in the overall number of papers published in *JPP*. Next, Kazak (2002) indicated that articles during her term as editor continued to focus predominantly on chronic illnesses and evidenced many of the same trends as before. In her concluding remarks, she noted the need for additional papers on professional practice issues, as well as for research on the impact of families and other systems on the child. During Brown's recent term as editor (2002–2007), conditions such as obesity and asthma received greater attention; there was also an increase in methodology and assessment articles (Brown, 2007). Although Brown (2007) reported a greater than 50% increase in intervention articles over the previous 5 years, he noted the continued need for work in this area—a call that is an ongoing goal for the journal under the present editor, Dennis Drotar.

Considerations for Future Research

Wright (1967) stated that the pediatric psychologist should serve as a scientist-clinician and ground his or her work in empirical research. We affirm Kronenberger's (2006) statement that research within the field of pediatric psychology provides the field with credibility within the multidisciplinary health care system. The field of pediatric psychology has matured and is ready to experimentally validate previous correlational research (Brown, 2007). As research in the field continues to influence the progress of the field, articles on prevention, clinical trial interventions, and professional issues will continue to be important areas of research in the future (Brown, 2007). In the end, the research efforts of scientists can provide the field with increased understanding of the relationship between psychological and medical issues and with more effective prevention and intervention systems, thereby aiding practitioners in providing more adequate services to children and their families (Roberts, 1993).

Training in Pediatric Psychology

When Logan Wright first coined the term "pediatric psychology" in 1967, he stressed the importance of developing specialized professional training as integral to the development of the field. An early examination of the SPP membership roster revealed that 58% of members were trained in clinical psychology, followed by 10% in educational psychology, 8% in developmental psychology, 7% in counseling psychology, and 5% in general psychology (see Routh, 1977). A number of archival articles have detailed training opportunities and setting characteristics in pediatric psychology (e.g., see Ottinger & Roberts, 1980; Routh, 1969; Stabler & Mesibov, 1984; Tuma, 1977; Tuma & Grabert, 1983). Training in the field of pediatric psychology has undergone substantial expansion, and the formal organization of the field, SPP, accommodates a variety of diverse activities and backgrounds (Roberts et al., 2003). This section highlights historical developments and important future directions in training in the field of pediatric psychology. Overviews of practice patterns and settings, as well as of evidence-based treatments, are provided elsewhere (see Buckloh & Greco, Chapter 3, and Nelson & Steele, Chapter 7, this volume).

Early Practice and Training

Within the literature, there are few written records of psychologists working in pediatric settings in the early years. Routh (1994) documented the practice of Jean W. MacFarlane as a psychologist at a children's hospital in San Francisco in 1917–1918, as well as that of S. I. Franz in Los Angeles beginning in 1946. Recognizing the psychosocial needs of children seen in pediatric clinics, Wilson (1964) stated in his presidential address to the American Pediatric Society (APS) that "one of the things I would do if I could control the practice of pediatrics would be to encourage groups of pediatricians to employ their own clinical psychologists" (p. 988). Relatedly, Smith, Rome, and Freedheim (1967) documented a general and data-based description of a half-day-a-week practice model, involving collaboration between two pediatricians and a psychologist. The authors mentioned that this collaborative clinical practice improved access for psychological services for children and their families, and that it reduced parental resistance to referral. However, this working relationship was not without its challenges. For example, Fischer and Engeln (1972) documented early collaborative difficulties, such as setting practice fees and finding ample space for psychological clinical work.

In 1966, the first formal doctoral training program in pediatric psychology was started by the Departments of Pediatrics and Psychology at the University of Iowa under the direction of pediatrician Gerald Solomons. This graduate program was initiated by a psychologist and a pediatrician, and was initially designed to train pediatricians in child development; however, no pediatricians were identified who expressed interest in the training. The program did, however, aid in the career development of several psychologists, involving them in clinical training in an interdisciplinary clinical setting. During the 5 years of the program, approximately 10 graduate fellows were trained; Routh (1975) stated that these fellows were "clearly identifiable as pediatric psychologists since their graduation" (p. 7).

Current Trends in Training

As highlighted above, specialized training was not formalized early in the field's development; however, training opportunities in pediatric psychology are becoming more abundant (Prinstein & Roberts, 2006). In an official training brochure for SPP, La Greca, Stone, Drotar, and Maddux (1987) stated that "there is no single path to becoming a psychologist" (p. 2). Accordingly, a survey of the 1999 SPP membership list found that although the majority of pediatric psychologists had graduated from a clinical psychology doctoral program (Mullins, Hartman, Chaney, Balderson, & Hoff, 2003), a number of the psychologists surveyed had diverse backgrounds in such areas as counseling, developmental, school, and educational psychology, among others. The development and refinement of several sets of training recommendations, targeting professionals who work with children, adolescents, and their families in general (see La Greca & Hughes, 1999; Roberts et al., 1998), provided a groundwork for understanding part of the professional development of pediatric psychologists.

A SPP Task Force on training utilized previous recommendations to develop a list of 12 basic training domains pertinent to developing a specialty in pediatric psychology (Spirito et al., 2003): (1) lifespan development; (2) lifespan developmental psychopathology; (3) child, adolescent, and family assessment; (4) intervention strategies; (5) research methods and systems evaluation; (6) professional, ethical, and legal issues pertaining to children, adolescents, and families; (7) diversity issues and multicultural competence; (8) the role of multiple disciplines in service delivery systems; (9) prevention, family support, and health promotion; (10) social issues affecting children, adolescents, and families; (11) consultation–liaison (CL) roles; and (12) disease process and medical management. According to La Greca and Hughes (1999), the first 10 domains encompass three basic themes, including having a strong focus on development and developmental theories, emphasizing the ability to use interdisciplinary models and work within various disciplines that support children, and fostering an understanding of multicultural perspectives. Although these first 10 domains are pertinent to clinical child psychology training, CL roles as well as knowledge of disease processes and medical management are unique competencies recommended specifically for psychologists interested in working with children who have health-related problems (see Carter, Kronenberger, Scott, & Ernst, Chapter 8, this volume, for a further review of inpatient pediatric CL).

In addition to providing guidelines for training in pediatric psychology, the SPP Task Force (Spirito et al., 2003) defined three levels of training. First, "exposure" refers primarily to didactic training, such as classes and observations; second, "experience" refers to the practice of newly acquired skills; third, "expertise" involves mastery and the ability to practice skills and apply knowledge independently. In keeping with these levels of exposure, it is clear that training in graduate school alone is rarely sufficient. Thus training in pediatric psychology generally moves from basic exposure, and possibly some experiential learning, in graduate school to more specialized experiences and the development of expertise during internship and postdoctoral training (La Greca, Stone, & Swales, 1989).

Training Sequence for Pediatric Psychologists

Undergraduate Training

Because pediatric psychology is rarely introduced to undergraduate students as a subspecialty in general undergraduate psychology courses, it is important that members of the field work to foster undergraduate interest by providing opportunities for exposure (Drotar, Palermo, & Landis, 2003). Such opportunities include becoming a student member of SPP, joining the SPP mentorship program, and attending regional and national conferences in child health psychology. Once an interest is sparked, students considering applying to graduate school should be encouraged to gain research experience and work or volunteer in child-focused settings. Information on programs offering training in pediatric psychology can be found on the APA Division 54 webpage (*www.societyofpediatricpsychology.org/~division54/students*).

Graduate Training

Over the approximately 4–6 years that students are obtaining training onsite, the primary focus is to teach the general clinical child competencies outlined by the SPP Task Force through a combination of exposure (i.e., coursework) and experience (i.e., practicum placements). Some graduate programs accomplish these goals by offering elective courses, directed readings, and research and practicum experiences, as well as by encouraging involvement in relevant professional organizations. In general, these programs' specialty tracks in pediatric psychology emphasize competencies in multidisciplinary work by collaborating with local hospitals and medical schools to provide multiple mentors, practicum experiences with a variety of pediatric populations, and opportunities for clinical research (for examples of training programs, see Drotar, 1998; Roberts & Steele, 2003). Although research opportunities are frequently offered (i.e., publications, conference attendance, journal reviews), faculty members have also reported several challenges to providing students with experience in pediatric psychology research, such as collaborating with faculty and staff in pediatric settings and developing specialized research design and data analysis skills (Drotar, Palermo, & Landis, 2003). Although these examples certainly do not encompass all the potential methods of graduate school training in pediatric psychology, each offers insight into valuable methods of providing exposure and experience at the graduate school level.

Predoctoral Internship Training

Although only about half of SPP members surveyed in 1999 completed an internship with a major rotation in pediatrics, there is a trend toward more students' completing internships with a primary focus in pediatrics (Mullins et al., 2003). These sites tend to be at university-affiliated hospitals or children's hospitals (Mackner, Swift, Heidgerken, Stalets, & Linscheid, 2003) because such locations offer prime opportunities for addressing CL, disease processes, and medical management skills. Indeed, all 35 internship sites surveyed by Mackner and colleagues (2003) indicated that they had opportunities for CL, which frequently included rotations with hematology/oncology, diabetes, and pain management. For instance, the University of Alabama–Birmingham provides training in these areas by having students observe mentors, attend seminars, and assist with case conceptualization (Madan-Swain & Wallander, 2003).

Postdoctoral Fellowship Training

There was a threefold increase in the number of SPP members who completed a postdoctoral fellowship in pediatric psychology between the 1960s and 1990s (Mullins et al., 2003). This increase may indicate a greater desire to build expertise within pediatric psychology by taking time to focus training on clinical skills with specific populations, treatment methods, and/or research skills (Drotar, Palermo, & Ievers-Landis, 2003). The increases in the knowledge base of the specialty and the necessary time to master it also probably play a role, as do licensure requirements in many states for postdoctoral experiences. This 1- to 2-year period of highly specialized training often meets trainees' needs by providing flexible opportunities for interdisciplinary teaching and supervision of psychology and medical students and staff, grant and manuscript writing, and mentorship in work-related tasks (i.e., scheduling, networking, career advice).

Licensure and Board Certification

After successfully completing a graduate program and acquiring the minimum number of supervised hours, psychologists are eligible for licensure. Licensure is required by all states in order to be able to provide psychological services to the public. The final phases of obtaining licensure include passing the Examination of Professional Practice in Psychology (EPPP) and demonstrating sufficient knowledge of state and provincial statutes regarding mental health practices. Beyond licensure, advanced credentials from the American Board of Professional Psychology (ABPP) identify psychologists' specialties within the field, similar to the way a medical doctor pursues board certification in pediatrics, surgery, or internal medicine. In the past, pediatric psychologists frequently chose the specialty of "clinical psychology"; however, pediatric psychologists now comprise about half of those board-certified by the American Board of Clinical Child and Adolescent Psychology (*www.clinicalchildpsychology.com*; *www.abpp.org*). In order to receive this credential, psychologists provide verification of their abilities in the specialty area by submitting tapes of their clinical skills and participating in a 3-hour oral examination (Finch, Simon, & Nezu, 2006). Similar to several of the SPP Task Force recommendations, this verification attempts to assess competency in professional knowledge; assessment; intervention; interpersonal relations with clients; ethical and legal standards of behavior; commitment to the specialty and awareness of current issues in the field; and supervision and consultation. Benefits of demonstrating specialty competencies include safeguards for the public, financial incentives from institutions and insurance, and license mobility (American Board of Clinical Child and Adolescent Psychology, *www. clinicalchildpsychology.com*). This orientation to competency complements the national movement toward establishing competency standards in professional psychology, including not only attention to the training sequence, but continual postlicensure assessment of competence (Roberts, Borden, Christiansen, & Lopez, 2005; Rubin et al., 2007).

Future Directions in Training

Due to these developments in training, it is now possible to specify a more focused and formalized pathway for gaining exposure, experience, and expertise in pediatric psychology. However, as evidenced by the diverse educational backgrounds of pediatric psychologists, there is no single route to becoming a pediatric psychologist (Kaslow & David, 2003). In fact, some flexibility has been encouraged, so that students and training programs can develop tracks that best fit their interests, needs, and resources. In the future, it will be important to consider ways to incorporate new training ideas and tasks, such as program evaluation research skills, without overburdening both students and faculty (Drotar, Palermo, & Landis, 2003). It will also be necessary to discuss how to respond to constant changes and advances in the medical field that affect education in pediatric psychology (Brown, 2003).

The Future of Pediatric Psychology

A Delphic poll was conducted by Brown and Roberts (2000) to highlight pertinent issues that individuals identified as having the most significant impact on the future of pediatric psychology. The results indicated that the field needed to focus on demonstration of its viability, increased collaboration and integration of pediatric psychologists into primary care, and issues related to reimbursement. Although there has been progress in some areas, several issues still remain ongoing priorities for guiding the field. The future will require (1) adjustment to changing reimbursement patterns; (2) continual proof of the "worth" or value added by pediatric psychology services; and (3) adjustment to changes in medical treatments and new technologies in the world at large, including the application and potential effectiveness of new technology products (e.g., cell phones, computers, iPods, text messaging) in treatment outcomes. The use of these technologies in the health domain is obviously increasing, and additional investigations will be necessary as these products break into the marketplace (see also Drotar, 2006; Palermo, 2008; Palermo & Wilson, Chapter 15, this volume). Not all new technology and products will be of value for application in pediatric psychology applications and research, therefore these methodologies need to be carefully evaluated.

Predicting the future of the field of pediatric psychology necessitates examining what pediatric psychology has done well in the past and maintaining those gains. An examination of articles published in the late 1970s versus today would probably reveal many of the same general topics and concerns. Although some of the methodologies and foci in the field have changed (e.g., cancer treatments and outcomes; neonatal intensive care unit treatments and outcomes), issues such as adjustment and coping, adherence (compliance), and treatment side effects have remained somewhat steady in the literature. Although *JPP* has broadened its perspective, several areas still merit attention (Brown, 2007). For example, public health issues (e.g., health disparities, access to care) and the psychosocial impact of chronic illnesses are in need of continued examination. Professional practice issues are also relatively underrepresented (Kazak, 2002). Thus much more information is needed on the actual practice of pediatric psychology. Such issues as gaining acceptance and respect from pediatric colleagues, reimbursement, and ethical and legal issues require the same amount of attention today as when the field was just developing. The field of pediatric psychology was an innovation in its development, and the field has continued to be innovative and to adapt over time. The field's vibrant history predicts a dynamic future of fulfilling the needs of children through research and application.

Concluding Remarks

Early collaborations between pediatricians and psychologists paved the way for the emergence of pediatric psychology. Over time, the field has clearly evolved. Although it is a relatively young field compared to other psychology and health-related disciplines, pediatric psychology has matured and has been recognized both within the broad discipline of psychology and across various health care environments (Kazak, 2000). Roberts (1993) observed that progress in the field is due to the "strength of early conceptualization, the vision of its pioneers, the clear need for better understanding of relationships, and the quality of interventions serving children and families" (p. 23). Moreover, the early scientific research and clinical practice in the field has helped increase our present understanding of the various factors related to working with children and adolescents with health-related conditions. While working to develop the future of the field, SPP has also recognized the importance of preserving its history. The executive committee now includes a position for a historian and space is devoted on the SPP website to the field's history (*www.societyofpediatricpsychology.org*).

In the early years of the emergence of pediatric psychology and health psychology as concepts, Schofield (1969) stated that "the opportunities for psychology to play a much expanded and valuable role among all the health-related disciplines are so many and so varied as to defy cataloguing" (p. 574). This is no less true today, and the parameters of the field of pediatric psychology continue to expand through scientific research and clinical practice. Identifying new questions of interest and using new research designs, methodologies, and technology will continue to increase our understanding of the interaction of children and families in pediatric settings and healthy development.

As the other chapters in this *Handbook* demonstrate, pediatric psychology represents a wide range of topics. Indeed, according to the official definition of the field,

> Areas of expertise within the field include, but are not limited to: psychosocial, developmental and contextual factors contributing to the etiology, course and outcome of pediatric medical conditions; assessment and treatment of behavioral and emotional concomitants of illness, injury, and developmental disorders; prevention of illness and injury; promotion of health and health-related behaviors; education, training and mentoring of psychologists and providers of medical care; improvement of health care delivery systems and advocacy for public policy that serves the needs of children, adolescents, and their families. (Society of Pediatric Psychology, n.d.)

Most individual pediatric psychologists, however, have a narrower set of interests and activities. Ultimately, the breadth of activities of the researchers and clinicians in the field of pediatric psychology cannot be captured by one single topic. This edition of the *Handbook of Pediatric Psychology* represents the vitality of the field by highlighting continued and emerging research and practice, and by expanding and encompassing the many areas the field covers for children, families, and professionals.

References

Anderson, J. E. (1930). Pediatrics and child psychology. *Journal of the American Medical Association*, 95, 1015–1018.

Aylward, B. S., Roberts, M. C., Colombo, J., & Steele, R. G. (2008). Identifying the classics: An examination of articles published in the *Journal of Pediatric Psychology* from 1976–2006. *Journal of Pediatric Psychology*, 33, 576–589.

Brennemann, J. (1933). Pediatric psychology and the child guidance movement. *Journal of Pediatrics*, 2, 1–26.

Brown, K. J., & Roberts, M. C. (2000). Future issues in pediatric psychology: Delphic survey. *Journal of Clinical Psychology in Medical Settings*, 7, 5–15.

Brown, R. T. (2003). Introduction to the special issue: Training in pediatric psychology. *Journal of Pediatric Psychology*, 28, 81–83.

Brown, R. T. (2007). *Journal of Pediatric Psychology (JPP)*, 2003–2007: Editor's vale dictum. *Journal of Pediatric Psychology*, 32, 1165–1178.

Buck, R. L. (1961). Behavioral scientists in schools of medicine. *Journal of Health and Human Behavior*, 2, 59–64.

Caecae, E. (1936). The need for psychological training for pediatricians and of child psychology in pediatric schools. *Atti Soieta Italiana per il Progresso Delle Scienze*, 3, 250–252.

Cassell, S., & Paul, M. H. (1967). The role of puppet therapy on the emotional responses of children hospitalized for cardiac catheterization. *Journal of Pediatrics, 71,* 233–239.

Cushna, B. (1968). Psychology and pediatrics. *American Psychologist, 23,* 288.

Drotar, D. (1995). *Consulting with pediatricians.* New York: Plenum Press.

Drotar, D. (1998). Training students for careers in medical settings: A graduate program in pediatric psychology. *Professional Psychology: Research and Practice, 29,* 402–404.

Drotar, D. (2006). Innovations in the use of new technologies in research and clinical care for children and adolescents with chronic health conditions. *Children's Health Care, 35,* 1–3.

Drotar, D., Palermo, T., & Ievers-Landis, C. (2003). Commentary: Recommendations for the training of pediatric psychologists: Implications for postdoctoral training. *Journal of Pediatric Psychology, 28,* 109–113.

Drotar, D., Palermo, T., & Landis, C. (2003). Training graduate-level pediatric psychology researchers at Case Western Reserve University: Meeting the challenges of the new millennium. *Journal of Pediatric Psychology, 28,* 123–134.

Duff, R. S., Rowe, D. S., & Anderson, F. P. (1973). Patient care and student learning in a pediatric clinical. *Pediatrics, 50,* 839–846.

Elkins, P. D., & Roberts, M. C. (1988). *Journal of Pediatric Psychology:* A content analysis of articles over its first 10 years. *Journal of Pediatric Psychology, 13,* 575–594.

Fernberger, S. W. (1932). The American Psychological Association: A historical summary, 1892–1930. *Psychological Bulletin, 29,* 1–89.

Finch, A., Simon, N., & Nezu, C. (2006). The future of clinical psychology: Board certification. *Clinical Psychology: Science and Practice, 13,* 254–257.

Fischer, H. L., & Engeln, R. G. (1972). How goes the marriage? *Professional Psychology, 3,* 73–79.

Friedman, R. (1972). Some characteristics of children with "psychogenic" pain. *Clinical Pediatrics, 11,* 331–333.

Gesell, A. (1919). The field of clinical psychology as an applied science: A symposium. *Journal of Applied Psychology, 3,* 81–84.

Gesell, A. (1926). Normal growth as a public health concept. *Transactions of the American Child Health Association, 3,* 48.

Kagan, J. (1965). The new marriage: Pediatrics and psychology. *American Journal of Diseases of Children, 110,* 272–278.

Kaslow, N., & David, C. (2003). Commentary: Training in pediatric psychology: A survey of predoctoral internship programs. *Journal of Pediatric Psychology, 28,* 443–445.

Kazak, A. E. (2000). *Journal of Pediatric Psychology:* A brief history (1969–1999). *Journal of Pediatric Psychology, 25,* 463–470.

Kazak, A. E. (2002). *Journal of Pediatric Psychology (JPP),* 1998–2002: Editor's vale dictum. *Journal of Pediatric Psychology, 27,* 653–663.

Kenny, T. J. (1975). Pediatric psychology: A reflective approach. *Pediatric Psychology, 3,* 8.

Kronenberger, W. G. (2006). Commentary: A look at ourselves in the mirror. *Journal of Pediatric Psychology, 31,* 647–649.

La Greca, A., & Hughes, J. (1999). United we stand, divided we fall: The education and training needs of clinical child psychologists. *Journal of Clinical Child Psychology, 28,* 435–447.

La Greca, A., Stone, W., & Swales, T. (1989). Pediatric psychology training: An analysis of graduate, internship, and postdoctoral programs. *Journal of Pediatric Psychology, 14,* 103–116.

La Greca, A. M. (1997). Reflections and perspectives on pediatric psychology: Editor's vale dictum. *Journal of Pediatric Psychology, 22,* 759–777.

La Greca, A. M., Stone, W. L., Drotar, D., & Maddux, J. (1987). *Pediatric psychology: Some common questions about training.* Washington, DC: Society of Pediatric Psychology, American Psychological Association.

Mackner, L., Swift, E., Heidgerken, A., Stalets, M., & Linscheid, T. (2003). Training in pediatric psychology: A survey of predoctoral internship programs. *Journal of Pediatric Psychology, 28*, 433–441.

Madan-Swain, A., & Wallander, J. (2003). Commentary: Internship training. *Journal of Pediatric Psychology, 28*, 105–107.

Matarazzo, J. D., & Daniel, R. S. (1957). Psychologists in medical schools. *Neuropsychiatry, 4*, 93–107.

McClelland, C. Q., Staples, W. P., Weisberg, I., & Berger, M. E. (1973). The practitioner's role in behavioral pediatrics. *Journal of Pediatrics, 82*, 325–331.

Mensh, I. N. (1953). Psychology in medical education. *American Psychologist, 8*, 83–85.

Mesibov, G. B. (1984). Evolution of pediatric psychology: Historical roots to future trends. *Journal of Pediatric Psychology, 2*, 15–17.

Moll, W. (1968). History of American medical education. *British Journal of Medical Education, 2*, 173–181.

Mullins, L., Hartman, V., Chaney, J., Balderson, B., & Hoff, A. (2003). Training experiences and theoretical orientations of pediatric psychologists. *Journal of Pediatric Psychology, 28*, 115–122.

Ottinger, D. R., & Roberts, M. C. (1980). A university-based predoctoral practicum in pediatric psychology. *Professional Psychology, 11*, 707–713.

Palermo, T. M. (2008). Editorial: Section on innovations in technology in measurement, assessment, and intervention. *Journal of Pediatric Psychology, 33*, 35–38.

Prinstein, M. J., & Roberts, M. C. (2006). The professional adolescence of clinical child and adolescent psychology and pediatric psychology: Grown up and striving for autonomy. *Clinical Psychology: Science and Practice, 13*, 263–268.

Richmond, J. B. (1967). Child development: A basic science for pediatrics. *Pediatrics, 39*, 649–658.

Roberts, M., Carson, C., Erickson, M., Friedman, R., La Greca, A., Lemanek, K., et al. (1998). A model for training psychologists to provide services for children and adolescents. *Professional Psychology: Research and Practice, 29*, 293–299.

Roberts, M. C. (1986). *Pediatric psychology: Psychological interventions and strategies for pediatric problems.* New York: Pergamon Press.

Roberts, M. C. (1992). Vale dictum: The editor's view of the field of pediatric psychology. *Journal of Pediatric Psychology, 17*, 785–805.

Roberts, M. C. (1993). Introduction to pediatric psychology: An historical perspective. In M. C. Roberts, G. P. Koocher, D. K. Routh, & D. Willis (Eds.), *Readings in pediatric psychology* (pp. 1–21). New York: Plenum Press.

Roberts, M. C., Borden, K. A., Christiansen, M. D., & Lopez, S. J. (2005). Fostering a culture shift: Assessment of competence in the education and careers of professional psychologists. *Professional Psychology: Research and Practice, 36*(4), 355–361

Roberts, M. C., Maddux, J., Wurtele, S. K., & Wright, L. (1982). Pediatric psychology: Health care psychology for children. In T. Millon, C. J. Green, & R. B. Meagher (Eds.), *Handbook of clinical health care psychology* (pp. 191–226). New York: Plenum Press.

Roberts, M. C., Mitchell, M. C., & McNeal, R. (2003). The evolving field of pediatric psychology: Critical issues and future challenges. In M. C. Roberts (Ed.), *Handbook of pediatric psychology* (3rd ed., pp. 3–18). New York: Guilford Press.

Roberts, M. C., & Steele, R. G. (2003). Predoctoral training in pediatric psychology at the University of Kansas Clinical Child Psychology Program. *Journal of Pediatric Psychology, 28*, 99–103.

Routh, D. K. (1969). Graduate training in pediatric psychology: The Iowa program. *Pediatric Psychology, 1*, 5–6.

Routh, D. K. (1970). Psychological training in medical school departments of pediatrics: A survey. *Professional Psychology, 1*, 469–472.

Routh, D. K. (1975). The short history of pediatric psychology. *Journal of Clinical Child Psychology, 4,* 6–8.

Routh, D. K. (1977). Postdoctoral training in pediatric psychology. *Professional Psychology, 8,* 245–250.

Routh, D. K. (1982). Pediatric psychology as an area of scientific research. In J. M. Tuma (Ed.), *Handbook for the practice of pediatric psychology* (pp. 290–320). New York: Wiley.

Routh, D. K. (1990). Psychology and pediatrics. The future of the relationship. In A. M. Gross & R. S. Drabman (Eds.), *Handbook of clinical behavioral pediatrics* (pp. 403–414). New York: Plenum Press.

Routh, D. K. (1994). *Clinical psychology since 1917: Science, practice, and organization.* New York: Plenum Press.

Routh, D. K., & Mesibov, G. B. (1979). The editorial policy of the *Journal of Pediatric Psychology. Journal of Pediatric Psychology, 4,* 1–3.

Rubin, N. J., Bebeau, M., Leigh, I. W., Lichtenberg, J. W., Nelson, P. D., Portnoy, S., et al. (2007). The competency movement within psychology: An historical perspective. *Professional Psychology: Research and Practice, 38*(5), 452–462.

Rubin-Rabson, G. (1948). Psychology in pediatrics. *Journal of Pediatrics, 33,* 128–135.

Salk, L., Hilgartner, M., & Granich, B. (1972). The psycho-social impact of hemophilia on the patient and his family. *Social Science and Medicine, 6,* 491–505.

Schofield, W. (1969). The role of psychology on the delivery of health services. *American Psychologist, 24,* 565–584.

Smith, E. E., Rome, L. P., & Freedheim, D. K. (1967). The clinical psychologist in the pediatric office. *Journal of Pediatrics, 21,* 48–51.

Society of Pediatric Psychology. (n.d.). *Who we are.* Retrieved March 5, 2009, from *www.society ofpediatricpsychology/org/~division54/who/index.shtml*

Spirito, A., Brown, R., D'Angelo, E., Delamater, A., Rodrigue, J., & Siegel, L. (2003). Society of Pediatric Psychology Task Force report: Recommendations for the training of pediatric psychologists. *Journal of Pediatric Psychology, 28,* 85–98.

Stabler, B., & Mesibov, G. B. (1984). Role functioning of pediatric and health psychologists in health care settings. *Professional Psychology, 15,* 142–151.

Steele, M. M., Graves, M. M., Roberts, M. C., & Steele, R. G. (2007). Examining the influence of the *Journal of Pediatric Psychology*: An empirical approach. *Journal of Pediatric Psychology, 32,* 150–153.

Tuma, J. M. (1977). Practicum, internship, and postdoctoral training in pediatric psychology: A survey. *Journal of Pediatric Psychology, 2,* 9–12.

Tuma, J. M., & Grabert, J. (1983). Internship and postdoctoral training in pediatric and clinical child psychology: A survey. *Journal of Pediatric Psychology, 8,* 245–268.

Wilson, J. L. (1964). Growth and development of pediatrics. *Journal of Pediatrics, 65,* 984–991.

Wright, L. (1967). The pediatric psychologist: A role model. *American Psychologist, 22,* 323–325.

Wright, L., & Jimmerson, S. (1971). Intellectual sequelae of *Hemophilus influenzae* meningitis. *Journal of Abnormal Psychology, 77,* 181–183.

Wright, L., Nunnery, A., Eichel, B., & Scott, R. (1968). Application of conditioning principles to problems of tracheostomy addiction in children. *Journal of Consulting and Clinical Psychology, 32,* 603–606.

Wright, L., Woodcock, J. M., & Scott, R. (1970). Treatment of sleep disturbance in a young child by conditioning. *Southern Medical Journal, 44,* 969–972.

CHAPTER 2

Ethical and Legal Issues in Pediatric Psychology

WILLIAM A. RAE
DONALD BRUNNQUELL
JEREMY R. SULLIVAN

Pediatric psychologists must always engage in ethical and professional practice. However, the ethics code of the American Psychological Association (APA, 2002) does not always provide explicit guidance for the unique ethical dilemmas encountered by pediatric psychologists. In fact, the APA ethics code was deliberately written to accomplish the following two objectives: (1) to avoid rigid dictums that might soon become obsolete, and (2) to allow professional judgment to influence decision making in unforeseeable situations. Pediatric psychologists must interpret the ethics code in a manner that reflects their particular practice environment, including health care settings.

Pediatric psychologists represent a distinctive stratum within professional psychology, so special considerations are necessary in applying ethical principles to their practice. Like other professional psychologists, pediatric psychologists have expertise in assessment, intervention, and consultation, but the application of these proficiencies is complicated by the fact that they work with children, adolescents, and families in medical contexts. These complexities, along with the special vulnerabilities of minors, mean that pediatric psychologists should constantly strive to maintain the highest ethical and legal standards. Moreover, pediatric psychologists often work within institutions where they engage in institutional interventions as a way of improving the psychosocial environment. These institutional settings require special ethical considerations that place special demands on pediatric psychologists. For example, pediatric psychologists often engage in professional practice that requires frequent interdisciplinary interactions. In fact, it is common for the pediatric psychologist to be the lead professional in the health care setting. In such cases, they are typically responsible for appropriately communicating mental health information, often tempered by input from other disciplines (e.g., pediatrics, psychiatry, occupational therapy, social work, speech pathology) in a way that can be understood and accepted by children and families. These issues greatly

19

complicate the ethical decision-making process. The Health Insurance Portability and Accountability Act (HIPAA) contributes yet another layer of complexity (e.g., medical records vs. psychotherapy notes) that influences important ethical decisions encountered by pediatric psychologists.

The purpose of this chapter is to describe ethical and legal issues that may affect pediatric psychologists in their multiple professional roles as mental health practitioners, as members of the health care team, and as researchers. The chapter is organized into four sections that accomplish this aim. The first section addresses emerging ethical issues in pediatric psychology. The second section describes general mental health issues, such as informed consent, confidentiality, and record keeping. The third section outlines bioethics within the context of practical problems confronted by pediatric psychologists in hospital settings. Lastly, research ethics for pediatric psychologists are discussed.

Emerging Ethical Issues in Pediatric Psychology

Evidence-Based Treatment

During the last two decades, the managed care movement has provided a strong impetus for providing support for the effectiveness of psychological treatments (see Nelson & Steele, Chapter 7, this volume). The APA (2002) ethics code clearly states that interventions must be effective and not detrimental, or treatment should be discontinued. Although evidence-based treatment is currently considered the optimal standard of practice, considerable confusion occurred in previous iterations of the concept. In the mid-1990s, the term "empirically supported treatments" (Chambless & Hollon, 1998; Task Force on Promotion and Dissemination of Psychological Procedures, 1995) was used, which implied there should be demonstrated empirical research showing that the treatment worked. More recently, the standard conceptualization of "evidence-based practice" integrates research evidence with clinical judgment, while also taking into account patients' culture, preferences, and other characteristics that could potentially improve outcomes (APA Presidential Task Force, 2006). Making an informed judgment about what intervention to apply to each case is often complicated. Ethical decision making under these circumstances can be especially fraught with difficulty, since the appropriate "standard of practice" is not always clearly defined. The ethical pediatric psychologist must evaluate existing treatment literature within the context of the patient's characteristics and developmental level, and then use professional judgment to decide on a course of treatment.

Telehealth and Electronically Mediated Practice

"Telehealth," the use of telecommunication to provide health services across distance, is an emerging area in pediatric psychology that has the potential to increase access to specialized services and enhance community-based services for underserved pediatric populations (Farmer & Muhlenbruck, 2001; Liss, 2005). Telehealth interventions for pediatric problems have been shown to reduce pain and anxiety (Holden et al., 2003), and also have been used to treat distress in radiation therapy as part of the Starbright program (Klosky et al., 2004). Telehealth service providers struggle with several ethical challenges, including confidentiality, inherent risks, safety concerns, and therapeutic value (Reed, McLaughlin, & Milholland, 2000). (See Palermo & Wilson, Chapter 15, this volume, for a complete discussion of telehealth/eHealth issues.)

Cultural Competency

Professional pediatric psychologists must recognize the multiethnic and multicultural nature of pediatric populations, and, in doing so, make it an ethical priority to incorporate training to facilitate awareness of cultural issues that could influence their practice. The pediatric psychology training guidelines clearly mandate the importance of training for culturally diverse populations (Spirito et al., 2003). Training for cultural competency is a responsibility that should be an ethical imperative for all pediatric psychologists (Clay, Chapter 6, this volume).

Mental Health Ethics for Pediatric Psychologists

Informed Consent

The purpose of gaining informed consent from patients is to ensure that each patient is provided with sufficient information to make an informed decision about participating in a professional activity. Within the context of pediatric psychology, informed consent usually means "parental permission," since most patients seen by pediatric psychologists are minors. Permission from a parent or other legal guardian is therefore required for a child's or adolescent's participation in clinical services or research, with assent or agreement obtained from the young patient. Informed consent should be obtained by describing the procedures in a way that is clearly understandable to the patient or parent. This includes using developmentally appropriate language when working with children, and using an interpreter in order to provide information in the patient's native language if proficiency in English is limited (APA, 2002). Consent or assent should be documented in writing, and patients should have an opportunity to ask questions and gather additional information about the professional activity. The extent to which psychologists may legally provide services to minors in the absence of parental permission varies from state to state, with many states allowing for such services under explicitly defined and urgent circumstances (e.g., suicidal ideation, abuse, drug counseling).

Informed consent is obtained within the context of research, assessment, intervention, and consultation services provided by pediatric psychologists. Assessment includes the use of traditional assessment measures, such as intelligence and personality tests; it may also include more specialized evaluation tools, such as measures of treatment adherence, pain, health beliefs, coping skills, family stress, and other issues related to medical treatments and outcomes (Spirito et al., 2003). Specific considerations in obtaining informed consent for assessment include explaining the purpose of the assessment in language the patient or parent can understand, accurately describing fees for the assessment, detailing the types and lengths of assessment procedures, and explaining the limits of confidentiality of assessment results (APA, 2002).

Intervention services provided by pediatric psychologists may include individual, group, or family therapy based on a range of theoretical perspectives (Spirito et al., 2003). Within the context of intervention services, the APA (2002) ethics code states that informed consent should cover the nature and likely course of the services, fees and payment procedures, situations that would limit confidentiality, and the experimental nature of the intervention if a new or developing treatment will be used. Parents consenting to intervention services for their children should have an idea of what the services will "look like." The more information psychologists can provide, the more prepared and informed parents will be when deciding to grant permission for participation in the intervention services.

Within the context of pediatric psychology, consultation involves working with other professionals on behalf of child and adolescent patients and their families. The pediatric psychologist is often part of a multidisciplinary team of professionals who work together to provide a comprehensive program of care for a child and family (Spirito et al., 2003). Other service providers may include pediatricians, psychiatrists, nurses, and other medical specialists, as well as nonmedical professionals (e.g., teachers, counselors, psychologists, administrators, and social workers). With all of these consultative relationships, information about the patient must be shared among professionals in order to develop informed treatment approaches. The informed consent process should attempt to describe the purpose of consultation, to identify anticipated interactions (e.g., among treatment team members such as physicians, nurses, specialists, and teachers), and to explain the need for such interactions. The APA (2002) ethics code does not address consultation as a distinct treatment modality, but it does note that psychologists engaging in consultation with colleagues should first obtain consent from the patient, and should share the minimal amount of information necessary to help the patient. As the consultative services change in response to the characteristics or needs of the child (e.g., an additional specialist is added to the treatment team because of changes to the child's diagnosis or prognosis), parents should continually be apprised of the interactions between the psychologist and other service providers.

Evaluation of Capacity to Consent

Miller, Drotar, and Kodish (2004) have defined competence for informed consent as follows: "a person is generally viewed as competent if she or he can understand the therapy or research procedure, consider major risks and benefits, and make an informed decision based on this deliberation" (p. 257). Thus competence to consent involves elements of comprehension and decision-making capacity. As noted by Collogan and Fleischman (2005), adults are generally presumed to be legally competent to make decisions on behalf of themselves and their children unless proven otherwise (e.g., due to severe deficits in cognitive functioning). Children, on the other hand, are presumed to lack competence or decisional capacity simply as a function of their developmental status as minors. These presumptions, however, have recently been met with some criticism, leading experts to call for more empirically based efforts to operationalize and assess these abilities. Collogan and Fleischman (2005) describe several relevant standards that psychologists can use when assessing decisional capacity for participation in research or psychological services. Included are patients' ability to actively reach a decision or express a preference; their understanding of the factors that contribute to the decision (e.g., risks and benefits of participation); their ability to manipulate information; and their ability to apply information to their own circumstances. These abilities may be assessed via interview and observational methods, the use of hypothetical scenarios and checking for understanding, or more formal methods (such as relevant subtests from intelligence tests to estimate overall cognitive capacity).

Confidentiality

Confidentiality is the cornerstone of the therapeutic relationship (Koocher & Keith-Spiegel, 2008). Many patients and families would not divulge private information to a pediatric psychologist unless they were assured that the information would remain confidential, which could lead to spurious assessments and interventions. Protecting confidentiality is a primary obligation for all psychologists. Confidentiality practices are not only legally grounded, but are also established by institutions. Yet some professionals dealing with issues of confidentiality continue to be confused about how the ethical and legal aspects should be interpreted (Fisher, 2008). A discussion of confidentiality issues should take place during the informed consent process at the initiation of the professional contact, although this discussion is not always feasible in the chaotic medical environment. During the informed consent procedure, a pediatric psychologist should discuss the limits to confidentiality and should describe how confidential information will be used.

Confidentiality issues for children and adolescents are different from those with adults. Adults expect that private information obtained from a mental health professional will be kept confidential except when they give their written consent to have information released. By contrast, young children usually do not expect broad confidentiality for private information, since parents are knowledgeable about many of these details anyway. On the other hand, adolescents require more assurances of confidentiality, because they are often suspicious of parental motives and intentions. Many psychologists who treat adolescents require that confidentiality be maintained from parents, even though there is no legal basis for doing so. The pediatric psychologist must weigh an adolescent's right to confidentiality versus the need for the parents to obtain confidential information about their child.

Determining the limits of confidentiality can be problematic for pediatric psychologists. Conflicting expectations often exist for the patient, parent, referral agent (e.g., physician), and institution (e.g., hospital). In the same way, conflicting expectations may also occur for pediatric psychologists who work with families, because a patient, parents, siblings, and extended family members can all have different expectations about what information should be shared with whom. Before initiating professional services, the pediatric psychologist should attempt to clarify the confidentiality issues for all the stakeholders involved. Even when these issues are clarified, there may still be different expectations. For example, primary care pediatricians commonly expect to be privy to the most confidential information, but patients may not want certain private information divulged, even to their physician. Ultimately, the parents and the child have to decide how information is shared with family members or health care providers.

Breaking confidentiality is legally mandated in the United States under three circumstances. First, in all 50 states, the District of Columbia, Puerto Rico, and the U.S. Virgin Islands, psychologists are among the professionals required to break confidentiality if they suspect that a child is being neglected or physically, emotionally, or sexually abused. In actual practice, the timing and manner of breaking this confidence can be influenced by statute and by circumstantial variables that may affect the welfare of the patient. Second, psychologists must divulge confidential information if ordered to do so by a court. Finally, pediatric psychologists should always break confidentiality to report imminent danger to the patient or to others. The pediatric psychologist must evaluate the potential of danger and disclose that information only to appropriate public authorities, professional workers, potential victims, and/or parents as required by law. Pediatric psychologists appear to have little ambivalence about breaking confidentiality if a child or adolescent appears to be suicidal or homicidal, but they have considerable ambivalence when judging risky adolescent behaviors in such areas as sexual behavior and substance use, as these are affected by intensity, frequency, and duration of the behavior (Rae, Sullivan, Razo, George, & Ramirez, 2002).

Record Keeping

The APA (2002) ethical principles state that psychologists must document the services they perform; must maintain accurate, current, and pertinent records of services; and must maintain appropriate confidentiality in the creating, storing, accessing, transferring, and disposition of records. This requirement includes written, recorded, or computerized records. The records should be sufficiently detailed to permit the continued provision of services by the psychologists themselves or by other professionals. Any documentation of services should only include information germane to the purposes of that documentation.

In actual practice, a pediatric psychologist's records can vary widely, depending on the setting and institutional requirements. For example, an ethical dilemma can occur for a hospital-based pediatric psychologist who must write chart notes in the hospital record. HIPAA makes a distinction between routine chart notes in the medical record and psychotherapy notes, which are kept separate and are not routinely disclosed by the mental health professional. The pediatric psychologist should strive to document thoroughly and accurately, but should also be sensitive to the potentially harmful effects of revealing confidential information in the routine chart notes. In medical centers, other health care providers want access to information in order to provide comprehensive care, but the pediatric psychologist should continually assess the potential harm in revealing that information.

Another conflict can occur when confidential information about a patient is revealed to parents. Legally, parents have the right to obtain copies of all medical records on their minor children. However, parental access to records could be detrimental to the therapeutic process, particularly if the privacy promised to a minor patient is infringed by inquisitive parents. For example, if information about nonlethal substance use or sexual activity were revealed, it could destroy the cooperative relationship between the patient and the pediatric psychologist. In a similar way, when patients reach the age of legal majority, they can request copies of all records. Because of the trend toward increased patient access to records, all written documentation should be maintained with the assumption that children or families will eventually see the records (Koocher & Keith-Spiegel, 2008).

Bioethics for Children and Adolescents

Bioethics at its heart is an application of philosophical efforts to discern the roots of moral values and to determine how those values apply to individual cases. A basic understanding of these approaches in health care and medical practice is essential. A pediatric psychologist can have a unique voice and role in a bioethics discussion.

Ethics Committees and Ethics Consultation

Cranford and Doudera (1984) defined an ethics committee as "a multidisciplinary group of health care professionals within a health care institution that has been specifically established to address the ethical dilemmas that occur within the institution" (p. 6). They outlined the goals of an ethics committee's work as education, development of policies and guidelines, and consultation/case review. In addition to clinical ethics, committees and consultants have begun in the past decade to become more involved with organizational ethics and to attempt to assess the effects of organizational decisions and policies on individuals and groups of patients. Organizational ethics is a major emphasis of the Joint Commission on Accreditation of Healthcare Organizations (JCAHO, 2001), and is listed in the areas of emphasis in many recent hospital inspections. The clear trend is to assess the impact of the organization on patient care.

Ethics consultation in individual cases may be carried out by full committees, subcommittees, or individual consultants who are part of an ethics committee or acting independently. No standard format for consultation exists, although a task force of the American Society for Bioethics and Humanities (1998) has attempted to outline core competencies for consultation. They call for core knowledge in the following areas: bioethical issues and concepts, such as ethical theory, end-of-life decision making, and advance care planning; the health care system; the local institution and its policies; beliefs and perspectives of patients and staff members; and relevant professional ethics codes and health care laws. Active engagement with their institutional ethics committees should be a goal of pediatric psychologists.

Medical Decision Making for Children

The important issues of informed consent and assent are discussed in this chapter, but the discussion of who makes medical decisions for children is especially essential. Clearly, once children become legal guardians of their own persons, they decide for themselves. Until that point (generally 18 years of age), their legal guardians, usually parents, are responsible for the consent to treatment. Because children's lives are their own, the children should be involved in medical decisions to the extent of their capacity, even when they are not capable of understanding the entire situation or recognized as legally competent. The most comprehensive review of children's understanding in the context of medical treatment and research decisions shows that there are no simple answers to these questions, and that age is not a sufficient standard for true understanding (Miller et al., 2004). Such factors as prior experience, cognitive and academic abilities, psychological problems, and the context of the decision must be examined carefully on a case-by-case basis.

For instance, in their qualitative study of elementary-school-age children in diabetes care, Alderson, Sutcliffe, and Curtis (2006) have argued that children openly involved in the care of their chronic disease can take significant responsibility for their treatment and decision making in their disease. There is no legal requirement for assent to medical treatment, although, pragmatically speaking, treatment without assent is difficult as a child enters adolescence. The parents are charged with the duty to act on their understanding of the best interests of the child, but it is the child's rights and interests that should determine the decision, not the parents' interests or preferences. One formulation of this duty includes the responsibility to defend the child's right to an open future—the idea of maintaining a broad range of choices for the child until the child can make decisions for him- or herself (Feinberg, 1980). Although parents are presumed to have the legal authority to act on their child's behalf, this is not an unlimited authority. The concept of children's inclusion in decisions to the extent of their capacity is broadly supported (American Academy of Pediatrics, 1995).

Potential conflicts can arise when the parents' religious or cultural views limit the treatment options for the child. A fairly common situation of this sort occurs with the families of Jehovah's Witnesses, who specifically request that blood products from one person not be given to another (Watchtower Bible and Tract Society of New York, 1992). State laws and local judicial practices differ with regard to cases where the parents are Jehovah's Witnesses. This results in using the courts to override parents' judgment to refuse blood transfusion for their children in life-threatening situations, while at the same time recognizing the decision of legally competent patients to decline the treatment (Layon, D'Amico, Caton, & Mollet, 1990). These issues become even more complex when adolescents with emerging capacity to decide on their own preferences and life goals become involved. The laws of each state bear on the status of emancipated minors, but to the extent that they are capable, the basic principle of autonomy suggests that adolescents should control their own decision making. Even in such areas as forgoing life-sustaining treatment (see below), many ethicists argue that mature minors should have the right, in most circumstances, to refuse treatment (Derish & Vanden Heuvel, 2000).

Forgoing Life-Sustaining Treatment

Decisions to withhold or withdraw life-sustaining treatment have most often been discussed with regard to cardiopulmonary resuscitation (CPR), the so-called "do not resuscitate" (DNR) orders, and the issue of fluids and nutrition. General attempts to address this question (American Thoracic Society, 1991; Hastings Center, 1987; President's Commission for the Study of Ethical Problems, 1983) indicate that there is no logical, philosophical distinction between withholding and withdrawing treatment. Those working in the situation confirm almost universally, however, that there is an emotional difference between the two situations. Exploration of this perceived difference is often helpful in discussions of particular cases.

The right to refuse resuscitation and other treatments is now among those guaranteed by the regulations of JCAHO (2001) and the federal government's Centers for Medicare and Medicaid Services. The right to refuse or have treatments withdrawn extends to all medical treatments, not only DNR orders about resuscitation. Such issues as the invasiveness of the treatment, the pain and suffering entailed in the treatment, the short- and long-term prognosis for the patient, and the quality of life that can be achieved are all relevant to the decisions (Youngner, 1987). Other issues, such as the role of family members when patients are not legally competent (as is true of most children), patients' and families' fears of abandonment if a DNR order is instituted, and the use of DNR orders as a cost containment method, are also raised. These decisions are more complex for children, for whom a surrogate (such as a parent) must make the decisions, but generally the right to refuse treatment on behalf of someone else is recognized in law and ethics (Paris & Fletcher, 1987; Weir & Gostin, 1990). As members of the health care team not directly involved in providing these services, psychologists can play an important role in assisting families to ask questions and clarify the options open to them in the decision-making process.

The issue of withholding or withdrawing medical nutrition and hydration is even more contentious, especially when children are involved. The symbolic importance of food, its place in human ritual, and the dependence of young children complicate decisions about the provision of medical nutrition and hydration. In general, there is agreement that in cases where the goals of the patient and purposes of life are not served, it is possible to overcome the presumption favoring the provision of treatment in order to withhold or discontinue nutrition and hydration (Brodeur, 1991); however, a consensus regarding the requirement to provide nutrition and hydration does not exist. Smith (1991), for example, has argued that withholding feeding and fluids is in most cases a decision to kill another person. Several authors have discussed acceptable grounds for discontinuing medical nutrition and hydration (Chrastek, Brunnquell, & Hasse, 2002; Johnson & Mitchell, 2000; Nelson et al., 1995). One central point of the discussion is the fact that feeding by tube is a medical treatment, quite different from the obligation to provide oral sustenance. Another central concern surrounds the invasive and coercive aspects of feedings in which a person does not willingly participate. It is important to note that the life prospects of some children may be very similar to those of debilitated older adults, for whom a general consensus exists that forced feedings are not required. Forcing treatments on children that are optional for adults compromises the rights of children.

A related topic in the discussion on forgoing life-sustaining treatment entails the control of pain and suffering at the end of life. There is general agreement that relief of pain and suffering in all medical care is an obligation. In fact, it is now required in hospitals (JCAHO, 2001) and is subject to malpractice claims if not properly addressed (Furrow, 2001). However, in end-of-life situations, there are concerns that medications used to control pain can lead to a diminished respiratory drive and other side effects that may hasten death. This concern, often referred to as the "double effect," balances the unintended effects of the treatment with the intended effect of pain control. Although no absolute consensus exists in our society, most people take the view that emphasizes patient autonomy and quality of life. This view holds that the double effect is acceptable if (1) the patient is in a terminal phase, and there is no alternative to control the pain and suffering; (2) the medications are used in response to symptoms; and (3) the patient or proxy is fully informed and consents to the course of treatment (Sulmasy, 2000).

Disability, Discrimination, and Perspective

Within the health care environment, there is a growing bioethical discussion about the status of those with disabilities; this discussion is especially relevant to psychologists, who are often involved in both assessment and intervention for persons with cognitive or multiple disabilities. The question of the social versus the medical model of disability has been broadly debated. According to the social formulation, disability is not a characteristic of the individual person, but rather a characteristic of society's adaptation to the typical person. Vehemas (2004) has defined "disability" as a disadvantage or restriction of activity caused by a contemporary social organization that does not account for impairment. In this view, the obligation of the professional is to fight against the discrimination of society in general, and to advocate for the rights and well-being of persons with disabilities. In contrast, the medical model identifies a defect in the individual that should be corrected by medical treatment.

In juxtaposition to the social model, the medical model is criticized as seeing disability as a unitary category that does not recognize individual differences (Haimowitz, 2001). Silvers (2001) has criticized the presumption that "normal" or "species-typical" is good, and that people must be cured of their differences. The debate extends to genetic screening for disabilities, and whether such screening in fact represents an attempt to limit suffering, a eugenic movement, or a form of genocide against people with differences (Scott, 2005; Shakespeare, 1998). Using the phrase "the expressivist objection," they hold that using medical technology to avoid pregnancies that lead to disabilities or to alter the expression of traits considered disabilities demonstrate overt hostility and discrimination against all persons with disabilities.

Neuroethics

"Neuroethics" is the exploration of the ethics of new neuroimaging, neuromanipulative technologies, and neurosurgery. Early publications (Marcus, 2002; Roskies, 2002) set out to include ethical consideration of emerging information and practice. Although some note that these are variants of ethical issues in other technologies, such as genetics and general bioethics (Wachbroit, 2008), the robust literature is relevant to psychologists. One key issue is the appearance of abnormal results that are not the target of the investigation, but could have clinical significance. Kim, Illes, Kaplan, Reiss, and Atlas (2002) noted that 9% of children in neuroimaging studies were referred for further evaluation due to incidental findings. The ethical issues of the impact of such findings on parents and children, the likelihood of further invasive studies, and the potential for harmful treatment are significant (Illes et al., 2004). Similarly, Ford and Henderson (2006) have discussed surgical interventions for neurological problems, the increased burden of informed consent, and the requirement of practitioners to refuse to provide treatment when inappropriately demanded or if it is of uncertain benefit.

The use of functional magnetic resonance imaging (fMRI) in determining the status of behavior and functioning of the mind is also controversial. There are several scientific reports, used and exaggerated by the popular press, that identify specific functions related to particular areas of the brain. The reports speculate about the use of fMRI in legal settings, such as determining the veracity of testimony or memory, establishing the age at which one can be held accountable for criminal behavior, or maintaining the privacy of thought. Tovino's (2007) review of this area and subsequent discussions generally agree that fMRI and other new technologies are not ready for clinical use, and by implication, certainly not legal use.

The use of medications to change the emotional valence of events is also under discussion. For example, the use of propranalol to stop consolidation of negative emotional aspects of trauma and minimize posttraumatic stress disorder raises serious questions about the relative harms and benefits of minimizing future suffering and changing the nature of human experience. Effects on memory formation in general have been reported with its use (Henry, Fishman, & Youngner, 2007). Until the effects of such interventions are more clearly understood in research with competent adults, and the ethics more fully explored, the use of such measures for children should be avoided.

Enhancement

The use of health care technologies to enhance normal traits (as opposed to treating states of illness and disease) is not new, but has taken on an increasingly high profile for psychologists in health care settings. Questions include the use of growth hormone therapy for children without a hormonal deficiency (American Academy of Pediatrics, 1997); the use of surgical techniques for leg lengthening, correcting craniofacial anomalies, or creating genitalia that are normal in appearance (Parens, 2006); behavioral enhancements, such as the use of antidepressants or stimulants for attention-deficit/hyperactivity disorder (Singh, 2005); and neurocognitive enhancements in general (Dees, 2007; Farah et al., 2004). At its broadest level, the ethical debate about enhancement begins with arguments about the legitimate scope of medical practice, and whether it should be limited to treating disease and disorder, or should more broadly focus on enhancing well-being in every circumstance. It also addresses freedom of choice as it relates to control over one's body and experience. This debate is even more complex for children, who cannot make decisions for themselves, but whose developmental experiences are affected as they grow up. The safety profile and the long- and short-term risks for each enhancement technology must be fully explored and discussed with the decision maker. The precautionary principle argues for restraining such use until good data exist for both the efficacy of benefit and minimization of risks.

Research Ethics for Children and Adolescents

Many of the issues related to informed consent and confidentiality within the contexts of assessment, intervention, and consultation are also relevant with research in pediatric psychology. At the same time, the world of research also presents some unique ethical issues and challenges, which are addressed briefly here. For a more thorough discussion of these issues, the reader is referred to Drotar and colleagues (2000), Kodish (2005), and Rae and Sullivan (2003). Fisher (2004) has delineated some of the issues related to informed consent for research in light of HIPAA regulations.

The institutional review board (IRB) acts as an important checking and monitoring system in order to ensure that research is conducted in an ethical manner. Institutions that conduct research, such as universities and health science centers, have their own IRBs that govern research conducted by their faculty members. At such an institution, researchers must submit a proposal to the IRB that describes the research in detail, including procedures for selecting participants, obtaining informed consent/parental permission, maintaining confidentiality, assigning participants to experimental groups, and analyzing data. The IRB functions as a gatekeeper, so that the only research projects receiving institutional approval are those that meet high ethical and legal standards and protect the welfare of participants. The IRB approval process also provides an opportunity for the proposed research to be evaluated by an objective and external source that has no vested interest in the research; this presents the possibility for identifying ethical issues that a researcher may have missed.

Within the context of intervention research, it is important for the informed consent process to describe the nature of the interventions that will be provided during the research study, in terms of such factors as time commitments (e.g., weekly sessions), potentially sensitive nature of topics discussed, procedures used to assign participants to different groups, and other characteristics of the intervention and research that could influence willingness to participate. A beneficial side effect (for the researcher) of this process may be high retention rates once the study begins, as participants are more likely to stick with the study if there are no surprises or unanticipated consequences of participating (Drotar, 2006). Conversely, participants who do encounter surprises or unexpected consequences may withdraw from the study and develop a sense of distrust toward psychologists and psychological research.

An issue receiving increased attention in the literature is that of "incidental findings" in research. This term refers to discoveries that are not significant to the research study, but that do hold significance for participants' health (see Wolf et al., 2008). Wolf and colleagues (2008) provide the example of detecting a potentially harmful mass in a participant's brain during an MRI study; this discovery may be completely unrelated to the research questions, but clearly is important to the participant. Thus researchers should recognize the possibility of incidental findings, and informed consent processes should describe the procedures that researchers will follow if such findings should arise.

The informed consent process should also describe any incentives or compensation that participants will receive for their commitment to the study. In order for consent to be truly voluntary, incentives for participation must not be so great as to coerce participation among prospective children and families who would not participate in the absence of such incentives. This issue is especially salient when researchers are recruiting families who have scant financial resources, and therefore are more vulnerable to coerced participation that may be an attempt to collect compensation. At the same time, researchers and IRBs must understand that research projects demanding great time commitments from participants, or posing numerous inconveniences (e.g., multiple visits to a hospital or clinic, invasive procedures), may have difficulty recruiting participants if some type of compensation is not offered (Diekema, 2005). One solution has been to offer a small amount of payment at each point of data collection rather than a large one-time payment, so that incentives are spread out over the course of the study and therefore less likely to contribute to coerced participation (Rice & Broome, 2004).

Collogan and Fleischman (2005) have noted one of the complicating factors in securing informed consent for research: Giving this consent requires an understanding that a child or family may or may not benefit from participation (depending on the efficacy of standard care and experimental interventions). This is very different from consenting to psychological services such as therapy or consultation, in which there is a clear expectation of benefit because of the clinician's obligation to act in the best interest of the patient's therapeutic progress. Thus researchers must make clear the possibility (or, in some cases, the probability) that participation in the research project will not result in any direct benefit to the child or family, although their participation may benefit society at large if the study provides generalizable results. In a related issue, researchers must take care not to overestimate the potential benefits of an experimental intervention just to increase the number of participants (Rae & Sullivan, 2003). Finally, parents and children should feel safe to decline participation, and must receive assurance that they will still be provided appropriate treatment if they elect to decline participation in a research project.

As noted by Fisher (2004), a pediatric psychologist who conducts research often faces the dilemma of functioning in dual roles: researcher and service provider. This dual relationship becomes problematic when the psychologist's role as service provider interferes with the voluntary nature of research participation, thereby leading to potential exploitation of patients (APA, 2002). For example, children and families working with a psychologist in assessment or intervention services may feel pressure to participate in clinical research conducted by the psychologist. Such pressure may be related to a desire to please the psychologist, or to the concern that quality of services would be reduced if consent to participate in the research study is withheld. Similarly, the psychologist's desire to recruit participants and successfully complete the research study may influence his or her interactions with patients. Thus this dual relationship should be closely monitored, or avoided altogether, if it can potentially cloud the psychologist's objectivity or unduly influence individuals' ability to provide consent voluntarily.

Children and adolescents constituting the control group in intervention studies should have access to standard care or treatment-as-usual interventions following the data collection phase, so that they are not harmed by their participation in research (Drotar, 2006). That is, participants should not be denied treatment as a result of consenting to participate in research. Standard care or treatment-as-usual control groups are preferable to no-treatment control groups, as the former provide participants with services other than the experimental intervention, thereby ensuring that these participants do not go untreated as a result of participating.

Conclusions

Applying ethical and legal standards to the care and treatment of children, adolescents, and families can be very complex for pediatric psychologists. It is critical for pediatric psychologists to recognize that children represent a vulnerable population, and therefore that assessment, intervention, consultation, and research in pediatric psychology require special care and sensitivity to the participants' welfare. In addition, the context of practice (e.g., hospital, clinic, inpatient) and other professionals involved must be considered. All psychologists must strive to be ethical, but pediatric psychologists should be held to an even higher standard, given their role as advocate for pediatric patients and their families.

References

Alderson, P., Sutcliffe, K., & Curtis, K. (2006). Children's competence to consent to medical treatment. *Hastings Center Report, 36*, 25–34.

American Academy of Pediatrics. (1995). Informed consent, parental permission, and assent in pediatric patients. *Pediatrics, 95*, 314–317.

American Academy of Pediatrics. (1997). Considerations related to the use of recombinant human growth hormone in children. *Pediatrics, 99*, 122–129.

American Psychological Association (APA). (2002). Ethical principles of psychologists and code of conduct. *American Psychologist, 57*, 1060–1073.

American Psychological Association (APA) Presidential Task Force on Evidence-Based Practice. (2006). Evidence-based practice in psychology. *American Psychologist, 61*, 271–285.

American Society for Bioethics and Humanities, Task Force on Standards for Bioethics Consultation. (1998). *Core competencies for health care ethics consultation*. Glenview, IL: Author.

American Thoracic Society. (1991). Withholding and withdrawing life-sustaining therapy. *American Review of Respiratory Disease, 144*, 726–731.

Brodeur, D. (1991). Is a decision to forego tube feeding for another a decision to kill? *Issues in Law and Medicine, 6*(4), 395–406.

Chambless, D. L., & Hollon, S. D. (1998). Defining empirically supported therapies. *Journal of Consulting and Clinical Psychology, 66*, 7–18.

Chrastek, J., Brunnquell, D., & Hasse, S. (2002). Letting nature take its course. *American Journal of Nursing, 102*, 24CC–24JJ.

Collogan, L. K., & Fleischman, A. R. (2005). Adolescent research and parental permission. In E. Kodish (Ed.), *Ethics and research with children: A case-based approach* (pp. 77–99). New York: Oxford University Press.

Cranford, R., & Doudera, E. (Eds.). (1984). *Institutional ethics committees and health care decision-making*. Ann Arbor, MI: Health Care Administration Press.

Dees, R. H. (2007). Better brains, better selves?: The ethics of neuroenhancements. *Kennedy Institute of Ethics Journal, 17*, 371–395.

Derish, M. T., & Vanden Heuvel, K. (2000). Mature minors should have the right to refuse life-sustaining medical treatment. *Journal of Law, Medicine and Ethics, 28*, 109–124.

Diekema, D. S. (2005). Payments for participation of children in research. In E. Kodish (Ed.), *Ethics and research with children: A case-based approach* (pp. 143–160). New York: Oxford University Press.

Drotar, D. (2006). *Psychological interventions in childhood chronic illness*. Washington, DC: American Psychological Association.

Drotar, D., Overholser, J. C., Levi, R., Walders, N., Robinson, J. R., Palermo, T. M., et al. (2000). Ethical issues in conducting research with pediatric and clinical child populations in applied settings. In D. Drotar (Ed.), *Handbook of research in pediatric and clinical child psychology: Practical strategies and methods* (pp. 305–326). New York: Kluwer Academic/ Plenum.

Farah, M. J., Illes, J., Cook-Deegan, R., Gardner, H., Kandel, E., King, P., et al. (2004). Neurocognitive enhancement: What can we do and what should we do? *Nature Reviews: Neuroscience, 5*, 421–425.

Farmer, J. E., & Muhlenbruck, J. (2001). Telehealth for children with special health care needs: Promoting comprehensive systems of care. *Clinical Pediatrics, 42*(2), 93–98.

Feinberg, J. (1980). The child's right to an open future. In W. Aiken & H. Lafollette (Eds.), *Whose child?: Children's rights, parental authority, and state power* (pp. 124–153). Totowa, NJ: Littlefield, Adams.

Fisher, C. B. (2004). Informed consent and clinical research involving children and adolescents: Implications of the revised APA ethics code and HIPAA. *Journal of Clinical Child and Adolescent Psychology, 33*, 832–839.

Fisher, M. A. (2008). Protecting confidentiality rights: The need for an ethical practice model. *American Psychologist, 63*, 1–13.

Ford, P. J., & Henderson, J. M. (2006). Ethics of neuromodulation. *NANS News, 1*, 6.

Furrow, B. R. (2001). Pain management and provider liability: No more excuses. *Journal of Law, Medicine and Ethics, 29*, 28–51.

Haimowitz, S. (2001). Disability matters: Differences and rights. *American Journal of Bioethics, 1*, 53–54.

Hastings Center. (1987). *Guidelines on the termination of life-sustaining treatment and the care of the dying*. Briarcliff Manor, NY: Author.

Henry, M., Fishman, J. R., & Youngner, S. J. (2007). Propranolol and the prevention of post-traumatic stress disorder: Is it wrong to erase the "sting" of bad memories? *American Journal of Bioethics, 7*, 12–20.

Holden, G., Bearison, D. J., Rode, D. C., Fishman-Kapiloff, M., Rosenberg, G., & Onghena, P.

(2003). Pediatric pain and anxiety: A meta-analysis of outcomes for a behavioral telehealth intervention. *Research on Social Work Practice, 13*, 693–704.

Illes, J., Kirschen, M. P., Karetsy, K., Kelly, M., Saha, A., Desmond, J. E., et al. (2004). Discovery and disclosure of incidental findings in neuroimaging research. *Journal of Magnetic Resonance Imaging, 20*, 743–747.

Johnson, J., & Mitchell, C. (2000). Responding to parental requests to forego pediatric nutrition and hydration. *Journal of Clinical Ethics, 11*, 128–135.

Joint Commission on Accreditation of Healthcare Organizations (JCAHO). (2001). *Hospital accreditation standards*. Oakbrook Terrace, IL: Author.

Kim, B. S., Illes, J., Kaplan, R. T., Reiss, A., & Atlas, S. W. (2002). Incidental findings on pediatric MR images of the brain. *American Journal of Neuroradiology, 23*, 1674–1677.

Klosky, J. L., Tyc, V. L., Srivastava, D. K., Tong, X., Kronenberg, M., Booker, Z. J., et al. (2004). Brief report: Evaluation of an interactive intervention designed to reduce pediatric distress during radiation therapy procedures. *Journal of Pediatric Psychology, 29*, 621–626.

Kodish, E. (Ed.). (2005). *Ethics and research with children: A case-based approach*. New York: Oxford University Press.

Koocher, G. P., & Keith-Spiegel, P. (2008). *Ethics in psychology and the mental health professions: Standards and cases* (3rd ed.). New York: Oxford University Press.

Layon, A. J., D'Amico, R., Caton, D., & Mollet, C. J. (1990). And the patient chose: Medical ethics and the case of the Jehovah's Witness. *Anesthesiology, 73*, 1258–1262.

Liss, H. (2005). Telehealth/Internet services for children, adolescents, and families. In R. C. Steele & M. C. Roberts (Eds.), *Handbook of mental health services for children, adolescents, and families* (pp. 293–303). New York: Kluwer.

Marcus, S. (2002). *Neuroethics: Mapping the field*. New York: Dana Foundation.

Miller, V. A., Drotar, D., & Kodish, E. (2004). Children's competence for assent and consent: A review of empirical findings. *Ethics and Behavior, 14*, 255–295.

Nelson, L., Rushton, C. H., Cranford, R. E., Nelson, R. M., Glover, J. J., & Truog, R. D. (1995). Forgoing medically provided nutrition and hydration in pediatric patients. *Journal of Law, Medicine and Ethics, 23*, 33–46.

Parens, E. (2006). *Surgically shaping children: Technology, ethics, and the pursuit of the normal*. Baltimore: Johns Hopkins University Press.

Paris, J. J., & Fletcher, A. B. (1987). Withholding of nutrition and fluids in the hopelessly ill patient. *Clinics in Perinatology, 14*, 367–377.

President's Commission for the Study of Ethical Problems in Medicine and Biomedical and Behavioral Research. (1983). *Deciding to forego life-sustaining treatment: Ethical, medical, and legal issues in treatment decisions*. Washington, DC: U.S. Government Printing Office.

Rae, W. A., & Sullivan, J. R. (2003). Ethical considerations in clinical psychology research. In M. C. Roberts & S. S. Ilardi (Eds.), *Handbook of research methods in clinical psychology* (pp. 52–70). Malden, MA: Blackwell.

Rae, W. A., Sullivan, J. R., Razo, N. P., George, C. A., & Ramirez, E. (2002). Adolescent health risk behavior: When do pediatric psychologists break confidentiality? *Journal of Pediatric Psychology, 27*, 541–549.

Reed, G. M., McLaughlin, C. J., & Milholland, K. (2000). Ten interdisciplinary principles for professional practice in telehealth: Implications for psychology. *Professional Psychology: Research and Practice, 31*, 170–178.

Rice, M., & Broome, M. E. (2004). Incentives for children in research. *Journal of Nursing Scholarship, 36*, 167–172.

Roskies, A. (2002). Neuroethics for the new millenium. *Neuron, 35*, 21–23.

Scott, R. (2005). Prenatal testing, reproductive autonomy, and disability interests. *Cambridge Quarterly of Healthcare Ethics, 14*, 65–82.

Shakespeare, T. (1998). Choices and rights: Eugenics, genetics, and disability equality. *Disability and Society, 13,* 665–681.

Silvers, A. (2001). A neutral ethical framework for understanding the role of disability in the life cycle. *American Journal of Bioethics, 1,* 57–58.

Singh, I. (2005). Will the real boy please behave: Dosing dilemmas for parents of boys with ADHD. *American Journal of Bioethics, 5,* 34–47.

Smith, W. B. (1991). Is a decision to forgo tube feeding for another a decision to kill? *Issues in Law and Medicine, 6,* 384–395.

Spirito, A., Brown, R. T., D'Angelo, E., Delamater, A., Rodrigue, J., & Siegel, L. (2003). Society of Pediatric Psychology Task Force report: Recommendations for the training of pediatric psychologists. *Journal of Pediatric Psychology, 28,* 85–98.

Sulmasy, D. P. (2000). Commentary: Double effect-intention is the solution, not the problem. *Journal of Law, Medicine and Ethics, 28,* 26–29.

Task Force on Promotion and Dissemination of Psychological Procedures. (1995). Training in and dissemination of empirically-validated psychological treatments. *The Clinical Psychologist, 48*(1), 3–23.

Tovino, S. (2007). Functional neuroimaging and the law: Trends and directions for future scholarship. *American Journal of Bioethics, 7,* 44–56.

Vehemas, S. (2004). Ethical analysis of the concept of disability. *Mental Retardation, 42,* 209–222.

Wachbroit, R. (2008). The prospects for neuro-exceptionalism: Transparent lies, naked minds. *American Journal of Bioethics, 8,* 3–8.

Watchtower Bible and Tract Society of New York. (1992). *Family care and medical management for Jehovah's Witnesses.* Brooklyn, NY: Author.

Weir, R. F., & Gostin, L. (1990). Decisions to abate life-sustaining treatment for nonautonomous patients: Ethical standards and legal liability for physicians after *Cruzan. Journal of the American Medical Association, 264,* 1846–1853.

Wolf, S. M., Lawrenz, F. P., Nelson, C. A., Kahn, J. P., Cho, M. K., Clayton, E. W., et al. (2008). Managing incidental findings in human subjects research: Analysis and recommendations. *Journal of Law, Medicine and Ethics, 36,* 219–248.

Youngner, S. J. (1987). Do-not-resuscitate orders: No longer secret, but still a problem. *Hastings Center Report, 17,* 24–33.

CHAPTER 3

Professional Development, Roles, and Practice Patterns

LISA M. BUCKLOH
PEGGY GRECO

Pediatric psychology as a field continues to evolve to encompass a wider variety of clinical settings, as well as to emphasize the consideration of the larger social context of the child—including parents, peers, and the community. Pediatric psychologists work in a variety of settings, and there is significant variability in the nature of their positions, the administrative models under which they function, and the activities for which they are responsible. Revenue-generating activities include patient care, research, teaching, training, administrative activities, consultation, honoraria, service contracts, and book royalties (Opipari-Arrigan, Stark, & Drotar, 2006). In addition to integrating practice changes that reflect empirical advances in assessment and treatment, the successful pediatric psychologist must monitor and respond to changes brought about in the practice of psychology by market forces, such as managed care and increased accountability for generating revenue.

In the first half of this chapter, we focus on the professional roles and practice patterns of pediatric psychologists in inpatient and outpatient settings, considering the broad environmental context of the child. We then review professional development issues that affect the practice of pediatric psychology, including training, licensure/certification, and coding and billing.

Overview of Practice Settings

As part of a study to establish benchmarks for performance for pediatric psychologists (Opipari-Arrigan et al., 2006), members of the Society of Pediatric Psychology (SPP) were surveyed about their primary work settings. The majority of the 356 respondents (63%) indicated that they worked in hospitals, with half of that group working in academic medical centers and the remainder in various hospital-based settings, such as hospitals not affiliated with medical schools. Private practice settings also accounted for a significant number of respondents (22%). Supporting the perception that pediatric psychologists function as scientists-practitioners, the majority of hospital-based respondents indicated that they held an academic appointment, and over half of the psychologists indicated that they were involved jointly in clinical service and research. Other settings endorsed by respondents as their primary work setting were academic departments of psychology (5%), mental health service agencies (3%), outpatient clinics (3%), school systems (2%), academic departments other than psychology (1%), and other (1%).

Professional Roles and Practice Patterns

Inpatient Settings

Overview of Hospital-Based Services

Hospital-based pediatric psychologists may work in many different types of hospitals, including general hospitals, children's hospitals, and children's specialty hospitals (e.g., rehabilitation hospitals). Hospital-based practice may include clinical care, research, teaching, training, and administration. Adhering to the scientist-practitioner model of practice, most pediatric psychologists within hospital-based settings conduct research as well as clinical care, usually with the same chronic illness group.

Inpatient clinical work may be problem-focused, such as responding to a call to intervene with behavioral or emotional difficulties that are either preexisting, or caused by and/or exacerbating an acute or chronic medical condition. However, heeding the call to prevention (Roberts, 1986), pediatric psychologists provide a significant proportion of clinical services that include facilitating adaptation to diagnosis and treatment, and promoting a positive transition of prevention skills and adaptive coping to the home environment.

Although the transition to home and the larger environmental context of the child (family, peers, school, and community) must be considered even while a child is hospitalized, the hospital milieu should also be taken into account, in order to ensure a comprehensive assessment and effective interdisciplinary intervention. The child's hospital environment includes parents; fellow patients as peers; and physicians, nurses, and therapists from other disciplines (child life, education, physical therapy, respiratory therapy, etc.) as members of the community. Multiple members of the hospital team can provide invaluable assistance in both assessing the child and implementing an intervention. For example, child life specialists may promote some of the same therapeutic goals in sessions with a child, or physicians may accommodate scheduling relaxation training and anxiety reduction prior to painful procedures or aversive medical therapies.

Within the hospital environment, the pediatric psychologist may take a lead role in coordinating care across disciplines, such as in case conferences; engaging parents, siblings, and peers in such interventions as support groups; encouraging collaborative, interdisciplinary relationships with other medical professionals; and remaining an educational resource for the medical staff, such as by participating in grand rounds lectures.

Consultation–Liaison

Clinical care in a hospital setting typically involves consultation–liaison with children who have been admitted for management of acute or chronic conditions. The psychologist in this role must conduct a diagnostic assessment, conceptualize the presenting problem, devise and communicate recommendations through written chart notes and/ or dictation into an electronic medical record, and implement interventions—all in an expeditious manner.

In one of the few published studies of the characteristics of inpatient consultations, Carter and colleagues (2003) found that pediatric inpatients referred for psychological consultation typically had significantly more internalizing and externalizing disturbances than did nonreferred hospitalized peers. Psychological intervention consisted of coping strategies interventions, cognitive and behavioral therapies, and case management, and resulted in overall improvement in management of health concerns and adjustment, as rated by both physicians and parents.

Critical Care Settings

In addition to working with general pediatric inpatients, pediatric psychologists in a hospital-based setting may work within a specific care environment, such as the neonatal intensive care unit, the pediatric intensive care unit, the burn unit, or the bone marrow transplant unit. Clinical services in these environments may encompass individual clinical work, such as consultation–liaison or inpatient follow-up, family-based therapy or supportive services, and interdisciplinary case management and treatment. Furthermore, psychologists may establish collaborative relationships with other disciplines within this specialized care setting, to develop environmental or procedural modifications to inpatient settings. For example, psychologists may design, implement, and evaluate interventions to decrease stress caused by painful procedures, excessive stimulation, lack of diurnal variation, and frequently changing caregivers—all problems that are inherent in intensive care settings. Promoting adaptive coping and enhancing parent–child relationships are also primary goals of clinicians in critical care settings.

Specialized Care Settings

Pediatric psychologists working within hospital-based settings may also work in departments that treat children with specific chronic illnesses, such as oncology, cardiology, endocrinology, or pulmonology. Often a specific psychologist is designated to work with a particular group of children and their families through a continuum of care, encompassing both inpatient and outpatient care. This model of care is especially beneficial for children in chronic illness groups for which periodic hospitalizations are the standard. Pediatric psychologists within specialized care settings typically assess, treat, and conduct research in areas relevant for each particular disease group. Examples include managing procedural pain and distress in children with cancer undergoing frequent bone marrow aspirations, and assessing and treating noncompliance in children with diabetes who have multiple regimen demands. The interventions that are designed, implemented, and evaluated may often be interdisciplinary in nature. For example, Greer, Gulotta, Masler, and Laud (2008) assessed the impact of an intensive inpatient interdisciplinary feeding program. Child health outcomes such as weight and caloric intake, as well as caregiver stress, improved significantly after treatment in the program.

Pediatric psychologists have begun shifting from a deficit-based to a competence-based conceptualization of individual and family reactions to chronic illness. Kazak (2006) has proposed a conceptual model to guide prevention and intervention activities: the "pediatric psychosocial preventative health model." This model serves as a guide to prevention and intervention services based on three levels of patient risk: "universal" for families at lowest risk of distress; "targeted" for families in acute distress; and "clinical treatment" for those families at highest risk of clinically significant levels of distress.

Emergency Departments

In a joint report, the American Academy of Pediatrics, the American College of Emergency Physicians, Dolan, and Mace (2006) emphasized the vital position of the emergency department (ED) in managing pediatric mental health emergencies, due to the fragmentation of the mental health infrastructure. Both of the organizations indicated the necessity of managing pediatric patients with mental illness, developmental delays, and behavioral and emotional disorders. Pediatric psychologists may thus play a vital role in emergency consultation, which typically may involve assessment and intervention with patients presenting with risk of harm to self or others; consultation for victims of or witnesses to assault; or consultation for medical crises in pediatric patients. Psychologists may also be involved in research concerning programmatic aspects of the ED setting. In their multidisciplinary consensus report to identify mental health needs of children and their families related to pediatric medical emergencies, Horowitz, Kassam-Adams, and Bergstein (2001) proposed a range of practice strategies and research strategies regarding the mental health needs of children in the ED, such as developing brief screening tools for identifying children at highest risk of continued psychological distress.

Psychologists are also involved in research that identifies factors associated with ED utilization. For example, a study of children with sickle cell disease found that poorer psychological adjustment of caregivers and communication patterns among children were associated with a higher frequency of ED visits, even after disease severity and demographic factors were controlled for (Brown, Connelly, Rittle, & Clouse, 2006). Health care utilization, such as number of ED visits, is often used as an outcome variable to assess the impact of specific interventions with pediatric populations (e.g., multisystemic therapy [MST]—Ellis, Naar-King, et al., 2005; behavioral family systems therapy [BFST]—Wysocki et al., 2006).

Rehabilitation Hospitals

Pediatric psychologists are also actively involved in rehabilitation settings, which typically provide comprehensive long-term treatment for children with chronically impairing medical conditions or conditions involving permanent physical and/or mental disabilities, such as traumatic or congenital brain injury. Psychology involvement in rehabilitation settings tends to be focused on long-term patient needs, rather than the crisis-oriented focus typical of acute inpatient settings or ED settings. Pediatric psychology services encompass comprehensive assessment and treatment planning for rehabilitation, home and school placement, behavioral treatment, environmental manipulation, and ongoing monitoring of psychological progress and consultation with staff (Singer & Drotar, 1989).

Outpatient Settings

Twenty-two percent of pediatric psychologists surveyed about their primary work settings indicated that they worked in a private practice settings, and 3% indicated working in outpatient clinics (Opipari-Arrigan et al., 2006). However, it is likely that more than the resulting total of 25% of pediatric psychologists worked in outpatient settings, as many hospital-based psychologists (63% of respondents) described themselves as working in a combination of inpatient and outpatient settings. Discharge from an inpatient setting to appropriate outpatient services may be complicated by limited availability of qualified clinicians in outpatient settings (Kronenberger, 2006), but it also indicates an opportunity for future growth.

Outpatient settings can be diverse: outpatient clinics housed within a hospital or medical center; outpatient clinics within or closely associated with a primary care practice; private outpatient clinics that assess and treat children and their families with a wide variety of presenting problems; or creative permutations of settings, such as the Outpatient Developmental Services Project (Armstrong et al., 1999), an integration of pediatric psychology services and primary medical care of children seen in a special immunology program.

Studies examining referral characteristics of patients referred to outpatient clinics within hospitals or medical centers indicate that the most frequent referral problems are not medically related. Common reasons for referral include noncompliance with parental requests, tantrums, and aggression (Charlop, Parrish, Fenton, & Cataldo, 1987); evaluation of cognitive difficulties and externalizing behavior problems (Rodrigue et al., 1995); and assessment of school problems and behavior problems (Sobel, Roberts, Rayfield, Barnard, & Rapoff, 2001).

Collaboration with pediatricians is a central component of pediatric psychology, and pediatric psychology involvement in primary care can result in effective resolution of the referred problem, as well as decreased rates of health care utilization (e.g., Finney, Riley, & Cataldo, 1991). Primary care is an ideal setting for screening and identifying psychological problems (e.g., social phobia—Bailey, Chavira, Stein, & Stein, 2006), as well as implementing nurse-led or psychologist-led interventions for common childhood psychological disorders (e.g., oppositional defiant disorder—Lavigne et al., 2008). In addition to assessment and treatment, psychologists are involved in training (e.g., training pediatric residents to discuss behavioral and emotional problems—Applegate, Kelley, Applegate, Jayasinghe, & Venters, 2003), and program development and treatment evaluation (e.g., Chapel Hill Pediatric Psychology Practice—Schroeder, 2004).

Relationships between pediatric psychologists and pediatricians may evolve further as prescription privileges for psychologists are debated. In a recent survey of opinions on this issue, the majority of pediatricians indicated that they are opposed to psychologists having prescription privileges, and a third believed that their professional relationships with psychologists would be damaged as a result (Rae, Jensen-Doss, Bowden, Mendoza, & Banda, 2008).

Community Settings

Although primarily based within hospital, clinic, or academic settings, pediatric psychologists are becoming increasingly active within community settings. The following discussion of the broader context of professional roles and practice settings is in the form of an overview, as all of these settings are discussed in more detail in subsequent chapters.

Family Context and Home Settings

Many critical psychological and health outcomes can be affected by family influences. Family-based research and family-centered interventions are highlighted in a special issue of the *Journal of Pediatric Psychology* (Fiese, 2005). In addition to integrating and considering family influences, pediatric psychologists have begun to implement trials of home-based therapies. Harris, Harris, and Mertlich (2005) pioneered in-home BFST for adolescents with poorly controlled diabetes. Although immediate follow-up assessment demonstrated decreases in conflict and behavior problems, these improvements were not maintained 6 months later. Ellis and colleagues have evaluated MST—a home-based, intensive, problem-focused therapy that seeks to engage the multiple systems of family, peers, school, and the health care system—as a treatment modality for adolescents with diabetes. Their randomized controlled treatment trials have shown that MST yields durable effects on adherence (Ellis, Frey, et al., 2005) and reduces health care utilization (Ellis, Naar-King, et al., 2005).

Social Context

Pediatric psychologists are increasingly focusing on the social context of chronic illness from the perspectives of (1) the role of peers as a source of support, (2) peer influence on treatment adherence, and (3) peers' impact on health-promoting and health risk behaviors (La Greca, Bearman, & Moore, 2002). Social relationships have direct implications for health care utilization. For example, Brown and colleagues (2006) note that the friendship quality of children with sickle cell disease influenced children's use of the ED.

For a child or adolescent with a chronic illness, positive peer support may help to strengthen adherence to medical regimens and have a positive impact on health management. Pediatric psychologists are developing tools to assess social support from friends (e.g., the Diabetes Social Support Inventory; La Greca et al., 1995), and devising interventions to engage peers in management of chronic illness in a productive and supportive fashion (e.g., Greco, Pendley, McDonell, & Reeves, 2001).

Conversely, negative peer influence may also have a direct impact on physical functioning. In adolescence, accommodating peers becomes even more important than complying with regimen demands (Thomas, Peterson, & Goldstein, 1997). Thus it is important for health promotion and prevention efforts to take into account adolescent peer networks, which influence not only social acceptance, but also health benefits and risks. For example, adolescents who belong to "burnout" and "nonconformist" groups tend to have the highest level of health risk behaviors, whereas adolescents belonging to the "brains" group engage in very low levels of health risk behaviors (La Greca, Prinstein, & Fetter, 2001).

School

Pediatric psychologists also advocate for the needs of children with chronic illness in the school setting. Research and clinical work in this area focuses on such areas as assessing and increasing teachers' knowledge of chronic illness care, evaluating and reducing barriers to care in school, and assessing and improving social competence and peer support. For example, Wagner, Heapy, James, and Abbott's (2006) study indicates that greater flexibility in regard to performing diabetes self-care in the school setting can result in better metabolic control.

Health Care Settings

Pediatric psychologists may also be involved in programmatic evaluation of interventions within a health care system. For example, Svoren, Butler, Levine, Anderson, and Laffel (2003) designed a Care Ambassador intervention: Families of children newly diagnosed with diabetes were offered support, guidance, and assistance in negotiating clinic visits, in addition to psychoeducational modules during clinic visits. Positive health benefits, including lower rates of health care utilization, were noted as a consequence of the intervention.

Professional Development

Training, Licensing, and Credentialing

Pre- and Postdoctoral Training

There is a movement toward competency-based education, training, and credentialing in psychology (e.g., Rubin et al., 2007), including in pediatric psychology. Roberts and colleagues (1998) and La Greca and Hughes (1999) have provided comprehensive guidelines for training psychologists to provide services to children and adolescents and their families; these two sets of guidelines are considered the foundation for developing skills and expertise in pediatric psychology. Based on these guidelines, an SPP Task Force developed specific recommendations for the training of pediatric psychologists (Spirito et al., 2003). (For a further review of these training recommendations, please see Aylward, Bender, Graves, & Roberts, Chapter 1, this volume.) In addition, examples of specific training programs for pediatric psychologists may be found in a special issue of the *Journal of Pediatric Psychology* on training in pediatric psychology (Brown, 2003), including predoctoral training in pediatric psychology (Roberts & Steele, 2003); training graduate-level researchers in pediatric psychology (Drotar, Palermo, & Landis, 2003); and preparing professionals to link health, school, and family systems (Power, Shapiro, & DuPaul, 2003). Commentary also may be found on the implications of the SPP Task Force's recommendations on pediatric psychology internships (Madan-Swain & Wallander, 2003) and postdoctoral training (Drotar, Palermo, & Ievers-Landis, 2003).

Predoctoral internship and postdoctoral training are generally required in the United States and Canada for licensure. The Association for Psychology Postdoctoral and Internship Centers (APPIC; *www.appic.org*) generates an online directory of internships and postdoctoral programs; this directory can be searched by using different parameters (e.g., location, rotations), and it includes information such as populations served, major rotations, and treatment modalities. In a survey of internship programs offering a major rotation in "pediatrics," Mackner, Swift, Heidgerken, Stalets, and Linscheid (2003) reported substantial variability in the structure of internship programs and supports for interns. Most of these internships were found in major metropolitan areas (85%) and were housed in university-affiliated hospitals (72%) or free-standing children's hospitals (52%). Regarding the training domains recommended by the SPP Task Force, most sites offered training in empirically supported treatments, opportunities to work with a range of developmental levels and ethnic minority populations, consultation–liaison services, and professional issues. Training in research, prevention, and health promotion was less well represented.

Licensure

Pediatric psychologists practicing in the United States and Canada are required to be licensed in their specific state or province in order to provide clinical services (Reaves, 2006). The general purpose of licensing is to protect the public from incompetent practitioners by ensuring that professionals meet the minimum standards of competency needed to protect the public health, safety, and welfare. In some states, another level of certification is tied to third-party reimbursement; this is termed the "health service provider," and is typically for graduates in clinical, counseling, or school psychology (Reaves, 2006).

Each state in the United States and each province/territory of Canada has its own psychology licensing board and requirements. The Association of State and Provincial Psychology Boards (ASPPB) is the alliance of these licensing boards. Although the ASPPB does not govern the process of psychology licensing, it coordinates the cooperative efforts of the boards, facilitates communication among boards, maintains responsibility for the standardized written Examination for Professional Practice in Psychology (EPPP), and facilitates mobility for psychologists (Kim & VandeCreek, 2003; Van Horne, 2006). The ASPPB also maintains a Disciplinary Data Bank and a Credentials Bank, and provides the EPPP Score Transfer Service (Van Horne, 2006).

The most stringent requirements for psychology licensure in the United States and Canada include (1) a doctoral degree in psychology from a program accredited by the American Psychological Association (APA), the Canadian Psychological Association (CPA), or an equivalent; (2) 4,000 hours of supervised clinical experiences (2,000 hours in an APA- or CPA-accredited internship and 2,000 hours postdoctoral training); and (3) passage of the EPPP (ASPPB, n.d.-d; Vaughn, 2006). Delaware, the District of Columbia, and Michigan require 2 years of postdoctoral training for licensure (Vaughn, 2006). Most state and provincial licensing boards require additional oral or written examinations on ethics, areas of practice, and/or the specific laws and rules of their jurisdictions (e.g., Melnyk & Vaughn, 2006). Specific requirements for licensure for each state, province, and territory, including information on the EPPP, can be found in a database entitled *The ASPPB Handbook of Licensing and Certification Requirements* (ASPPB, n.d.-e).

Continuing Education

Most U.S. states require licensed individuals to complete a certain number of continuing education (CE) hours per licensing period. These hours range from 6 to 30 per year, with most states requiring an average of 20 per year (APA, n.d.). Some states require CE credits in specific topic areas, such as reducing medical errors, ethics and legal issues, and domestic violence (ASPPB, n.d.-a). Seven states do not require any CE credits for relicensure (Colorado, Connecticut, Hawaii, Illinois, Michigan, New Jersey, and New York; ASPPB, n.d.-a). CE is an important part of maintaining competence in the ever-changing field of pediatric psychology. In a literature review of CE research, Vande-Creek, Knapp, and Brace (1990) concluded that CE activities enhance practitioners' performance and competence, especially if the learning objectives are made clear, the format requires active participation, and there are opportunities for supervised practice beyond the training period.

Credentialing/Mobility

Several resources are available to aid pediatric psychologists in the process of credentialing and to enhance their mobility within the United States and Canada. There are three distinct avenues to enhancing mobility: (1) the ASPPB Certificate of Professional Qualification in Psychology (CPQ; *www.asppb.org*); (2) the National Register of Health Service Providers in Psychology (NR; *www.nationalregister.org*) or the Canadian Register of Health Service Providers in Psychology (CR; *www.crhspp.ca*); and (3) the American Board of Professional Psychology (ABPP) specialty certification (*www.abpp.org*; reviewed in the "Board Certification" section below) (DeLeon & Hinnefeld, 2006; Wise, Hall, Ritchie, & Turner, 2006).

The CPQ is individual certification by ASPPB, documenting that the individual has met educational requirements, has had supervised experience, has passed the EPPP (has a current license to practice psychology), has a record of practicing psychology independently for at least 5 years, and has no history of disciplinary actions in any jurisdiction (ASPPB, n.d.-b). At this writing, 39 jurisdictions accept the CPQ, and 13 others are in the process of making legislative changes to accept it (ASPPB, n.d.-c).

The NR is a nonprofit credentialing organization for licensed psychologists that aids mobility, guides psychology students toward credentialing, and promotes credentialed psychologists to consumers (NR, n.d.-a). To qualify to become credentialed as a Health Service Provider in Psychology with the NR, one must have (1) a doctoral degree in psychology from an accredited program; (2) at least 2 years (3,000 hours) of supervised experience in health services; (3) an active, unrestricted psychology license at the independent practice level; and (4) no disciplinary action (NR, n.d.-c). At this writing, 35 jurisdictions accept this credential to enhance licensure mobility, and 10 jurisdictions are in the process of accepting it (NR, n.d.-b). The CR is similar in its mission to the NR, but does have some differences in eligibility requirements and the review process (Wise et al., 2006). For more detailed information about the CR, please go to its website (*www.crhspp.ca*).

Board Certification

Pediatric psychologists have the opportunity to identify their specialty by becoming board-certified by the ABPP. Eligibility requirements for ABPP specialty certification include (1) a doctoral degree from an APA- or CPA-accredited program in professional psychology, and (2) an active psychology license at the independent practice level (ABPP, n.d.-b). Of the 13 specialty boards, the American Board of Clinical Child and Adolescent Psychology, the American Board of Clinical Health Psychology, and the American Board of Clinical Psychology (ABPP, n.d.-b) are the most relevant for pediatric psychologists. In addition to the general requirements, each specialty board has specific requirements, such as predoctoral and postdoctoral training in the specialty area (ABPP, n.d.-a; Packard & Simon, 2006).

There are several reasons why board certification for psychologists is essential. With the exponential growth of psychological knowledge and skills, specialization has become a necessity (Packard & Simon, 2006). Practice environments require specialization, given work demands and reimbursement policies, and the generic nature of licensing in North America requires additional specialty credentialing to protect consumers. There is a movement toward credentialing all qualified psychologists in specialty areas—much as with physicians, of whom 90% seek board certification (American Board of Medical Specialties, 2000). In addition, board certification aids in the mobility process, with most licensing jurisdictions recognizing ABPP certification in reciprocity for licensure (ABPP, n.d.-c).

Work Performance

Benchmarks/Salaries

Since pediatric psychologists work in a variety of settings, there are significant variations in appointment, work expectations, and salary structures. The financial infrastructure for pediatric psychology services has changed over the 40-year history of the field, and some are calling reimbursement issues in pediatric psychology a "crisis" (Rae, 2004). Rae (2004) has suggested that pediatric psychologists focus on several areas to improve financial viability, including treatment of subclinical psychiatric disorders (see discussion of health and behavior codes below), prevention and reduction of risk factors, consultation with medical staff, and focus on how psychological care can reduce medical costs.

Koocher (2004) has added that pediatric psychologists must integrate psychological services into primary care and pediatric subspecialty settings, in addition to using sound clinical interventions and demonstrating clinical effectiveness. Although managed care has had an effect on the practice of pediatric psychology (see Tynan, Stehl, & Pendley, Chapter 5, this volume), Mitchell and Roberts (2004) have argued that pediatric psychologists have the opportunity to be a link between medical and psychological functioning and "experts in the future of competent and high-quality health care" (p. 58).

Drotar (2004) suggests other creative avenues for income generation, including specialized managed care contracts, contracts with schools, subsidy of services with hospitals or departments, government and foundation grants and training grants, and fundraising/private donations. Drotar also suggests strategies for advocacy, such as working with the APA to meet the goals of more comprehensive reimbursement codes, legal and health care reform, increased coverage from managed care contracts, and increased government funding.

Opipari-Arrigan and colleagues (2006) provided data on benchmarks of work performance for pediatric psychologists in their survey of members of the SPP ($N = 356$). An average annual salary of $78,984 was reported, with an average 4.6% raise over the past 5 years. Males reported a significantly higher average annual salary ($91,548) as compared with females ($71,431). Participants reported that the main activities contributing to their total professional revenue generated were patient care (83%), research (55%), teaching (43%), administrative activities (42%), consultation (20%), honoraria (14%), service contracts (10%), and book and other royalties (4%). On average, participants were held directly accountable for about half their salaries; sources that covered the remaining salaries were hospitals (27%), departments of pediatrics (16%), medical schools (10%), departments of psychiatry (7%), and universities (4%). Over two-thirds of the respondents reported clear productivity expectations—a finding consistent with the increasing demands for financial accountability and viability in hospital settings. The authors noted that the clinical demands within hospital settings were high, with over 80% of the sample participating in clinical work. However, consistent with the scientist-practitioner model valued by the SPP, research also was reported as a revenue-generating activity by over 50% of the sample (Berry, 2006). Opipari-Arrigan and colleagues have concluded that there is a great deal of variability in the administrative models under which pediatric psychology exists, and that this makes it difficult to define the best practice models for success in hospital settings.

Coding and Billing

Current Procedural Terminology Testing Codes. As of January 2006, psychologists must use new Current Procedural Terminology (CPT) psychological and neuropsychological testing codes, designed as part of the APA Practice Directorate's effort to obtain "professional work value" for assessment and testing codes and appropriate compensation for psychologists' time and effort in providing these services (APA Practice Directorate, 2005). These codes now distinguish between testing services provided by a professional or technician, and testing services that are computer-based, for both psychological and neuropsychological testing (American Medical Association [AMA], 2007). More information on the revised CPT testing codes can be found in APA Federal Regulatory Affairs (2006).

Health and Behavior Codes. Pediatric psychologists now have the opportunity to use additional billing codes included in the CPT system—health and behavior codes (H & B codes), which may be more accurate than using psychiatric diagnoses and billing codes for children with medical problems. These H & B assessment and intervention codes have been approved by the AMA and the Centers for Medicaid and Medicare Services, and became active in January 2002 (Noll & Fischer, 2004). The six approved codes are billed in 15-minute increments and are associated with a child's medical diagnosis, not a psychiatric diagnosis. The H & B assessment and intervention codes can be found in the CPT manual (AMA, 2007).

H & B codes can be used for such issues as pain management, improving adherence to medical regimen, treating adjustment problems related to a medical condition, and enhancing health-promoting behaviors or reducing health-related risk behaviors (APA Practice Directorate, n.d.-a; Noll & Fischer, 2004). They can be used in inpatient or outpatient settings and are appropriate for consultation–liaison services. These codes cannot be used when patients are assessed or treated solely for psychiatric diagnoses. Furthermore, patients who require both psychiatric service codes and H & B codes cannot receive both types of services on the same day; pediatric psychologists should bill for the primary service provided for the day (AMA, 2007; APA Practice Directorate, n.d.-a). Psychologists must bill these codes in conjunction with the patient's primary physical diagnosis code; they are not expected to make the diagnosis, but rather to use the existing medical diagnosis by a physician (APA Practice Directorate, n.d.-b). It is important to recognize that chart notes using H & B codes to document assessment or treatment services are not considered psychotherapy notes and can be included in a child's medical record (Noll & Fischer, 2004).

There are several advantages of using H & B codes with pediatric populations. These include improving the accuracy of billing; expanding the range of services provided to children with health problems; and increasing requests for psychological services by health care providers by increasing the comfort level of parents, children, and members of the medical team, since psychiatric codes are not used (Noll & Fischer, 2004). Moreover, use of H & B codes may improve reimbursement for pediatric psychologists, as these services are paid from a patient's medical insurance benefits rather than mental health benefits, and therefore are not subjected to "carve-out" provisions or higher outpatient copayments (APA Practice Directorate, n.d.-a).

There are also several insurance-related benefits to psychologists' use of H & B codes. Providers who use billing codes the most frequently usually become the lead organizations for the service code, and the more frequently providers use these codes, the more likely they are to be recognized by private third-party insurers (Noll & Fischer, 2004). The APA's (2006) update on the use of H & B codes from 2002 to 2004 indicated that psychologists are meeting the goal of more frequent use of the codes. From 2002 to 2003, the number of H & B services billed by psychologists has more than tripled, and psychologists provided over 95% of the H & B services furnished to Medicare beneficiaries (APA, 2006).

Conclusions

As the field of pediatric psychology continues to mature, professional roles and development issues will continue to evolve. The successful pediatric psychologist must be ready to face the challenges of the changing health care needs of children, adolescents, and families, as well as the broader market forces that influence this field. We, as professional psychologists, must become active participants in shaping the future of our practice through developing exemplary training programs; supporting specialty credentialing and enhancing mobility efforts; advocating for appropriate reimbursement and expansion of our services in health care; conducting cutting-edge applied research; and implementing empirically supported assessment and intervention protocols. To continue to enhance the field's financial viability, we pediatric psychologists will need to continue to be flexible, creative, and collaborative, and to seek out new opportunities for reimbursement and income generation.

References

American Academy of Pediatrics, American College of Emergency Physicians, Dolan, M. A., & Mace, S. E. (2006). Pediatric mental health emergencies in the emergency medical services system. *Annals of Emergency Medicine, 48*, 484–486.

American Board of Medical Specialties. (2000). *Annual report and reference handbook.* Evanston, IL: Author.

American Board of Professional Psychology (ABPP). (n.d.-a). *Certification: Procedures.* Retrieved April 7, 2008, from *www.abpp.org/abpp_certification_procedures.htm*

American Board of Professional Psychology (ABPP). (n.d.-b). *Specialty board certification in professional psychology.* Retrieved March 13, 2009, from *www.abpp.org/abpp_certification_overview.htm*

American Board of Professional Psychology (ABPP). (n.d.-c). *Why should a qualified psychologist attain specialty certification?* Retrieved April 7, 2008, from *www.abpp.org/abpp_certification_why.htm*

American Medical Association (AMA). (2007). *Current procedural terminology: CPT 2008, standard edition.* Chicago: Author.

American Psychological Association (APA). (n.d.). *APA 2008 independent study catalog.* Retrieved April 6, 2008, from *www.apa.org/ce/conted_catalog08.pdf.*

American Psychological Association. (APA). (2006, August). *Health and behavior codes update.* Retrieved March 31, 2008, from *www.div40.org/Committee_Activities_Pages/Advisory_Committee/Practice/H_B_update.doc*

American Psychological Association (APA) Federal Regulatory Affairs. (2006, January 19). Questions and answers about the 2006 revised CPT testing codes. Retrieved March 30, 2008, from *www.apapractice.org/apo/Q_A.html*

American Psychological Association (APA) Practice Directorate. (2005). Psychology gains new CPT testing codes for 2006. *APA Monitor on Psychology, 36,* 24.

American Psychological Association (APA) Practice Directorate. (n.d.-a). APA Practice Directorate announces new health and behavior CPT codes. Retrieved March 30, 2008, from *www.apa.org/practice/cpt_2002.html*

American Psychological Association (APA) Practice Directorate. (n.d.-b). APA Practice Directorate answers frequently asked questions about the new health and behavior CPT codes. Retrieved March 30, 2008, from *www.apa.org/practice/cpt_faq.html*

Applegate, H., Kelley, M., Applegate, B. W., Jayasinghe, I. K., & Venters, C. L. (2003). Clinical case study: Pediatric residents' discussions of and interventions for children's behavioral and emotional problems. *Journal of Pediatric Psychology, 28,* 315–321.

Armstrong, F. D., Harris, L. L., Thompson, W., Semrad, M. M., Jensen, D. Y., Lee, K. et al. (1999). The Outpatient Developmental Services Project: Integration of pediatric psychology with primary medical care for children infected with HIV. *Journal of Pediatric Psychology, 24,* 381–391.

Association of State and Provincial Psychology Boards (ASPPB). (n.d.-a). *Continuing education requirements by jurisdiction.* Retrieved April 6, 2008, from *www.asppb.org/Handbook-Public/reports/default.aspx?ReportType=ContinuingEducation.*

Association of State and Provincial Psychology Boards (ASPPB). (n.d.-b). *CPQ: General CPQ requirements.* Retrieved April 6, 2008, from *www.asppb.org/mobility/cpq/requirements.aspx*

Association of State and Provincial Psychology Boards (ASPPB). (n.d.-c). *CPQ: List of accepting jurisdictions and maps.* Retrieved April 6, 2008, from *www.asppb.org/mobility/cpq/states.aspx*

Association of State and Provincial Psychology Boards (ASPPB). (n.d.-d). *Supervised experience required by jurisdiction.* Retrieved April 6, 2008, from *www.asppb.org/HandbookPublic/reports/default.aspx?ReportType=SupervisedExperience*

Association of State and Provincial Psychology Boards (ASPPB). (n.d.-e). *The ASPPB handbook of licensing and certification requirements.* Retrieved April 5, 2008, from *www.asppb.org./HandbookPublic/handbookreview.aspx*

Bailey, K. A., Chavira, D. A., Stein, M. T., & Stein, M. B. (2006). Brief measures to screen for social phobia in primary care pediatrics. *Journal of Pediatric Psychology, 31,* 512–521.

Berry, S. (2006). Commentary: Benchmarks for work performance of pediatric psychologists. *Journal of Pediatric Psychology, 31,* 865–867.

Brown, R. T. (Ed.). (2003). Training in pediatric psychology [Special issue]. *Journal of Pediatric Psychology, 28*(2), 81–83.

Brown, R. T., Connelly, M., Rittle, C., & Clouse, B. (2006). A longitudinal examination predicting emergency room use in children with sickle cell disease and their caregivers. *Journal of Pediatric Psychology, 31,* 163–173.

Carter, B. D., Kronenberger, W. G., Baker, J., Grimes, L. M., Crabtree, V. M., Smith, C., et al. (2003). Inpatient pediatric consultation–liaison: A case-controlled study. *Journal of Pediatric Psychology, 28,* 423–432.

Charlop, M. H., Parrish, J. M., Fenton, L. R., & Cataldo, M. F. (1987). Examination of hospital-based outpatient pediatric psychology services. *Journal of Pediatric Psychology, 12,* 485–503.

DeLeon, P. H., & Hinnefeld, B. J. (2006). Licensure mobility. In T. J. Vaughn (Ed.), *Psychology licensure and certification: What students need to know* (pp. 97–105). Washington, DC: American Psychological Association.

Drotar, D. (2004). Commentary: We can make our own dime or two, help children and their families, and advance science while doing so. *Journal of Pediatric Psychology, 29,* 61–63.

Drotar, D., Palermo, T., & Ievers-Landis, C. E. (2003). Commentary: Recommendations for the training of pediatric psychologists: Implications for postdoctoral training. *Journal of Pediatric Psychology, 28,* 109–113.

Drotar, D., Palermo, T., & Landis, C. E. (2003). Training graduate-level pediatric psychology researchers at the Case Western Reserve University: Meeting the challenges of the new millennium. *Journal of Pediatric Psychology, 28,* 123–134.

Ellis, D. A., Frey, M., Naar-King, S., Templin, T., Cunningham, P., & Cakan, N. (2005). Use of multisystemic therapy to improve regimen adherence among adolescents with Type 1 diabetes in chronic poor metabolic control: A randomized controlled trial. *Diabetes Care, 28,* 1604–1610.

Ellis, D. A., Naar-King, S., Frey, M., Templin, T., Rowland, M., & Cakan, N. (2005). Multisystemic treatment of poorly controlled Type 1 diabetes: Effects on medical resource utilization. *Journal of Pediatric Psychology, 30,* 656–666.

Fiese, B. H. (Ed.). (2005). Family-based interventions in pediatric psychology [Special issue]. *Journal of Pediatric Psychology, 30*(8).

Finney, J. W., Riley, A. W., & Cataldo, M. F. (1991). Psychology in primary health care: Effects of brief targeted therapy on children's medical care utilization. *Journal of Pediatric Psychology, 16,* 447–461.

Greco, P., Pendley, J., McDonell, K., & Reeves, G. (2001). A peer group intervention for adolescents with Type 1 diabetes and their best friends. *Journal of Pediatric Psychology, 26,* 485–490.

Greer, A. J., Gulotta, C. S., Masler, E. A., & Laud, R. B. (2008). Caregiver stress and outcomes of children with pediatric feeding disorders treated in an intensive interdisciplinary program. *Journal of Pediatric Psychology, 33,* 612–620.

Harris, M. A., Harris, B., & Mertlich, D. (2005). In-home family therapy for adolescents with poorly-controlled diabetes: Failure to maintain benefits at 6-month follow-up. *Journal of Pediatric Psychology, 30,* 683–688.

Horowitz, L., Kassam-Adams, N., & Bergstein, J. (2001). Mental health aspects of emergency medical services for children: Summary of a consensus conference. *Journal of Pediatric Psychology, 26,* 491–502.

Kazak, A. (2006). Pediatric psychosocial preventative health model (PPPHM): Research, practice and collaboration in pediatric family systems medicine. *Families, Systems, and Health*, 24, 381–395.

Kim, E., & VandeCreek, L. (2003). Facilitating mobility for psychologists: Comparisons with and lessons from other health care professions. *Professional Psychology: Research and Practice, 34*, 480–488.

Koocher, G. P. (2004). Commentary: First, AIDE for pediatric psychology. *Journal of Pediatric Psychology, 29*, 53–54.

Kronenberger, W. G. (2006). Commentary: A look at ourselves in the mirror. *Journal of Pediatric Psychology, 31*, 647–649.

La Greca, A. M., Auslander, W. F., Greco, P., Spetter, D., Fisher, E. B., & Santiago, J. V. (1995). I get by with a little help from my family and friends: Adolescents' support for diabetes care. *Journal of Pediatric Psychology, 21*, 449–476.

La Greca, A. M., Bearman, K. J., & Moore, H. (2002). Peer relations of youths with pediatric conditions and health risks: Promoting social support and healthy lifestyles. *Journal of Developmental and Behavioral Pediatrics, 23*, 271–280.

La Greca, A. M., & Hughes, J. N. (1999). United we stand, divided we fall: The education and training needs of clinical child psychologists. *Journal of Clinical Child Psychology, 28*, 435–447.

La Greca, A. M., Prinstein, M. J., & Fetter, M. D. (2001). Adolescent peer crowd affiliation: Linkages with health-risk behaviors and close friendships. *Journal of Pediatric Psychology, 26*, 131–143.

Lavigne, J. V., LeBailly, S. A., Gouze, K. R., Cicchetti, C., Pochyly, J., Arend, R., et al. (2008). Treating oppositional defiant disorder in primary care: A comparison of three models. *Journal of Pediatric Psychology, 33*, 449–461.

Mackner, L. M., Swift, E. E., Heidgerken, A. D., Stalets, M. M., & Linscheid, T. M. (2003). Training in pediatric psychology: A survey of predoctoral internship programs. *Journal of Pediatric Psychology, 28*, 433–441.

Madan-Swain, A., & Wallander, J. (2003). Commentary: Internship training. *Journal of Pediatric Psychology, 28*, 105–107.

Melnyk, W. T., & Vaughn, K. S. (2006). Complementary examinations. In T. J. Vaughn (Ed.), *Psychology licensure and certification: What students need to know* (pp. 55–72). Washington, DC: American Psychological Association.

Mitchell, M. C., & Roberts, M. C. (2004). Commentary: Financing pediatric psychology services: "Look what they've done to my song, ma" or "The sun'll come out tomorrow"? *Journal of Pediatric Psychology, 29*, 55–59.

National Register of Health Service Providers in Psychology (NR). (n.d.-a). *About the National Register*. Retrieved March 31, 2008, from *www.nationalregister.org/about_NR.html*

National Register of Health Service Providers in Psychology (NR). (n.d.-b). *Licensure mobility*. Retrieved March 13, 2009, from *www.nationalregister.org/benefits_mobility.html*

National Registers of Health Service Providers in Psychology (NR). (n.d.-c). *National Register credentialing requirements*. Retrieved March 31, 2008, from *www.nationalregister.org/ criteriaforhspp.html*

Noll, R. B., & Fischer, S. (2004). Commentary: Health and behavior CPT codes: An opportunity to revolutionize reimbursement in pediatric psychology. *Journal of Pediatric Psychology, 29*, 571–578.

Opipari-Arrigan, L., Stark, L., & Drotar, D. (2006). Benchmarks for work performance of pediatric psychologists. *Journal of Pediatric Psychology, 31*, 630–642.

Packard, T., & Simon, N. P. (2006). Board certification by the American board of professional psychology. In T. J. Vaughn (Ed.), *Psychology licensure and certification: What students need to know* (pp. 117–126). Washington, DC: American Psychological Association.

Power, T. J., Shapiro, E. S., & DuPaul, G. J. (2003). Preparing psychologists to link systems of care in managing and preventing children's health problems. *Journal of Pediatric Psychology*, 28, 147–155.

Rae, W. A. (2004). 2000 SPP Salk Award address: Financing pediatric psychology services: Buddy, can you spare a dime? *Journal of Pediatric Psychology*, 29, 47–52.

Rae, W. A., Jensen-Doss, A., Bowden, R., Mendoza, M., & Banda, T. (2008). Prescription privileges for psychologists: Opinions of pediatric psychologists and pediatricians. *Journal of Pediatric Psychology*, 33, 176–184.

Reaves, R. P. (2006). The history of licensure of psychologists in the United States and Canada. In T. J. Vaughn (Ed.), *Psychology licensure and certification: What students need to know* (pp. 17–26). Washington, DC: American Psychological Association.

Roberts, M. C. (1986). Health promotion and problem prevention in pediatric psychology: An overview. *Journal of Pediatric Psychology*, 11, 147–161.

Roberts, M. C., Carlson, C. L., Erickson, M. T., Friedman, R. M., La Greca, A. M., Lemanek, K. L., et al. (1998). A model for training psychologists to provide services for children and adolescents. *Professional Psychology: Research and Practice*, 29, 293–299.

Roberts, M. C., & Steele, R. G. (2003). Predoctoral training in pediatric psychology at the University of Kansas clinical child psychology program. *Journal of Pediatric Psychology*, 28, 99–103.

Rodrigue, J. R., Hoffmann, R. G., Rayfield, A., Lescano, C., Kubar, W., Streisand, R., et al. (1995). Evaluating pediatric psychology consultation services in a medical setting: An example. *Journal of Clinical Psychology in Medical Settings*, 2, 89–107.

Rubin, N. J., Bebeau, M., Leigh, I. W., Lichtenberg, J. W., Nelson, P. D., Portnoy, S., et al. (2007). The competency movement within psychology: An historical perspective. *Professional Psychology: Research and Practice*, 38, 452–462.

Schroeder, C. S. (2004). A collaborative practice in primary care: Lessons learned. In B. Wildman & T. Stancin (Eds.), *New directions for research and treatment of pediatric psychosocial problems in primary care* (pp. 1–34). Kent, OH: Kent University Press.

Singer, L., & Drotar, D. (1989). Psychological practice in a pediatric rehabilitation hospital. *Journal of Pediatric Psychology*, 14, 479–489.

Sobel, A. B., Roberts, M. C., Rayfield, A. D., Barnard, M. U., & Rapoff, M. A. (2001). Evaluating outpatient pediatric psychology services in a primary care setting. *Journal of Pediatric Psychology*, 26, 395–405.

Spirito, A., Brown, R. T., D'Angelo, E. J., Delamater, A. M., Rodrigue, J. R., & Siegel, L. J. (2003). Society of Pediatric Psychology task force report: Recommendations for the training of pediatric psychologists. *Journal of Pediatric Psychology*, 28, 85–98.

Svoren, B. M., Butler, D., Levine, B. S., Anderson, B. J., & Laffel, L. (2003). Reducing acute adverse outcomes in youths with Type 1 diabetes: A randomized, controlled trial. *Pediatrics*, 112(4), 914–922.

Thomas, A. M., Peterson, L., & Goldstein, D. (1997). Problem solving and diabetes regimen adherence by children and adolescents with IDDM in social pressure situations: A reflection of normal development. *Journal of Pediatric Psychology*, 22, 541–561.

VandeCreek, L., Knapp, S., & Brace, K. (1990). Mandatory continuing education for licensed psychologists: Its rationale and current implementation. *Professional Psychology: Research and Practice*, 21, 135–140.

Van Horne, B. A. (2006). Resources available from the association of state and provincial psychology boards. In T. J. Vaughn (Ed.), *Psychology licensure and certification: What students need to know* (pp. 27–38). Washington, DC: American Psychological Association.

Vaughn, T. J. (2006). Overview of licensure requirements to meet "high standard" in the United States and Canada. In T. J. Vaughn (Ed.), *Psychology licensure and certification: What students need to know* (pp. 7–15). Washington, DC: American Psychological Association.

Wagner, J., Heapy, A., James, A., & Abbott, G. (2006). Glycemic control, quality of life, and school experiences among students with diabetes. *Journal of Pediatric Psychology, 31,* 764–769.

Wise, E. H., Hall, J. E., Ritchie, P. L. J., & Turner, L. C. (2006). The National Register of Health Service Providers in Psychology and the Canadian Register of Health Service Providers in Psychology. In T. J. Vaughn (Ed.), *Psychology licensure and certification: What students need to know* (pp. 127–137). Washington, DC: American Psychological Association.

Wysocki, T., Harris, M. A., Buckloh, L. M., Mertlich, D., Lochrie, A. S., Taylor, A., et al. (2006). Effects of behavioral family systems therapy for diabetes on adolescents' family relationships, treatment adherence, and metabolic control. *Journal of Pediatric Psychology, 31,* 928–938.

CHAPTER 4

Research Design and Statistical Applications

GRAYSON N. HOLMBECK
KATHY ZEBRACKI
KATIE McGORON

What is the role of research in the field of pediatric psychology? To answer this question, it is useful to imagine what clinical practice would be like if we had no research foundation for our work. Without such a foundation, practitioners would have no basis for suggesting specific interventions or understanding why some interventions are successful and why others fail. Similarly, without a research foundation, assessments conducted with children would be based on unstandardized assessment methods, and no normative data would be available. Clearly, most of us would agree that scientific research is the foundation of pediatric psychology, including all activities in which pediatric psychologists are engaged (Noll, 2002; Roberts & Ilardi, 2003).

The purpose of this chapter is to review research designs and methods in the field of pediatric psychology. We begin with a focus on the importance of *theory* as a basis for conducting pediatric psychology research, and then move on to a discussion of research questions often posed by pediatric psychologists. Next, we provide an overview of research designs commonly used in pediatric psychology, including a review of challenges faced by pediatric psychologists who conduct research in pediatric settings. Moreover, we discuss several methodological and statistical issues that are important to consider in designing research and conducting data analyses. We conclude with a look to the future, discussing recommendations for research in the field of pediatric psychology.

The Importance of Theory in Pediatric Psychology Research

A conceptual model or theoretical framework facilitates the development of a program of research (as opposed to a set of unrelated studies) and drives all aspects of the research endeavor (Riekert & Drotar, 2000; Thompson & Gustafson, 1996). Influential theories in the field of pediatric psychology tend to share many features: (1) a clarity of focus; (2) a developmental emphasis; (3) the ability to address limitations of previous research; (4) specification of predictors (i.e., independent variables) and outcomes (i.e., dependent variables), with a clear rationale for each; (5) a clear articulation of links between predictors and outcomes (which sometimes involves specification of mediational and moderational effects), with accompanying testable hypotheses; and (6) clear implications for interventions.

Types of Research Questions

After articulating the theory, framework, or model that will be the basis for their investigations, researchers express their research interests in the form of research questions and hypotheses. Kazdin (1999) has outlined several general types of research questions from the field of clinical psychology, and these are the focus of this section.

What Is the Relationship between the Variables of Interest?

Although the first question may be the simplest type of research question, it is also a very common one that has been employed in a variety of research areas. This type of research question incorporates most cross-sectional and longitudinal correlational designs. Although the designs and data analyses used to answer such questions can be quite sophisticated, the *correlation* is the basis for all of these research questions. In some cases (i.e., cross-sectional designs), one can merely document a statistical association between two variables; in other cases (i.e., longitudinal designs), one may be able to determine which variables temporally precede the onset of other variables or changes over time.

What Factors Influence the Magnitude of the Relationship between the Variables?

Variables that have an impact on the association between two or more other variables are typically referred to as "moderator" variables (Baron & Kenny, 1986; Holmbeck, 1997, 2002). A moderator is a variable that influences the strength or the direction of a relationship between a predictor variable and a criterion variable (Figure 4.1). Sup-

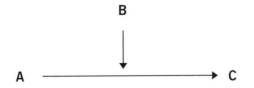

FIGURE 4.1. Moderated relationship among variables (A, predictor; B, moderator; C, criterion/outcome). From Rose, Holmbeck, Coakley, and Franks (2004). Copyright 2004 by Lippincott Williams and Wilkins. Reprinted by permission.

pose a researcher is interested in examining whether the relationship between familial stress and child adjustment to a chronic condition depends on the level of uncertainty that characterizes a child's condition. That is, a significant association between stress and adjustment may emerge *only* when there is considerable uncertainty regarding the child's illness status. By testing "level of uncertainty" as a moderator of the relationship between stress and outcome, the researcher can specify certain conditions under which family stress predicts child adjustment.

Pediatric psychologists often posit moderational processes when conducting studies of risk, protective, and resilience factors (Rose, Holmbeck, Coakley, & Franks, 2004). "Resilience" refers to the process by which children successfully navigate stressful situations or adversity and attain developmentally relevant competencies (Masten, 2001). A "protective" factor either ameliorates negative outcomes or promotes adaptive functioning. The protective factor serves its protective role only in the context of adversity; it does not operate in low-adversity conditions. Protective factors are contrasted with "resource" factors, which have a positive impact regardless of the presence or absence of a stressor (Rutter, 1990; see Figure 4.2). It is also important to note that a protective factor represents a moderational effect (i.e., a statistically significant interaction effect), whereas a resource factor represents an additive effect (i.e., two main effects; Figure 4.2). Risk and vulnerability factors operate in much the same way as resource and protective factors, but in the opposite direction (Figure 4.3). A "vulnerability" factor is a moderator that increases the chances for maladaptive outcomes in the presence of adversity (Rutter, 1990) and only operates in the context of adversity. By contrast, a variable that negatively influences an outcome regardless of the presence or absence of adversity is a "risk" factor (Rutter, 1990; see Figure 4.3).

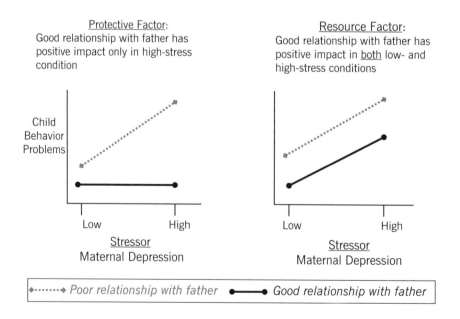

FIGURE 4.2. Protective and resource factors. From Rose, Holmbeck, Coakley, and Franks (2004). Copyright 2004 by Lippincott Williams and Wilkins. Reprinted by permission.

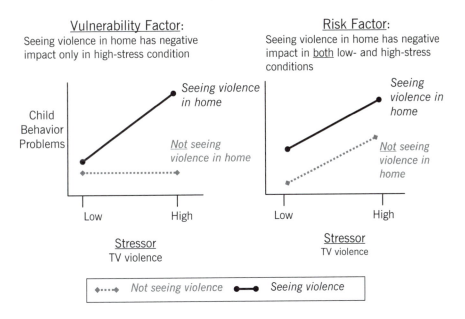

FIGURE 4.3. Vulnerability and risk factors. From Rose, Holmbeck, Coakley, and Franks (2004). Copyright 2004 by Lippincott Williams and Wilkins. Reprinted by permission.

What Mechanism Explains the Relationship between the Variables?

A mechanism that explains "why" two or more variables are associated is often referred to as a "mediator" variable. Often a mediator variable is conceptualized as the mechanism through which one variable (i.e., the predictor) influences another variable (i.e., the criterion; Baron & Kenny, 1986; Holmbeck, 1997, 2002; MacKinnon, 2008; see Figure 4.4). Suppose a researcher finds that parental intrusive behavior is negatively associated with child adherence to a medical regimen. Given these findings, a researcher could explore whether a third variable (e.g., child independence) might account for or explain the relationship between these variables. In this case, parental intrusiveness would have a negative impact on level of child independence, which in turn would contribute to poor medical adherence (Holmbeck, Johnson, et al., 2002; see Figure 4.4). Although the logic underlying meditational models is quite straightforward, several rather complex mediational models have recently been proposed (e. g., see Bauer, Preacher, & Gil's

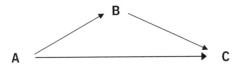

FIGURE 4.4. Mediated relationship among variables (A, predictor; B, mediator; C, criterion/outcome). From Rose, Holmbeck, Coakley, and Franks (2004). Copyright 2004 by Lippincott Williams and Wilkins. Reprinted by permission.

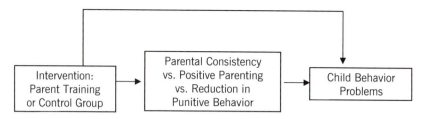

FIGURE 4.5. Mediators in intervention research: Parenting behaviors as mediators of the relationship between parent training (intervention) and child behavior (outcome). From Rose, Holmbeck, Coakley, and Franks (2004). Copyright 2004 by Lippincott Williams and Wilkins. Reprinted by permission.

[2006] discussion of mediation within the context of multilevel modeling, or Rose et al.'s [2004] discussion of mediated moderation and moderated mediation).

A research design that includes random assignment to treatment and control conditions provides a particularly powerful design for drawing conclusions about causal mediational relationships (i.e., "why" an intervention works; Kraemer, Wilson, Fairburn, & Agras, 2002; Weersing & Weisz, 2002). Such intervention/mediation models allow a researcher not only to test potential mediators within an experimental design, but also to examine the differential utility of several mediational variables. In other words, the researcher can determine which mediator best accounts for the effectiveness of a given treatment (e.g., see Figure 4.5; Forgatch & DeGarmo, 1999).

Are There Differences between Groups?

Research questions often focus on differences between groups—for example, whether children with a chronic condition have the same number of peer friendships as children without a chronic condition. Such research can be very complex, including questions of whether groups differ in adjustment trajectories over time. Although this type of research question is a variation on the correlational question posed above, group differences research tends to focus on the hypothesized differentiation of discrete groups, rather than on associations between two or more continuous variables. Perhaps the most compelling group differences research involves randomized controlled trials, where the investigators are interested in whether outcomes differ between a treatment group and a control condition after participants have been randomly assigned to the different groups. We turn to this type of research in the next section.

Research Designs in Pediatric Psychology

In this section, several types of designs and research strategies are discussed: (1) experimental and treatment outcome research, (2) quasi-experimental designs, (3) observational research designs, (4) single-participant designs, and (5) meta-analytic techniques. To conclude this section, we discuss several challenges that are specific to conducting research with pediatric populations.

Experimental and Treatment Outcome Designs

Well-designed and well-implemented randomized controlled trials (sometimes referred to as randomized clinical trials or RCTs) are considered the "gold standard" in evaluating the efficacy of behavioral interventions and ensuring unbiased comparisons across groups (Altman et al., 2001). Most importantly, they are the basis for determining whether an intervention can be classified as "empirically supported" (i.e., evidence-based; see Nelson & Steele, Chapter 7, this volume; see also Beale, 2006; Chambless & Ollendick, 2001; Kazdin & Weisz, 1998; Spirito, 1999). The most noteworthy feature of an RCT is that participants are randomly assigned to conditions—a design feature that addresses most of the threats to the internal validity of the study. RCTs, however, are not flawless; inadequate methodologies can lead to biased results, which misinform clinical practice and decision making in health care policy (Moher et al., 1998; Schulz, Chalmers, Hayes, & Altman, 1995). Moreover, given that participants are randomly *assigned* to conditions, such designs do not advance our knowledge of how individuals select, enter into, and engage in treatment.

Internal and External Validity

One of the strengths of RCTs is that they directly address issues related to the internal validity of the study. These threats to the validity of the findings have been discussed in detail in several texts that focus on research methodology (e.g., Kazdin, 2003). Briefly, the degree to which an experiment has internal validity relates to whether group differences (i.e., treatment vs. control) can be attributed to the intervention rather than to other extraneous factors (Kazdin, 1999, 2003). Another way to put it is that the investigators are interested in ruling out alternative explanations for their findings by eliminating all differences between the groups other than the intervention manipulation. Indeed, there are several types of confounds (or factors) that may operate differentially across groups (e.g., historical factors, the effects of assessment on the outcomes of interest, differential attrition; Kazdin, 1999). Threats to the external validity of the study focus on the degree to which the findings of the study can be generalized to circumstances that may differ from the experimental conditions characterizing a given study (Kazdin, 1999, 2003).

Control Groups

A critical decision in designing an RCT is the choice of a control condition (Kendall, Flannery-Schroeder, & Ford, 1999). If one is working in a relatively new area of research, one may ask whether an intervention is more effective than the absence of any form of intervention. In this case, one may be interested in including a no-treatment control group. A useful alternative to the no-treatment control condition is to include either an attention placebo control group or a standard care control condition (Kendall et al., 1999). These types of control groups address concerns related to "attention" from the interventionist. In the case of the attention placebo control group, the participants who have been randomly assigned to the control condition are exposed to a "treatment," which is expected to be ineffective in producing significant change in the outcome of interest. Standard care control groups can be employed when the population of interest is already exposed to some level of treatment because of a condition inherent to the population (e.g., standard clinic care in children with Type 1 diabetes). If a treatment has already been shown to be effective in prior work, investigators may choose to employ a waiting-list control condition, whereby the control group will receive the treatment *after* the study is completed (Kendall et al., 1999). There are two advantages of this strategy: (1) All participants in the study will eventually be given the opportunity to receive the treatment; and (2) the waiting-list condition can be assessed for treatment effects after they have been exposed to the intervention, thus providing a cross-validation of findings. Finally, in the case where there is already sufficient evidence that a treatment condition "works" better than no treatment, the treatment of interest can be compared to an alternative treatment that has been shown to be effective in past research.

Intent-to-Treat Analyses

In any longitudinal research, it is rare that all participants who begin a study complete all components of the study over time. The same could be said for an RCT, which is a type of longitudinal study (given the use of pretesting, posttesting, and follow-up assessments). In many studies, there are differences between participants who complete the study and those who do not, which can undermine the external validity of the investigation.

This issue of attrition takes on added importance in RCTs. In an RCT, if one examines treatment effects only for those who completed the study, such effects may be exaggerated (or biased), because those who were not benefiting from the treatment may be the same participants who dropped out of the study. Those who conduct RCTs have developed a method for managing this problem—namely, intent-to-treat analyses (Hollis & Campbell, 1999; LaValley, 2003). When conducting data analyses, an investigator includes all participants from the groups to which they were randomized, regardless of whether they dropped out of the study. Several approaches to intent-to-treat analyses have been employed (Hollis & Campbell, 1999). Some use the last-observation-carried-forward (LOCF) strategy to manage missing values in the context of a longitudinal study (including RCTs) (LaValley, 2003; Streiner, 2002). With this approach, the last value reported for a respondent who has dropped out of the study is carried forward and is used for all subsequent "missing" data points. As suggested by Streiner (2002), multiple-imputation analyses or growth curve analyses will be less biased than the LOCF approach. With multiple-imputation analyses, missing values are replaced with values that have been "imputed" (or estimated) from data provided by other participants in the data set (Little & Rubin, 2002). With growth curve analyses, missing values are not imputed; instead, all data from the participants are utilized, and a curve is generated for each participant based on all available data (Singer & Willett, 2003).

Clinical Significance

When conducting an RCT, one may find statistical differences between the groups at posttesting; however, if the sample sizes are quite large, the actual differences between the groups may be very slight. As discussed by Kendall and colleagues (1999), the clinical significance of an intervention is important to assess as an adjunct to an evaluation of statistical significance. With clinical significance, one is assessing the degree to which the participants no longer suffer from the condition that made them eligible for the RCT. Several strategies can be used to document clinical significance (e.g., the number of participants whose scores on the outcome of interest have moved into the normative range, or whether participants continue to meet diagnostic criteria for the condition of interest; Kazdin, 2003).

The CONSORT Criteria

Reporting findings from an RCT in a clear and comprehensive manner is essential for determining the internal and external validity of the intervention. The Consolidated Standards of Reporting Trials (CONSORT) statement, published in 1996 (Begg et al., 1996) and revised in 2001 (Altman et al., 2001), was designed to facilitate critical review and understanding of RCTs by guiding authors on how to report trials and guiding reviewers on how to systematically evaluate the findings of RCTs. The CONSORT statement includes a 22-item checklist (Figure 4.6) and flow diagram (Figure 4.7) of essential data to be included when reporting on an RCT. Readers are referred to *www.consort-statement.org* for the full statement and a detailed explanation of the checklist items.

The CONSORT statement was initially developed for use with a two-group, parallel-design medical intervention trial; however, modifications and extensions for use with other designs, types of interventions, and data have been made (Moher, Altman, Schulz, & Elbourne, 2004). Stinson, McGrath, and Yamada (2003) found that CONSORT items are applicable to psychological interventions; however, Drotar (2002) found that most reports of pediatric RCTs failed to provide the information necessary to assess the studies' validity and to apply the interventions in clinical practice. Most recently, the CONSORT Group developed an extension for trials assessing nonpharmacological treatments, such as behavioral interventions (Boutron, Moder, Altman, Schulz, & Ravaud, 2008). Moreover, the Transparent Reporting of Evaluations with Nonrandomized Designs (TREND) statement was developed to provide guidelines for nonrandomized designs similar to those that CONSORT provides for RCTs (Des Jarlais, Lyles, Crepaz, & TREND Group, 2004). Readers are referred to *www.trend-statement.org* for a copy of the TREND checklist.

In addition to the standard CONSORT checklist and flowsheet, Davidson and colleagues (2003) suggest that investigators report on the five following items when conducting RCTs in behavioral medicine: (1) background training and professional credentials of the treatment providers; (2) type, duration, and form of supervision of the treatment providers; (3) treatment preference or allegiance of the treatment providers and patients; (4) manner of testing and treatment delivery; and (5) treatment fidelity. Furthermore, Wysocki (2008) recommends that the following additional elements be considered by those submitting manuscripts reporting RCTs to the *Journal of Pediatric Psychology*: (1) attention to ethical issues, (2) verification of treatment integrity, (3) attention to cost effectiveness and dissemination of the intervention, and (4) registration of the clinical trial (e.g., *www.clinicaltrials.gov*).

PAPER SECTION and topic	Item	Descriptor	Reported on page #
TITLE & ABSTRACT	1	How participants were allocated to interventions (e.g., "random allocation," "randomized," or "randomly assigned").	
INTRODUCTION Background	2	Scientific background and explanation of rationale.	
METHODS Participants	3	Eligibility criteria for participants, and the settings and locations where the data were collected.	
Interventions	4	Precise details of the interventions intended for each group, and how and when they were actually administered.	
Objectives	5	Specific objectives and hypotheses.	
Outcomes	6	Clearly defined primary and secondary outcome measures, and, when applicable, any methods used to enhance the quality of measurements (e.g., multiple observations, training of assessors).	
Sample size	7	How sample size was determined, and, when applicable, explanation of any interim analyses and stopping rules.	
Randomization— Sequence generation	8	Method used to generate the random allocation sequence, including details of any restrictions (e.g., blocking, stratification)	
Randomization— Allocation concealment	9	Method used to implement the random allocation sequence (e.g., numbered containers or central telephone), clarifying whether the sequence was concealed until interventions were assigned.	
Randomization— Implementation	10	Who generated the allocation sequence, who enrolled participants, and who assigned participants to their groups.	
Blinding (masking)	11	Whether or not participants, those administering the interventions, and those assessing the outcomes were blinded to group assignment. If done, how the success of blinding was evaluated.	
Statistical methods	12	Statistical methods used to compare groups for primary outcome(s); methods for additional analyses, such as subgroup analyses and adjusted analyses.	
RESULTS Participant flow	13	Flow of participants through each stage (a diagram is strongly recommended). Specifically, for each group, report the numbers of participants randomly assigned, receiving intended treatment, completing the study protocol, and analyzed for the primary outcome. Describe protocol deviations from study as planned, together with reasons.	
Recruitment	14	Dates defining the periods of recruitment and follow-up.	
Baseline data	15	Baseline demographic and clinical characteristics of each group.	

(cont.)

FIGURE 4.6. CONSORT statement checklist: Items to include in reporting an RCT. From *www.consort-statement.org*. Copyright by The CONSORT Group. Reprinted by permission. The CONSORT Statement is a document that is periodically updated to account for the evolving nature of the research that supports it. It is currently being updated, with an anticipated publication date of late 2009. Upon publication of this next revision, the CONSORT 2001 checklist and flow diagram being used in this chapter will become outdated. Please refer to *www.consort-statement.org* to ensure that you are always using the most updated version of the CONSORT Statement.

PAPER SECTION and topic	Item	Descriptor	Reported on page #
Numbers analyzed	16	Number of participants (denominator) in each group included in each analysis and whether the analysis was by "intention to treat." State the results in absolute numbers when feasible (e.g., 10/20, not 50%).	
Outcomes and estimation	17	For each primary and secondary outcome, a summary of results for each group, and the estimated effect size and its precision (e.g., 95% confidence interval).	
Ancillary analyses	18	Address multiplicity by reporting any other analyses performed, including subgroup analyses and adjusted analyses, indicating those prespecified and those exploratory.	
Adverse events	19	All important adverse events or side effects in each intervention group.	
DISCUSSION Interpretation	20	Interpretation of the results, taking into account study hypotheses, sources of potential bias or imprecision, and the dangers associated with multiplicity of analyses and outcomes.	
Generalizability	21	Generalizability (external validity) of the trial findings.	
Overall evidence	22	General interpretation of the results in the context of current evidence.	

FIGURE 4.6. *(cont.)*

Quasi-Experimental Designs

As discussed by Greenhoot (2003), the primary difference between experimental and quasi-experimental intervention designs is that the former designs involve random assignment of participants to levels of the independent variable (e.g., intervention vs. control in an RCT), whereas the latter do not involve random assignment. Quasi-experimental designs are often the method of choice when random assignment to conditions is not possible. The most common quasi-experimental design is the nonequivalent control group design. For example, suppose one is interested in comparing outcomes of two camp programs for children with attention-deficit/hyperactivity disorder, and random assignment to camps is not feasible. Of course, the potential limitation of this type of design is that there are selection differences between the camp programs (e.g., there may be demographic differences between the children who select one program vs. the other program). The use of a pretest is an important feature of this design, and demographic differences between groups can be controlled as covariates.

Observational Research Designs

Most research in pediatric psychology employs observational research designs and methods. Kazdin (2003) and Mann (2003) have reviewed different types of designs that fall into this category, including (1) cohort studies and (2) case–control studies. Cohort studies are used to examine variables that precede the development of some outcome. They can also be used to determine the "incidence" of a condition (i.e., the number of new cases of a condition over time within a specified population of interest). For exam-

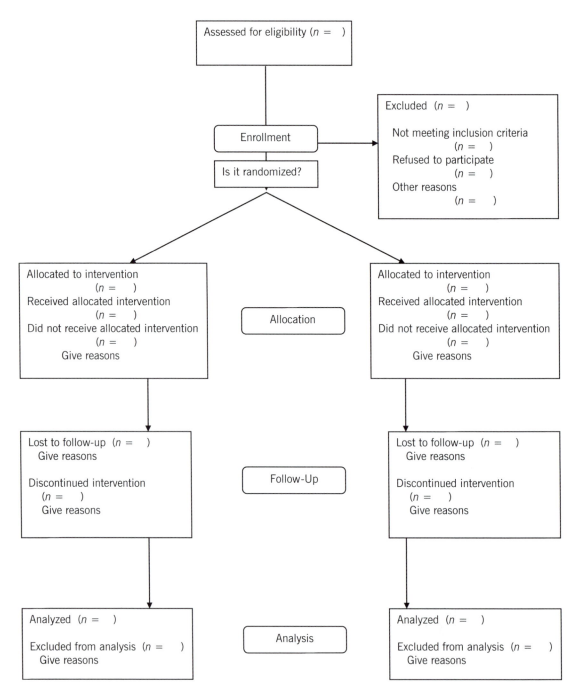

FIGURE 4.7. The CONSORT flowchart. From *www.consort-statement.org*. Copyright by The CONSORT Group. Reprinted by permission. The CONSORT Statement is a document that is periodically updated to account for the evolving nature of the research that supports it. It is currently being updated, with an anticipated publication date of late 2009. Upon publication of this next revision, the CONSORT 2001 checklist and flow diagram being used in this chapter will become outdated. Please refer to *www.consort-statement.org* to ensure that you are always using the most updated version of the CONSORT Statement.

ple, one might examine a cohort of individuals over time to determine what variables are associated with the occurrence of lung cancer or a heart attack (Mann, 2003). Or one might conduct a longitudinal study of children exposed to a hurricane to determine what variables are associated prospectively with the onset of posttraumatic stress disorder symptoms (Kazdin, 2003). The advantage of cohort designs is that they allow one to establish a time line that precedes the outcome of interest with predictors that are not biased by the occurrence of the outcome (Kazdin, 2003). In a case–control study, the investigator identifies samples that do or do not exhibit the outcome of interest (e.g., depression, divorce, a traumatic brain injury). Such a design can also be used to determine the "prevalence" of a condition (i.e., the frequency of a condition's occurrence at a certain point in time). An important difference between case–control studies and cohort studies is that cohort studies follow a group of participants who have not yet exhibited the outcome of interest to determine who will and who will not exhibit the outcome of interest (Kazdin, 2003; Mann, 2003). In case–control studies, those who already have the outcome are compared with those who do not. The most common case–control design is cross-sectional, in which two groups are compared on variables of interest.

Single-Participant Designs

Single-participant designs have long been used in measuring intervention effects at the individual level (Barlow & Hersen, 1984; Kazdin, 1982) and have significantly contributed to our knowledge base in pediatric psychology (Rapoff & Stark, 2008). Single-participant designs are fundamentally similar to group comparison approaches; however, participants are used as their own controls. Although there are several design options for single-participant techniques, all designs share at least four common characteristics: (1) objective data/baseline assessment, (2) continuous assessment, (3) change in only one variable at a time, and (4) replication across individuals or dependent variables.

There are several single-participant design options, with the most common being (1) A-B designs, (2) reversal designs, (3) multiple-baseline designs, and (4) changing-criterion designs (Barlow & Hersen, 1984; Kazdin, 1982). The simplest method, the A-B design, allows comparison of baseline behavior (i.e., "A," usual care or no treatment) and behavior after an intervention or treatment (i.e., "B"); it is most suitable for use when a return to a baseline condition is unethical, impractical, or undesired. Reversal designs, also known as A-B-A or A-B-A-B, are extensions of the A-B design with baseline and intervention phases repeated. One strength of such designs (relative to the A-B design) is the ability to show a functional relationship between the intervention and outcome over time. A multiple-baseline design consists of a series of A-B designs that can be implemented within the same individual across different behaviors, within the same individual across different settings, or within the same behavior across different individuals. Finally, a changing-criterion design is an A-B design involving multiple interventions following an initial baseline, with the criterion for successful outcomes becoming more stringent over time.

Single-participant designs have several advantages. First, they allow for examination of interparticipant and intraparticipant variability in outcomes. Second, single-participant designs can accommodate small sample sizes, such as those in studies of rare conditions, and can be used when withholding treatment is unpractical or unethical. Third, these designs may enhance clinical practice by allowing clinicians to monitor and assess real-time change and to modify interventions accordingly. Finally, single-participant studies can serve as an initial step in developing empirically validated treatments and evidence-based practices. There are also limitations to using single-participant designs. Lack of generalizability is the most prominent threat to external validity; however, this can be addressed by replication (e.g., repeating the same procedures with several additional patients). There are also several threats to internal validity that need to be considered, such as the impact of extraneous events, maturation effects, carryover effects, and multiple-intervention inference.

Meta-Analytic Techniques

Meta-analysis is a technique used to summarize and pool results from multiple studies to produce aggregated outcomes (Durlak, 1999; Lipsey & Wilson, 2001). Because a major obstacle in conducting research in the field of pediatric psychology is the recruitment of large samples, meta-analysis may have a higher level of utility in this field (by aggregating data across multiple small-sample studies). Within the literature on intervention, meta-analysis can highlight successful treatments as well as promising new directions. At the most general level, a meta-analysis is conducted as follows: (1) A research question is formulated, and hypotheses are clearly stated; (2) a comprehensive sample of studies is obtained (i.e., one conducts a thorough literature review of both published and unpublished studies and selects studies based on explicit inclusionary criteria); (3) information from individual research reports is coded; (4) analyses are conducted with statistics specially designed for meta-analyses; and (5) conclusions are drawn, and recommendations for future research are provided.

Researchers employ measures of effect size to convey results in meta-analysis. Although different studies may make use of different measures of effect size, one common index is Cohen's d. In the context of an RCT, this effect size is calculated by subtracting the mean of the control group from the mean of the target group, divided by a pooled standard deviation (other statistics often used in meta-analysis are the product–moment correlation [r] and odds ratios). Simply put, effect sizes express the magnitude of difference between two groups in standard deviation units, which allows results across studies to be compared and pooled.

Challenges in Conducting Research with Pediatric Populations

Several research issues pertain specifically to the study of pediatric populations. First, it is important to determine the setting in which the data will be collected. Because many pediatric populations regularly attend hospital clinics, clinic-based data collections may be a relatively efficient strategy. On the other hand, there are certain drawbacks to this strategy: (1) Children and/or parents may be particularly stressed during clinic visits; (2) a child is often accompanied by only one caregiver, making it difficult to assess all family members; and (3) clinic settings are busy environments, which may be distracting to research participants. Data collections from children with a chronic condition may also be complicated if there are cognitive impairments accompanying the condition or if there is a temporary exacerbation of the condition. In a longitudinal study with a pediatric population, a researcher is studying a physical condition that may change over time (with respect to presentation or severity). Moreover, treatments for the condition may also change over time, which could have an impact on the severity of the condition. In such work, whether cross-sectional or longitudinal, sample sizes are another very important concern. Studies in pediatric populations are often underpowered (even when there is a low level of attrition); thus multisite trials are common.

Methodological and Statistical Issues

In this section, we discuss several issues relevant to data collection and statistical analyses in the field of pediatric psychology.

Multisource, Multimethod Data in Pediatric Settings

Once a researcher has formulated a particular research question, decisions need to be made concerning the research design, including the nature of the data to be collected. For instance, what sources or informants will provide the data? And what methods will be used to collect the data? Answers to these questions are critical, because they will have an impact on the ability to rule out alternative explanations for the findings (see Holmbeck, Li, Schurman, Friedman, & Coakley, 2002, for an extended discussion of issues related to the collection and management of multisource, multimethod data; see also Palermo & Wilson, Chapter 15, this volume, for information on methods of collecting data electronically).

Strategies for Managing Attrition and Retention of Participants

In conducting an RCT or any type of longitudinal study, attending to issues of attrition and retention is critical. Several strategies are available to reduce attrition. First, it is helpful to foster the participants' commitment to the study. This can be accomplished by sending project newsletters to participants, although it is critical that the primary hypotheses of the study not be revealed in such newsletters. Second, it is important to develop a tracking system to keep participants' contact information current. Third, at each data collection point, it is important to gather all current contact information (including email addresses), as well as contact information for individuals who will always know the whereabouts of a given participant. Finally, if researchers have funds to compensate participants for their work, they can increase the compensation at each data collection point, with a "bonus" provided to those who complete all data collections (although researchers should avoid making such inducements coercive).

Cleaning Data

Using strategies to ensure the integrity of data is critical (Farrell, 1999). For example, after data have been entered, it is important to run frequency analyses on all variables to check for out-of-range values. Moreover, it is useful to employ double-data-entry procedures to detect errors in data entry. It is beneficial to enter data at the item level, rather than at the scale level, so that psychometrics can be examined (e.g., alpha coefficients). One also needs to be attentive to when items need to be recoded (in cases where the item is keyed in a direction opposite to that of the scale of which it is a part). Moreover, one also has to make decisions about how to handle missing values (Farrell, 1999; Little & Rubin, 2002). Once the data have been cleaned and decisions have been made about missing values, it is useful to examine the data for "univariate outliers" (i.e., values that fall outside the typical range for one's sample), as well as for "multivariate outliers" (i.e., unusual combinations of scores across variables for given participants) (see Tabachnick & Fidell, 2007). If a variable is significantly skewed, it is useful to consider data transformations (e.g., log transformations) (Farrell, 1999; Tabachnick & Fidell, 2007).

Cultural and Ethnic Factors

The field of pediatric psychology has witnessed a shift of emphasis to multiculturalism and diversity (Clay, Mordhurst, & Lehn, 2002). Prevalence rates of many diseases vary by race and ethnicity (e.g., obesity, sickle cell disease, spina bifida, Tay–Sachs disease) (Clay et al., 2002), and treatment success is often moderated by cultural and ethnic variables (Clay et al., 2002). Interestingly, Clay and colleagues (2002) conducted a review of 71 empirically supported treatments in pediatric psychology (the reports were published in 1965–1997), and found that only 27% of the studies reported the racial or ethnic composition of the sample and only 18% reported the socioeconomic status (SES) of the sample. These authors recommended that investigators take the following issues into consideration when conducting culturally oriented research in pediatric psychology: (1) the influence of culturally relevant family constructs; (2) the degree to which health care beliefs, practices, and utilization may be influenced by culture; (3) ways in which treatments can address the unique barriers faced by low-SES families and those from underrepresented groups; (4) the independent and interactional effects of health and minority status; (5) ways in which some cultural variables may be protective; (6) the cultural appropriateness of assessment measures; and (7) the degree to which cultural issues are considered in interpreting research results.

Power, Effect Sizes, and Confidence Intervals

As of 2007, the *Journal of Pediatric Psychology* has required that investigators include effect sizes and confidence intervals in their submitted manuscripts, when appropriate (see also Wilkinson & Task Force on Statistical Inference, 1999). Given that studies in the field of pediatric psychology usually have small sample sizes, these recommendations are particularly relevant. If investigators were to focus only on statistical significance, a correlation coefficient of .30, for example, might be significant in one sample but nonsignificant in another sample, depending on the sample size. But the effect size for an r of .30 would be identical across the two studies (in fact, r is a measure of effect size). Several papers have appeared that demonstrate methods for computing effect sizes (e.g., Rosenthal, 1994). To determine the sample size necessary to detect an effect of a given size, one typically conducts a power analysis prior to collecting data (Wilkinson & Task Force, 1999). Finally, confidence intervals provide "margins of error" around a statistical value; in other words, it is a measure of the precision of a statistical value. For example, one might compute confidence intervals around a mean, which is computationally a function of (but not equivalent to) the standard error (Cumming & Finch, 2005). One then plots one's findings with confidence intervals (or error bars).

Suggestions for Conducting Data Analyses and Protecting Statistical Conclusion Validity

Perhaps the best advice that can be given about data analyses is the following: "Although complex designs and state-of-the-art methods are sometimes necessary to address research questions effectively, simpler classical approaches can often provide elegant and sufficient answers to important questions. Do not choose an analytic method to impress your readers or to deflect criticism" (Wilkinson & Task Force, 1999, p. 598). More generally, Kazdin (2003) discusses several possible threats to statistical conclusion validity, or the statistical evaluation component of the study, that have an impact on the quality of the study's conclusions: (1) low statistical power, (2) violated assumptions of statistical tests, (3) a lack of reliability for some or all of the measures, (4) running large numbers of analyses, and (5) random heterogeneity in the respondents.

Conclusions and Recommendations: The State of the Art and a Look to the Future

The purpose of this chapter has been to highlight issues for investigators to consider when designing research in the field of pediatric psychology. We have intentionally begun our discussion with a focus on theory, because we believe that the process of theory generation drives all other aspects of the research endeavor. We now offer several directions for future research in the field of pediatric psychology, based on our review. First, we recommend that more research be longitudinal and developmentally oriented (Holmbeck, Bruno, & Jandasek, 2006). Second, we recommend that researchers go beyond examining bivariate associations between predictors and outcomes in single pediatric samples. Third, we recommend that scholars attempt to specify and examine the influence of moderator variables; in this way, they should be able to determine to whom the effects apply or do not apply. Fourth, for findings that have considerable support in the literature, we suggest that researchers begin to theorize about variables that may explain (or mediate) such associations. Fifth, we recommend careful attention to issues of internal and external validity in designing a study, to rule out alternative explanations for the findings. Finally, we suggest that researchers take good care of their data by minimizing missing data, cleaning the data prior to conducting data analyses, attending to issues of data integrity (data distributions, outliers), and attempting to increase retention. With advances in research on pediatric populations, we will understand better the impact of chronic conditions as these conditions unfold over time. With such understanding, we will be able to design developmentally relevant intervention strategies for such youths and their families.

Acknowledgment

Completion of this chapter was supported by a research grant from the National Institute of Child Health and Human Development (No. R01-HD048629).

References

Altman, D. G., Schulz, K. F., Moher, D., Egger, M., Davidoff, F., Elbourne, D., et al. (2001). The revised CONSORT statement for reporting randomized trials: Explanation and elaboration. *Annals of Internal Medicine, 134,* 663–694.

Barlow, D. H., & Hersen, M. (1984). *Single case experimental designs* (2nd ed.). New York: Pergamon Press.

Baron, R. M., & Kenny, D. A. (1986). The moderator–mediator variable distinction in social psychological research: Conceptual, strategic, and statistical considerations. *Journal of Personality and Social Psychology, 51,* 1173–1182.

Bauer, D. J., Preacher, K. J., & Gil, K. M. (2006). Conceptualizing and testing random indirect effects and moderated mediation in multilevel models: New procedures and recommendations. *Psychological Methods, 11,* 142–163.

Beale, I. L. (2006). Scholarly literature review: Efficacy of psychological interventions for pediatric chronic illnesses. *Journal of Pediatric Psychology, 31,* 437–451.

Begg, C., Cho, M., Eastwood, S., Horton, R., Moher, D., Olkin, I., et al. (1996). Improving the quality of reporting randomized controlled trials: The CONSORT statement. *Journal of the American Medical Association, 276,* 637–639.

Boutron, I., Moher, D., Altman, D., Schulz, K., & Ravaud, P. (2008). Extending the CONSORT statement for randomized trials of nonpharmacologic treatment: Explanation and elaboration. *Annals of Internal Medicine, 148,* 295–309.

Chambless, D. L., & Ollendick, T. H. (2001). Empirically supported psychological interventions: Controversies and evidence. *Annual Review of Psychology, 52,* 685–716.

Clay, D. L., Mordhurst, M. J., & Lehn, L. (2002). Empirically supported treatments in pediatric psychology: Where is the diversity? *Journal of Pediatric Psychology, 27,* 325–337.

Cumming, G., & Finch, S. (2005). Inference by eye: Confidence intervals and how to read pictures of data. *American Psychologist, 60,* 170–180.

Davidson, K., Goldstein, M., Kaplan, R., Kaufmann, P., Knatterud, G., Orleans, C. T., et al. (2003). Evidence-based behavioral medicine: What is it and how do we achieve it? *Annals of Behavioral Medicine, 26,* 161–171.

Des Jarlais, D., Lyles, C., Crepaz, N., & TREND Group. (2004). Improving the reporting quality of nonrandomized evaluations of behavioral and public health interventions: The TREND statement. *American Journal of Public Health, 94,* 361–366.

Drotar, D. (2002). Enhancing reviews of psychological treatments with pediatric populations: Thoughts on next steps. *Journal of Pediatric Psychology, 27,* 167–176.

Durlak, J. A. (1999). Meta-analytic research methods. In P. C. Kendall, J. N. Butcher, & G. N. Holmbeck (Eds.), *Handbook of research methods in clinical psychology* (2nd ed., pp. 419–428). New York: Wiley.

Farrell, A. D. (1999). Statistical methods in clinical research. In P. C. Kendall, J. N. Butcher, & G. N. Holmbeck (Eds.), *Handbook of research methods in clinical psychology* (2nd ed., pp. 72–106). New York: Wiley.

Forgatch, M. S., & DeGarmo, D. S. (1999). Parenting through change: An effective prevention program for single mothers. *Journal of Consulting and Clinical Psychology, 67,* 711–724.

Greenhoot, A. F. (2003). Design and analysis of experimental and quasi-experimental investigations. In M. C. Roberts & S. S. Ilardi (Eds.), *Handbook of research methods in clinical psychology* (pp. 92–114). Oxford, UK: Blackwell.

Hollis, S., & Campbell, F. (1999). What is meant by intention to treat analysis?: Survey of published randomized controlled trials. *British Medical Journal, 319,* 670–674.

Holmbeck, G. N. (1997). Toward terminological, conceptual, and statistical clarity in the study of mediators and moderators: Examples from the child-clinical and pediatric psychology literatures. *Journal of Consulting and Clinical Psychology, 65,* 599–610.

Holmbeck, G. N. (2002). Post-hoc probing of significant moderational and mediational effects in studies of pediatric populations. *Journal of Pediatric Psychology, 27,* 87–96.

Holmbeck, G. N., Bruno, L. F., & Jandasek, B. (2006). Longitudinal research in pediatric psychology: An introduction to the special issue. *Journal of Pediatric Psychology, 31,* 995–1001.

Holmbeck, G. N, Johnson, S. Z., Wills, K. E., McKernon, W., Rose, B., Erklin, S., et al. (2002). Observed and perceived parental overprotection in relation to psychosocial adjustment in preadolescents with a physical disability: The mediational role of behavioral autonomy. *Journal of Consulting and Clinical Psychology, 70,* 96–110.

Holmbeck, G. N., Li, S. T., Schurman, J. V., Friedman, D., & Coakley, R. M. (2002). Collecting and managing multisource and multimethod data in studies of pediatric populations. *Journal of Pediatric Psychology, 27,* 5–18.

Kazdin, A. E. (1982). *Single-case research designs: Methods for clinical and applied settings.* New York: Oxford University Press.

Kazdin, A. E. (1999). Overview of research design issues in clinical psychology. In P. C. Kendall, J. N. Butcher, & G. N. Holmbeck (Eds.), *Handbook of research methods in clinical psychology* (2nd ed., pp.3–30). New York: Wiley.

Kazdin, A. E. (2003). *Research design in clinical psychology* (4th ed.). Boston: Allyn & Bacon.

Kazdin, A. E., & Weisz, J. R. (1998). Identifying and developing empirically supported child and adolescent treatments. *Journal of Consulting and Clinical Psychology, 66,* 19–36.

Kendall, P. C., Flannery-Schroeder, E. C., & Ford, J. D. (1999). Therapy outcome research methods. In P. C. Kendall, J. N. Butcher, & G. N. Holmbeck (Eds.), *Handbook of research methods in clinical psychology* (2nd ed., pp. 330–363). New York: Wiley.

Kraemer, H. C., Wilson, T., Fairburn, C. G., & Agras, W. S. (2002). Mediators and moderators of treatment effects in randomized clinical trials. *Archives of General Psychiatry, 59,* 877–883.

LaValley, M. P. (2003, October). *Intent-to-treat analysis of randomized clinical trials.* Paper presented at the meetings of the American College of Rheumatology and the Association of Rheumatology Health Professionals, Orlando, FL.

Lipsey, M. W., & Wilson, D. B. (2001). *Practical meta-analysis.* Thousand Oaks, CA: Sage.

Little, R. J. A., & Rubin, D. B. (2002). *Statistical analysis with missing data.* New York: Wiley.

MacKinnon, D. P. (2008). *Introduction to statistical mediation analysis.* New York: Erlbaum.

Mann, C. J. (2003). Observational research methods. Research design II: Cohort, cross-sectional, and case control studies. *Emergency Medicine Journal, 20,* 54–60.

Masten, A. S. (2001). Ordinary magic: Resilience processes in development. *American Psychologist, 56,* 227–238.

Moher, D., Altman, D. G., Schulz, K. F., & Elbourne, D. (2004). Opportunities and challenges for improving the quality of reporting clinical research: CONSORT and beyond. *Canadian Medical Association Journal, 171,* 349–350.

Moher, D., Pham, B., Jones, A., Cook, D. J., Jadad, A. R., Moher, M., et al. (1998). Does quality of reports of randomised trials affect estimates of intervention efficacy reported in meta-analyses? *Lancet, 352,* 609–613.

Noll, R. B. (2002). How to build a better mousetrap: Introduction to the special issue on methodology and design. *Journal of Pediatric Psychology, 27,* 1–3.

Rapoff, M., & Stark, L. (2008). Editorial: *Journal of Pediatric Psychology* statement of purpose: Section on single-subject studies. *Journal of Pediatric Psychology, 33,* 16–21.

Riekert, K. A., & Drotar, D. (2000). Adherence to medical treatment in pediatric chronic illness: Critical issues and answered questions. In D. Drotar (Ed.), *Promoting adherence to medical treatment in chronic childhood illness* (pp. 3–32). Mahwah, NJ: Erlbaum.

Roberts, M. C., & Ilardi, S. S. (Eds.). (2003). *Handbook of research methods in clinical psychology.* Oxford, UK: Blackwell.

Rose, B. M., Holmbeck, G. N., Coakley, R. M., & Franks, E. A. (2004). Mediator and moderator effects in developmental and behavioral pediatric research. *Journal of Developmental and Behavioral Pediatrics*, 25, 58–67.

Rosenthal, R. (1994). Parametric measures of effect size. In H. Cooper & L. V. Hedges (Eds.), *The handbook of research synthesis* (pp. 231–244). New York: Sage.

Rutter, M. (1990). Psychosocial resilience and protective mechanisms. In J. Rolf, A. S. Masten, D. Cicchetti, K. H. Nuechterlein, & S. Weintraub (Eds.), *Risk and protective factors in the development of psychopathology* (pp. 181–214). New York: Cambridge University Press.

Schulz, K. F., Chalmers, I., Hayes, R. J., & Altman, D. G. (1995). Empirical evidence of bias: Dimensions of methodological quality associated with estimates of treatment effects in controlled trials. *Journal of the American Medical Association*, 273, 408–412.

Singer, J. D., & Willett, J. B. (2003). *Applied longitudinal data analysis: Modeling change and event occurrence*. Oxford, UK: Oxford University Press.

Spirito, A. (1999). Introduction [to special series of papers on empirically supported treatments in pediatric psychology]. *Journal of Pediatric Psychology*, 24, 87–89.

Stinson, J., McGrath, P., & Yamada, J. (2003). Clinical trials in the *Journal of Pediatric Psychology*: Applying the CONSORT statement. *Journal of Pediatric Psychology*, 28, 159–167.

Streiner, D. L. (2002). The case of the missing data: Methods of dealing with dropouts and other research vagaries. *Candian Journal of Psychiatry*, 47, 68–75.

Tabachnick, B. G., & Fidell, L. S. (2007). *Using multivariate statistics* (5th ed.). Boston: Pearson.

Thompson, R. J., & Gustafson, K. E. (1996). *Adaptation to chronic childhood illness*. Washington, DC: American Psychological Association.

Weersing, V. R., & Weisz, J. R. (2002). Mechanisms of action in youth psychotherapy. *Journal of Child Psychology and Psychiatry*, 43, 3–29.

Wilkinson, L., & Task Force on Statistical Inference. (1999). Statistical methods in psychology journals: Guidelines and explanations. *American Psychologist*, 54, 594–604.

Wysocki, T. (2008). Editorial: *Journal of Pediatric Psychology*—Statement of purpose section on randomized trials. *Journal of Pediatric Psychology*, 33, 12–15.

CHAPTER 5

Health Insurance and Pediatric Psychology Services

WILLIAM DOUGLAS TYNAN
MEREDITH LUTZ STEHL
JENNIFER SHROFF PENDLEY

Mental health insurance and reimbursement of services are of utmost concern to pediatric psychology and its practice. Reviewing the history of private and federal insurance makes it possible to gain a better understanding of the system that guides insurance and reimbursement models that function today. Moreover, the everyday practice of pediatric psychology requires an understanding of managed care, as well as of how to use mental health codes and health and behavior (H & B) codes. Finally, it is important to attend to more specific insurance-related issues that have an impact on pediatric psychology, including integrated care, the use of bundling, and employee assistance programs.

A Brief History of Health Insurance

Payment for health care by government and private insurers has a history that dates back to the 19th century in both the United States and Europe, with the earliest plans emphasizing secondary costs (e.g., loss of patient income, social costs, indirect costs to society) rather than those of direct care. Whereas Europe focused on national systems for compulsory sickness insurance, the United States relied on other means, due to a decentralized federal government and a vast rural population (Starr, 1982). Unions, lodges or societies based on national origin, and other benevolent societies filled the local needs. During this period, Americans also bought accident and life insurance to cover indirect costs for injured workers. Today in the United States, the government and employers are the largest insurers for health—providing coverage to specific populations, but still leaving nearly 46 million people without coverage (Assistant Secretary for Planning and Evaluation, 2005). Employers in this country have a history of furnishing medical care to employees in an effort to maintain a healthier work force, recruit work-ers, and instill loyalty. In an effort to fund care for specific groups of patients, unions, other fraternal societies, state governments, and agencies of the federal government (e.g., the former Veterans Administration, now the Department of Veterans Affairs) have fol-lowed suit. However, the relationship between payers and providers is, by definition and design, a source of conflict. Insurers place an emphasis on cost containment, with the ultimate goal of financial gains for shareholders, whereas providers place an emphasis on care for patients and revenue for practice. In general, providers resisted health insur-ance plans for many years, in favor of the direct therapeutic and financial relationship between healers and patients that existed prior to the rise of third-party payers. In fact, the American Medical Association (AMA) opposed many private and public insurance plans during the 20th century because of this potential intrusion, as well as the possible loss of control by clinicians over how patient care would be provided (Starr, 1982).

Issues surrounding third-party payment—particularly in regard to cost containment, as well as issues surrounding the uninsured—have been evident for decades. Beginning in 1933, President Franklin D. Roosevelt considered attaching national health insurance to the initial Social Security legislation, and in 1938 he convened a National Health Conference to review possible plans. In the postwar period, during a phase of rapid economic growth, President Harry Truman attempted to revive the 1938 plan as part of a package to increase research and medical training, as well as to provide universal coverage. President Lyndon Johnson, as part of the 1960s Great Society program, also attended to the needs of the uninsured by introducing Medicare for older Americans and Medicaid for those in poverty. These programs addressed the comprehensive health care needs of children through the Early and Periodic Screening, Diagnostic, and Treat-ment (EPSDT) section, which was introduced in the original Medicaid plan of 1972. Next, President Richard Nixon explored the possibility of building on existing govern-ment programs to provide universal health care coverage, with a health maintenance organization (HMO) model based on the Kaiser program in California. All of these proposed plans, from Roosevelt's to Nixon's, faced strong opposition from provider groups and existing insurance companies, in addition to political opposition from those opposed to the expansion of government (Starr, 1982). During President William Clin-ton's administration, an attempt was made to expand health care coverage and make coverage more affordable by comprehensively overhauling health care. However, despite detailed discussion and planning, no legislative changes occurred. Recently, health care has become the focus of state government intervention; some states (e.g., Massachusetts) have enacted their own universal coverage plans, while other states are discussing such plans.

Initiation of Private Health Insurance

Whereas the national debate on federal insurance has continued for decades, private health plans began growing in the 1930s (Starr, 1982). These private insurers devel-oped three types of medical benefits: indemnity plans (i.e., payment or reimbursement to a patient for certain medical expenses, but not usually the entire amount, based on individual contract between the insurance and insured); service benefits (i.e., guarantees of direct payment to a provider, often in full); and direct services (e.g., HMO plans, which provide the clinic or service with the providers as employees of the insurer). The first private health insurer, the Blue Cross network, began in 1929—essentially selling prepaid hospital services, which helped to fund financially strapped hospitals during the depression. These plans eventually merged to form the statewide Blue Cross or Blue Shield plans of today, while other private insurance companies emerged in the postwar period. With the national wage and price freezes in effect in the late 1940s, many major corporations started to offer health insurance plans as a benefit to attract employees. Initially, most plans only covered hospital stays, but over time they came to include doctors' fees (both inpatient and outpatient), and eventually prescription coverage and other health services.

With more widespread insurance coverage and the development of more sophisticated medical technology and treatment, health care costs rose dramatically from the early 1950s through the 1980s. Fees were often set by a standard of "usual and customary rates" (UCRs); that is, the insurers agreed to what doctors generally charged in a region for a service. However, because there were no caps on those fees, they rose gradually, due to the rising cost of providing health care services. As a result, UCRs increased, with no apparent limit. In response, insurers attempted in the 1980s to control rising health care costs by developing managed care plans of various types, in which the insurers would contract with providers to discount the cost of services and with members to use the contract providers. Management of care included not only price reductions, but also active management by clinicians employed by insurers to review cases and to approve or disapprove procedures.

Managed Care

Insurance companies that choose to manage care, with the overall purpose of decreasing costs by monitoring and limiting certain types of care, have three major options: becoming an HMO, becoming a preferred provider organization (PPO), or using capitation. Each option has had an impact on health care by potentially limiting access to services (Kent & Hersen, 2003) and reducing provider income (Roberts & Hurley, 1997), but possibly increasing access through lower copayments. The first option for managed payment is an HMO, which entails a company owning its own outpatient clinics with psychologists as employees of the HMO. For psychologists in these organizations, incentives are different than in private practice; the emphasis is on using available resources to treat a patient population, rather than on generating billable hours. These organizations have also begun emphasizing preventive services and patient incentives to maintain health, as well as providing care through an integration of medical specialties with mental health, rather than focusing on urgent care (Vogt, Lafata, Tolsma, & Greene, 2004).

The second and most frequently used option for a third-party payer is to become a PPO. In a PPO, providers submit credentials to be included, agree to a specified lower fee and copayment per session, and then submit treatment plans and apply for authorization for sessions. In exchange, the PPO sends patients to the provider. The third option is capitation, which rarely involves psychology and mental health services. In a capitation model, a primary care provider, such as a large primary care pediatric group, may contract to provide all primary care services for a fixed member-per-month fee. Backup insurance usually covers catastrophic illness or injuries in this type of plan. In capitated plans, mental health services are usually provided via a large group of salaried providers—a managed behavioral health organization (MBHO).

Managed Behavioral Health Organizations: Carve-Out Companies

Many large health insurance companies choose to manage mental health benefits by utilizing "carve-out" companies. Carve-outs are segments of insurance risk, defined by services or disease, that are separated from overall health risk, and are then covered in a separate contract between an insurer or employer and a carve-out vendor. Thus one insurance company may manage medical health services for an individual, while a specialized MBHO manages the mental health services. Approximately 150 million Americans are covered by MBHO companies. In recent years, MBHOs have expanded from being used only by private insurers to competing for contracts for public (Medicaid) insurance. MBHOs have expanded because they reportedly increase cost savings by approximately 20% (Feinberg, 2004), compared to health insurance companies that manage their own mental health services as part of a general medical insurance package. The savings are achieved largely by offering lower reimbursement rates, reducing inpatient hospitalization days, and limiting outpatient visits while hypothetically improving access. However, these savings primarily come from the reduction in direct costs of mental health services, not necessarily from a reduction in overall health care costs.

MBHOs have no financial incentive to capture overall health cost offsets. For example, for a child with a chronic illness whose emotional and behavioral difficulties affect medication adherence, a MBHO may refuse to authorize additional mental health sessions, because the MBHO has little incentive to spend resources on additional sessions when it does not bear the cost of hospitalizing that child for the consequences of poor medication adherence. Similarly, if an MBHO refuses to pay for psychiatric or psychological treatment for a child with attention-deficit/hyperactivity disorder (ADHD), the costs to the MBHO decrease. However, the child may then be treated by a neurologist, who is likely to be more expensive than a psychiatrist or psychologist. Furthermore, managed care health insurance companies have little incentive to pursue savings from coordinating care with the MBHO because of the substantial investment needed to develop the expertise to identify patient populations with high potential cost offset (Olfson, Sing, & Schlesinger, 1999). Potentially, when all costs are reviewed, there are few or no savings by MBHO companies, particularly for individuals who have chronic illness or risk conditions.

For some children, these issues become even more complex. For example, if a child attending a public school is covered under a state Medicaid plan with an MBHO managing mental health care, the child may receive services through his or her public school, health insurance, and mental health plan, all of which are paid for by the state. In this situation, the state realizes no savings, as costs are simply shifted from one insurer to the other and back to the school system—particularly when a child has complex, special needs. The solution is to provide coordinated and efficient care so that the child is served well and resources are most efficiently utilized. Only service coordination will achieve that goal, not a system in which different payers compete to save money, and providers compete for reimbursement.

An additional challenge to providing integrated care with MBHOs occurs frequently in pediatric hospitals when health care providers (e.g., physicians) are paneled with a health insurance company, but the psychologists are not paneled by the MBHO used by that health insurer. As a result, integrated psychological and pediatric care is obstructed by the funding system. For example, an endocrinologist may refer a patient to the hospital's psychologist, but the psychologist is not able to see the patient because that psychologist is not paneled by the MBHO. The patient is subsequently referred to a provider in the community and often does not follow through or care is not coordinated. In 2000, the AMA adopted a resolution calling for the end of carve-outs (Klein, 2000), but to date these companies still manage the majority of mental health and behavioral health care benefits.

Provider Choice and Managed Care

For some families, provider choice is an important variable, and certainly the goodness of fit between a therapist and family can strongly influence the success of treatment (Sussman, Steinmetz, & Peterson, 1999). In an HMO plan or a prepaid health plan with an MBHO, choice is limited, as services are provided from a limited pool of in-network health care professionals. For those who have a point-of-service plan (also known as a fee-for-service plan), a family is able to see any licensed provider, and its insurance company will cover service for some of the fees, but only up to the amount that the insurer considers reasonable. Finally, if a family has a PPO plan, it must again select from a limited number of providers who have agreed to lower fees in exchange for referrals. For example, in some PPO plans, a provider may only charge $90 for an appointment and collect an $18 (20%) copay from a family, even though the standard rate for that service is $125 per hour. Some PPO plans offer increased flexibility regarding choice of providers by providing "out-of-network" benefits, but families may be required to pay higher out-of-pocket fees. For example, if a patient chooses to see an out-of-network provider who charges $125 per hour, and the insurer states that $90 per hour is reasonable with a 20% copayment, then that insurer will only reimburse for 80% of $90 (in this case, $72), causing the patient to be liable for the other $53.

Coverage and Providers of Mental Health Services

Provision of mental health services for individuals with certain types of severe impairment have been covered by government in the form of asylums and residential institutions since the colonial era. In the post–World War II period, successful mental health and substance abuse treatment of adults, particularly veterans, helped return employees to the work force. These successful outcomes resulted in employers' continued willingness to pay for such benefits, in the form of either employee assistance programs or mental health benefits attached to health insurance. Although some treatments, such as inpatient benefits, were costly, the benefit to corporations in retaining skilled employees was considered to be worth these costs.

As with any other coverage, mental health coverage is usually part of a health care insurance package that is purchased by an employer or other group for its members. Each state, through its insurance commissioner, based on state laws and in conjunction with any related federal laws, may mandate specific items and services that must be included, but mandated services are considered to be the minimum. A purchaser (i.e., a large employer or a group that contracts with the insurance company on behalf of the members) may choose to buy various services as a part of the basic contract; alternatively, it can set up a system allowing members to pay an extra premium that gives them a higher level of coverage, access to other providers, or other desired services. Therefore, it is possible that a specific insurance company can cover the employees of two different companies in the same town and provide very different health and mental health benefits. Moreover, two employees within the same company may have the same "basic" insurance but have two different "plans" that provide different benefits. Payment for services is based on three factors: participation of the provider in the insurance plan, the procedure provided, and the diagnosis of the patient.

To be a participating provider for a health insurance plan, the psychologist must complete an application to the insurer, which includes information on education, licensure, any board certification (e.g., that of the American Board of Professional Psychology), any past claims of misconduct, malpractice insurance, office hours, and availability. Once accepted and approved by the insurer, the provider is considered "paneled," and is now a participating provider. This process varies among insurance companies; some companies may have unique limitations and restrictions that a provider must meet prior to approval (e.g., some insurers will only approve psychologists with postlicensure experience).

Procedure Codes: Mental Health Codes and Health and Behavior Codes

The Current Procedural Terminology (CPT) codes, originally developed in 1966 by the AMA, provide a universal way of defining and documenting medical procedures and services. This has evolved into a method by which third-party reimbursement is obtained. Psychologists use a variety of CPT codes to delineate the services they provide; the two major categories are (1) mental health codes and (2) health and behavior (H & B) codes.

Mental health codes are the most common types of codes utilized by psychologists and are indicated when the primary service provided is due to a mental or personality disorder that meets the criteria of the *Diagnostic and Statistical Manual of Mental Disorders*, fourth edition, text revision (American Psychiatric Association, 2000). All DSM-IV-TR diagnoses have been assigned numerical codes that are based directly on the *International Classification of Diseases*, Ninth Revision, Clinical Modification (ICD-9-CM) classification system (see National Center for Health Statistics, 2003).

Mental health CPT codes encompass both evaluation and treatment. For evaluation, insurers cover a diagnostic interview (CPT 90801) of the patient or caregiver, for purposes of obtaining history and current symptoms. A second code for an "interactive" evaluation (CPT 90802) exists. One can also request two evaluation sessions (a history from a parent and a second hour of interacting with a child); however, most companies will not pay for the second (interactive) session. The American Psychological Association (APA) Practice Directorate (2006) notes that psychological testing (CPT 96101) for the purposes of cognitive evaluation and screening for learning disabilities is rarely covered. Such testing is usually considered to be within the domain of public school special education services. Psychological testing for the purposes of clarifying diagnosis or documenting functioning in specific domains is sometimes allowed, though it usually requires preauthorization. Neuropsychological evaluations (CPT 96118) administered to assess the impact of a physical illness or injury on functioning are sometimes covered under mental health benefits (APA Practice Directorate, 2006), or, alternatively, are sometimes covered under health benefits; regardless, they almost always must be precertified on a case-by-case basis. This distinction regarding which benefits will cover the evaluation (medical health vs. mental health) can be very confusing for the provider as well as for the insurance representative, sometimes resulting in the provider being transferred back and forth between the mental health and medical sides of the insurance company.

Regarding therapy, the modality of therapy covered varies among insurance plans. Routinely, 25- or 50-minute individual therapy sessions are covered (CPT 90804 or 90806). Group therapy (CPT 90853) is often, but not always, covered. Family therapy with the identified patient present in the session (CPT 90847) is sometimes covered, but family services are less likely to be covered if the patient is not present (CPT 90846) (e.g., a meeting with parents only). Multifamily group therapy (CPT 90849), in which several families or caregivers are seen together, is often not covered. At this time there is no specific CPT code for parent or caregiver therapy groups (e.g., parent training groups), but some plans will cover these as multifamily groups. As a general rule, if a therapy service is delivered directly to the patient, there is more likely to be coverage compared to therapy where the service is delivered to the parent.

If a patient does not meet DSM-IV-TR psychiatric criteria, but is treated for other types of services (including those related to adherence, medical symptom management, health-promoting behaviors, health-related risk-taking behaviors, procedural distress, and/or adjustment to medical illness), psychologists can use H & B codes to bill for these services. These newer CPT codes were adopted by the AMA to document services rendered within medical contexts. They were approved by the AMA for inclusion in the CPT after an initial proposal to the AMA was made jointly by the APA Practice Directorate and the APA Interdivisional Healthcare Committee (Divisions 17, 22, 38, 40, and 54). They were accepted by the Centers for Medicare and Medicaid Services (CMS) and were activated in January 2002 (APA Practice Directorate, 2002).

H & B codes include assessment and treatment services. Assessment codes are primarily used for health-focused interviews, behavioral observations, and the use of questionnaires to determine treatment focus. There are codes for two types of assessment: an initial assessment (96150) that focuses on the biological, psychological, and social factors that may affect health and intervention; and a reassessment (96151) that reevaluates a condition and assesses need for further treatment (APA Practice Directorate, 2002). Treatment codes include codes for individual intervention (96152), focusing on behavioral, cognitive, or social factors that affect an individual's health, as well as group intervention (96153), which includes group-based services that provide educational information, cognitive-behavioral intervention, or social support. Two other H & B codes cover family-based intervention with the patient present (96154) and such intervention without the patient present (96155) (APA Practice Directorate, 2002).

The importance of the new H & B codes within the field of pediatric psychology cannot be underestimated. The new codes allow psychologists to bill and receive reimbursement for services often provided within medical settings or with chronic illness populations. In essence, these codes allow for pediatric psychologists to document and bill for services already being provided, yet not previously recognized; they have been reported to increase psychologists' revenue, which is essential to the profession's longevity in fiscally stressed hospital or clinic environments (Brosig & Zahart, 2006). Prior to the introduction of these codes, services provided by pediatric psychologists had to be documented by using the mental health CPT codes for psychological assessment or psychotherapy (90801–90899), which required the patient to meet criteria for a mental health diagnosis. Psychologists who provided services focused on prevention (e.g., addressing adjustment issues in a child newly diagnosed with cancer), health-promoting behaviors (e.g., weight management), or other medically related services (e.g., adherence concerns) were often unable to bill accurately for these services when patients did not meet psychiatric criteria. Moreover, empirical data support the use of group-based models for treatment of chronic health conditions, including parenting groups focused on asthma education or family-based group models for weight management; however, the mental health codes do not allow for group-based treatment focusing on these issues. The H & B codes now afford psychologists the opportunity to describe services accurately and to bill appropriately when working with patients to improve their health status with psychological interventions.

H & B codes cannot be used when a psychologist is treating psychiatric illness or providing preventive counseling (e.g., counseling for patients at risk for obesity) (e.g., counseling patients at risk for obesity) (Leichter, Dreelin, & Moore, 2004; Robert Wood Johnson Foundation, 2008). Instead, the psychologist can use these codes when seeing a patient for a specific medical diagnosis that has been documented by a physician. In the case of a patient with multiple illnesses, the psychologist should bill for the primary medical diagnosis being treated or the one that requires health psychology intervention. In situations where patients are receiving different types of services (e.g., health-related interventions focusing on adherence, as well as mental health services for a psychiatric condition), both services can be provided, but should not be disseminated or billed for on the same day (APA Practice Directorate, 2002). In these circumstances, H & B codes should be used when the predominant service provided is specific to the medical condition, and mental health codes should be utilized when the service is primarily provided because of a psychiatric condition.

H & B codes can be used by a wide variety of professionals, including physicians and nurse practitioners; however, data from 2004 revealed that psychologists were using these codes far more often than other providers, with 95% of such billing completed by psychologists (Delamater, 2004). Not surprisingly, the more consistent and accurate use of these codes leads to increased compensation and reimbursement.

Documentation of all services provided by psychologists is critical. Generally, documentation takes place in the form of treatment plans and session notes. Documentation for services billed under H & B codes is distinctively different from that for mental health codes: Billing is coded in 15-minute increments instead of 1-hour increments. Unlike psychotherapy or mental health notes, documentation should be concise and is kept in the patient's medical record—and, although it is protected by the Health Insurance Portability and Accountability Act (HIPAA), it generally does not have the special protection provided to mental health notes (Nicholson, 2002).

Use of Mental Health Codes versus H & B Codes

Mental health codes are widely used in pediatric psychology, and clinicians generally bill under these procedures. As yet, the use of H & B codes is significantly lower. A Web-based study conducted to evaluate the use of H & B codes (Delamater, 2004) suggested that 90% of psychologists (N = 177) sampled were aware of these codes, with 44% indicating that they utilized the codes in practice. Out of those billing with the codes, many reported that insurance companies would deny claims over 50% of the time. A majority of denied claims (73%) were reportedly denied because psychologists used a medical diagnosis. A higher level of reimbursement was seen when psychologists communicated their intent to use the codes with insurance companies prior to filing a claim. Delamater (2004) also surveyed 45 pediatric psychologists. Out of those who responded ($N = 12$), approximately half reported that they were not using H & B codes because of prearranged contracts with their hospital that did not require them to bill for services, or because these codes had not been reimbursed in the past (Delamater, 2004).

Reimbursement rates vary according to the type of codes being utilized. In a typical mental health plan, patients are covered for approximately 20–30 sessions per year and are expected to pay 20–50% of the charges. This level of copayment is significantly higher than for general health care, where copayments are flat fees of $10 to $25. To note a specific example, Medicare, the federal health insurance program for Americans age 65 and older, covers 50% of most outpatient care, with unlimited visits. The most recent federal legislation related to this (the Paul Wellstone Mental Health and Addictions Equity Act of 2007, H.R. 1424) was passed by the House of Representatives and the Senate and signed by President George W. Bush on October 3, 2008. (Attached to this legislation was a much larger appropriation bill to stabilize U.S. financial markets.) The Wellstone Act is intended to ensure mental health parity. That is, it would require insurance companies to provide the same level of care (i.e., copayment, number of visits) for mental health services as for other services. It is too soon to tell how the federal laws will be applied; however, this legislation and prior parity acts (e.g., the Mental Health Parity Act of 1996), which have eliminated caps on lifetime benefits, should reduce copayments.

Unlike reimbursement for mental health codes, payment for H & B codes is derived from medical (vs. mental health) insurance funds. This alters reimbursement rates because there are no outpatient mental health treatment limitations, and often medical insurance funds are more extensive than mental health funds (Noll & Fischer, 2004). Even if a medical insurer has carved out mental health services to an MBHO, H & B services are still billed to the medical insurer. The provider needs to remember to bill for a health service and not a mental health service. Reimbursement rates through Medicare are determined by local costs. Medicare generally reimburses all of the H & B codes, with the exception of the code for family treatment without the patient (96155). The amount of money reimbursed by Medicare for H & B codes appears to be increasing; in 2002, Medicare reimbursed $1.5 million, and in 2004, reimbursement reached $10 million (American Psychological Association, 2005). Medicaid is also increasingly reimbursing for the use of H & B codes. The number of private insurance companies who reimburse for these codes varies. As of July 2006, the APA reported that approximately 50 private payers were reimbursing the codes. Increased awareness of the codes, as well as more focus on reimbursement for these codes with private payers, is necessary in order for this trend to continue (APA Practice Directorate, 2006).

Increased Implementation of H & B Codes: Trials and Troubleshooting

One of the paradoxes of modern child mental health (and mental health in general) is that insurance companies typically have a policy endorsing the use of evidence-based treatments, but sometimes there is no specific CPT code for such a treatment or for a treatment format (e.g., a group of parents). Although a given number of visits or dollar amount may be covered in a policy, the policy is still limited to the codes specified *in that particular contract*. Thus, in a situation where a less expensive, more effective group therapy is a more appropriate treatment, a psychologist may find that group therapy is not a covered benefit and that the only covered treatment option is individual therapy. Verifying insurance benefits, and knowing which diagnostic and treatment modalities are covered, are essential for reimbursement.

In addition to issues related to the use of mental health codes, there are issues related to implementation of H & B codes in the practice of pediatric psychology. The primary ones are lack of awareness of these codes and difficulty in obtaining reimbursement for them. To increase the use of these codes, insurers within a provider's area should be asked about their knowledge of the codes and reimbursement policies. Much of this correspondence can be tracked via email and phone, and it should be recorded. For those providers working in larger hospital-based systems, the use of billing or insurance verification specialists can be exceptionally helpful during this process. After learning about insurers' knowledge, those involved can begin to educate insurers about code use. Previous groups have written letters that use data collected from APA to provide education about the services the codes cover, the rules for code use, and the ability of psychologists to bill for these particular codes. In addition, such letters should ask for insurance companies' assistance in creating policies that allow for reimbursement.

Once this information has been disseminated, it is important to test the use of the H & B codes in clinical practice. Finding clinical areas where the codes can be widely used (e.g., where treatment is less focused on psychiatric illness), and where medical teams are open to a test of the codes, is important. Many find that in this process providers will need to work with families and their larger organizations to develop a plan for how denied claims will be handled. Throughout this process, providers or those in support roles will need to track which payers have reimbursed the codes and what the reasons for denied claims are. Readdressing denied claims is important, as is reeducation if a payer is consistently not reimbursing. In conducting these test cases, many obstacles are potentially encountered. Appeals should be submitted if a payer denies a code, and reimbursement for H & B codes should be explicitly negotiated when insurance contracts are entered/reviewed. Another common issue that presents is that psychologists are not paneled with the medical side of the insurance carrier, and instead are only paneled on the mental health insurance side (see the earlier discussion of carve-out companies).

Continued collaboration with others who have an investment in seeing these codes used—including adult health psychologists, national organizations, state psychology boards, and families—is important to advance the use and reimbursement of these billing codes. Finally, it is important to use the resources readily available to members of APA if difficulties arise (APA, 2002). Medicare and Medicaid currently should reimburse these codes and a provider's regional CMS office or the APA Practice Directorate's Government Relations Office should be contacted if claims are denied.

Models of Implementation of H & B Codes

Brosig and Zahart (2006) published a study on the implementation of H & B codes at the Medical College of Wisconsin, where an insurance verification specialist for the inpatient consultation service tracked information on the rate of reimbursement. Findings suggested that reimbursement for mental health codes averaged 40–50% over the 4-year study period, whereas reimbursement for H & B codes averaged 58–80% over this period. Reasons for denials of H & B claims included the following: Claims were not covered by Medicaid (75%); there was no referral/prior authorization (10%); the provider was not eligible under the plan (13%); and the service rendered was considered part of another service provided at the same time (2%). The authors suggested that the hiring of an insurance verification specialist increased reimbursement after initial denial via the appeals process (2.8% in 2002 to 32.4% in 2005) and improved the revenue generation by providers. A potential obstacle to utilizing insurance verification specialists is that larger hospitals may not choose to devote these resources to mental health, because they may prefer to focus on higher yields in other medical specialties (e.g., surgery). As we have described here, implementation is not simple and direct; it is a process involving contracting and billing, working with the denials to educate insurers, and ultimately getting most (if not all) claims paid.

Diagnoses

Along with limitations for services as defined by procedure codes, companies will restrict coverage on the basis of diagnoses. Typically, insurance companies cover problems ranging from anxiety and depression to relationship difficulties. However, they often do not cover developmental disabilities, including most autism spectrum disorders, because they regard these problems as being in the education domain. In addition, companies routinely do not cover disorders that they deem can be managed by other agencies or providers. For example, a company may choose not to cover ADHD under mental health benefits, stating that it is a brain-based disorder best treated with medication by a primary care provider, rather than a psychiatric condition. These attempts to limit cost and access to mental health providers by referring some patients to primary care providers are usually the result of carve-out companies managing mental health benefits (see the earlier discussion). Carve-outs are often the most misunderstood part of the mental health system, creating confusion for providers and patients.

Primary Care Referral and Integrated Care

As part of the rise of managed care in mental health, a trend toward making primary care providers "gatekeepers" of health care started in the 1980s. As gatekeepers, these providers were required to provide written referrals in order for children to receive any mental health services. Recently, data have demonstrated that restrictive management of outpatient services costs more than simply delivering the service and thus, this policy has changed. However, data have also indicated that integrating health and mental health care can lower health care costs. For example, Delta Air Lines found that coordinating health and mental health care without requiring referrals from a primary care provider both reduced costs and resulted in improved employee health (Robinson, Chimeto, Bush, & Papay, 2001). Aetna (2007) has further developed the concept of an integrated health team to address the needs of adult patients who have complex chronic illnesses, and who as a result are at higher risk for mental health disorders. Although there are still annual limits to sessions, a referral from a primary care provider is not needed. Outcome data from this integrated care package demonstrated both improved functioning and reduced costs. As a strategy both to improve care and to reduce costs in adult health care, integrated care models are a major set of initiatives (Frank, McDaniel, Bray, & Heldring, 2003; Klapow, Pruitt, & Epping-Jordan, 1997; Robinson & Reiter, 2007)

Research examining integrated care in pediatrics is in its infancy. A review by the Substance Abuse and Mental Health Services Administration (Dorfman, 2000) found only a handful of studies showing significant cost savings in pediatrics by improved access to mental health care. Reduced medical costs were not clearly indicated, but were inferred as a function of improved parent and child behaviors. In a study evaluating management of common behavior problems in preschool and school-age children, results showed decreased behavior problems and reduced subsequent primary care visits after a brief intervention by psychologists in the primary pediatric offices (Finney, Riley, & Cataldo, 1991). Other program evaluations, not specifically designed to evaluate cost offsets, also suggest that an integrated care model improves health and reduces costs. For example, Glasgow and colleagues (1991) reported a 47% decrease in readmissions for diabetic ketoacidosis in children with Type 1 diabetes over a 5-year period following the implementation of a comprehensive multidisciplinary program. Although other variables certainly may have influenced this outcome, these types of data suggest that programs that address the comprehensive needs of families, including psychological needs, improve health while lowering costs. These results are impressive to third-party payers interested in reducing costs while maintaining the health of the patient population.

Public Insurance

Medicaid was originally set up in 1966 as a state and federal partnership to provide health care insurance for those in poverty. Qualifications for Medicaid are directly related to income levels, with those at 100% of the federal poverty level for a given region qualifying for coverage. Although there are very specific guidelines for each state on the provision of care, states have the option of requesting a waiver to provide care in a different manner. If such a waiver is granted, a state can proceed with its own coverage plan that must be approved by the federal agency. Coverage of psychological services varies widely from state to state. In some states, psychologists are not reimbursed, or are reimbursed at a very low rate. In other states, such reimbursement is actually at a higher level than that provided by commercial insurers. In many areas, states have contracted with one or more PPOs, HMOs, or MBHOs to manage and provide care, and psychologists may participate as they would with any other managed care group.

Along with Medicaid, the State Children's Health Insurance Program (SCHIP) was created in 1997 to insure children whose families had too high an income to qualify for Medicaid, but still could not afford private coverage (Kenney & Chang, 2004). Under SCHIP, families making up to 200% (or, in some states, 400%) of the federal poverty level can qualify or "buy in" for coverage. In most states, enrollment in Medicaid or SCHIP is coordinated with a common application and income verification process. In the first 5 years of SCHIP, nearly 5% of all children were covered (Kenney & Chang,

2004; Kenney & Yee, 2007). Although both Medicaid and SCHIP are intended to provide insurance for all children living in low-income families, additional provisions of the Medicaid law have allowed other children to be covered (Long & Coughlin, 2005). Currently, under the provisions of the Family Opportunity Act of 2005 (see National Conference of State Legislators, 2008), the majority of states also cover disabled children (i.e., children receiving Supplemental Social Security for disabilities, or children identified through other procedures as having chronic disabling conditions). Some states provide this coverage for all children, while others require that higher-income families pay some premium.

Among the most important aspects of Medicaid (in some states, extended to SCHIP programs) are the Early and Periodic Screening, Diagnostic, and Treatment (EPSDT) provisions, which apply only to children. EPSDT services and benefits are mandatory for all individuals under age 21 who are enrolled in Medicaid. First promulgated in 1972, the EPSDT rules require periodic health examinations, including comprehensive developmental assessment, appropriate immunizations, laboratory tests, and health education. In addition, dental, vision, and hearing services are required, including appropriate screening, diagnostic, and treatment services. The treatment component of EPSDT is broadly defined in federal law as including treatments to ameliorate conditions that are detected early in life (Rosenbaum & Wise, 2007); such treatments fall within the federal definition of medical assistance (as described in Section 1905(a) of the Social Security Act) that is needed to "correct or ameliorate defects and physical and mental illnesses and conditions discovered by the screening services." All medically necessary diagnostic and treatment services included within this federal definition must be covered, regardless of whether or not such services are otherwise covered under the state Medicaid plan for adults ages 21 and older.

EPSDT benefits are designed to help ensure access to needed services, including assistance in scheduling appointments and transportation to keep appointments. As described in federal rules, the EPSDT program consists of two mutually supportive operational components: (1) assuring the availability and accessibility of required health care resources, and (2) helping Medicaid recipients and their parents or guardians use health care resources effectively. Although psychologists have not generally availed themselves of the EPSDT provisions, largely because the services must be deemed "medically necessary," recent efforts to improve developmental and behavioral screening by primary care providers (Assuring Better Child Health and Development, 2008; Halfon, DuPlessis, & Inkelas, 2007) have resulted in Medicaid offices clearly supporting payment for developmental screening questionnaires and other primary care counseling services. In states where this is occurring, there may be opportunities for pediatric psychologists to become more involved in the diagnostic and treatment aspects of the EPSDT program.

Employee Assistance Programs

Employee assistance programs are set up by employers to help workers identify and resolve personal problems, emotional struggles, family difficulties, or legal problems. The visits are confidential and often free, but limited in the number of available sessions and often only available through a small number of designated provider groups. Despite limitations, these programs can be a valuable resource for parents or guardians who need to engage in short-term therapy in the face of stress caused by a child's illness or condition. The programs' providers can also help direct families in the direction of other services or providers covered by their mental health benefits if additional services are needed.

Bundling

All of the examples given so far assume that psychologists are billing as independent health or mental health professionals for their specific identifiable services. However, in many locations psychologists work as part of a team (either outpatient or inpatient), and services may be billed and are reimbursed as part of a "bundle" or package (Rae, 2004). For example, a hematology/oncology clinic may have specific fees for clinic visits that incorporate funds to pay a psychologist, social worker, or other providers. Sometimes specialty clinics work out a rate with an insurer that assumes multidisciplinary services will be available, including psychological services. At many hospitals, psychological inpatient consultations are not billed to outside insurers. The hospital absorbs the cost of these services into the room daily rate, similar to inpatient nursing services. Bundling can be an important source of revenue, but only if it is identified and defined in the departmental budget, and if the department is appropriately credited for the services that it provides as part of the bundle.

Summary

This chapter has shown that the current status of reimbursement for psychological services can be considered confusing, at best. However, the future does hold promise. Many health organizations recognize the utility, value, and importance of psychological services, and allow departments either to operate at a loss or to bundle their services within a package. Many administrators know that psychological services are valuable and endeavor to include them, but improvement of reimbursement remains a priority. Moreover, along with the traditional mental health CPT codes, H & B CPT codes now offer potential new sources of revenue. The ever-increasing emphasis on health may result in greater reimbursement for prevention and early intervention, as long as efficacy and cost effectiveness are demonstrated. Traditionalists—those who mourn the "good old days" of simply submitting bills to an indemnity plan and getting reimbursed—should recall that the good old days lasted less than 25 years, and that ultimately all health care providers must prove their utility and worth. With its emphasis on empirical measurement of outcome, psychology will stand in a better position in the future, as long as psychologists document the services they provide; the outcomes in terms of patient improvement; and the cost savings over having services provided by other, more expensive providers.

References

Aetna. (2007). Aetna Behavioral Health Med Psych program shows improvement in quality of life and productivity. *Aetna Behavioral Health Insights: Behavioral Health Newsletter*, 2(7), 1–2.

American Psychiatric Association. (2000). *Diagnostic and statistical manual of mental disorders* (4th ed., text rev.). Washington, DC: Author.

American Psychological Association (APA). (2002). Need help in using the new health and behavior CPT codes? Retrieved January 3, 2008, from *www.apa.org/monitor/sep02/cpt-codes.html*

American Psychological Association (APA). (2002). Practice Directorate announces new health and behavior codes. Retrieved January 3, 2008, from *www.apapractice.org/cpt_2002.html*

American Psychological Association (APA). (2005). *Practitioners find benefits using health and behavior codes.* Retrieved from *www.apapractice.org/apo/health_and_behavior/practitioners_find.html*

American Psychological Association (APA) Practice Directorate. (2006). Testing codes toolkit. Retrieved April 7, 2008, from *www.apapractice.org/apo/toolkit.html#*

Assistant Secretary for Planning and Evaluation. (2005). Estimating the number in U.S. without health insurance. Retrieved February 15, 2008, from *aspe.hhs.gov/health/re[prts/est-uninsured/index.htm*

Assuring Better Child Health and Development. (2008). Retrieved September 25, 2008, from *www.abcdresources.org/index.html*

Brosig, C. L., & Zahart, D. M. (2006). Evolution of an inpatient pediatric psychology consultation service: Issues related to reimbursement and the use of Health and Behavior codes. *Journal of Clinical Psychology in Medical Settings, 13*(4), 425–429.

Delamater, A. (2004, August). *Health and Behavior code surveys.* Paper presented at the 112th Annual Convention of the American Psychological Association, Honolulu, HI.

Dorfman, S. (2000). *Preventive interventions under managed care: Mental health and substance abuse services.* Rockville, MD: Substance Abuse and Mental Health Services Administration.

Feinberg, D. T. (2004). Are "carve-outs" in or out? *Journal of Child and Adolescent Psychopharmacology, 14*(2), 161–163.

Finney, J. W., Riley, A. W., & Cataldo, M. F. (1991). Psychology in primary health care: Effects of brief targeted therapy on medical care utilization. *Journal of Pediatric Psychology, 16,* 447–461.

Frank, R. G., McDaniel, S. H., Bray, J. H., & Heldring, M. (2003, August). *Primary care psychology.* Paper presented at the 111th Annual Convention of the American Psychological Association, Washington, DC.

Glasgow, A., Benchell, J., Tynan, W. D., Turek, J., Driscoll, C., Epstein, S., et al. (1991). Readmissions of children with insulin dependent diabetes mellitus. *Pediatrics, 88*(1), 98–104.

Halfon, N., DuPlessis, H., & Inkelas, M. (2007). *Transforming the U.S. child health system.* Retrieved March 23, 2008, from *www.commonwealthfund.org/publications/publications_show.htm?doc_id=469557*

Kenney, G., & Chang, D. (2004). The State Children's Health Insurance Program: Successes, shortcomings, and challenges. *Health Affairs, 23*(5), 51–62.

Kenney, G., & Yee, J. (2007). SCHIP at a crossroads: Experiences to date and challenges ahead. *Health Affairs, 26*(2), 356–369.

Kent, A. J., & Hersen, M. (2000). *A psychologist's guide to managed mental health care.* Mahwah, NJ: Erlbaum.

Klapow, J. C., Pruitt, S. D., & Epping-Jordan, J. E. (1997). Rehabilitation psychology in primary care: Preparing for a changing health care environment. *Rehabilitation Psychology, 42*(4), 325–335.

Klein, P. G. (2000). *Elimination of mental health and chemical dependency carve-outs.* American Medical Association. (House of Delegates Resolution No. 702).

Leichter, S. B., Dreelin, E., & Moore, S. (2004). Integration of clinical psychology in the comprehensive diabetes care team. *Clinical Diabetes, 22*(3), 129–131.

Long, S. K. C., & Couglin, T. A. (2005). Access to care for disabled children under Medicaid. *Health Care Financing Review, 26*(2), 89–103.

Mental Health Parity Act of 1996. (1996). Retrieved October 7, 2008, from *www.cms.hhs.gov/ healthinsreformforconsume/04_thementalhealthparityact.asp*

National Center for Health Statistics. (2003). *ICD-9, clinical modification.* Retrieved March 3, 2008, from *www.cdc.gov/nchs/icd9.htm*

National Conference of State Legislatures. (2005). *Family Opportunity Act.* Retrieved March 1, 2008, from *www.ncsl.org/statefed/health/famopact.htm*

Nicholson, R. (2002). The dilemma of psychotherapy notes and HIPAA. *Journal of the American Health Information Management Association, 73*(2), 38–39.

Noll, R. B., & Fischer, S. (2004). Commentary: Health and behavior CPT codes: An opportunity to revolutionize reimbursement in pediatric psychology. *Journal of Pediatric Psychology, 29,* 571–578.

Olfson, M., Sing, M., & Schlesinger, H. J. (1999). Mental health/medical care cost offsets: Opportunities for managed care. *Health Affairs, 18*(2), 79–90.

Paul Wellstone Mental Health and Addictions Equity Act of 2007, H.R. 1424. (2008). Retrieved October 7, 2008, from *thomas.loc.gov/cgi-bin/bdquery/z?d110:h.r.01424:*

Rae, W. A. (2004). Financing pediatric psychology services: Buddy, can you spare a dime? *Journal of Pediatric Psychology, 29*(1), 47–52.

Robert Wood Johnson Foundation. (2008). *Childhood obesity.* Retrieved March 15, 2008, from *www.rwjf.org/programareas/programarea.jsp?pid=1138*

Roberts, M. C., & Hurley L. K. (1997). *Managing managed care.* New York: Plenum Press.

Robinson, G., Chimeto, L., Bush, S., & Papay, J. (2001). *Comprehensive mental health insurance benefits: Case studies.* Rockville, MD: Substance Abuse and Mental Health Services Administration.

Robinson, P., & Reiter, J. (2007). *Behavioral consultation and primary care: A guide to integrating services.* New York: Springer.

Rosenbaum, S., & Wise, P. H. (2007). Crossing the Medicaid–private insurance divide: The case of EPSDT. *Health Affairs, 26*(2), 382–393.

Starr, P. (1982). *The social transformation of American medicine: The rise of a sovereign profession and the making of a vast industry.* New York: Basic Books.

Sussman, M. B., Steinmetz, S. K., & Peterson, G. W. (1999). *Handbook of marriage and the family* (2nd ed.). New York: Springer.

Vogt, T. M., Lafata, J. E., Tolsma, D. D., & Greene, S. M. (2004). The role of research in integrated health care systems: The HMO Research Network. *American Journal of Managed Care, 10*(9), 643–648.

PART II

Cross-Cutting Issues

CHAPTER 6

Cultural and Diversity Issues in Research and Practice

DANIEL L. CLAY

The importance of cultural and diversity issues in pediatric psychology has now been well established. Census data reveal that of the 5.2 million to 8.2 million children in the United States with significant chronic health problems, more than 50% will be from an ethnic minority and/or of low socioeconomic status (SES) within the next couple of decades (Clay, 2007; U.S. Bureau of the Census, 2008). Race, ethnicity, culture, and SES have been empirically linked to health disorders and outcomes in hundreds of studies (Adler & Rehkopf, 2008). For example, racial and ethnic health disparities in prevalence, morbidity, and mortality have been demonstrated in the most common pediatric conditions—including cancer, diabetes, obesity, asthma, sickle cell disease, and heart disease, among others (Clay, Mordhorst, & Lehn, 2002). Consequently, the National Institutes of Health have been focusing on the identification of factors associated with these disparities and in approaches to address them. With the increasing numbers of children with chronic medical problems from minority and/or low-SES backgrounds seeking medical services, and the link of cultural variables to treatment processes and outcomes, it is critical for pediatric psychologists and other health care providers to understand the impact of cultural variables. This chapter focuses on cultural issues specific to research and practice. An emphasis is placed on examining how best to apply empirically supported manualized approaches to assessment and treatment, to ensure cultural relevance and effectiveness with a diverse clientele.

Definitions

Many researchers and practitioners have a general idea of what "race," "ethnicity," and "culture" mean when they are referring to such constructs in conversation. However, these nebulous terms are often difficult to define operationally in research, resulting in problems in measurement and assessment, as discussed below. A thorough discussion of definitional issues in the context of research is provided by Walders and Drotar (2000); some definitional issues are presented here to clarify how these terms are used in this chapter.

Race is commonly used as a defining cultural characteristic, but is problematic because its superficial categories are based on physical characteristics of people, such as skin and eye color, hair color, and texture (Williams, 2007). Over time, definitions of "race" have varied widely, resulting in categories ranging from 3 to 34 based on geography, physical characteristics, and genetic analyses (Kato, 1996). More recent genetic studies (e.g., Williams, 2007) have resulted in little evidence for the distinct racial categories traditionally used in psychosocial research.

Use of the term "ethnic group" began nearly 50 years ago to avoid the derogatory connotations of "race"; this term implies membership in a socially defined group instead of a biologically defined group (Williams, 2007). Ethnicity is also used to indicate national origin (e.g., Mexican American), but it does not account for important within-group variations and those found within geographic regions (Kato, 1996). For example, many cultural groups, which have very prominent and important distinctions, can reside in one specific region.

"Culture" is a broader term that incorporates the mores, traditions, customs, rituals, language, and other patterns specific to a distinct group of people (Williams, 2007). Cultural variables go well beyond race and ethnicity to include such defining aspects of people as age, gender, sexual orientation, religion, geographic location (e.g., urban vs. rural), and SES. These variables are often the ones that relate to important processes and outcomes in illnesses and their treatment.

Research on Applying Evidence-Based Practice to Diverse Populations

The role of scientific evidence in supporting treatment approaches has increased dramatically over the last 10 years, in response to the demand that the efficacy of treatments be demonstrated through sound scientific inquiry. Professional organizations such as the American Psychological Association have responded by establishing criteria for evidence-based practice. This relatively recent emphasis has created a great deal of dialogue among scientists and practitioners as clinical approaches are increasingly linked back to empirical data demonstrating their effectiveness, particularly for interventions provided to those with a culturally diverse background (Clay et al., 2002). This dialogue has helped the research literature evolve to address problems in applying evidence-based practices to diverse populations.

At the root of these initial discussions are two related concerns. The first concern relates to the use in scientific research of randomized clinical trials that focus almost exclusively on high internal validity. This emphasis on high internal validity results in highly structured and highly controlled studies that aim to eliminate any potential confounding variables or explanations for the outcome of a study. However, the contexts in which clinical services are provided are anything but highly controlled and structured. Patients or clients often choose their provider instead of getting assigned one; they often seek additional or complementary treatments while receiving services; and therapists often change the course of treatment in midstream, based on what is working and what is not working—to name only a few examples. Consequently, many practicing clinicians have characterized randomized controlled trials (the "gold standard" for treatment research) as having little or no applicability to their practice (Sue, 1999). This is especially true when practitioners are providing treatments for persons with low-SES and/or culturally diverse backgrounds, as the limited resources of such clients often place additional demands on the treatment environment.

A second major concern in these initial discussions is that most evidence-based treatments are supported by research that does not take into account many of the diversity issues we now know are critically related to treatment process and outcome (Bernal & Scharron Del Rio, 2001; Hall, 2001). For example, my colleagues and I (Clay et al., 2002) reviewed 71 original studies used to support evidence-based treatments in pediatric diseases known to be linked to race/ethnicity/culture (e.g., asthma, cancer, diabetes, obesity). Only 27% of the studies reported race or ethnicity; only 18% reported the SES of participants; and only 6% discussed potential moderating cultural variables. These data supported the criticisms that existing research did not adequately address issues specific to diverse children and their families.

These initial concerns have been addressed more recently, despite this slow start. A second generation of empirical research has aimed at determining the extent to which evidence-based manualized treatments are effective for minority populations and those from low-SES backgrounds. These studies have utilized various methodologies, including having some therapists use manualized treatments with minority samples without adapting the intervention, while having others utilize adaptations of standard manualized approaches (e.g., Martinez & Eddy, 2005). Others have employed a manualized approach and compared minority participants with European American participants, to determine whether the effect sizes for the intervention would differ (e.g., Ferrell, Beidel, & Turner, 2004). Discussion of these issues and their effect on the evolving empirical literature, as well as on research and treatment models, continues to be a major topic in psychology (Whaley & Davis, 2007). In general, this research has been encouraging: It has demonstrated that both adapted and nonadapted manualized treatments have positive effects on diverse populations with a variety of presenting problems, although additional research is much needed.

Huey and Polo (2008) reviewed treatment outcome studies published through 2006 for children and adolescents in several diagnostic groups and conducted a meta-analysis. Outcome studies with ethnic minority youths were evaluated according to accepted criteria for evidence-based treatments (e.g., Chambless & Hollon, 1998; Nathan & Gorman, 2007). They found that ethnicity and culture-responsive treatment status did not moderate treatment outcomes. Although no "well-established" treatments for ethnic minority youths were identified, "probably efficacious" and "possibly efficacious" treatments were found for many disorders, including anxiety-related conditions, depression, substance abuse, conduct problems, trauma-related syndromes, attention-deficit/hyperactivity disorder, and other clinical problems. However, these authors noted that very few studies tested the effects of cultural adaptations of interventions, and that culturally validated outcomes were lacking. They also noted numerous methodological weaknesses of these studies, especially low statistical power and poor representation of less acculturated youths. Numerous suggestions for improving research are provided in this comprehensive article.

Miranda and colleagues (2005) published an extensive literature review on psychosocial interventions for ethnic minorities. These authors have concluded that there is a growing literature supporting the effectiveness of evidence-based mental health interventions for ethnic minorities. They conclude that in general, evidence-based approaches to

mental health treatment are largely generalizable to the African American and Latino/
Latina populations. Likewise, although the current literature is sparse, there appears
to be promise for Asian Americans as well. A significant question remains, however,
regarding whether evidence-based interventions must be adapted to be effective. These
authors do state that consideration of culture and context is essential; this is consistent
with published guidelines on culturally competent care.

In addition to these reviews of randomized controlled trials, clinicians have published case studies that illustrate the principles relevant to culturally competent care.
Martinez-Taboas (2005) presents a case study of a Latina woman with psychogenic
seizures, and describes a modified, culturally specific approach to treatment. Castro-
Blanco (2005) provides an alternative view of the cultural issues in the case, recommending additional culturally sensitive adaptations to existing treatment models. These
two papers provide an excellent example of how important cultural issues and adaptations to treatment can influence treatment planning and implementation.

Some scientist-practitioners have developed and tested manualized treatments specifically for use with diverse populations. Munoz and Mendelson (2005) discuss the
creation of theory-driven, evidence-based treatment approaches for persons of color by
persons of color who are familiar with the diverse communities for which the interventions are intended. Multisite randomized clinical trials have revealed the effectiveness
of such approaches with diverse populations. These results are very encouraging, and
such approaches are models for further development of new and adapted evidence-based
approaches for diverse populations.

Methodological Issues

Walders and Drotar (2000) and Hall (2001) provide extensive discussions of the methodological issues summarized here. Much of the early research examining issues in
culturally diverse samples used a between-groups design. With this design, researchers
compared group means for groups of differing racial or ethnic composition (e.g., African American and European American participants). This kind of research has had both
positive and negative consequences. On the positive side, these early studies provided
empirical evidence that the unique characteristics of specific racial or ethnic subgroups
deserved additional research attention, because differences between groups were found
for many process and outcome variables. It was no longer adequate simply to assume
that research done with middle-class European American subjects was generalizable
to populations of persons from other racial, ethnic, or SES backgrounds. The research
helped to spawn numerous theories about why such group differences exist, which have
been catalysts for culturally specific research examining within-group differences associated with culture (e.g., Martinez & Eddy, 2005). For example, such constructs as
racial identity, cultural identity, cultural affiliation, acculturation, and individualism–
collectivism have helped to illuminate ways in which individuals within groups may
vary and why. In addition to enhancing the empirical research base, consideration of
these constructs can be useful to inform clinical practice.

Beyond the specific form or method that culturally sensitive research takes, recruitment of participants, their families, and their health care providers for such research can
be challenging, for many reasons. Those with histories of oppression or coercion often
distrust researchers—and with good cause. Some researchers have studied tradition-

ally oppressed groups (e.g., Native Americans) without giving back to these groups in meaningful ways. Collaborative partnerships in research should result in tangible and immediate benefits for communities of underrepresented groups, and it is our ethical obligation to ensure these benefits (Hall, 2001).

Research with cultural minorities presents additional logistical barriers associated with low SES. In the United States, ethnic minorities are overrepresented among the lowest-SES groups, and poverty is a worldwide issue that affects health care and health outcomes. Lower SES creates difficulties for intervention research (particularly studies of interventions for medical problems) because of a lack of transportation, day care, and/or means of communication, as well as inability to miss work. The additional demands or burdens of research participation may just be too much for families with limited financial resources (Clay, 2000).

Numerous measurement issues have been the focus of much debate in the scientific literature. The problems with definitions discussed earlier can make measuring race, ethnicity, culture, or cultural affiliation very difficult. The research typically uses self-report of these factors, which relies on participants' self-identification with a particular group. However, many people are of mixed race or ethnicity, and their self-identity may depend on context. For example, people of mixed race may identify with one culture more during spiritual worship and another culture when receiving medical or psychological treatments. Asking children of mixed race to identify themselves with a racial, ethnic, or cultural group may be especially difficult (Walders & Drotar, 2000).

Okazaki and Sue (1995) and Walders and Drotar (2000) also discuss the importance of linguistic and conceptual equivalence in research of differing cultures. "Linguistic" equivalence refers to the translation of research instruments in such a way that the different language versions retain equivalent psychometric properties. "Conceptual" equivalence refers to the meaning of a concept or construct across cultures. For example, a common term like "depression" or "sadness" may have different meanings across cultures. Similarly, terms or concepts may have pejorative connotations or other associations in some cultures but not in others.

Recommendations for Future Research

The emphasis on evidence-based treatments in pediatric psychology, and the increasing number of culturally diverse children and families needing intervention, underscore the need to conduct rigorous treatment efficacy research that appropriately incorporates cultural variables. Several researchers and theorists have made recommendations for improving the quality of psychological and health research that incorporates such variables (Bernal & Scharron Del Rio, 2001; Clay et al., 2002; Hall, 2001; Huey & Polo, 2008; Sue, 1999; Walders & Drotar, 2000). Table 6.1 contains a summary of recommendations for research in pediatric psychology intended to advance the evidence base in support of treatments for diverse children and their families. In addition, it is important to include stakeholders from diverse communities in developing such research; this will ensure cultural sensitivity and relevance, improve access to communities, and improve the external validity of research findings. Some researchers have argued that community participation is essential in developing adaptable interventions that will fit specific needs of diverse communities while maintaining their fidelity (Castro, Berrera, & Martinez, 2004).

TABLE 6.1. Recommendations for Research Incorporating Cultural Issues

1. Examine family factors associated with culture and their relationships to treatment.

2. Explore how culture influences health care beliefs, practices, health care utilization, and adherence.

3. Focus research on developing treatments that address unique barriers faced by families with low SES.

4. Examine the independent and interactional effects of health and minority status on development and health.

5. Identify cultural variables that may serve as protective factors or as strengths that enhance treatment effects and outcome.

6. Include a discussion of cultural assumptions or biases when reporting treatments used in efficacy research with diverse populations.

7. Address the cultural appropriateness of measures and methodologies when conducting research with diverse populations or examining variables related to culture.

8. Consider the influence of culture when evaluating and interpreting results.

9. Focus research to aid in the development of evidence-based treatments for specific populations.

Note. Data from Clay, Mordhorst, and Lehn (2002).

In general, research has increasingly incorporated recent advances in theory and methodologies to benefit diverse populations. The national focus on these issues, and the subsequent funding from federal agencies such as the National Institutes of Health and the Centers for Disease Control and Prevention, have resulted in a more systematic approach to these ideas. For example, the National Center on Minority Health and Health Disparities (*www.ncmhd.nih.gov*) has funded research centers studying health disparities, has developed special programs to mentor minority researchers investigating health disparities issues, and has offered loan repayment for health disparities research.

Clinical Implications

The progress of theory and research in cultural diversity issues related to health, mental health, and psychological intervention has had a profound impact on clinical services and training. Better understanding of how such issues are associated with health disparities, treatment processes, and treatment outcomes has resulted in a dialogue on cultural competency and standards for culturally competent care at both institutional and individual levels.

Cultural Competency

Prominent scholars have called for specific areas of clinical competency for culturally appropriate care for well over a decade (Sue, Arredondo, & McDavis, 1992), and the issue of cultural competency was being discussed for decades before that. More recently, entire volumes have been dedicated to cultural competency in psychological interventions (e.g., Fouad & Arredondo, 2007; Pederson, Draguns, Lonner, & Trimble,

2002; Pope-Davis & Coleman, 1997; Pope-Davis, Coleman, Liu, & Toporek, 2003) and health care (Srivastava, 2006). Likewise, professional associations like the Association for American Medical Colleges (*www.aamc.org*) and the American Psychological Association (*www.apa.org*) have enacted standards for cultural competency for physicians and psychologists (e.g., American Psychological Association, 2003). Training programs for medical and allied health care providers now focus on systematic training experiences to ensure that graduates are trained to provide culturally competent care, and credentialing agencies are requiring proof of such competency as a prerequisite to licensure or certification.

What does "cultural competency" mean? A culturally competent provider has been defined as one who (1) is aware of his or her own biases, assumptions, and values related to ethnic minorities and to those who differ from him- or herself; (2) strives to understand the worldview of all individuals in a manner that is free of negative judgments; and (3) develops and implements culturally sensitive interventions (Sue et al., 1992). Cultural competency is then seen as comprising three domains: (1) beliefs and attitudes, (2) knowledge, and (3) skills. The first domain refers to an individual's understanding of him- or herself as a cultural being with beliefs, assumptions, biases, prejudices, and attitudes based on experience and learning. It also refers to the clinician developing a positive orientation toward multicultural perspectives (Pope-Davis et al., 2003). The second domain refers to the knowledge one has of other cultures, including the beliefs, assumptions, tendencies, and characteristics of those cultures. For example, it is helpful to understand which cultures tend to be more collectivist than individualistic, or what customary practices exist in some cultures. Finally, the third domain refers to specific abilities to work effectively with diverse clients, such as choosing and modifying interventions to maximize their positive effects with such clients.

Miranda and colleagues (2005) have discussed cultural competency and the extent to which evidence-based approaches need to be adapted for use with minority or culturally diverse populations. They state that "[k]nowledge of the culture and context and the capacity to distinguish between what may be culturally adaptive versus pathological are minimal considerations of culturally competent care" (p. 134).

Cultural competency involves numerous aspects of clinical care, including selection and use of assessment measures, as well as selection and implementation of treatments. The focus here is on the selection and implementation of interventions, because many of the same issues apply to the assessment process. General guidelines for cultural competency in work with children are discussed elsewhere (Clay, 2007; Liu & Clay, 2002). These guidelines are easily adapted to working with children with health problems and their families. Four guidelines in particular can help clinicians make decisions about which treatments to use and how to adapt them to accommodate cultural issues: (1) Evaluate which, if any, cultural aspects are relevant; (2) determine the level of skills and information necessary for competent treatment (and seek additional resources or refer if necessary); (3) examine potential evidence-based interventions and understand the cultural assumptions or biases of each; and (4) draw on cultural strengths in choosing and implementing the treatment.

First, culturally competent care requires knowledge about which cultural issues are salient and relevant. What are the child's and family's beliefs about the illness, its cause, their role in treatment and in treatment decision making, and so on? Are there cultural rituals or beliefs that are important to recognize? Are spiritual or religious issues prominent?

The second step is to determine the skills and information necessary to provide competent treatment. Does the family speak English? Is a translator needed? Would a service provider of another gender be more acceptable to the family? Should a clergyperson be involved? Are specialized skills and knowledge necessary, and if so, who can be enlisted to assist? In many cases, referral to an individual who speaks the family's language or shares the family's religious affiliation may not be possible, so clinicians must provide the best options available given limited resources and options.

The third step is to examine the available evidence-based treatment options to determine which would be most appropriate, beneficial, and consistent with the family's cultural beliefs. What evidence-based approaches exist to address the identified condition? What are the potential biases and assumptions of these approaches? What cultural issues may affect the client's and family's ability to engage in and benefit from the treatment approach? What cultural strengths or beliefs are particularly salient to the treatment methods and content? To what extent can the evidence-based approach be modified, if necessary, while still maintaining the therapeutic ingredients?

The final step is to select the best available treatment option and, if necessary, modify it to maximize the cultural strengths. Should interventions include parents and extended family members? Should alternative treatment approaches based on cultural norms, rituals, and practices be employed? Including family and community members in treatment approaches with clients from highly collectivistic cultures can be very effective, even when such use of these extended family or group members is not necessarily included in the manualized treatment protocol. Use of cultural practices or rituals, in combination with traditional manualized treatment approaches, can be very important in gaining the support and trust of the patient and the family.

In sum, it is critical that individual clinicians possess the attitudes/beliefs, knowledge, and skills to provide competent care to a pediatric psychology clientele of ever-increasing diversity. This is now the standard for best practices (American Psychological Association, 2003). Training programs for advanced practitioners are now systematically addressing cultural competency. Implementing culturally competent interventions can be very difficult for pediatric psychologists, however, because they are often members of an interdisciplinary treatment team that may consist of other clinicians with different attitudes, skill levels, and commitments to culturally competent care.

Institutional Standards

In addition to cultural competency at the individual level, institutions are being held accountable for providing resources and services to ensure optimal care for patients from diverse backgrounds. The Office of Minority Health (*www.omhrc.gov*) has established national standards for culturally and linguistically appropriate services (CLAS). These standards are directed primarily at health care organizations, although individual service providers are also encouraged to use the standards to ensure the cultural and linguistic accessibility of their services. These standards include both mandates and guidelines. The mandates are current federal requirements for all recipients of federal funds; current guidelines within these standards have been recommended for adoption as mandates. The Office of Minority Health website is an excellent resource, and readers are encouraged to consult the site to access its many resources for providing CLAS.

The 14 standards encompass three general categories: culturally competent care, language and accessible services, and organizational support for cultural competency.

Issues addressed include recruitment of a diverse staff; education of all staff on cultural issues; language assistance services (including proficient interpreters and/or bilingual staff, as well as documents and signage available in languages of commonly encountered groups); a strategic plan that includes oversight and accountability for CLAS; and a culturally sensitive grievance process for addressing cross-cultural conflicts. Health care organizations are also encouraged to make information about their progress on implementing CLAS standards available to the public. Indeed, these standards represent a bold move forward in efforts to ensure appropriate services to the increasingly diverse population in need of such services.

Summary

The increasing diversity of the population in the United States, combined with the link between health outcomes and cultural variables, demands that pediatric psychologists incorporate and address cultural issues. Preliminary research on application of evidence-based treatments with ethnic minority and low-SES populations is promising, but much more research is still needed. Published guidelines now exist to address multicultural education, training, research, practice, and organizational change. With an emphasis on cultural competency, the evolving body of research is guiding professionals in training, research, and service provision to address the unique needs, strengths, and barriers of the ever-diversifying U.S. population. Best practices and ethical guidelines require that institutions and individual practitioners provide culturally sensitive and competent care.

References

Adler, N. E., & Rehkopf, D. H. (2008). U.S. disparities in health: Descriptions, causes, and mechanisms. *Annual Review of Public Health, 29,* 235–252.

American Psychological Association. (2003). Guidelines on multicultural education, training, research, practice, and organizational change for psychologists. *American Psychologist, 58,* 377–402.

Bernal, G., & Scharron Del Rio, M. R. (2001). Are empirically supported treatments valid for ethnic minorities?: Toward an alternative approach for treatment research. *Cultural Diversity and Ethnic Minority Psychology, 7,* 328–342.

Castro, F. G., Berrera, M., & Martinez, C. R. (2004). The cultural adaptation of prevention interventions: Resolving tensions between fidelity and fit. *Prevention Science, 5,* 41–45.

Castro-Blanco, D. R. (2005). Cultural sensitivity in conventional psychotherapy: A comment on Martinez-Taboas (2005). *Psychotherapy: Theory, Research, Practice, Training, 42,* 14–16.

Chambless, D. L., & Hollon, S. D. (1998). Defining empirically supported therapies. *Journal of Consulting and Clinical Psychology, 66,* 7–18.

Clay, D. L. (2000). Commentary: Rethinking our interventions in pediatric chronic pain and treatment research. *Journal of Pediatric Psychology, 25,* 53–55.

Clay, D. L. (2007). Culturally competent interventions in schools for children with physical health problems. *Psychology in the Schools, 44,* 389–396.

Clay, D. L., Mordhorst, M. J., & Lehn, L. (2002). Empirically supported treatments in pediatric psychology: Where is the diversity? *Journal of Pediatric Psychology, 27,* 325–337.

Ferrell, C. B., Beidel, D. C., & Turner, S. M. (2004). Assessment and treatment of socially phobic children: A cross cultural comparison. *Journal of Clinical Child and Adolescent Psychology, 33,* 260–268.

Fouad, N. A., & Arredondo, P. (2007). *Becoming culturally oriented: Practical advice for psychologists and educators.* Washington, DC: American Psychological Association.

Hall, G. C. N. (2001). Psychotherapy research with ethnic minorities: Empirical, ethical, and conceptual issues. *Journal of Consulting and Clinical Psychology, 69,* 502–510.

Huey, S. J., & Polo, A. J. (2008). Evidence-based psychosocial treatments for ethnic minority youth. *Journal of Clinical Child and Adolescent Psychology, 37,* 262–301.

Kato, P. M. (1996). On nothing and everything: The relationship between ethnicity and health. In P. M. Kato & T. Mann (Eds.), *Handbook of diversity issues in health psychology* (pp. 287–299). New York: Plenum Press.

Liu, W. M., & Clay, D. L. (2002). Multicultural counseling competencies: Guidelines in working with children and adolescents. *Journal of Mental Health Counseling, 24,* 177–175.

Martinez, C. R., & Eddy, J. M. (2005). Effects of culturally adapted parent management training on Latino youth behavior health outcomes. *Journal of Consulting and Clinical Psychology, 73,* 841–851.

Martinez-Taboas, A. (2005). Psychogenic seizures in an *espiritismo* context: The role of culturally sensitive psychotherapy. *Psychotherapy: Theory, Research, Practice, Training, 42,* 6–16.

Miranda, J., Bernal, G., Lau, A., Kohn, L., Hwang, W.-C., & LaFromboise, T. (2005). State of the science on psychosocial interventions for ethnic minorities. *Annual Review of Clinical Psychology, 1,* 113–142.

Munoz, R. F., & Mendelson, T. (2005). Toward evidence-based interventions for diverse populations: The San Francisco General Hospital Prevention and Treatment Manuals. *Journal of Consulting and Clinical Psychology, 73,* 790–799.

Nathan, P. E., & Gorman, J. M. (Eds.). (2007). *A guide to treatments that work* (3rd ed.). New York: Oxford University Press.

Okazaki, S., & Sue, S. (1995). Methodological issues in assessment research with ethnic minorities. *Psychological Assessment, 7,* 367–375.

Pedersen, P. B., Draguns, J. G., Lonner, W. J., & Trimble, J. E. (Eds.). (2002). *Counseling across cultures* (5th ed.). Thousand Oaks, CA: Sage.

Pope-Davis, D. B., & Coleman, H. L. K. (Eds.). (1997). *Multicultural counseling competencies: Assessment, education and training, and supervision.* Thousand Oaks, CA: Sage.

Pope-Davis, D. B., Coleman, H. L. K., Liu, W. M., & Toporek, R. L. (Eds.). (2003). *Handbook of multicultural competencies in counseling and psychology.* Thousand Oaks, CA: Sage.

Srivastava, R. H. (2006). *The healthcare professional's guide to clinical cultural competence.* New York: Elsevier.

Sue, D. W., Arredondo, P., & McDavis, R. J. (1992). Multicultural counseling competencies and standards: A call to the profession. *Journal of Counseling and Development, 70,* 477–486.

Sue, S. (1999). Science, ethnicity, and bias: Where have we gone wrong? *American Psychologist, 54,* 1070–1077.

U.S. Bureau of the Census. (2008). 2007 population estimates. Retrieved July 25, 2008, from *www.census.gov.*

Walders, N., & Drotar, D. (2000). Understanding cultural and ethnic influences in research with child clinical and pediatric psychology populations. In D. Drotar (Ed.), *Handbook of research in pediatric and clinical child psychology: Practical strategies and methods* (pp. 165–188). New York: Kluwer Academic/Plenum.

Whaley, A. L., & Davis, K. A. (2007). Cultural competence and evidence-based practice in mental health services. *American Psychologist, 62,* 563–574.

Williams, R. A. (2007). Cultural diversity, health care disparities, and cultural competency in American medicine. *Journal of the American Academy of Orthopedic Surgeons, 15,* S52–S58.

CHAPTER 7

Evidence-Based Practice in Pediatric Psychology

TIMOTHY D. NELSON
RIC G. STEELE

"Evidence-based practice (EBP) in psychology" is defined as "the integration of the best available research with clinical expertise in the context of patient characteristics, culture, and preferences" (American Psychological Association [APA] Presidential Task Force on Evidence-Based Practice, 2006, p. 273). Implicit in this definition is the assumption that science and service complement each other, and that the lessons of both are essential in producing the best clinical practice. The relative weight of empirical findings and clinical expertise has been the subject of considerable debate (Beutler, 2004; Levant, 2004); however, a prevailing notion that research evidence should inform clinical practice and vice versa has begun to emerge. The current definition and emerging consensus on EBP in psychology has developed out of a long-standing discussion of the role of science in clinical practice, as well as similar developments in medicine (e.g., Institute of Medicine [IOM], 2001). In an attempt to place our discussion of EBP in pediatric psychology within a broader context, we briefly discuss the history of the EBP movement and its influences, before exploring the current challenges facing the field of pediatric psychology as it moves toward greater implementation of EBP in the future.

History of the EBP Movement

As noted in the APA Presidential Task Force (2006) report, clinical psychology has a long history of considering issues related to EBP, both in applied practice (e.g., Witmer, 1907/1996) and clinical training (e.g., Shakow et al., 1947). The struggle to define the role of science in clinical practice moved to the forefront of professional psychology in the 1990s with the controversial "empirically supported treatment" (EST) movement. In an attempt to bridge the perceived gap between science and practice, in 1995 the APA's Division 12 (Clinical Psychology) created (1) the Task Force on Promotion and Dissemination of Psychological Procedures and (2) the Task Force on Psychological Interventions, to identify treatments with the best empirical support and encourage their use in clinical practice. The Division 12 Task Force specified criteria for various levels of empirical support, and then the criteria were subsequently used to create lists of treatments that met these criteria (e.g., Chambless & Hollon, 1998; Chambless et al., 1996). Although these early lists focused primarily on adult treatments, efforts to identify and highlight ESTs for children and adolescents soon followed. For example, reviews (e.g., Chambless & Ollendick, 2001) and special issues and sections of the *Journal of Clinical Child Psychology* (Vol. 27, No. 2) and the *Journal of Pediatric Psychology* (Vols. 24–26) have focused on ESTs for children and adolescents with a variety of disorders.

The movement toward ESTs in clinical psychology was driven by a number of factors from within psychology, as well as influences from outside the field. Within psychology, the accumulation of rigorous research demonstrating the efficacy and effectiveness of specific psychological treatments for a variety of conditions (see Kazdin & Weisz, 2003) precipitated a growing sentiment that psychological practice could and should be placed on a firm empirical footing. However, despite the accumulating evidence for the efficacy of certain approaches, it became clear that many clinicians in the field did not utilize these validated interventions, but rather opted for treatments with little empirical support (Kazdin, Siegel, & Bass, 1990). Indeed, Aarons (2004) reported that clinicians in his survey were relatively unfamiliar with the terms "evidence-based practice" and "empirically supported treatments." This science–practice gap was a discouraging reality for a field claiming to be scientific and aspiring to provide optimal care based on existing knowledge of best practices.

The EST movement was also influenced by a number of factors outside professional psychology. The growing presence and influence of managed care organizations provided an impetus in several ways for examining the state of the field with regard to the quality of clinical services provided. The Division 12 Task Force and the entire EST movement were largely responses to calls for greater accountability in clinical practice (Weisz, Hawley, Pilkonis, Woody, & Follette, 2000) and part of an attempt to demonstrate the value of psychotherapy to consumers and managed care organizations (Steele & Roberts, 2003). Many in the field were especially eager to combat the notion that psychological treatments were less effective than or secondary to pharmacological interventions (Barlow, 1996), and aimed to highlight the effects of the most efficacious psychological treatments to the general public.

A related factor influencing psychology's attempts to encourage ESTs was the movement toward evidence-based approaches in other health care fields. Most notably, the idea of evidence-based medicine (IOM, 2001; Sackett, Rosenberg, Gray, Haynes, & Richardson, 1996) influenced psychology not only in its desire to integrate science and practice, but also in the methods used to establish an empirical base to guide clinical decisions (e.g., randomized clinical trials, or RCTs). Although some have challenged the wisdom of following a "medical model" of clinical research and service delivery (e.g., Messer & Wampold, 2002), the influence of medicine's movement toward evidence-based principles on professional psychology in general, and pediatric psychology specifically, has been considerable.

Despite the many compelling reasons for the EST movement, a significant backlash on the part of some practitioners emerged and divided the field (Beutler, Williams, Wakefield, & Entwistle, 1995). The movement's identification and listing of ESTs were attacked on a number of grounds. Opponents of ESTs criticized the emphasis on RCTs as the "gold standard" of clinical research (e.g., Havik & VandenBos, 1996; Persons & Silberschatz, 1998), and some argued that the research base, although expanding, was still insufficient as a foundation for practice (e.g., Garfield, 1996; Levant, 2004). Still others claimed that the therapeutic process is too complex to be captured by simplistic outcome research (Strupp, 2001), and that factors such as the therapeutic relationship should be studied instead of different treatment protocols (Norcross, 2001).

In an attempt to reach some consensus and move beyond the often divisive rhetoric surrounding the EST controversy, the APA Presidential Task Force (2006) defined and endorsed EBP in psychology. This definition highlighted three critical components— best research evidence, clinical expertise, and patient context—as the foundation of EBP in psychology, and paralleled earlier statements on evidence-based medicine (IOM, 2001; Sackett et al., 1996). The Task Force's statement on EBP in psychology provides a broad blueprint for research and clinical endeavors aimed at facilitating EBP, and is a logical starting point for discussions of EBP in pediatric psychology.

The Evolution of EBP in Pediatric Psychology

Although the evolution of EBP in pediatric psychology was undoubtedly influenced by the broader EBP movement in professional psychology, the road traveled was perhaps less contentious. For years, the field of pediatric psychology has embraced EBP through official Society of Pediatric Psychology (SPP) publications and in the writings of leaders in the field (e.g., Spirito, 1999; Spirito & Kazak, 2006). In fact, the current discussion in the field is not so much *whether* the philosophy of EBP should be adopted, but rather *how* its ideals can be pursued most effectively. Therefore, we forgo the arguments for EBP in pediatric psychology—they have been made convincingly elsewhere (see Kazak, 2006)—and focus on how to facilitate EBP in years to come.

We believe that the promotion of EBP in pediatric psychology will require the field to move beyond lists of treatments and focus on ways to facilitate (1) the continued development and dissemination of a strong evidence base; (2) training of pediatric psychologists who are prepared to contribute to the evidence base and competently deliver evidence-based interventions; and (3) adaptation of evidence-based protocols to the unique values, preferences, and cultural contexts of patients and families. In the remainder of this chapter, we focus on pediatric psychology's progress in each of these areas, as well as recommendations for addressing these issues and moving forward.

Development of Evidence Base

Treatment Outcome Research

EBP is founded on solid science and the ability to identify best treatments through rigorous research. The intervention literature in pediatric psychology has grown considerably in recent years, and a strong empirical base has been established for many pediatric conditions (see Spirito, 1999; Spirito & Kazak, 2006). The majority of this research has taken the form of "efficacy" studies (e.g., clinical trials) that examine treatment effects under tightly controlled conditions. Often considered the "gold standard" of clinical research, RCTs have demonstrated positive treatment outcomes for numerous present-ing problems often encountered by pediatric psychologists. Signaling the centrality of such trials to the future of pediatric psychology, the *Journal of Pediatric Psychology* (*JPP*) has created an ongoing special section focused on publishing RCTs (Wysocki, 2008). Validating pediatric psychology interventions in RCTs is especially important, given the emphasis on this kind of evidence in medical settings and the potential impli-cations of RCT evidence on reimbursement practices in those settings.

Although the continuation and expansion of efficacy research in pediatric psychol-ogy are essential, there has been increasing recognition in recent years that the scope of treatment research must be broadened to address relevant questions pertaining to the transportability, cost-effectiveness, and acceptability of well-supported interven-tions (Nelson & Steele, 2006). So-called "effectiveness" studies, which examine treat-ment outcomes with clinical populations in clinical settings, have been highlighted and are beginning to emerge in the pediatric psychology literature (e.g., Hayes, Matthews, Copley, & Welsh, 2008; Johnston & Steele, 2007). Although this kind of intervention research is often challenging to conduct, it is necessary to understanding how treat-ments work under "real-world" conditions.

Recognizing the need for high-quality effectiveness research, *JPP* has recently solicited papers for a special issue on clinical effectiveness, noting a gap in knowledge regarding the generalizability of interventions tested in RCTs. The transportability of efficacious interventions "from bench to bedside" (Stark, 2008) will be crucial to pedi-atric psychology's attempts to demonstrate the value of services provided by pediatric psychologists in a variety of settings (Brown & Roberts, 2000). In addition to evaluating RCT-tested interventions in clinical settings, EBP in pediatric psychology will require researchers to draw from the growing literature on innovation dissemination (e.g., Stir-man, Crits-Christoph, & DeRubeis, 2004), to better understand the process by which innovations in pediatric psychology treatment can be most efficiently disseminated into practice settings.

In an attempt to improve the clinical impact of pediatric psychology treatment research, various authors have proposed that treatment researchers demonstrate the *clinical significance* of pediatric psychology interventions (e.g., Drotar & Lemanek, 2001; Kazdin, 2008). Rather than simply indicating that a treatment has a statistically significant effect, researchers are increasingly encouraged to show the magnitude of treatment effects (e.g., using effect sizes), as well as effects on functional outcomes. As discussed more fully below, increasing the representation of ethnic minorities and cul-turally diverse populations in treatment samples has also been highlighted as an impor-tant step to making the treatment literature more relevant to clinical practice (Clay, Mordhorst, & Lehn, 2002). Finally, the need to synthesize the rapidly growing treat-ment literature in pediatric psychology has led to calls for meta-analyses and critical reviews to pool findings from multiple studies and offer insights regarding best research evidence (e.g., Drotar & Lemanek, 2001).

Cost-Effectiveness Research

Another important, but often neglected, area of research for pediatric psychology with respect to EBP is cost-effectiveness (Wysocki, 2008). Treatments that are clinically effec-tive but not cost-effective may not be viable in many settings, due to limited resources and/or reimbursement considerations. Demonstrating the financial implications of an intervention—including both costs of treatment and *costs of nontreatment*—is rare within the pediatric psychology literature, but will be necessary in facilitating widespread adoption of treatments with strong research support (see Buckloh & Greco, Chapter 3, this volume; Rae, 2004). Such investigations can be integrated into ongoing effectiveness trials (Nelson & Steele, 2006) and have emerged in other areas of health care (Detsky & Laupacis, 2007) and psychology (Yates, 1994). Evaluation of both short- and long-term costs should be broadly conceptualized to include costs to children and families (e.g., time, effort, payment), costs to institutions and providers (e.g., human and financial resources of providing treatment), and costs to the broader community (e.g., support of community institutions providing care). The concept of medical cost offset, which proposes that some pediatric psychology interventions can reduce medically related expenditures by improving child health (e.g., interventions for adherence to medications), is of particular interest to pediatric psychology (Roberts, Mitchell, & McNeal, 2003). Research on the cost-effectiveness of pediatric psychology prevention and treatment programs will be integral in demonstrating the value—both clinical and financial—of the services pediatric psychologists provide. Establishing the cost-effectiveness of well-supported interventions will also support EBP by demonstrating the financial benefits of best practices.

Evidence-Based Assessment

Although much of the literature on EBP has focused on psychological interventions, EBP principles are equally important in assessment procedures. The concept of "evidence-based assessment" (EBA) has emerged in recent years and is being increasingly recognized as an essential component of EBP (Cohen et al., 2008). Valid and sensitive assessments are necessary in determining the most appropriate treatment approaches and in evaluating progress during the course of treatment. Strong measures of clinical outcomes are also essential to demonstrating positive effects in intervention research.

Assessment with children and adolescents presents numerous challenges related to the developmental appropriateness of instruments and reliability of reports obtained from multiple informants (e.g., child, parent, peer, and teacher reports). In light of these issues, the *Journal of Clinical Child and Adolescent Psychology* (Mash & Hunsley, 2005) published a special issue on EBA in clinical child psychology, detailing assessment methods for various types of child psychopathology. These reviews can be extremely helpful in guiding pediatric psychologists; however, caution must be exercised in translating the literature on child assessment to pediatric populations. In their introduction to the *JPP*'s special issue on EBA in pediatric psychology, Cohen and colleagues (2008) noted that many measures used with pediatric populations were originally developed for and normed on samples of healthy children or children with psychopathology. To address this issue, the SPP Assessment Task Force facilitated critical reviews of measures across eight areas of particular interest to pediatric psychology that classified measures in each area into "well-established," "approaching well-established," and "promising" categories of evidence (see Cohen et al., 2008). These reviews constitute an important step for the field in fostering EBA; however, much work remains to validate many instruments with a variety of pediatric populations. Areas for future research include establishing norms for pediatric populations, determining the clinical value of various measures with specific illness groups, establishing measurement invariance across populations (e.g., healthy and ill; different medical conditions), directly comparing the performance of competing measures, and developing new measures for specific populations. Such studies will be helpful in identifying the best assessment procedures, refining existing protocols, and encouraging their use in clinical practice.

Training of Pediatric Psychologists in EBP

The continued promotion of EBP in pediatric psychology will require a commitment to training the next generation of pediatric psychologists in the skills essential to EBP. More than simply "teaching ESTs" (Collins, Leffingwell, & Belar, 2007), such training must include a multifaceted approach to producing both excellent researchers and competent clinicians grounded in the guiding framework of EBP. As discussed above, EBP in pediatric psychology requires a strong and continually expanding empirical base, and training researchers who can meet this need with innovative and rigorous research will be essential to the field. Likewise, clinicians who can effectively evaluate the treatment literature, make evidence-based decisions, and deliver appropriately tailored interventions will be crucial to the integration of science and practice in pediatric clinical settings.

Research Training

A rigorous and informative literature is the foundation of EBP in pediatric psychology. Training programs are charged with producing pediatric researchers who can provide the next generation of evidence for the field and create new intervention and prevention programs to be tested. If clinical researchers are to provide the evidence for EBP (Frick, 2007), they will need to be equipped with certain skills in order to conduct research that is relevant to clinical practice. Perhaps most apparent is the need to train researchers who can effectively conduct intervention studies in clinical settings (Bauer, 2007). Drotar and Lemanek (2001) noted the importance of obtaining hands-on experience in intervention research during graduate school and postdoctoral training as preparation for careers in pediatric psychology research.

Such training and experience should reflect the breadth of research methods in order to generate findings that can be easily translated into effective therapies. For example, the low prevalence of many pediatric conditions often requires pediatric psychology researchers to conduct large multisite trials in order to obtain adequate sample sizes (Spirito et al., 2003). Such trials present a number of challenges, including standardization of procedures and quality control across sites, as well as statistical challenges in analyzing data nested within multiple settings.

Equally important (but often neglected) are single-subject methodologies such as A-B-A, multiple-baseline, and changing-criterion designs, each of which provides rigorous options for contributing to the evidence base for a specific treatment. Despite the value and advantages that such methodologies offer the field, many graduate programs do not currently offer intensive training in these approaches (Rapoff & Stark, 2008); however, an investment in such training could greatly contribute to the field's understanding of treatment effectiveness. As noted by Rapoff and Stark, research conducted with these methods often produces results that are easily understood by clinicians, and may represent methods with the greatest likelihood of being used by clinicians to contribute to the research literature.

At a broader level, the field is increasingly recognizing the value of alternative research methodologies in establishing evidence for clinical practice (e.g., focus groups; see Holmbeck, 2008), and training programs will need to keep students abreast of new developments in methodology. In addition, as the treatment literature and research methods in pediatric psychology continue to grow, methods for rigorously synthesizing the literature will become increasingly important areas for training. Meta-analyses and systematic reviews have been identified as useful ways of summarizing the state of knowledge in specific areas of pediatric psychology (Drotar & Lemanek, 2001), although training in these methodologies is not yet integrated into the core of many training programs.

Hand in hand with methodological considerations is the issue of providing adequate statistical training to the next generation of pediatric psychologists. Although a strong foundation in traditional statistical techniques (e.g., analysis of variance, multiple regression) will continue to be essential, training in more sophisticated analytic strategies will expand the range of questions pediatric researchers can ask and answer. Multilevel modeling techniques to handle nested data (e.g., from multisite trials), structural equation modeling to test complex models (Nelson, Aylward, & Steele, 2008), and longitudinal analyses to investigate change over time (Holmbeck, Bruno, & Jandasek, 2006) are some of the areas that will become increasingly valuable to researchers in pediatric psychology. Familiarity with these analytic techniques will be important not only for researchers, but also for clinicians, who will need to critically evaluate studies employing these analyses in determining best research evidence.

Clinical Training

Much of the discussion of EBP training in the literature has focused on graduate clinical training. Despite increasing consensus that graduate students should be trained in EBP, the optimal methods for such training in psychology (and pediatric psychology specifically) are unclear. Other health care disciplines, such as medicine, nursing, and social work, have developed guidelines for EBP training that may be informative to psychology (Spring, 2007). Training in EBP for pediatric psychology (as in EBP for other health care professions) will require learning not only which treatment protocols have research support, but also how to integrate research evidence with clinical judgment and to deliver interventions in a way that is tailored to the individual client's unique context. Rather than simply teaching a list of specific treatments, EBP-focused training programs teach students a *process* (Leffingwell & Collins, 2008; Straus, Richardson, Glasziou, & Haynes, 2005) that they will apply each time they provide clinical services. This is an important distinction, as recent survey data have shown that many graduate students (and professionals) still mistakenly equate EBP with ESTs (Luebbe, Radcliffe, Callands, Green, & Thorn, 2007). In reality, ESTs constitute a necessary but ultimately not sufficient component of EBP in psychology.

In contrast to the limited view of EBP as synonymous with EST, the APA definition of EBP in psychology requires not only that clinicians can identify the treatments with the strongest evidence base, but also demonstrate expertise in the delivery of those interventions. Unfortunately, recent evidence has suggested that although students generally receive didactic training in interventions with empirical support, hands-on experience with such treatments during training is lacking (Woody, Weisz, & McLean, 2005). The situation may be particularly worrisome in pediatric psychology, given that trainees often specialize in the discipline later in their training and may have limited exposure to pediatric psychology interventions during graduate school. Assessing competence in clinical skills that are central to EBP—including assessment, diagnosis, conceptualization, and treatment competencies—is an essential (but challenging) component of effective training (Leffingwell & Collins, 2008). As the field shifts to an increasing emphasis on continual assessment of these competencies (Roberts, Borden, Christiansen, & Lopez, 2005), measurement strategies will begin to emerge and should be implemented systematically in clinical training programs.

Within the broader clinical psychology literature, some examples of EBP training are available (e.g., Collins, Leffingwell, & Belar, 2007; DiLillo & McChargue, 2007). These examples, which highlight the importance of integrating EBP training into both didactic and practicum experiences, provide a useful starting point in considering training issues for EBP in pediatric psychology. Collins and colleagues (2007) describe specific recommendations for teaching trainees to evaluate the literature critically, using summary sources such as Cochrane Reviews and meta-analyses rather than relying on clinical supervisors to provide treatment plans. Furthermore, they discuss the role of faculty members and advanced students in modeling the EBP process on vertical clinical practicum teams. DiLillo and McChargue (2007) describe how standard training clinic procedures (e.g., format of termination reports) can be adapted to help promote the process of EBP. A common theme across descriptions of EBP training programs is that a concerted effort must be made to specifically foster EBP principles and applications throughout a variety of training endeavors; simply endorsing EBP without integrating the EBP process throughout the curriculum is unlikely to have an impact on trainees' practice patterns.

Because the evidence base in pediatric psychology treatments continues to expand, training in the process of EBP, rather than teaching lists of effective treatments, will be crucial. Current and future pediatric psychologists will need to sort efficiently through growing psychological and medical literatures to remain informed about the most up-to-date research findings. They must also competently adapt best practices to individual cases and implement interventions within the unique cultures of the various settings where pediatric psychologists practice (e.g., medical centers, schools, primary care). Although familiarity with specific interventions—a kind of *crystallized knowledge*—will be important, a more *fluid knowledge* of how to identify best practices and adapt those to specific cases within specific settings will be required. Opportunities to gain experience and skills with this process during training should occur in a graduated fashion, as trainees progress from observing faculty and advanced trainees modeling the process to more hands-on experiences with conceptualizing and implementing interventions within an evidence-based framework.

Assessment of Professional Competencies

Mirroring the recognition of the importance of more thorough competencies assessment in graduate training programs, there is growing concern that psychology has lagged behind other professions in terms of required periodic assessments of post-entry-level competencies (Leigh et al., 2007). Professional psychology has long endorsed the idea of professional competencies, as evidenced by the APA ethics code as well as numerous accreditation standards, credentialing bodies, registries, specialty boards, and continuing education requirements (Rubin et al., 2007). However, as noted by Roberts and colleagues (2005), acceptance of the idea of periodic post-entry-level competencies assessment will require a major ideological shift within the profession.

Although perhaps inherent in some of the core competencies identified by writers in the area—for example, "selection of *the best* strategy for intervention" (Kaslow, 2004, p. 776; emphasis added)—explicit discussions of post-entry-level competencies related to EBP principles and processes are rare. If EBP is to move beyond identification of a list of treatments for which there is adequate empirical support, then assessment of competencies related to the processes of identifying, selecting, adapting (see below), and implementing "the best" strategies for assessment and intervention is necessary. As in evaluation of other professional competencies, difficult questions about the nature and form of the ongoing assessments must be answered (Barber, Sharpless, Klostermann, & McCarthy, 2007; Leigh et al., 2007). Doing so will ensure the vitality of the profession (and of the professionals) as new assessment tools and interventions are developed.

Patient Values, Preferences, and Cultural Context of EBP

A critical, although often neglected, component of EBP in psychology requires that treatments with the best available evidence be implemented with expertise "*in the context of patient characteristics, culture, and preferences*" (APA Presidential Task Force, 2006, p. 273; emphasis added). As we have noted elsewhere (Steele, Mize Nelson, & Nelson, 2008), this question is most frequently addressed in terms of client ethnicity, and speaks to the question of "for whom" interventions are most effective (see Paul, 1967, and more recently Elkin, Roberts, & Steele, 2008).

Despite recent calls for greater attention to diversity issues in pediatric psychology (Clay et al., 2002; Tucker, 2002; see also Clay, Chapter 6, this volume), intervention studies examining treatments within ethnic minority samples are still relatively rare. In his editorial vale dictum, Brown (2007) identified 23 intervention studies that were published in *JPP* between 2003 and 2007. In preparing this chapter, we observed that of these 23 intervention studies, 6 (27.3%[1]) reported study sample ethnic minority representation of at least 25% (including 1 case study and 2 RCTs conducted in predominately African American samples); 2 studies (9.1%) examined completion rates by ethnic group; 1 study (4.6%) examined differential treatment outcomes across ethnic groups; and 2 studies (9.1%) failed to report even basic sample characteristics related to ethnicity (see also Raad, Bellinger, McCormick, Roberts, & Steele, 2008). Although these data indicate that the majority of treatment studies (91%) in *JPP* at least reported ethnic group/racial characteristics, these numbers nevertheless suggest that current research

---

[1] One study was conducted within a sample of children with cystic fibrosis. Given the demographic characteristics of the population of children affected by this disease (i.e., almost entirely European American), we did not include this study in the denominators when we examined the reporting of ethnic group differences and outcomes.

published in *JPP* is not adequately examining possible ethnic group differences in treatment processes (e.g., completion) or treatment outcomes from emerging evidence-based treatments (EBTs).

Within the clinical child psychology literature, more empirical research has been conducted on ethnicity as a moderator of treatment outcome. For example, Miranda and colleagues (2005) recently reviewed the psychotherapy outcome literature for ethnic minority youths, and found that ethnicity was not a significant moderator of effectiveness in the studies reviewed. Rather, limited evidence was found for socioeconomic disadvantage as a moderator of treatment outcome. Similarly, Huey and Polo (2008) recently conducted a meta-analysis of psychosocial treatment outcomes within ethnic minority samples of children and adolescents; they found overall treatment effects of medium magnitude ($d = 0.44$), and no evidence that youths' ethnicity moderated treatment effects. However, Huey and Polo noted that these results were limited by low statistical power to detect differences, possible underrepresentation of less acculturated youths in study samples, and inadequate numbers of effectiveness studies (i.e., studies conducted in "real-world" clinical settings). These authors recommended additional empirical research to further examine whether and how ethnicity and related factors moderate treatment efficacy in children and adolescents.

Although the phrase "More research is necessary" is certainly justified by the current literature in clinical child and pediatric psychology, it does little to help the clinician struggling to find an EBT for use with an ethnic minority client. Based on the results of their meta-analysis, Huey and Polo (2008) recommended the use of EBTs that are "well established" or "probably efficacious" in minority samples (p. 263). However, in the absence of research specifically demonstrating efficacy in minority samples, Huey and Polo still recommended that EBTs be considered "first-line" interventions in the treatment of minority youths, noting that the use of EBTs with such youths (even when interventions have not been specifically tested in minority samples) is preferable to the use of alternative interventions with no known empirical support. This recommendation is consistent with suggestions by Kotchick and Grover (2008), who have recommended (1) using EBTs whenever available; (2) flexibly adhering to the treatment manual to address the needs of the client, (3) addressing diversity issues within sessions, and (4) collecting quantitative or qualitative data to assess symptom reduction and client satisfaction.

Questions about the relative efficacy of culturally adapted interventions have recently received attention in the general clinical and the clinical child literatures (Bernal, 2006; Huey & Polo, 2008; Kotchick & Grover, 2008; Whaley & Davis, 2007). For example, Matos, Torres, Santiago, Jurado, and Rodriguez (2006) recently adapted the general parent–child interaction therapy (PCIT) model (Brinkmeyer & Eyberg, 2003) for use with Puerto Rican families. Beyond translation of the manual into local (i.e., Puerto Rican) Spanish, adaptations included greater attention to key cultural variables (e.g., *personalismo, familism*), incorporation of extended family members into therapy, and greater attention given to family issues not directly related to the child's behavior. Although results from this pilot study supported the utility of the adapted PCIT model, the investigation did not evaluate the adapted model in comparison to the original PCIT model. More generally, Miranda and colleagues (2005) have commented that "no data are available to determine to what extent culturally adapting the interventions would improve outcomes for minority youths beyond that achieved with a more generic intervention" (p. 125). Furthermore, Huey and Polo note that the results from their meta-analysis provided little evidence that minority youths benefited more from "culturally adapted therapies" than from standard EBTs. Because of this, Huey and Polo urge caution in the use of cultural adaptations of therapies, instead recommending that therapists provide EBTs in their original forms in the context of culturally informed therapeutic relationships, being particularly sensitive to culturally relevant variables that present barriers to treatment goals. Until data regarding moderators of treatment outcomes are available for interventions developed in the child health arena, the evidence-based guidelines from the clinical child literature appear warranted for our discipline.

Certainly, ethnic diversity is only one aspect of patient characteristics that should be taken into account. Other factors that could potentially moderate treatment effects include gender, age, family or social context, socioeconomic status, religious beliefs, sexual orientation, treatment preference, and numerous other individual and contextual considerations (APA Presidential Task Force, 2006). Indeed, Kazdin (2008) notes that his research group has identified more than 10 moderators of therapeutic change among children presenting for outpatient therapy for conduct problems. Among these moderators are variables from multiple ecological systems, including parent childrearing practices, parent quality of life, family life events, severity of child dysfunction, and child scholastic variables. Given its intrinsic systems orientation (see Steele & Aylward, Chapter 43, this volume), the field of pediatric psychology may naturally include various ecological systems in its interventions (Spirito & Kazak, 2006). Doing so may increase the social validity of its interventions, and thereby increase the likelihood of favorable treatment outcomes for participants across a wide array of individual differences. However, this remains a largely untested supposition. Further examination of treatment outcomes within and across diverse patient groups seems necessary for continued growth in the field.

Conclusions

EBP is a concept that has gained increasing support in recent years within both pediatric psychology and the broader field of clinical psychology. It has become the predominant overarching philosophical framework guiding clinicians and researchers alike in the pursuit of rigorous evidence to support interventions, as well as in the effective and broad deployment of those interventions within clinical settings where children, adolescents, and families are served. Although the movement to promote EBP in clinical psychology has at times stirred considerable controversy, EBP has been widely endorsed within pediatric psychology, and its principles have been held up as the standard to which the field should aspire.

Given its strong and long-standing commitment to the integration of science and practice, pediatric psychology is well positioned to pursue an agenda that promotes EBP. As we have argued in this chapter, achieving this goal will require not only lists of treatments, but strategic commitments to the continued development of a rigorous research base, training of scientists and practitioners in EBP, and creative and flexible adaptation of effective treatments to individual client contexts. As reflected in the relative coverage of topics in this chapter, the greatest strides toward EBP in pediatric psychology have been made with regard to identifying treatments that can and do work in clinical settings. What remains much less developed is an adequate research base into the processes that moderate the efficacy of treatments (e.g., clinical expertise; therapeutic relationship issues; client/patient characteristics, preferences, values; etc). Continued progress toward the goal of EBP, including more research into implementation processes (e.g., client expertise, client values/preferences, dissemination) and cost-effectiveness, will be essential to the future of pediatric psychology as EBP principles exert increasing influence on professional psychology, medicine, and other related fields in the years to come.

References

Aarons, G. A. (2004). Mental health provider attitudes toward adoption of evidence-based practice: The Evidence-Based Practice Attitude Scale (EBPAS). *Mental Health Services Research*, 6, 61–74.

American Psychological Association (APA) Presidential Task Force on Evidence-Based Practice. (2006). Evidence-based practice in psychology. *American Psychologist*, 61, 271–285.

Barber, J. P., Sharpless, B. A., Klostermann, S., & McCarthy, K. S. (2007). Assessing intervention competence and its relation to therapy outcome: A selected review derived from the outcome literature. *Professional Psychology: Research and Practice*, 38, 493–500.

Barlow, D. H. (1996). The effectiveness of psychotherapy: Science and policy. *Clinical Psychology: Science and Practice*, 3, 236–240.

Bauer, R. M. (2007). Evidence-based practice in psychology: Implications for research and research training. *Journal of Clinical Psychology*, 63, 685–694.

Bernal, G. (2006). Intervention development and cultural adaptation research with diverse families. *Family Process*, 45, 143–151.

Beutler, L. E. (2004). The empirically supported treatments movement: A scientist-practitioner response. *Clinical Psychology: Science and Practice*, 11, 225–229.

Beutler, L. E., Williams, R. E., Wakefield, P. J., & Entwistle, S. R. (1995). Bridging scientist and practitioner perspectives in clinical psychology. *American Psychologist*, 50, 984–994.

Brinkmeyer, M., & Eyberg, S. M. (2003). Parent–child interaction therapy for oppositional children. In A. E. Kazdin & J. R. Weisz (Eds.), *Evidence-based psychotherapies for children and adolescents* (pp. 204–223). New York: Guilford Press.

Brown, K. J., & Roberts, M. C. (2000). Future issues in pediatric psychology: Delphic survey. *Journal of Clinical Psychology in Medical Settings*, 7, 5–15.

Brown, R. T. (2007). *Journal of Pediatric Psychology* (*JPP*), 2003–2007: Editor's vale dictum. *Journal of Pediatric Psychology*, 32, 1165–1178.

Chambless, D. L., & Hollon, S. D. (1998). Defining empirically supported therapies. *Journal of Consulting and Clinical Psychology*, 66, 7–18.

Chambless, D. L., & Ollendick, T. H. (2001). Empirically supported psychological interventions: Controversies and evidence. *Annual Review of Psychology*, 52, 685–716.

Chambless, D. L., Sanderson, W. C., Shoham, V., Bennett-Johnson, S. B., Pope, K. S., Crits-Christoph, P., et al. (1996). An update on empirically validated therapies. *The Clinical Psychologist*, 49, 5–18.

Clay, D. L., Mordhorst, M. J., & Lehn, L. (2002). Empirically supported treatments in pediatric psychology: Where is the diversity? *Journal of Pediatric Psychology*, 27, 325–337.

Cohen, L. L., La Greca, A. M., Blount, R. L., Kazak, A. E., Holmbeck, G. N., & Lemanek, K. L. (2008). Introduction to special issue: Evidence-based assessment in pediatric psychology. *Journal of Pediatric Psychology*, 33, 911–915.

Collins, F. L., Leffingwell, T. R., & Belar, C. D. (2007). Teaching evidence-based practice: Implications for psychology. *Journal of Clinical Psychology*, 63, 657–670.

Detsky, A. S., & Laupacis, A. (2007). Relevance of cost-effectiveness analysis to clinicians and policy makers. *Journal of the American Medical Association, 298*, 221–224.

DiLillo, D., & McChargue, D. (2007). Implementing elements of evidence-based practice into scientist-practitioner training at the University of Nebraska–Lincoln. *Journal of Clinical Psychology, 63*, 671–685.

Drotar, D., & Lemanek, K. (2001). Steps toward a clinically relevant science of interventions in pediatric settings: Introduction to the special issue. *Journal of Pediatric Psychology, 26*, 385–394.

Elkin, T. D., Roberts, M. C., & Steele, R. G. (2008). Emerging issues in the evolution of evidence-based practice. In R. G. Steele, T. D. Elkin, & M. C. Roberts (Eds.), *Handbook of evidence-based therapies for children and adolescents* (pp. 569–575). New York: Springer.

Frick, P. J. (2007). Providing the evidence for evidence-based practice. *Journal of Clinical Child and Adolescent Psychology, 36*, 2–7.

Garfield, S. L. (1996). Some problems associated with "validated" forms of psychotherapy. *Clinical Psychology: Science and Practice, 3*, 218–229.

Havik, O. E., & VandenBos, G. R. (1996). Limitations of manualized psychotherapy for everyday practice. *Clinical Psychology: Science and Practice, 3*, 264–267.

Hayes, L., Matthews, J., Copley, A., & Welsh, D. (2008). A randomized controlled trial of mother–infant or toddler parenting program: Demonstrating effectiveness in practice. *Journal of Pediatric Psychology, 33*, 473–486.

Holmbeck, G. N. (2008). *Journal of Pediatric Psychology* statement of purpose: Section on methodology. *Journal of Pediatric Psychology, 33*, 9–11.

Holmbeck, G. N., Bruno, E. F., & Jandasek, B. (2006). Longitudinal research in pediatric psychology: An introduction to the special issue. *Journal of Pediatric Psychology, 31*, 995–1001.

Huey, S. J., & Polo, A. J. (2008). Evidence-based psychosocial treatments for ethnic minority youth. *Journal of Clinical Child and Adolescent Psychology, 37*, 262–301.

Institute of Medicine (IOM). (2001). *Crossing the quality chasm: A new health system for the 21st century*. Washington, DC: National Academy Press.

Johnston, C. A., & Steele, R. G. (2007). Treatment of pediatric overweight: An examination of feasibility and effectiveness in an applied clinical setting. *Journal of Pediatric Psychology, 32*, 106–110.

Kaslow, N. J. (2004). Competencies in professional psychology. *American Psychologist, 59*, 774–781.

Kazak, A. E. (2006). The president's message: Research into practice in pediatric psychology. *Progress Notes, 30*, 1.

Kazdin, A. E. (2008). Evidence-based treatment and practice: New opportunities to bridge clinical research and practice, enhance the knowledge base, and improve patient care. *American Psychologist, 63*, 146–159.

Kazdin, A. E., Siegel, T. C., & Bass, D. (1990). Drawing upon clinical practice to inform research on child and adolescent psychotherapy: A survey of practitioners. *Professional Psychology: Research and Practice, 21*, 189–198.

Kazdin, A. E., & Weisz, J. R. (2003). Introduction: Context and background of evidence-based psychotherapies for children and adolescents. In A. E. Kazdin & J. R. Weisz (Eds.), *Evidence-based psychotherapies for children and adolescents* (pp. 3–20). New York: Guilford Press.

Kotchick, B. A., & Grover, R. L. (2008). Implementing evidence-based treatments with ethnically diverse clients. In R. G. Steele, T. D. Elkin, & M. C. Roberts (Eds.), *Handbook of evidence-based therapies for children and adolescents* (pp. 487–504). New York: Springer.

Leffingwell, T. R., & Collins, F. L. (2008). Graduate training in evidence-based practice in psychology. In R. G. Steele, T. D. Elkin, & M. C. Roberts (Eds.), *Handbook of evidence-based therapies for children and adolescents* (pp. 551–568). New York: Springer.

Leigh, I. W., Smith, I. L., Bebeau, M. J., Lichtenberg, J. W., Nelson, P. D., Portney, S., et al. (2007). Competency assessment models. *Professional Psychology: Research and Practice, 38,* 463–473.

Levant, R. F. (2004). The empirically validated treatments movement: A practitioner's perspective. *Clinical Psychology: Science and Practice, 11,* 219–224.

Luebbe, A. M., Radcliffe, A. M., Callands, T. A., Green, D., & Thorn, B. E. (2007). Evidence-based practice in psychology: Perception of graduate students in scientist-practitioner programs. *Journal of Clinical Psychology, 63,* 643–655.

Mash, E. J., & Hunsley, J. (2005). Evidence-based assessment of child and adolescent disorders: Issues and challenges. *Journal of Clinical Child and Adolescent Psychology, 34,* 362–379.

Matos, M., Torres, R., Santiago, R., Jurado, M., & Rodriguez, I. (2006). Adaptation of parent–child interaction therapy for Puerto Rican families: A preliminary study. *Family Process, 45,* 205–222.

Messer, S. B., & Wampold, B. E. (2002). Let's face facts: Common factors are more potent than specific therapy ingredients. *Clinical Psychology: Science and Practice, 9,* 21–25.

Miranda, J., Guillermo, B., Lau, A., Kohn, L., Hwang, W., & LaFromboise, T. (2005). State of the science on psychosocial interventions for ethnic minorities. *Annual Review of Clinical Psychology, 1,* 113–142.

Nelson, T. D., Aylward, B. S., & Steele, R. G. (2008). Structural equation modeling in pediatric psychology: Overview and review of applications. *Journal of Pediatric Psychology, 33,* 679–687.

Nelson, T. D., & Steele, R. G. (2006). Beyond efficacy and effectiveness: A multifaceted approach to treatment evaluation. *Professional Psychology: Research and Practice, 37,* 389–397.

Norcross, J. C. (2001). Purposes, processes, and products of the Task Force on Empirically Supported Therapy Relationships. *Psychotherapy: Theory, Research, Practice, Training, 38,* 345–356.

Paul, G. L. (1967). Outcome research in psychotherapy. *Journal of Consulting Psychology, 31,* 109–118.

Persons, J. B., & Silberschatz, G. (1998). Are results of randomized controlled trials useful to psychotherapists? *Journal of Consulting and Clinical Psychology, 66,* 126–135.

Raad, J. M., Bellinger, S., McCormick, E., Roberts, M. C., & Steele, R. G. (2008). Brief report: An update of reporting practices of demographic, methodological, and ethical procedures in journals of pediatric and child psychology. *Journal of Pediatric Psychology, 33,* 688–693.

Rae, W. A. (2004). 2000 SPP Salk Award Address: Financing pediatric psychology services: Buddy, can you spare a dime? *Journal of Pediatric Psychology, 29,* 47–52.

Rapoff, M., & Stark, L. (2008). Editorial: *Journal of Pediatric Psychology* statement of purpose: Section on single-subject studies. *Journal of Pediatric Psychology, 33,* 16–21.

Roberts, M. C., Borden, K. A., Christiansen, M. D., & Lopez, S. J. (2005). Fostering a culture shift: Assessment of competence in the education and careers of professional psychologists. *Professional Psychology: Research and Practice, 36,* 355–361.

Roberts, M. C., Mitchell, M. C., & McNeal, R. (2003). The evolving field of pediatric psychology: Critical issues and future challenges. In M. C. Roberts (Ed.), *Handbook of pediatric psychology* (3rd ed., pp. 3–18). New York: Guilford Press.

Rubin, N. J., Bebeau, M., Leigh, I. W., Lichtenberg, J. W., Nelson, P. D., Portnoy, S., et al. (2007). The competency movement within psychology: An historical perspective. *Professional Psychology: Research and Practice, 38,* 452–462.

Sackett, D. L., Rosenberg, W. M., Gray, J. A., Haynes, R. B., & Richardson, W. S. (1996). Evidence-based medicine: What it is and what it isn't. *British Medical Journal, 312,* 71–72.

Shakow, D., Hilgard, E. R., Kelly, E. L., Luckey, B., Sanford, R. N., & Shaffer, L. F. (1947). Recommended graduate training program in clinical psychology. *American Psychologist, 2,* 539–558.

Spirito, A. (1999). Introduction: Special series on empirically supported treatments in pediatric psychology. *Journal of Pediatric Psychology, 24,* 87–90.

Spirito, A., Brown, R. T., D'Angelo, E., Delamater, A., Rodrigue, J., & Siegel, L. (2003). Society of Pediatric Psychology Task Force report: Recommendations for training pediatric psychologists. *Journal of Pediatric Psychology, 28,* 85–98.

Spirito, A., & Kazak, A. E. (2006). *Effective and emerging treatments in pediatric psychology.* New York: Oxford University Press.

Spring, B. (2007). Evidence-based practice in clinical psychology: What it is, why it matters; what you need to know. *Journal of Clinical Psychology, 63,* 611–631.

Stark, L. (2008). The president's message. *Progress Notes, 32,* 1–2.

Steele, R. G., Mize Nelson, J. A., & Nelson, T. D. (2008). Methodological issues in the evaluation of therapies. In R. G. Steele, T. D. Elkin, & M. C. Roberts (Eds.), *Handbook of evidence-based therapies for children and adolescents* (pp. 25–43). New York: Springer.

Steele, R. G., & Roberts, M. C. (2003). Therapy and interventions research with children and adolescents. In M. C. Roberts & S. S. Ilardi (Eds.), *Handbook of research methods in clinical psychology* (pp. 307–326). Oxford, UK: Blackwell.

Stirman, S. W., Crits-Christoph, P., & DeRubeis, R. J. (2004). Achieving successful dissemination of empirically supported psychotherapies: A synthesis of dissemination theory. *Clinical Psychology: Science and Practice, 11,* 343–359.

Straus, S. E., Richardson, W. S., Glasziou, P., & Haines, R. B. (2005). *Evidence-based medicine: How to practice and teach EBM* (3rd ed.). Edinburgh, UK: Elsevier/Churchill Livingstone.

Strupp, H. H. (2001). Implications of the empirically supported treatment movement for psychoanalysis. *Psychoanalytic Dialogues, 11,* 615–619.

Tucker, C. M. (2002). Expanding pediatric psychology beyond hospital walls to meet the health care needs of ethnic minority children. *Journal of Pediatric Psychology, 27,* 315–323.

Weisz, J. R., Hawley, K. M., Pilkonis, P. A., Woody, S. R., & Follette, W. C. (2000). Stressing the (other) three Rs in the search of empirically supported treatments: Review procedures, research quality, relevance to practice and the public interest. *Clinical Psychology: Science and Practice, 7,* 243–258.

Whaley, A. L., & Davis, K. E. (2007). Cultural competence and evidence-based practice in mental health services. *American Psychologist, 62,* 563–574.

Witmer, L. (1996). Clinical psychology. *American Psychologist, 51,* 248–251. (Original work published 1907)

Woody, S. R., Weisz, J., & McLean, C. (2005). Empirically-supported treatments: 10 years later. *The Clinical Psychologist, 58,* 5–11.

Wysocki, T. (2008). Editorial: *Journal of Pediatric Psychology* statement of purpose: Section on randomized trials. *Journal of Pediatric Psychology, 33,* 12–15.

Yates, B. T. (1994). Toward the incorporation of costs, cost-effectiveness analysis, and cost–benefit analysis into clinical research. *Journal of Consulting and Clinical Psychology, 62,* 729–736.

CHAPTER 8

Inpatient Pediatric Consultation–Liaison

BRYAN D. CARTER
WILLIAM G. KRONENBERGER
ERIC SCOTT
MICHELLE M. ERNST

Pediatric consultation–liaison (hereafter referred to as CL) represents perhaps the most active form of collaboration between pediatric psychologists and pediatric health care specialists, and is directed toward the alleviation of suffering, distress, and disease management challenges in childhood illness. In its most narrow definition, CL involves a psychologist providing assessment and guidance to a pediatrician colleague on the management of a circumscribed clinical problem with a specific patient. In its most broad application, the CL psychologist becomes a systems-level catalyst—in educating and empowering multiple interacting components of the health care system in providing a responsive environment that maximizes the overall psychological adjustment and quality of life for patients and their families.

This multifaceted role extends beyond helping a patient to cope with emotional adjustments of illness or addressing internalizing or acting-out behaviors that may ensue. Interventions may include addressing physical symptoms, helping to manage physical pain, teaching coping skills, and evaluating side effects of medication, among others. Thus the consultant's role goes beyond the needs of the child and encompasses providing support and education for families, as well as serving as a liaison among the patient, the family, and the medical team (Shaw & DeMaso, 2006).

Characterization and Prevalence of CL Services in Children's Hospitals

Pediatric CL services vary considerably in size and composition. In its most basic form, a CL service may consist of a part-time psychologist providing generalist services to a wide array of pediatric subspecialties (Drotar, 1976). At the other end of the spectrum are large multidisciplinary teams consisting of a combination of pediatric psychologists, child psychiatrists, psychology postdoctoral fellows, psychology predoctoral interns, child psychiatry fellows, general psychiatry residents, developmental/behavioral pediatric residents, general pediatric residents, psychiatric nurses, and trainees in a variety of professions in practica arrangements.

There are few reviews of the models, characteristics, and prevalence of inpatient pediatric CL services in children's hospitals. In a recent survey of 144 children's hospital-based child psychiatry CL services in the United States (Shaw, Wamboldt, Bursch, & Stuber, 2006), returned surveys (33%) indicated that the average psychologist on the service was a .27 full-time equivalent (FTE), while the average child psychiatrist was a .44 FTE. Although pediatric CL services may vary in professional composition, their primary role within hospitals typically encompasses evaluating children and their families for mental health concerns; recommending and providing treatments; and educating families, staff, and referring physicians on a wide array of factors associated with adjustment to medical illness and injury.

The few published studies on reasons for referrals to a pediatric CL service indicate that common referral questions include adaptation and adjustment to medical illness; resolution of behavioral problems; evaluation of developmental delays; abatement of psychological crisis; assessment of depression and suicidality (Drotar, Spirito, & Stancin, 2003; Olson et al., 1988); and neuropsychological testing and evaluation to determine illness/injury-associated cognitive deficits (Rodrique et al., 1995). In the only case-controlled study of an inpatient pediatric CL service, Carter and colleagues (2003) reported a wide diversity of referral sources, including equal distributions from hematology/oncology, surgery/trauma, pulmonology, and several other services. The most common reasons for referral included requests for assisting a child in coping with physical illness/injury, improving treatment adherence, assessing and treating depression and anxiety, teaching pain management techniques, assistance with parent coping, helping with adjustment to a new medical diagnosis, and resolving family conflict. In the Shaw and colleagues (2006) survey, the most common referral concerns included patient depression, anxiety, suicide risk assessment, and medication evaluation.

Variation across referral questions may exist due to several factors (including the needs of the specific patient populations within given hospitals, specific consultants' interests and expertise, familiarity between a referring physician and a consultant, etc.). Most CL services provide diagnostic assessment, psychotherapy for patients/parents, psychotropic medication, referrals for postdischarge outpatient interventions, facilitation of transfer to psychiatric hospitals, and liaison education to referring physicians.

Models of CL

Consultation versus Liaison Emphasis

The terms "consultation" and "liaison" are often mistakenly assumed to be synonymous with one another. However, there are important distinctions between being a consultant and functioning in a liaison role, even though many psychologists provide both services. As hospital consultants, pediatric psychologists become directly involved in patient care only upon the request of a referring professional or service. Encountering a circumscribed problem with a particular patient often prompts a physician to request a pediatric psychologist to perform an evaluation and propose treatment recommendations. Strain (2002) has characterized a consultant as a "firefighter" intervening in problematic cases, performing timely and efficient problem-focused interventions, but rarely expected to educate health care staff about preventive "fireproofing" or informing and empowering staff to treat similar problems that are likely to arise in the future. In such an arrangement, there may or may not be a long-term relationship between the consultant and the treating physician. Once recommendations are made, the relationship may end.

Whereas a consultant is called only after clear concerns arise, a pediatric psychologist in a liaison role is more likely to be involved in the day-to-day workings of a particular hospital service or unit (e.g., attending daily rounds and patient case conferences, making independent decisions to see patients without an attending referral). The psychologist is also often formally embedded within a department or working service. For example, he or she may be employed by or have a portion of time formally dedicated to a division of hematology/oncology. The psychologist in such a liaison role is likely to be involved in all of the systemic and mental health concerns on the unit, not just with those of referred patients. In the consultant role, the psychologist is likely to see only a fraction of the patients on any particular unit; in the liaison role, the psychologist conceptualizes systems-level changes that can enhance the coping and adjustment of all patients, families, and health care staff members (Strain, 2002).

Patient-Centered versus Systems-Centered Focus

Consultation models have also been differentiated according to whether the focus of the consultation is primarily on the patient ("patient-centered") or on the larger system upon which the patient and family must rely for medical care ("systems-centered") (Strain, 2002). In patient-centered consultation, the primary goal is to evaluate the patient in order to provide direct treatment, together with relevant management recommendations to the referring health care team. In contrast, systems-centered (also known as "consultee-centered") consultation occurs when the focus of the consultation is on creating change in the professional and/or health care team members requesting the consultation, in order to make them more effective in the intervention with the case in question, as well as other cases with similar profiles or characteristics (Alpert & Spencer, 1986; Strain, 2002).

Relationships with Psychiatry and Pediatrics Specialties: Integrated versus Parallel Services

Just as there is variability in models of CL, the formal appointment and employment of psychologists on CL services can vary considerably. Psychologists may be employed directly by hospitals; may have appointments in various departments (psychiatry, pediatrics, neurology, and subspecialties within those areas, such as behavioral pediatrics and hematology/oncology); or may be organized into departments of psychology within the hospital. Because psychologists may be housed within various "home" departments, "parallel" or "overlapping" services may arise across different departments. Steiner, Sanders, Canning, and Litt (1994) attempted to reduce redundancy of services by integrating psychiatric services into clinical pediatric activities. This model for having psychologists within a pediatric psychiatry CL service was a joint venture between the division of pediatric psychiatry (within a department of psychiatry) and the department of pediatrics. An alternative model is the "bridge model" of consultation, which involves a psychologist or psychiatrist, usually affiliated with a department of psychiatry, being assigned to a pediatric specialty clinic (Strain, 2002). This "bridge" is meant to span the lack of access to psychiatric services among patients in the pediatric clinic, as well as to supplement the knowledge base of the agency members. Although the psychologist may have direct patient care responsibilities, often his or her primary role is to provide structured pedagogical courses for staff, students (medical students or residents), and physicians. Psychologists also may practice in a setting where a "hybrid" model is adopted. In this model, the psychologist is embedded within a department of a hospital unaffiliated with psychiatry or psychology (Strain, 2002). Employment is often fully within the department, with clinical, teaching, and research responsibilities dedicated exclusively to that department.

The Process of Pediatric CL

Referral

Requests for inpatient pediatric consultations are made for a wide array of presenting problems and referral questions (Carter et al., 2003; Fritz, 1993; Kremer & Wasserman, 1994; Lewandowski & Baranoski, 1994; Olson, Mullins, Chaney, & Gilman, 1993). Some CL services provide protocol consultations, whereby the consultant is expected to evaluate all new patients on a particular service as a matter of routine, to screen for psychosocial needs. This arrangement is most likely when patients have a serious chronic illness such as cystic fibrosis or diabetes. Frequently the CL psychologist working with these specialty services will be available to see patients in other clinical settings such as the outpatient clinic.

The referral process can vary from service to service and from case to case. A staff member or provider on the hospital unit (e.g., unit secretary, medical student, resident or fellow, nurse, social worker, or attending physician) typically calls in the referral. The attending physician often delegates this responsibility to the resident or medical student in teaching hospital settings. Increasingly, consultation requests are entered electronically into the hospital computer system and received by the CL service without any direct contact. These various methods of receiving referrals can promote potential distortion of the referral problem(s) in the busy daily schedule of the medical team; therefore, consultants must carefully screen and manage referrals in their system (Carter et al., 2003; Drotar, 1995; Mullins, Gillman, & Harbeck, 1992). Perhaps most importantly, the success of any consultation is highly dependent on the consultant and consultee coming to a consensus on the specific definitions of the referral problem and desired or expected outcomes from the consultation. Unless this is successfully attained, it is likely that the consultee will be dissatisfied with the process and outcome of the consultation (Carter & von Weiss, 2005). Thus, consultation assumes a shared responsibility for problem solution, involving a collaborative alliance of the patient and family, health care team, and the consultant.

Importance of Goal Setting

It is important for the referring physician to discuss the reasons for requesting the consultation with the family and patient before the initial contact. At times the patient and/or parent/guardian have limited input into the referral process and may have anxieties and objections to being evaluated by a psychologist. It is usually not helpful for the referring physician to state only that the patient needs psychological or psychiatric assistance, even in cases where there is a high likelihood of a primarily functional basis for the patient's symptoms (e.g., as in conversion or somatization disorders). More appropriately, the referring professional should be guided in framing the referral as a frequently employed mechanism for helping all parties better understand the patient's problems, in order to enhance diagnostic and treatment effectiveness and minimize the patient's distress.

Ideally, after the CL psychologist and family complete the assessment process, there is general agreement about one or more concerns that need to be addressed in the consultation, which will lead to further delineation of realistically achievable goals for the assessment and disposition. Pediatric CL goals are typically specific, problem-focused, and designed to be met within achievable time frames. Clear delineation of consultation goals at the outset of the process has been shown to be associated with positive referring professional ratings of consultation goal attainment, as well as with professional and patient/family satisfaction with the CL services (Carter et al., 2003).

Assessment

Drotar and colleagues (2003) have described inpatient consultations as generally following a medical model, wherein the consultant conducts an assessment of the referred pediatric patient in order to advise the referring physician about the management of psychosocial aspects of the patient's care. The assessment process often involves multiple clinical interviews with the child, family, and staff, history taking, repeated behavioral observations, and occasionally formal psychological assessment. Time and logistical constraints often demand a problem-focused assessment process. The assessment findings are communicated to the hospital staff via written, phone, and face-to-face contacts (Drotar, 1995).

Parent-Based Information

Parents or other guardians are key sources of information about a child's history, behavior, personality, and family environment. In addition to clinical interview with parents, measurement of various factors (child adjustment and behavioral problems, quality of life, regimen adherence, etc.) with structured rating scales may assist the CL psychologist in obtaining norm-referenced data on more pervasive difficulties in adjustment that may contribute to the child's presentation in the hospital. For example, Carter and colleagues (2003) found that prehospitalization behavioral difficulties assisted in predicting the need for referral.

Patient-Based Information

In addition to obtaining information from parents, observation, interview, and sometimes formal testing of the patient are important components of the CL assessment process. However, factors such as the patient's physical condition, absence from the room for diagnostic tests and treatments, nonadherence, and stressful aspects of being in the hospital environment can interfere with this portion of the assessment. It is important for the consultant to be creative and flexible in assessing the pediatric patient, with a major emphasis on establishing rapport and determining basic mental status parameters. Such sources of patient information as drawings, play observation, and the like can be most informative to the evaluation.

Nursing-Based Observations

The nursing staff, by virtue of having frequent contact with the child and family on the medical unit, can often provide very revealing information to the consultant about the actual meaning behind the medical record entries and the dynamics that have led to the referral (Drotar, 1995). In addition to review of nursing notes and direct interview of nurses, a nurse-completed behavior checklist such as the Pediatric Inpatient Behavior Scale (PIBS; Kronenberger, Carter, & Thomas, 1997) can provide a quick, structured assessment of a variety of internalizing and externalizing behavioral problems that may adversely affect the child's functioning in the hospital setting.

Assessing Family and Systems Factors

There has been an increasing emphasis on family-centered perspectives in conceptualizing and treating chronic illness in children (Kazak, Simms, & Rourke, 2002; Wysocki et al., 2000). From a systems-based perspective, the reciprocal interaction of the patient/family with the health care and other systems requires a broad-based collaborative approach (McDaniel, Hepworth, & Doherty, 1992). A useful protocol for conducting pediatric consultations from a family systems-based model has been provided by Kazak and colleagues (2002).

Communication of Findings and Recommendations

The consultant's methods of communicating findings and recommendations to the referring physician, health care team, parents, and child are determined by a number of factors. Communications to the referring professional and hospital staff are routinely provided via a consultation report or progress note entry in the patient's medical chart. CL reports tend to be brief, specific, and problem-focused, with brief descriptions of the presenting problems, developmental and medical history, a review of current treatments and medications, a summary of the consultant's evaluation of the patient as related to the referral problem, and specific recommendations for intervention and disposition. More complex referral questions, involving such issues as formal psychological testing or complex child protective issues (e.g., pretransplant evaluations, pediatric condition falsification), often require more extensive and detailed written reports.

Face-to-face discussion with a colleague, with the increased interpersonal communication it provides, may be necessary to maximize the usefulness of the consultation, lead to role clarification for arranging referral disposition, and even provide opportunities for informal teaching (Drotar, 1995). Although it is not always the case, on occasion the patient and/or their parents may request information about the findings and recommendations of the consultation evaluation. In those cases where the consultant is going to be involved in providing treatment services during the patient's hospital stay or in outpatient follow-up, the careful sharing of this information can be an important part of the trust-building phase of a therapeutic relationship.

Intervention: The Five C's of Pediatric CL

Carter and von Weiss (2005) characterize CL activities according to the arenas of practice/intervention into which most case referrals can be categorized, by way of an alliterative mnemonic device they call the "five C's" of consultation: crisis, coping, compliance (adherence), communication, and collaboration.

Crisis

When children are diagnosed with a potentially serious illness or injury, they and their families are often in a state of shock and disbelief, and may have difficulty coping with the bewildering details and decisions of medical evaluation and treatment (Drotar & Zagorski, 2001). In such situations, families are in need of highly focused interventions that provide a sense of understanding and control. Pollin (1994, 1995) has developed a medical crisis counseling model that is particularly suited to pediatric trauma situations. In this model, the consultant primarily focuses on the patient's medical condition, with interventions aimed at normalizing the patient's and family's state of emotional distress while also mobilizing the family to engage in highly concrete actions that facilitate more effective coping.

Coping

There are many stressors associated with acute and chronic childhood illness and injury (Harbeck-Weber, Fisher, & Dittner, 2003). These include acute procedure-related experiences (e.g., injections, venipunctures, intravenous line placements, minor surgeries), as well as more lengthy procedures (hospitalizations, major surgeries, chemotherapy, repeated painful dressing changes, etc.). Chronic illnesses such as cystic fibrosis, malignancies, diabetes, chronic renal disease, or sickle cell disease present a child and family with months, years, or even a lifetime of stressful and hassling procedures that require major changes in expectations and lifestyle modifications, often with an uncertain outcome.

In designing interventions to facilitate child and family coping, the CL psychologist must be cognizant of both developmental and individual factors; for example, younger children's limited linguistic and cognitive abilities may limit their understanding of health concepts and ability to utilize coping resources and external supports. Differences in coping styles are associated with adaptation to hospitalization and surgery, physiological stress response (salivary cortisol production), and child cooperation with pre- and postsurgery procedures (Harbeck-Weber & Peterson, 2003). Evidence suggests that strategies whereby a child modifies the objective situation ("primary control" strategies) are most effective when employed to cope with stressors over which the child has control, whereas strategies involving the child modifying his or her emotional and behavioral reactions to the stressor ("secondary control" strategies) are most effective with uncontrollable stressors (Compas, Malcarne, & Banez, 1992; Rothbaum, Weisz, & Snyder, 1982). All of these efforts to facilitate child coping occur in the context of the "social ecology" of the hospital and health care team (Thompson & Gustafson, 1996; Wallander, Varni, Babani, Banis, & Wilcox, 1989). In addition, family environment variables, such as parental psychopathology, adaptability, cohesion, emotional expressiveness, communication skills, and conflict resolution skills, have an impact on the child's coping with illness and treatment; problems in those areas may necessitate the use of family-based interventions (Kazak et al., 1999; Kell, Kliewer, Erichson, & Ohene-Frempong, 1998; Sanders, Shepherd, Cleghorn, & Woolford, 1994; Wallander & Thompson, 1995; Wysocki et al., 2000).

Compliance (Adherence)

With more children surviving medical conditions that were once considered fatal, and requiring complex treatment plans that call for long-term behavior changes in the children and their caretakers, problems with nonadherence have become major pediatric health concerns with serious and far-reaching consequences for patient morbidity, mortality, and health care utilization (La Greca & Bearman, 2003; Rapoff, 1999; Spirito & Kazak, 2006). Rates of noncompliance with medical regimens of 50% and higher have been found for patients with chronic illness (Rapoff, 1999).

Poor adherence to prescribed medical regimens may adversely affect health, leading to an inpatient admission to address both the disease process and adherence issues. Patients and their families may fail to administer medications in the appropriate doses or on schedule, fail to follow dietary guidelines, defy physical activity restrictions, or be openly uncooperative with invasive or noxious medical procedures, even within the closely controlled confines of the inpatient unit. In fact, the very process of monitoring adherence presents methodological challenges for the patient, family, and health care team. Multiple methods may need to be employed, such as direct observations of the patient's behavior, self-report logs/diaries, provider ratings, counting remaining medications, and use of monitoring devices and assays (La Greca & Bearman, 2003).

Although not all approaches are supported by empirical evidence, Carter and von Weiss (2005) report the following interventions as being frequently employed in facilitating patient and family adherence in the inpatient pediatric setting: education; teaching mastery skills (role play, rehearsal); behavioral contracting; removing barriers to adherence; monitoring and charting performance of medical treatment components; altering family/health care system dynamics; normalizing/reframing the patient's condition; altering patient/family lifestyle behaviors; and altering expectations of family/health care providers to coincide with realistic developmental needs.

Communication

Under the conditions of lengthy hospitalization, patient and family lack of control over uncomfortable diagnostic and treatment procedures, demanding staff caseloads and schedules, and complex medical decision making, there are significant risks for miscommunication between patient/family and medical staff. A CL psychologist often receives referrals because the staff is encountering behavioral difficulties with a child and/or family that prove disruptive to the functioning of the hospital unit. In such potentially volatile situations, the CL psychologist must employ strong skills in communication and diplomacy, and must demonstrate sensitivity to patient, family, and medical team issues (Brown & Macias, 2001). The psychologist often must diffuse patient and family defensiveness, particularly if they have not been made aware of the referral. Such factors as the psychologist maintaining a regular presence at service rounds and team meetings, engaging in ongoing collaborative relationships with hospital staff, assisting with increasing cultural sensitivity, and respectfully reframing patient/family and staff behaviors to facilitate understanding can help prevent miscommunication (Carter & von Weiss, 2005).

Collaboration

The importance of the collaborative relationship between the pediatric psychologist and the referring services cannot be overemphasized. Historically, this relationship has evolved out of shared goals in the areas of service, teaching, and research (Drotar, 1995). Many CL psychologists in academic medical center settings report that some of the most rewarding service collaborations with their pediatric colleagues have evolved out of investigative research collaborations. Close collaborations with other members of the medical team, the patient, and the family can have a critically important impact on clinical care.

Operational and Organizational Challenges to Inpatient Pediatric Psychology CL Services

Inpatient pediatric psychology CL services face a number of unique organizational challenges, stemming from differences between these services and a traditional outpatient psychology service. Scheduling and referrals for CL services, for example, are less predictable and less regulated. Types of patient encounters, diagnostic coding, and billing also differ from traditional mental health services. In addition, systems/milieu issues are different for CL services than for other psychology services.

Financial Challenges and Institutional Support

Like other clinical services, CL services require financial and/or institutional support in order to function. In addition to funding for personnel, CL services need space, materials, support staff, and other resources to provide appropriate evaluations and interventions. As a result, most CL services rely on a blend of clinical billing, clinical contracts, and administrative contracts to generate revenue. Clinical billing for CL services can be problematic if it does not generate sufficient revenue to cover a target amount of costs. Several characteristics of CL services can interfere with adequate income from clinical billing. First, CL referrals are often for emergent situations that must be resolved within a tight time frame; this sometimes requires that clinical services be provided prior to receiving authorization from insurance. In some cases, attempts to obtain authorization fail because insurance utilization review specialists cannot fit a CL authorization request into a system that was designed to accommodate only traditional mental health authorizations.

A second set of challenges to CL clinical billing is denial of claims, which can occur more frequently for CL services because of confusion on the part of the insurance company about receiving a "psychology" bill for a patient who is hospitalized for a "medical" reason. Alternatively, claims may be rejected because of restrictions on the number or type of consultations allowed by an insurance product. Claims may also be denied because CL psychologists are not a part of a patient's insurance network or because mental health benefits are often carved out of a patient's general insurance plan. This can occur even when the hospital and/or the pediatric service are in the network for the patient. (See Tynan, Stehl, & Pendley, Chapter 5, this volume.)

Even when insurance does pay for services, payment rates for CL services can be less than half of the amount that can be billed and collected for outpatient psychological services, because CL providers must spend considerable time performing nonbillable services (e.g., communication with referral sources, communication with social services, milieu work, waiting time, service provided by multiple members of the team on the same day). Such services often account for 50–100% of service provision time (Kronenberger, 2004). Moreover, as most major pediatric hospitals provide needed services to patients regardless of ability to pay, CL consultants see a disproportionately high number of families who cannot pay for the part of their bill that is not covered by insurance.

The traditional structure of billing for mental health services is ill suited for the CL setting, because most children referred to CL services do not fit easily into a classic psychiatric diagnosis, and because CL evaluations and interventions do not match most of the classic mental health procedure codes as defined in the Current Procedural Terminology (CPT; American Medical Association, 2007). In 2002, new health and behavior (H & B) CPT codes became accepted by key governmental payers. Because these codes allow psychologists to bill for services provided to children who have a physical illness but no formal or classic mental health diagnosis (Noll & Fischer, 2004), they are ideally suited for use in the provision of CL services. H & B codes are often (but not always) covered by the medical portion of a child's insurance, with billing reflecting the child's medical diagnosis as the main diagnostic code. This can help to eliminate some of the problems with mental health codes and with misunderstanding and/or denial of the service by a mental health insurance carrier. (Again, see Tynan et al., Chapter 5.)

As a result of billing and reimbursement challenges, many CL services rely on institutional support to meet shortfalls in funding, material, and personnel. The simplest form of institutional support is the clinical contract or grant, in which a hospital, department, or teaching institution provides the CL service with an annual stipend to supplement the clinical collections raised by the service. Other models of institutional support for CL services are coverage of certain personnel costs (e.g., covering the salary of a nurse or social worker), providing space without rent charge, including the CL service in a larger grant or contract, or reducing other productivity requirements of CL personnel. In some cases, CL services are supported by research or training grants.

Multiple Roles and Role Strain

Along with financial challenges, role challenges are among the most common and significant strains encountered by CL psychologists. CL psychologists must learn to distinguish their role from that of professionals in related services, such as child life, social work, and chaplaincy. For example, use of psychological scales by social workers, pain management performed by child life specialists, and family therapy conducted by a chaplain may create disagreement about boundaries between disciplines and services. Addressing these boundaries requires a mixture of collaborative interaction, problem solving, education, flexibility, tolerance, and limit setting.

CL psychologists often also experience role challenges in their "home" department (usually pediatrics, psychology, or psychiatry). One of the more common challenges is defining a role that fits with CL duties while also contributing to the department's over-all mission and resources. CL psychologists often have other productivity expectations (e.g., outpatient services, teaching, and research) in addition to their CL role. Balancing these demands is critical for having sufficient time and energy for CL activities, and rea-sonable productivity demands of the CL service by the home department are required.

Beyond Clinical Services: Challenges in Training and Research

In addition to clinically related role demands, many CL psychologists juggle training and research expectations. However, the high visibility of CL services in the hospital, and the unique and often urgent demands of medically hospitalized pediatric patients, requires a steep learning curve for trainees and close monitoring by the attending psy-chologist. Referring physicians expect uniformly high-quality service on each request, regardless of who is providing the consultation.

Research about inpatient CL services is crucial for understanding, enhancing, and supporting CL work. However, the opportunities for research are limited by influences ranging from recruitment difficulties to measurement challenges. Even large CL stud-ies have relatively few subjects within each illness type, raising questions about the appropriateness and methodology of combining illness conditions for statistical analy-sis (Carter et al., 2003). Recruitment for inpatient CL studies is also hindered because potential subjects are hospitalized and therefore under significant strain, and they may be reluctant or unable to participate. As a result of these challenges, relatively little research has been performed on general inpatient CL populations.

Opportunities and Innovations in Pediatric CL Work

Opportunities

The field of pediatric psychology has long recognized the importance of demonstrating the viability of our research and clinical services to other child health care profession-als (Brown & Roberts, 2000). Pediatric psychologists can be instrumental in designing interventions that minimize hospital costs by facilitating discharge planning, as well as working with high-health-care-utilization families to address psychosocial concerns that may contribute to extended or frequent hospitalizations (Aoki, Sato, & Hosaka, 2004). Establishing clear discharge goals, addressing child and family psychological issues affecting health care use, arranging for focused follow-up services, and mitigat-ing barriers to adherence can contribute to more efficient and effective use of medical services (Finney, Riley, & Cataldo, 1991; Janicke & Finney, 2000).

The field of pediatric psychology has a long-standing history of developing and uti-lizing knowledge-based clinical interventions to address common behavioral health concerns (Powers, Jones, & Jones, 2005). In addition, current pediatric psychology models emphasize system-focused approaches, encouraging the assessment of multiple factors in conceptualizing, intervening, and making multidisciplinary treatment recommendations (Kazak, 2006; McDaniel & LeRoux, 2007). Pediatric CL psychologists are in contact with multiple care providers and are uniquely trained to provide systems-based conceptualizations and interventions (e.g., developing a unit-wide behavioral program to improve the adherence of adolescents with cystic fibrosis to best-practice airway clearance protocols).

The CL psychologist is often present for multiple communication events (e.g., medical service rounds, psychosocial rounds, team meetings, care conferences, etc.) and can affect collaboration through both team and family interventions, as well as by modeling helpful communication and negotiation strategies to enhance family–team partnership. Thus, both by virtue of clinical training and research contributions, pediatric psychologists working in the inpatient medical setting may have unique expertise that can enhance their institution's multisystem collaboration and family-centered care—not only in the formulation and implementation of case-based interventions, but also in facilitating institutional efforts to enhance family-centered care.

Advances in Clinical Interventions

Other exciting advances are also occurring in a number of areas that fit well within the family-centered movement and have been successful in addressing common CL referral concerns. These areas include motivational interviewing (Erickson, Gerstle, & Feldstein, 2005; Miller & Rollnick, 2002) and acceptance and commitment therapy (Gregg, Callaghan, Hayes, & Glenn-Lawson, 2007; Murrell, Coyne, Wilson, Hayes, & Strosahl, 2005). These promising interventions can be used in conjunction with, or perhaps as alternatives to, more traditional cognitive-behavioral approaches in addressing crucial pediatric CL issues such as treatment adherence.

Among the challenges of pediatric CL work can be time limitations on such challenging tasks as defining roles, establishing rapport, conducting assessment, conceptualizing treatment/formulation plans, conducting intervention, and providing or arranging for follow-up, all within two to three sessions (or less). Fortunately, there are some technologies that can enhance effectiveness under such demanding time constraints. For example, one of us has developed a mobile multimedia "Coping Cart" at Kosair Children's Hospital, which the pediatric CL psychologist can use in establishing rapport and enhancing patient adherence (Carter, Bowersox, & Kronenberger, 2008). The Coping Cart is a kid-friendly decorated cart that carries a computer, video camera, digital still camera, and printer/scanner; a biofeedback unit; medical toys and puppets/dolls; books; videos for viewing; and wireless Internet access to bookmarked child-, teen-, and family-friendly informative and interactive websites. Pediatric patients using the Coping Cart can participate in making videos of procedures, coping strategies, and the like; these videos (with appropriate signed consent) are archived into a video library used to facilitate coping, understanding, and adherence with other patients.

Improvements in biofeedback equipment that employ interactive video games or that convert physiological indices into appealing computer animation (e.g., balloons blowing across the sky, or shooting bows and arrows) make this technology much more portable and attractive to pediatric patients. Often biofeedback software programs can be utilized on laptop computers for easy transportation to hospitalized patients. Use of digital voice recording for facilitating coping or relaxation scripts can allow patients to download these resources onto MP3 players for easier, inconspicuous use. Finally, use of telehealth and other electronic means (see Palermo & Wilson, Chapter 15, this volume) can facilitate follow-up services for patients in need of care who are without local resources.

Future Directions

We pediatric psychologists are increasingly playing a role both in the provision of CL services and in developing and researching innovative evidence-based interventions to improve our patients' quality of life, along with the quality of care within the pediatric hospital setting. The many challenges of the current health care environment demand that we continue to demonstrate the value of our roles to the hospital and health care system through the provision of highly competent services, while continuing to recruit a new generation of pediatric psychologists into this exciting specialization.

References

Alpert, J. L., & Spencer, J. B. (1986). Consultation. In G. Tryon (Ed.) *The professional practice of psychology* (pp. 106–129). Norwood, NJ: Ablex.

American Medical Association. (2007). *Current Procedural Terminology: CPT 2008, Standard Edition.* Chicago: Author.

Aoki, T., Sato, T., & Hosaka, T. (2004). Role of consultation–liaison psychiatry toward shortening of length of stay for medically ill patients with depression. *International Journal of Psychiatry in Clinical Practice, 8,* 71–76.

Brown, K. J., & Roberts, M. (2000). Future issues in pediatric psychology. *Journal of Clinical Psychology in Medical Settings, 7,* 5–15.

Brown, R. T., & Macias, M. (2001). Chronically ill children and adolescents. In J. N. Hughes, A. M. La Greca, & J. C. Conoley (Eds.), *Handbook of psychological services for children and adolescents* (pp. 353–372). New York: Oxford University Press.

Carter, B. D., Bowersox, S., & Kronenberger, W. G. (2008, April). *Case studies in the utility of a mobile multimedia "Coping Cart" to facilitate coping, adjustment and adherence in hospitalized pediatric patients.* Poster presented at the National Conference on Child Health Psychology, Miami Beach, FL.

Carter, B. D., Kronenberger, W. G., Baker, J., Grimes, L. M., Crabtree, V. M., Smith, C., et al. (2003). Inpatient pediatric consultation–liaison: A case-controlled study. *Journal of Pediatric Psychology, 28,* 425–432.

Carter, B. D., & von Weiss, R. (2005). Pediatric consultation–liaison: Applied child health psychology. In R. Steele & M. Roberts (Eds.), *Handbook of mental health services for children and adolescents* (pp. 63–77). New York: Kluwer Academic/Plenum Press.

Compas, B., Malcarne, V., & Banez, G. (1992). Coping with psychological stress: A developmental perspective. In B. Carpenter (Ed.), *Personal coping: Theory, research and application* (pp. 47–64). Westport, CT: Praeger.

Drotar, D. (1976). Psychological consultation in a pediatric hospital. *Professional Psychology, 7,* 77–83.

Drotar, D. (1995). *Consulting with pediatricians: Psychological perspectives*. New York: Plenum Press.

Drotar, D., Spirito, A., & Stancin, T. (2003). Professional roles and practice patterns. In M. C. Roberts (Ed.), *Handbook of pediatric psychology* (3rd ed., pp. 50–66). New York: Guilford Press.

Drotar, D., & Zagorski, L. (2001). Providing psychological services in pediatric settings in an era of managed care. In J. N. Hughes, A. M. La Greca, & J. C. Conoley (Eds.), *Handbook of psychological services for children and adolescents* (pp. 89–104). New York: Oxford University Press.

Erickson, S. J., Gerstle, M., & Feldstein, S. W. (2005). Brief interventions and motivational interviewing with children, adolescents, and their parents in pediatric health care settings: A review. *Archives of Pediatrics and Adolescent Medicine, 159*, 1173–1180.

Finney, J. W., Riley, A. W., & Cataldo, M. F. (1991). Psychology in primary health care: Effects of brief targeted therapy on children's medical care utilization. *Journal of Pediatric Psychology, 16*, 447–461.

Fritz, G. K. (1993). Common clinical problems in pediatric consultation. In G. K. Fritz, R. E. Mattison, B. Nurcombe, & A. Spirito (Eds.), *Child and adolescent mental health consultation in hospitals, schools, and courts* (pp. 47–65). Washington, DC: American Psychiatric Press.

Gregg, J. A., Callaghan, G. M., Hayes, S. C., & Glenn-Lawson, J. L. (2007). Improving diabetes self-management through acceptance, mindfulness, and values: A randomized controlled trial. *Journal of Consulting and Clinical Psychology, 75*, 336–343.

Harbeck-Weber, C., Fisher, J. L., & Dittner, C. A. (2003). Promoting coping and enhancing adaptation to illness. In M. C. Roberts (Ed.), *Handbook of pediatric psychology* (3rd ed., pp. 99–118). New York: Guilford Press.

Harbeck-Weber, C., & Peterson, L. (1993). Children's conception of illness and pain. In R. Vasta (Ed.), *Annals of child development* (pp. 133–163). Bristol, PA: Jessica Kingsley.

Janicke, D. M., & Finney, J. W. (2000). Determinants of children's primary health care use. *Journal of Clinical Psychology in Medical Settings, 7*, 29–39.

Kazak, A., Simms, S., Barakat, L., Hobbie, W., Foley, B., Golomb, V., et al. (1999). Surviving Cancer Competently Interventions Program (SCCIP): A cognitive-behavioral and family therapy intervention for adolescent survivors of childhood cancer and their families. *Family Process, 38*, 175–192.

Kazak, A. E. (2006). Pediatric psychosocial preventative health model (PPPHM): Research, practice, and collaboration in pediatric family systems medicine. *Families, Systems and Health: The Journal of Collaborative Family HealthCare, 24*, 381–395.

Kazak, A. E., Simms, S., & Rourke, M. T. (2002). Family systems practice in pediatric psychology. *Journal of Pediatric Psychology, 27*, 133–143.

Kell, R. S., Kliewer, W., Erichson, M. T., & Ohene-Frempong, M. (1998). Psychological adjustment of adolescents with sickle cell disease: Relations with demographic, medical, and family competence variables. *Journal of Pediatric Psychology, 23*, 301–312.

Kremer, P. K. G., & Wasserman, A. L. (1994). Diagnostic dilemmas in pediatric consultation. *Child and Adolescent Psychiatric Clinics of North America, 3*, 485–512.

Kronenberger, W. G. (2004, August). *Pediatric psychiatry/psychology services at a large tertiary care children's hospital*. Poster presented at the annual conference of the American Psychological Association, Honolulu, HI.

Kronenberger, W. G., Carter, B. D., & Thomas, D. (1997). Assessment of behavior problems in pediatric inpatient settings: Development of the Pediatric Inpatient Behavior Scale (PIBS). *Children's Health Care, 26*, 211–232.

La Greca, A. M., & Bearman, K. J. (2003). Adherence to pediatric treatment regimens. In M.

C. Roberts (Ed.), *Handbook of pediatric psychology* (3rd ed., pp. 99–118). New York: Guilford Press.

Lewandowski, L. A., & Baranoski, M. V. (1994). Psychological aspects of acute trauma. *Child and Adolescent Psychiatric Clinics of North America, 3,* 513–529.

McDaniel, S. H., Hepworth, J., & Doherty, W. (1992). *Medical family therapy: A biopsychosocial approach to families with health problems.* New York: Basic Books.

McDaniel, S. H., & LeRoux, P. (2007). An overview of primary care family psychology. *Journal of Clinical Psychology in Medical Settings, 14,* 23–32.

Miller, W. R., & Rollnick, S. (2002). *Motivational interviewing: Preparing people for change* (2nd ed.). New York: Guilford Press.

Mullins, L. D., Gillman, J., & Harbeck, C. (1992). Multiple-level interventions in pediatric psychology settings: A behavioral systems perspective. In A. M. La Greca, L. J. Siegel, J. L. Wallander, & C. E. Walker (Eds.), *Stress and coping in child health* (pp. 371–399). New York: Guilford Press.

Murrell, A. R., Coyne, L. W., Wilson, K. G., Hayes, S. C., & Strosahl, K. D. (2005). ACT with children, adolescents, and their parents. In S. C. Hayes & K. Strosahl (Eds.), *A practical guide to acceptance and commitment therapy* (pp. 249–273). New York: Springer Science + Business Media.

Noll, R. B., & Fischer, S. (2004). Commentary: Health and behavior CPT codes: An opportunity to revolutionize reimbursement in pediatric psychology. *Journal of Pediatric Psychology, 29,* 571–578.

Olson, R. A., Holden, E. W., Friedman, A., Faust, J., Kenning, M., & Mason, P. J. (1988). Psychological consultation in a children's hospital: An evaluation of services. *Journal of Pediatric Psychology, 13,* 479–492.

Olson, R. A., Mullins, L., Chaney, J. M., & Gillman, J. B. (1993). The role of the pediatric psychologist in a consultation–liaison service; In R. A. Olson, L. L. Mullins, J. B. Gillman, & J. M. Chaney (Eds.), *The sourcebook of pediatric psychology* (pp. 1–8). Boston: Allyn & Bacon.

Pollin, I. (1994). *Taking charge: Overcoming the challenges of long-term illness.* New York: Times Books.

Pollin, I. (1995). *Medical crisis counseling: Short-term therapy for long-term illness.* New York: Norton.

Powers, S. W., Jones, J. S., & Jones, B. A. (2005). Behavioral and cognitive-behavioral interventions with pediatric populations. *Clinical Child Psychology and Psychiatry, 10,* 65–77.

Rapoff, M. A. (1999). *Adherence to pediatric medical regimens.* New York: Kluwer Academic.

Rodrigue, J., Hoffmann, R. G., Rayfield, A., Lescano, C., Kubar, W., Streisand, R., et al. (1995). Evaluating pediatric psychology consultation services in a medical setting: An example. *Journal of Clinical Psychology in Medical Settings, 2,* 89–107.

Rothbaum, F., Weisz, J. R., & Snyder, S. S. (1982). Changing the world and changing the self: A two-process model of perceived control. *Journal of Personality and Social Psychology, 42,* 5–37.

Sanders, M., Shepherd, R., Cleghorn, G., & Woolford, H. (1994). The treatment of recurrent abdominal pain in children: A controlled comparison of cognitive-behavioral family interventions and standard pediatric care. *Journal of Consulting and Clinical Psychology, 62,* 306–314.

Shaw, R. J., & DeMaso, D. R. (2006). *Clinical manual of pediatric psychosomatic medicine: Mental health consultation with physically ill children and adolescents.* Washington, DC: American Psychiatric Publishing.

Shaw, R. J., Wamboldt, M., Bursch, B., & Stuber, M. (2006). Practice patterns in pediatric consultation–liaison: A national survey. *Psychosomatics, 47,* 43–49.

Spirito, A., & Kazak, A. (2006). *Effective and emerging treatments in pediatric psychology.* New York: Oxford University Press.

Steiner, H., Sanders, M., Canning, E. H., & Litt, I. (1994). A model for managing clinical and personnel issues in C-L psychiatry. *Psychosomatics, 35,* 73–79.

Strain, J. S. (2002). Consultation psychiatry. In M. G. Wise & J. R. Rundell (Eds.), *The American Psychiatric Publishing textbook of consultation–liaison psychiatry: Psychiatry in the medically ill* (pp. 123–150). Washington, DC: American Psychiatric Publishing.

Thompson, R. J., & Gustafson, K. (1996). *Adaptation to chronic childhood illness.* Washington, DC: American Psychological Association.

Wallander, J., & Thompson, R. J. (1995). Psychosocial adjustment of children with chronic physical conditions. In M. C. Roberts (Ed.), *Handbook of pediatric psychology* (2nd ed., pp. 124–141). New York: Guilford Press.

Wallander, J., Varni, J., Babani, L., Banis, H., & Wilcox, K. (1989). Family resources as resistant factors for psychological maladjustment in chronically ill and handicapped children. *Journal of Pediatric Psychology, 14,* 23–42.

Wysocki, T., Harris, M., Greco, P., Bubb, J., Danda, C., Harvey, L., et al. (2000). Randomized controlled trial of behavioral therapy for families of adolescents with insulin-dependent diabetes mellitus. *Journal of Pediatric Psychology, 25,* 23–33.

CHAPTER 9

Adherence to Pediatric Treatment Regimens

ANNETTE M. LA GRECA
ELEANOR RACE MACKEY

Adherence to pediatric treatment regimens is a major public health concern. Estimates suggest that the overall treatment adherence rate is about 50% for pediatric populations (Rapoff, 1999), although rates of nonadherence have been reported to be over 90% for dietary aspects of regimens for youths with HIV infection (Marhefka, Tepper, Farley, Sleasman, & Mellins, 2006), or for regular use of inhaled steroids for low-income youths with asthma (Piecoro, Potoski, Talbert, & Doherty, 2001). Furthermore, pediatric nonadherence contributes to high rates of health care utilization (e.g., Piecoro et al., 2001), and to preventable morbidity and mortality (Bauman et al., 2002; DiMatteo, 2004; Shemesh et al., 2004). In fact, the annual U.S. health care costs resulting from nonadherence may be as high as $300 billion (DiMatteo, 2004).

Furthermore, it is likely that pediatric adherence will continue to be a major health concern in the foreseeable future, as newer, more complex treatments are developed. For example, because of life-saving antiretroviral therapy for pediatric HIV infection, this disease is now considered a chronic condition. However, antiretroviral therapy requires an intensive and complicated medication regimen, coupled with dietary restrictions and potential drug side effects (Steele & Grauer, 2003). Thus medical advances bring new challenges for youngsters' adherence.

Not surprisingly, pediatric adherence is also a complex issue, and both children and families must be viewed as active participants in the medical decision-making process. Although adherence is essential for disease management, it does not always guarantee symptom relief or illness recovery (DiMatteo, Giordani, Lepper, & Croghan, 2002; Steele & Grauer, 2003). Thus families must decide how to balance children's health care needs with efforts to achieve a "normal life."

The present chapter provides an overview of pediatric adherence and is divided into three major sections. The first focuses on issues of definition and measurement; the second focuses on the multiple factors associated with adherence; and the third section reviews interventions to improve pediatric treatment adherence.

Definition and Measurement Issues

Definitions of Adherence

Investigators have used widely divergent definitions of "adherence," even among those examining the same illness or regimen, Typically, adherence refers to "the extent to which a person's behavior ... coincides with medical or health advice" (Haynes, 1979, pp. 2–3). This statement implies that the individual's behaviors can be compared against some defined criteria. However, most measures of adherence do not measure a person's behavior *in relation to a prescribed medical regimen* (La Greca, 1990); in fact, different treatment regimens may be prescribed for individuals with the same disease. To deal with this issue, some investigators examine adherence in relation to an ideal regimen (e.g., Johnson, Silverstein, Rosenbloom, Carter, & Cunningham, 1986). Others measure the frequency of health behaviors without comparisons to standards or prescriptions (Davis et al., 2001), and use the term "self-care behaviors" instead of "adherence."

Operational definitions of adherence have varied. Initially, many investigators used a categorical approach, specifying criteria or cutoff scores for successful adherence, and then using the criteria to define groups of "adherent" and "nonadherent" patients (e.g., Phipps & DeCuir-Whalley, 1990). Although this approach continues to be used (e.g., Carter & Ananthakrishnan, 2003), it has limitations. One concern with the categorical approach is the arbitrary nature of the cutoff criteria, as it is not known what constitutes an adequate level of adherence for most medical problems. As a further drawback, the nonstandard use of cutoff scores makes it difficult to compare adherence levels across studies, across different aspects of a regimen, or across different diseases (La Greca, 1990). Studies that examine the sensitivity and specificity of adherence cutoff scores might enhance the utility of the categorical approach to adherence, but until such data are collected, it may be more practical to view adherence on a continuum (Quittner, Modi, Lemanek, Ievers-Landis, & Rapoff, 2008; Steele & Grauer, 2003).

Recent approaches to adherence also consider the multiple aspects involved in a given treatment regimen, rather than viewing adherence as a unitary construct. For example, some investigators compute adherence rates by dividing the number of adherence behaviors completed by the number prescribed, and doing this for multiple tasks (see Rapoff, 1999). Others use interviews or self-reports to obtain indices of adherence for multiple aspects of a treatment regimen (e.g., Harris et al., 2000). Combinations of approaches (e.g., percentages of adherence behaviors completed and self-reports) have also been used to evaluate adherence for multicomponent regimens (Quittner et al., 2008; Steele & Grauer, 2003). Such approaches avoid the use of arbitrary cutoff scores and allow a comparison of adherence levels across different behaviors, studies, and conditions, although they may not address the *relative importance* of some adherence behaviors compared to others.

Methods for Measuring Adherence

Perhaps the most difficult question confronting pediatric researchers is how to measure adherence (La Greca, 1990). Most methods overestimate adherence. In fact, it is often difficult to obtain *any* assessment of adherence from the most nonadherent youngsters, as they may not comply with the requirements of the assessment method (e.g., completing written logs).

Several considerations are important in selecting a measure. First, measures that are appropriate for short-term regimens (e.g., drug assays) may not be practical or appropriate for chronic diseases with complex regimens. Second, regimens that involve multiple, complex behaviors may need a variety of strategies for comprehensive assessment, keeping in mind that adherence to one aspect of a regimen does not imply adherence to others. Third, many measures focus on self-care behaviors without regard for how well the behaviors match the prescribed treatment. In such cases, efforts to assess the prescribed regimen from the patients' and providers' perspectives may be useful to determine the extent to which patients' behaviors correspond to medical recommendations. What appears to be nonadherent behavior may instead be a patient's inaccurate knowledge of the regimen, or a health care provider's inexact specification of the desired health care behaviors. Finally, it is important to recognize that adherence behaviors and *health outcomes* are not synonymous, and may only be moderately related. For example, Johnson (1994) found that more than a third of the youngsters with "good" adherence to a diabetes regimen's requirements for testing/eating frequency had poor disease control, and that about a third of those with "poor" adherence had good disease control. Studies that include separate measures of adherence and health outcomes may be the most informative, and may help to detect ineffective regimens.

Drug Assays

Assays are among the most direct, objective, reliable, and easily quantifiable methods for assessing adherence to medication regimens. Assays involve obtaining blood, urine, or saliva samples to determine the presence or concentration of a drug that has been prescribed.

Drug assays may be best for evaluating adherence to short-term medication regimens, although they may also be useful for long-term regimens when repeated measurements have been obtained (e.g., Shemesh et al., 2004). Unfortunately, many regimens cannot be monitored by an assay, and even when assays are feasible, they often assess adherence over short time periods and may not represent adherence over longer intervals. Pharmacokinetic variations, or individual variability in rates of drug absorption, metabolism, distribution, and excretion within the body, can affect the efficacy of a drug and thus also influence drugs assay results (Lemanek, 1990).

Self-Reports, Structured Interviews, and Diaries

Child, adolescent, and/or parent reports are often used for assessing adherence, as they are easy and inexpensive to obtain and can assess a complex array of behaviors (e.g., amount and timing of medications, frequency and duration of exercise). Self-reports have been widely used for evaluating adherence to complex regimens (La Greca & Bearman, 2003; Rapoff, 1999). According to a recent analysis of psychometric support for measures of pediatric adherence (Quittner et al., 2008), well-established self-report and structured interview measures include the Self-Care Inventory (for diabetes; La Greca, Swales, Klemp, & Madigan, 1988; Lewin et al., in press), the Diabetes Regimen Adherence Scale (Brownlee-Duffeck et al., 1987), and the Disease Management Interview—Cystic Fibrosis (Quittner et al., 2000). (See Quittner et al., 2008, for a list of promising and "nearly established" adherence measures.)

Self-reports are more accurate when recall periods are brief and when answers to detailed objective questions, rather than subjective judgments, are requested (Quittner et al., 2008). Thus having children or parents rate their overall adherence since the last office visit may be less accurate than requesting specific information on a variety of regimen behaviors (e.g., number of times blood testing is completed).

Furthermore, patients' recall over the previous 24 hours will be more accurate than for extended, retrospective time periods. For this reason, investigators have developed "cued-recall" diary measures to evaluate adherence behaviors over a 24-hour period (e.g., Freund, Johnson, Silverstein, & Thomas, 1991; Modi & Quittner, 2006b). Typically, children and parents are interviewed separately regarding management tasks; two to three assessments may be averaged to estimate adherence over an extended time period. Evidence suggests that the 24-hour recall method for diabetes (Freund et al., 1991) and the Daily Phone Diary for chronic illnesses (Modi & Quittner, 2006b) have well-established psychometric support (Quittner et al., 2008). The main drawback to these procedures is the labor-intensive nature of data collection and scoring.

Technological advances may lead to even greater sophistication in diary methods for assessing adherence. For example, ecological momentary assessment (EMA; Stone & Shiffman, 1994) allows youths to report their adherence behaviors in real time, via personal digital assistants (PDAs). Dunton, Whalen, Jamner, and Floro (2007) utilized EMA in a study of youths' physical activity by programming PDAs for each adolescent's specific sleep and wake time. The PDAs prompted a diary entry with an auditory signal every 30 (± 10) minutes, for up to 25–30 entries per day, so that adolescents could enter their current activity, social company, and location. EMA may thus provide a more accurate view of adherence behaviors than other diary methods.

In general, self-reports have been useful for evaluating adherence, as those who admit problems have been found to be nonadherent by other methods (Quittner et al., 2008). However, self-reports overestimate adherence and also are influenced by social desirability (Rapoff, 1999).

Ratings by Health Care Professionals

Ratings by health care providers have been used to assess adherence (e.g., DiMatteo, 2004; Witherspoon & Drotar, 2006), although they are subject to the same limitations as self-reports. In addition, health care providers' ratings may be influenced by patients' prior nonadherence, problems with disease control, or poor cooperation with medical staff (La Greca, 1990). Finney, Hook, Friman, Rapoff, and Christophersen (1993) also found that health care providers greatly overestimated parents' adherence. On the positive side, health care providers see a wide range of patients and may be able to detect extremes in adherence.

Pill Counts

Although pill counts have been widely used to assess adherence to medication regimens (DiMatteo, 2004), they have been supplanted by the use of electronic monitoring devices (see section below) (Quittner et al., 2008). Pill counts compare the amount of medication remaining in a container with the amount that would be left if the person consumed all that was prescribed. Pharmacy refill records have also been used to determine the extent to which patients adhere to medication prescriptions (see Quittner et al., 2008; Steele & Grauer, 2003). However, pill counts and pharmacy refill records overestimate adherence, as youngsters may remove the pills or refill a prescription but may not ingest the medication. These measures also cannot track other related behaviors, such as the timing or amount of medication ingested.

Electronic Monitoring Devices

Technological advances have improved the quality of data that can be obtained from daily monitoring activities or pill counts. For example, glucose reflectance meters for evaluating daily blood samples in youngsters with diabetes can be equipped with memory chips to record the date, time, and results of glucose testing (Wilson & Endres, 1986). Devices have also been developed for pill bottle openings, such as the Medication Event Monitor System, which embeds a microprocessor in a standard medication vial cap to record the date and time of vial openings and closings (Cramer, 1995). In addition, electronic monitors for metered-dose inhalers (used to evaluate adherence to asthma medications) appear to provide more accurate estimates of adherence than parent or child reports or diaries (Quitter et al., 2008). At the same time, a primary drawback to such electronic devices is their cost. Other drawbacks include that a medication may not have been taken even though pill removal was recorded (or the inhaler was activated), and that the devices sometimes malfunction, leading to missing data and inexact estimates of adherence (Quittner et al., 2008).

Factors That Affect Adherence

Multiple factors can affect adherence. This section briefly reviews four major areas related to pediatric adherence: (1) developmental issues, (2) characteristics of the child and family, (3) characteristics of the health care system, and (4) characteristics of the disease or regimen. The issues raised in this section are important, as they may be used to inform interventions for pediatric adherence or may suggest risk factors to help identify problematic adherence.

Developmental Issues

Developmental status (often indexed by age) refers to the youngsters' level of cognitive, motor, social, emotional, and physiological functioning, all of which may affect the course and management of disease. For example, children's developmental status may affect their reactions to physical illness, their degree of involvement in disease management, and the types of interventions that may be most effective (see La Greca & Bearman, 2003, for more details).

In general, pediatric adherence rates are lower than those for adults (e.g., DiMatteo, 2004), and adolescents have been found to be less adherent with medical treatments than children (La Greca & Bearman, 2003; Rapoff, 1999). There are some exceptions, however, as adolescents may be more adherent than younger children with invasive treatments, such as bone marrow aspiration (Phipps & DeCuir-Whalley, 1990). Multiple factors may contribute to these age-related differences, such as age-related shifts in a child's responsibility for disease management, increasing pressures from peers to be accepted and "fit in," and biological changes associated with development; these issues are discussed below. Children's cognitive maturity also may play a role in their understanding of the disease (see La Greca & Bearman, 2003).

Responsibility

Responsibility for disease management varies as a function of youngsters' age and developmental level. Parents (especially mothers) often assume responsibility for implementing medical regimens for young children and preadolescents (De Civita & Dobkin, 2004). However, a gradual shift in responsibility occurs over the course of development, and this may vary by the type of regimen task (La Greca, 1998; Shemesh et al., 2004). For example, adolescents may have primary responsibility for taking medication, whereas parental involvement may remain high for dietary management tasks (La Greca, 1998; La Greca, Follansbee, & Skyler, 1990). To understand adherence, one needs to know *who* assumes responsibility for the various and diverse aspects of the treatment regimen, and *how* that responsibility is shared within the family. Greater family involvement and shared responsibility have been associated with better adherence for youths with diabetes (Helgeson, Reynolds, Siminerio, Escobar, & Becker, 2008) and HIV (Martin et al., 2007; Naar-King et al., 2008).

Social-Emotional Development

Children's social-emotional development is an important consideration. Children progress from a state of dependent, close attachment to parents during early childhood, to an expanding awareness of and desire for friendships and peer contacts during the elementary school years, and later to a preoccupation with peer acceptance and personal independence during adolescence (La Greca & Prinstein, 1999). These varying social-emotional needs (autonomy, affiliation) can affect adherence. For example, some adolescents neglect their medical care in order to avoid appearing different from peers, particularly if the treatment produces undesirable cosmetic side effects (e.g., Schroder, Crabtree, & Lyall-Watson, 2002; Simons & Blount, 2007). Thus efforts to improve adolescents' adherence might address ways to cope with peer pressure and social demands.

Physical Development

Physical development also influences disease management. Some chronic diseases, like diabetes or asthma, are more difficult to control during periods of rapid growth and metabolic fluctuation, such as puberty (e.g., Bloch, Clemons, & Sperling, 1987). Puberty also changes the distribution of body fat and muscle mass, which can affect drug absorption rates (Brooks-Gunn & Graber, 1994). These biological factors are important to consider, because if the prescribed regimen is ineffective, adolescents may disengage entirely from self-care efforts.

Child and Family Characteristics

Demographic variables, such as race, gender, religion, and maternal educational level, have not been consistent predictors of adherence in pediatric populations (Lemanek, 1990). However, evidence suggests that children and adolescents of lower socioeconomic status, from minority backgrounds, and from single-parent families may be less adherent to complex, chronic disease regimens (e.g., Berquist et al., 2006; Jacobson et al., 1997; La Greca & Bearman, 2003).

Knowledge and Skills

Children's and families' disease knowledge and skills for managing the disease are critical for adherence. Active knowledge goes beyond understanding the illness process; it includes an accurate understanding of the tasks that are involved in treatment management, and the ability to execute such tasks/skills accurately and to make adjustments when problems arise. Disease knowledge and skills are essential for complex disease regimens.

For very young children, *parents'* disease knowledge and skills are important because of their active involvement in the treatment regimen. For instance, among infants and very young children with sickle cell disease, Witherspoon and Drotar (2006) found that parents' knowledge of the risk of infection was positively related to their children's treatment adherence. In contrast, *children's* disease knowledge and skills are critical when they are responsible for disease management, as may be the case with children's use of inhalers for asthma treatment (e.g., Boccuti, Celano, Geller, & Phillips, 1996). Many of the intervention programs described in this chapter include educational components, although it is important to keep in mind that knowledge alone may be insufficient to promote adequate levels of adherence.

Psychosocial Adjustment

Most pediatric problems affect heterogeneous groups of youngsters, with varied levels of coping and adjustment. Because of this, studies have examined linkages between youngsters' emotional functioning and their treatment adherence. A common assumption is that youngsters' psychosocial functioning influences their disease management.

In general, positive psychosocial adaptation has been associated with good treatment adherence, particularly for youths with chronic disease (Brownbridge & Fielding, 1994; Jacobson et al., 1990). However, youths with serious emotional difficulties, such as depression, often have problems with adherence (Kovacs, Goldston, Obrosky, & Iyengar, 1992) or disease control (DeMore, Adams, Wilson, & Hogan, 2005; La Greca, Swales, Klemp, Madigan, & Skyler, 1995). Thus health care providers might consider screening youths for depressed mood or other emotional problems that could interfere with treatment adherence.

Family Support, Communication, and Conflict

Family members represent a primary source of instrumental and emotional support for children and adolescents (Cauce, Reid, Landesman, & Gonzales, 1990), and thus play a critical role in treatment management. For example, families who provide more support for diabetes care activities have adolescents who are more adherent with their treatment regimen (La Greca & Bearman, 2002). Similar findings have been obtained for youths with cystic fibrosis (Delambo, Ievers-Landis, Drotar, & Quittner, 2004). In fact, one of the challenges facing parents of adolescents is finding ways that they can remain supportive and involved in treatment, while also encouraging adolescents to take greater self-responsibility for health care (La Greca, 1998; La Greca, Auslander, et al., 1995).

Family communication, especially in regard to issues of disease management, is also related to treatment adherence (La Greca & Bearman, 2003; Rapoff, 1999). Several interventions discussed later in this chapter include strategies for enhancing family communication.

Although family support and communication are beneficial, problems with adherence are almost certain to emerge when there is family conflict. Numerous studies have found that family conflict is inversely related to youngsters' adherence (e.g., Lewandowski & Drotar, 2007). In addition, managing pediatric conditions can also contribute to family stress, as treatments may disrupt the family's routine and lifestyle (La Greca, 1998). For example, regimens requiring dietary modifications (e.g., for hypertension, phenylketonuria [PKU], diabetes, or obesity) can alter family eating habits. Other medical protocols may require frequent hospital-based treatments, as is the case for renal dialysis or chemotherapy, or unexpected emergency room visits, as can occur with asthma, sickle cell disease, or seizure disorders. Such treatments can seriously interfere with the parents' or family's daily routine, and represent barriers to successful treatment adherence. In turn, parental or family stress can adversely influence youngsters' adherence (La Greca, 1998).

Biological Functioning

Although it is an understudied factor, individual variability in physiological functioning and in responsiveness to medical interventions is also important for adherence. For example, the therapeutic dose for chemotherapy is determined by its *typical* effect; yet there is marked variability in the frequency and magnitude of aversive side effects, such as nausea and vomiting (Barofsky, 1984). Children and adolescents who have a suboptimal response to medical treatment may be at risk for problems with adherence.

Child and Family Barriers to Adherence

In addition to the issues described above, children and families vary in their reports of barriers to treatment adherence. For instance, child or parent forgetfulness has been found to be a significant barrier to adherence for many children with cystic fibrosis, asthma, and sickle cell disease (Modi & Quittner, 2006a; Witherspoon & Drotar, 2006). Other barriers include difficulties with time management (Modi & Quittner, 2006a), running out of medication (Witherspoon & Drotar, 2006), and child oppositional behaviors (Modi & Quittner, 2006a). In addition, some youths or families may *choose* nonadherence (this is also known as "volitional nonadherence" or "adaptive nonadherence"; see La Greca & Bearman, 2003), because they feel that a regimen task is unnecessary or that the treatment plan is undesirable. Cultural and religious beliefs may also contribute to volitional nonadherence and should be considered in any evaluation of barriers to adherence (Spirito & Kazak, 2006).

The Health Care System

Little attention has been devoted to the influence of the health care system on youngsters' treatment adherence. Yet, with major changes in health care delivery, it is critical to understand how the health care system may affect children's and families' participation in treatment.

Personal and Contextual Aspects

Aspects of the physician–patient relationship have been associated with adherence. Specifically, parents and adolescents are more likely to adhere to medical recommendations when they are satisfied with the medical care provided (e.g., Naar-King, Podolski, Ellis, Frey, & Templin, 2006). Also important for adherence are doctor–patient rapport and perceptions of the medical provider as friendly, warm, and empathic (De Civita & Dobkin, 2004); support and encouragement from health care providers (Kyngas, 2007; Schroder et al., 2002); and continued contact with the same physician (Litt & Cuskey, 1980).

Unfortunately, a health care system that emphasizes cost containment makes it difficult for health professionals to provide personal care. One consequence of cost containment has been reduced time available for direct patient contact (Walders, Nobile, & Drotar, 2000), which can result in communication problems and poor quality of care (Emanuel & Dubler, 1995).

Other aspects of the medical setting also affect adherence, such as the convenience of medical care (e.g., closeness to home, accessible location, short waiting-room time) (Hazzard, Hutchinson, & Krawiecki, 1990). Providing transportation and child care may also enhance families' participation in their youngsters' treatment (Saylor, Elksnin, Farah, & Pope, 1990).

Health Care Communication

Effective health care communication is essential for developing a successful treatment plan and for facilitating adherence (see Levetown & Committee on Bioethics, 2008). In many cases, medical advice may be inconsistent or unclear, especially with complex regimens (Freund et al., 1991). One index of effective communication is the parents' or patients' ability to recall the specifics of the regimen (Ievers-Landis & Drotar, 2000). In this regard, De Civita and colleagues (2007) found that parents of youths (average age 10 years) with juvenile arthritis were less able to recall health care providers' recommendations for exercise than for medications. Poor recall may contribute to inadvertent nonadherence.

Disease and Regimen Considerations

Chronicity

Pediatric conditions vary on a continuum from acute, short-term problems to chronic conditions involving lifelong management. Even with acute conditions, adherence rates for medication fall off dramatically over time (see Rapoff, 1999). However, adherence difficulties abound with long-term regimens. Youngsters with diabetes (Naar-King et al., 2006), renal disease (Brownbridge & Fielding, 1994), and orthodontic problems (Albino, Lawrence, Lopes, Nash, & Tedesco, 1991), all display significant declines in adherence over the course of treatment. Such findings suggest that it is unrealistic to expect *consistently* good adherence with a chronic disease regimen, especially without strong incentives for health care behaviors. Health care providers might focus on supporting adherence before problems arise, and providing encouragement when inevitable difficulties occur.

Complexity

Multifaceted or intrusive regimens—ones that require dietary changes, blood monitoring, or physical therapy, for example—have poorer rates of adherence than medication regimens (Lemanek, Kamps, & Chung, 2001; Quittner, Espelage, Ievers-Landis, & Drotar, 2000). Treatments for HIV are especially challenging, as they require multidrug regimens and the medications have varied side effects (Johnson, 2000); yet failure to comply can result in new drug-resistant strains, producing individual and society-wide threats (Wainberg & Friedland, 1998). Regimens that involve activity limitations or lifestyle changes are also challenging. For instance, youths with diabetes have higher rates of adherence for insulin injections than for the eating- and exercise-related aspects of their regimen (La Greca et al., 1990; Quittner et al., 2000).

Consequences of Adherence

Fewer problems are observed when adherence brings immediate, positive results, as in the case of pain relief or symptom reduction (e.g., Arnhold et al., 1970). In contrast, regimens that provide no immediate consequences for adherence, are of uncertain efficacy, or have aversive side effects are often problematic (Blowey et al., 1997; Roberts, 2005).

For asymptomatic diseases, the benefits of adherence are often associated with *future* outcomes. For example, with Type 1 diabetes, efforts to achieve good metabolic control can prevent or forestall serious disease complications such as retinopathy (Diabetes Control and Complications Trial Research Group, 1994), although good control does not *guarantee* future good health. These future-oriented, preventive goals are often insufficient motivators for daily adherence behaviors, and are outweighed by the immediate and ongoing efforts needed to comply. In fact, adherence to preventive health regimens is also poor (e.g., Teach, Lillis, & Grossi, 1998). Regimens with few or no immediate positive consequences for adherence may require the use of motivational strategies (e.g., incentives, motivational interviewing) to promote adequate levels of adherence.

Models of Medical Adherence

Although studies have identified numerous correlates of adherence in pediatric populations, they have not always considered the multiple factors that influence youngsters' health behaviors. Multivariate conceptualizations of health care behaviors are critical for future advances in the field (see also La Greca & Bearman, 2003, and Rapoff, 1999, for more details).

Health Belief Model

The health belief model (HBM; Becker, Maiman, Kirscht, Haefner, & Drachman, 1977) focuses on the individual's perceptions of susceptibility to illness or illness complications; severity or seriousness of the disease or its complications; and the benefits of prescribed health care actions. Perceived barriers to health care (e.g., financial cost, risk, limitations on activities) serve as negative predictors of adherence. In theory, adherent individuals are those who perceive that they are vulnerable to an illness (or its complications), view the illness as serious, believe that the regimen will produce positive results, and are not hindered by treatment obstacles.

Tests of the HBM among youths with HIV (Steele et al., 2001), asthma (DePaola, Roberts, Blaiss, Frick, & McNeal, 1997), or obesity (Becker et al., 1977) have obtained mixed results. Consistent with the HBM, higher perceived barriers to treatment have been linked with poorer adherence (e.g., Bond, Aiken, & Somerville, 1992). However, perceived threat (susceptibility, disease severity) has been associated with poorer adherence (Bond et al., 1992). Studies of minority children have found limited support for the HBM with regard to regimen adherence for Type 1 diabetes (Patino, Sanchez, Eidson, & Delamater, 2005) and HIV (Steele et al., 2001). Such findings indicate the need for further refinement of the HBM for chronic pediatric conditions.

Transtheoretical Model of Change

Prochaska, DiClemente, and Norcross (1992) developed the transtheoretical model (TTM) of behavior change to identify the best fit between an individual's characteristics and health care interventions. The TTM postulates five stages of change: precontemplation (not thinking about making changes), contemplation (considering change in the future), preparation (considering change in the immediate future), action (changing behavior), and maintenance (continued change over time). Progression through the stages is not linear; individuals may relapse and recycle back through previous stages (Ruggiero & Prochaska, 1993). This model also suggests that individuals may be at different stages for different health care tasks.

An important feature of the TTM is that it matches different stages in the model with different types of intervention strategies. For example, an adolescent with diabetes who has not been monitoring blood glucose (BG) levels, but has good future intentions (i.e., is in the contemplation stage), might respond well to efforts from health care professionals that emphasize the benefits of such monitoring. Not until the action stage, however, will this adolescent be ready for intensive interventions to improve BG monitoring. In contrast, youngsters with good BG-monitoring skills (i.e., maintenance stage) may need support for monitoring activities to prevent relapse. The TTM also may identify individuals who are likely to drop out of interventions. Individuals in the precontemplation or contemplation stages, for example, are not likely to follow through with interventions to improve adherence behaviors. Preliminary work on the prevention of adolescent obesity (Mauriello et al., 2006) is promising, although the TTM awaits confirmation with other pediatric conditions.

Interventions for Pediatric Adherence

Given the challenges of adhering to medical regimens, interventions to improve treatment adherence are an important area of interest for researchers and practitioners. This section contains a brief overview of strategies for facilitating treatment adherence, including educational, behavioral, psychosocial, and multicomponent approaches. These intervention approaches build on the known correlates of adherence behaviors (as discussed earlier), such as enhancing knowledge and skills for disease management, increasing social support, reducing family conflict, and so on. (For additional details on adherence interventions, see Kahana, Drotar, & Frazier, 2008; La Greca & Bearman, 2003; Rapoff, 1999; Suarez & Mullins, 2008.)

Educational Interventions

Educational approaches that teach children and their families about the nature of the disease and the basic skills involved in disease management are important at the time of initial diagnosis, and also when adolescents begin to assume increased responsibility for their own regimen (La Greca & Bearman, 2003). At these time points, it is essential that youths and families have the necessary knowledge and skills to implement the regimen effectively. Supporting educational interventions, a recent review and meta-analysis of educational interventions for asthma self-management concluded that educational programs were associated with improved lung function, reduced school absenteeism, fewer days of restricted activity, and fewer visits to the emergency department (Guevara, Wolf, Grum, & Clark, 2003).

Nevertheless, it seems unrealistic to expect that education alone will be sufficient to ensure adherence to complex, chronic regimens. For example, Butz and colleagues (2006) found that a home-based asthma education program had no effect on nebulizer use or asthma morbidity. As another example, Singh, Kable, Guerrero, Sullivan, and Elsas (2000) found that an educational intervention for youths with PKU resulted in initial improvement in adherence to dietary recommendations, but this effect was not maintained at 1 year postintervention. Such findings are consistent with a recent meta-analysis of adherence interventions for chronic pediatric conditions (Kahana et al., 2008), which found a small effect size (mean $d = 0.16$) for educational interventions. Overall, it appears that education may be a necessary, but not a sufficient, condition for good treatment adherence.

Behavioral Interventions

Behavioral interventions address the antecedents of adherence behaviors, such as supervision or reminders, or the consequences of adherence, such as incentives. Behavioral interventions are discussed below.

Supervision and Reminders/Cues

Medical supervision may take the form of frequent medical visits, phone calls to discuss treatment, or monitoring of medications through assays of drug levels. Reminders (such as calendars, postcards, and phone calls) or visual cues (such as signs on the refrigerator or bathroom mirror) may prompt the performance of regimen tasks. For example, reminders, such as labels on inhalers, have been found to improve inhaler technique and asthma outcomes in youths (Basheti, Armour, Bosnic-Antichevich, & Reddel, 2008). In addition, Puccio and colleagues (2006) found that brief daily phone contacts via cell phone improved adherence to medication regimens among adolescents and young adults with HIV/AIDS over the course of 12 weeks, although that time frame was insufficient to ensure long-term change. Although reminders may help over short intervals, they appear to be insufficient to improve adherence over long periods and may be best utilized as part of broader multicomponent programs (e.g., Burkhart, Dunbar-Jacob, Fireman, & Rohay, 2002).

Self-Monitoring

Self-monitoring of disease symptoms or adherence behaviors may be useful for acute illnesses with short-term medication regimens (see La Greca & Bearman, 2003). For complex regimens, self-monitoring interventions have not been promising. Wysocki, Green, and Huxtable (1989) found that self-monitoring alone was *not* an effective intervention strategy for improving BG testing among adolescents with Type 1 diabetes, although self-monitoring was more effective when paired with monetary incentives for BG testing.

Incentives/Reinforcement

Incentives have been useful for enhancing adherence to medication regimens (Rapoff, 1999), and for improving patient follow-up after acute episodes of illness (Smith et al., 2004). Incentives have also been used to improve appointment keeping (e.g., Finney, Lemanek, Brophy, & Cataldo, 1990) and BG testing for youths with diabetes (Wysocki et al., 1989), although in some cases improvements only lasted as long as the reinforcement was available. Incentives may be useful as part of a multicomponent approach to improving adherence, but are not likely to be useful alone.

Family and Peer Interventions (Enhancing Support and Communication; Reducing Conflict)

Below we review adherence interventions that focus on enhancing social support and communication, reducing family conflict, and/or increasing skills that are important for disease management (see La Greca & Bearman, 2003, for additional studies). Kahana and colleagues (2008) considered some of the interventions described below as "behavioral," finding medium effect sizes (mean $d = 0.54$) for such interventions. It is important to note that the interventions described below focus on family or peer issues that pertain to disease management and not to efforts to improve psychosocial functioning more generally, which are less effective (Kahana et al., 2008).

Family Interventions

Family interventions for chronic disease conditions may have beneficial effects on youngsters' adherence and/or disease control. In an early study, Satin, La Greca, Zigo, and Skyler (1989) examined the effects of a 6-week multifamily intervention for adolescents with Type 1 diabetes. Multifamily sessions stressed communication about diabetes-specific situations, problem-solving strategies for diabetes management, and family support for self-care. Adolescents who participated in the multifamily groups demonstrated significant improvements in self-care and metabolic control at 6 months posttreatment, relative to control youngsters.

As another example, Anderson, Ho, Brackett, and Caffel (1999) conducted a randomized clinical trial to improve parental involvement in youngsters' (ages 10–15 years) diabetes care, aimed at maintaining family involvement and improving glycemic control. Youths were randomly assigned to a "teamwork" condition, attention control, or standard care. "Teamwork" was integrated into routine medical visits over 12 months. The teamwork approach kept parents involved in their children's diabetes care, reduced family conflict, and improved the youngsters' glycemic control.

Recently, Wysocki and colleagues (2006, 2008) conducted randomized controlled trials of behavioral family systems therapy (BFST) with families of adolescents with diabetes. BFST targets "family communication and problem-solving, extreme beliefs of parents and adolescents that impede communication, and systemic barriers to problem solving" (Wysocki et al., 2006, p. 928). Findings revealed significant changes in youngsters' metabolic control and treatment adherence after BFST, as compared to standard care or an educational condition (Wysocki et al., 2006, 2008).

Peer Support and Involvement

Youngsters' adherence may also benefit from peer support (La Greca et al., 1995). Greco, Pendley, McDonell, and Reeves (2001) developed a four-session intervention for adolescents with diabetes and their best friends, which encouraged friends to become involved with diabetes management. Sessions covered descriptive information about diabetes; reflective listening skills and problem solving; ways that friends could be supportive and assist with diabetes care; and stress management skills. At postintervention, adolescents and their friends reported greater diabetes knowledge and support; parents also reported less diabetes-related conflict with their adolescents. Adolescents' treatment adherence was not evaluated directly.

Summary

Including families in treatment, and focusing on ways to reduce family conflict and improve communication and support, may have a significant effect on adherence. Efforts to involve youngsters' close friends may also be beneficial, but are not well studied as yet.

Multicomponent Interventions

Multicomponent interventions have been developed to address the complexity of treatments for chronic pediatric conditions and the multiple factors that contribute to adherence. Multicomponent interventions may combine educational, behavioral, and/or psychosocial strategies for improving adherence. Examples of multicomponent interventions are described below (see La Greca & Bearman, 2003, for additional studies). Kahana and colleagues (2008) defined multicomponent interventions for pediatric adherence as ones combining educational and behavioral strategies, and found a medium effect size for their effectiveness (mean $d = 0.51$).

Powers and colleagues (2005) designed a multicomponent intervention to improve nutritional intake and growth in young children with cystic fibrosis. This intervention included nutritional education as well as child behavior management skills that focused on mealtime behaviors and nutrition. All interventions were conducted in an individual therapy format, and the intervention was compared to usual care. Although the sample size was small (N = 10), the children assigned to the multicomponent intervention showed significant improvements in growth and in energy intake compared with the children receiving usual care.

As another example, Stark and colleagues (2005) combined "dietary counseling" and a "behavioral intervention for parents and youth[s]" to improve dietary calcium intake among youths with juvenile rheumatoid arthritis. The combined program improved children's dietary calcium intake, compared to an enhanced "standard care" condition.

Finally, in a recent series of studies, Ellis and colleagues (Ellis et al., 2007; Ellis, Naar-King, Cunningham, & Secord, 2006) adapted an intensive, home-based psychotherapy (multisystemic therapy, or MST), previously shown to be effective with adolescent problem behaviors, for adolescents who had poorly controlled diabetes or HIV infection. MST addresses potential barriers to adherence in multiple settings, including family, medical, community, and individual. Findings from this line of research have been somewhat mixed. Specifically, for HIV-infected adolescents, improvements in caregiver knowledge and adolescents' viral load were found, but there were no changes in caregiver-reported adherence following treatment (Ellis et al., 2006). For adolescents with diabetes, MST reduced hospital admissions for diabetes ketoacidosis (which typically results from poor adherence) at postintervention and at 6-month follow-up, but initial improvements in adolescents' diabetes control were not maintained at follow-up, and adherence to BG testing only improved for adolescents from two-parent families (Ellis et al., 2007). Although MST seems promising, further research on it is indicated.

In summary, multicomponent interventions for adherence appear promising, although the relative effectiveness of the treatment components are not known, and the long-term effects on adherence and disease control have been mixed (or not well studied). Nevertheless, given the complex demands of many treatment regimens, the development of adherence interventions that include multiple strategies will continue to be important for research and clinical practice, as it may be unrealistic to expect that a single intervention strategy will lead to successful adherence.

Emerging Interventions

Motivational Interviewing

A recent innovation has been the use of motivational interviewing (MI) in health care settings. MI is a goal-directed, client-centered counseling approach that helps individuals increase their motivation for change (see Suarez & Mullins, 2008, for a review). MI has been shown to improve adults' adherence to regimens for diabetes, asthma, hypertension, and heart disease (Knight, McGowan, Dickens, & Bundy, 2006), but has only recently been applied to pediatric populations. Early results are promising. In one of the few studies, Channon and colleagues (2007) conducted a randomized controlled trial of MI with adolescents who had Type 1 diabetes. Compared to a control condition, MI resulted in improvements in adolescents' metabolic control and psychosocial functioning at 24 months postintervention. Additional studies that examine MI in pediatric populations would be desirable.

Technology-Based Interventions

Advances in technology have opened up new avenues for improving adherence in youth. Telehealth/eHealth (see Palermo & Wilson, Chapter 15, this volume, for a full discussion) is the delivery of information and services via telecommunications devices, such as the phone, text messaging, or the Internet. The limited research available to date in this area shows promise. For instance, Franklin, Waller, Pagliari, and Greene (2006) found that sending daily text messages to youths with Type 1 diabetes to remind them of individual self-management goals improved their treatment adherence. Other researchers have developed promising interventions for asthma that integrate Web-based education programs and education phone calls from a case manager (e.g., Wise et al., 2007). As youths increasingly rely on computers and cell phones, this is an important area for interventions. However, on the cautionary side, Kahana and colleagues (2008) found that the effect size for the few available studies on technology-based interventions was not significantly different from zero (mean $d = 0.08$).

General Summary and Conclusions

Adherence to pediatric medical regimens is complex and challenging. Understanding the parameters underlying adherence to pediatric regimens will be advanced by greater attention in future research to developmental, family, and individual differences in adherence; to aspects of the health care environment that play a role in adherence; and to conceptual models of adherence behaviors that take into account multiple individual and contextual factors. Systematic analysis of these and other factors may enable clinicians and researchers to tailor intervention efforts more effectively to the specific needs of individual children, adolescents, and families. In particular, multiwave studies that examine the course of chronic illness and disease management *over time* (e.g., Helgeson et al., 2008) are especially needed.

In terms of interventions to improve pediatric adherence, effective strategies for acute illnesses with short-term medication regimens include providing verbal and written instructions, providing visual cues or reminders, and increasing medical supervision. However, treatments for chronic, complex regimens remain a challenge. Thus far, evidence suggests that the strongest intervention effects are observed for family-based and multicomponent interventions.

Future intervention studies would benefit from evaluating intervention effects for specific adherence behaviors, so that the impact of an intervention might be better appreciated. Moreover, further attention to intervention development and evaluation in areas other than diabetes or pulmonary disease would be desirable. For example, Kahana and colleagues' (2008) review of interventions for pediatric adherence illustrates that the vast majority of studies (83%) have focused on asthma, diabetes, or cystic fibrosis, with substantially less attention to HIV infection, juvenile rheumatoid arthritis, or other pediatric conditions. To some extent, this reflects the very low rates of adherence that have been found for diabetes and pulmonary disease (DiMatteo, 2004) compared with other conditions. Nevertheless, extending the intervention work to other pediatric conditions is critically important.

Several additional issues are noteworthy. First, in terms of measuring adherence, it appears that many investigators are using multiple assessment strategies (e.g., monitoring devices for medication usage plus diaries for dietary adherence), and that advances in technology are likely to further improve the accuracy of assessing methods. Adherence measures for HIV infection, pulmonary diseases, and diabetes (see Quittner et al., 2008; Steele & Grauer, 2003) are the most well developed at this time, and thus may serve as models for other areas of pediatric adherence.

Second, as newer treatment regimens are developed for pediatric conditions, it will be useful to evaluate their impact on adherence. For example, do children's adherence rates vary as a function of the type of asthma medication prescribed (Carter & Ananthakrishnan, 2003), or the type of insulin delivery system or dietary plan prescribed for Type 1 diabetes?

In addition, intervention studies would benefit from greater attention to the developmental, family, and individual differences that might *moderate* treatment responsiveness. Possible moderators to examine include children's developmental level, the severity and duration of the pediatric condition, the availability of family and peer support, comorbidity with other problems, and the degree of parental involvement in treatment. Studies that incorporate motivational interviewing or new technologies into comprehensive, multicomponent interventions are also of interest, especially studies that elucidate the active ingredients of the intervention. Finally, attention to the cost-effectiveness of adherence interventions will be essential if they are to be useful in today's managed health care environment (Walders et al., 2000).

References

Albino, J. E., Lawrence, S. D., Lopes, C. E., Nash, L. B., & Tedesco, L. A. (1991). Cooperation of adolescents in orthodontic treatment. *Journal of Behavioral Medicine, 14*, 53–70.

Anderson, B. J., Ho, J., Brackett, J., & Laffel, L. M. B. (1999). An office-based intervention to maintain parent–adolescent teamwork in diabetes management. *Diabetes Care, 22*, 713–721.

Arnhold, R. G., Adebonojo, F. O., Callas, E. R., Callas, J., Carte, E., & Stein, R. C. (1970). Patients and prescriptions: Comprehension and compliance with medical instructions in a suburban pediatric practice. *Clinical Pediatrics, 9*, 648–651.

Barofsky, I. (1984). Therapeutic compliance and the cancer patient. *Health Education Quarterly, 10*(Spec. Suppl.), 43–56.

Basheti, I. A., Armour, C. L., Bosnic-Antichevich, S. Z., & Reddel, H. K. (2008). Evaluation of a novel educational strategy, including inhaler-based reminder labels, to improve asthma inhaler technique. *Patient Education and Counseling, 72*(1), 26–33.

Bauman, L. J., Wright, E., Leickly, F. E., Crain, E., Kruszon-Moran, D., Wade, S. L., et al. (2002). Relationship of adherence to pediatric asthma morbidity among inner-city children. *Pediatrics, 111*(1), e6. Retrieved October 28, 2008, from *www.pediatrics.org/cgi/content/full/110/1/e6*

Becker, M. H., Maiman, L. A., Kirscht, J. P., Haefner, D. P., & Drachman, R. H. (1977). The health belief model and prediction of dietary compliance: A field experiment. *Journal of Health and Social Behavior, 18*, 348–366.

Berquist, R. K., Berquist, W. E., Esquivel, C. O., Cox, K. L., Wayman, K. I., & Litt, I. F. (2006). Adolescent non-adherence: Prevalence and consequences in liver transplant recipients. *Pediatric Transplant, 10*, 304–310.

Bloch, C. A., Clemons, P., & Sperling, M. A. (1987). Puberty decreases insulin sensitivity. *Journal of Pediatrics, 110*, 481–487.

Blowey, D. L., Hebert, D., Arbus, G. S., Pool, R., Korus, M., & Koren, G. (1997). Compliance with cyclosporine in adolescent renal transplant recipients. *Pediatric Nephrology, 11,* 547–551.

Boccuti, L., Celano, M., Geller, R. J., & Phillips, K. M. (1996). Development of a scale to measure children's metered dose inhaler and spacer technique. *Annals of Allergy, Asthma, and Immunology, 77,* 217–221.

Bond, G. G., Aiken, L. S., & Somerville, S. C. (1992). The health belief model and adolescents with insulin-dependent diabetes mellitus. *Health Psychology, 11,* 190–198.

Brooks-Gunn, J., & Graber, J. A. (1994). Puberty as a biological and social event: Implications for research on pharmacology. *Journal of Adolescent Health, 15,* 663–671.

Brownbridge, G., & Fielding, D. M. (1994). Psychosocial adjustment and adherence to dialysis treatment regimens. *Pediatric Nephrology, 8,* 744–749.

Brownlee-Duffeck, M., Peterson, L., Simonds, J. F., Goldstein, D., Kilo, C., & Hoette, S. (1987). The role of health beliefs in the regimen adherence and metabolic control of adolescents and adults with diabetes mellitus. *Journal of Consulting and Clinical Psychology, 55,* 139–144.

Burkhart, P. V., Dunbar-Jacob, J. M., Fireman, P., & Rohay, J. (2002). Children's adherence to recommended asthma self-management. *Pediatric Nursing, 28*(4), 409–414.

Butz, A. M., Tsoukleris, M. G., Donighan, M., Hsu, V. D., Zuckerman, I., Mudd, K. E., et al. (2006). Effectiveness of nebulizer use-targeted asthma education on underserved children with asthma. *Archives of Pediatrics and Adolescent Medicine, 160,* 622–628.

Carter, E. R., & Ananthakrishnan, M. (2003). Adherence to montelukast versus inhaled corticosteroids in children with asthma. *Pediatric Pulmonology, 36*(4), 301–304.

Cauce, A. M., Reid, M., Landesman, S., & Gonzales, N. (1990). Social support in young children: Measurement, structure, and behavioral impact. In B. R. Sarason, I. G. Sarason, & G.R. Pierce (Eds.), *Social support: An interactional view* (pp. 64–94). New York: Wiley.

Channon, S. J., Huws-Thomas, M. V., Rollnick, S., Hood, K., Cannings-John, R. L., Rigers, C., et al. (2007). A multicenter randomized controlled trial of motivational interviewing in teenagers with diabetes. *Diabetes Care, 30,* 1390–1395.

Cramer, J. A. (1995). Microelectric systems for monitoring and enhancing patient compliance with medication regimens. *Drugs, 49,* 321–327.

Davis, C. L., Delamater, A. M., Shaw, K. H., La Greca, A. M., Eidson, M. S., Perez-Rodriguez, J. E., et al. (2001). Parenting styles, regimen adherence, and glycemic control in 4- to 10-year-old children with diabetes. *Journal of Pediatric Psychology, 26,* 123–129.

De Civita, M., & Dobkin, P. L. (2004). Pediatric adherence as a multidimensional and dynamic construct, involving a triadic partnership. *Journal of Pediatric Psychology, 29*(3), 157–169.

De Civita, M., Feldman, D. E., Meshefedjian, G. A., Dobkin, P. L., Malleson, P., & Duffy, C. M. (20070. Caregiver recall of treatment recommendations in juvenile idiopathic arthritis. *Arthritis and Rheumatology, 15,* 226–233.

Delambo, K. E., Ievers-Landis, C., Drotar, D., & Quittner, A. L. (2004). Association of observed family relationship quality and problem-solving skills with treatment adherence in older children and adolescents with cystic fibrosis. *Journal of Pediatric Psychology, 29,* 343–353.

DeMore, M., Adams, C., Wilson, N., & Hogan, M. B. (2005). Parenting stress, difficult child behavior, and use of routines in relation to adherence in pediatric asthma. *Children's Health Care, 34*(4), 245–259.

DePaola, L. M., Roberts, M. C., Blaiss, M. S., Frick, P. J., & McNeal, R. E. (1997). Mothers' and children's perceptions of asthma medication. *Children's Health Care, 26*(4), 265–283.

Diabetes Control and Complications Trial Research Group. (1994). Effect of intensive diabetes treatment on the development and progression of long-term complications in adolescents with insulin-dependent diabetes mellitus: Diabetes Control and Complications Trial. *Journal of Pediatrics, 125*, 177–188.

DiMatteo, M. R. (2004). Variations in patients' adherence to medical recommendations: A quantitative review of 50 years of research. *Medical Care, 42*(3), 200–209.

DiMatteo, M. R., Giordani, P. J., Lepper, H. S., & Croghan, T. W. (2002). Patient adherence and medical treatment outcomes: A meta-analysis. *Medical Care, 40*(9), 794–811.

Dunton, G. F., Whalen, C. L., Jamner, L. D., & Floro, J. N. (2007). Mapping the social and physical contexts of physical activity across adolescence using ecological momentary assessment. *Annals of Behavioral Medicine, 34*(2), 144–153.

Ellis, D. A., Naar-King, S., Cunningham, P. B., & Secord, E. (2006). Use of multisystemic therapy to improve antiretroviral adherence and health outcomes in HIV-infected pediatric patients: Evaluation of a pilot program. *AIDS Patient Care and STDs, 20*(2), 112–121.

Ellis, D. A., Yopp, J., Templin, T. N., Naar-King, S., Frey, M. A., Cunningham, P. B., et al. (2007). Family mediators and moderators of treatment outcomes among youths with poorly controlled Type 1 diabetes: Results from a randomized controlled trial. *Journal of Pediatric Psychology, 32*, 194–205.

Emanuel, E. J., & Dubler, N. N. (1995). Preserving the physician–patient relationship in the era of managed care. *Journal of the American Medical Association, 273*, 323–329.

Finney, J. W., Hook, R. J., Friman, P. C., Rapoff, M. A., & Christophersen, M. F. (1993). The overestimation of adherence to pediatric medical regimens. *Children's Health Care, 22*, 297–304.

Finney, J. W., Lemanek, K. L., Brophy, C. J., & Cataldo, M. F. (1990). Pediatric appointment keeping: Improving adherence in a primary care allergy clinic. *Journal of Pediatric Psychology, 15*, 571–579.

Franklin, V. L., Waller, A., Pagliari, C., & Greene, S. A. (2006). A randomized controlled trial of Sweet Talk, a text-messaging system to support young people with diabetes. *Diabetic Medicine, 23*, 1332–1338.

Freund, A., Johnson, S. B., Silverstein, J., & Thomas, J. (1991). Assessing daily management of childhood diabetes using 24-hour recall interviews: Reliability and stability. *Health Psychology, 10*, 200–208.

Greco, P. Pendley, J. S., McDonell, K., & Reeves, G. (2001). A peer group intervention for adolescents with Type 1 diabetes and their best friends. *Journal of Pediatric Psychology, 26*, 485–490.

Guevara, J. P., Wolf, F. M., Grum, C. M., & Clark, N. M. (2003). Effects of educational interventions for self management of asthma in children and adolescents: Systematic review and meta-analysis. *British Medical Journal, 326*, 1308–1309.

Harris, M. A., Wysocki, T., Sadler, M., Wilkinson, K., Harvey, L. M., Buckloh, L. M., et al. (2000). Validation of a structured interview for the assessment of diabetes self-management. *Diabetes Care, 23*, 1301–1304.

Haynes, R. B. (1979). Introduction. In R. B. Haynes, D. W. Taylor, & D. L. Sackett (Eds.), *Compliance in health care* (pp. 1–7). Baltimore: Johns Hopkins University Press.

Hazzard, A., Hutchinson, S. J., & Krawiecki, N. (1990). Factors related to adherence to medication regimens in pediatric seizure patients. *Journal of Pediatric Psychology, 15*, 543–555.

Helgeson, V. S., Reynolds, K. A., Siminerio, L., Escobar, O., & Becker, D. (2008). Parent and adolescent distribution of responsibility for diabetes self care: Links to health outcomes. *Journal of Pediatric Psychology, 33*, 497–508.

Ievers-Landis, C. E., & Drotar, D. (2000). Parental and child knowledge of the treatment regimen for childhood chronic illnesses: Related factors and adherence to treatment. In D. Drotar (Ed.), *Promoting adherence to medical treatment in chronic childhood illness: Concepts, methods, and interventions* (pp. 259–282). Mahwah, NJ: Erlbaum.

Jacobson, A. M., Hauser, S. T., Lavori, P., Wolfsdorf, J. I., Herskowitz, R. D., Milley, J. E., et al. (1990). Adherence among children and adolescents with insulin-dependent diabetes mellitus over a four-year longitudinal follow-up: I. The influence of patient coping and adjustment. *Journal of Pediatric Psychology, 15*, 511–526.

Jacobson, A. M., Hauser, S. T., Willett, J. B., Wolfsdorf, J. I., Dvorak, R., Herman, L., et al. (1997). Psychological adjustment to IDDM: 10-year follow-up of an onset cohort of child and adolescent patients. *Diabetes Care, 20*, 811–818.

Johnson, S. B. (1994). Health behavior and health status: Concepts, methods, and applications. *Journal of Pediatric Psychology, 19*, 129–141.

Johnson, S. B. (2000). Compliance behavior in clinical trials: Error or opportunity? In D. Drotar (Ed.), *Promoting adherence to medical treatment in chronic childhood illness: Concepts, methods, and intervention* (pp. 307–321). Mahwah, NJ: Erlbaum.

Johnson, S. B., Silverstein, J., Rosenbloom, A., Carter, R., & Cunningham, W. (1986). Assessing daily management of childhood diabetes. *Health Psychology, 5*, 545–564.

Kahana, S., Drotar, D., & Frazier, T. (2008). Meta-analysis of psychological interventions to promote adherence to treatment in pediatric chronic health conditions. *Journal of Pediatric Psychology, 33*, 590–611.

Knight, K. M., McGowan, L., Dickens, C., & Bundy, C. (2006). A systematic review of motivational interviewing in physical health care settings. *British Journal of Health Psychology, 11*, 319–332.

Kovacs, M., Goldston, D., Obrosky, D. S., & Iyengar, S. (1992). Prevalence and predictors of pervasive noncompliance with medical treatment among youths with insulin-dependent diabetes mellitus. *Journal of the American Academy of Child and Adolescent Psychiatry, 31*, 1112–1119.

Kyngas, H. A. (2007). Predictors of good adherence of adolescents with diabetes (insulin dependent diabetes mellitus). *Chronic Illness, 3*(1), 20–28.

La Greca, A. M. (1990). Issues in adherence with pediatric regimens. *Journal of Pediatric Psychology, 15*, 423–436.

La Greca, A. M. (1998). It's "all in the family": Responsibility for diabetes care. *Journal of Pediatric Endocrinology and Metabolism, 11*(Suppl. 2), 379–385.

La Greca, A. M., Auslander, W. F., Greco, P., Spetter, D., Fisher, E. B., & Santiago, J. V. (1995). I get by with a little help from my family and friends: Adolescents' support for diabetes care. *Journal of Pediatric Psychology, 20*, 449–476.

La Greca, A. M., & Bearman, K. J. (2002). The Diabetes Social Support Questionnaire—Family Version: Evaluating adolescents' diabetes-specific support from family members. *Journal of Pediatric Psychology, 27*, 665–676.

La Greca, A. M., & Bearman, K. J. (2003). Adherence to pediatric regimens. In M. C. Roberts (Ed.), *Handbook of pediatric psychology* (3rd ed., pp. 119–140). New York: Guilford Press.

La Greca, A. M., Follansbee, D., & Skyler, J. S. (1990). Developmental and behavioral aspects of diabetes management in youngsters. *Children's Health Care, 19*, 132–137.

La Greca, A. M., & Prinstein, M. J. (1999). Peer group. In W. K. Silverman & T. H. Ollendick (Eds.), *Developmental issues in the clinical treatment of children* (pp. 171–198). Needham Heights, MA: Allyn & Bacon.

La Greca, A. M., Swales, T., Klemp, S., & Madigan, S. (1988). Self care behaviors among adolescents with diabetes. *Proceedings of the Ninth Annual Sessions of the Society of Behavioral Medicine, Boston*, A42.

La Greca, A. M., Swales, T., Klemp, S., Madigan, S., & Skyler, J. S. (1995). Adolescents with diabetes: Gender differences in psychosocial functioning and glycemic control. *Children's Health Care, 24*, 61–78.

Lemanek, K. (1990). Adherence issues in the medical management of asthma. *Journal of Pediatric Psychology, 15*, 437–458.

Lemanek, K. L., Kamps, J., & Chung, N. B. (2001). Empirically supported treatments in pediatric psychology: Regimen adherence. *Journal of Pediatric Psychology, 26*(5), 253–275.

Levetown, M., & Committee on Bioethics. (2008). Communicating with children and families: From everyday interactions to skill in conveying distressing information. *Pediatrics, 121*, e1441–e1460.

Lewandowski, A., & Drotar, D. (2007). The relationship between parent-reported social support and adherence to medical treatment in families of adolescents with Type 1 diabetes. *Journal of Pediatric Psychology, 32*, 427–436.

Lewin, A. B., La Greca, A. M., Geffken, G. R., Williams, L. B., Duke, D. C., Storch, E. A., et al. (in press). Validity and reliability of adolescent and parent rating scale of Type 1 diabetes adherence behaviors: The Self-Care Inventory (SCI). *Journal of Pediatric Psychology.*

Litt, I. F., & Cuskey, W. R. (1980). Compliance with medical regimens during adolescence. *Pediatric Clinics of North America, 27*, 1–15.

Marhefka, S. L., Tepper, V. J., Farley, J. J., Sleasman, J. W., & Mellins, C. A. (2006). Brief report: Assessing adherence to pediatric antiretroviral regimens using the 24-hour recall interview. *Journal of Pediatric Psychology, 31*(9), 989–994.

Martin, S., Elliott-DeSorbo, D. K., Wolters, P. L., Toledo-Tamula, M. A., Roby, G., Zeichner, S., et al. (2007). Patient, caregiver and regimen characteristics associated with adherence to highly active antiretroviral therapy among HIV-infected children and adolescents. *Journal of Pediatric Infectious Diseases, 26*, 61–67.

Mauriello, L. M., Driskell, M. M. H., Sherman, K. J., Johnson, S. S., Prochaska, J. M., & Prochaska, J. O. (2006). Acceptability of a school-based intervention for the prevention of adolescent obesity. *Journal of School Nursing, 22*(5), 269–277.

Modi, A. C., & Quittner, A. L. (2006a). Barriers to treatment adherence for children with cystic fibrosis and asthma: What gets in the way? *Journal of Pediatric Psychology, 31*(8), 846–858.

Modi, A. C., & Quittner, A. L. (2006b). Utilizing computerized phone diary procedures to assess health behaviors in family and social contexts. *Children's Health Care, 35*, 29–45.

Naar-King, S., Montepiedra, G., Nichols, S., Farley, J., Garvie, P. A., Kammerer, B., et al. (2008). Allocation of family responsibility for illness management in pediatric HIV. *Journal of Pediatric Psychology, 34*, 187–194.

Naar-King, S., Podolski, C. L., Ellis, D. A., Frey, M. A., & Templin, T. (2006). Social ecological model of illness management in high-risk youths with Type 1 diabetes. *Journal of Consulting and Clinical Psychology, 74*(4), 785–789.

Patino, A. M., Sanchez, J., Eidson, M., & Delamater, A. M. (2005). Health beliefs and regimen adherence in minority adolescents with type 1 diabetes. *Journal of Pediatric Psychology, 30*, 503–512.

Phipps, S., & DeCuir-Whalley, S. (1990). Adherence issues in pediatric bone marrow transplantation. *Journal of Pediatric Psychology, 15*(4), 459–475.

Piecoro, L. T., Potoski, M., Talbert, J. C., & Doherty, D. E. (2001). Asthma prevalence, cost, and adherence with expert guidelines on the utilization of health care services and costs in a state Medicaid population. *Health Services Research, 36*(2), 351–371.

Powers, S. W., Jones, J. S., Ferguson, K. S., Piazza-Waggoner, C., Daines, C., & Acton, J. D. (2005). Randomized clinical trial of behavioral and nutrition treatment to improve energy intake and growth in toddlers and preschoolers with cystic fibrosis. *Pediatrics, 116*, 1442–1450.

Prochaska, J. O., DiClemente, C. C., & Norcross, J. C. (1992). In search of how people change: Applications to addictive behaviors. *American Psychologist, 47*, 1102–1114.

Puccio, J. A., Belzer, M., Olson, J., Martinez, M., Salata, C., & Tucker, D. (2006). The use of cell phone reminder calls for assisting HIV-infected adolescents and young adults to adhere to highly active antiretroviral therapy: A pilot study. *AIDS Patient Care and STDs, 20,* 438–444.

Quittner, A. L., Espelage, D. L., Ievers-Landis, C. E., & Drotar, D. (2000). Measuring adherence to medical treatments in childhood chronic illness: Considering multiple methods and sources of information. *Journal of Clinical Psychology in Medical Settings, 7,* 41–54.

Quittner, A. L., Modi, A. C., Lemanek, K. L., Ievers-Landis, C. E., & Rapoff, M. A. (2008). Evidence-based assessment of adherence to medical treatments in pediatric psychology. *Journal of Pediatric Psychology, 33,* 916–936.

Rapoff, M. A. (1999). *Adherence to pediatric medical regimens.* New York: Kluwer Academic.

Roberts, K. J. (2005). Barriers to antiretroviral medication adherence in young HIV infected children. *Youth and Society, 37*(2), 230–245.

Ruggiero, L., & Prochaska, J. (1993). Introduction: Application of the transtheoretical model to diabetes. *Diabetes Spectrum, 6,* 22–24.

Satin, W., La Greca, A. M., Zigo, M. A., & Skyler, J. S. (1989). Diabetes in adolescence: Effects of multifamily group intervention and parent simulation of diabetes. *Journal of Pediatric Psychology, 14,* 259–275.

Saylor, C. F., Elksnin, N., Farah, B. A., & Pope, J. A. (1990). Depends on who you ask: What maximizes participation of families in early intervention programs? *Journal of Pediatric Psychology, 15,* 557–569.

Schroder, N., Crabtree, M. J., & Lyall-Watson, S. (2002). The effectiveness of splinting as perceived by the parents of children with juvenile idiopathic arthritis. *British Journal of Occupational Therapy, 65,* 75–80.

Shemesh, E., Shneider, B. L., Savitzky, J. K., Arnott, L., Gondolesi, G. E., Krieger, N. R., et al. (2004). Medication adherence in pediatric and adolescent liver transplant recipients. *Pediatrics, 113,* 825–832.

Simons, L. E., & Blount, R. L. (2007). Identifying barriers to medication adherence in adolescent transplant recipients. *Journal of Pediatric Psychology, 32*(7), 831–844.

Singh, R. H., Kable, J. A., Guerrero, N. V., Sullivan, K. M., & Elsas, L. J. (2000). Impact of a camp experience on phenylalanine levels, knowledge, attitudes, and health beliefs relevant to nutrition management of phenylketonuria in adolescent girls. *Journal of the American Dietetic Association, 100,* 797–803.

Smith, S. R., Jaffe, D. M., Fisher, E. B., Trinkaus, K. M., Highstein, G., & Strunk, R. C. (2004). Improving follow-up for children with asthma after an acute emergency department visit. *Journal of Pediatrics, 145,* 772–777.

Spirito, A., & Kazak, A. E. (2006). *Effective and emerging treatments in pediatric psychology.* Oxford, UK: Oxford University Press.

Stark, L. J., Janicke, D. M., McGrath, A. M., Mackner, L. M., Hommel, K. A., & Lovell, D. (2005). Prevention of osteoporosis: A randomized clinical trial to increase calcium intake in children with juvenile rheumatoid arthritis. *Journal of Pediatric Psychology, 30*(5), 377–386.

Steele, R. G., Anderson, B., Rindel, B., Dreyer, M. L., Perrin, K., Christensen, R., et al. (2001). Adherence to antiretroviral therapy among HIV-positive children: Examination of the role of caregiver health beliefs. *AIDS Care, 13*(5), 617–629.

Steele, R. G., & Grauer, D. (2003). Adherence to antiretroviral therapy for pediatric HIV infection: Review of the literature and recommendations for research. *Clinical Child and Family Psychology Review, 6*(1), 17–30.

Stone, A. A., & Shiffman, S. (1994). Ecological momentary assessment (EMA) in behavioral medicine. *Annals of Behavioral Medicine, 16,* 199–202.

Suarez, M., & Mullins, S. (2008). Motivational interviewing and pediatric health interventions. *Journal of Developmental and Behavioral Pediatrics, 29,* 417–428.

Teach, S. J., Lillis, K. A., & Grossi, M. (1998). Compliance with penicillin prophylaxis in patients with sickle cell disease. *Archives of Pediatrics and Adolescent Medicine, 152,* 274–278.

Wainberg, M., & Friedland, G. (1998). Public health implications of antiretroviral therapy and HIV drug resistance. *Journal of the American Medical Association, 279,* 1977–1983.

Walders, N., Nobile, C., & Drotar, D. (2000). Promoting treatment adherence in childhood chronic illness: Challenges in a managed care environment. In D. Drotar (Ed.), *Promoting adherence to medical treatment in chronic childhood illness: Concepts, methods, and interventions* (pp. 201–236). Mahwah, NJ: Erlbaum.

Wise, M., Gustafson, D. H., Sorkness, C. A., Molfenter, T., Staresinic, A., Meis, T., et al. (2007). Internet telehealth for pediatric asthma case management: Integrating computerized and case manager features for tailoring a Web-based asthma education program. *Health Promotion and Practice, 8*(3), 282–291.

Witherspoon, D., & Drotar, D. (2006). Correlates of adherence to prophylactic penicillin therapy in children with sickle cell disease. *Children's Health Care, 35*(4), 281–296.

Wysocki, T., Green, L., & Huxtable, K. (1989). Blood glucose monitoring by diabetic adolescents: Compliance and metabolic control. *Health Psychology, 8,* 267–284.

Wysocki, T., Harris, M. A., Buckloh, L. M., Mertlich, D., Lochrie, A. S., & Taylor, A. (2006). Effects of behavioral family systems therapy for diabetes on adolescents' family relationships, treatment adherence, and metabolic control. *Journal of Pediatric Psychology, 31*(9), 928–938.

Wysocki, T., Harris, M. A., Buckloh, L. M., Mertlich, D., Lochrie, A. S., & Taylor, A. (2008). Randomized, controlled trial of behavioral family systems therapy for diabetes: Maintenance and generalization of effects on parent–adolescent communication. *Behavior Therapy, 39,* 33–46.

CHAPTER 10

Chronic and Recurrent Pain

LYNNDA M. DAHLQUIST
MARNI SWITKIN NAGEL

Few psychologists or pediatricians today would dispute the idea that children experience pain. However, widespread appreciation of the need to study and effectively manage children's pain developed relatively recently. Prior to the late 1980s, many pediatric textbooks did not even discuss pain management (Schechter, Berde, & Yaster, 2003). Children were thought to have a limited capacity to experience pain because of their immature neurological systems. As a result, chronic pain was viewed as an adult rather than a pediatric problem. In contrast, today's professionals are much more sensitive to the pain experiences of children and infants, and to the impact that pain can have on their developing nervous systems. Pain management strategies are now typically a standard part of the specialty care of children with chronic or recurrent pain conditions, such as abdominal pain, arthritis, and headaches (Schechter et al., 2003).

Despite this progress, dualistic views of pain (i.e., either it is "real" or it is "all in the child's head") are still common (Robbins, Smith, Gluting, & Bishop, 2005). Unfortunately, such misperceptions can lead professionals to discount children's pain complaints (especially when they are not clearly tied to physical pathology), or to label children as psychologically disturbed if their pain appears excessive. In the worst-case scenarios, children may be subjected to unnecessary medications and surgeries, rather than receiving potentially beneficial psychological interventions (Masters, 2006).

The goal of this chapter is to provide an overview of the variables that influence the experience of chronic and recurrent pain in children, and to summarize empirically supported approaches to treatment. Our review is selective rather than comprehensive, highlighting studies that examine etiology, illustrate treatment strategies, or critically review the literature.

Defining Chronic and Recurrent Pain

Pain is considered to be "chronic" and/or "recurrent" when it persists for 3–6 months, either continuously (chronic pain) or intermittently (recurrent pain) (Harden, 2005; Zeltzer, Tsao, Bursch, & Myers, 2006). Although definitions in the literature vary, depending on the pain diagnosis and research group, a frequently used definition of recurrent pain is at least three pain episodes that interfere with functioning within a 3-month period (e.g., Robbins et al., 2005). Chronic or recurrent pain is estimated to affect 25–30% of children and adolescents (Perquin et al., 2000; Zeltzer et al., 2006). The most common pediatric chronic and recurrent pain conditions (and their corresponding estimated prevalence rates) include headaches (10–28%), abdominal pain (10–20%), back pain (12–30%), limb pain (10%), and juvenile fibromyalgia/fatigue (6%) (Degotardi et al., 2006; Hicks, von Baeyer, & McGrath, 2006; Olsson, 1999; Van Epps, Zempsky, Schechter, Pescatello, & Lerer, 2007; Vervoort, Goubert, Eccleston, Bijttebier, & Crombez, 2006).

Biological Bases of Pain

Pain sensation initially results from injury to tissue adjacent to specific nerve fibers (Rosenzweig, Breedlove, & Leiman, 2002). Following tissue damage, chemical substances (e.g., neuropeptides, serotonin, and histamines) are released, which then activate specialized receptors (called nociceptors) that respond to noxious stimulation during the process of inflammation (Covington, 2000; Rosenzweig et al., 2002). The quality of pain sensation reflects the type of nociceptor activated. Stimulation of cutaneous Aδ nociceptors (large-diameter, myelinated, high-threshold receptors) results in sharp, pricking pain; stimulation of cutaneous C nociceptors (thin, unmyelinated fibers) results in burning or dull pain; and stimulation of nociceptors in muscle nerves results in aching pain (Rosenzweig et al., 2002).

Nociceptive versus Neuropathic Pain

"Nociceptive" pain arises when nerve endings in the peripheral tissue, which alert the body to potential or actual tissue damage, are activated (Nicholson, 2006; Zieglgansberger, Berthele, & Tolle, 2005). Nociceptive pain can be acute or chronic in nature (Harden, 2005). "Neuropathic" pain is triggered by changes in the peripheral or central nervous system; these changes cause low-threshold sensory fibers that previously would have generated innocuous sensations to begin producing painful sensations (Scholz & Woolf, 2007; Zieglgansberger et al., 2005). According to Harden (2005), stimulus-evoked neuropathic pain includes "hyperalgesia," an exaggerated pain response produced by a painful stimulus (e.g., pinprick), and "allodynia," a pain response produced by a stimulus that is not typically painful (e.g., light touch). Stimulus-independent neuropathic pain occurs spontaneously, without provocation, and is usually described as persistent shooting, electrical, or burning pain that may be constant or intermittent (Harden, 2005). Neuropathic pain syndromes tend to become more severe over time, as the efficiency with which neurons process sensory information increases with repetitive stimulation, resulting in lower pain thresholds (Zieglgansberger et al., 2005).

Type I complex regional pain syndrome (CRPS-I, formerly known as reflex sympathetic dystrophy or neurovascular dystrophy) is one of the most common types of neuropathic pain in children (Olsson, 1999). This disorder usually involves pain in the distal portion of an arm or leg, which may begin after an injury but persists long after the injury appears to have healed. In addition to spontaneous pain and allodynia or hyperalgesia, children also show signs of autonomic dysfunction (e.g., the affected foot may be significantly colder or warmer than the other foot). Secondary muscle weakness and other motor impairments often develop as a result of inactivity or attempts to guard the limb (Olsson, 1999).

Variables That Modulate Pain Perception

Gate Control Theory

Melzack and Wall (1965, 1982) proposed that pain perception depends on a complex "gating" mechanism in the dorsal horn of the spinal cord, through which both sensory and pain fibers relay signals. If the "gate" is open, pain sensations are transmitted to the cortex, where they are recognized as pain. If the "gate" is closed, no signal is sent to the brain, and no pain is perceived. Thus, if an impulse from a sensory fiber reaches the "gate" before an impulse from a pain fiber, the connecting neuron will be activated by the sensory fiber and thus be unresponsive to the pain impulse. In other words, the sensory stimulation will close the "gate." These authors also proposed that descending messages from central cognitive variables can open or close the "gate," and thus that cognition and emotion play a role in all pain experiences. Although recent research suggests that the processes involved in pain processing are more complex than originally proposed by Melzack and Wall (e.g., Vowles, McNeil, Sorrell, & Lawrence, 2006), imaging studies confirm the interrelated roles of sensory, affective, cognitive, and attentional processes in the perception of pain (Zieglansberger et al., 2005).

Stress and Negative Emotions

Stress and negative emotions are particularly important influences on chronic and recurrent pain conditions in children and adolescents (Martin-Herz, Smith, & McMahon, 1999). Mothers' reports of stressful life events (e.g., Walker, Garber, & Greene, 1994) and children's reports of daily stressors (Varni et al., 1996; Walker, Garber, Smith, Van Slyke, & Claar, 2001; White & Farrell, 2006), as well as negative emotional states such as anxiety and depression (Carlsson, Larsson, & Mark, 1996; Levy & Walker, 2005; Lewandowski, Palermo, & Peterson, 2006; Powers, Gilman, & Hershey, 2006; Vowles et al., 2006), have been shown to be are associated with more frequent and more intense headache and abdominal pain symptoms. These findings suggest that chronic pain conditions may be caused, at least in part, by physiological vulnerability to stress (Powers et al., 2006) or problems with recovery from stress (Compas, 1999). It has also been proposed that individuals who are high in negative affect may report greater pain because they are more prone to complain about negative events in general, or because they are more likely to monitor physical sensations and perceive innocuous sensations as indicative of pathology or pain (Vervoort et al., 2006). On the other hand, the experience of pain can also increase negative affect, and can itself serve as a stressor (Compas,

1999). Moreover, negative emotions can moderate the relation between stress and pain, making the effects of stress on pain more severe during negative mood states (Walker et al., 2001).

Emotional states also are related to the level of functional impairment or disability that can result from chronic pain (Langeveld, Koot, & Passchier, 1999; Lewandowski et al., 2006). For example, depressive symptoms may result from the loss of access to positive activities caused by the pain problem (e.g., Lewandowski et al., 2006). Alternatively, emotional symptoms may exacerbate pain-related disability if a child avoids activities that might improve functional outcome because of depression or fear of pain (Martin, McGrath, Brown, & Katz, 2007).

Coping Strategies

The way in which an individual copes with pain can exacerbate pain-related symptoms (Compas et al., 2006). Individuals who demonstrate negative thinking or catastrophize when faced with pain report more intense pain (Crombez et al., 2003; Vervoort et al., 2008) and psychological distress (Gil et al., 2001), exhibit lower pain tolerance (Piira, Taplin, Goodenough, & von Baeyer, 2002), and experience greater activity reduction and disability (Gil, Williams, Thompson, & Kinney, 1991). Passive coping strategies, such as denial, wishful thinking, isolation, and behavioral disengagement, have also been shown to be associated with greater pain intensity, somatic symptoms, disability, and depression (Compas et al., 2006; Walker, Smith, Garber, & Van Slyke, 1997).

Predictability and Perceived Controllability

Predictability and perceived controllability have been shown to affect pain perception. For example, when children were told when a cold-pressor trial would end, they reported less pain than children who underwent a cold-pressor trial of the same duration without any temporal information (Coldwell et al., 2002). When individuals believe that they can adjust the intensity of a painful stimulus (even though they actually have no control over the intensity), they rate the pain as less aversive and habituate to it more rapidly than when they are not given the perception of control (Staub, Tursky, & Schwartz, 1971).

Sleep

Although pain-induced sleep deprivation is widely acknowledged as one of many variables contributing to the suffering of patients with chronic pain, sleep also affects pain perception and coping skills (Lewin & Dahl, 1999). By causing irritability, emotional lability, and impaired attention and behavioral control, sleep deprivation interferes with children's efforts to divert their attention from pain sensations (Lewin & Dahl, 1999). Sleep deprivation also appears to have neurobiological effects on pain perception—causing increased sensitivity to thermal and muscle pain (Lautenbacher, Kundermann, & Krieg, 2006; Roehrs, Hyde, Blaisdell, Greenwald, & Roth, 2006), and interfering with the analgesic effects of opioids and with the ability of monoamines to potentiate the effects of opioids (Lautenbacher et al., 2006).

To date, most of the sleep research pertaining to child and adolescent pain conditions has been descriptive, documenting that children with chronic and recurrent pain are at greater risk for disordered sleep (Huntley, Campo, Dahl, & Lewin, 2007; Long, Krishnamurthy, & Palermo, 2008). Sleep problems are particularly prominent in juvenile primary fibromyalgia syndrome, a chronic pain condition associated with musculoskeletal pain, depression, and fatigue (Degotardi et al., 2006). In addition to daytime sleepiness and fatigue, disturbed sleep is associated with greater pain intensity, poorer health-related quality of life, and greater functional disability (Huntley et al., 2007; Long et al., 2008; Palermo & Kiska, 2005).

Using a structured sleep intervention targeting sleep hygiene, stimulus control, relaxation strategies, and maladaptive cognitions, as part of a larger cognitive-behavioral treatment package, Degotardi and colleagues (2006) were able to improve the sleep quality of children with fibromyalgia. Research is needed to determine the degree to which other chronic and recurrent pain symptoms can be improved via interventions that specifically target sleep.

Sociocultural Considerations

Pain perception and expression are tied to cultural backgrounds and beliefs, family traditions and values, and an individual's worldview (Sobraiske, 2006). Sociocultural variables that have been found to influence children's pain experiences, include age, gender, religion, cultural background, and socioeconomic status (Cheng, Foster, & Hester, 2003). Age, for example, influences children's understanding of pain and their expression of pain, with younger children more likely than older children to demonstrate overt behavioral expressions of distress when in pain (Cheng et al., 2003). With respect to gender, there is some evidence that girls report more frequent, longer-duration, and higher pain intensity for headaches, migraines, facial pain, upper back pain, and sickle cell disease (Unruh & Campbell, 1999), although some studies demonstrate no differences (Cheng et al., 2003). Culture appears to influence how children are expected to respond to painful stimuli, to whom they should report pain, the words they use to describe pain, and under what circumstances (if any) one should admit to feeling pain (Banoub-Baddour & Laryea, 1991).

Assessment of Chronic/Recurrent Pain

One of the early pediatric measures of chronic/recurrent pain, the Pediatric Pain Questionnaire (PPQ; Varni, Thompson, & Hanson, 1987), measures pain intensity and location (through visual analogue scale ratings and coloring in body diagrams), sensory and affective aspects of the child's pain (through a list of pain descriptors), and the child's and family's pain histories. Although originally designed for children with arthritis, the PPQ has been used with a number of illness populations. (For examples of other structured interviews or multicomponent questionnaires, see Budd, Workman, Lemsky, & Quick, 1994; McGrath et al., 2000; Mikkelsson, Salminen, & Kautiainen, 1997.)

Because of the error that often accompanies retrospective recall, and the fact that more severe pain episodes are more easily recalled, prospective monitoring of recurrent pain symptoms through daily pain diaries is often recommended (Hunfeld et al., 2001). The format of pain diaries varies widely—from noting the occurrence of pain only when it happens, to recording the presence or absence of pain at regular, fixed intervals. Some diaries also require intensity ratings and calculation of duration, as well as pain triggers, coping strategies employed, and use of medication (Cohen et al., 2008). Newly developed electronic diaries may prove to be especially useful for chronic and recurrent pain conditions by offering convenient real-time assessment of pain and related variables, and by making it impossible for children to fake compliance by filling in several days' worth of ratings at one time (Stinson et al., 2008).

In keeping with a biopsychosocial model of pain, assessment of chronic and recurrent pain should not be limited to the physical/perceptual aspects of a child's pain (i.e., quality, frequency, intensity and duration of pain sensations). It is also important to evaluate attentional and emotional variables that may influence the child's experience, efforts to cope with pain, the reactions of others to the child's pain, and the degree of disability that has resulted from the pain condition (Eccleston, Yorke, Morley, Williams, & Mastroyannopoulou, 2003; Zeltzer et al., 2006).

Structured interviews with children and their parents are among the main vehicles for assessing historical and contextual variables contributing to chronic and recurrent pain experiences (Allen & Matthews, 1998). Other standard behavioral assessment strategies, such as behavioral observations and parent and teacher daily records, can be used to identify possible contingencies (Allen & Matthews, 1998).

Pain diaries can also be used to document the important aspects of functional disability that are often associated with chronic and recurrent pain conditions (e.g., withdrawal from typical activities or social interactions, or number of school absences) (Allen & Matthews, 1998; Cohen et al., 2008; Gil et al., 2001). Specific questionnaires, such as the Functional Disability Inventory (Walker & Greene, 1991), are available as well to assess the degree to which a child's pain interferes with daily activities. (See also the recent review by McGrath et al., 2008.)

In a recent review of the literature, Eccleston, Jordan, and Crombez (2006) identified 43 measures that have been used to assess chronic pain in adolescents, the majority of which were created for other populations and then adapted for a population with chronic pain. All of the instruments utilized self-report in a questionnaire or structured interview format, with some including adolescent, parent, and/or teacher report versions. Other reviews provide information about the assessment of pain via self-report (Stinson, Kavanagh, Yamada, Gill, & Stevens, 2006), observational methods (von Baeyer & Spagrud, 2007), and functional outcomes (McGrath et al., 2008).

Pharmacological Interventions

Non-Narcotic Analgesics

Nonsteroidal anti-inflammatory drugs (NSAIDs—e.g., aspirin, ibuprofen [Motrin]) are widely used to reduce inflammation and treat mild to moderate pain (e.g., joint, bone, muscle, and headache pain). Acetaminophen (Tylenol) also has analgesic effects, but does not reduce inflammation (Maunuksela & Olkkola, 2003). Side effects typically involve gastrointestinal, kidney, liver, and blood system (reduced platelets) effects. Orally administered NSAIDs achieve an analgesic effect slowly, about 1 hour after ingestion, making timing of doses important. NSAIDs also have an "opioid-sparing" effect (Maunuksela & Olkkola, 2003, p. 178); that is, when used in combination with narcotics, they can reduce the amount of narcotic needed.

Narcotic Agents

Narcotic pain medications (opioids) include such drugs as codeine and morphine. These affect the central nervous system, rather than the peripheral nervous system, relieving pain by "inhibiting the release of excitatory neurotransmitters from nerve terminals transmitting nociceptive stimuli" (Yaster, Kost-Byerly, & Maxwell, 2003, p. 182). They are most often used for moderate to severe pain. Dizziness, sedation, and nausea are common side effects. Higher doses of morphine can cause respiratory depression (Yaster et al., 2003). Over time, tolerance can develop, so that a child will require higher doses of the drug in order to obtain the same level of pain control. Narcotics also can cause physical dependence, meaning that the child's body will react with withdrawal symptoms if the medications are discontinued abruptly. However, the presence of tolerance or withdrawal does not mean that the child is addicted to narcotics. "Addiction" refers to the psychological need for a drug and is extremely rare in children treated for chronic pain (Walco, Burns, & Cassidy, 2003).

Unconventional Analgesics

Antidepressants are commonly used in conjunction with other pain medications (Sethna, 1999). For patients who are both depressed and experiencing chronic pain, there is evidence that their pain improves when their depression remits. However, tricyclic antidepressants also have been shown to have benefits for children with neuropathic pain who do not demonstrate depression (Sethna, 1999). Tricyclic antidepressants appear to potentiate the effectiveness of opioids when used in combination, thus enabling better pain control to be achieved at lower doses of narcotics. Finally, tricyclic antidepressants can improve sleep in patients whose sleep cycles have been disrupted by pain (Sethna, 1999). Although empirical studies with children are limited, anticonvulsants, such as gabapentin (Neurontin), appear to reduce neuropathic pain (e.g., CRPS-I) in children (Low, Ward, & Wines, 2007).

Medication Schedules

Pain medications are most effective when administered around the clock (i.e., at regular intervals), rather than on an "as-needed" (p.r.n.) basis (Maunuksela & Olkkola, 2003). Regular schedules maintain a constant level of medication in the body and help prevent the recurrence of pain.

Physical Interventions

Nerve Stimulation and Physical Therapy

Transcutaneous electrical nerve stimulation (TENS) therapy involves electrical stimulation of large afferent nerve fibers (A fibers) near the site of a child's pain in such a way that nociceptive C fiber input is inhibited (McCarthy, Shea, & Sullivan, 2003). Thus the child feels a tingling or vibration sensation rather than an aching pain sensation. TENS also may relieve pain by activating endogenous opioids (McCarthy et al., 2003). Although there has been little research on the effectiveness of TENS for chronic pain in children, available data suggest that it can help reduce the pain associated with CRPS-I, sickle cell crises, and chronic back pain (Van Epps et al., 2007).

Physical therapy is used to is used to mobilize a child's limbs to prevent or to restore muscle and joint function, and is a crucial element of treatment for chronic pain conditions such as juvenile rheumatoid arthritis or CRPS-I, in which the child is likely to (1) lose muscle strength or joint motility because of pain-related inactivity, and/or (2) develop secondary pain problems because of muscle weakness or protective posturing (Wilder, 2003). In cases of severe neuropathic pain, surgical procedures (e.g., nerve blocks) may be used to provide enough pain relief so that the child can engage in physical therapy (Dadure et al., 2005; Wilder, 2003).

Although some families of children with sickle cell disease (Yoon & Black, 2006) and arthritis or arthralgia (Zebracki, Holzman, Bitter, Feehan, & Miller, 2007) report using massage for pain control, there are few randomized controlled trials testing the effectiveness of massage for pediatric chronic pain. Emerging research suggests that massage may improve morning stiffness and pain in children with arthritis, and that acupuncture may be effective in reducing the frequency and severity of migraine headaches (Tsao & Zeltzer, 2005).

Biofeedback

Biofeedback training involves monitoring and quantifying a physiological response, and conveying this information to the patient in such a way that the child perceives minute changes in his or her physiological status. Muscle tension (typically measured in the frontalis muscle or at the site of the child's pain) and skin temperature are the most common physical functions monitored for pain relief (Holden, Deichmann, & Levy, 1999).

The nature of the actual feedback provided to children varies across studies. Simple feedback may involve a tone that increases or decreases in pitch, digital finger temperature readings, temperature strips that change color, or lights that turn on or off to signal changes in temperature or muscle tension. More complex computer game-like feedback systems involve animals or objects that change speed or position in response to changes in the child's muscle tension (Culbert, Kajander, & Reaney, 1996).

Depending on the pain application, biofeedback is used as a means either to achieve a heightened state of relaxation (Holden et al., 1999; Lavigne, Ross, Berry, Hayford, & Pachman, 1992), or to alter a physiological process thought to cause the pain sensations (Gauthier, Ivers, & Carrier, 1996). For example, tension headaches are thought to be caused in part by sustained tension in pericranial muscles; consequently, electromyographic (EMG) biofeedback is used to teach patients to relax the frontalis muscle (Gauthier et al., 1996; Hermann & Blanchard, 2002). Migraine headaches, on the other hand, are thought to be caused by constriction of intra- and extracranial arteries (Gauthier et al., 1996). Therefore, biofeedback procedures for migraines typically target vascular activity by teaching children to warm their index finger (Gauthier et al., 1996; Hermann & Blanchard, 2002).

Biofeedback has been shown to be effective for migraines and for tension headache (Hermann & Blanchard, 2002; Holden et al., 1999), with results being maintained through 6- to 12-month follow-up periods (Hermann & Blanchard, 2002). Preliminary findings suggest that biofeedback also may be useful in reducing reduce overall sympathetic nervous system arousal in other chronic pain conditions, such as recurrent abdominal pain (Humphreys & Gevirtz, 2000; Masters, 2006). However, the magnitude of improvement that children show in biofeedback studies is not necessarily highly correlated with the degree of control the children show over the targeted physiological process (e.g., hand temperature; Hermann & Blanchard, 2002), leading some researchers to propose that biofeedback involves "more complex therapeutic processes than simple physiologic retraining" (Rains, Penzien, McCrory, & Gray, 2005, p. S95).

Cognitive-Behavioral Pain Management Strategies

Because cognitive-behavioral interventions for chronic pain conditions are most often provided in a package format—that is, children are taught several different pain management skills as part of a comprehensive pain management intervention—there are limited outcome data for the individual components of intervention. Consequently, except where otherwise noted, the following sections describe the different components of treatment programs that have been included in effective treatment packages.

Relaxation

Progressive muscle relaxation training teaches children to tense and then relax specific groups of muscles. If more than one session of relaxation training is conducted, the number of muscle groups is gradually reduced until a more rapid, cue-controlled strategy is taught, in which the entire body is relaxed at once while a child subvocalizes a relaxation cue word (e.g., Dahlquist, 1999; Larsson, Carlsson, Fichtel, & Melin, 2005). Children are taught to use relaxation in response to stress or pain symptoms, and are typically expected to practice relaxation outside of therapy sessions (Larsson et al., 2005). Some programs also include deep breathing exercises (e.g., Robbins et al., 2005).

A series of randomized controlled trials of relaxation therapy for adolescents with headaches conducted by Larsson and colleagues (2005) demonstrated that relaxation therapy was more effective than a variety of attention control conditions, resulting in fewer headache days and lower headache intensity. Relaxation/stress management strategies have been incorporated into a number of cognitive-behavioral pain management programs for a variety of other chronic pain conditions, including sickle cell disease, recurrent abdominal pain (Levy & Walker, 2005), and joint pain (Walco, Varni, & Ilowite, 1992).

Imagery

Imagery is often integrated into cognitive-behavioral treatment programs as a tool to enhance relaxation. Children may be encouraged to imagine themselves in a setting that is very peaceful or incompatible with pain (Dahlquist, 1999; Robbins et al., 2005), or in a setting in which they have personally been pain-free (Walco et al., 1992). Imagery strategies that acknowledge pain but then transform it in some way to make it less noxious may be particularly useful for high-intensity pain, which may be too difficult to ignore. For example, Walco and colleagues (1992) taught children with arthritis to imagine turning off "pain switches" throughout their bodies, or to imagine joint pain as a blowtorch being extinguished.

Hypnosis involves imagery in combination with suggestions of heightened relaxation and/or a change in the experience of pain (Jensen & Patterson, 2006). Although randomized controlled trials with adequate controls for patient expectancy are lacking (Jensen & Patterson, 2006; Saadat & Kain, 2007), emerging evidence suggests that hypnosis may be useful in the treatment of headaches and recurrent abdominal pain (Hammond, 2007; Saadat & Kain, 2007).

Self-Statements

Cognitive interventions specifically target negative and catastrophizing thoughts, replacing them with encouraging self-statements (e.g., "Be brave, hang in there"; Sanders et al., 1989, p. 297) and efforts to relax and/or divert attention from the pain (Sanders, Shepherd, Cleghorn, & Woolford, 1994). Robbins and colleagues (2005) recently evaluated a five-session cognitive-behavioral intervention for children with recurrent abdominal pain that focused heavily on helping children identify negative cognitions, challenge negative predictions, and use positive self-statements. Their program, which also included relaxation training and parent training in ways to minimize sick role behaviors and encourage adaptive coping, resulted in greater reductions in pain symptoms and greater improvements in school attendance than standard medical care. Improvements were maintained at 3- and 6- to 12-month follow-ups.

Operant Interventions

In contrast to interventions designed to decrease a child's subjective experience of pain, operant interventions focus on modifying the child's overt manifestations of pain and other illness-related behaviors that may be inadvertently maintained by intermittent positive or negative reinforcement (Allen & Matthews, 1998; Dahlquist, 1999; Levy & Walker, 2005). Simple actions, such as lying down, keeping a part of the body still, or restricting activities often reduce pain intensity in the short term (even though they have little impact on long-term pain frequency), and are thus negatively reinforced (Allen & Matthews, 1998). Illness behaviors may result in comfort, expressions of sympathy, or opportunities to spend extra time with parents or other family members, or may allow a child to escape or avoid chores, academic tasks, or other stressful peer or family interactions (Dahlquist, 1999; Vervoort et al., 2006). Walker (1999) proposed that children who are having difficulty accomplishing normal developmental tasks, who experience or anticipate failure, and who perceive themselves to be incompetent are especially at risk for activity restriction and social withdrawal in response to pain. This tendency is likely to be exacerbated in highly competitive academic environments or in highly critical home environments. Consequently, operant strategies are often integrated into cognitive-behavioral pain management programs that also target stress triggers and pain symptoms (Allen & Shriver, 1998; Banez & Gallagher, 2006; Palermo & Chambers, 2006; Robbins et al., 2005).

Competing contingencies also may interfere with parents' management of their children's pain behavior. Providing comfort and pain relief may make some parents feel closer to their children or may allow them to avoid aversive situations, such as work or marital conflict (Dahlquist, 1999; Walker, 1999). In such cases, the contingencies that maintain the parents' behavior should also be targeted in the pain management intervention. Moreover, when parents decrease their activity level or do not fulfill responsibilities when they are ill or in pain, children are likely to demonstrate similar behaviors when they are in pain (Levy & Walker, 2005). However, only a few researchers (e.g., Sanders et al., 1994) have specifically targeted parental modeling of sick role behaviors as part of their behavior management program. Other aspects of family functioning that may be relevant to chronic pain include family communication patterns, autonomy and conflict in parent–adolescent relationships, and parenting style (Palermo & Chambers, 2006).

If contextual factors are not addressed in a timely fashion, children with chronic pain can develop what some gastroenterologists and developmental pediatricians have recently termed "pain-associated disability syndrome" (PADS) (Bursch, Joseph, & Zeltzer, 2003; Zeltzer et al., 2006). These children demonstrate serious deterioration in functioning (i.e., school absenteeism and/or severe restrictions in other aspects of functioning) lasting at least 2 months (Bursch et al., 2003). A comprehensive approach to pain management, incorporating medical treatment, physical therapy, and psychological intervention, is needed in order to help these children regain healthy functioning.

Bursch and colleagues (2003) identify several aspects of the way medical care is provided to children with chronic pain that can either help or hinder the recovery progress. Although their recommendations are geared toward children with pain-associated disability syndrome, they are applicable to children with less severe chronic pain problems as well.

1. All of the members of the team should present a consistent conceptualization of the child's pain problem, and should use similar terminology in order to prevent confusion. Providers should stress that the child's pain is real, explain the process of nociception and the sensitization of the perceptual and central nervous system, and help families understand the role of the environment in pain and disability.

2. The professionals working with the child need to be in agreement regarding when to stop an evaluation. If one physician continues to pursue more diagnostic evaluations, the child and family will remain focused on finding a physical cause rather than on rehabilitation.

3. Maximizing the child's level of functioning in physical social, academic, and daily living activities, rather than the complete elimination of pain, should be the goal of treatment. To keep the focus on functioning, team members should avoid frequent assessment of the child's pain. Instead, assessment should concentrate on small weekly improvements in functioning, and treatment should be geared toward helping the child improve his or her coping skills and remediate areas of deficiencies (e.g., academics, stamina).

Future Directions

Topics for Future Research

Despite the considerable evidence that cognitive-behavioral, operant, and biofeedback pain management programs are effective, little is known about the essential components of treatment packages (Eccleston et al., 2003). Component analyses of intervention programs are needed in order to develop more cost-effective pain management strategies. At a more theoretical level, the mechanisms underlying successful treatment outcome also warrant further study. For example, interviews with children following successful cognitive-behavioral treatment for fibromyalgia (Degotardi et al., 2006), and the work of others (Hermann & Blanchard, 2002), suggest that changes in perceived control over pain may mediate improvements in pain and functional status.

Future studies also should pay greater attention to moderators of treatment outcome, in order to begin to identify the children and/or families who may be best suited for certain interventions (Cvengros, Harper, & Shevell, 2007; Larsson et al., 2005). Sanders, Cleghorn, Shepherd, and Patrick (1996) found that their combination of cognitive–behavioral pain management techniques and parent training in behavior management was most effective with children with recurrent abdominal pain whose parents believed their pain to be stress- rather than illness-related and were already encouraging independent pain management at baseline. Emerging research also suggests that active engagement with the therapy process (e.g., willingness to comply with baseline self-monitoring procedures, behavior management recommendations, and home practice) may be important determinants of success (Allen & McKeen, 1991; Cvengros et al., 2007; Larsson et al., 2005). Future research should address the challenge of what to offer families with poorer behavior management skills, less psychological views of their children's pain, and/or poor adherence to treatment protocols.

Finally, a number of pediatric chronic pain problems remain relatively understudied. Some 12–30% of adolescents experience chronic back pain (Van Epps et al., 2007), for example, but we found no studies of biopsychosocial treatments for chronic back pain in children or adolescents. Cognitively impaired and/or noncommunicating children are particularly at risk for having pain that is inadequately assessed and controlled (Hunt, Mastroyannopoulou, Goldman, & Seers, 2003; Stallard, Williams, Velleman, Lenton, & McGrath, 2002). However, the chronic pain experiences of children with developmental disabilities have received relatively little empirical attention (Oberlander & Symons, 2006). Considerably more research is needed in order to address the unique challenges involved in the assessment and treatment of chronic and recurrent pain in children with developmental disabilities.

Innovations in Service Delivery

As the work of Larsson and colleagues (2005) demonstrates, chronic pain does not need to be treated in purely medical settings. Some aspects of chronic pain management, such as relaxation training, can be conducted by school nurses in school settings during the school day. Although the school nurses in the Larsson et al. studies were not as effective as the professionally trained therapists, the nurse-executed school-based program was superior to attention control and self-monitoring in reducing tension headaches in adolescents. It may also be possible to offer some aspects of pain management intervention via CD-ROM programs, such as the Headstrong program for headaches (Connelly, Rapoff, Thompson, & Connelly, 2006), or via Internet-based cognitive-behavioral treatment programs coupled with email and phone contact (e.g., Hicks et al., 2006). Preliminary studies of computer-based interventions are very encouraging, with treatment subjects showing significantly greater improvements in self-reported headache pain, compared with waiting-list controls (Connelly et al., 2006; Hicks et al., 2006).

These innovative programs provide enhanced pain management without the cost and inconvenience often associated with extensive professional involvement. Moreover, and, perhaps most importantly, they have the potential to improve the quality of the lives of children who might not otherwise have received any treatment at all.

References

Allen, K. D., & Matthews, J. R. (1998). Behavior management of recurrent pain in children. In T. S. Watson & F. M. Gresham (Eds.), *Handbook of child behavior therapy* (pp. 263–285). New York: Plenum Press.

Allen, K. D., & McKeen, L. R. (1991). Home-based multi-component treatment of pediatric migraine. *Headache, 31,* 467–472.

Allen, K. D., & Shriver, M. D. (1998). Role of parent-mediated pain behavior management strategies in biofeedback treatment of childhood migraines. *Behavior Therapy, 29,* 477–490.

Banez, G. A., & Gallagher, H. M. (2006). Recurrent abdominal pain. *Behavior Modification, 30,* 50–71.

Banoub-Baddour, S., & Laryea, M. (1991). Children in pain: A culturally sensitive perspective for child care professionals. *Journal of Child and Youth Care, 6,* 19–24.

Budd, K. S., Workman, D. E., Lemsky, C. M., & Quick, D. M. (1994). The Children's Headache Assessment Scale (CHAAS): Factor structure and psychometric properties. *Headache, 17,* 159–179.

Bursch, B., Joseph, M. H., & Zeltzer, L. K. (2003). Pain-associated disability syndrome. In N. Schechter, C. Berde, & M. Yaster (Eds.), *Pain in infants, children, and adolescents* (2nd ed., pp. 841–848). Philadelphia: Lippincott Williams & Wilkins.

Carlsson, J., Larsson, B., & Mark, A. (1996). Psychosocial functioning in school children with recurrent headaches. *Headache, 36,* 77–82.

Cheng, S., Foster, R. L., & Hester, N. O. (2003). A review of factors predicting children's pain experiences. *Issues in Comprehensive Nursing, 26,* 203–216.

Cohen, L., Lemanek, K., Blount, R., Dahlquist, L., Lim, C., Palermo, T., et al. (2008). Evidence-based assessment of pediatric pain. *Journal of Pediatric Psychology, 33,* 939–955.

Coldwell, S. E., Kaakko, T., Gaertner-Makihara, A. B., Williams, T., Milgrom, P., Weinstein, P., et al. (2002). Temporal information reduces children's pain reports during a multiple-trial cold pressor procedure. *Behavior Therapy, 33,* 45–63.

Compas, B. (1999). Coping and responses to stress among children with recurrent abdominal pain. *Journal of Developmental and Behavioral Pediatrics, 20,* 323–324.

Compas, B., Boyer, M., Stanger, C., Colletti, R. B., Thomsen, A. H., Dufton, L. M., et al. (2006). Latent variable analysis of coping, anxiety/depression, and somatic symptoms in adolescents with chronic pain. *Journal of Consulting and Clinical Psychology, 74,* 1132–1142.

Connelly, M., Rapoff, M., Thompson, N., & Connelly, W. (2006). Headstrong: A pilot study of a CD-ROM intervention for recurrent pediatric headache. *Journal of Pediatric Psychology, 31,* 737–747.

Covington, E. C. (2000). The biological basis of pain. *International Review of Psychiatry, 12,* 128–147.

Crombez, G., Bijttebier, P., Eccleston, C., Mascagni, T., Mertens, G., Goubert, L., et al. (2003). The child version of the Pain Catastrophizing Scale (PSC-C): A preliminary version. *Pain, 104*(3), 639–646.

Culbert, T. P., Kajander, R. L., & Reaney, J. B. (1996). Biofeedback with children and adolescents: Clinical observations and patient perspectives. *Journal of Developmental and Behavioral Pediatrics, 17,* 342–350.

Cvengros, J. A., Harper, D., & Shevell, M. (2007). Pediatric headache: An examination of process variables in treatment. *Journal of Child Neurology, 22*, 1172–1181.

Dadure, C., Motais, F., Ricard, C., Raux, O., Troncin, R., & Capdevilla, X. (2005). Continuous peripheral nerve blocks at home for treatment of recurrent complex regional pain syndrome I in children. *Anesthesiology, 102*, 387–391.

Dahlquist, L. M. (1999). *Pediatric pain management.* New York: Kluwer Academic.

Degotardi, P. J., Klass, E. S., Rosenberg, B. S., Fox, D. G., Gallelli, K. A., & Gottlieb, B. S. (2006). Development and evaluation of a cognitive-behavioral intervention for juvenile fibromyalgia. *Journal of Pediatric Psychology, 31*, 714–723.

Eccleston, C., Jordan, A. L., & Crombez, G. (2006). The impact of chronic pain on adolescents: A review of previously used measures. *Journal of Pediatric Psychology, 31*, 684–697.

Eccleston, C., Yorke, L., Morley, S., Williams, A. C. deC., & Mastroyannopoulou, K. (2003). Psychological therapies for the management of chronic and recurrent pain in children and adolescents. *Cochrane Database of Systematic Reviews*, Issue 1 (Article No. CD003968), DOI: 10.1002/14651858.CD003968.

Gauthier, J. G., Ivers, H., & Carrier, S. (1996). Nonpharmacological approaches in the management of recurrent headache disorders and their comparison and combination with pharmacotherapy. *Clinical Psychology Review, 16*, 543–571.

Gil, K. M., Anthony, K. K., Carson, J. W., Redding-Lallinger, R., Daeschner, C. W., & Ware, R. E. (2001). Daily coping practice predicts treatment effects in children with sickle cell disease. *Journal of Pediatric Psychology, 26*, 163–173.

Gil, K. M., Williams, D. A., Thompson, R. J., & Kinney, T. R. (1991). Sickle cell disease in children and adolescents: The relation of child and parent pain coping strategies to adjustment. *Journal of Pediatric Psychology, 16*, 643–663.

Harden, R. N. (2005). Chronic neuropathic pain: Mechanisms, diagnosis, and treatment. *The Neurologist, 11*, 111–122.

Hammond, D. C. (2007). Review of the efficacy of clinical hypnosis with headaches and migraines. *International Journal of Clinical and Experimental Hypnosis, 55*, 207–219.

Hermann, C., & Blanchard, E. B. (2002). Biofeedback in the treatment of headache and other childhood pain. *Applied Psychophysiology and Biofeedback, 27*, 143–162.

Hicks, C. L., von Baeyer, C. L., & McGrath, P. J. (2006). Online psychological treatment for pediatric recurrent pain: A randomized evaluation. *Journal of Pediatric Psychology, 31*, 724–736.

Holden, E. W., Deichmann, M. M., & Levy, J. D. (1999). Empirically supported treatments in pediatric psychology: Recurrent pediatric headache. *Journal of Pediatric Psychology, 24*, 91–109.

Humphreys, P. A., & Gevirtz, R. N. (2000). Treatment of recurrent abdominal pain: Components analysis of four treatment protocols. *Journal of Pediatric Gastroenterology and Nutrition, 31*, 47–51.

Hunfeld, J. A. M., Perquin, C. W., Duivenvoorden, H. J., Hazebroek-Kampschreur, A. A. J. M., Passchier, J., van Suijlekom-Smit, L. W. A., et al. (2001). Chronic pain and its impact on quality of life in adolescents and their families. *Journal of Pediatric Psychology, 26*, 145–153.

Hunt, A., Mastroyannopoulou, K., Goldman, A., & Seers, K. (2003). Not knowing: The problem of pain in children with severe neurological impairment. *International Journal of Nursing Studies, 40*, 171–183.

Huntley, E. D., Campo, J. V., Dahl, R. E., & Lewin, D. S. (2007). Sleep characteristics of youth with functional abdominal pain and a health comparison group. *Journal of Pediatric Psychology, 32*, 938–949.

Jensen, M., & Patterson, D. R. (2006). Hypnotic treatment of chronic pain. *Journal of Behavioral Medicine, 29*, 95–124.

Langeveld, J. H., Koot, H. M., & Passchier, J. (1999). Do experienced stress and trait negative affectivity moderate the relationship between headache and quality of life in adolescents? *Journal of Pediatric Psychology, 24,* 1–11.

Larsson, B., Carlsson, J., Fichtel, A., & Melin, L. (2005). Relaxation treatment of adolescent headache sufferers: Results from a school-based replication series. *Headache, 45,* 692–704.

Lautenbacher, S., Kundermann, B., & Krieg, J. (2006). Sleep deprivation and pain perception. *Sleep Medicine Reviews, 10,* 357–369.

Lavigne, J. V., Ross, C. K., Berry, S. L., Hayford, J. R., & Pachman, L. M. (1992). Evaluation of a psychological treatment package for treating pain in juvenile rheumatoid arthritis. *Arthritis Care and Research, 5,* 101–110.

Levy, R., & Walker, L. (2005). Cognitive behavior therapy for the treatment of recurrent abdominal pain. *Journal of Cognitive Psychotherapy, 19,* 137–149.

Lewandowski, A. S., Palermo, T. M., & Peterson, C. C. (2006). Age-dependent relationships among pain, depressive symptoms, and functional disability in youth with recurrent headaches. *Headache, 46,* 656–662.

Lewin, D. S., & Dahl, R. E. (1999). The importance of sleep in the management of pediatric pain. *Journal of Developmental and Behavioral Pediatrics, 20,* 244–252.

Long, A. C., Krishnamurthy, V., & Palermo, T. M. (2008). Sleep disturbances in school-age children and chronic pain. *Journal of Pediatric Psychology, 33,* 258–268.

Low, A., Ward, K., & Wines, A. (2007). Pediatric complex regional pain syndrome. *Journal of Pediatric Orthopedics, 27,* 567–572.

Martin, A. L., McGrath, P. A., Brown, S. C., & Katz, J. (2007). Anxiety sensitivity, fear of pain, and pain-related disability in children and adolescents with chronic pain. *Pain Research and Management, 12,* 267–272.

Martin-Herz, S. P., Smith, M. S., & McMahon, R. J. (1999). Psychosocial variables associated with headache in junior high school students. *Journal of Pediatric Psychology, 24,* 13–23.

Masters, K. S. (2006). Recurrent abdominal pain, medical intervention, and biofeedback: What happened to the biopsychosocial model? *Applied Psychophysiology and Biofeedback, 31,* 155–165.

Maunuksela, E., & Olkkola, K. (2003) Non-steroidal anti-inflammatory drugs in pediatric pain management. In N. L. Schechter, C. B. Berde, & M. Yaster (Eds.), *Pain in infants, children, and adolescents* (2nd ed., pp. 171–180). Philadelphia: Lippincott Williams & Wilkins.

McCarthy, C. F., Shea, A. M., & Sullivan, P. (2003). Physical therapy management of pain in children. In N. L. Schechter, C. B. Berde, & M. Yaster (Eds.), *Pain in infants, children, and adolescents* (2nd ed., pp. 434–448). Philadelphia: Lippincott Williams & Wilkins.

McGrath, P. A., Speechley, K. N., Siefert, C. E., Biehn, J. T., Cairney, A. E. L., Gorodzinsky, F. P., et al. (2000). A survey of children's acute, recurrent, and chronic pain: Validation of the pain experience interview. *Pain, 87,* 59–73.

McGrath, P. J., Walco, G. A., Turk, D. C., Dworkin, R. H., Brown, M. T., Davidson, K., et al. (2008). Core outcome domains and measure for pediatric acute and chronic/recurrent pain clinical trials: PedIMMPACT recommendations. *Journal of Pain, 9,* 771–783.

Melzack, R., & Wall, P. D. (1965). Pain mechanisms: A new theory. *Science, 150,* 971–979.

Melzack, R., & Wall, P. D. (1982). *The challenge of pain.* New York: Basic Books.

Mikkelsson, M., Salminen, J. J., & Kautiainen, H. (1997). Non-specific musculoskeletal pain in preadolescents: Prevalence and 1-year persistence. *Pain, 73,* 29–35.

Nicholson, B. (2006). Differential diagnosis: Nociceptive and neuropathic pain. *American Journal of Managed Care, 12,* 256–262.

Oberlander, T., & Symons, F. (2006). *Pain in children and adults with developmental disabilities.* Baltimore: Brookes.

Olsson, G. L. (1999). Neuropathic pain in children. In P. J. McGrath & G. A. Finley (Eds.),

Progress in pain research and management: Vol. 13. Chronic and recurrent pain in children and adolescents (pp. 75–98). Seattle, WA: International Association for the Study of Pain (IASP) Press.

Palermo, T. M., & Chambers, C. T. (2006). Parent and family factors in pediatric chronic pain and disability: An integrative approach. *Pain, 119,* 1–4.

Palermo, T. M., & Kiska, R. (2005). Subjective sleep disturbances in adolescents with chronic pain: Relationship to daily functioning and quality of life. *Journal of Pain, 6,* 201–207.

Perquin, C. W., Hazebroek-Kampschreur, A. A., Hunfeld, J. A., Bohnen, A. M., van Suijlekom-Smit, L. W., Passchier, J., et al. (2000). Pain in children and adolescents: A common experience. *Pain, 87,* 51–58.

Piira, T., Taplin, J. E., Goodenough, B., & von Baeyer, C. L. (2002). Cognitive-behavioural predictors of children's tolerance of laboratory-induced pain: Implications for clinical assessment and future directions. *Behaviour Research and Therapy, 40,* 571–584.

Powers, S. W., Gilman, D. K., & Hershey, A. D. (2006). Headache and psychological functioning in children and adolescents. *Headache, 46,* 1404–1415.

Rains, J., Penzien, D., McCrory, D., & Gray, R. (2005). Behavioral headache treatment: History, review of the empirical literature, and methodological critique. *Headache, 45*(Suppl. 2), S92–S109.

Robbins, P. M., Smith, S. M., Glutting, J. J., & Bishop, C. T. (2005). A randomized controlled trial of a cognitive-behavioral family intervention for pediatric recurrent abdominal pain. *Journal of Pediatric Psychology, 30,* 397–408.

Roehrs, T., Hyde, M., Blaisdell, B., Greenwald, M., & Roth, T. (2006). Sleep loss and REM sleep loss are hyperalgesic. *Sleep, 29,* 145–151.

Rosenzweig, M. R., Breedlove, S. M., & Leiman, A. L. (2002). *Biological psychology: An introduction to behavioral, cognitive, and clinical neuroscience* (3rd ed.). Sunderland, MA: Sinauer.

Saadat, H., & Kain, Z. (2007). Hypnosis as a therapeutic tool in pediatrics. *Pediatrics, 120,* 179–181.

Sanders, M. R., Cleghorn, G., Shepherd, R., & Patrick, M. (1996). Predictors of clinical improvement in children with recurrent abdominal pain. *Behavioural and Cognitive Psychotherapy, 24,* 27–38.

Sanders, M. R., Rebgetz, M., Morrison, M., Bor, W., Gordon, A., Dadds, M., et al. (1989). Cognitive-behavioral treatment of recurrent nonspecific abdominal pain in children: An analysis of generalization, maintenance and side effects. *Journal of Consulting and Clinical Psychology, 57,* 294–300.

Sanders, M. R., Shepherd, R. W., Cleghorn, G., & Woolford, H. (1994). The treatment of recurrent abdominal pain in children: A controlled comparison of cognitive-behavioral family intervention and standard pediatric care. *Journal of Consulting and Clinical Psychology, 62,* 306–314.

Schechter, N. L., Berde, C. B., & Yaster, M. (2003). Pain in infants, children, and adolescents: An overview. In N. Schechter, C. Berde, & M. Yaster (Eds.), *Pain in infants, children, and adolescents* (2nd ed., pp. 3–18). Philadelphia: Lippincott Williams & Wilkins.

Scholz, J., & Woolf, C. (2007). The neuropathic pain triad: Neurons, immune cells and glia. *Nature Neuroscience, 10,* 1361–1368.

Sethna, N. F. (1999). Pharmacotherapy in long-term pain. In P. J. McGrath & G. A. Finley (Eds.), *Progress in pain research and management: Vol. 13. Chronic and recurrent pain in children and adolescents* (pp. 243–266). Seattle, WA: IASP Press.

Sobraiske, M. (2006). Machismo sustains health and illness beliefs of Mexican American men. *Journal of the American Academy of Nurse Practitioners, 18,* 348–350.

Stallard, P., Williams, L., Velleman, R., Lenton, S., & McGrath, P. (2002). Brief report: Behaviors identified by caregivers to detect pain in non-communicating children. *Journal of Pediatric Psychology, 27,* 209–214.

Staub, E., Tursky, B., & Schwartz, G. E. (1971). Self-control and predictability: Their effects on reactions to aversive stimulation. *Journal of Personality and Social Psychology, 18,* 157–162.

Stinson, J., Stevens, B., Feldman, B., Streiner, D., McGrath, P., Dupuis, A., et al. (2008). Construct validity of a multidimensional electronic pain diary for adolescents with arthritis. *Pain, 136,* 281–292.

Stinson, J. N., Kavanagh, T., Yamada, J., Gill, N., & Stevens, B. (2006). Systematic review of the psychometric properties, interpretability and feasibility of self-report pain intensity measures for use in clinical trials in children and adolescents. *Pain, 125,* 143–157.

Tsao, J., & Zeltzer, L. (2005). Complementary and alternative medicine approaches for pediatric pain: A review of the state-of-the-science. *eCAM, 2,* 149–159.

Unruh, A. M., & Campbell, M. A. (1999). Gender differences in children's pain experiences. In P. J. McGrath & G. A. Finley (Eds.), *Progress in pain research and management: Vol. 13. Chronic and recurrent pain in children and adolescents* (pp. 199–241). Seattle, WA: IASP Press.

Van Epps, S., Zempsky, W., Schechter, N., Pescatello, L. S., & Lerer, T. (2007). The effects of a two-week trial of transcutaneous electrical nerve stimulation for pediatric chronic back pain [Letter to the editor]. *Journal of Pain and Symptom Management, 34,* 115–117.

Varni, J. W., Rapoff, M. A., Waldron, S. A., Gragg, R. A., Bernstein, B. H., & Lindsley, C. B. (1996). Effects of perceived stress on pediatric chronic pain. *Journal of Behavioral Medicine, 19,* 515–528.

Varni, J. W., Thompson, K. L., & Hanson, V. (1987). The Varni/Thompson Pediatric Pain Questionnaire: I. Chronic musculoskeletal pain in juvenile rheumatoid arthritis. *Pain, 28,* 27–38.

Vervoort, T., Craig, K., Goubert, L., Dehoorne, J., Joos, R., Matthys, D., et al. (2008). Expressive dimensions of pain catastrophizing: A comparative analysis of school children and children with clinical pain. *Pain, 134,* 59–68.

Vervoort, T., Goubert, L., Eccleston, C., Bijttebier, P., & Crombez, G. (2006). Catastrophic thinking about pain is independently associated with pain severity, disability, and somatic complaints in school children and children with chronic pain. *Journal of Pediatric Psychology, 31,* 674–683.

von Baeyer, C. L., & Spagrud, L. J. (2007). Systematic review of observational (behavioral) measures of pain for children and adolescents aged 3 to 18 years. *Pain, 127,* 140–150.

Vowles, K. E., McNeil, D. W., Sorrell, J. T., & Lawrence, S. M. (2006). Fear and pain: Investigating the interaction between aversive states. *Journal of Abnormal Psychology, 115,* 821–833.

Walco, G., Burns, J., & Cassidy, R. (2003). The ethics of pain control in infants and children. In N. Schechter, C. Berde, & M. Yaster (Eds.), *Pain in infants, children, and adolescents* (2nd ed., pp. 157–168). Philadelphia: Lippincott Williams & Wilkins.

Walco, G. A., Varni, J. W., & Ilowite, N. T. (1992). Cognitive-behavioral pain management in children with juvenile rheumatoid arthritis. *Pediatrics, 89,* 1075–1079.

Walker, L. S. (1999). The evolution of research on recurrent abdominal pain: History, assumptions, and a conceptual model. In P. J. McGrath & G. A. Finley (Eds.), *Progress in pain research and management: Vol. 13. Chronic and recurrent pain in children and adolescents* (pp. 141–172). Seattle, WA: IASP Press.

Walker, L. S., Garber, J., & Greene, J. W. (1994). Somatic complaints in pediatric patients: A prospective study of the role of negative life events, child social and academic competence, and parental somatic symptoms. *Journal of Consulting and Clinical Psychology, 62,* 1213–1221.

Walker, L. S., Garber, J., Smith, C. A., Van Slyke, D. A., & Claar, R. L. (2001). The relation of daily stressors to somatic and emotional symptoms in children with and without recurrent abdominal pain. *Journal of Consulting and Clinical Psychology*, *69*, 85–91.

Walker, L. S., & Greene, J. W. (1991). The Functional Disability Inventory: Measuring a neglected dimension of child health-status. *Journal of Pediatric Psychology*, *16*, 39–58.

Walker, L. S., Smith, C. A., Garber, J., & Van Slyke, D. A. (1997). Development and validation of the Pain Response Inventory for children (PRI). *Psychological Assessment*, *9*, 392–405.

White, K., & Farrell, A. (2006). Anxiety and psychological stress as predictors of headache and abdominal pain in urban early adolescents. *Journal of Pediatric Psychology*, *31*, 582–596.

Wilder, R. T. (2003). Regional anesthetic techniques for chronic pain management. In N. Schechter, C. Berde, & M. Yaster (Eds.), *Pain in infants, children, and adolescent* (2nd ed., pp. 396–416). Philadelphia: Lippincott Williams & Wilkins.

Yaster, M., Kost-Byerly, S., & Maxwell, L. G. (2003). Opioid agonists and antagonist. In N. L. Schecter, C. B. Berde, & M. Yaster (Eds.), *Pain in infants, children, and adolescents* (2nd ed., pp. 181–224). Philadelphia: Lippincott Williams & Wilkins.

Yoon, S., & Black, S. (2006). Comprehensive, integrative management of pain for patients with sickle-cell disease. *Journal of Alternative and Complementary Medicine*, *12*, 995–1001.

Zebracki, K., Holzman, K., Bitter, K., Feehan, K., & Miller, M. (2007). Brief report: Use of complementary and alternative medicine and psychological functioning in Latino children with juvenile idiopathic arthritis or arthralgia. *Journal of Pediatric Psychology*, *32*, 1006–1010.

Zeltzer, L. K., Tsao, J. C. I., Bursch, B., & Myers, C. D. (2006). Introduction to the special issue on pain: From pain to pain-associated disability syndrome. *Journal of Pediatric Psychology*, *31*, 661–666.

Zieglgansberger, W., Berthele, A., & Tolle, T. R. (2005). Understanding neuropathic pain. *CNS Spectrums*, *10*, 298–308.

CHAPTER 11

Management of Pediatric Pain and Distress Due to Medical Procedures

RONALD L. BLOUNT
WILLIAM T. ZEMPSKY
TIINA JAANISTE
SUBHADRA EVANS
LINDSEY L. COHEN
KATIE A. DEVINE
LONNIE K. ZELTZER

From birth to the grave, painful medical procedures are a fact of life. Many procedures promote fear—both of the pain they may produce, and of the possible implications for the patient's health and well-being. For example, the Centers for Disease Control and Prevention (2008) recommends 24 immunization doses to be administered through multiple injections by age 15 months. This is in conjunction with other sticks, circumcision for males, and other procedures routinely performed on healthy infants. Prematurity, accidents, injuries, or disease necessitate additional care, almost always with concomitant painful procedures. The nature of early experiences may predispose better or worse reactions to later health care challenges. It is encouraging that there is a strong scientific foundation available for assisting people facing these and other potentially frightening and painful medical situations.

This chapter provides an evidence-based review of interventions for children's procedural pain. We focus briefly on correlated factors and assessment, and cover in greater depth psychological and pharmacological interventions. Special attention is devoted to pain in infants, as a vulnerable population for whom unique interventions have been developed. We also separately address preparation for surgery. Surgery is an area in which anxiety peaks during exposure to frightening but not painful stimuli in the operating room, particularly mask placement for anesthesia. Pharmacological approaches for pain and sedation are then reviewed.

Individual Differences and Correlated Factors

Pain responses vary widely among children. Some correlated and possibly causal factors include age and sex, temperament, experience, and parents' and medical staff members' behavior.

Age and Sex Differences

Younger children tend to report greater pain intensity and to show more behavioral distress than older children (Kleiber et al., 2007). Although results are equivocal, some research shows that girls report greater pain intensity. Piira, Taplin, Goodenough, and von Baeyer (2002) found that older boys (10–14 years old) demonstrated greater pain tolerance than girls during a cold-pressor task, but no sex differences were found for younger children (7–9 years old). Sex differences may become more pronounced in adolescence.

Temperament

A review by Ranger and Campbell-Yeo (2008) found that certain aspects of temperament were consistently associated with higher pain response, including low adaptability, low mood, low approach, and high emotionality. Pain-sensitive temperament was linked to higher distress during lumbar punctures (LPs), and children who were more pain-sensitive benefited more over time from an intervention to decrease distress during LPs (Chen, Craske, Katz, Schwartz, & Zeltzer, 2000).

Experience

The International Association for the Study of Pain (IASP) recognizes that pain is in part a learned experience (IASP Subcommittee on Taxonomy, 1979). Learning may occur through classical conditioning of external (e.g., medical equipment) and internal (e.g., cognitions, arousal) stimuli present during a painful procedure. Taddio, Shah, Gilbert-MacLeod, and Katz (2002) found that 24- to 36-hour-old newborns can develop classically conditioned anticipatory distress to alcohol swabs that precede heel lances. With repeated procedures, these classically conditioned stimuli may come to elicit distress and avoidance, leading to potential negative reinforcement, and consequently to greater fear and distress in medical contexts (Blount, Piira, & Cohen, 2003). Parent-rated child distress during prior medical treatments significantly predicted distress during preschoolers' immunization injections (Frank, Blount, Smith, Manimala, & Martin, 1995). Also, anticipatory distress prior to painful procedures is highly predictive of distress during subsequent painful phases of a medical procedure, although this relationship is not necessarily due to learning processes. For example, anticipatory distress several minutes before bone marrow aspirations (BMAs) was correlated ($r = .86$) with distress during the BMAs (Blount, Sturges, & Powers, 1990).

Whether because of learning, innate predispositions, or a combination of the two, the degree of distress experienced during injections children received while they were kindergarteners was predictive of children's somatization 7 years later (Rocha & Prkachin, 2007). Also, in a retrospective study, young adults' reports of their medical fear, procedural pain, and coping effectiveness during medical procedures they experienced as children were predictive of current self-reported procedural fear and pain (Pate, Smith, Blount, & Cohen, 1996). Furthermore, medical fear as children was predictive of avoidance of medical situations (e.g., clinic visits) as adults. Therefore, providing effective treatments to children in need may yield lifetime benefits.

Parents' and Medical Staff's Behavior

Through correlational and experimental studies, some parent and medical staff behaviors have been shown to be helpful to children (coping-promoting: nonprocedural talk, humor, and coaching), whereas others have been found to be detrimental (distress-promoting: reassurance, empathy, apologies, giving control, and criticism) (Blount et al., 1989, 1990; Blount, Landolf-Fritsche, Powers, & Sturges, 1991; Schechter et al., 2007). Distress-promoting comments focus children's attention on their own distress or on threatening aspects of the procedure, thereby heightening the children's distress, whereas coping promoting comments redirect attention elsewhere. For preschoolers receiving immunization injections, parent and nurse coping-promoting behaviors predicted 40% of the variance in child coping. Parent behavior accounted for 53% of the variance in child distress, with parent distress-promoting behavior being the significant predictor (Frank et al., 1995). Similar adult influences on infants' reactions to injections are described later in this chapter. In addition, training parents (Blount, Powers, Cotter, Swan, & Free, 1994) and nurses (Cohen, Blount, Cohen, Schaen, & Zaff, 1999) to distract children has yielded more child coping and less distress. Evidence for the detrimental effects of reassurance has been provided in at least two experimental investigations (Chambers, Craig, & Bennett, 2002; Manimala, Blount, & Cohen, 2000). There is also evidence for generalization of coping-promoting behaviors from trained parents to untrained nurses (Blount et al., 1992) and from trained nurses to untrained parents (Cohen, Blount, & Panopoulos, 1997).

The influential pattern of adult–child interactions appears to have generalizability across ages, medical procedures, and types of pain or discomfort. For example, Walker and colleagues (2006) used a water-loading procedure, in which patients with functional abdominal pain or healthy peers were instructed to drink as much water as they could. After that, both groups spent time with their mothers, who were instructed to interact with them in one of three ways. Either they engaged their children in attending conversation, which focused on sensations of fullness or discomfort; they engaged the children in distracting conversation, which directed attention to topics other than fullness, pain, or discomfort; or they were in a control condition where they could talk about any topic. Results indicated that the symptom complaints of healthy children and patients with pain were twice as high in the attention condition and half as high in the distraction condition. The adverse effects of attention were greater for girls than for boys. Also, children in the distraction condition rated parents as making them feel better, compared to ratings by children who were in the attention condition.

In summary, although age, sex, temperament, prior experience, and high anticipatory distress can help identify those who may be in need of training, they do not indicate what to do to assist the children. In contrast, low rates of adults' coping-promoting behaviors and high rates of distress-promoting behaviors, as well as low rates of child coping behaviors, are associated with higher child distress and indicate targets for intervention. Furthermore, there are effective coping skills training interventions to enhance adults' use of coping-promoting behaviors (e.g., Blount et al., 1994). For this reason, we strongly advocate teaching adults to use coping-promoting behaviors. If they do so, distress-promoting behaviors will naturally decrease. Training only parents or nurses to use coping-promoting prompts may be adequate for some children to increase their coping and lower their distress. If not, a child training component can be added.

Assessment

Methods for assessing procedural pain and distress include children's self-reports, reports by others, observational measures, and (less frequently) physiological monitoring. We do not believe that there is a "gold standard," with one assessment method clearly superior to others. Each approach has unique strengths and weaknesses. Rather than recommending particular instruments, we refer the reader to scholarly reviews by the Society of Pediatric Psychology's Evidence-Based Assessment (SPP-EBA) Task Force on Pain Assessment (Cohen et al., 2008) and by the Pediatric Initiative on Methods, Measurement, and Pain Assessment in Clinical Trials (Stinson, Kavanagh, Yamada, Gill, & Stevens, 2006; von Baeyer & Spagrud, 2007). There are both overlaps and differences in these two groups' findings. Some overlaps and differences in the reviews of observational measures are discussed by Blount and Loiselle (2009).

In addition to assessing pain and distress, we recommend measuring children's coping behaviors and adults' behaviors during the procedures. These malleable child and adult behaviors help determine the amount of pain and distress children will experience. A recent review of coping inventories by the SPP-EBA Task Force's Workgroup on Coping and Stress should aid in instrument selection (Blount, Simons, et al., 2008).

Preparing Children for Painful Procedures: Information Provision

Children who are better informed generally have lower distress and are better adjusted during and after the procedure. Timely, age-appropriate information may provide a degree of exposure that reduces anxiety to potentially frightening medical situations, as well as help the child and parents correctly anticipate what the procedure entails. Also, coping skills training may be conducted in conjunction with information provision (Jaaniste, Hayes, & von Baeyer, 2007b).

The type of preparation program is important. O'Byrne, Peterson, and Saldana (1997) surveyed hospital professionals, who rated coping skills, relaxation, and film as the most effective preparation procedures, and tours, printed materials, and narrative preparation as least effective. Of note, the least effective preparation procedures were endorsed as most frequently used, probably due to their ease of administration and low cost.

Regardless of the method used, preparatory information should be specific rather than general, and should include procedural (what will be done) and sensory (what the patient will experience or feel) information. The optimal timing of preparation may depend on the child's age and the nature of the procedure. Children need earlier and more extensive preparation for lengthier and more painful procedures, especially those requiring hospitalization or high levels of child cooperation. Kain, Mayes, and Caramico (1996) found that children age 6 years and older were least anxious if prepared 5–7 days prior to surgery, and most anxious if presented information within 24 hours of surgery. Younger children may benefit from preparatory information closer to the time of surgery. The effects of information were enhanced by the addition of a distraction intervention for children during an analogue pain induction procedure (Jaaniste, Hayes, & von Baeyer, 2007a). A clinical example of combining information with a multicomponent coping skills intervention is described below in the section on surgery preparation (Kain et al., 2007).

Attention Manipulation

Attention is the primary mechanism through which painful stimulation reaches awareness. Effective psychological interventions for acute pediatric pain and distress have in common the element of focusing patients' attention *away from* unpleasant sensory stimuli and/or distressing emotions, and *toward* relatively more pleasant and engaging alternative stimuli (Blount et al., 2003). Following is a review of attentional coping techniques, including sensory focusing, distraction, and other cognitive-behavioral therapy (CBT) techniques, as well as hypnosis.

Sensory Focusing

Sensory focusing involves directing attention to the physical sensations of the medical procedure, including pain or discomfort, in a nondistressing way. Attending to sensory aspects in a nonemotional manner has the possibility of disrupting sensation–distress associations. However, a study by Fanurik, Zeltzer, Roberts, and Blount (1993) found distraction to be more effective than sensory focusing (e.g., "Focus on the air bubbles on your arm") in a sample of 8- to 10-year-olds who had their arms in cold water during the cold-pressor pain task. Although Piira, Hayes, Goodenough, and von Baeyer (2006) also found distraction to be more effective for children age 9 years or younger, coping interventions that closely matched a child's coping style resulted in longer cold-pressor pain tolerance than mismatched interventions for older children. Thus the literature suggests that sensory focusing may prove useful for older children who prefer an approach coping style, in which they would focus on, rather than away from, the stressor. Otherwise, distraction techniques have more support. The effectiveness of sensory focusing also needs to be investigated in clinical contexts that involve acute pain.

Distraction and Multicomponent Cognitive-Behavioral Interventions

As part of the work of the SPP Empirically Supported Treatment Task Force, Powers (1999) reviewed CBT interventions for procedure-related pain. He noted that various approaches were used (often in combination), including distraction (Elliott & Olson, 1983; Kazak et al., 1996), breathing exercises (Jay, Elliott, Katz, & Siegel, 1987), behavioral rehearsal (Blount et al., 1994), relaxation and positive self-talk (Dahlquist, Gil, Armstrong, Ginsberg, & Jones, 1985), emotive imagery (Jay et al., 1987), reinforcement for cooperation (Elliott & Olson, 1983), training parents to coach their children to use coping behaviors (Blount et al., 1994), and having nurses prompt children to watch cartoon videos (Cohen et al., 1997). These CBT procedures led to increased use of coping skills, parents' and medical staff members' coaching the children, and reduced pain and distress. Some investigations that included comparisons with pharmacological agents found CBT to be as effective as, or more effective than, such agents as diazepam (Valium) (Jay et al., 1987) or EMLA cream (discussed later) (Cohen et al., 1999). Also, the combination of CBT with midazolam (Versed) was better than midazolam alone on some outcome variables (Kazak et al., 1996). Powers (1999) concluded that CBT met criteria to be considered as a "well-established treatment" for procedural pain in children and adolescents.

The beneficial effects of distraction have also been supported in a meta-analysis (Kleiber & Harper, 1999). Furthermore, in a Cochrane Database review, Uman, Chambers, McGrath, and Kisely (2006) studied psychosocial interventions for 2- to 19-year-olds undergoing needle procedures. The largest effect sizes for treatment versus control conditions existed for distraction and multicomponent CBT interventions, with hypnosis being promising. Promising evidence was also found for other interventions, including information/preparation procedures and nurse coaching to promote child distraction. It is encouraging that the data converge to support the effectiveness of distraction in particular, as well as multicomponent CBT interventions.

Virtual reality (VR) is a novel technique for promoting distraction. VR equipment typically consists of a head-mounted visual display with auditory input. In a review, Lange, Williams, and Fulton (2006) concluded that the evidence for the use of VR was strongest for burns. As an intervention for the pain caused by treating burn injuries, Hoffman, Doctor, Patterson, Carrougher, and Furness (2000) designed Snow World, in which a patient moves through an ice world with a video-game-like atmosphere. Pain was reduced in several studies (see *www.hitl.washington.edu/projects/vrpain*; Hoffman et al., 2000). Some limitations of VR include the cost and technical expertise required; the necessity of proper head orientation, which makes it difficult for patients in prone positions to use; and possible impaired communication with the patient.

Effective Use of Distraction Procedures

Regardless of the techniques for promoting distraction, the stimuli or activity should be highly engaging, should be easily performed, and should require an observable response. Observable responses confirm that the coping behavior is being performed. In addition, prompts by adults can help facilitate children's coping and redirect their attention as needed away from compelling painful or frightening medical procedures. There is some evidence that coping/distracting activities should be matched to the demands of different medical phases (Blount et al., 1990). For example, in one study, distracting conversations or toy play helped to lower anticipatory distress, but these techniques were replaced with prompted use of a party blower during painful LPs (Blount et al., 1994). Using a party blower is simple, is distracting, and requires less thought by the child than nonprocedural talk during painful LPs would require. During painful procedures, simple distraction techniques that do not exceed a patient's limited attentional capacity at that time are probably more effective.

Hypnosis

Hypnosis involves a state of increased suggestibility, attention, and relaxation. Although the exact mechanism of its action is not well understood, neuroimaging techniques show that hypnosis is associated with activation of brain areas consistent with decreased arousal, visual imagery, and possible reinterpretation of perceptual experiences (Wood & Bioy, 2008). Hypnosis has been used with children experiencing BMAs (Liossi & Hatira, 2003), fracture pain (Iserson, 1999), and postoperative pain and anxiety (Lambert, 1996). Uman and colleagues (2006) found hypnosis to be a promising intervention for self-reported pain in children and adolescents. However, hypnosis may be less effective for children under 5 years of age, and some people are not easily hypnotized (Liossi, White, & Hatira, 2006). Challenges in the area include the lack of agreement over operational definitions of hypnosis, as well as the heterogeneity of techniques that have been used (hypnotherapy, guided imagery, imagery). Future research should establish standardized treatment manuals and should attempt to understand efficacy as a function of child age and pain type.

Combining Information Provision and Attention Manipulation

A revised version of our prescriptive model of medical and coping interventions by phase of medical procedure (Blount et al., 2003) is presented in Table 11.1. Information provision including both sensory and procedural components should be presented to both child and parent during Phase 1, the time prior to the procedure. Most studies indicate that preparation should occur about a week to several days before the procedure, at least for older children (Jaaniste et al., 2007b; Kain et al., 1996). This duration may allow a child to mentally prepare for the event or give time for anxiety to diminish via prolonged exposure to the information. Preparation is also a time for training parents in coping promoting skills and training children to use coping behaviors before and during medical treatments. Home practice can also be incorporated.

During Phase 2, the child and parent are in the medical setting anticipating the procedure. Rather than introducing new information or dwelling on the upcoming event, playful nonprocedural activities and conversation should be used. These activities help to lower the child's fear and anxiety before the procedure, and therefore predispose him or her to lower distress during the next phase (Blount et al., 1990). As the procedure becomes imminent and preprocedural instructions are given (e.g., "Climb on the table"), parents and staff should continue to provide distracting prompts, albeit allowing for necessary procedural comments (e.g., "a little stick").

Phase 3 includes encounter with the painful procedure. Active coaching should continue. For less painful procedures, distraction techniques such as a continuation of Phase 2's use of interactive cartoon viewing (Cohen et al., 1999) may suffice. For more painful procedures, such as LPs, prompted use of simple coping behaviors that require little cognitive processing (e.g., deep breathing or use of distracting party blowers) may be preferable. If so, practice during the preparation phase may be necessary to facilitate a child's performance of the desired behaviors. Alternatively, if a trained therapist is available, hypnosis may be used (Uman et al., 2006).

TABLE 11.1. Prescriptive Model of Medical and Coping Interventions by Phase of Medical Procedure

	Phase1	Phase 2	Phase 3	Phase 4	Phase 5
Temporal proximity to procedure	Approach of the procedure	Anticipatory phase (in the setting prior to medical procedure)	Procedure (during the procedure)	Postprocedure (immediately after the procedure)	Completion (minutes to hours or more after the procedure)
Child experiences	Preparation for upcoming event	Anticipation of imminent event	Encounter with the stimulus and stress	Recovery from pain and distress	Recollection and return to normal daily activities
Proportion of information provision to distraction	• Offer age-appropriate sensory and procedural information to child and parents about the upcoming procedure. • Provide opportunities to ask questions. • Simple, less painful procedures require less preparation.	• Decrease both information provision and the child's focus on the upcoming procedure. • Increase distraction.	• Provide primarily distraction and minimal information as needed. • Distraction is greatest and information provision lowest in this phase.	• Continue mild forms of distraction. • Begin resumption of normal activities as appropriate.	• Continue resumption of normal life activities.
Coping interventions	• Train child and adults in specific coping and coping-promoting behaviors, as well as when to use them. • Anxiety reduction occurs via exposure to aspects of the stressor, perhaps through coping skills practice. • These factors increase child's and parents' sense of mastery.	• Have parents/staff prompt child's use of coping strategies. • Coping behaviors may include movies, nonprocedural talk, toy play, and other engaging activities. • Use problem-focused, not emotion-focused, coping. • Supportive, skilled parents and staff instill confidence.	• Coach/prompt child to use coping behaviors. Coping behaviors during painful procedures are often simple, such as breathing or using a party blower. • Minimize avoidance. • Lower distress/pain should lead to less classical conditioning.	• Distracting activity or talk can speed reductions in distress, but allow child to recover if needed. Be sensitive to child's lead and receptiveness to efforts. • Focus on successful coping and instill sense of achievement.	• Focus child's attention on positive coping efforts to prompt memory encoding of successful coping and nonexaggeration of distress. • If pain persists, continue engaging activities (e.g., movie, talk) as needed if child is receptive.
Medical factors to consider and interventions to use	• Assess the child's history with procedures, physical condition, painfulness, and other aspects of the medical procedure. Child may be shown and allowed to handle simple versions of equipment, such as placing mask for anesthesia.	• Use topical or other anesthetics and, if necessary, sedation and analgesics. • Use less threatening or painful medical instruments, such as small-gauge needles. • Maintain child-friendly environment if possible.	• Use less painful medical equipment (e.g., smaller needles) and topical anesthesia. • Keep unexpected events to a minimum.	• Use pain-reducing medications as needed.	• Use pain-reducing medications if needed.

178

Distress diminishes during Phase 4, and less intense attentional redirection activities can be used to help speed the child's recovery. It is important to be sensitive to the child's state, as children may be less responsive after highly painful and distressing events. Attempting to engage children when they are not likely to be responsive can increase frustration and distress.

During Phase 5, when the procedure is over and the child has recovered, adults should praise the child for his or her coping attempts and emphasize the good things the child did. This may help the child remember the event as less distressing and the coping efforts as more beneficial. Chen, Zeltzer, Craske, and Katz (1999) have used a prompted and selective memory-encoding procedure similar to this to help children who must undergo repeated painful procedures.

Preparation for Surgery

Children's perioperative anxiety is predictive of adverse postsurgical outcomes, including more pain, increased emergence delirium, and negative postoperative behaviors (Kain et al., 2007). Methods for reducing perioperative anxiety include (1) sedative administration before surgery, (2) parental presence, (3) preparation and coping skills, and (4) hypnosis (Kain et al., 2007; Wright, Stewart, Finley, & Buffett-Jerrott, 2007). Midazolam is a commonly used sedative administered prior to surgery. Doses in the range of 0.25 to 0.50 mg/kg are effective for reducing anxiety within 20–30 minutes (Wright et al., 2007). However, in some patients midazolam has resulted in longer time to discharge, longer recovery times, and some maladaptive postsurgical behaviors, such as nightmares (Wright et al., 2007).

Parental presence during mask anesthesia induction has also been investigated. Although most children prefer a parent to be with them, well-controlled randomized trials have not found evidence supporting the benefit of parental presence for reducing children's presurgical anxiety (Piira, Sugiura, Champion, Donnelly, & Cole, 2005; Wright et al., 2007). Instead, it is probable that *what* parents do is more critical than their mere presence (Caldwell-Andrews, Blount, Mayes, & Kain, 2005; Piira et al., 2005). Investigations are currently underway to assess the impact of adults' behaviors on children's coping and distress during anesthesia induction.

Preparation programs for surgery have included information provision, modeling to convey what to expect and how to cope, and training of the child and others in coping procedures (Blount, McCormick, MacLaren, & Kain, 2008; Jaaniste et al., 2007a). Kain and colleagues (2007) used a randomized clinical trial to evaluate the effectiveness of standard care, parental presence, oral midazolam at 0.50 mg/kg, and the multicomponent ADVANCE program. ADVANCE includes techniques for anxiety reduction, distraction, video modeling and education, avoiding excessive reassurance, incorporating parents, parent coaching of the child in the holding area through induction, and a parent-directed home-based exposure/shaping component to promote mask familiarity and acceptance. Children in the ADVANCE group exhibited lower anxiety in the holding area; similar anxiety to that of children in the midazolam condition, and lower anxiety than that of the other two groups during mask induction; and less emergence delirium, less need for fentanyl for pain relief, and quicker discharge than children in the other three groups following surgery.

Calipel, Lucas-Polomeni, Wodey, and Ecoffey (2005) compared hypnosis to oral midazolam. Results indicated lower anxiety during mask induction and fewer postsurgical behavior problems for children receiving hypnosis versus midazolam. Although this approach appears useful, replication would benefit from clearer operational definitions for the intervention.

Interventions for Infants

There is a growing body of literature documenting behavioral approaches for acute pain relief in infants. Many of these interventions are primarily physical or sensory in nature, including massage, holding and rocking, providing pacifiers, and providing skin-to-skin contact. For example, Johnston and colleagues (2002) found that having parents hold neonates against their chests and providing skin-to-skin contact for 30 minutes prior to heel lancing resulted in significant reductions in pain behavior. This technique, called "kangaroo care," is becoming a widely accepted method of providing comfort and minimizing pain for premature infants.

A review by Stevens, Yamada, and Ohlsson (2004) supports the use of sucrose water (12–50%) given immediately prior to a medical event to minimize pain for young infants. It is typically given by either dipping a pacifier into a sucrose solution or instilling it directly into an infant's mouth with a syringe. Sucrose may work primarily via the mechanism of attention redirection; infants may be particularly attentive to sweet, pleasant taste sensations.

Cohen (2002) found that nurse-led movie distraction for 2- to 36-month-olds receiving immunizations led to lower pain during the anticipatory and recovery phases than was found in a control condition. Cohen and colleagues (2006) replicated these findings with 1- to 26-month-olds. However, Cramer-Berness and Friedman (2005) found no benefit for distraction provided by parents using toys for 2- to 24-month-olds undergoing immunizations. In contrast, infants whose parents offered supportive care using strategies they had found helpful in the past were less distressed than those in the typical care condition. In combination, these studies provide support for distraction for lowering infants' distress, provided that sufficiently distracting stimuli are used. Cramer-Berness and Friedman's results also indicate that some as yet unidentified parental behaviors may result in lower infant distress. Bustos, Jaaniste, Salmon, and Champion (2008) provide some illumination to this issue, finding that parents who were instructed to use coping promoting behaviors (nonprocedural talk and humor) had 4- to 6-month-olds who were less distressed during immunizations than infants in a standard care condition were.

As they do with older children, parents play a critical role in helping manage infants' medical distress. Piira, Champion, Bustos, Donnelly, and Lui (2007) examined parent–infant interactions with the Child–Adult Medical Procedure Interaction Scale—Revised (CAMPIS-R; Blount et al., 1997), and found that maternal coping-promoting behaviors were correlated negatively with infant distress and the duration of crying following injections. Using the Measure of Adult and Infant Soothing and Distress (MAISD), Cohen, Bernard, Mcclellan, and MacLaren (2005) showed that infants engaged in distraction when parents or nurses attempted to engage them or offered toys. Distress was positively associated with parent and nurse reassurance. Blount, Devine, Cheng,

Simons, and Hayutin (2008) used the Infant Version of the CAMPIS (CAMPIS-IV) to conduct a sequential analytic investigation of parent, nurse, and infant behaviors that influenced 2- to 20-month-olds' level of crying following immunizations. Strong support was found for the benefits of sucking a bottle or pacifier, holding an infant in a belly-to-belly position, nonprocedural talk to the infant, and having the infant play with objects. Some support was found for bouncing, rocking, and patting the baby. No support was found for adults' reassurance, apologies, or empathic statements to an infant; there was even some indication that reassurance might be detrimental. Behavioral observation studies using such instruments as the CAMPIS-IV and the MAISD may inform the development of new interventions or refine existing ones.

Pharmacological Management of Procedural Pain and Distress

When choosing pharmacological interventions for procedural pain and anxiety, the patient's age as well as the invasiveness, painfulness, and duration of the procedure must be considered. Some procedures, such as venous access, routinely require local or topical anesthetics; others, whether painful (e.g., LP) or nonpainful (e.g., magnetic resonance imaging, or MRI), may require potent sedatives and analgesics. It is important for psychologists and other nonmedical professionals working in the area of acute pain management to have a basic familiarity with pharmacological approaches.

Topical and Local Anesthetics

Topical and local anesthetics are the drugs of choice for simple procedures such as venipuncture, venous access, laceration repair, subcutaneous port access, and dermatological procedures (Zempsky, 2006). Among these agents, lidocaine injected subcutaneously is effective for decreasing pain from venous access, dermatological procedures, and laceration repair. Lidocaine can be injected with little pain if the technique includes buffering with bicarbonate, warming it before injecting, and injecting slowly with a small-gauge needle.

Topical anesthetics allow for needleless dermal anesthesia. However, each topical agent has some shortcoming, such as the time required to work or lack of adaptability to different procedures (Zempsky, 2006). The most extensively studied of these agents, Eutectic Mixture of Local Anesthetics (EMLA) cream, has been shown to be effective for a variety of procedures, including venous cannulation, venipuncture, immunization, subcutaneous port access, and LPs (Uhari, 1993). EMLA is safe when used appropriately, even in premature infants. Unfortunately, EMLA requires 60 minutes to provide adequate anesthesia. EMLA can be used for nonemergent procedures when properly anticipated (Zempsky, 2006).

LMX4 is a liposomal lidocaine cream-based formulation similar to EMLA; however, it provides efficacy in only 30 minutes. LMX4 has not been well studied for procedures other than venous access, and its safety in children under age 3 has not been established. In many centers, it is used interchangeably with EMLA (Kleiber, Sorenson, Whiteside, Gronstal, & Tannous, 2002).

Synera, a patch containing lidocaine and tetracaine, includes a heating system that accelerates transcutaneous delivery and analgesic effect within 20–30 minutes. Synera is safe and effective for venous access and dermatological procedures (Sethna et al., 2005). Tetracaine and heat both cause vasodilatation, which may facilitate venous access.

Iontophoresis promotes the rapid transfer of lidocaine, which is positively charged, into the skin under the influence of electric current (Zempsky, Anand, Sullivan, Fraser, & Cucina, 1998). Lidocaine iontophoresis is superior to EMLA as a topical anesthetic for venous access and does not produce systemic lidocaine levels during routine use. However, some patients experience tingling, itching, or burning with this technology, which has limited its acceptance.

Vapocoolant sprays, such as ethyl chloride and flourimethane, work in about 30 seconds and are inexpensive. However, the evidence regarding their efficacy for injection pain and venous access procedures is conflicting (Costello, Ramundo, Christopher, & Powell, 2006; Reis & Holubkov, 1997). Also, some children find their cold sensation unpleasant.

Zingo is a product that utilizes a prefilled needleless compressed helium gas system to accelerate powdered lidocaine into the skin. Zingo is safe, and anesthesia is achieved painlessly in about 1 minute. Studies of Zingo have not been done for injections, but show efficacy for both venipuncture and venous access procedures (Zempsky, Robbins, Leong, & Schechter, 2008).

LET, used exclusively for laceration repair, is a combination of lidocaine, epinephrine, and tetracaine that can be made by a hospital pharmacy. When placed in a wound 20–30 minutes prior to laceration repair, LET provides excellent anesthesia for facial lacerations, and can be used to reduce the pain of lidocaine infiltration for extremity lacerations (Ernst et al., 1995). LET is safe, but should not be used on mucous membranes or digits.

Procedural Sedation

In choosing sedation agents, it is important to consider whether the procedure will be painful (e.g., BMA, fracture reduction), less painful but anxiety-producing (e.g., voiding cystourethrogram [VCUG], laceration repair with local anesthesia), or nonpainful but requiring motionlessness (e.g., MRI). Guidelines describe the appropriate monitoring a child should receive during and after procedural sedation (American Academy of Pediatrics Committee on Drugs, 2002; American Society of Anesthesiologists Task Force, 2002). Sedation carries risks that include hypoventilation, apnea, airway obstruction, aspiration, laryngospasm, and cardiopulmonary impairment. Although any of the commonly used agents described below can result in deep sedation, they are presented in order of targeted endpoint from minimal to deep sedation. For a full review, see Krauss and Green (2006).

Midazolam (Versed) is an anxiolytic agent that can be given intravenously, orally, nasally, or rectally. It can be used alone (VCUG, preoperative anxiety), as an adjunct with a local or topical anesthetic (laceration repair, LP), or with an analgesic (fracture reduction, BMA) to reduce anxiety. It does not provide motionlessness and can lead to disinhibition. Side effects include respiratory depression, airway obstruction, and paradoxical excitement.

Nitrous oxide has anxiolytic and analgesic properties that make it useful alone or in conjunction with a local or topical anesthetic for a variety of procedures (dental, VCUG, laceration repair, sexual abuse exam). It is inhaled via a mask. Side effects include respiratory and myocardial depression. Nitrous oxide may be a teratogen, and therefore a scavenger system must be available for collecting waste gases.

Chloral hydrate is a hypnotic agent given orally or rectally. It has no analgesic action, but does provide motionlessness for diagnostic imaging or electroencephalography. Problems with chloral hydrate include its inconsistent action, a high percentage of sedation failures, and a long duration of action. Side effects include respiratory depression and agitation.

Barbiturates (methohexital, pentobarbital), usually reserved for diagnostic imaging procedures, provide sedation and motionlessness, but no analgesic action. Side effects include respiratory depression, hypotension, paradoxical excitement, and impaired mood.

Opiates (fentanyl, sufentinyl, morphine, hydromorphone) are excellent analgesics that can be used along with such agents as propofol or midazolam during sedation. Fentanyl, a semisythetic opioid, is the most commonly used of these agents for this purpose. It has a shorter onset and half-life and is more potent than morphine or hydromorphone. Side effects of opiates include respiratory depression, nausea, vomiting, and itching.

Ketamine is a dissociative and an excellent anesthetic. It is used for painful procedures such as fracture reduction, large or complex laceration repairs, and chest tube placements. Ketamine causes nystagmus and a trance-like appearance, which often scare parents observing the procedure. Potential side effects include laryngospasm, raised intracranial pressure and intraocular pressure, disinibition, and agitation.

Propofol is an anesthetic agent with a rapid onset and offset that is increasingly being used for various procedures (e.g., fracture reduction, imaging, colonoscopy) by nonanesthesiologists. It has no analgesic action, so it must be used in conjunction with an analgesic during painful procedures. Side effects include respiratory depression and hypotension.

Integration of Psychological and Pharmacological Approaches

Pediatric procedural pain and distress include both psychological and physiological components, and it is often necessary to approach this area in an integrated way. In the prescriptive model presented in Table 11.1, we describe the medical factors to consider, along with interventions that are appropriate at the different phases. In addition to assessment during Phase 1, medical management of procedural pain and distress occurs primarily in the time periods in close temporal proximity before and after (and, of course, during) procedures. For simple procedures, topical anesthesia is sufficient, whereas for more complicated interventions, sedation may be required. Effective psychological intervention may reduce the need for or amount of anesthetic or sedative agents, primarily through lowering preprocedural anxiety and distracting attention from painful stimuli. As noted earlier, several studies have shown psychological approaches in some cases to be as effective as, or more effective than, such pharmacological agents as EMLA (Cohen et al., 1999), diazepam (Jay et al., 1987), and midazolam (Kain et al., 2007). There is also evidence that combined psychological and pharmacological approaches are more effective than pharmacological agents alone (Kazak et al., 1996). Conversely, effective topical anesthesia that reduces pain may reduce children's anxiety about subsequent procedures. Developing optimal combinations of medical and psychological approaches to managing procedural pain and distress will be a priority for future research.

Commentary and Future Directions

Perhaps because pediatric procedural pain and distress are so compelling, considerable research attention has been devoted to this area over the last three to four decades. Pioneering researchers have made notable advances in both psychosocial and medical approaches to addressing this problem. In many ways, this is one of the more developed areas of pediatric psychology: Technologies for assessment and treatment of pain now exist for populations from premature infants through adolescents, and across a host of painful or frightening procedures.

As any field matures, new frontiers for research may shift from stunning innovation to more precise refinement of assessment and intervention techniques, as well as better application and dissemination of established principles. In many ways, the field of procedural pain management is at that juncture. A firm foundation has been laid and should be built upon. Creativity is needed, and often this may take the form of pulling together different bodies of existing knowledge in unique ways or implementing what is known into additional areas of pediatric health care.

Future research should include additional attention to social influences on preprocedural pain and anxiety in different populations of children. For example, research is currently being conducted on how voice quality or intonation may interface with vocal content (e.g., reassuring comments) to facilitate distress. In addition, the influence of social interactions is being assessed in new populations, including patients with functional abdominal pain (Walker et al., 2006), those undergoing mask anesthesia induction (Kain et al., 2007), and infants (e.g., Piira et al., 2007). Results from these studies can help inform research with additional pediatric populations whose acute, episodic, and persistent pain may be influenced by similar factors.

Dissemination of medical and psychosocial approaches for procedural pain management from research to applied clinical settings is an ongoing issue. As in many other fields, bringing about enduring change in health care practices in applied settings can be problematic, or at the very least, gradual. Collaboration with medical professionals in applied settings, publishing in different psychological and medical journals to reach a wider audience, and presenting new research at local meetings that may be more likely to attract practitioners may help facilitate translation of research into practice. Also, it is possible that pediatric pain researchers may benefit from collaboration with industrial–organizational psychologists in their dissemination efforts. Furthermore, the use of novel methods of intervention, such as interactive computer programs for training basic coping skills to parents and children seeking medical treatment, may be a way to circumvent logistical obstacles in busy clinic settings.

References

American Academy of Pediatrics Committee on Drugs. (2002). Guidelines for monitoring and management of pediatric patients during and after sedation for diagnostic and therapeutic procedures: Addendum. *Pediatrics, 110,* 836–838.

American Society of Anesthesiologists Task Force on Sedation and Analgesia by Nonanesthesiologists. (2002). Practice guidelines for sedation and analgesia by nonanesthesiologists. *Anesthesiology, 96,* 1004–1017.

Blount, R. L., Bachanas, P. J., Powers, S. W., Cotter, M., Franklin, A., Chaplin, W., et al. (1992). Training children to cope and parents to coach them during routine immunizations: Effects on child, parent and staff behaviors. *Behavior Therapy*, 23, 689–705.

Blount, R. L., Cohen, L. L., Frank, N. C., Bachanas, P. J., Smith, A. J., Manimala, M. R., et al. (1997). The Child–Adult Medical Procedure Interaction Scale—Revised: An assessment of validity. *Journal of Pediatric Psychology*, 22, 73–88.

Blount, R. L., Corbin, S. M., Sturges, J. W., Wolfe, V. V., Prater, J. M., & James, L. D. (1989). The relationship between adults behavior and child coping and distress during BMA/LP procedures: A sequential analysis. *Behavior Therapy*, 20, 585–601.

Blount, R. L., Devine, K. A., Cheng, P. S., Simons, L. E., & Hayutin, L. (2008). The influence of adult behaviors and vocalizations on infant distress during immunizations. *Journal of Pediatric Psychology*, 33, 1163–1174.

Blount, R. L., Landolf-Fritsche, B., Powers, S. W., & Sturges, J. W. (1991). Differences between high and low coping children and between parent and staff behaviors during painful medical procedures. *Journal of Pediatric Psychology*, 16, 795–809.

Blount, R. L., & Loiselle, K. A. (2009). Behavioural assessment of pediatric pain. *Pain Research and Management*, 14, 47–52.

Blount, R. L., McCormick, M. L., MacLaren, J. E., & Kain, Z. (2008). Preparing children for invasive procedures and surgery. In G. A. Walco & K. R. Goldschneider (Eds.). *Pain in children: A practical guide for primary care* (pp. 93–99). Totowa, NJ: Humana Press.

Blount, R. L., Piira, T., & Cohen, L. L. (2003). Management of pediatric pain and distress due to medical procedures. In M. C. Roberts (Ed.), *Handbook of pediatric psychology* (3rd ed., pp. 216–233). New York: Guilford Press.

Blount, R. L., Powers, S. W., Cotter, M. W., Swan, S. C., & Free, K. (1994). Making the system work: Training pediatric oncology patients to cope and their parents to coach them during BMA/LP procedures. *Behavior Modification*, 18, 6–31.

Blount, R. L., Simons, L. E., Devine, K. A., Jaaniste, T., Cohen, L. L., Chambers, C., et al. (2008). Evidence-based assessment of coping and stress in pediatric psychology. *Journal of Pediatric Psychology*, 33, 1021–1045.

Blount, R. L., Sturges, J. W., & Powers, S. W. (1990). Analysis of child and adult behavioral variations by phase of medical procedure. *Behavior Therapy*, 21, 33–48.

Bustos, T., Jaaniste, T., Salmon, K., & Champion, G. D. (2008). Evaluation of a brief parent intervention teaching coping-promoting behavior for the infant immunization context. *Behavior Modification*, 32, 450–467.

Caldwell-Andrews, A. A., Blount, R. L., Mayes, L. C., & Kain, Z. N. (2005). Behavioral interactions in the perioperative environment: A new conceptual framework an the development of the Perioperative Child–Adult Medical Procedure Interaction Scale. *Anesthesiology*, 103(6), 1130–1135.

Calipel, S., Lucas-Polomeni, M., Wodey, E., & Ecoffey, C. (2005). Premedication in children: Hypnosis versus midazolam. *Pediatric Anesthesia*, 15, 275–281.

Centers for Disease Control and Prevention. (2008). Recommended immunization schedules for persons aged 0–18 years—United States, 2008. *Morbidity and Mortality Weekly Report*, 56(51–52), Q1–Q4.

Chambers, C. T., Craig, K. D., & Bennett, S. M. (2002). The impact of maternal behavior on children's pain experiences: An experimental analysis. *Journal of Pediatric Psychology*, 27, 293–301.

Chen, E., Craske, M. G., Katz, E. R., Schwartz, E., & Zeltzer, L. K. (2000). Pain-sensitive temperament: Does it predict procedural distress and response to psychological treatment among children with cancer? *Journal of Pediatric Psychology*, 25, 269–278.

Chen, E., Zeltzer, L. K., Craske, M. G., & Katz, E. R. (1999). Alternation of memory in the reduction of children's distress during repeated aversive medical procedures. *Journal of Consulting and Clinical Psychology, 67,* 481–490.

Cohen, L. L. (2002). Reducing infant immunization distress through distraction. *Health Psychology, 21,* 207–211.

Cohen, L. L., Bernard, R. S., McClellan, C. B., & MacLaren, J. E. (2005). Assessing medical room behavior during infants' painful medical procedures: The Measure of Adult and Infant Soothing and Distress (MAISD). *Children's Health Care, 34,* 81–94.

Cohen, L. L., Blount, R. L., Cohen, R. J., Schaen, E. R., & Zaff, J. F. (1999). A comparative study of distraction versus topical anesthesia for pediatric pain management during immunizations. *Health Psychology, 18,* 591–598.

Cohen, L. L., Blount, R. L., & Panopoulos, G. (1997). Nurse coaching and cartoon distraction: An effective and practical intervention to reduce child, parent, and nurse distress during immunizations. *Journal of Pediatric Psychology, 22,* 355–370.

Cohen, L. L., Lemanek, K., Blount, R. L., Dahlquist, L. M., Lim, C. S., Palermo, T. M., et al. (2008). Evidence-based assessment of pediatric pain. *Journal of Pediatric Psychology, 33,* 939–955.

Cohen, L. L., MacLaren, J. E., Fortson, B. L., Friedman, A., DeMore, M., Lim, C. S., et al. (2006). Randomized clinical trial of distraction for infant immunization pain. *Pain, 125,* 165–171.

Costello, M., Ramundo, M., Christopher, N. C., & Powell, K. R. (2006). Ethyl vinyl chloride vapocoolant spray fails to decrease pain associated with intravenous cannulation in children. *Clinical Pediatrics, 45,* 628–632.

Cramer-Berness, L. J., & Friedman, A. J. (2005). Behavioral interventions for infant immunizations. *Children's Health Care, 34,* 95–111.

Dahlquist, L. M., Gil, K. M., Armstrong, F. D., Ginsberg, A., & Jones, B. (1985). Behavioral management of children's distress during chemotherapy. *Journal of Behavior Therapy and Experimental Psychiatry, 16,* 325–329.

Elliott, C., & Olson, R. (1983). The management of children's distress in response to painful medical treatment for burn injuries. *Behaviour Research and Therapy, 12,* 675–683.

Ernst, A. A., Marvez, E., Nick, T. G., Chin, E., Wood, E., & Gonzaba, W. T. (1995). Lidocaine adrenaline tetracaine gel versus tetracaine adrenaline cocaine gel for topical anesthesia in linear scalp and facial lacerations in children aged 5 to 17 years. *Pediatrics, 95,* 255–258.

Fanurik, D., Zeltzer, L., Roberts, M., & Blount, R. L. (1993). The relationship between children's coping styles and psychological interventions for cold pressor pain. *Pain, 53,* 213–222.

Frank, N. C., Blount, R. L., Smith, A. J., Manimala, M. R., & Martin, J. K. (1995). Parent and staff behavior, previous child medical experience, and maternal anxiety as they relate to child distress and coping. *Journal of Pediatric Psychology, 20,* 277–289.

Hoffman, H. G., Doctor, J. N., Patterson, D. R., Carrougher, G. J., & Furness, T. A. (2000). Virtual reality as an adjunctive pain control during burn wound care in adolescent patients. *Pain, 85,* 305–309.

International Association for the Study of Pain (IASP) Subcommittee on Taxonomy. (1979). Pain terms: A list with definitions and notes on usage. *Pain, 6,* 249–252.

Iserson, K. V. (1999). Hypnosis for pediatric fracture reduction. *Journal of Emergency Medicine, 17,* 53–56.

Jaaniste, T., Hayes, B., & von Baeyer, C. L. (2007a). Effects of preparatory information and distraction on children's cold-pressor pain outcomes: A randomized controlled trial. *Behaviour Research and Therapy, 45,* 2789–2799.

Jaaniste, T., Hayes, B., & von Baeyer, C. L. (2007b). Providing children with information about forthcoming medical procedures: A review and synthesis. *Clinical Psychology: Science and Practice, 14,* 124–143.

Jay, S. M., Elliott, C. H., Katz, E., & Siegel, S. E. (1987). Cognitive-behavioral and pharmacologic interventions for children's distress during painful medical procedures. *Journal of Consulting and Clinical Psychology, 55,* 860–865.

Johnston, C. C., Stevens, B., Pinelli, J., Gibbins, S., Filion, F., Jack, A., et al. (2002). Kangaroo care is effective in diminishing pain response in preterm neonates. *Archives of Pediatrics and Adolescent Medicine, 157* (11), 1084–1088.

Kain, Z. N., Caldwell-Andrews, A. , Mayes, L. C., Weinberg, M. E., Wang, S., MacLaren, J. E., et al. (2007). Family-centered preparation for surgery improves perioperative outcomes in children: A randomized controlled trial. *Anesthesiology, 106,* 65–74.

Kain, Z. N., Mayes, L. C., & Caramico, L. A. (1996). Preoperative preparation in children: A cross-sectional study. *Journal of Clinical Anesthesia, 8,* 508–514.

Kazak, A. E., Penati, B., Boyer, B. A., Himelstein, B., Brophy, P., Waibel, M. K., et al. (1996). A randomized controlled prospective study of a psychological and pharmacological intervention protocol for procedural distress in pediatric leukemia. *Journal of Pediatric Psychology, 21,* 615–631.

Kleiber, C., & Harper, D. C. (1999). Effects of distraction on children's pain and distress drug medical procedures: A meta-analysis. *Nursing Research, 48,* 44–49.

Kleiber, C., Schutte, D., McCarthy, A., Floria-Santos, M., Murray, J., & Hanrahan, K. (2007). Predictors of topical anesthetic effectiveness in children. *Journal of Pain, 8,* 168–174.

Kleiber, C., Sorenson, M., Whiteside, K., Gronstal, B. A., & Tannous, R. (2002). Topical anesthetics for intravenous insertion in children: A randomized equivalency study. *Pediatrics, 110,* 758–761.

Krauss, B., & Green, S. M. (2006). Procedural sedation and analgesia in children. *Lancet, 367,* 766–780.

Lambert, S. A. (1996). The effects of hypnosis/guided imagery on the postoperative course of children. *Journal of Developmental and Behavioral Pediatrics, 17*(5), 307–310.

Lange, B., Williams, M., & Fulton, I. (2006). Virtual reality distraction during pediatric medical procedures. *Pediatric Pain Letter, 8*(1), 6–10.

Liossi, C., & Hatira, P. (2003). Clinical hypnosis in the alleviation of procedure-related pain in pediatric oncology patients. *International Journal of Clinical and Experimental Hypnosis, 51*(1), 4–28.

Liossi, C., White, P., & Hatira, P. (2006). Randomized clinical trial of local anesthetic versus a combination of local anesthetic with self-hypnosis in the management of pediatric procedure-related pain. *Health Psychology, 25*(3), 307–315.

Manimala, R., Blount, R. L., & Cohen, L. L. (2000). The effects of parental reassurance versus distraction on child distress and coping during immunizations. *Children's Health Care, 29,* 161–177.

O'Byrne, K., Peterson, L., & Saldana, L. (1997). Survey of pediatric hospitals' preparation programs: Evidence of the impact of health psychology research. *Health Psychology, 16,* 147–154.

Pate, J. T., Smith, A. J., Blount, R. L., & Cohen, L. L. (1996). Childhood medical experience and temperament as predictors of adult functioning in medical situations. *Children's Health Care, 25,* 281–296.

Piira, T., Champion, G. D., Bustos, T., Donnelly, N., & Lui, K. (2007). Factors associated with infant pain response following an immunization injection. *Early Human Development, 83,* 319–326.

Piira, T., Hayes, B., Goodenough, B., & von Baeyer, C. L. (2006). Effects of attentional direction, age, and coping style on cold-pressor pain. *Behaviour Research and Therapy, 44,* 835–848.

Piira, T., Sugiura, T., Champion, G. D., Donnelly, N., & Cole, A. S. (2005). The role of parental presence in the context of children's medical procedures: A systematic review. *Child: Care, Health, and Development, 31,* 233–243.

Piira, T., Taplin, J. E., Goodenough, B., & von Baeyer, C. L. (2002). Cognitive-behavioural predictors of children's tolerance of laboratory-induced pain: Implications for clinical assessment and future directions. *Behaviour Research and Therapy, 40*, 571–584.

Powers, S. W. (1999). Empirically supported treatments in pediatric psychology: Procedure-related pain. *Journal of Pediatric Psychology, 24*, 131–145.

Ranger, M., & Campbell-Yeo, M. (2008). Temperament and pain response: a review of the literature. *Pain Management Nursing, 9*(1), 2–9.

Reis, E. C., & Holubkov, R. (1997). Vapocoolant spray is equally effective as EMLA cream in reducing immunization pain in school aged children. *Pediatrics, 100*, e5.

Rocha, E. M., & Prkachin, K. M. (2007). Temperament and pain reactivity predict health behavior seven years later. *Journal of Pediatric Psychology, 32*, 393–399.

Schechter, N. L., Zempsky, W. T., Cohen, L. L., McGrath, P. J., McMurtry, M., & Bright, N. S. (2007). Pain reduction during pediatric immunizations: Evidence-based review and recommendations. *Pediatrics, 119*, e1184–e1198.

Sethna, N. F., Verghese, S. T., Hannallah, R. S., Solodiuk, J. C., Zurakowski, D., & Berde, C. B. (2005). A randomized controlled trial to evaluate S-Caine patch for reducing pain associated with vascular access in children. *Anesthesiology, 102*, 403–408.

Stevens, B., Yamada, J., & Ohlsson, A. (2004). Sucrose for analgesia in newborn infants undergoing painful procedures. *Cochrane Database of Systematic Reviews*, Issue 3 (Article No. CD001069), DOI: 10.1002/14651858.CD001069.pub2.

Stinson, J. N., Kavanagh, T., Yamada, J., Gill, N., & Stevens, B. (2006). Systematic review of the psychometric properties, interpretability and feasibility of self-report pain intensity measures for use in clinical trials in children and adolescents. *Pain, 125*, 143–157.

Taddio, A., Shah, V., Gilbert-MacLeod, C., & Katz, J. (2002). Conditioning and hyperalgesia in newborns exposed to repeated heel lances. *Journal of the American Medical Association, 288*, 857–861.

Uhari, M. (1993). A eutectic mixture of lidocaine and prilocaine for alleviating vaccination pain in infants. *Pediatrics, 92*, 719–721.

Uman, L. S., Chambers, C. T., McGrath, P. J., & Kisely, S. R. (2006). Psychological interventions for needle-related procedural pain and distress in children and adolescents. *Cochrane Database of Systematic Reviews*, Issue 4 (Article No. CD005179), DOI: 10.1002/14651858. CD005179.pub2.

von Baeyer, C. L., & Spagrud, L. J. (2007). Systematic review of observational (behavioral) measures of pain for children and adolescents aged 3–18 years. *Pain, 127*, 140–150.

Walker, L. S., Williams, S. E., Smith, C. A., Garber, J., Van Slyke, D. A., & Lipani, T. A. (2006). Parent attention versus distraction: Impact on symptom complaints by children with and without chronic functional abdominal pain. *Pain, 122*, 43–52.

Wood, C., & Bioy, A. (2008). Hypnosis and pain in children. *Journal of Pain and Symptom Management, 35*(4), 437–446.

Wright, K. D., Stewart, S. H., Finley, G. A., & Buffett-Jerrott, S. E. (2007). Prevention and intervention strategies to alleviate preoperative anxiety in children: A critical review. *Behavior Modification, 31*, 52–79.

Zempsky, W. T. (2006). Topical anesthetics for procedural pain in children: What does the future hold? *Current Drug Therapy, 1*, 283–290.

Zempsky, W. T., Anand, K. S., Sullivan, K. M., Fraser, D., & Cucina K. (1998). Lidocaine iontophoresis for topical anesthesia prior to intravenous line placement in children. *Journal of Pediatrics, 132*, 1061–1063.

Zempsky, W. T., Robbins, B., Leong, M., & Schechter, N. L. (2008). A novel needlefree powder lidocaine delivery system for rapid local analgesia. *Journal of Pediatrics, 152*, 405–411.

CHAPTER 12

Pediatric Pharmacology and Psychopharmacology

RONALD T. BROWN
BRIAN P. DALY
JOHANNA L. CARPENTER
JEREMY S. COHEN

Nearly every pediatric psychologist has encountered a child who is prescribed medication for either a chronic health condition or a behavioral or mood disorder. There has been a significant increase in the prescription of psychotropic medications for preschoolers (Delate, 2004) and older children (Medco Health Solutions, 2004) over time. Factors that have accounted for this increase include a greater public awareness of childhood psychological disorders (Riddle, Kastelic, & Frosch, 2001); expansions of existing diagnostic criteria, which have led to increases in the incidence of children with childhood psychiatric disorders (Gadow, 1997); advances in the identification of the biological bases of childhood psychopathology, and the increasing availability of newer pharmacological agents with more favorable side effect profiles (Brown & Sawyer, 1998); and, finally, a systematic effort to contain and drive down the costs of health care (Brown & Freeman, 2003).

Although there have been tremendous advances in psychopharmacology, the clinical use of most psychotropic medications for children far exceeds the data available regarding safety and efficacy (Brown & Sammons, 2002). Research pertaining to psychotropic medications for children is progressing at a much slower rate than investigations of the same medications prescribed for adult use (Werry & Aman, 1999). The prescription of many psychotropic agents for children and adolescents is often based on information gathered from research with adults, and such agents are not necessarily sanctioned for use with pediatric populations.

Differences between Pediatric and Adult Pharmacology

Pediatric pharmacology differs markedly from pharmacotherapy with adults in a number of ways. First, the rates at which medications are absorbed, distributed in the body, and metabolized by children differ greatly from those for adults (Werry & Aman, 1999). In addition, many medications have shorter half-lives in children and adolescents than in adults, and therefore may require more frequent dosing (Brown & Sammons, 2002). Age also plays a significant role in predicting the effects of medication, with younger children typically having more unpredictable responses than their older counterparts. Finally, when considering additional medications, prescribing physicians must take into account any adverse medication interactions that may occur in polypharmacy (the use of more than one pharmaceutical agent simultaneously)—a frequent occurrence among children with chronic illnesses.

Adherence to pharmacological regimens is another critical factor that influences the efficacy of treatment. Because caregivers typically take responsibility for administration of children's medication, parental attitudes invariably influence children's use of medication. Caregivers may be ambivalent about using psychotropic medication in particular, particularly when a child's behavior is not deemed to be a problem at home or when symptoms are not overtly visible. For a more complete review of adherence to treatment regimens, the interested reader is referred to LaGreca and Mackey (Chapter 9, this volume).

Pediatric Psychopharmacology

We now turn our review to those psychotropic agents that are used to manage various forms of externalizing, internalizing, psychotic, developmental, and tic disorders in children and adolescents.

Attention-Deficit/Hyperactivity Disorder

Of the pharmacological options available, central nervous system stimulant medications are the most widely studied and most commonly prescribed medications for the management of attention-deficit/hyperactivity disorder (ADHD) in school-age children and adolescents (Zito et al., 2003). The stimulants most frequently prescribed to pediatric populations are methylphenidate (e.g., Ritalin), dextroamphetamine (e.g., Adderall), and amphetamines. There is more compelling evidence to support the safety, dosing, and efficacy of stimulants than any other psychotropic agent for pediatric populations (Greenhill, 2002). Approximately 65–75% of children with an ADHD diagnosis will respond positively to an initial trial of stimulant medication (Pliszka, 2007). Nonetheless, if a child fails the initial stimulant trial, the response rate is up to 85% if the child is switched to another class of stimulants (e.g., from methylphenidate to amphetamines) (Arnold, 2000).

It is noteworthy, though, that while stimulants work well in managing ADHD symptoms (e.g., attention, impulsivity, overactivity), they are less effective in enhancing functional outcomes (e.g., academic skills, social skills) (Runnheim, Frankenberger, & Hazelkorn, 1996). Moreover, the literature provides no evidence to suggest that the stimulants enhance the guarded long-term prognosis for children with the disorder

(MTA Cooperative Group, 1999). In clinical trials with preschool children, low-dose methylphenidate was found to be effective, safe, and generally tolerable; however, stimulant response was lower than in school-age children, and more adverse side effects (e.g., emotionality and/or irritability) were reported among preschoolers than among older children (Greenhill et al., 2006; Wigal et al., 2006).

The most frequently reported adverse effects of stimulant drug therapy are decreased appetite, headaches, abdominal discomfort, problems falling asleep, irritability, motor tics, nausea, fatigue, and social withdrawal (McMaster University Evidence-Based Practice Center, 1999; Pliszka et al., 2000). Overall, the adverse effects are generally similar for all stimulants; are transient; and are linearly related to dose, with higher doses associated with a greater frequency of adverse effects (Santosh & Taylor, 2002).

The only nonstimulant medication approved by the Food and Drug Administration (FDA) for the treatment of ADHD is atomoxetine (Strattera), a norepinephrine reuptake inhibitor. It is noteworthy that the FDA recommended in 2005 that a "black box" warning be provided with Strattera, due to the rare possibility of hepatotoxicity and increased suicidal thinking in children and adolescents (FDA, 2005).

Oppositional Defiant Disorder and Conduct Disorder

The evidence for the psychopharmacological treatment of oppositional defiant disorder (ODD) is limited, unless the children have a comorbid diagnosis of ADHD. In those instances when comorbid ADHD is present, combined treatment with a stimulant medication and clonidine, or with atomoxetine alone, may lead to the reduction of both ADHD and ODD symptoms (Hazell & Stuart, 2003; Newcorn, Spencer, Biederman, Milton, & Michelson, 2005).

The classes of medications most frequently employed to manage the symptoms of aggression and mood disturbance associated with conduct disorder include stimulants, mood stabilizers, and typical and atypical antipsychotics. Some evidence indicates that stimulants (e.g., methylphenidate) are effective in the management of aggression in adolescents with conduct disorder (Klein, Abikoff, Ganeles, Seese, & Pollack, 1997). However, a review of other studies suggests more variable results, with effect sizes ranging from small to moderately large (Aman & Lindsay, 2002). The mood stabilizer lithium has been effective in reducing aggression in hospitalized children with conduct disorder (Gerardin, Cohen, Mazet, & Flament, 2002). However, potential adverse side effects associated with the use of lithium include thyroid-stimulated hormone elevations, hypothyroidism, polydipsia and polyuria, and possible lethality in an overdose situation (Kutcher et al., 2004). Of the typical antipsychotics, haloperidol (Haldol) has demonstrated efficacy in reducing aggression and disruptive behaviors (Campbell et al., 1984). Again, significant adverse side effects such as extrapyramidal symptoms (e.g., tics and tremors that are not reversible) are associated with haloperidol. Results from several controlled trials indicate that the atypical antipsychotic risperidone (Risperdal) is generally safe and effective in treating children with disruptive behavior disorders (Findling, Aman, De Smedt, & Derivan, 2002; Turgay, Snyder, Binder, Fisman, & Carrol, 2002).

Obsessive–Compulsive Disorder

For the treatment of obsessive–compulsive disorder (OCD) in children and adolescents, the FDA has approved several medications for certain age groups: the selective serotonin reuptake inhibitors (SSRIs), which include sertraline (Zoloft) (for ages 6 and older), flu-oxetine (Prozac) (for ages 7 and older), and fluvoxamine (Luvox) (for ages 8 and older); and clomipramine (Anafranil), a serotonin reuptake inhibitor (for children ages 10 and older). Results of a meta-analysis reveal that clomipramine, sertraline, fluoxetine, flu-voxamine, and paroxetine (Paxil) demonstrate a strong and significant effect over pla-cebo, with a moderate effect size of 0.46 (Geller et al., 2003). In research examining the efficacy of the various SSRI medications, there are no statistically significant differences between agents, suggesting that treatment strategies should be guided by considerations of adverse side effects and medication half-lives (Geller et al., 2003).

Other Anxiety Disorders

Separation anxiety disorder, generalized anxiety disorder (GAD), and social phobia are frequently studied together in pharmacotherapy trials, due to their frequently occur-ring comorbidity. Since several randomized controlled trials (RCTs) have supported the short-term efficacy of SSRIs in the treatment of these disorders in youths, the Ameri-can Academy of Child and Adolescent Psychiatry (AACAP) recommends that SSRIs be considered part of the multimodal approach to the treatment of these anxiety disorders (AACAP, 2007a). It is noteworthy that the use of benzodiazepines, buspirone, and tricy-clic antidepressants for the management of separation anxiety is not currently supported in the literature (Waslick, 2006). Among youths with separation anxiety disorder or GAD, fluvoxamine was associated with significant improvement in anxiety symptoms compared to placebo, although the presence of depressive symptoms and social phobia predicted a worse response to pharmacotherapy in both groups (Research Units on Pediatric Psychopharmacology [RUPP] Anxiety Disorders Study Group, 2001). Data from a 6-month open-label extension trial suggest that the acute effects of fluvoxamine can be maintained over a longer time period (Walkup et al., 2002). It is noteworthy that few pharmacological recommendations are available for children and adolescents with posttraumatic stress disorder or acute stress disorder (Waslick, 2006).

Major Depressive Disorder

SSRIs have generally been found to be efficacious in treating pediatric major depres-sion (40–70% response rate), but a high placebo response rate also has been reported (30–60%; AACAP, 2007b). RCTs of fluoxetine, the only SSRI to be FDA-approved for the treatment of child and adolescent depression, have demonstrated pronounced dif-ferences between placebo and medication response (Emslie et al., 1997, 2002). A recent meta-analysis of 13 RCTs of SSRI treatment for child and adolescent depression found that only fluoxetine was associated with moderately significant effects on depression (Usala, Clavennab, Zuddasa, & Bonati, 2008).

Other SSRIs that have been shown to be more efficacious than placebo in at least one RCT include citalopram (Celexa) (Wagner et al., 2004), sertraline (Wagner et al., 2003), and paroxetine (Emslie et al., 2006), although several studies reported small or no effect of the agents, due to the large placebo response (AACAP, 2007c). In addition, significant effects of these SSRIs (not including fluoxetine) may only be seen in adoles-cent populations and not child populations (Bridge et al., 2007). It is noteworthy that tricyclic antidepressants are not efficacious in the treatment of pediatric depression and are not recommended as an initial pharmacotherapy (AACAP, 2007c).

The most common adverse side effects of SSRIs in children and adolescents include sedation, weight gain, agitation, sleep disruption, gastrointestinal problems, and sexual problems (Murphy, Segarra, Storch, & Goodman, 2008). It is noteworthy that all antidepressant medications carry a "black box" warning about behavioral activation and increased risk of suicidal thinking and behavior in children and adolescents with major depressive disorder and other psychiatric disorders (e.g., anxiety or eating disorders) (FDA, 2005). The FDA decided to include this warning after analyzing pooled data from trials that suggested an average risk of suicidality of 4% while on medication, as compared to 2% while on placebo (Brown et al., 2008). The first few months of treatment are considered the time of greatest concern for behavioral activation and suicidality.

Bipolar Disorder

Mood stabilizers and/or atypical antipsychotics are generally recommended as first-line treatments in pediatric populations who meet formal diagnostic criteria for a manic episode (AACAP, 2007b). The FDA has approved risperidone for the short-term treatment of manic or mixed episodes in youths ages 10–17 years; aripiprazole (Abilify) for the acute treatment of mania in adolescents; and lithium for bipolar disorder in children and adolescents ages 12 years and older. Weight gain is a particularly problematic adverse side effect of treatment with antipsychotics.

Schizophrenia Spectrum Disorders

Antipsychotic medication is the primary pharmacological treatment for schizophrenia and associated disorders in youths, given its established efficacy in adults. Atypical antipsychotic agents, rather than traditional neuroleptics, are considered first-line treatments, because the atypical agents have demonstrated better efficacy in treating negative symptoms associated with schizophrenia and at least equal efficacy in treating positive symptoms of the disorder (Meltzer, Lee, & Ranjan, 1994). Only risperidone and aripiprazole are currently approved by the FDA for the management of schizophrenia in adolescents ages 13–17. For treatment-refractory schizophrenia, clozapine (Clozaril) is the most efficacious agent, although this agent's adverse side effect profile (including seizures and agranulocytosis) precludes its use as a first-line treatment (AACAP, 2001; Sporn et al., 2007).

Serious adverse side effects occur at higher rates among children and adolescents taking antipsychotics than among adults. They include abnormal involuntary movements, prolactin elevation, intracardiac conduction effects, hematological and neurological adverse events, and neuroleptic malignant syndrome (a flu-like syndrome with high fevers that is potentially fatal).

Autism Spectrum Disorders

Findings from studies reveal that psychotropic medications employed in the treatment of autism and other pervasive developmental disorders (PDDs) are not efficacious in alleviating the disorders' core deficits (e.g., impaired social interaction and communication) (see Campbell, Segall, & Dommestrup, Chapter 34, this volume). However, pharmacotherapy is frequently used to manage secondary symptoms (e.g., disruptive behaviors) and comorbid conditions (e.g., anxiety disorders) among children and adolescents with autism or other PDDs, particularly those symptoms that interfere with children's functioning in social and educational settings (King, 2000). Risperidone is FDA-approved for the treatment of irritability, aggression, self-injury, temper tantrums, and affective lability associated with autism for children and adolescents ages 5–16. Risperidone has also demonstrated efficacy in managing restricted, stereotyped motor behaviors and interests among children and adolescents with autism (McDougle et al., 2005).

In the treatment of moderate to severe co-occurring overactivity, methylphenidate was found to be superior to placebo for children with autism, PDD not otherwise specified, or Asperger's disorder, although effect sizes were smaller and adverse events more common than in general pediatric populations (RUPP Autism Network, 2005). Results from open trials for sertraline, citalopram, and escitalopram (Lexapro) all indicate support for reducing the anxiety, agitation, and/or stereotypies associated with PDDs (Namerow, Thomas, Bostic, Prince, & Monuteaux, 2003; Owley et al., 2003).

Mental Retardation

Psychiatric diagnoses are frequently comorbid with intellectual disability in children and adolescents. Research on the pharmacological treatment of mental health conditions in this population has been limited, due to difficulty in making valid diagnoses and tracking symptom improvement (Shedlack, Hennen, Magee, & Cheron, 2005). The use of psychotropic medication in persons with mental retardation is common for the treatment of self-injurious behaviors, stereotyped behaviors, and aggression. Several trials have found risperidone to be superior to placebo in treating disruptive behaviors among children with subaverage intelligence (Reyes, Croonenberghs, Augustyns, & Eerdekens, 2006). For the treatment of depression and anxiety in individuals with mental retardation, SSRIs are frequently used because of their relatively mild side effect profile, whereas tricyclic antidepressants may have a negative impact on cardiac rhythm, seizure threshold, and cognition (AACAP, 1999). Benzodiazepines, clonidine, and β-blockers are not recommended as first-line or long-term treatments for anxiety, due to the potential for cognitive side effects. Antiepileptic drugs (e.g., valproic acid) are recommended as first-line treatments for bipolar disorder in children and adolescents diagnosed with mental retardation, given the potential for lithium to cause cognitive dulling among these individuals (AACAP, 1999). Because individuals with mental retardation are more sensitive to the adverse side effects of conventional neuroleptics, including tardive dyskinesia (Gualtieri, Quade, Hicks, Mayo, & Schroeder, 1984), atypical antipsychotics are appropriate first-line treatments for schizophrenia and associated disorders.

Tic Disorders

Although multiple classes of psychotropic medications have been employed to control or minimize tics, only the typical neuroleptics (haloperidol and pimozide), atypical neuroleptics (risperidone and ziprazidone), and α_2-adrenergic agonists (clonidine and guanfacine) have received empirical support (for a review, see Brown et al., 2008). The α_2-adrenergic agonists (clonidine and guanfacine) may be considered the first-choice medications in the management of tics, because they have relatively low rates of adverse side effects and because they also may be of benefit in ameliorating comorbid ADHD

(Gaffney et al., 2002; Sandor, 2003). In comparison, the typical and atypical neuroleptics, while effective, are associated with significant adverse side effects.

Pharmacotherapies for Chronic Health Conditions

We now turn our review to those chronic pediatric illnesses for which various pharmacotherapies are employed, many of which exert cognitive or behavioral toxicities that frequently affect learning in the classroom setting and social functioning among peers.

Toxicities

Behavioral and emotional toxicities associated with medication use in children and adolescents may be difficult to identify. Acute symptoms can include intoxication, delirium, psychosis, hallucinations, depression, mania, and anxiety (Arnold, Janke, Waters, & Milch, 1999). Longer-term reactions, including neuropsychological and resultant learning impairments, are also possible. Changes in behavior and emotion may occur for myriad reasons; these include the disease itself, normal variations of behavior, dosage, interaction with other medications, developmental change, or psychosocial factors (Arnold et al., 1999).

Asthma

Although asthma medications are able to remediate or prevent bronchial smooth muscle constriction and airway inflammation (Zdanowicz, 2007), current pharmacotherapy for asthma is not curative (Barnes, 2006). Effective medications include β_2 agonists (e.g., albuterol, alsmeterol), corticosteroids (e.g., beclomethasone, budesonide), methylxanthines (e.g., theophylline), cromloyn/nedrocromil, leukotriene modifiers (e.g., zafirlukast, montelukast), muscarinic antagonists (e.g., ipratropium), and monoclonal antibodies (e.g., omalizumab). The most frequent treatment consists of an inhaler with a combination of a long-acting β_2 agonist and corticosteroid (Barnes, 2006). Adverse side effects of asthma medications may include physiological reactions, such as increased heart rate or shaking (Bender, 1999). Although asthma medications do not demonstrate a significant adverse impact on cognitive functioning, changes in sleep should be monitored, due to the potential effects on attention and concentration (Bender, 1999).

The most effective and fast-acting bronchodilators are the β_2 agonists (Barnes, 2006). Short-acting β_2 agonists can be used to treat intermittent asthma symptoms or may be used as preventive measures prior to exercise (Szefler, 2000). Adverse side effects for these agents are generally limited. Long-acting β_2 agonists (e.g., salmeterol) are often used with inhaled corticosteroids in the management of moderate to severe persistent asthma. These agents also can be used to control breakthrough and nighttime symptoms (Szefler, 2000). It is noteworthy that long-acting β_2 agonists may be associated with an increased risk for serious adverse effects, such as severe asthma episodes, and their use should be monitored carefully (Zdanowicz, 2007).

Corticosteroids are considered the most effective anti-inflammatory medications available for the treatment of asthma and have been found to reduce the frequency and severity of asthma attacks (Zdanowicz, 2007). However, corticosteroid use in children may be associated with growth suppression (Zdanowicz, 2007), and thus these agents are only used for a short period of time in the management of pediatric asthma.

Theophylline acts as a bronchodilator and can be used to control intermittent and nighttime symptoms in combination with corticosteroids. Theophylline should not be considered a first treatment option, and at high levels may increase the risk of drug toxicity (Zdanowicz, 2007).

Leukotriene modifiers reduce bronchoconstriction and also have some anti-inflammatory effects (Szefler, 2000). These agents are generally less effective than inhaled corticosteroids, but as add-ons they may reduce the need for high doses of corticosteroids (Barnes, 2006). These agents also can be used as a preventive treatment in mild asthma.

Cancer

The most frequently occurring types of cancers in children are leukemia, brain tumors, and lymphomas (Jemal et al., 2006). Typical treatment options include chemotherapy, radiation therapy, their combination, and surgery. Treatment protocols depend on multiple factors, including type of cancer, stage of the disease, and whether there is a risk of central nervous system infiltration of the cancer cells. Because antineoplastic medications not only kill cancer cells, but also damage normal cells, several short-term adverse side effects are associated with these medications. In addition to the short-term effects, late effects (i.e., diseases encountered in adult survivors of cancer that are associated with treatment of the cancer during childhood) also have been associated with radiation and chemotherapy treatment (Duffner, 2006). For example, the use of anthracyclines, a common class of drugs used for childhood cancers, has been associated with risk of cardiac problems among survivors of childhood cancer (Galderisi et al., 2007). Growth suppression, endocrine dysfunction, and infertility may also result from various chemotherapies used during childhood or adolescence (Oeffinger, Ford, & Sklar, 2009).

Neurocognitive late effects may be present as well, particularly as a result of aggressive radiation therapy or chemotherapy—particularly those therapies that are used in the central nervous system either to treat cancers or to prevent cancer cells from infiltrating the central nervous system (i.e., prophylactic therapy) (Moore, 2005). In addition to treatment modality, disease characteristics (i.e., location), age at time of diagnosis, gender, preexisting neurological conditions, and time since treatment may contribute to the neurocognitive late effects associated with pediatric cancer (Moore, 2005). Given that attentional difficulties are part of the neurocognitive sequelae observed in survivors of acute lymphoblastic leukemia and brain tumors, investigators have begun to examine the efficacy of methylphenidate among this population. Initial studies indicate preliminary support for the efficacy and safety of the stimulants for survivors of these cancers; however, there is scant evidence for the long-term effects of the stimulants among cancer survivors (Daly & Brown, 2007).

Diabetes

Treatment of Type 1 insulin-dependent diabetes mellitus involves injection of insulin, with the goal of maintaining normal blood glucose levels. Many different insulin brands are available, and these differ in onset, peak time, and duration of action. Long-acting insulins may increase the difficulty of managing blood glucose levels, due to unpredictable absorption (Barnett, 2006). Neurocognitive effects associated with poor metabolic control include deficits in attention, processing speed, and memory (Holmes, Cant, Fox, Lampert, & Greer, 1999).

Although Type 2 diabetes usually begins in adulthood, it is an increasing problem in children and adolescents (American Diabetes Association, 2000). If exercise and nutritional changes are not sufficient, pharmacological treatments include insulin and oral medications. The newest drugs for the treatment of Type 2 diabetes are incretins (e.g., Exenatide); these are synthetic hormones injected at mealtime that increase insulin secretion (Modi, 2007). Oral medications, including sulfonylureas, meglitinides, biguanides, thiazolidinediones, and alpha-glucosidase inhibitors, act to decrease blood glucose levels.

Sickle Cell Disease

Treatment for sickle cell disease is typically targeted at the management of disease-related complications and prevention of infections (Steinberg, 1999). Penicillin prophylaxis in early childhood, and immunization against *Streptococcus pneumoniae* and influenza, have significantly improved life expectancy rates for individuals with sickle cell disease (Steinberg, 1999). In severe cases of the disease, blood transfusions or bone marrow transplantation may be required. Repeated transfusions have reduced the risk of stroke in children with sickle cell anemia (Steinberg, 1999). Although pain management is frequently pervasive in the care of children and adolescents with sickle cell disease, there is currently no standard method of care. Acute pain is often caused by vaso-occlusion and requires parenterally administered opiates and hydration (Claster & Vichinsky, 2003). Nonsteroidal anti-inflammatory agents can also be used to manage milder types of pain, thereby avoiding some of the adverse effects associated with narcotic analgesia, which can include sedation and anticholinergic effects (e.g., dry mouth, constipation).

Hydroxyurea, a ribonucleotide reductase inhibitor, is an orally administered chemotherapy that increases hemoglobin F concentrations in the blood. Use of this agent is associated with decreased morbidity and mortality among children, adolescents, and adults with sickle cell disease (Steinberg, 2006). Hydroxyurea is also used as a preventive treatment for disease complications, but not for management of acute symptoms (Claster & Vichinsky, 2003). Given that long-term effects of hydroxyurea are unknown, it is primarily indicated for use in patients experiencing severe complications associated with sickle cell disease (Steinberg, 1999).

Pediatric Pain

Pediatric pain is categorized as pain associated with disease or trauma, pain resulting from medical procedures, and pain without physical etiology (Varni, 1983). For mild to moderate pain, treatment frequently includes the use of non-narcotic analgesia. Aspirin is an antipyretic agent that reduces inflammation (Brown, Tanaka, & Donegan, 1998), but is contraindicated for children with liver disease, hemophilia, and Vitamin K deficiency (Brown et al., 1998). Adverse side effects of aspirin include gastrointestinal bleeding. Acetaminophen is prescribed more often in children because of its milder adverse side effect profile, although it does not have anti-inflammatory effects (Dahlquist &

Switkin, 2003). The use of nonsteroidal anti-inflammatory drugs (e.g., ibuprofen) is limited for children and adolescents, due to controversies regarding safety in pediatric populations (e.g., postoperative bleeding, exacerbated respiratory disease) (Anderson & Palmer, 2006).

For severe and chronic pain, opioid analgesics (e.g., morphine, codeine) are typically administered. Synthetic analogues include meperdine (Demerol), hydromorphone (Dilaudid), fentanyl citrate (Sublimaze), oxycodone (Percocet, Percodan), and pentazocine (Talwin) (Dahlquist & Switkin, 2003). Morphine is the standard opioid analgesic administered during acute pain episodes. Adverse side effects include respiratory depression, dizziness, sweating, nausea, and vomiting (Dahlquist & Switkin, 2003). Tramadol is now being used with increasing frequency in children, because it poses a lower risk for respiratory depression than morphine does (Anderson & Palmer, 2006). Finally, narcotic analgesia has significant sedating properties, thereby dulling cognition; this can have a significant impact on children's learning and behavior in classroom and social settings.

Seizures

For the management of pediatric seizure disorders, the most commonly prescribed medications are the antiepileptic drugs, including phenobarbital, valproic acid (Depakene, Depakote), phenytoin (Dilantin), carbamazepine (Tegretol), felbamate (Felbatol), lamotrigine (Lamictal), and topiramate (Topamax). The use of these agents is frequently tailored to the specific type of seizure. For example, in the case of generalized seizure disorders, valproic acid is the most commonly prescribed first-line treatment (Oka et al., 2004), whereas the treatments of choice for absence (petit mal) seizures are ethosuximide, valproate sodium or valproic acid, and lamotrigine (Sullivan & Dlugos, 2004). Medications commonly used in the management of generalized tonic–clonic (grand mal) seizures include valproic acid, phenytoin, and phenobarbital, whereas partial seizures are treated with carbamazepine, phenytoin, and valproate. It is important for practitioners to monitor school performance among children with seizures, as the use of antiepileptic medication may impair cognitive performance. For example, phenobarbital is associated with a particularly high risk of cognitive side effects, including IQ decline (Farwell et al., 1990) and diminished achievement even after the drug is discontinued (Sulzbacher, Farwell, Temkin, Lu, & Hirtz, 1999). The cognitive side effects of carbamazepine, phenytoin, valproate sodium, and topiramate are similar; they include psychomotor slowing and decreased attention and memory (Loring & Meador, 2004). With the exception of topiramate, newer agents are generally associated with a more positive neuropsychological profiles (e.g., gabapentin, lamotrigine), although additional RCTs are warranted.

Conclusions and Recommendations

There is a particular need for the expertise that pediatric psychologists bring to clinical and research settings, including knowledge with regard to developmental issues; attitudes of caregivers, teachers, and children about medication; and issues related to the assessment of the safety and efficacy of various pharmacotherapies in children and adolescents. Of course, pediatric psychologists' expertise in the area of research and measurement has allowed a much broader understanding of psychotropic medications in pediatric populations and the effects of these agents on behavior and learning.

We are of the opinion that the use of these psychotropic agents in pediatric populations has far exceeded the available data pertaining to efficacy and safety. With the exception of the stimulants, the safety and efficacy of most psychotropic medications in pediatric populations have received scant attention. Moreover, issues of medication adherence, developmental effects on medication efficacy and safety, and attitudes about medication are important areas in which pediatric psychologists can make viable contributions over the next several years.

There is no doubt that the use of medication has revolutionized the care of and practice for children and adolescents in pediatric inpatient and outpatient settings. Nearly all children and adolescents who come to our attention will be receiving some type of pharmacotherapy that affects learning, behavior, or both. Pediatric psychologists have many of the skills necessary to make important contributions to the extant research literature, including a broad knowledge of issues related to adherence; the skills to assess both the efficacy and the adverse effects of pharmacological agents; and an understanding of how cognitive and social development may interact with the influence of medication to affect children's cognition, behavior, and socialization among peers. Finally, with numerous clinical trials underway and the promise of the National Institute of Mental Health to launch RCTs of psychotropic agents for pediatric populations, there remain future employment opportunities for pediatric psychologists in their efforts to enhance the quality of life for ill children and adolescents in the years to come.

References

Aman, M. G., & Lindsay, R. L. (2002). Psychotropic medicines and aggressive behavior: Part I. Psychostimulants. *Child and Adolescent Psychopharmacology News, 7*, 1–6.

American Academy of Child and Adolescent Psychiatry (AACAP). (1999). Practice parameters for the assessment and treatment of children, adolescents, and adults with autism and other pervasive developmental disorders. *Journal of the American Academy of Child and Adolescent Psychiatry, 38*(12, Suppl.), 32S–54S.

American Academy of Child and Adolescent Psychiatry (AACAP). (2001). Practice parameter for the assessment and treatment of children and adolescents with schizophrenia. *Journal of the American Academy of Child and Adolescent Psychiatry, 40*(7, Suppl.), 4S–23S.

American Academy of Child and Adolescent Psychiatry (AACAP). (2007a). Practice parameter for the assessment and treatment of children and adolescents with anxiety disorders. *Journal of the American Academy of Child and Adolescent Psychiatry, 46*, 267–283.

American Academy of Child and Adolescent Psychiatry (AACAP). (2007b). Practice parameter for the assessment and treatment of children and adolescents with bipolar disorder. *Journal of the American Academy of Child and Adolescent Psychiatry, 46*, 107–125.

American Academy of Child and Adolescent Psychiatry (AACAP). (2007c). Practice parameter for the assessment and treatment of children and adolescents with depressive disorders. *Journal of the American Academy of Child and Adolescent Psychiatry, 46*, 1503–1526.

American Diabetes Association. (2000). Type 2 diabetes in children and adolescents. *Diabetes Care, 23*, 381–389.

Anderson, B. J., & Palmer, G. M. (2006). Recent pharmacological advances in paediatric analgesics. *Biomedicine and Pharmacotherapy, 60*, 303–309.

Arnold, L. E. (2000). Methylphenidate vs. amphetamine: A comparative review. *Journal of Attention Disorders, 3,* 200–211.

Arnold, L. E., Janke, I., Waters, B., & Milch, A. (1999). Psychoactive effects of medical drugs. In J. S. Werry & M. G. Aman (Eds.), *Practitioner's guide to psychoactive drugs for children and adolescents* (2nd ed., pp. 387–412). New York: Plenum Press.

Barnes, P. J. (2006). Drugs for asthma. *British Journal of Pharmacology, 147,* S297–S303.

Barnett, A. H. (2006). Insulin glargine in the treatment of Type I and Type 2 diabetes. *Vascular Health and Risk Management, 2,* 59–67.

Bender, B. G. (1999). Learning disorders associated with asthma and allergies. *School Psychology Review, 28,* 204–214.

Bridge, J. A., Iyengar, S., Salary, C. B., Barbe, R. P., Birmaher, B., Pincus, H. A., et al. (2007). Clinical response and risk for reported suicidal ideation and suicide attempts in pediatric antidepressant treatment: A meta-analysis of randomized controlled trials. *Journal of the American Medical Association, 297,* 1693–1696.

Brown, R. T., Antonuccio, D. O., DuPaul, G. J., Fristad, M. A., King, C. A., Leslie, L., et al. (2008). *Childhood mental health disorders: Evidence base and contextual factors for psychosocial, psychopharmacological, and combined interventions.* Washington, DC: American Psychological Association.

Brown, R. T., & Freeman, W. S. (2003). Primary care. In D. Marsh & M. Fristad (Eds.), *Handbook of serious emotional disturbance in children and adolescents* (pp. 428–444). New York: Wiley.

Brown, R. T., & Sammons, M. T. (2002). Pediatric psychopharmacology: A review of new developments and recent research. *Professional Psychology: Research and Practice, 33,* 135–147.

Brown, R. T., & Sawyer, M. G. (1998). *Medications for school-age children: Effects on learning and behavior.* New York: Guilford Press.

Brown, R. T., Tanaka, O. F., & Donegan, J. E. (1998). Pain management. In L. Phelps (Ed.), *Health-related disorders in children and adolescents: A guidebook for understanding and educating* (pp. 501–513). Washington, DC: American Psychological Association.

Campbell, M., Small, A. M., Green, W. H., Jennings, S. J., Perry, R., Bennett, W. G., et al. (1984). Behavioral efficacy of haloperidol and lithium carbonate: A comparison in hospitalized aggressive children with conduct disorder. *Archives of General Psychiatry, 41,* 650–656.

Claster, S., & Vichinsky, E. P. (2003). Managing sickle cell disease. *British Medical Journal, 327,* 1151–1155.

Dahlquist, L. M., & Switkin, M. C. (2003). Chronic and recurrent pain. In M. C. Roberts (Ed.), *Handbook of pediatric psychology* (3rd ed., pp. 198–215). New York: Guilford Press.

Daly, B. P., & Brown, R. T. (2007). Management of neurocognitive late effects with stimulant medication. *Journal of Pediatric Psychology, 32,* 1111–1126.

Delate, T. (2004). Child antidepressant use skyrockets. *Psychiatric Services, 55*(4).

Duffner, P. K. (2006). The long term effects of chemotherapy on the central nervous system. *Journal of Biology, 5,* 21–24.

Emslie, G. J., Heiligenstein, J. H., Wagner, K. D., Hoog, S. L., Ernest, D. E., Brown, E., et al. (2002). Fluoxetine for acute treatment of depression in children and adolescents: A placebo-controlled randomized clinical trial. *Journal of the American Academy of Child and Adolescent Psychiatry, 41,* 1205–1214.

Emslie, G. J., Rush, J., Weinberg, W. A., Kowatch, R. A., Hughes, C. W., Carmody, T., et al. (1997). A double-blind, randomized, placebo-controlled trial of fluoxetine in children and adolescents with depression. *Archives of General Psychiatry, 54,* 1031–1037.

Emslie, G. J., Wagner, K. D., Kutcher, S., Krulewicz, S., Fong, R., Carpenter, D. J., et al. (2006).

Paroxetine treatment in children and adolescents with major depressive disorder: A random-ized, multicenter, double-blind, placebo-controlled trial. *Journal of the American Academy of Child and Adolescent Psychiatry, 45*, 709–719.

Farwell, J. R., Lee, Y. J., Hirtz, D. G., Sulzbacher, S. I., Ellenberg, J. H., & Nelson, K. B. (1990). Phenobarbital for febrile seizures: Effects on intelligence and on seizure recurrence. *New England Journal of Medicine, 322*, 364–369.

Findling, R. L., Aman, M. G., De Smedt, G., & Derivan, A. (2002). Risperidone in children with conduct problems and subaverage IQ. *European Journal of Psychiatry, 17*, 118–118.

Food and Drug Administration (FDA). (2005). FDA alert [09/05]: Suicidal thinking in children and adolescents. Retrieved May 5, 2008, from *www.fda.gov/cder/drug/infopage/atomox-etine/default.htm*

Gadow, K. D. (1997). An overview of three decades of research in pediatric psychopharmacoepi-demiology. *Journal of Child and Adolescent Psychopharmacology, 7*, 219–236.

Gaffney, G. R., Perry, P. J., Lund, B. C., BeverStille, K. A., Arndt, S., & Kuperman, S. (2002). Risperidone versus clonidine in the treatment of children and adolescents with Tourette's syndrome. *Journal of the American Academy of Child and Adolescent Psychiatry, 41*, 330–336.

Galderisi, M., Marra, F., Esposito, R., Lomoriello, V. S., Pardo, M., & de Devitiis, O. (2007). Cancer therapy and cardiotoxicity: The need of serial Doppler echocardiography. *Cardio-vascular Ultrasound, 5*, 4–17.

Geller, D. A., Biederman, J., Stewart, S. E., Mullin, B., Martin, A., Spencer, T., et al. (2003). Which SSRI?: A meta-analysis of pharmacotherapy trials in pediatric obsessive–compulsive disorder. *American Journal of Psychiatry, 160*, 1919–1928.

Gerardin, P., Cohen, D., Mazet, P., & Flament, M. F. (2002). Drug treatment of conduct disor-der in young people. *European Neuropsychopharmacology, 12*, 361–370.

Greenhill, L., Kollins, S., Abikoff, H., McCracken, J., Riddle, M., Swanson, J., et al. (2006). Efficacy and safety of immediate-release methylphenidate treatment for preschoolers with ADHD. *Journal of the American Academy of Child and Adolescent Psychiatry, 45*, 1284–1293.

Greenhill, L. L. (2002, October). *Efficacy and safety of OROS MPH in adolescents with ADHD.* Paper presented at the 49th annual meeting of the American Academy of Child and Adolescent Psychiatry, San Francisco.

Gualtieri, C. T., Quade, D., Hicks, R. E., Mayo, J. P., & Schroeder, S. R. (1984). Tardive dyski-nesia and other clinical consequences of neuroleptic treatment in children and adolescents. *American Journal of Psychiatry, 141*, 20–23.

Hazell, P. L., & Stuart, J. E. (2003). A randomized controlled trial of clonidine added to psy-chostimulant medication for hyperactive and aggressive children. *Journal of the American Academy of Child and Adolescent Psychiatry, 42*, 886–894.

Holmes, C. S., Cant, M. C., Fox, M. A., Lampert, N. L., & Greer, T. (1999). Disease and demo-graphic risk factors for disrupted cognitive functioning in children with insulin-dependent diabetes mellitus (IDDM). *School Psychology Review, 28*, 215–227.

Jemal, A., Siegel, R., Ward, E., Murray, T., Xu, J., Smigal, C., et al. (2006). Cancer statistics, 2006. *CA: A Cancer Journal for Clinicians, 56*, 106–130.

King, B. H. (2000). Pharmacological treatment of mood disturbances, aggression, and self-injury in persons with pervasive developmental disorders. *Journal of Autism and Developmental Disorders, 30*, 439–445.

Klein, R. G., Abikoff, H., Ganeles, D., Seese, L. M., & Pollack, S. (1997). Clinical efficacy of methylphenidate in conduct disorder with and without attention-deficit hyperactivity disor-der. *Archives of General Psychiatry, 54*, 1073–1080.

Kutcher, S., Aman, M., Brooks, S. J., Buitelaar, J., van Daalen, E., Fegert, J. et al. (2004).

International consensus statement on attention-deficit/hyperactivity disorder (ADHD) and disruptive behaviour disorders (DBDs): Clinical implications and treatment practice suggestions. *European Journal of Neuropsychopharmacology, 14,* 11–28.

Loring, D. W., & Meador, K. J. (2004). Cognitive side effects of antiepileptic drugs in children. *Neurology, 62,* 872–877.

McDougle, C. J., Scahill, L., Aman, M. G., McCracken, J. T., Tierney, E., Davies, M., et al. (2005). Risperidone for the core symptom domains of autism: Results from the study by the Autism Network of the Research Units on Pediatric Psychopharmacology. *American Journal of Psychiatry, 162,* 1142–1148.

McMaster University Evidence-Based Practice Center. (1999). *Treatment of attention-deficit hyperactivity disorder.* (Evidence Report/Technology Assessment No. 11, AHCPR Publication No. 99-E018). Rockville, MD: Agency for Health Care Policy and Research.

Medco Health Solutions. (2004). Drug trends. Retrieved May 9, 2008, from *www.drugtrend. com/medco/consumer/drugtrend/trends/jsp*

Meltzer, H. Y., Lee, M. A., & Ranjan, R. (1994). Recent advances in the pharmacotherapy of schizophrenia. *Acta Psychiatrica Scandinavica,* 384(Suppl.), 95–101.

Modi, P. (2007). Diabetes beyond insulin: Review of new drugs for treatment of diabetes. *Current Drug Discovery Technologies, 4,* 39–47.

Moore, B. D. (2005). Neurocognitive outcomes in survivors of childhood cancer. *Journal of Pediatric Psychology, 30,* 51–63.

MTA Cooperative Group. (1999). A 14-month randomized clinical trial of treatment strategies for attention-deficit hyperactivity disorder (ADHD). *Archives of General Psychiatry, 56,* 1073–1086.

Murphy, T. K., Segarra, E., Storch, E. A., & Goodman, W. K. (2008). SSRI adverse events: How to monitor and manage. *International Review of Psychiatry, 20,* 203–208.

Namerow, L. B., Thomas, P., Bostic, J. Q., Prince, J., & Monuteaux, M. C. (2003). Use of citalopram in pervasive developmental disorders. *Journal of Developmental and Behavioral Pediatrics, 24,* 104–108.

Newcorn, J. H., Spencer, T. J., Biederman, J., Milton, D. R., & Michelson, D. (2005). Atomoxetine treatment in children and adolescents with attention-deficit/hyperactivity disorder and comorbid oppositional defiant disorder. *Journal of the American Academy of Child and Adolescent Psychiatry, 44,* 240–248.

Oeffinger, K. C., Ford, J. S., & Sklar, C. A. (2009). Fertility and sexuality. In L. S. Wiener, M. Pao, A. E. Kazak, M. J. Kupst, & A. F. Patemnaude (Eds.), *Quick reference for pediatric oncology clinicians: The pediatric and psychological dimensions of pediatric cancer symptom management* (pp. 236–244). Charlottesville, VA: American Psychosocial Oncology Society.

Oka, E., Murakami, N., Ogino, T., Kobayashi, K., Ohmori, I., Akiyama, T., et al. (2004). Initiation of treatment and selection of antiepileptic drugs in childhood epilepsy. *Epilepsia, 45,* 17–19.

Owley, T., Walton, L., Salt, J., Guter, S. J., Winnega, M., Leventhal, B. L., et al. (2005). An open-label trial of escitalopram in pervasive developmental disorders. *Journal of the American Academy of Child and Adolescent Psychiatry, 44,* 343–348.

Pliszka, S. R. (2007). Pharmacologic treatment of attention-deficit/hyperactivity disorder: Efficacy, safety, and mechanisms of action. *Neuropsychology Review, 17,* 61–72.

Pliszka, S. R., Greenhill, L. L., Crimson, M. L., Sedillo, A., Carlson, C., Conners, K. C., et al. (2000). The Texas children's medication algorithm project: Report of the Texas consensus conference panel on medication treatment of childhood attention-deficit/hyperactivity disorder. Part I. *Journal of the American Academy of Child and Adolescent Psychiatry, 39,* 908–919.

Research Units on Pediatric Psychopharmacology (RUPP) Anxiety Disorders Study Group.

(2001). Fluvoxamine for the treatment of anxiety disorders in children and adolescents. *New England Journal of Medicine, 344,* 1279–1285.

Research Units on Pediatric Psychopharmacology (RUPP) Autism Network. (2005). Randomized, controlled, crossover trial of methylphenidate in pervasive developmental disorders with hyperactivity. *Archives of General Psychiatry, 62,* 1266–1274.

Reyes, M., Croonenberghs, J., Augustyns, I., & Eerdekens, M. (2006). Long-term use of risperidone in children with disruptive behavior disorders and subaverage intelligence: Efficacy, safety, and tolerability. *Journal of Child and Adolescent Psychopharmacology, 16,* 260–272.

Riddle, M. A., Kastelic, E. A., & Frosch, E. (2001). Pediatric psychopharmacology. *Journal of Child Psychology and Psychiatry, 42,* 73–90.

Runnheim, V. A., Frankenberger, W. R., & Hazelkorn, M. N. (1996). Medicating students with emotional and behavioral disorders and ADHD: A state survey. *Behavioral Disorders, 21,* 306–314.

Sandor, P. (2003). Pharmacological management of tics in patients with TS. *Journal of Psychosomatic Research, 55,* 41–48.

Santosh, P. J., & Taylor, E. (2002). Stimulant drugs. *European Journal of Child and Adolescent Psychiatry, 9,* 27–43.

Shedlack, K. J., Hennen, J., Magee, C., & Cheron, D. M. (2005). Assessing the utility of atypical antipsychotic medication in adults with mild mental retardation and comorbid psychiatric disorders. *Journal of Clinical Psychiatry, 66,* 52–62.

Sporn, A. L., Vermani, A., Greenstein, D. K., Bobb, A. J., Spencer, E. P., Clasen, L. S., et al. (2007). Clozapine treatment of childhood-onset schizophrenia: Evaluation of effectiveness, adverse effects, and long-term outcome. *Journal of the American Academy of Child and Adolescent Psychiatry, 46,* 1349–1356.

Steinberg, M. H. (1999). Management of sickle cell disease. *Drug Therapy, 340,* 1021–1030.

Steinberg, M. H. (2006). Pathophysiologically based drug treatment of sickle cell disease. *Trends in Pharmacological Sciences, 27,* 204–210.

Sullivan, J. E., & Dlugos, D. J. (2004). Idiopathic generalized epilepsy. *Current Treatment Options in Neurology, 6,* 231–242.

Sulzbacher, S., Farwell, J. R., Temkin, N., Lu, A. S., & Hirtz, D. G. (1999). Late cognitive effects of early treatment with phenobarbital. *Clinical Pediatrics, 38,* 387–394.

Szefler, J. K. (2000). Asthma: The new advances. *Advances in Pediatrics, 47,* 273–308.

Turgay, A., Snyder, R., Binder, C., Fisman, S., & Carrol, A. (2002). Risperidone in children with subaverage IQ and behavior disorders. *European Journal of Psychiatry, 17,* 118–118.

Usala, T., Clavennab, A., Zuddasa, A., & Bonati, M. (2008). Randomised controlled trials of selective serotonin reuptake inhibitors in treating depression in children and adolescents: A systematic review and meta-analysis. *European Neuropsychopharmacology, 18,* 62–73.

Varni, J. W. (1983). *Clinical behavioral pediatrics: An interdisciplinary biobehavioral approach.* New York: Pergamon Press.

Wagner, K. D., Ambrosini, P., Rynn, M., Wohlberg, C., Yang, R., Greenbaum, M. S., et al. (2003). Efficacy of sertraline in the treatment of children and adolescents with major depressive disorder: Two randomized controlled trials. *Journal of the American Medical Association, 290,* 1033–1041.

Wagner, K. D., Robb, A. S., Findling, R. L., Jin, J., Gutierrez, M. M., & Heydorn, W. E. (2004). A randomized, placebo-controlled trial of citalopram for the treatment of major depression in children and adolescents. *American Journal of Psychiatry, 161,* 1079–1083.

Walkup, J., Labellarte, M., Riddle, M. A., Pine, D. S., Greenhill, L., Fairbanks, J., et al. (2002). Treatment of pediatric anxiety disorders: An open label extension of the Research Units on Pediatric Psychopharmacology anxiety study. *Journal of Child and Adolescent Psychopharmacology, 12,* 175–188.

Waslick, B. (2006). Psychopharmacology interventions for pediatric anxiety disorders: A research update. *Child and Adolescent Psychiatric Clinics of North America, 15,* 51–71.

Werry, J. S., & Aman, M. G. (Eds.). (1999). *Practitioner's guide to psychoactive drugs for children and adolescents* (2nd ed.). New York: Plenum Press.

Wigal, T., Greenhill, L., Chuang, S., McGough, J., Vitiello, B., Skrobala, A., et al. (2006). Safety and tolerability of methylphenidate in preschool children with ADHD. *Journal of the American Academy of Child and Adolescent Psychiatry, 45,* 1294–1303.

Zdanowicz, M. M. (2007). Pharmacotherapy of asthma. *American Journal of Pharmaceutical Education, 71,* 1–12.

Zito, J. M., Safer, D. J., DosReis, S., Gardner, J. F., Magder, L., Soeken, K., et al. (2003). Psychotropic practice patterns for youth: A 10-year perspective. *Archives of Pediatrics and Adolescent Medicine, 157,* 17–25.

CHAPTER 13

Pediatric Medical Traumatic Stress

ANNE E. KAZAK
STEPHANIE SCHNEIDER
NANCY KASSAM-ADAMS

Pediatric illnesses, injuries, and treatments are potentially traumatic events (PTEs) with both short- and long-term consequences for patients and family members. In the past decade, there has been significant research documenting traumatic stress responses in pediatric patients and their parents across multiple illness and injury samples, with prevalence rates estimated to be 19% for injured children and 12% for ill children (Kahana, Feeny, Youngstrom, & Drotar, 2006). "Pediatric medical traumatic stress" (PMTS) is defined as "a set of psychological and physiological responses of children and their families to pain, injury, serious illness, medical procedures, and invasive or frightening treatment experiences" (National Child Traumatic Stress Network, 2004). Although it includes acute stress disorder (ASD) and posttraumatic stress disorder (PTSD), PMTS is broader and generally measured not by diagnosis but by a cluster of posttraumatic stress symptoms—particularly arousal, reexperiencing, and avoidance—linked to medical events. PMTS is common in pediatric settings, and although many children and families experience symptoms of posttraumatic stress, they show low overall rates of psychopathology. Many initially distressed children and families are resilient and appear to adapt and cope effectively with the aid of short-term, supportive interventions.

Many aspects of pediatric illness, injury, and treatment may be traumatic. PTEs, such as being intubated, learning that one's child has a life-threatening illness, or seeing a sibling hit by a car, may be perceived as traumatic by many if not most people. However, it is the *subjective experience of the PTE* that renders it traumatic. Objective characteristics of the illness (e.g., staging, severity, complexity) and related treatments (e.g., intensity, duration, type) are not frequently related to subsequent symptoms. Similarly, although the occurrence of a physical injury increases risk of PTSD, the objective severity of the injury is not necessarily related to the severity of subsequent PTSD symptoms. Although there is some evidence that the severity or intensity of medical procedures, and scarring or disfigurement with some injures, can be associated with more severe PMTS, evidence suggests that the perception of life threat, and the subjective appraisal of the severity of the injury/illness and intensity of treatment, are what moderate traumatic stress reactions.

PMTS is a relatively new concept. The first large multisite study in 320 survivors of childhood cancer and their parents, using a never-ill comparison group, was completed by Stuber, Kazak, and colleagues in the mid-1990s and highlighted the importance of traumatic responses for mothers and fathers (Kazak et al., 1998). The first studies documenting traumatic stress symptoms after pediatric injury were conducted in the late 1990s (Daviss et al., 2000; DeVries et al., 1999; Di Gallo, Barton, & Parry-Jones, 1997; see also reviews by Bruce, 2006; O'Donnell, Creamer, Bryant, Schnyder, & Shalev, 2003).

Model of the Phases of Medical Trauma

Our model of the phases of medical trauma (Kazak et al., 2006) is a conceptual framework that guides assessment and intervention based on the course of response to traumatic illness or injury. It postulates three phases: peritrauma; early and evolving responses; and longer-term responses. The timing and duration of each phase vary, depending on the nature and course of the medical event, as well as the possibility of recurrent, cyclical, or subsequent episodes of trauma.

Phase I: Peritrauma (During and Immediately Following the Medical PTE)

Child and parent responses immediately after the PTE can predict the course of PMTS. For example, child and adolescent ASD symptoms that emerge within a few hours of a road traffic injury have been linked with later severity of PMTS (Bryant, Salmon, Sinclair, & Davison, 2007; Meiser-Stedman, Yule, Smith, Glucksman, & Dalgleish, 2005). Early aspects of the medical condition or resulting treatment have also been linked to PMTS. Early physiological arousal in injured children (e.g., elevated heart rate in the emergency department) has been linked to child PTSD outcome (De Young, Kenardy, & Spence, 2007; Kassam-Adams, García-España, Fein, & Winston, 2005). For children in intensive care, length of hospitalization (Connolly, McClowry, Hayman, Mahony, & Artman, 2004), younger child age, severity of illness, and intensity of treatment are associated with PMTS 6 months after discharge (Rennick, Johnson, Dougherty, Platt, & Ritchie, 2002). For parents in one study, the presence and severity of ASD during admission were predictive of later PTSD, as was the subjective appraisal of life threat (Balluffi et al., 2004). There is also evidence that separation anxiety and social interactions may help explain PMTS responses for young children with burns (Saxe et al., 2005) and their parents (Hall et al., 2006).

Several preexisting child, parental, or family factors are associated with the emergence of PMTS. For children, prior psychopathology is associated with PTSD outcomes after traumatic injury (Daviss et al., 2000). Two studies of parents show similar associations: Preexisting anxiety and/or other psychological difficulties appear to predict PMTS in parents of cancer survivors (Kazak et al., 1998; Manne et al., 2004) and PTSD in parents of traumatically injured children (Daviss et al., 2000). Parents' coping style (Phipps, Larson, Long, & Rai, 2006), attitudes toward health care services, and perceptions of their children's health (Young et al., 2003) may also be related to PMTS. Social support is also related to PMTS in survivors of childhood cancer and their parents, as well as parents of organ transplantation survivors (Kazak et al., 1998; Young et al., 2003).

Phase II: Early, Ongoing, and Evolving Responses

After initial diagnosis of illness or injury, PTEs continue to occur during treatment and can elicit traumatic stress responses. Evolving traumatic stress responses during this second stage can have negative health and functional outcomes, including medication nonadherence (Mintzer et al., 2005) and lower quality of life (Holbrook et al., 2005). In general, higher levels of PMTS occur in children and parents closer to the time of diagnosis (Phipps, Long, Hudson, & Rai, 2005). More than 80% of injured children and their parents report at least one severe ASD symptom within a month of injury (Winston et al., 2002). For parents of children newly diagnosed with cancer, 50% of mothers and 40% of fathers met formal diagnostic criteria for ASD (Patino-Fernandez et al., 2008). In an independent sample, two-thirds of mothers and one-half of fathers reported PMTS in the moderate to severe range (Kazak, Boeving, Alderfer, Hwang, & Reilly, 2005). The severity of an individual's early responses may help predict longer-term outcomes. ASD symptom severity in the first month after injury is consistently correlated with later PMTS severity (Kassam-Adams & Winston, 2004).

Specific experiences and perceptions during medical care have been associated with PMTS. Cancer survivors with upsetting memories of treatment experiences and anxiety during treatment have a greater chance of developing long-term traumatic stress. Parental anxiety during medical care, related to fears that their children would die and to worry about relapse, was related to later PMTS (Best, Streisand, Catania, & Kazak, 2001). The importance of life threat as an early precipitant of PTSD is evidenced across pediatric populations, including youths with asthma, diabetes, and cancer. Adolescents with asthma who had a life-threatening attack had PTSD at a higher rate (20%) than those who did not have a life-threatening incident (11%). Parallel findings for parents show the impact on the family, with 29% of parents of children with a life-threatening incident meeting diagnostic criteria, relative to 14% of parents of control children with asthma (Kean, Kelsay, Wamboldt, & Wamboldt, 2006). These data are consistent with other reports of PTSD in parents of children with diabetes (Horsch, McManus, Kennedy, & Edge, 2007; Landolt, Vollrath, Laimbacher, Gnehm, & Sennhauser, 2005). There is also evidence that parental PMTS is specifically associated with cancer relapse (Jurbergs, Long, Ticona, & Phipps, 2009). Children and parents can have different responses to the same PTE during this phase. Six weeks after the accidents or diagnoses (diabetes, cancer), children with accident-related injuries had higher PMTS than those with diabetes or cancer, whereas parents of patients with cancer had significantly higher rates of PMTS than the other groups (Landolt, Vollrath, Ribi, Gnehm & Sennhauser, 2003).

Phase III: Longer-Term PMTS

Long-term PMTS has been reported in pediatric cancer, transplantation, and burns many years after the onset of the illness and the end of treatment. The most robust evidence exists for child cancer survivors and injured children. Higher rates of PMTS (including significant differences from controls), and elevated rates of PTSD (12–20%), are found in older samples of survivors of childhood cancer; these findings suggest a developmental influence, as well as the association of persistent PMTS with other psychosocial concerns in young adulthood (Rourke, Hobbie, Schwartz, & Kazak, 2007). The prevalence of PTSD in longer-term studies of children with injuries ranges from 6 to 25%, with additional children experiencing PMTS and functional impairment (DeVries et al., 1999, Kassam-Adams & Winston, 2004). Several smaller studies suggest the occurrence of longer-term PMTS and PTSD in children with other conditions, such as liver transplantation (Walker, Harris, Baker, Kelly, & Houghton, 1999) and burns (Stoddard, Norman, Murphy, & Beardslee, 1989). Burn survivors have also been shown to have elevated PMTS and PTSD, with related associations with poorer quality of life (Landolt, Buehlmann, Maag, & Schiestl, 2009).

Longer-term PMTS or PTSD has been well documented in families of childhood cancer survivors (Kazak, Alderfer, Rourke, et al., 2004; Kazak et al., 1997; Manne et al., 2004), parents of transplant recipients (Farley et al., 2007; Young et al., 2003), parents of children with epilepsy (Iseri, Ozten, & Aker, 2006), parents of patients with burns (Rizzone, Stoddard, Murphy, & Kruger, 1994), and parents of injured children (DeVries et al., 1999). The prevalence of these symptoms can be marked; for example, in a study of 150 families of adolescent survivors of childhood cancer, nearly all families (99%) had at least one parent meet symptom criteria for reexperiencing, and 20% of the families had at least one parent with current PTSD (Kazak, Alderfer, Rourke, et al., 2004). Specific dyadic patterns of PMTS in couples (parents) can be identified (Alderfer, Cnaan, Annunziato, & Kazak, 2005). PMTS is also relevant for siblings of cancer survivors (Alderfer, Labay, & Kazak, 2003).

Assessment and Treatment of PMTS

Assessment of PMTS

Now that the prevalence and impact of PMTS have been clearly established, it is essential to develop evidence-based assessment and intervention approaches for PMTS for children, adolescents, young adults, and family members. As a start, screening to identify those at greatest risk for long-term PMTS is a key goal in Phase I. The Screening Tool for Early Predictors of PTSD (Winston, Kassam-Adams, García-España, Ittenbach, & Cnaan, 2003) and the Child Trauma Screening Questionnaire (Kenardy, Spence, & Macleod, 2006) have each demonstrated good sensitivity and specificity in predicting child PTSD symptoms and impairment 6 months after injury.

Measures of PTSD most commonly used to assess medical trauma in Phases II and III include the Impact of Events Scale (Weiss & Marmar, 1997), the Child PTSD Reaction Index (Pynoos, Frederick, Nader, & Arroyo, 1987), the Child PTSD Symptom Scale (Foa, Johnson, Feeny, & Treadwell, 2001), and the Clinician-Administered PTSD Scale for Children (Newman et al., 2004), along with their adult counterparts for parents. Recent measures validated in samples with PMTS include the Acute Stress Checklist for

Children (Kassam-Adams, 2006), and the Child Stress Disorders Checklist (Saxe et al., 2003).

Intervention by Phase

Phase I

A goal of interventions during or immediately after a PTE (Phase I) is to modify the subjective experience of the PTE so that is less likely to be perceived as traumatic or lead to persistent traumatic stress symptoms. Consistent with family-centered medical practice, preventative interventions that skillfully address both child and parent needs during the course of a potentially traumatic medical event can be integrated into pediatric care. The Pediatric Medical Traumatic Stress Toolkit (Stuber, Schneider, Kassam-Adams, Kazak, & Saxe, 2006; available at *www.NCTSN.org/medtoolkit*) provides a "D-E-F" framework (distress, emotional support, and family involvement) for guiding professionals' trauma-informed assessment and intervention at the point of care.

Preliminary evidence exists regarding the effectiveness of interventions in this phase. Mothers of premature infants in a neonatal intensive care unit who participated in a structured, trauma-focused intervention showed significant improvements in posttraumatic stress symptoms compared to a control group (Jotzo & Poets, 2005). Some evidence also suggests that the dose of morphine administered to pediatric burn patients is inversely associated with PMTS 6 months later (Saxe et al., 2001).

Phase II

The goal of intervention during Phase II is to reduce or prevent PMTS. A three-session manualized intervention for parents/caregivers of children newly diagnosed with cancer, the Surviving Cancer Competently Intervention Program—Newly Diagnosed, has preliminary data supporting its ability to reduce PMTS (Kazak, Simms, et al., 2005). A stepped model of preventive intervention aimed at reducing PMTS following pediatric injury has been developed for the acute care setting and is being evaluated in a randomized trial (Kassam-Adams & Winston, 2004). Individual (child) cognitive-behavioral therapy may be helpful for youths after motor vehicle accidents (Smith et al., 2007).

Phase III

During Phase III, the goal of intervention is to treat symptoms of PTSD. To our knowledge, the only empirically evaluated intervention for medical trauma is the Surviving Cancer Competently Intervention Program, tested in a randomized clinical trial of 150 families (Kazak, Alderfer, Streisand, et al., 2004). This program integrates cognitive-behavioral and family therapy approaches to address posttraumatic stress symptoms in adolescent childhood cancer survivors and their mothers, fathers, and siblings.

Key Issues and Future Directions

PMTS has emerged as an important "marker" of psychosocial distress and one that may help clarify processes of coping and adaptation associated with pediatric illness and injury, as well as point to effective treatment approaches. Research on PMTS has increased dramatically in the past 10–15 years, with clear empirical support for the presence of traumatic stress symptoms across patient groups and across treatment phases (i.e., from acute stress associated with diagnosis or injury, to distress that continues years after the treatments end).

PMTS is an understandable, "normal," and not necessarily pathological, reaction to events that are nearly universal in their potential to elicit extreme responses from children and parents. There is still much to be learned about how traumatic events are experienced and about the potential for positive (growth) outcomes. Posttraumatic growth and posttraumatic stress can occur together (Barakat, Alderfer, & Kazak, 2006; Salter & Stallard, 2004). Viewing the response to a PTE as having both positive and negative outcomes helps patients and families balance their understanding and experience of it, and allows for interventions that build on individual and family strengths, while facilitating discussion of more upsetting aspects.

There is empirical evidence for PMTS across multiple members of the family. This is most evident for parents, and the literature provides important data on fathers in particular. Parents and children are not highly congruent in their reports of medically related trauma symptoms (Kassam-Adams, García-España, Miller, & Winston, 2006; Shemesh et al., 2005), although child and parent symptoms are related (Landolt, Vollrath, Timm, Gnehm, & Sennhauser, 2005; Meiser-Steadman et al., 2006). It is important to expand on some of the early findings regarding family-level effects, and particularly to understand differences among family members' experiences of PTEs and their ongoing communication about events and responses.

PMTS may be related to biopsychosocial outcomes that impact psychosocial functioning, quality of life and health, and ongoing utilization of health care. It is important to understand and address how symptoms of arousal and/or avoidance may affect these outcomes, particularly short- and long-term follow-up care as pediatric patients make the transition to adult health care systems. A methodological challenge will be to develop creative ways to include representative samples in research when avoidance is one of the symptoms under investigation.

A traumatic stress framework can be helpful for informing clinical care and research documenting the effectiveness of this care. In the more acute phases of treatment, the concept of traumatic stress is one that health care providers appreciate, and one that can be used to orient those involved in the patient's care to common PTEs in medical settings. Continued research documenting the effectiveness of nonpathologizing, competence-enhancing brief interventions to prevent or reduce PMTS is necessary. In addition, existing evidence-based treatments for child traumatic stress could be suitably adapted (and evaluated) for use with those children and families who experience persistent distress.

Medical trauma can also present challenges to the conceptualization of trauma. It may be difficult to distinguish specific traumatic events during an extended period of time when recurrent stress and distress are common. Medical trauma may be compounded and/or made more complex by recurrent events; the child's age and prior medical history; the type of setting in which treatment is delivered; a complicated treatment course; unexpected hospitalizations; or preexisting psychosocial difficulties. Organ transplantation has been described as an "anticipated trauma" (Emre, 2006), prompting consideration of how traumatic stress responses might be also anticipated. There is consensus in the broader trauma literature about the extent to which the perception of an event is more essential to a PTE than the actual objective event. The literature in medical trauma suggests that subjective appraisal is key, and potential targets for intervention may include beliefs about uncertainty (Santacroce & Lee, 2006), future threats (Stoppelbein, Greening, & Elkin, 2006), or ongoing health concerns (Wiener et al., 2006).

Summary

A traumatic stress framework has emerged in the past two decades, with substantial evidence supporting the occurrence of PMTS in patients and parents, across illness groups, and from the point of injury or disease onset and early treatment through long-term follow-up. Current and ongoing efforts linking PMTS with other individual, family and systemic factors are important next steps, along with the development of evidence-based assessment and intervention.

Acknowledgments

Preparation of this chapter was supported by the Center for Pediatric Traumatic Stress at The Children's Hospital of Philadelphia, a Treatment and Services Administration Center of the National Child Traumatic Stress Network (No. SM058139). We thank Branlyn Werba, PhD, for her thoughtful comments.

References

Alderfer, M., Labay, L., & Kazak, A. (2003). Brief report: Does posttraumatic stress apply to siblings of childhood cancer survivors? *Journal of Pediatric Psychology, 28*, 281–286.

Alderfer, M. A., Cnaan, A., Annunziato, R. A., & Kazak, A. (2005). Patterns of posttraumatic stress symptoms in parents of childhood cancer survivors. *Journal of Family Psychology, 19*, 430–440.

Balluffi, A., Kassam-Adams, N., Kazak, A., Tucker, M., Dominguez, T., & Helfaer, M. (2004). Traumatic stress in parents of children admitted to the pediatric intensive care unit. *Pediatric Critical Care Medicine, 5*, 547–553.

Barakat, L., Alderfer, M., & Kazak, A. (2006). Posttraumatic growth in adolescent survivors of cancer and their families. *Journal of Pediatric Psychology, 31*, 413–419.

Best, M., Streisand, R., Catania, L., & Kazak, A. (2001). Parental distress during pediatric leukemia and parental posttraumatic stress symptoms after treatment ends. *Journal of Pediatric Psychology, 26*, 299–307.

Bruce, M. (2006). A systematic and conceptual review of posttraumatic stress in childhood cancer survivors and their parents. *Clinical Psychology Review, 26*, 233–256.

Bryant, R. A., Salmon, K., Sinclair, E., & Davidson, P. (2007). The relationship between acute stress disorder and posttraumatic stress disorder in injured children. *Journal of Traumatic Stress, 20*, 1075–1079.

Connolly, D., McClowry, S., Hayman, L., Mahony, L., & Artman, M. (2004). Posttraumatic stress disorder in children after cardiac surgery. *Journal of Pediatrics, 144*, 480–484.

Daviss, W., Mooney, D., Racusin, R., Ford, J., Fleischer, A., & McHugo, G. (2000). Predicting posttraumatic stress after hospitalization for pediatric injury. *Journal of the American Academy of Child and Adolescent Psychiatry, 39,* 576–583.

De Young, A., Kenardy, J., & Spence, S. (2007). Elevated heart rate as a predictor of PTSD six months following accidental pediatric injury. *Journal of Traumatic Stress, 20,* 751–756.

DeVries, A. P. J., Kassam-Adams, N., Cnaan, A., Sherman Slate, E., Gallagher, P., & Winston, F. K. (1999). Looking beyond the physical injury: Posttraumatic stress disorder in children and parents after pediatric traffic injury. *Pediatrics, 104,* 1293–1299.

Di Gallo, A., Barton, J., & Parry-Jones, W. L. (1997). Road traffic accidents: Early psychological consequences in children and adolescents. *British Journal of Psychiatry, 170,* 358–362.

Emre, S. (2006). Posttraumatic stress disorder in posttransplant children: Creating a clinical program to address their needs. *CNS Spectrums, 11,* 118, 120–126.

Farley, L. M., DeMaso, D. R., D'Angelo, E., Kinnamon, C., Bastardi, H., Hill, C. E., et al. (2007). Parenting stress and parental post-traumatic stress disorder in families after pediatric heart transplantation. *Journal of Heart and Lung Transplantation, 26,* 120–126.

Foa, E., Johnson, K., Feeny, N., & Treadwell, K. (2001). The Child PTSD Symptom Scale: A preliminary examination of its psychometric properties. *Journal of Clinical Child Psychology, 30,* 376–384.

Hall, E., Saxe, G., Stoddard, F., Kaplow, J., Koenen, K., Chawla, N., et al. (2006). Posttraumatic stress symptoms in parents of children with acute burns. *Journal of Pediatric Psychology, 31,* 403–412.

Holbrook, T. L., Hoyt, D. B., Coimbra, R., Potenza, B., Sise, M., & Anderson, J. P. (2005). Long-term posttraumatic stress disorder persists after major trauma in adolescents: New data on risk factors and functional outcome. *Journal of Trauma–Injury Infection and Critical Care, 58,* 764–769.

Horsch, A., McManus, F., Kennedy, P., & Edge, J. (2007). Anxiety, depressive, and posttraumatic stress symptoms in mothers of children with Type 1 diabetes. *Journal of Traumatic Stress, 20,* 881–891.

Iseri, P. K., Ozten, E., & Aker, A. T. (2006). Posttraumatic stress disorder and major depressive disorder is common in parents of children with epilepsy. *Epilepsy and Behavior, 8,* 250–255.

Jotzo, M., & Poets, C. (2005). Helping parents cope with the trauma of premature birth: An evaluation of a trauma-preventative psychological intervention. *Pediatrics, 115,* 915–919.

Jurbergs, N., Long, A., Ticona, L., & Phipps, S. (2009). Symptoms of posttraumatic stress in parents of children with cancer: Are they elevated relative to parents of healthy children? *Journal of Pediatric Psychology, 34,* 4–13.

Kahana, S. Y., Feeny, N. C., Youngstrom, E. A., & Drotar, D. (2006). Posttraumatic stress in youth experiencing illnesses and injuries: An exploratory meta-analysis. *Traumatology, 12,* 148–161.

Kassam-Adams, N. (2006). Development and validation of the Acute Stress Checklist for Children (ASC-Kids). *Journal of Traumatic Stress, 19,* 129–139.

Kassam-Adams, N., García-España, J. F., Fein, J., & Winston, F. (2005). Heart rate and posttraumatic stress in injured children. *Archives of General Psychiatry, 62,* 335–340.

Kassam-Adams, N., García-España, J. F., Miller, V. A., & Winston, F. (2006). Parent–child agreement regarding children's acute stress: The role of parent acute stress reactions. *Journal of the American Academy of Child and Adolescent Psychiatry, 12,* 1485–1493

Kassam-Adams, N., & Winston, F. K. (2004). Predicting child PTSD: The relationship between ASD and PTSD in injured children. *Journal of the American Academy of Child and Adolescent Psychiatry, 43,* 403–411.

Kazak, A., Alderfer, M., Rourke, M., Simms, S., Streisand, R., & Grossman, J. (2004). Posttraumatic stress symptoms (PTSS) and posttraumatic stress disorder (PTSD) in families of adolescent childhood cancer survivors. *Journal of Pediatric Psychology, 29,* 211–219.

Kazak, A., Alderfer, M., Streisand, R., Simms, S., Rourke, M., Barakat, L., et al. (2004). Treatment of posttraumatic stress symptoms in adolescent survivors of childhood cancer and their families: A randomized clinical trial. *Journal of Family Psychology, 18,* 493–504.

Kazak, A., Barakat, L., Meeske, K., Christakis, D., Meadows, A., Casey, R., et al. (1997). Posttraumatic stress, family functioning, and social support in survivors of childhood leukemia and their mothers and fathers. *Journal of Consulting and Clinical Psychology, 65,* 120–129.

Kazak, A., Boeving, A., Alderfer, M., Hwang, W. T., & Reilly, A. (2005). Posttraumatic stress symptoms in parents of pediatric oncology patients during treatment. *Journal of Clinical Oncology, 23,* 7405–7410.

Kazak, A., Kassam-Adams, N., Schneider, S., Zelikovsky, N., Alderfer, M., & Rourke, M. (2006). An integrative model of pediatric medical traumatic stress. *Journal of Pediatric Psychology, 31,* 343–355.

Kazak, A., Simms, S., Alderfer, M., Rourke, M., Crump, T., McClure, K., et al. (2005). Feasibility and preliminary outcomes from a pilot study of a brief psychological intervention for families of children newly diagnosed with cancer. *Journal of Pediatric Psychology, 30,* 644–655.

Kazak, A., Stuber, M., Barakat, L., Meeske, K., Guthrie, D., & Meadows, A. (1998). Predicting posttraumatic stress symptoms in mothers and fathers of survivors of childhood cancer. *Journal of the American Academy of Child and Adolescent Psychiatry, 37,* 823–831.

Kean, E. M., Kelsay, K., Wamboldt, F., & Wamboldt, M. Z. (2006). Posttraumatic stress in adolescents with asthma and their parents. *Journal of the American Academy of Child and Adolescent Psychiatry, 45,* 78–86.

Kenardy, J. A., Spence, S. H., & Macleod, A. C. (2006). Screening for posttraumatic stress disorder in children after accidental injury. *Pediatrics, 118,* 1002–1009.

Landolt, M., Buehlmann, C., Maag, T., & Schiestl, C. (2009). Brief report: Quality of life is impaired in pediatric burn survivors with posttraumatic stress disorder. *Journal of Pediatric Psychology, 34,* 14–21.

Landolt, M., Vollrath, M., Ribi, K., Gnehm, H., & Sennhauser, F. (2003). Incidence and associations of parental and child posttraumatic stress symptoms in pediatric patients. *Journal of Child Psychology and Psychiatry, 44,* 1199–1207.

Landolt, M. A., Vollrath, M., Laimbacher, J., Gnehm, H. E., & Sennhauser, F. H. (2005). Prospective study of posttraumatic stress disorder in parents of children with newly diagnosed Type 1 diabetes. *Journal of the American Academy of Child and Adolescent Psychiatry, 44,* 682–689.

Landolt, M. A., Vollrath, M., Timm, K., Gnehm, H. E., & Sennhauser, F. H. (2005). Predicting posttraumatic stress symptoms in children after road traffic accidents. *Journal of the American Academy of Child and Adolescent Psychiatry, 44,* 1276–1283.

Manne, S., DuHamel, K., Ostroff, J., Parsons, S., Martini, D., Williams, S., et al. (2004). Anxiety, depressive, and posttraumatic stress disorders among mothers of pediatric hematopoietic stem cell transplantation. *Pediatrics, 113,* 1700–1708.

Meiser-Stedman, R., Yule, W., Smith, P., Glucksman, E., & Dalgleish, T. (2005). Acute stress disorder and posttraumatic stress disorder in children and adolescents involved in assaults or motor vehicle accidents. *American Journal of Psychiatry, 162,* 1381–1383.

Mintzer, L. L., Stuber, M. L., Seacord, D., Castaneda, M., Mesrkhani, V., & Glover, D. (2005). Traumatic stress symptoms in adolescent organ transplant recipients. *Pediatrics, 115,* 1640–1649.

National Child Traumatic Stress Network. (2004, October). Pediatric Medical Traumatic Stress Toolkit. Retrieved January 10, 2008, from *www.NCTSN.org/medtoolkit*

Newman, E., Weathers, F. W., Nader, K., Kaloupek, D. G., Pynoos, R. S., Blake, D. D., et al.

(2004). *Clinician-Administered PTSD Scale for Children and Adolescents (CAPS-CA)*. Los Angeles: Western Psychological Services.

O'Donnell, M., Creamer, M., Bryant, R., Schnyder, U., & Shalev, A. (2003). Posttraumatic stress disorders following injury: An empirical and methodological review. *Clinical Psychology Review, 23*, 587–603.

Patino-Fernandez, A., Pai, A., Alderfer, M. A., Hwang, W. T., Reilly, A., & Kazak, A. (2008). Acute stress in parents of children newly diagnosed with cancer. *Pediatric Blood and Cancer, 50*, 289–292.

Phipps, S., Larson, S., Long, A., & Rai, S. N. (2006) Adaptive style and symptoms of posttraumatic stress in children with cancer and their parents. *Journal of Pediatric Psychology, 31*, 298–309.

Phipps, S., Long, A., Hudson, M., & Rai, S. N. (2005). Symptoms of post-traumatic stress in children with cancer and their parents: Effects of informant and time from diagnosis. *Pediatric Blood and Cancer, 45*, 952–959.

Pynoos, R., Frederick, S., Nader, K., & Arroyo, W. (1987). Life threat and posttraumatic stress in school age children. *Archives of General Psychiatry, 44*, 1057–1063.

Rennick, J., Johnston, C., Dougherty, G., Platt, R., & Ritchie, J. (2002). Children's psychological responses to illness and exposure to invasive technology. *Journal of Developmental and Behavioral Pediatrics, 23*, 133–144.

Rizzone, L., Stoddard, F., Murphy, M., & Kruger, L. (1994). Posttraumatic stress disorder in mothers of children and adolescents with burns. *Journal of Burn Care and Rehabilitation, 15*, 158–163.

Rourke, M., Hobbie, W., Schwartz, L., & Kazak, A. (2007). Posttraumatic stress disorder (PTSD) in young adult survivors of childhood cancer. *Pediatric Blood Cancer, 49*, 177–182.

Salter, E., & Stallard, P. (2004). Posttraumatic growth in child survivors of a road traffic accident. *Journal of Traumatic Stress, 17*, 335–340.

Santacroce, S. J., & Lee, Y. L. (2006). Uncertainty, posttraumatic stress, and health behavior in young adult childhood cancer survivors. *Nursing Research, 55*, 259–266.

Saxe, G., Chawla, N., Stoddard, F., Kassam-Adams, N., Courtney, D., Cunningham, K., et al. (2003). Child Stress Disorders Checklist: A measure of ASD and PTSD in children. *Journal of the American Academy of Child and Adolescent Psychiatry, 42*, 972–978.

Saxe, G., Stoddard, F., Courtney, D., Cunningham, K., Chawla, N., Sheridan, R., et al. (2001). Relationship between acute morphine and the course of PTSD in children with burns. *Journal of the American Academy of Child and Adolescent Psychiatry, 40*, 915–921.

Saxe, G. N., Stoddard, F., Hall, E., Chawla, N., Lopez, C., Sheridan, R., et al. (2005). Pathways to PTSD, Part I: Children with burns. *American Journal of Psychiatry, 162*, 1299–1304.

Shemesh, E., Newcorn, J. H., Rockmore, L., Schneider, B. L., Emre, S., Gelb, B. D., et al. (2005). Comparison of parent and child reports of emotional trauma symptoms in pediatric outpatient settings. *Pediatrics, 115*, e582–e589.

Smith, P., Yule, W., Perrin, S., Tranah, T., Dalgleish, T., & Clark, D. (2007). Cognitive-behavioral therapy for PTSD in children and adolescents: A preliminary randomized controlled trial. *Journal of the American Academy of Child and Adolescent Psychiatry, 46*, 1051–1061.

Stoddard, F., Norman, D., Murphy, J. M., & Beardslee, W. (1989). Psychiatric outcome of burned children and adolescents. *Journal of the American Academy of Child and Adolescent Psychiatry, 28*, 589–595.

Stoppelbein, L. A., Greening, L., & Elkin, T. D. (2006). Risk of posttraumatic stress symptoms: A comparison of child survivors of pediatric cancer and parental bereavement. *Journal of Pediatric Psychology, 31*, 367–376.

Stuber, M. L., Schneider, S., Kassam-Adams, N., Kazak, A. E., & Saxe, G. (2006). The Medical Traumatic Stress Toolkit. *CNS Spectrums, 11*, 137–142.

Walker, A., Harris, G., Baker, A., Kelly, D., & Houghton, J. (1999). Posttraumatic stress responses following liver transplantation in older children. *Journal of Child Psychology and Psychiatry, 40,* 363–374.

Weiss, D. S., & Marmar, C. R. (1997). The Impact of Event Scale—Revised. In J. P. Wilson & T. M. Keane (Eds.), *Assessing psychological trauma and PTSD* (pp. 399–411). New York: Guilford Press.

Wiener, L., Battles, H., Bernstein, D., Long, L., Derdak, J., Mackall, C. L., et al. (2006). Persistent psychological distress in long-term survivors of pediatric sarcoma: The experience at a single institution. *Psycho-Oncology, 15,* 898–910.

Winston, F., Kassam-Adams, N., García-España, J. F., Ittenbach, R., & Cnaan, A. (2003). Screening for risk of persistent posttraumatic stress in injured children and their parents. *Journal of the American Medical Association, 290,* 643–649.

Winston, F., Kassam-Adams, N., Vivarelli-O'Neill, C., Ford, J., Newman, E., Baxt, C., et al. (2002). Acute stress disorder symptoms in children and their parents after pediatric traffic injury. *Pediatrics, 109,* e90.

Young, G., Mintzer, L., Seacord, D., Castaneda, M., Mesrkhani, V., & Stuber, M. (2003). Symptoms of posttraumatic stress disorder in parents of transplant recipients: Incidence, severity and related factors. *Pediatrics, 111,* e725–e731.

CHAPTER 14

Palliative Care, End of Life, and Bereavement

CYNTHIA A. GERHARDT
AMY E. BAUGHCUM
TAMMI YOUNG-SALEME
KATHRYN VANNATTA

A child's death is one of the most traumatic events a family may experience, and one that parents hope they never have to face. However, each year over 50,000 children under age 20 die in the United States (Heron, 2007), and over 500,000 have a life-threatening condition (Arias, MacDorman, Strobino, & Guyer, 2003). Half of all deaths occur in the first year of life, often from prematurity, birth complications, congenital anomalies, or sudden infant death syndrome (Heron, 2007). For children ages 1–19, unintentional injury and homicide are the leading causes of death (accounting for 30%), while cancer is the leading cause of death by disease (accounting for 4%). Although many childhood deaths are unexpected, an estimated 15,000 children die from conditions that might benefit from supportive or palliative care (Feudtner et al., 2001). At any point in time, about 5,000 children are living within the last 6 months of their lives (Feudtner et al., 2001).

The terms "palliative care," "end-of-life care," and "hospice" are often used interchangeably, but there are key differences. Palliative care prevents, relieves, or reduces physical and psychosocial suffering associated with a serious medical condition or treatment (Field & Behrman, 2003). Pain management and antiemetics are examples of palliative therapies. Core components of palliation include maintenance of quality of life, as well as interdisciplinary care that extends to the entire family. Palliative and curative therapies should coexist throughout an illness, with palliation increasing as curative therapies become less effective, to facilitate the transition to end-of-life care and/or hospice. End-of-life care refers to preparation for an anticipated death and managing the last stage of a fatal condition (e.g., decisions about mechanical support); hospice is a program or facility that provides palliative, end-of-life, and bereavement care for families of individuals, usually within the last 6 months of life (Field & Behrman, 2003).

Unfortunately, all of these terms are frequently considered taboo in pediatrics. The death of a child is out of the natural order of events and may be preceded by heroic efforts to save the child despite all odds and costs. Pediatric providers have reported inadequate training, poor hospital support, and discomfort in managing end-of-life care (Contro, Larson, Scofield, Sourkes, & Cohen, 2004; Hilden et al., 2001). The transition to end-of-life care is often late or abrupt in pediatrics, which can lead to poor symptom management and significant suffering (Field & Behrman, 2003; Wolfe, Grier, et al., 2000). For some children, death is an inevitable outcome, but one that can be managed with sensitivity as an ongoing phase of the illness. Acknowledging a child's impending death can provide opportunities to ease anxiety, maximize comfort, increase family communication, and complete advance care planning.

The Institute of Medicine and the American Academy of Pediatrics have called for improvements in our care of children with life-limiting illnesses (Field & Behrman, 2003). Education and research regarding pediatric palliative care is limited, and multiple factors may complicate pediatric end-of-life care: ethical and legal issues, financial barriers, illness types and trajectories, and availability or access (particularly outside of tertiary care centers). Pediatric psychologists have many important roles in the care of children with life-limiting illnesses. They can facilitate communication between health care providers and families; assist with coping and adjustment; aid in decision making and advance care planning; provide staff support and education; conduct research to inform clinical practice; and participate in advocacy and policy making. Some pediatric psychologists provide palliative care as part of an interdisciplinary team that often has long-term contact with families, while others provide consultation or crisis intervention near the time of death or after. These different approaches can affect treatment goals and intervention strategies, as well as expectations of success in working with families.

Care of Children and Families at the End of Life

Although research on pediatric end-of-life care is limited, most of it has focused on children with cancer and relies heavily on medical charts or retrospective parent reports. Patterns of care have suggested that half of children who die of cancer die at home (Bradshaw, Hinds, Lensing, Gattuso, & Razzouk, 2005; Klopfenstein, Hutchison, Clark, Young, & Ruymann, 2001; Wolfe, Grier, et al., 2000). Of children who die in the hospital, 50% or more are in an intensive care unit (ICU), and one-half to two-thirds have "do not resuscitate" (DNR) orders, written on average in the last month of life (Bradshaw et al., 2005; Drake, Frost, & Collins, 2003; Klopfenstein et al., 2001; Wolfe, Grier, et al., 2000).

Despite having access to specialized care (e.g., ICU, hospice), many children experience considerable suffering at the end of life (Collins et al., 2000; Drake et al., 2003; Jalmsell, Kreicbergs, Onelov, Steineck, & Henter, 2006; Wolfe, Grier, et al., 2000), reflecting the difficulty inherent in balancing length and quality of life. The most prevalent physical symptoms among children with life-limiting illnesses include fatigue, pain, respiratory problems, decreased appetite, nausea/vomiting, and drowsiness (Hongo et al., 2003; Jalmsell et al., 2006; Wolfe, Grier, et al., 2000). Fatigue and pain are the most frequent and distressing symptoms, occurring in nearly all children at the end of life (Drake et al., 2003; Theunissen et al., 2007; Wolfe, Grier, et al., 2000). The most common psychological symptoms include sadness, anxiety, and irritability (Collins et al., 2000; Hongo et al., 2003). Complete or partial resolution of symptoms is low, with children having an average of 11 symptoms in the last week of life (Drake et al., 2003). In several studies, fatigue was undertreated at the end of life, whereas pain was treated nearly 80% of the time but usually without success (Drake et al., 2003; Theunissen et al., 2007; Wolfe, Grier, et al., 2000). Although complete resolution of symptoms may be unrealistic at the end of life, symptom management and children's quality of life can be vastly improved.

Given the significant symptom burden experienced by children with life-limiting conditions, concern for family members is also warranted as they accommodate the illness and its treatment within the family system (Kazak, 1992). In addition to coping with the illness, families must manage a child's medical care, communication among health care providers and family members, disruptions in family roles and routines, financial costs, and the imminent probability of the child's death. Parents must handle their own distress, while simultaneously managing their child's distress and making difficult treatment decisions in a limited amount of time.

Parents, particularly mothers, of children with chronic illnesses are at risk for psychosocial difficulties (Pai et al., 2007; Wallander & Varni, 1998). Caring for a seriously ill child can have significant effects on parental mood, sleep, and fatigue, with fear of the child's death and physical symptoms frequently reported at the end of life (Gedaly-Duff, Lee, Nail, Nicholson, & Johnson, 2006; Theunissen et al., 2007). There is minimal research on family adjustment and caregiver strain during the palliative and end-of-life phases, but pediatric psychologists can provide invaluable support during this time, as discussed below.

Communication and Decision Making

During a child's illness, parents must have ongoing communication with medical staff and their child about his or her health. Pediatric psychologists can facilitate communication, but parents bear the primary responsibility for making decisions, as well as explaining and filtering information for their child. Unfortunately, parents may not understand important aspects of their child's condition, which can complicate communication (Levi, Marsick, Drotar, & Kodish, 2000). Understanding of medical information may be hindered by the frequent use of euphemisms and implicit language by health care providers. Anxiety and reluctance on behalf of physicians to prognosticate, deliver bad news, and diminish hope can also play a role (Meyer, Burns, Griffith, & Truog, 2002).

As a result, many parents have reported dissatisfaction with their children's care and medical communication at the end of life (Contro, Larson, Scofield, Sourkes, & Cohen, 2002; Meyer et al., 2002). In one study, over half of parents felt they had little or no control during their children's final days (Meyer et al., 2002). Approximately 25% did not feel fully informed of their children's prognoses and stated they would have made different decisions had they received better information. Another study noted that physicians realized children's illnesses were terminal an average of more than 3 months before parents did, suggesting significant gaps in communication between families and health care providers (Wolfe, Klar, et al., 2000).

Although it is generally accepted that school-age children should be informed of their illness and should assent to treatment, health care providers and parents struggle with how much to tell children and how to include them in decision making. Communication should be based on children's stages of cognitive and emotional development. Understandably, parents provide more information to older children (Eiser & Havermans, 1992; Graham-Pole, Wass, Eyberg, Chu, & Olejnik, 1989). Age-related changes in the ability to comprehend complex and abstract concepts, as well as previous experience with death, increase children's understanding of illness and death (Eiser & Havermans, 1992; Rushforth, 1999). By age 5 or 6, most children understand the universality of death; however, a fully formulated concept of death, particularly a sense of personal mortality, is usually not evident until after age 8 or 9 (Oltjenbruns, 2001).

Information provided to children with life-limiting conditions has typically focused on treatment and procedural details, and less on disease severity or prognosis (Eiser & Havermans, 1992). Chesler and Barbarin (1987) found that only 30% of parents talked to their children about all or almost all aspects of the children's cancer. In a study of parents whose children died of cancer, 34% had talked about death with their children, and none of the parents regretted it (Kreicbergs, Valdimarsdottir, Onelov, Henter, & Steineck, 2004b). However, 27% of parents who did not talk with their children had regrets. Parents were more likely to talk with their children and surviving siblings if they sensed that the ill children were aware of their imminent death, the children were older, and the families were more religious (Graham-Pole et al., 1989; Kreicbergs et al., 2004b).

Children want to know about their disease, treatment, and prognosis. Ellis and Leventhal (1993) surveyed 50 children with cancer ages 8–17 and found that 95% wanted to be told if they were dying. Most felt that physicians should make treatment decisions, but 28% of children and 63% of adolescents wanted to be involved. Children with more severe disease and side effects may request and receive more information from parents (Cohen, Friedrich, Copeland, & Pendergrass, 1989). Although difficulty talking to parents about death and fear of being alone have been reported at the end of life (Theunissen et al., 2007), some children are aware that they are dying and may feel isolated if they are unable to talk about it (Hilden, Watterson, & Chrastek, 2000).

Psychologists can play a key role in communication with the medical team and a child's family. This may include assessing family beliefs about death and previous losses; helping parents talk about death with the ill child and siblings; giving the child a chance to ask questions and express feelings through developmentally appropriate means (e.g., journal, artwork); allowing the family members to share feelings for one another; and preparing them to say goodbye. Some children may wish to give gifts or will belongings to loved ones, participate in funeral planning, and make special requests for after their death (Foster et al., in press). These discussions, though difficult, have the potential to promote healing, provide closure, and minimize guilt and regrets after the death.

Advance care planning should consider the cultural, spiritual, and moral values of the child and family (Kirkwood, 2005; Matlins & Magida, 2003), as well as ethical and legal guidelines. Consensus building and assessing family preferences for end-of-life care, such as life-sustaining treatment, mechanical support, DNR status, and place of death, is important. For patients over age 18, advance directives (e.g., living will, durable power of attorney) should be addressed. Advance care plans should include the family and medical team and should be documented in writing. They may also require periodic revision, depending on changes in the child's status and reevaluation of family needs and preferences.

Bereavement and Grief Theory

"Bereavement" is the objective loss of someone significant, whereas "grief" is an individual's reaction to the loss (Stroebe, Hansson, Stroebe, & Schut, 2001). Symptoms can include affective, cognitive, behavioral, and physiological features, such as despair, anger, crying, agitation, sleep disruption, and thoughts of the deceased. Prolonged, severe, or atypical reactions have prompted attempts to distinguish normal grief from complicated or traumatic grief. There is some evidence for traumatic grief as a distinct disorder in adulthood (Prigerson & Jacobs, 2001), but it is unclear whether this is applicable to children. There has also been a conceptual shift from a pathological framework to one that recognizes grief as a normal reaction to loss, which can also be associated with positive outcomes or growth experiences (Schaeffer & Moos, 2001).

Contemporary theory suggests that differences in grief outcomes may be best accounted for by models that integrate more than one theoretical approach. This is in contrast to individual theories that emphasize the need to break emotional bonds with the deceased or progress through fixed stages (e.g., shock, denial, acceptance) for recovery. The dual-process model suggests that individuals must oscillate between loss-oriented tasks to deal with the death (e.g., crying, remembering) and restoration-oriented tasks to manage ongoing responsibilities (e.g., work, parenting) (Stroebe & Schut, 1999). An overemphasis on either type of task may lead to difficulties, whereas a balance may promote better adaptation. Bereaved individuals may also develop an ongoing attachment or continuing bond with the deceased (Klass, Silverman, & Nickman, 1996), allowing them to maintain a "sense of presence" with their loved one (e.g., "my guardian angel," "still a part of me"). Recent work has shown that bereaved adults form continuing bonds with the deceased (Field, Eval, & Bonanno, 2003), but less is known about bereaved children (Hogan & DeSantis, 1996).

A child and family may experience anticipatory grief over the child's loss of functioning and/or impending death (Coor & Coor, 2000). Some individuals may distance themselves from the child before death. If possible, it is important to determine whether family members have any special requests (e.g., baptism) and whether they wish to be together before or during the death. Not all family members can or want to be present at the time of death, but this should be addressed with the wishes of both the child and family in mind. Family members should be prepared for physical responses to death (e.g., changes in respiration) if they are present. Some may want to hold the child, take pictures, or prepare the body (e.g., bathing, dressing) following death. Families should be allowed as much time as needed to say goodbye during these last moments.

Parental Grief

Although relatively understudied, the death of a child is one of the most difficult and profound experiences for surviving parents and siblings. It has been described as more painful than any other loss (Cleiren, Diekstra, Kerkhof, & van der Wal, 1994). Parental grief can persist for years, and recovery is more an acceptance of a fluctuation in pain than the total disappearance of pain (Hazzard, Weston, & Gutterres, 1992). The death is not a single event that is mourned; it represents a series of hopes and dreams that are repeatedly lost. As such, it can intensify during significant periods (e.g., holidays, graduation), resulting in "regrief." Despite the intensity of their grief, bereaved parents have also reported significant personal growth and positive outcomes after the death (Hogan & Schmidt, 2002).

Not surprisingly, the impact on bereaved parents is substantial. Bereaved parents are at risk for depression, anxiety, guilt, posttraumatic stress, and anger (Hazzard et al., 1992; Kreicbergs, Valdimarsdottir, Onelov, Henter, & Steineck, 2004a; Murphy et al., 1999; Vance et al., 1995). They routinely score worse on most standardized scales of adjustment, especially internalizing problems, than normative populations and controls do (Lehman, Wortman, & Williams, 1987; Moore, Gilliss, & Martinson, 1988). Families may undergo significant change, with less family cohesion and more strain (Lehman, Lang, Wortman, & Sorenson, 1989; Martinson, McClowry, Davies, & Kuhlenkamp, 1994). Bereaved parents have also reported less marital satisfaction and sexual intimacy, more thoughts about separation, and higher divorce rates than nonbereaved parents (Gottlieb, Lang, & Amsel, 1996; Lang & Gottlieb, 1991; Najman et al., 1993). Bereaved parents may be preoccupied with their grief and "overlook" surviving children (Rosen, 1985), or, alternatively, they may become closer and overprotective (Lehman et al., 1989). Bereaved parents have reported more parenting stress than controls (Lehman et al., 1987), and their children have reported less communication, availability, and support from them (Rosen, 1985).

Sibling Grief

Siblings of children with chronic illnesses may be at risk for multiple difficulties before the death and after (Sharpe & Rossiter, 2002). In many pediatric illnesses, the death may have been preceded by years of stressful treatments, when much of the family's attention and resources were directed toward the ill child. Older siblings may have even participated in caring for their ailing brother or sister. Because siblings share many experiences, they have a unique and powerful bond, and its loss can cause significant grief and emotional pain (Davies, 1999).

Research on sibling bereavement is limited, partly due to the lack of standardized measures of grief in children (Niemeyer & Hogan, 2001). Hogan and Greenfield (1991) have reported the presence of grief symptoms in bereaved siblings, as well as positive growth, such as having a better outlook on life and being kinder, compassionate, and more tolerant. Most research has noted that siblings' grief and psychosocial difficulties abate over time, but it is not unusual for them to have symptoms years later (Davies, 1999). Siblings may also experience "regrief" when they process the death from a different vantage point as they mature (Oltjenbruns, 2001).

Retrospective, qualitative studies suggest that surviving siblings may have feelings of isolation and social withdrawal both at home and with peers (Davies, 1991; Martinson & Campos, 1991). Compared to norms, bereaved siblings may have significantly less social competence and more social withdrawal within 2 years of the death (Birenbaum, Robinson, Phillips, Stewart, & McCown, 1989; Hutton & Bradley, 1994). Both internalizing and externalizing problems have also been reported (Birenbaum et al., 1989; Hutton & Bradley, 1994; McCown & Davies, 1995). Siblings have reported feeling guilty, anxious, and depressed (Fanos & Nickerson, 1991; Rosen, 1985); parents have noted similar problems, including anxiety, trouble sleeping, and posttraumatic stress symptoms, in their children (Applebaum & Burns, 1991; Powell, 1991).

Interventions

There are few empirically based interventions for families of children at end of life or after bereavement, as well as for health care providers. Although a recent review of several meta-analyses did not find strong support for the efficacy of bereavement interventions (Jordan & Neimeyer, 2003), there is ongoing debate about this conclusion (Larson & Hoyt, 2007). Issues regarding the target audience, content, structure, and timing of interventions remain challenging. Some families may find support groups, books, Web-based resources, or therapy helpful. For staff members, stress management, maintenance of professional boundaries, peer support, and debriefings may be useful. However, grief is personal and unique. It should not be presumed that all interventions are beneficial or benign, as some may intensify grief or be perceived negatively by families and staff. Allowing a natural course for grief may be better for some individuals.

Summary and Future Directions

Pediatric psychologists play important roles in the care of families of children with life-limiting illness. Early work indicates that children and families experience significant symptom burden at end of life and after bereavement. Increased research in this area can provide direction for improvements in care to reduce morbidity for children and families. Attention to education, training, and policy is also paramount. Unfortunately, the sensitive nature of pediatric palliative care and bereavement has made clinical care and research a delicate and challenging process. Furthermore, research funding has been difficult to obtain, as there are few organizations dedicated solely to supporting palliative care.

There is substantial room for methodological improvements in this area. First, there is a lack of standardized measures for use at end of life; as a result, there is an overreliance on chart review and retrospective parental reports. Although prospective studies with multiple informants are ideal, they are often absent from the literature. Children may not be able to provide self-perceptions near the end of life, but it is important to begin to include their perspective when possible. Controlled studies to prospectively examine the adjustment of bereaved families are also needed. Lastly, the early state of research in this area supports the use of both qualitative and quantitative strategies as we continue to try to understand the experiences of these families. With careful and continued progress, we can achieve the ultimate goal of improving care and reducing suffering in both children and parents affected by life-limiting illnesses.

Acknowledgment

This work was supported in part by grants from the National Institutes of Health (Nos. R01 CA098217 and R01 CA118332).

References

Applebaum, D. R., & Burns, B. G. (1991). Unexpected childhood death: Post-traumatic stress disorder in surviving siblings and parents. *Journal of Clinical Child Psychology, 20,* 114–120.

Arias, E., MacDorman, M. F., Strobino, D. M., & Guyer, B. (2003). Annual summary of vital statistics—2002. *Pediatrics, 112,* 1215–1230.

Birenbaum, L. K., Robinson, M. A., Phillips, D. S., Stewart, B. J., & McCown, D. E. (1989). The response of children to the dying and death of a sibling. *Omega, 20,* 213–228.

Bradshaw, G., Hinds, P. S., Lensing, S., Gattuso, J. S., & Razzouk, B. I. (2005). Cancer-related deaths in children and adolescents. *Journal of Palliative Medicine, 8,* 86–95.

Chesler, M. A., & Barbarin, O. (1987). *Childhood cancer and the family: Meeting the challenge of stress and support.* New York: Brunner/Mazel.

Cleiren, M., Diekstra, R. F., Kerkhof, A. J., & van der Wal, J. (1994). Mode of death and kinship in bereavement: Focusing on "who" rather than "how." *Crisis, 15,* 22–36.

Cohen, D. S., Friedrich, W. N., Copeland, D. R., & Pendergrass, T. W. (1989). Instruments to measure parent–child communication regarding pediatric cancer. *Children's Health Care, 18,* 142–145.

Collins, J. J., Byrnes, M. E., Dunkel, I. J., Lapin, J., Nadel, T., Thaler, H. T., et al. (2000). The measurement of symptoms in children with cancer. *Journal of Pain and Symptom Management, 19,* 363–377.

Contro, N., Larson, J., Scofield, S., Sourkes, B., & Cohen, H. (2002). Family perspectives on the quality of pediatric palliative care. *Archives of Pediatrics and Adolescent Medicine, 156,* 14–19.

Contro, N. A., Larson, J., Scofield, S., Sourkes, B., & Cohen, H. J. (2004). Hospital staff and family perspectives regarding quality of pediatric palliative care. *Pediatrics, 114,* 1248–1252.

Coor, C. A., & Coor, D. M. (2000). Anticipatory mourning and coping with dying: Similarities, differences, and suggested guidelines for helpers. In T. A. Rando (Ed.), *Clinical dimensions of anticipatory mourning* (pp. 223–252). Champaign, IL: Research Press.

Davies, B. (1991). Long-term outcomes of adolescent sibling bereavement. *Journal of Adolescent Research, 6,* 83–96.

Davies, B. (1999). *Shadows in the sun: The experiences of sibling bereavement in childhood.* Philadelphia: Brunner/Mazel.

Drake, R., Frost, J., & Collins, J. J. (2003). The symptoms of dying children. *Journal of Pain and Symptom Management, 26,* 594–603.

Eiser, C., & Havermans, T. (1992). Children's understanding of cancer. *Psycho-Oncology, 1,* 169–181.

Ellis, R., & Leventhal, B. (1993). Information needs and decision-making preferences of children with cancer. *Psycho-Oncology, 2,* 277–284.

Fanos, J. H., & Nickerson, B. G. (1991). Long-term effects of sibling death during adolescence. *Journal of Adolescent Research, 6,* 70–82.

Feudtner, C., Hays, R. M., Haynes, G., Geyer, J. R., Neff, J. M., & Koepsell, T. D. (2001). Deaths attributed to pediatric complex chronic conditions: National trends and implications for supportive care services. *Pediatrics, 107,* e99.

Field, M. J., & Behrman, R. E. (Eds.). (2003). *When children die: Improving palliative and end-of-life care for children and their families.* Washington, DC: Institute of Medicine, National Academies Press.

Field, N. P., Eval, G. O., & Bonanno, G. A. (2003). Continuing bonds and adjustment 5 years after the death of a spouse. *Journal of Consulting and Clinical Psychology, 71,* 110–117.

Foster, T. L., Gilmer, M. J., Davies, B., Barrera, M., Compas, B. E., Fairclough, D. L., et al. (in press). Parent and sibling perspectives of the legacies of children dying of cancer. *Journal of Pediatric Oncology Nursing.*

Gedaly-Duff, V., Lee, K. A., Nail, L. M., Nicholson, H. S., & Johnson, K. P. (2006). Pain, sleep disturbance, and fatigue in children with leukemia and their parents: A pilot study. *Oncology Nursing Forum, 33,* 614–646.

Gottlieb, L., Lang, A., & Amsel, R. (1996). The long-term effects of grief on marital intimacy following infant death. *Omega, 33,* 1–19.

Graham-Pole, J., Wass, H., Eyberg, S., Chu, L., & Olejnik, S. (1989). Communicating with dying children and their siblings: A retrospective analysis. *Death Studies, 13,* 465–483.

Hazzard, A., Weston, J., & Gutterres, C. (1992). After a child's death: Factors related to parental bereavement. *Journal of Developmental and Behavioral Pediatrics, 13,* 24–30.

Heron, M. P. (2007). *Deaths: Leading causes for 2004* (No. 56). Hyattsville, MD: National Center for Health Statistics.

Hilden, J. M., Emanuel, E. J., Fairclough, D. L., Link, M. P., Foley, K. M., Clarridge, B. C., et al. (2001). Attitudes and practices among pediatric oncologists regarding end-of-life care: Results of the 1998 American Society of Clinical Oncology survey. *Journal of Clinical Oncology, 19,* 205–212.

Hilden, J. M., Watterson, J., & Chrastek, J. (2000). Tell the children. *Journal of Clinical Oncology, 18,* 3193–3195.

Hogan, N. S., & DeSantis, L. (1996). Adolescent sibling bereavement: Toward a new theory. In C. A. Corr & D. E. Balk (Eds.), *Handbook of adolescent death and bereavement* (pp. 173–195). New York: Springer.

Hogan, N. S., & Greenfield, D. B. (1991). Adolescent sibling bereavement: Symptomatology in a large community sample. *Journal of Adolescent Research, 6,* 97–112.

Hogan, N. S., & Schmidt, L. A. (2002). Testing the grief to personal growth model using structural equation modeling. *Death Studies, 26,* 615–634.

Hongo, T., Watanabe, C., Okada, S., Inoue, N., Yajima, S., Fujii, Y., et al. (2003). Analysis of the circumstances at the end of life in children with cancer: Symptoms, suffering and acceptance. *Pediatrics International, 45,* 60–64.

Hutton, C. J., & Bradley, B. S. (1994). Effects of sudden infant death on bereaved siblings: A comparative study. *Journal of Child Psychology and Psychiatry, 35,* 723–732.

Jalmsell, L., Kreicbergs, U., Onelov, E., Steineck, G., & Henter, J. I. (2006). Symptoms affecting children with malignancies during the last month of life: A nationwide follow-up. *Pediatrics, 117,* 1314–1320.

Jordan, J. R., & Neimeyer, R. A. (2003). Does grief counseling work? *Death Studies, 27,* 765–786.

Kazak, A. E. (1992). The social context of coping with childhood chronic illness: Family systems and social support. In A. M. La Greca, L. J. Siegel, J. L. Wallander, & C. E. Walker (Eds.), *Stress and coping in child health* (pp. 262–278). New York: Guilford Press.

Kirkwood, N. A. (2005). *A hospital handbook on multiculturalism and religion.* Harrisburg, PA: Morehouse.

Klass, D., Silverman, P. R., & Nickman, S. L. (1996). *Continuing bonds: New understandings of grief.* Washington, DC: Taylor & Francis.

Klopfenstein, K. J., Hutchison, C., Clark, C., Young, D., & Ruymann, F. B. (2001). Variables influencing end-of-life care in children and adolescents with cancer. *Journal of Pediatric Hematology/Oncology, 23,* 481–486.

Kreicbergs, U., Valdimarsdottir, U., Onelov, E., Henter, J. I., & Steineck, G. (2004a). Anxiety and depression in parents 4–9 years after the loss of a child owing to a malignancy: A population-based follow-up. *Psychological Medicine, 34,* 1431–1441.

Kreicbergs, U., Valdimarsdottir, U., Onelov, E., Henter, J.-I., & Steineck, G. (2004b). Talking about death with children who have severe malignant disease. *New England Journal of Medicine, 351,* 1175–1186.

Lang, A., & Gottlieb, L. (1991). Marital intimacy in bereaved and nonbereaved couples: A comparative study. In D. Papadatou & C. Papadatos (Eds.), *Children and death* (pp. 267–275). New York: Hemisphere.

Larson, D. G., & Hoyt, W. T. (2007). What has become of grief counseling?: An evaluation of the empirical foundations of the new pessimism. *Professional Psychology: Research and Practice, 38*, 347–355.

Lehman, D. R., Lang, E. R., Wortman, C. B., & Sorenson, S. B. (1989). Long-term effects of sudden bereavement: Marital and parent–child relationships and children's reactions. *Journal of Family Psychology, 2*, 344–367.

Lehman, D. R., Wortman, C. B., & Williams, A. F. (1987). Long-term effects of losing a spouse or child in a motor vehicle crash. *Journal of Personality and Social Psychology, 52*, 218–231.

Levi, R. B., Marsick, R., Drotar, D., & Kodish, E. D. (2000). Diagnosis, disclosure, and informed consent: Learning from parents of children with cancer. *Journal of Pediatric Hematology/Oncology, 22*, 3–12.

Martinson, I. M., & Campos, R. G. (1991). Adolescent bereavement: Long-term responses to a sibling's death from cancer. *Journal of Adolescent Research, 6*, 54–69.

Martinson, I. M., McClowry, S. G., Davies, B., & Kuhlenkamp, E. J. (1994). Changes over time: A study of family bereavement following childhood cancer. *Journal of Palliative Care, 10*, 19–25.

Matlins, S. M., & Magida, A. J. (2003). *How to be a perfect stranger: The essential religious etiquette handbook* (3rd ed.). Woodstock, VT: SkyLight Paths.

McCown, D. E., & Davies, B. (1995). Patterns of grief in young children following the death of a sibling. *Death Studies, 19*, 41–53.

Meyer, E. C., Burns, J. P., Griffith, J. L., & Truog, R. D. (2002). Parental perspectives on end-of-life care in the pediatric intensive care unit. *Critical Care Medicine, 30*, 226–231.

Moore, I. M., Gilliss, C. L., & Martinson, I. M. (1988). Psychosomatic symptoms in parents 2 years after the death of a child with cancer. *Nursing Research, 37*, 104–107.

Murphy, S. A., Braun, T., Tillery, L., Cain, K. C., Johnson, L. C., & Beaton, R. D. (1999). PTSD among bereaved parents following the violent deaths of their 12- to 28-year-old children: A longitudinal prospective analysis. *Journal of Trauma and Stress, 12*, 273–291.

Najman, J. M., Vance, J. C., Boyle, F., Embleton, G., Foster, B., & Thearle, J. (1993). The impact of a child death on marital adjustment. *Social Science and Medicine, 37*, 1005–1010.

Niemeyer, R. A., & Hogan, N. S. (2001). Quantitative or quantitative?: Measurement issues in the study of grief. In M. S. Stroebe, R. Hansson, W. Stroebe, & H. Schut (Eds.), *Handbook of bereavement research: Consequences, coping, and care* (pp. 89–118). Washington, DC: American Psychological Association.

Oltjenbruns, K. (2001). Developmental context of childhood: Grief and regrief phenomena. In M. S. Stroebe, R. Hansson, W. Stroebe, & H. Schut (Eds.), *Handbook of bereavement research: Consequences, coping, and care* (pp. 169–197). Washington, DC: American Psychological Association.

Pai, A. L. H., Lewandowski, A., Youngstrom, E., Greenley, R. N., Drotar, D., & Peterson, C. C. (2007). A meta-analytic review of the influence of pediatric cancer on parent and family functioning. *Journal of Family Psychology, 21*, 407–415.

Powell, M. (1991). The psychosocial impact of sudden infant death syndrome on siblings. *Irish Journal of Psychology, 12*, 235–247.

Prigerson, H. G., & Jacobs, S. C. (2001). Traumatic grief as a distinct disorder: A rationale, consensus criteria, and a preliminary empirical test. In M. S. Stroebe, R. Hansson, W. Stroebe, & H. Schut (Eds.), *Handbook of bereavement research: Consequences, coping, and care* (pp. 613–645). Washington, DC: American Psychological Association.

Rosen, H. (1985). Prohibitions against mourning in childhood sibling loss. *Omega, 15*, 307–316.

Rushforth, H. (1999). Practitioner review: Communicating with hospitalised children: Review and application of research pertaining to children's understanding of health and illness. *Journal of Child Psychology and Psychiatry, 40,* 683–691.

Schaeffer, J. A., & Moos, R. H. (2001). Bereavement experiences and personal growth. In M. S. Stroebe, R. Hansson, W. Stroebe, & H. Schut (Eds.), *Handbook of bereavement research: Consequences, coping, and care* (pp. 145–167). Washington, DC: American Psychological Association.

Sharpe, D., & Rossiter, L. (2002). Siblings of children with a chronic illness: A meta-analysis. *Journal of Pediatric Psychology, 27,* 699–710.

Stroebe, M. S., Hansson, R., Stroebe, W., & Schut, H. (2001). Introduction: Concepts and issues in contemporary research on bereavement. In M. Strobe, R. Hansson, W. Stroebe, & H. Schut (Eds.), *Handbook of bereavement research: Consequences, coping, and care* (pp. 3–22). Washington, DC: American Psychological Association.

Stroebe, M. S., & Schut, H. (1999). The dual process model of coping with bereavement. *Death Studies, 23,* 197–224.

Theunissen, J. M., Hoogerbrugge, P. M., van Achterberg, T., Prins, J. B., Vernooij-Dassen, M. J., & van den Ende, C. H. (2007). Symptoms in the palliative phase of children with cancer. *Pediatric Blood and Cancer, 49,* 160–165.

Vance, J., Najman, J., Thearle, M., Embelton, G., Foster, W., & Boyle, F. (1995). Psychological changes in parents eight months after the loss of an infant from stillbirth, neonatal death, or sudden infant death syndrome: A longitudinal study. *Pediatrics, 96,* 933–938.

Wallander, J. L., & Varni, J. W. (1998). Effects of pediatric chronic physical disorders on child and family adjustment. *Journal of Child Psychology and Psychiatry, 39*(1), 29–46.

Wolfe, J., Grier, H. E., Klar, N., Levin, S. B., Ellenbogen, J. M., Salem-Schatz, S., et al. (2000). Symptoms and suffering at the end of life in children with cancer. *New England Journal of Medicine, 342,* 326–333.

Wolfe, J., Klar, N., Grier, H. E., Duncan, J., Salem-Schatz, S., Emanuel, E. J., et al. (2000). Understanding of prognosis among parents of children who died of cancer: Impact on treatment goals and integration of palliative care. *Journal of the American Medical Association, 284,* 2469–2475.

CHAPTER 15

eHealth Applications in Pediatric Psychology

TONYA M. PALERMO
ANNA C. WILSON

Digital and electronic technologies are increasingly critical and integral to the research and clinical work conducted by pediatric psychologists (Palermo, 2008). Although the term "eHealth" is widely used in many fields of medicine, the precise definition varies among clinicians and researchers (Oh, Rizo, Enkin, & Jadad, 2005). The Robert Wood Johnson Foundation (2003) defines eHealth as the use of emerging interactive and communication technologies (e.g., the Internet, personal computers, voice recognition systems) to improve or enable health and health care. Within the field of pediatric psychology, we define eHealth as the application of interactive and communication technologies to improve or enable health and health care in children, adolescents, and families (Palermo, 2008). In this chapter, we review eHealth applications in pediatric psychology research and clinical settings, focusing on electronic devices and communication technologies that have been used in assessment, health promotion, and treatment delivery. The scope of this chapter is limited to an overview of eHealth technologies that are likely to have a direct impact on the ways in which pediatric psychologists educate children and families, conduct assessment and intervention, and interact with research participants. Thus we do not review technologies that are internal to health care systems, such as electronic medical records and in-hospital communication systems. Telemedicine is also not reviewed in this chapter, as these systems primarily facilitate communication between providers and patients within a health care system. We organize the chapter into four sections, covering (1) sampling and recruitment strategies, (2) assessment, (3) patient education, and (4) treatment, and we provide illustrative examples of the application of eHealth technologies to each.

Sampling and Recruitment Strategies

Pediatric psychologists are utilizing several technologies to reach broader populations, including Internet recruitment, Web surveys, and computer-assisted telephone interviews. Internet recruitment can be helpful in reaching large numbers of geographically diverse participants and children with low-base-rate disorders or rare conditions. Advertisements and information about studies can be distributed through websites that parents are likely to frequent, as well as through email distribution listservs. For example, in a recent study examining parental perceptions of children's mastery of diabetes self-care, participants were recruited via a specific website, *www.childrenwithdiabetes.com* (Weissberg-Benchell, Goodman, Antisdel Lomaglio, & Zebracki, 2007). Similarly, in a study focused on a rare condition, phenylketonuria (PKU), fathers' involvement in helping children cope with this disease was examined via recruitment on a PKU website (Wysocki & Gavin, 2004).

Similar to the advantages for sampling and recruitment, the Internet also offers researchers a convenient means for survey data collection. Several online programs, such as Zoomerang™ or SurveyMonkey™, offer simple survey design interfaces and allow survey creators to export data directly into software programs for analysis. For example, Web surveys have been used to collect information about sleep disturbances in children with early-onset bipolar disorder (Lofthouse et al., 2008), and to validate new survey measures of parental feeding practices (Musher-Eizenman & Holub, 2007).

Internet sampling and recruitment strategies have some limitations, including the possibility of sampling biases. Future research is needed to better understand how parents and children who access the Internet regularly, frequent certain websites, or choose to respond to online surveys may or may not differ from samples recruited through other methods of contact.

Assessment and Measurement of Health Behaviors and Outcomes

Various technologies have been used to enhance the assessment and monitoring of symptoms, behaviors, and perceptions among pediatric populations. Innovations in measurement technology have allowed pediatric psychologists to better understand complex health behaviors. Use of these assessment technologies can improve measurement objectivity and provide real-time information—both advantages over traditional retrospective self-report measures. The assessment technologies described in this section also offer researchers the advantage of convenience in data collection and extraction, as information from these devices can be directly exported for analysis with statistical software programs.

Electronic Devices in Assessment

Hand-held computers, personal digital assistant (PDA) devices, and cellular telephones have been used to obtain *in vivo* assessments for research purposes. These devices can be programmed to sound alarms that will prompt or remind participants to report on symptoms and behaviors at any time of day. Research indicates that PDA devices outperform pen-and-paper methods in the collection of patient diary data, and PDA diaries have been shown to increase compliance and accuracy in children's reporting of symptoms and behaviors (Dale & Hagen, 2007; Palermo, Valenzuela, & Stork, 2004). PDAs have been used to assess gastrointestinal symptoms (Walker & Sorrells, 2002), as well as chronic pain in children with arthritis (Stinson et al., 2006) and headache (Palermo et al., 2004).

Electronic devices have also been used to provide objective assessments of behaviors such as sleep and physical activity. One device, called an "actigraph," is a small watch-like device worn on the wrist to record body movements. It has been used to assess sleep in children and adolescents with chronic abdominal pain, headache, and musculoskeletal pain (Bruni, Russo, Violani, & Guidetti, 2004; Palermo, Toliver-Sokol, Fonareva, & Koh, 2007); among children undergoing outpatient surgery (MacLaren & Kain, 2008); and among children with leukemia (Gedaly-Duff, Lee, Nail, Nicholson, & Johnson, 2006).

Actigraphs and pedometers have also been used to assess physical activity levels among children. Actigraphy has been used to establish gender and age norms for moderate activity levels (e.g., Riddoch et al., 2004), to examine the effects of neighborhood features on activity (Jago, Baranowski, & Baranowski, 2006), and to examine the role of physical activity reduction in weight gain following adenotonsillectomy surgery among overweight children (Roemmich et al., 2006). Daytime physical activity levels have been examined via actigraphy in adolescents with chronic pain (Long, Palermo, & Manees, 2008). "Pedometers," portable electronic devices that count the number of steps taken, offer a less expensive alternative to actigraphy and have also been used in the study of sedentary and vigorous physical activity patterns in children (Roemmich, Gurgol, & Epstein, 2004).

Other small electronic sensor devices have been used to provide a more objective measure of adherence to medications in pediatric populations. These sensors are typically binary (e.g., open vs. closed), and provide information about the number of uses of a device or the number of times a bottle has been opened. Medication adherence has been evaluated in a number of pediatric studies with electronic devices such as the Medication Event Monitoring System SmartCaps. For example, in children and adolescents with cystic fibrosis, electronic devices have evaluated adherence to specific medications and have been shown to be more accurate than self-report measures (Modi et al., 2006). However, some limitations of using electronic devices for assessment can affect the reliability of data, including technological problems such as equipment or battery failure (Palermo et al., 2004), as well as improper usage of the devices. As new devices become available, further research is needed to investigate the reliability and validity of these data, particularly in comparison to data obtained via validated self-report and objective measures.

Patient Education and eHealth Literacy

A recent survey by the Pew Internet and American Life Project (2007) indicates that the majority of American adults (75%) and teens (90%) use the Internet almost daily, and that over half of American households now have broadband Internet access. This survey also shows that the rate of home broadband access has increased dramatically among rural, lower-income, and ethnic minority families in the past few years, and that most Americans have access through work, school, or public libraries. Consumers invest more time and resources in gaining access to health information than any other type of information available online (Powell, Lowe, Griffiths, & Thorogood, 2005), and parents report using the Internet frequently to obtain information about their children's health (D'Alessandro, Kreiter, Kinzer, & Peterson, 2004).

A plethora of health information is available on the Internet, including health information sites, chat rooms, and bulletin boards where parents can post questions and read responses. Unfortunately, poor quality of information on health is a common problem among Internet sites (Eysenbach, Powell, Kuss, & Sa, 2002), and only 25% of adults consistently report checking the source and date of health information found online (Pew Internet and American Life Project, 2006). Therefore, consumers need skills for evaluating the health information that they read. The skills needed to find, understand, appraise, and apply health information from electronic sources have been defined as "eHealth literacy" (Norman & Skinner, 2006). Some research has shown that health care providers can influence parental usage of and attitudes about Internet health information (D'Alessandro et al., 2004): When pediatricians provided specific websites for parents to use to look up child health information, most parents accessed these sites and often recommended them to others.

Efforts have been made to create online resources for reputable information that is created and reviewed by health care providers; many of these resources are commercial enterprises (e.g., WebMD™). Many children's hospitals now provide basic health and condition-specific information on hospital websites. Prevention and health promotion efforts have also utilized other computer-based technologies to deliver information to families. Computer kiosks have been used for child health promotion in various low-income urban locations, such as public libraries, Department of Motor Vehicles offices, and fast-food restaurants, and have been shown to increase knowledge and desire to change behaviors (Thompson, Lozano, & Christakis, 2007). Numerous opportunities remain for further research on child, adolescent, and parent patterns of Internet usage to acquire health information and make health-related decisions, as well as on ways to improve their abilities to access high-quality information.

Treatment Approaches

Applications of interactive and communication technologies to provide psychological or behavioral treatment to pediatric populations are burgeoning. This section is organized by the types of technologies used to deliver treatment: electronic devices, CD-ROMs, private computer networks, Internet interventions, and virtual reality technology.

Electronic Devices

Electronic devices have been used in treatment, primarily to increase adherence. For example, cell phone calls have been used to increase adherence to HIV medication regimens in adolescents (Puccio et al., 2006), and text messaging has been used to increase adherence and self-efficacy in youths with diabetes (Franklin, Waller, Pagliari, & Greene, 2006). Several studies have used feedback from devices to encourage behavior change. Examples include the use of physical activity feedback (in which data from an activity device must be determined to meet a certain threshold in order for a reinforcer to be provided) to increase youths' physical activity (Roemmich et al., 2004), and the use of wireless glucose monitors integrated with a website and game to increase diabetes treatment adherence (Kumar, Wentzell, Mikkelsen, Pentland, & Laffel, 2004).

CD-ROMs

Psychoeducational intervention programs that are delivered via CD-ROMs have the advantages of using interactive media to engage children in psychological treatments while being cheap and portable. One example in this category is a series of psychoeducational intervention programs called Starbright Explorer Series™, developed on CD-ROMs by the Starbright Foundation, a nonprofit organization focused on children and adolescents with serious illnesses. Starbright programs have been developed for children with asthma, sickle cell disease, diabetes, and cystic fibrosis. Many of these CD-ROMs have undergone evaluation. For example, one group of investigators evaluated the CD-ROM intervention developed for children with cystic fibrosis in a randomized controlled trial (Davis, Quittner, Stack, & Yang, 2004). In this study, 47 children with cystic fibrosis were randomly assigned to a CD-ROM treatment group or a waiting-list control group after a baseline assessment of knowledge and coping skills. Significant posttreatment improvements were found in knowledge and coping skills in the treatment group.

Investigators have also developed their own CD-ROM intervention programs to reach other pediatric populations. For example, Connelly, Rapoff, Thompson, and Connelly (2006) developed and evaluated a CD-ROM pain management program called Headstrong, which focused on relaxation training for children ages 7–12 years with recurrent headache. They found significant improvements in headache activity (less intense and frequent pain) in children who received the 4-week intervention versus children receiving standard care.

Primary disadvantages of CD-ROMs are the inability to update information or to communicate with users in real time, and increased difficulty in dissemination in comparison to publicly available resources such as the Internet.

Private Computer Networks

The Starbright Foundation has also developed a private, broadband, online computer network to connect children among numerous hospitals in the United States and Canada. Children's hospitals must purchase this network, called Starbright World™, to have access. The program includes a multimedia package to enhance communication and social support (e.g., chatrooms, email, video conferencing); to encourage self-expression (e.g., art activities, essay contests); to provide education and information (e.g., multimedia programs on health care conditions and procedures, "ask-a-doc" chats); and to provide distraction (e.g., games, websites). A special issue of *Children's Health Care* (Bush & Simonian, 2002) was devoted to research on two interventions developed by the Starbright Foundation, one of which was Starbright World. Several studies evaluated the impact of Starbright World on different populations of children in inpatient or outpatient settings, finding that coping with such common challenges as pain, anxiety, and loneliness could be enhanced in children with chronic health conditions including HIV, cancer, and chronic granulomatous disease (Battles & Wiener, 2002). In other research, Starbright World was found to have a positive impact on psychological adjustment, knowledge, coping, and social support in children and adolescents with cancer, sickle cell disease, and asthma (e.g., Hazzard, Celano, Collins, & Markov, 2002). A major expansion effort by the Starbright Foundation resulted in allowing home access to Starbright World to children who had used this multimedia program in the hospital, expanding the reach of and flexibility in using the intervention; future evaluation efforts are likely to focus on this remote, home access version of Starbright World.

Internet Interventions: Use of the World Wide Web

Although the adult Internet intervention literature has rapidly grown over the years, and a comprehensive book has recently been published to summarize computer-aided psychotherapy (Marks, Cavanaugh, & Gega, 2007), developing interventions for delivery via the Internet for pediatric populations is a smaller and more recent effort. Internet interventions are typically behaviorally based treatments that have been transformed for delivery via the Internet. The International Society for Research on Internet Interventions further describes these interventions as characteristically highly structured, self-guided, based on effective face-to-face interventions, personalized to the user, interactive, enhanced by multimedia features, and tailored to provide feedback and follow-up (Ritterband, Andersson, Christensen, Carlbring, & Cuijpers, 2006). These features distinguish Internet interventions from other websites that solely provide health information content, but are not interactive, personalized, or designed to achieve behavior change (Ritterband, Gonder-Frederick, et al., 2003). There have been randomized controlled trials to evaluate Internet interventions for pediatric populations, targeting health behaviors related to obesity (Williamson et al., 2005), encopresis (Ritterband, Cox, et al., 2003), recurrent pain (Hicks, von Baeyer, & McGrath, 2006), asthma (Krishna et al., 2003), smoking (Patten et al., 2006), and traumatic brain injury (Wade, Carey, & Wolfe, 2006). This research has found strong support for this mode of treatment delivery. Positive outcomes have also been found for cognitive-behavioral therapy interventions delivered via the Internet for health problems, across such outcomes as knowledge, behavior change, health symptoms, and health status (Cuijpers, van Straten, & Andersson, 2008).

Importantly, tests of Internet interventions with parents and children in urban areas and of diverse socioeconomic status have demonstrated their wide applicability (e.g., Joseph et al., 2007). Although there is significant variation across Internet interventions in the level of Internet interactivity and personalization, as well as in therapist involvement, the feasibility of using computer technologies to deliver cognitive-behavioral therapy to children with various health conditions has been demonstrated. Internet delivery of interventions will play a major role in future treatment developments in pediatric psychology.

As with all of the eHealth technologies, there are also limitations associated with Internet interventions. One limitation is that most Internet interventions to date have been designed to focus on a single problem, and may not detect or treat additional problems that may become important during the course of treatment (Marks et al., 2007). These programs also require high cost and effort in initial development, and once developed may not be widely available or feasible for use in all settings. Finally, individual differences in previous experience with computer technology have been shown to have an impact on the efficacy of Internet interventions (Carey, Wade, & Wolfe, 2008).

Virtual Reality Technology

Virtual reality (VR) technology provides a three-dimensional environment and allows users to engage in a video game or virtual world that may distract them from a painful experience, train them to move in certain ways, or provide exposure to feared events. VR often includes a head-mounted display that creates a three-dimensional environment in the visual field, adding a sensory blocking component to the engagement in a video game. In pediatric populations, this technology has been used primarily for distraction from acute painful procedures. Hoffman, Patterson, and colleagues pioneered the application of VR in adolescents and young adults undergoing burn debridement (Hoffman, Doctor, Patterson, Carrougher, & Furness, 2000). Other investigators have used distraction via VR in the context of invasive procedures such as intravenous line placement (Gold, Kim, Kant, Joseph, & Rizzo, 2006) and porta-cath placement (Gershon, Zimand, Pickering, Rothbaum, & Hodges, 2004). VR games have also been used to teach fire safety skills to children with fetal alcohol syndrome (Padgett, Strickland, & Coles, 2006), and to simulate an exercise environment in children with cerebral palsy to improve kinetics (Chen et al., 2007). Recent research in VR has evaluated the nature of the distracting stimulus (active vs. passive) on children's response to pain (e.g., Dahlquist et al., 2007). Because VR is costly in comparison to other distracting stimuli, future studies that provide direct comparisons between VR and other interventions will help direct efforts.

Conclusions and Future Directions

eHealth applications are emerging rapidly in pediatric psychology research and practice. These technologies have been successfully applied to sampling and recruitment in pediatric psychology research studies, to assessment and measurement of health behaviors and symptoms, to education of patients via the Internet, and to treatments delivered via computer applications. Over the next decade, new work in these areas will continue to expand.

Various challenges face pediatric psychologists who are engaged in eHealth applications. The costs (in time, money, and labor) of developing new computer applications such as Internet interventions are tremendous, and concerted efforts are needed to reduce duplication. Moreover, this is a rapidly changing field. A June 2, 2008, search of the National Institutes of Health's Computer Retrieval of Information on Scientific Projects database showed at least 35 ongoing funded studies of Internet interventions for pediatric populations. Collaboration among eHealth researchers will help pool knowledge and strategize efforts. There are also challenges inherent in trying to move applications from the research setting to clinical practice. In several countries in Europe, the government has supported eHealth interventions and has facilitated reimbursement for practitioners providing care to patients via Internet interventions (Ritterband et al., 2006). Issues of reimbursement have not yet been addressed in practice in the United

States. There are also challenges in dissemination that involve business and commercialism; this will be an important area of focus in order to sustain successful computer applications once research funding ends (Ritterband et al., 2006).

Future directions for interventions utilizing technology include the addition of home monitoring and feedback, using novel devices and sensors that can be integrated with Internet programs or linked with clinician feedback. These integrated systems will allow symptoms to be monitored in real time, and clinicians or the computer program can provide directive or reinforcing responses based on symptom levels. For example, in one treatment study, children monitored peak expiratory flow and daily asthma symptoms on the Internet and received an interactive clinical/therapeutic response (Jan et al., 2007). Studies such as this are critical for demonstrating that computer systems can be used for clinical monitoring of symptoms. New technological developments will lead to increased availability of these types of systems targeted toward different health and illness groups, and may prove to be cost-effective tools in the management of chronic conditions.

References

Battles, H. B., & Wiener, L. S. (2002). From adolescence through young adulthood: Psychosocial adjustment associated with long-term survival of HIV. *Journal of Adolescent Health, 30,* 161–168.

Bruni, O., Russo, P. M., Violani, C., & Guidetti, V. (2004). Sleep and migraine: An actigraphic study. *Cephalalgia, 24,* 134–139.

Bush, J. B., & Simonian, S. J. (Eds.). (2002). Research on STAR BRIGHT interventions [Special issue]. *Childrens Health Care, 31*(1).

Carey, J. C., Wade, S. L., & Wolfe, C. R. (2008). Lessons learned: The effect of prior technology use on Web-based interventions. *Cyberpsychology and Behavior, 11,* 188–195.

Chen, Y. P., Kang, L. J., Chuang, T. Y., Doong, J. L., Lee, S. J., Tsai, M. W., et al. (2007). Use of virtual reality to improve upper-extremity control in children with cerebral palsy: A single-subject design. *Physical Therapy, 87,* 1441–1457.

Connelly, M., Rapoff, M. A., Thompson, N., & Connelly, W. (2006). Headstrong: A pilot study of a CD-ROM intervention for recurrent pediatric headache. *Journal of Pediatric Psychology, 31,* 737–747.

Cuijpers, P., van Straten, A., & Andersson, G. (2008). Internet-administered cognitive behavior therapy for health problems: A systematic review. *Journal of Behavioral Medicine, 31,* 169–177.

Dahlquist, L. M., McKenna, K. D., Jones, K. K., Dillinger, L., Weiss, K. E., & Ackerman, C. S. (2007). Active and passive distraction using a head-mounted display helmet: Effects on cold pressor pain in children. *Health Psychology, 26,* 794–801.

Dale, O., & Hagen, K. B. (2007). Despite technical problems personal digital assistants outperform pen and paper when collecting patient diary data. *Journal of Clinical Epidemiology, 60,* 8–17.

D'Alessandro, D. M., Kreiter, C. D., Kinzer, S. L., & Peterson, M. W. (2004). A randomized controlled trial of an information prescription for pediatric patient education on the Internet. *Archives of Pediatrics and Adolescent Medicine, 158,* 857–862.

Davis, M. A., Quittner, A. L., Stack, C. M., & Yang, M. C. (2004). Controlled evaluation of the Starbright CD-ROM program for children and adolescents with cystic fibrosis. *Journal of Pediatric Psychology, 29,* 259–267.

Eysenbach, G., Powell, J., Kuss, O., & Sa, E. R. (2002). Empirical studies assessing the quality of health information for consumers on the World Wide Web: A systematic review. *Journal of the American Medical Association, 287,* 2691–2700.

Franklin, V. L., Waller, A., Pagliari, C., & Greene, S. A. (2006). A randomized controlled trial of Sweet Talk, a text-messaging system to support young people with diabetes. *Diabetic Medicine, 23,* 1332–1338.

Gedaly-Duff, V., Lee, K. A., Nail, L., Nicholson, H. S., & Johnson, K. P. (2006). Pain, sleep disturbance, and fatigue in children with leukemia and their parents: A pilot study. *Oncology Nursing Forum, 33,* 641–646.

Gershon, J., Zimand, E., Pickering, M., Rothbaum, B. O., & Hodges, L. (2004). A pilot and feasibility study of virtual reality as a distraction for children with cancer. *Journal of the American Academy of Child and Adolescent Psychiatry, 43,* 1243–1249.

Gold, J. I., Kim, S. H., Kant, A. J., Joseph, M. H., & Rizzo, A. S. (2006). Effectiveness of virtual reality for pediatric pain distraction during I.V. placement. *Cyberpsychology and Behavior, 9,* 207–212.

Hazzard, A., Celano, M., Collins, M., & Markov, Y. (2002). Effects of Starbright World on knowledge, social support, and coping in hospitalized children with sickle cell disease and asthma. *Children's Health Care, 31,* 69–86.

Hicks, C. L., von Baeyer, C. L., & McGrath, P. J. (2006). Online psychological treatment for pediatric recurrent pain: A randomized evaluation. *Journal of Pediatric Psychology, 31,* 724–736.

Hoffman, H. G., Doctor, J. N., Patterson, D. R., Carrougher, G. J., & Furness, T. A., 3rd. (2000). Virtual reality as an adjunctive pain control during burn wound care in adolescent patients. *Pain, 85,* 305–309.

Jago, R., Baranowski, T., & Baranowski, J. C. (2006). Observed, GIS, and self-reported environmental features and adolescent physical activity. *American Journal of Health Promotion, 20,* 422–428.

Jan, R. L., Wang, J. Y., Huang, M. C., Tseng, S. M., Su, H. J., & Liu, L. F. (2007). An Internet-based interactive telemonitoring system for improving childhood asthma outcomes in Taiwan. *Telemedicine Journal and e-Health, 13,* 257–268.

Joseph, C. L., Peterson, E., Havstad, S., Johnson, C. C., Hoerauf, S., Stringer, S., et al. (2007). A web-based, tailored asthma management program for urban African-American high school students. *American Journal of Respiratory Critical Care Medicine, 175,* 888–895.

Krishna, S., Francisco, B. D., Balas, E. A., Konig, P., Graff, G. R., & Madsen, R. W. (2003). Internet-enabled interactive multimedia asthma education program: A randomized trial. *Pediatrics, 111,* 503–510.

Kumar, V. S., Wentzell, K. J., Mikkelsen, T., Pentland, A., & Laffel, L. M. (2004). The DAILY (Daily Automated Intensive Log for Youth) trial: A wireless, portable system to improve adherence and glycemic control in youth with diabetes. *Diabetes Technology and Therapeutics, 6,* 445–453.

Lofthouse, N., Fristad, M., Splaingard, M., Kelleher, K., Hayes, J., & Resko, S. (2008). Web survey of sleep problems associated with early-onset bipolar spectrum disorders. *Journal of Pediatric Psychology, 33,* 349–357.

Long, A. C., Palermo, T. M., & Manees, A. M. (2008). Brief report: Using actigraphy to compare physical activity levels in adolescents with chronic pain and healthy adolescents. *Journal of Pediatric Psychology, 33,* 660–665.

MacLaren, J., & Kain, Z. N. (2008). A comparison of preoperative anxiety in female patients with mothers of children undergoing surgery. *Anesthesia and Analgesia, 106,* 810–813.

Marks, I. M., Cavanaugh, K., & Gega, L. (2007). *Hands-on help: Computer-aided psychotherapy.* New York: Psychology Press.

Modi, A. C., Lim, C. S., Yu, N., Geller, D., Wagner, M. H., & Quittner, A. L. (2006). A multimethod assessment of treatment adherence for children with cystic fibrosis. *Journal of Cystic Fibrosis, 5*, 177–185.

Musher-Eizenman, D., & Holub, S. (2007). Comprehensive Feeding Practices Questionnaire: Validation of a new measure of parental feeding practices. *Journal of Pediatric Psychology, 32*, 960–972.

Norman, C. D., & Skinner, H. A. (2006). Ehealth literacy: Essential skills for consumer health in a networked world. *Journal of Medical Internet Research, 8*, article e9.

Oh, H., Rizo, C., Enkin, M., & Jadad, A. (2005). What is ehealth (3): A systematic review of published definitions. *Journal of Medical Internet Research, 7*, article e1.

Padgett, L. S., Strickland, D., & Coles, C. D. (2006). Case study: Using a virtual reality computer game to teach fire safety skills to children diagnosed with fetal alcohol syndrome. *Journal of Pediatric Psychology, 31*, 65–70.

Palermo, T. M. (2008). Editorial: Section on innovations in technology in measurement, assessment, and intervention. *Journal of Pediatric Psychology, 33*, 35–38.

Palermo, T. M., Toliver-Sokol, M., Fonareva, I., & Koh, J. L. (2007). Objective and subjective assessment of sleep in adolescents with chronic pain compared to healthy adolescents. *Clinical Journal of Pain, 23*, 812–820.

Palermo, T. M., Valenzuela, D., & Stork, P. P. (2004). A randomized trial of electronic versus paper pain diaries in children: Impact on compliance, accuracy, and acceptability. *Pain, 107*, 213–219.

Patten, C. A., Croghan, I. T., Meis, T. M., Decker, P. A., Pingree, S., Colligan, R. C., et al. (2006). Randomized clinical trial of an Internet-based versus brief office intervention for adolescent smoking cessation. *Patient Education and Counseling, 64*, 249–258.

Pew Internet and American Life Project. (2006). Reports: Health, online health search. Retrieved February 1, 2008, from *www.pewinternet.org/pdfs/PIP_Online_Health_2006.pdf*

Pew Internet and American Life Project. (2007). Reports: Technology and media usage, home broadband adoption. Retrieved February 1, 2008, from *www.pewinternet.org/pdfs/PIP_Broadband2007.pdf*

Powell, J. A., Lowe, P., Griffiths, F. E., & Thorogood, M. (2005). A critical analysis of the literature on the Internet and consumer health information. *Journal of Telemedicine and Telecare, 11*(Suppl. 1), 41–43.

Puccio, J. A., Belzer, M., Olson, J., Martinez, M., Salata, C., Tucker, D., et al. (2006). The use of cell phone reminder calls for assisting HIV-infected adolescents and young adults to adhere to highly active antiretroviral therapy: A pilot study. *AIDS Patient Care and STDs, 20*, 438–444.

Riddoch, C. J., Bo Andersen, L., Wedderkopp, N., Harro, M., Klasson-Heggebo, L., Sardinha, L. B., et al. (2004). Physical activity levels and patterns of 9- and 15-yr-old European children. *Medicine and Science in Sports and Exercise, 36*, 86–92.

Ritterband, L. M., Andersson, G., Christensen, H. M., Carlbring, P., & Cuijpers, P. (2006). Directions for the International Society for Research on Internet Interventions (ISRII). *Journal of Medical Internet Research, 8*, article e23.

Ritterband, L. M., Cox, D. J., Walker, L. S., Kovatchev, B., McKnight, L., Patel, K., et al. (2003). An Internet intervention as adjunctive therapy for pediatric encopresis. *Journal of Consulting and Clinical Psychology, 71*, 910–917.

Ritterband, L. M., Gonder-Frederick, L. A., Cox, D. J., Clifton, A. D., West, R. W., & Borowitz, S. (2003). Internet interventions: In review, in use, and into the future. *Professional Psychology: Research and Practice, 34*, 527–534.

Roemmich, J. N., Barkley, J. E., D'Andrea, L., Nikova, M., Rogol, A. D., Carskadon, M. A., et al. (2006). Increases in overweight after adenotonsillectomy in overweight children with obstructive sleep-disordered breathing are associated with decreases in motor activity and hyperactivity. *Pediatrics, 117*, 200–208.

Roemmich, J. N., Gurgol, C. M., & Epstein, L. H. (2004). Open-loop feedback increases physical activity of youth. *Medicine and Science in Sports and Exercise, 36,* 668–673.

Robert Wood Johnson Foundation. (2003). Riding the wave of ehealth technologies. Retrieved February 1, 2008, from *www.rwjf.org*

Stinson, J. N., Petroz, G. C., Tait, G., Feldman, B. M., Streiner, D., McGrath, P. J., et al. (2006). E-ouch: Usability testing of an electronic chronic pain diary for adolescents with arthritis. *Clinical Journal of Pain, 22,* 295–305.

Thompson, D. A., Lozano, P., & Christakis, D. A. (2007). Parent use of touchscreen computer kiosks for child health promotion in community settings. *Pediatrics, 119,* 427–434.

Wade, S. L., Carey, J., & Wolfe, C. R. (2006). An online family intervention to reduce parental distress following pediatric brain injury. *Journal of Consulting and Clinical Psychology, 74,* 445–454.

Walker, L. S., & Sorrells, S. C. (2002). Brief report: Assessment of children's gastrointestinal symptoms for clinical trials. *Journal of Pediatric Psychology, 27,* 303–307.

Weissberg-Benchell, J., Goodman, S. S., Antisdel Lomaglio, J., & Zebracki, K. (2007). The use of continuous subcutaneous insulin infusion (CSII): Parental and professional perceptions of self-care mastery and autonomy in children and adolescents. *Journal of Pediatric Psychology, 32,* 1196–1202.

Williamson, D. A., Martin, P. D., White, M. A., Newton, R., Walden, H., York-Crowe, E., et al. (2005). Efficacy of an Internet-based behavioral weight loss program for overweight adolescent African-American girls. *Eating and Weight Disorders, 10,* 193–203.

Wysocki, T., & Gavin, L. (2004). Psychometric properties of a new measure of fathers' involvement in the management of pediatric chronic diseases. *Journal of Pediatric Psychology, 29,* 231–240.

PART III

Medical, Developmental, Behavioral, and Cognitive-Affective Conditions

CHAPTER 16

Neonatology, Prematurity, and Developmental Issues

GLEN P. AYLWARD

Pediatric, developmental, and clinical child psychologists are increasingly involved with children born prematurely or otherwise at biological risk. Activities include developmental assessment, infant stimulation, family consultation, referral for early intervention services, longitudinal follow-up, addressing psychosocial and family issues, and identification of later neurodevelopmental problems (Aylward, 1997).

Prematurity is not a defined disease or syndrome; rather, it is a condition with numerous aspects (Institute of Medicine, 2006). Preterm birth (<37 weeks gestational age) is the leading cause of perinatal mortality (75%) and morbidity (>50%). The frequency of preterm birth is approximately 12–13%. Approximately 5% of preterm births are at <28 weeks gestational age (extreme prematurity), 15% are born at 28–31 weeks (severe prematurity), 20% at 32–33 weeks (moderate prematurity), and 60–70% at 34–36 weeks gestational age (late prematurity/near term) (Goldenberg, Culhane, Iams, & Romero, 2008). The age of viability is 23–24 weeks gestational age.

Mortality rates in preterm infants have decreased by 45% from 1980 to 2000. Antenatal corticosteroids, assisted ventilation, surfactant, and other medical innovations have contributed to this decrease. Developmental morbidity is inversely related to gestational age and birthweight. For example, only 20–21% of those born at <26 weeks have no impairments (Marlow, Wolke, Bracewell, & Samara, 2002). Nonetheless, no gestational age (including term) is exempt from neurodevelopmental disabilities, recurrent or chronic health problems and their psychosocial sequelae, or stressful effects on the family (Drotar et al., 2006; Saigal & Doyle, 2008).

Similarly, with respect to birthweights, improved survival rates of babies with low birthweight (LBW; <2,500 g or 5.5 lb), very low birthweight (VLBW; <1,500 g or 3.3 lb), extremely low birthweight (ELBW; <1,000 g or 2.2 lb), and incredibly low birthweight (<750 g or 1.6 lb) have increased the need for services. LBW accounts for approximately 7.4% of births, and infants born at weights between 501 and 1,500 g contribute disproportionately to perinatal mortality and morbidity rates (Stevenson et al., 1998). Concerns are raised that the increase in the absolute number of surviving infants exposed to potential central nervous system (CNS) damage will produce a higher rate of neurodevelopmental morbidity.

Factors to Be Considered in Evaluation of Preterm Infants

Birthweight and Gestational Age

Birthweight is essentially a proxy for prematurity. Traditionally, infants were primarily grouped by birthweight rather than gestational age because of inaccurate obstetric estimation of gestational age and the questionable utility of postnatal assessment, particularly in very small infants (Hack & Fanaroff, 1999). However, fetal ultrasound has improved gestational age estimation, and gestational age is a stronger determinant of organ/system maturation and viability than is birthweight (Institute of Medicine, 2006). However, infants with VLBW or ELBW may be (1) extremely premature babies with average-for-gestational-age (AGA) birthweights, (2) less premature babies with small-for-gestational-age (SGA; <10th percentile) birthweights, or (3) older preterm and term infants with extremely SGA birthweights. This distinction is necessary, because the ultimate survival and outcome of infants included in these groups can vary markedly. Therefore, *both* birthweight and gestational age should be considered in work with high-risk infants, and particular care should be taken to ensure that only AGA infants are included in specific birthweight categories.

Other Factors

Numerous biological and environmental factors affect outcome of these at-risk infants, in addition to birthweight and gestational age. These influences span the pre-, peri-, and postnatal periods and beyond. Among the multiple factors associated with VLBW or extremely low gestational age are (1) severity of the neonatal course, (2) sociodemographic factors, and (3) subsequent illness (Aylward, 2002a, 2005). The major sources of morbidity in the neonatal period are intracranial events, pulmonary immaturity, and infections (McCormick, 1989). Therefore, severe ultrasound abnormality, septicemia, necrotizing enterocolitis, chronic lung disease or bronchopulmonary dysplasia, recurrent apnea and bradycardia, and signs of asphyxia (e.g., seizures) are indicators of increased risk for later problems. The number of days an infant remains hospitalized after birth is often considered a marker for biological risk; however, this measure is disproportionately affected by infants with extremely low gestational ages. Infants with the same birthweight or gestational age can differ markedly with respect to outcome. When one is evaluating outcome based on birthweight or gestational age, perinatal factors and physiological conditions of the *individual* infant must be considered.

Risk Scores

Various illness severity scores have been developed to quantify biomedical factors. These include the Score for Neonatal Acute Physiology (SNAP and SNAP-II), the Revised Score for Neonatal Acute Physiology Perinatal Extension (SNAPPE-II), the Vermont–

Oxford Network Risk Adjustment, the Neonatal Medical Index, and the Neurobiologic Risk Score (Brazy, Eckerman, Oehler, Goldstein, & O'Rand, 1991; Korner et al., 1993; Richardson, Gray, McCormick, Workman-Daniels, & Goldmann, 1993; Zupancic, Richardson, & Horbar, 2004). These scoring templates differ with respect to the number of items, the time period(s) when the data are collected, the types of items or events scored, and the weighting of variables. Predictions from perinatal risk scores to neurodevelopmental outcome frequently are weak, with prediction rates being better suited to survival.

Disabilities

A gradient of developmental sequelae exists in children that is inversely related to decreasing birthweight or gestational age. As a result, the smaller or younger the baby, the greater the likelihood of problems. The rates of major disabilities (which include moderate/severe mental retardation, sensorineural hearing loss/blindness, cerebral palsy, and epilepsy) are 6–8% in babies with LBW, 14–17% in infants with VLBW, and 20–25% in children with ELBW. In comparison, major disabilities occur in 5% of full-term infants (Bennett & Scott, 1997; Hack, Taylor, & Klein, 1995). These disability rates have remained relatively constant over the last decade. The nature of impairment may be changing, however, since problems are frequently being found in infants previously considered to be "nondisabled." These high-prevalence/low-severity dysfunctions include learning disabilities (LDs), borderline mental retardation, attention-deficit/hyperactivity disorder (ADHD), specific neuropsychological deficits, and behavioral problems. High-prevalence/low-severity dysfunctions occur in 50–70% of infants with VLBW, and, again, an inverse birthweight gradient is found (Goyen, Lui, & Woods, 1998; O'Callaghan et al., 1996; Taylor, Klein, & Hack, 2000). The situation is compounded by the fact that the social, ethnic, and educational backgrounds of mothers of these infants may also influence the prevalence of these disabilities. Whereas major disabilities are often identified during infancy, high-prevalence/low-severity dysfunctions become more obvious at school entry and later. Currently, there are no good behavioral predictors of these more subtle problems that can be identified during infancy or preschool age.

Correction for Prematurity

Age correction for prematurity (subtracting the weeks of prematurity from the child's chronological age) is applied when preterm infants are followed longitudinally; however, such correction is controversial. The general consensus is that correction should occur, arguably up to 2 years of age (Aylward, 2002a; Blasco, 1989; Lems, Hopkins, & Sampson, 1993). However, some investigators suggest that correction not be utilized; that correction continue throughout childhood or further; or that it be applied in an incremental fashion (e.g., partial correction), depending on an infant's gestational age, age at time of measurement, and area of function being assessed. Use of correction reflects a biological/maturational perspective, whereas adoption of chronological age represents an environmentally based orientation. Current arguments for incremental correction or total lack of correction are unconvincing.

Brain Developmental Issues

In infants born preterm, subsequent outcome is the result of an interchange among normal developmental processes, recovery of function from varying CNS insults, improvement in physical status, and environmental influences (Aylward, 1997). A supportive environment can facilitate self-righting in a child (Sameroff & Chandler, 1975). Therefore, characteristics of either the child or the environment can potentially be protective or risk-producing in nature. An accumulation of nonoptimal factors—child-related, environmental, or both—increases the draw toward less optimal outcome.

A background factor may be considered a "resource" (yields a positive benefit in the presence or absence of a stressor—e.g., early intervention helps both preterm and full-term infants); a "protective factor" (protective only in the presence of adversity—e.g., center-based preschool is beneficial only in children from lower-socioeconomic-status [lower-SES] households); a "risk factor" (negatively influences outcome regardless of presence or absence of adversity—e.g., severe intraventricular hemorrhage [IVH]); or a "vulnerability factor" (will produce poor outcome only in presence of adversity—e.g., LBW and low SES) (Rose, Holmbeck, Coakley, & Franks, 2004).

The Concept of Risk in Infancy

"Risk" refers to variables that have a potentially negative influence on development. There are three categories of risk: established, biological, and environmental. Established risks are medical conditions of a known etiology whose compromised developmental outcome is well documented (e.g., genetic disorders, HIV in infancy). Biological risks include exposure to potentially noxious prenatal, perinatal, or postnatal events, prematurity, or LBW. Environmental risks include the quality of the caregiver–infant interaction, opportunities for developmental/cognitive stimulation, and health care. Relationships among SES, perinatal complications, and cognitive development are complex. As a result, many children are exposed to both biological and environmental risks; this combination is referred to as "double jeopardy" (Parker, Greer, & Zuckerman, 1988). In these cases, nonoptimal biological and environmental factors work synergistically to affect later function negatively (Aylward, 1992). There is a ceiling effect, in which a severe degree of biological risk will minimize the impact of environmental influences.

Biological Risks

There are many causes for developmental problems in neonates and infants. These include infections and nutritional, metabolic, traumatic, intoxicant, maternal prenatal disease-related, anoxic–hypoxic, or idiopathic factors. The timing of exposure to these etiological agents is important (Aylward, 1997). A "critical period" is the time during which the action of a specific internal or external influence is necessary (critical) for normal CNS development. A "sensitive period" is the time during which the CNS is highly susceptible to the effects of harmful or deleterious internal or external conditions, which can lead to alterations, reorganization, and potential disruptions in the system. Critical periods generally are very circumscribed, whereas sensitive periods are more variable.

Disruptions

Disruption in cortical development (corticogenesis) and brain connectivity is inversely related to birthweight and/or gestational age (particularly in infants <33 weeks gestational age), even in the absence of other concomitant biomedical risks. This disruption may be related to birth or events occurring during several critical periods of brain development, such as (1) the migration phase (3–5 months of gestation); (2) organization/differentiation (6 months of gestation through 3 postnatal years); and (3) myelination (6 months of gestation onward) (Volpe, 1998). Even in the absence of identifiable non-optimal CNS events, preterm birth is characterized by a failure of brain structures to proceed in a predictable temporal and spatial sequence.

It can be quite difficult to separate biological risk that arises solely as a consequence of preterm birth from the specific effects attributable to perinatal insults such as IVH or hypoxic–ischemic encephalopathy (HIE). Neonatal ultrasounds may not be sensitive enough to detect subtle injury to gray or white matter, which becomes more apparent on magnetic resonance imaging (MRI) performed in adolescence (Stewart et al., 1999). These abnormalities are more prevalent in individuals born very preterm than in full-term controls. Therefore, the brain of a baby born prematurely may not be organized in the same manner as that of a full-term counterpart. There are also secondary effects, where uninjured areas of the cerebral cortex develop abnormally in the presence of focal lesions in parts of the brain to which the areas are reciprocally connected. This is termed "secondary cortical dysplasia" (Hack & Taylor, 2000). Moreover, prematurity itself may be a reflection of preexisting risk conditions that have affected the fetus prior to birth—conditions that negatively affect brain development of the fetus and cause the mother to deliver prematurely.

Asphyxia

The spectrum of CNS disorders following perinatal insults is determined by the brain's maturational stage at the time of the insult, as well as by the nature and severity of the insult (Aylward, 1997). As a result, the effects of a particular type of CNS event will differ in preterm and full-term infants. "Hypoxemia" is a reduction of oxygen in the blood (brain hypoxia is a reduction of oxygen to brain tissue). "Ischemia" is defined as reduced blood flow to the brain; "asphyxia" is a disturbed exchange of oxygen and carbon dioxide due to an interruption in respiration, which results in hypoxemia, hypercarbia (increased carbon dioxide), and acidemia (decreased blood pH). Asphyxia is accompanied by multisystem organ dysfunction (cardiovascular, gastrointestinal, pulmonary, and renal). HIE is caused by a deprivation of oxygen to the brain, due to the combined effects of hypoxemia and ischemia. "Anoxia" refers to complete lack of oxygen.

Asphyxia has traditionally been indexed as a low Apgar score (range 0–10, based on heart rate, respiratory effort, reflex irritability, muscle tone, and color). However, Apgar scores have been misused and are not predictive of subsequent outcome. A low 1-minute Apgar score is not correlated with later outcome (American Academy of Pediatrics Committee on Fetus and Newborn, 1996; Aylward, 1993), and even a low 5-minute score has limited utility. Therefore, caution should be exercised in considering low Apgar scores as indicators of later intellectual or academic problems in children; in fact, much of the injury could have occurred prior to birth.

In full-term infants, HIE produces cell death in the cerebral cortex, diencephalon, brainstem, and cerebellum. Injury to the basal ganglia and thalamus also occurs. Moderate or severe HIE in full-term infants is associated with high rates of cognitive and motor dysfunction, including microcephaly, mental retardation, epilepsy, and cerebral palsy. In preterm infants, HIE causes cell death deeper within the brain—namely, in the white matter behind and to the side of the lateral ventricles (periventricular leukomalacia; PVL); this occurs in 3–5% of infants with VLBW. There is less initial effect on gray matter in preterm than in full-term infants, and this insult is more often associated with spasticity, neurosensory problems, and motor problems than with cognitive deficits per se. IVH involves bleeding into the subependymal germinal matrix (site of cell proliferation); this occurs in 20–25% of infants <32 weeks gestational age, with higher percentages found in babies with lower gestational ages. Approximately 26% of those born weighing 501–750 g, and 12% of those born weighing 751–1,000 g, have severe (Grade III or IV) IVH. IVH is graded according to the amount of blood in the ventricles and degree of distention. Grade I involves subependymal/germinal matrix hemorrhage with no or minimal IVH; Grade II involves 10–50% of the ventricular area without ventricular dilatation; and Grade III involves >50% of the ventricular area, with distension of the lateral ventricles. Grade IV includes intracerebral involvement or other parenchymal lesions (with a 60% mortality rate), and it is thought not to be on a continuum, reflecting periventricular hemorrhagic infarction. This infarction involves death of periventricular white matter, is large and asymmetric, and involves frontal-parieto-occipital regions with alterations in hemispheric connectivity (see Aylward, 1997). The risk of disability at preschool and school age increases directly in relation to the grade of IVH: 5–10% with Grade I, 15–20% with Grade II, 35–55% with Grade III, and >90% with Grade IV.

A variety of CNS infections, often acquired *in utero*, can also produce adverse effects on an infant's development. These include cytomegalovirus (CMV), toxoplasmosis, congenital rubella, Type 2 herpes simplex virus, and HIV. Drugs may also have teratogenic effects on the CNS; however, here outcome is often affected by a complex matrix of environmental, physiological, and timing/chronicity issues. Frequently encountered drugs include cocaine hydrochloride, ethanol, antiepileptic medications, selective serotonin reuptake inhibitors, heroin, methadone, and methamphetamine.

Environmental Risk

Environmental risk is a powerful moderator of development. SES is defined in part by maternal educational and occupational status. Quantification of family income is also a significant component of the overall determination of SES (Bradley & Corwyn, 2002). Both race and SES should be regarded as markers of a myriad of associated environmental risk factors. SES also involves "capital"—financial, human (e.g., education), and social (Entwisle & Astone, 1994)—and SES indicators may also perform differently across different cultural groups. Social support includes both tangible components (e.g., housing) and intangible components (e.g., attitudes, encouragement to achieve).

The environment involves both process and status features. Process features are more proximal aspects of the environment that are experienced most directly (mother–infant interaction). Status features are distal and broader, involving more indirectly experienced environmental aspects (e.g., SES, location of residence). Environmental effects become increasingly apparent between 18 and 36 months, and are frequently reported at 24 months. Process or proximal environmental variables are more predictive of outcome at early ages; status or distal factors are more predictive at school age or later (Aylward, 1992, 1996). Occupational status or other distal variables in isolation may not accurately reflect the type of parenting to which a child is exposed, or either the day-to-day stresses or positive aspects of the environment that may serve to buffer the infant from the negative factors associated with global environmental risk.

Biomedical and Environmental Risk Interaction

Negative components of the environment have a synergistic or additive effect on infants who are biologically vulnerable, according to the transactional (Sameroff & Chandler, 1975) or "risk-route" models (Aylward & Kenny, 1979). Both models assume that a degree of plasticity exists in both the child and the environment.

Medical/biological factors have been found to determine whether a developmental problem occurs, but environmental factors have a tempering or exacerbating effect on the degree of the problem (Aylward, 1996). However, environmental effects may be minimized with more severe biological risk such as ELBW, probably because of the overwhelming impact of biomedical issues (Hack, Taylor, Klein, & Minich, 2000).

The biomedical–environmental risk interaction becomes highly complex when one considers school and functional outcomes. In general, biomedical variables are related to neurological, neuromotor, neuropsychological, and perceptual–performance functions. Environmental variables are more strongly associated with verbal, academic, and IQ measures. With regard to psychoeducational issues, perinatal variables are related to physical impairment, sensory impairment, and moderate to profound mental retardation; sociodemographic influences are associated with emotional disorders and speech/language impairment. Both biomedical and environmental risks are related to mild mental retardation and specific learning impairments (Resnick et al., 1998).

Outcomes

The question of possible later outcomes is a key issue faced by pediatric psychologists who work with children born prematurely. There exists an array of possible outcomes of interest: medical/physical, neurological, cognitive, academic, motor, neuropsychological, social, and behavioral (Aylward, 2002a, 2005). There is also an increased emphasis on functional and health-related quality of life.

Unfortunately, the follow-up literature contains methodological problems that make it difficult to distill findings and identify meaningful trends (Aylward, 2002b, 2005; Aylward, Pfeiffer, Wright, & Verhulst, 1989). There is no true "gold standard" in early developmental assessment. The Bayley Scales of Infant and Toddler Development, Third Edition (Bayley, 2006), has routinely been considered the best criterion measure during infancy; however, its endorsement is not universal. It is also estimated that mean intelligence quotient (IQ) or developmental quotient (DQ) on a given test increases up to 0.5 point per year or 3–5 points per decade (Flynn, 1999), and this increase may have an impact on longitudinal assessment.

Intelligence Quotients

Comparisons of infants born LBW or smaller and controls have consistently shown a 0.3 to 0.6 standard deviation decrease in IQ in the former. The decrement (excluding children with major disabilities) generally ranges from 3.8 to 9.3 IQ points, with some outlying studies showing 12- to 17-point differences (Aylward et al., 1989; Breslau, DelDotto, & Brown, 1994; Whitfield, Eckstein, & Grunau, 1997). Higher percentages of borderline IQ have been reported in the ELBW population, with estimates ranging from 13–15% (Whitfield et al., 1997) to as high as 37% at age 2 years (Hack et al., 2000; Taylor, Klein, & Hack, 2000; Vohr et al., 2000). In a cohort of infants born at <26 weeks in 1995, 21% had IQs two standard deviations or more below the mean, and 25% had borderline IQ (Marlow, Wolke, Bracewell, & Samara, 2002). Therefore, children born with ELBW or VLBW who do not have major disabilities have mean group IQ scores that fall in the borderline to average range of intelligence, typically being 8–11 points lower than those of controls (Aylward, 2002a, 2005; Bhutta, Cleves, & Casey, 2002). These children are at a distinct disadvantage when they compete with classmates, and IQ decrements do not occur in isolation. Moreover, many children born preterm with normal IQs have other, more specific problems (Aylward, 2002a).

Visual–Motor Skills

The majority of children born at the lowest gestational ages and birthweights manifest some type of visual–motor problem (Dewey, Crawford, Creighton, & Sauve, 1999; Goyen et al., 1998; Whitfield et al., 1997). Deficits are apparent on neuropsychological tasks involving copying, perceptual matching, spatial processing, finger tapping, pegboard performance, visual memory, and visual-sequential memory. Estimates of visual-perceptual and visual–motor integrative problems are in the 11–20% range, whereas rates of fine motor problems are as high as 71% in children with ELBW (Goyen et al., 1998). Indeed, fine motor problems are thought to be the basis for the visual–motor deficits. A higher percentage of prematurely born children are left-handed, and as a group they have poorer legibility and slower handwriting speed. More than one-third of those born moderately premature or younger require prescription glasses. It is possible that atypical visual experiences are associated with prematurity, and that these interfere with the normal developmental function of the visual system. In fact, the visual cortex of infants born preterm has accelerated development, while myelination of the optic radiations does not.

Language

Many language functions (particularly vocabulary, verbal fluency, and receptive language) are reasonably intact in children born prematurely. However, more complex verbal processes, such as understanding of syntax, abstract verbal skills, verb production, and mean length of utterance, have been found deficient in comparison to those of normal-birthweight peers (Le Normand & Cohen, 1999). These deficits are subtle, but critical in social and academic endeavors. They may be related to problems in verbal working memory (an executive function). Event-related potentials and fMRI data in both infants at term conceptional age and children at 8 years indicate neurofunctional differences between those born prematurely and full-term counterparts.

Academic Achievement

More than 50% of children with VLBW and 60–70% of those with ELBW require special assistance in school. By middle school age, children with ELBW are three to five times more likely to have a learning problem in reading, mathematics, spelling, or writing (O'Callaghan et al., 1996). By adolescence, there is an 8- to 10-fold increase in the necessity for remedial education resources or special educational needs, in comparison to full-term controls (Saigal, Stoskopf, Streiner, & Burrows, 2001; Taylor, Klein, Minich, & Hack, 2000). An inverse gradient is found with respect to learning difficulties (Breslau, 1995; Halsey, Collin, & Anderson, 1996; Taylor, Klein, & Hack, 2000). For example, diagnosable LDs occur in as many as 66% of children born <28 weeks; many of these children display nonverbal LDs (NVLD). Overall, 20% of children born at VLBW or ≤32 weeks are in self-contained LD classes; 16–29% repeat a grade; and 32% are in mainstream classes but are functioning more than one grade below their expected placement. Environment may have a moderating effect on LDs.

Behavioral Issues

Symptoms suggestive of ADHD are reported to occur 2.6–4 times more frequently in children born at VLBW/ELBW, with some estimates indicating a 6-fold increase; 9–10% of adolescents with ELBW are reported to have ADHD (Breslau, 1995; Saigal et al., 2001; Taylor, Hack, & Klein, 1998). It is hypothesized that prematurity and its effects act through association with health, cognitive function, and neuromotor function to explain behavioral and emotional problems at school age (e.g., Nadeau, Boivin, Tessier, LeFebvre, & Robacy, 2001). The link between extremely preterm birth and later internalizing and externalizing behavioral problems is also indirect. There are multiple reports of increased stress in the families of children born prematurely, and such stress is even higher if a child has a functional disability, increased medical concerns, or low developmental functioning. Parents frequently articulate concerns about such a child's self-esteem, acceptance by peers, and future, as well as the child's impact on other family members (Drotar et al., 2006; Taylor, Klein, & Hack, 2000).

Executive function, involved in planning, decision making, and behavioral regulation, is also affected in children born prematurely. Anderson and Doyle (2004) reported problems on the Initiate, Working Memory, Plan/Organize, and Monitor subscales of the Behavior Rating Inventory of Executive Function—all suggestive of problems with metacognition. Those with ELBW (in comparison to controls) were two to three times more likely to have trouble starting activities, displaying flexibility in generating ideas and strategies for problem solving, holding and manipulating information in short-term working memory, planning actions in advance, and organizing information. Executive function deficits have a substantial impact on cognitive, social, and academic functioning.

Outcome Status over Time

Of concern is the trend for the outcomes of children born at ELBW/VLBW or prematurely to worsen over time—the so-called "sleeper effect." In one study of children with ELBW, 52% were functioning in the normal range at 4 years of age; however, by age 8, only 31% did not have problems. The prevalence of so-called "minor disabilities" increased in this study from 31% at age 4 years to 53% by age 8 (Monset-Couchard, de Belhmann, & Kastler, 1996). As noted earlier, mild to moderate disabilities may be identified later because these less severe sequelae may only become apparent when demands for higher-level skills cannot be met because of preexisting subtle cognitive deficiencies.

Summary

Although the spectrum of sequelae found in children born at biological risk is similar to problems found in those born at normal birthweight/gestational age, the rates and complexity of these problems and profiles of deficits are disproportionately greater in the former group. This suggests the need for pediatric psychologists to be well versed in outcomes that are particularly associated with biomedical and environmental risk. Because summary scores may grossly underestimate the complex nature and long-range impact of these deficits on an individual child, we must consider improved assessment techniques to evaluate more specific functions.

Assessment must extend beyond traditional IQ and achievement testing, because these measures provide a limited overview of functional abilities, and do not identify more circumscribed deficits. Specific tests or rating scales that measure the following areas should also be considered: (1) attention and executive functions; (2) language; (3) sensory–motor functions; (4) visual–spatial processes; (5) memory and learning; and (6) ADHD and behavioral adjustment (Aylward, 2005; Institute of Medicine, 2006).

References

American Academy of Pediatrics Committee on Fetus and Newborn. (1996). Use and abuse of the Apgar score. *Pediatrics*, 98, 141–142.

Anderson, P. J., & Doyle, L. W. (2004). Executive functioning in school-aged children who were born very preterm or with extremely low birth weight. *Pediatrics*, 114, 50–57.

Aylward, G. P. (1992). The relationship between environmental risk and developmental outcome. *Journal of Developmental and Behavioral Pediatrics*, 13, 222–229.

Aylward, G. P. (1993). Perinatal asphyxia: Effects of biologic and environmental risks. *Clinics in Perinatology*, 20, 433–449.

Aylward, G. P. (1996). Environmental risk, intervention and developmental outcome. *Ambulatory Child Health*, 2, 161–170.

Aylward, G. P. (1997). *Infant and early childhood neuropsychology.* New York: Plenum Press.

Aylward, G. P. (2002a). Cognitive and neuropsychological outcome: More than IQ scores. *Mental Retardation and Developmental Disabilities Research and Reviews*, 8, 234–240.

Aylward, G. P . (2002b). Methodological issues in outcome studies of at-risk infants. *Journal of Pediatric Psychology*, 27, 37–45.

Aylward, G. P. (2005). Neurodevelopmental outcomes of infants born prematurely. *Journal of Developmental and Behavioral Pediatrics, 26,* 427–440.

Aylward, G. P., & Kenny, T. J. (1979). Developmental follow-up: Inherent problems and a conceptual model. *Journal of Pediatric Psychology, 4,* 331–343.

Aylward, G. P., Pfeiffer, S. I., Wright, A., & Verhulst, S. J. (1989). Outcome studies of low birth weight infants published in the last decade: A meta-analysis. *Journal of Pediatrics, 115,* 515–521.

Bayley, N. (2006). *The Bayley Scales of Infant and Toddler Development, Third Edition.* San Antonio, TX: Psychological Corporation.

Bennett, F. C., & Scott, D. T. (1997). Long-term perspective on premature infant outcome and contemporary intervention issues. *Seminars in Perinatology, 21,* 190–201.

Bhutta, A. T., Cleves, M. A., & Casey, P. H. (2002). Cognitive and behavioral outcomes of school-aged children who were born preterm. *Journal of the American Medical Association, 288,* 728–737.

Blasco, P. A. (1989). Preterm birth: To correct or not to correct. *Developmental Medicine and Child Neurology, 31,* 816–826.

Bradley, R. H., & Corwyn, R. F. (2002). Socioeconomic status and child development. *Annual Review of Psychology, 53,* 371–399.

Brazy, J. E., Eckerman, C. O., Oehler, J. M., Goldstein, R. F., & O'Rand, M. A. (1991). Nursery Neurobiologic Risk Score: Important factors in predicting outcome in very low birth weight infants. *Journal of Pediatrics, 118,* 783–792.

Breslau, N. (1995). Psychiatric sequelae of low birth weight. *Epidemiologic Reviews, 17,* 96–106.

Breslau, N., DelDotto, J. E., & Brown, G. (1994). A gradient relationship between low birth weight and IQ at age 6 years. *Archives of Pediatrics and Adolescent Medicine, 148,* 377–383.

Dewey, D., Crawford, S. G., Creighton, D. E., & Sauve, R. S. (1999). Long-term neuropsychological outcomes in very low birth weight children free of sensorineural impairments. *Journal of Clinical and Experimental Neuropsychology, 21,* 851–865.

Drotar, D., Hack, M., Taylor, G., Schulucher, M., Andreias, L., & Klein, N. (2006). The impact of extremely low birth weight on the families of school-aged children. *Pediatrics, 117,* 2006–2013.

Entwisle, D. R., & Astone, N. M. (1994). Some practical guidelines for measuring youths' race/ethnicity and socioeconomic status. *Child Development, 65,* 1521–1540.

Flynn, J. R. (1999). Searching for justice: The discovery of IQ gains over time. *American Psychologist, 54,* 5–20.

Goldenberg, R. L., Culhane, J. F., Iams, J. D., & Romero, R. (2008). Epidemiology and causes of preterm birth. *Lancet, 371,* 75–84.

Goyen, T., Lui, K., & Woods, R. (1998). Visual–motor, visual-perceptual, and fine-motor outcomes in very-low-birthweight children at 5 years. *Developmental Medicine and Child Neurology, 40,* 76–81.

Hack, M., & Fanaroff, A. A. (1999). Outcomes of children of extremely low birthweight and gestational age in the 1990's. *Early Human Development, 53,* 193–218.

Hack, M., & Taylor, H. G. (2000). Perinatal brain injury in preterm infants and later neurobehavioral function. *Journal of the American Medical Association, 284,* 1973–1974.

Hack, M., Taylor, H. G., & Klein, N. (1995). Long term developmental outcome of low birth-weight infants. In P. Shiono & R. Behrman (Eds.), *The future of children: Vol. 5. Low birth weight* (pp. 176–196). Los Altos, CA: Packard Foundation.

Hack, M., Taylor, H. G., Klein, N., & Minich, N. M. (2000). Functional limitations and special health care needs of 10- to 14-year-old children weighing less than 750 grams at birth. *Pediatrics, 106,* 554–559.

Halsey, C. L., Collin, M. F., & Anderson, C. L. (1996). Extremely low birth weight children and their peers. *Archives of Pediatrics and Adolescent Medicine, 150,* 790–794.

Institute of Medicine. (2006). *Preterm birth: Causes, consequences, and prevention* (R. E. Berman & A. Stith Butler, Eds.). Washington, DC: National Academies Press.

Korner, A. F., Stevenson, D. K., Kraemer, H. C., Spiker, D., Scott, D. T., Constantinou, J., et al. (1993). Prediction of the development of low birth weight preterm infants by a new Neonatal Medical Index. *Journal of Developmental and Behavioral Pediatrics, 14,* 106–111.

Lems, W., Hopkins, B., & Sampson, J. F. (1993). Mental and motor development in preterm infants: The issue of corrected age. *Early Human Development, 34,* 113–123.

Le Normand, M. T., & Cohen, H. (1999). The delayed emergence of lexical morphology in preterm children: The case of verbs. *Journal of Neurolinguistics, 12,* 235–246.

Marlow, N., Wolke, D., Bracewell, M. A., & Samara, M. (2002). Neurologic and developmental disability at six years of age after extremely preterm birth. *New England Journal of Medicine, 352,* 9–19.

McCormick, M. C. (1989). Long-term follow-up of infants discharged from neonatal intensive care units. *Journal of the American Medical Association, 261,* 1767–1772.

Monset-Couchard, M., de Belhmann, O., & Kastler, B. (1996). Mid- and long-term outcome of 89 premature infants weighing less than 1000g at birth, all appropriate for gestational age. *Biology of the Neonate, 70,* 328–338.

Nadeau, L., Boivin, M., Tessier, R., LeFebvre, F., & Robacy, P. (2001). Mediators of behavioral problems in 7-year-old children born after 24 to 28 weeks of gestation. *Journal of Developmental and Behavioral Pediatrics, 22,* 1–10.

O'Callaghan, M. J., Burns, Y. R., Gray, P. H., Harvey, J. M., Mohay, H., Rogers, Y. M., et al. (1996). School performance of ELBW children: A controlled study. *Developmental Medicine and Child Neurology, 38,* 917–926.

Parker, S., Greer, S., & Zuckerman, B. (1988). Double jeopardy: The impact of poverty on early child development. *Pediatric Clinics of North America, 35,* 1227–1240.

Resnick, M. B., Gomatam, S. V., Carter, R. L., Ariet, M., Roth, J., Kilgore, K. L., et al. (1998). Educational disabilities of neonatal intensive care graduates. *Pediatrics, 102,* 308–316.

Richardson, D. K., Gray, J. E., McCormick, M. C., Workman-Daniels, K., & Goldmann, D. A. (1993). Score for Acute Neonatal Physiology (SNAP): A physiologic severity index for neonatal intensive care. *Pediatrics, 91,* 617–623.

Rose, B. M., Holmbeck, G. N., Coakley, R., & Franks, E. A. (2004). Mediator and moderator effects in developmental and behavioral pediatric research. *Journal of Developmental and Behavioral Pediatrics, 25,* 58–67.

Saigal, S., & Doyle, L. W. (2008). An overview of mortality and sequelae of preterm birth from infancy to adulthood. *Lancet, 371,* 261–269.

Saigal, S., Stoskopf, B. L., Streiner, D. L., & Burrows, E. (2001). Physical growth and current health status of infants who were of extremely low birth weight and controls at adolescence. *Pediatrics, 108,* 407–415.

Sameroff, A. J., & Chandler, M. J. (1975). Reproductive risk and the continuum of caretaking casualty. In F. D. Horowitz (Ed.), *Review of child development research* (Vol. 4., pp. 187–244). Chicago: University of Chicago Press.

Stevenson, D. K., Wright, L. L., Lemons, J. A., Oh, W., Korones, S. B., Papile, L., et al. (1998). Very low birth weight outcomes of the National Institute of Child Health and Human Development Neonatal research Network, January 1993 through December, 1994. *American Journal of Obstetrics and Gynecology, 179,* 1632–1640.

Stewart, A. L., Rifkin, L., Amess, P. N., Kirkbride, V., Townsend, J. P., Miller, D. H., et al. (1999). Brain structure and neorcognitive and behavioral function in adolescents who were born very preterm. *Lancet, 353,* 1635–1657.

Taylor, H. G., Hack, M., & Klein, N. K. (1998). Attention deficits in children with <750 g birth weight. *Developmental Neuropsychology, 4*, 21–34.

Taylor, H. G., Klein, N., & Hack, M. (2000). School-age consequences of birth weight less than 750 g: A review and update. *Developmental Neuropsychology, 17*, 289–321.

Taylor, H. G., Klein, N., Minich, N. M., & Hack, M. (2000). Middle-school-age outcomes in children with very low birthweight. *Child Development, 71*, 1495–1511.

Vohr, B., Wright, L. L., Dusick, A. M., Mele, L., Verter, J., Steichen, J. J., et al. (2000). Neurodevelopmental and functional outcomes of extremely low birth weight infants in the National Institute of Child Health and Human Development Neonatal Research Network, 1993–1994. *Pediatrics, 105*, 1216–1226.

Volpe, J. J. (1998). Neurologic outcome of prematurity. *Archives of Neurology, 55*, 297–300.

Whitfield, M. F., Eckstein, R. V., & Grunau, L. H. (1997). Extremely premature (≤ 800 g) school children: Multiple areas of hidden disability. *Archives of Disease in Childhood, 77*, F85–F90.

Zupancic, J. A., Richardson, D. K., & Horbar, J. D. (2004). Revalidation of the Score for Neonatal Acute Physiology in the Vermont Oxford Network. *Pediatrics, 119*, e156–e163.

CHAPTER 17

Pediatric Asthma

ELIZABETH L. McQUAID
NATALIE WALDERS ABRAMSON

Asthma remains a leading public health challenge, and is the most common chronic illness facing children in the United States. The prevalence of asthma appears to have stabilized since the increases documented in the previous several decades, but rates remain at historically high levels (Moorman et al., 2007). An estimated 6.8 million children in the United States are affected by asthma, representing approximately 9.4% of all children (Bloom & Cohen, 2007).

Pediatric psychologists are uniquely positioned to help families optimize asthma management through educational and behavioral interventions, and are well suited to investigate the complex interplay between psychological factors and disease course. This chapter reviews the multiple points for successful intervention, interdisciplinary collaboration, and research endeavors to increase our understanding of psychosocial aspects of asthma.

Definition and Scope of the Problem

"Asthma" is characterized as a chronic inflammatory disorder of the airways that involves intermittent, recurring, and variable periods of airway obstruction (National Institutes of Health [NIH], 2007). The pathophysiology of asthma involves many pathways and processes, including chronic inflammation, airway hyperresponsiveness, bronchoconstriction, swelling of the airways, and mucus production. Asthma is characterized by chronic underlying inflammation, which may not produce noticeable symptoms, and exacerbations, which are characterized by active symptoms. Typically, asthma symptoms occur as a result of airway hyperresponsiveness to a variety of triggers, including airborne irritants (e.g., cigarette smoke), seasonal changes (e.g., cold weather), and respiratory infections, as well as allergens that elicit symptoms among individuals with specific immunological hypersensitivity (e.g., animal dander, dust mites). Triggers vary among individuals, and sensitivity can change over the course of illness. This complexity underscores the need for individualized treatment plans that highlight the specific profile of triggers, symptoms, and medication needs for a particular patient, depending on current symptom activity.

During an exacerbation, a range of processes may contribute to breathing difficulty; these include constriction of the bronchial smooth muscles, swelling of bronchial tissues, and increased mucus secretion (American Academy of Allergy, Asthma and Immunology [AAAAI], 2000). During such times, patients may experience a combination of coughing, wheezing, breathlessness, chest tightness, and reduced tolerance for activity (NIH, 2007). Although the airway obstruction is typically reversible without lung damage, more permanent "remodeling" of the airways may be a potential consequence of the disease. Airway remodeling is related to persistent untreated inflammation in the airway structures, which leads to permanent depletion in lung function. This underscores the need to optimally treat both the reversible airway obstruction during periodic exacerbations and the underlying chronic inflammation characteristic of asthma (Bibi, Feigenbaum, Hessen, & Shoseyov, 2006).

Asthma Prevalence and Morbidity

Although no clear single explanation exists for the increases in asthma prevalence in the late 20th century, some have theorized that they may have been due to greater exposure to indoor allergens due to overall lifestyle changes, such as more time spent inside engaged in sedentary activities (Platts-Mills, Blumenthal, Perzanowski, & Wood-folk, 2000). Others have proposed a "hygiene hypothesis," whereby frequent antibiotic use and decreased exposure to infections early in life may have altered the immune responses and, paradoxically, led to an increased likelihood of asthma onset (Mattes & Karmaus, 1999).

Although asthma-related deaths are relatively rare, asthma fatalities do occur. Nationally, the asthma mortality rate for individuals under age 19 years increased by nearly 80% between 1980 and 1993, whereas more recent estimates show a plateau (American Lung Association, 2007; Centers for Disease Control and Prevention [CDC], 1996). Asthma deaths have been linked to certain risk factors, including medication nonadherence and inadequate skills in perceiving symptom severity (Alvarez, Schulzer, Jung, & Fitzgerald, 2005).

The morbidity and mortality associated with pediatric asthma disproportionately affect ethnic minorities, urban communities, and low-income populations (Crain, Kercsmar, Weiss, Mitchell, & Lynn, 1998; Federico & Liu, 2003). Recent research underscores the complexity of the genetics of asthma. It also indicates that certain subgroups of ethnic minorities (e.g., African Americans, Puerto Ricans) have greater risk for asthma onset, more complicated illness course, increased exposure to environmental triggers, lower quality of care, and more fatalities (Hunninghake, Weiss, & Celedon, 2006; Inkelas, Garro, McQuaid, & Ortega, 2008; Lozano, Connell, & Koepsell, 1995). For example, African American youths with asthma are at increased risk of such adverse outcomes as emergency health care use and death (CDC, 2006). Greater negative consequences for asthma, such as poorly controlled symptoms, have also been identified among Puerto Ricans (Canino et al., 2006). Although some researchers caution that the disproportionate impact of asthma on ethnic minorities may reflect healthcare disparities associated with poverty and urban communities, higher asthma rates and risks have been identified among ethnic minorities even after these factors are controlled for (Joseph, Ownby, Peterson, & Johnson, 2000; Nelson et al., 1997), suggesting a complex interplay between genetic factors and conditions of urban living.

Measurement of Asthma Status

Numerous approaches are used to characterize asthma status, and disease presentation can vary widely within an individual over the course of the illness (Calhoun, Sutton, Emmett, & Dorinsky, 2003). Indicators of disease status can be grouped into several broad categories, including measures of symptom frequency, lung function measures, biological markers, and health care utilization measures.

Measures of symptom frequency, such as the Asthma Control Test (ACT; Nathan et al., 2004), are easily administered; they are designed to assess the frequency of both daytime and nocturnal symptoms, and the extent of reliance on quick-relief medications over a short time window. Although they provide a useful assessment of asthma status, they are limited by the accuracy of self-report or parent proxy report. Lung function measures typically involve the use of spirometry to measure the volume and flow of air movement through the lungs; this generates informative values, such as forced expiratory volume in the first second (FEV1), used to monitor disease severity and level of control. Biological indicators include such measures as exhaled nitric oxide (eNO), which is an indication of the extent of airway inflammation (Smith, Cowan, Brassett, Herbison, & Taylor, 2005), and airway resistance by forced oscillation (Ritz et al., 2002), which measures the amount of airflow resistance in the lungs. Although commonly used in research, these measures have yet to be adopted in routine clinical care, perhaps due to the expense of equipment and the extent of specialized expertise involved. Health care utilization measures, such as claims data indicating use of emergency services, provide information regarding asthma acuity, but they may also reflect local health care system resources or family response patterns.

Psychological Aspects

Before the advent of modern immunology and the recognition of allergic phenomena, asthma was considered primarily a "nervous disease" and was actually referred to in early medical textbooks as "asthma nervosa" (Alexander, 1950). Over the past several decades, transformations in the field have emphasized a complex, bidirectional integration of genetic, immunological, and psychosocial factors in both the onset and expression of asthma. For example, asthma onset is currently thought to be predicted by a combination of genetic factors (e.g., predisposition to allergy) (AAAAI, 2000), environmental variables (e.g., exposure to infections, allergens, or irritants) (Busse & Lemanske, 2001), and psychological influences such as maternal distress (Kozyrskyj et al., 2008) and stress (Mrazek & Klinnert, 1991).

Some parental behaviors have also been demonstrated to affect a child's risk for developing asthma. These include maternal smoking during pregnancy, as well as child exposure to environmental tobacco smoke (Environmental Protection Agency, 1992). Other research has suggested that such factors as difficulties in parenting may increase asthma risk (Klinnert & Mrazek, 1994; Klinnert et al., 2001). One prospective longitudinal study investigating risk factors for asthma onset indicated that two early indicators—an index of allergy and an index of global parenting difficulty at infant age 3 weeks—were independent predictors of asthma status between ages 6 and 8 years in children at genetic risk (Klinnert et al., 2001). The authors suggested that developmentally relevant stressful events and/or the quality of caregiving may in fact alter an infant's emotional and physiological regulation in the direction of increased allergic response.

Emotions and Asthma Course

There is a burgeoning literature regarding the association between emotions (typically conceptualized as stress) and asthma. A proportion of individuals with asthma (approximately 15–30%) identify stress and emotions as triggers for asthma episodes (Isenberg, Lehrer, & Hochron, 1992; Wright, Rodriguez, & Cohen, 1998). Early research in this area documented that a proportion of individuals with asthma react with bronchoconstriction when subjected to stressful experiences, such as performing mental arithmetic (Miklich, Rewey, Weiss, & Kolton, 1973), watching emotionally charged films (Miller & Wood, 1994), or speaking about an embarrassing event (McQuaid et al., 2000).

The psychophysiological mechanisms that link emotional processes to asthma disease process are not completely understood, although some models to explain this association have been posed. Early conceptualizations proposed that the autonomic nervous system mediates the effects of emotions on asthma. Specifically, for some individuals, increased activity of the vagus nerve and stimulation of the parasympathetic nervous system may result in bronchoconstriction in the large airways (see Isenberg et al., 1992, for a review). More recent theories attempt to integrate individual factors (such as psychophysiological reactivity) with broader contextual effects of both short-term and longer-term, chronic stress. Stress is thought to influence asthma course through multiple pathways, such as autonomic control of the airways, neuroendocrine function, and immune regulation (see Wright, 2005, for a review of this topic).

As an example, the work of Miller and Wood (Miller & Wood, 1994; Wood, Klebba, & Miller, 2000) proposes a pattern of emotional responsivity and physiological reactivity, linked through cholinergic pathways, which may affect airway function for some children with asthma. The risk for emotionally induced asthma is increased when a child's asthma is psychophysiologically reactive and when the child is exposed to significant life stress, negative family climate, or other emotional challenges. Later versions of this model (Wood et al., 2000, 2008) incorporate features of the parent–child relationship (e.g., relational security) as additional key factors. Alternative models hypothesize that exposure to chronic stressors (e.g., those associated with poverty and disadvantage) may affect changes in immunity and increase the inflammatory response, hence increasing risk for asthma exacerbations (Miller & Chen, 2007). Theories such as these that investigate the reciprocal influences among physiological processes, psychological vulnerability, and life circumstances in explaining the relationships between emotions and asthma are useful models for guiding future research and informing innovative prevention and intervention programs.

Behavioral Adjustment

The question of whether children with asthma have more behavior problems than their healthy peers has also been a topic of debate. Some early studies documented minimal behavioral differences between children with asthma and healthy controls (Graham, Rutter, Yule, & Pless, 1967), whereas more recent research indicates that children with asthma demonstrate more internalizing behavior problems than do either norm populations (Klinnert, McQuaid, McCormick, Adinoff, & Bryant, 2000; Wamboldt, Fritz, Mansell, McQuaid, & Klein, 1998) or comparative samples of healthy controls (Austin, Smith, Risinger, & McNelis, 1994). In addition, there is some evidence that children with more severe asthma have more behavior problems than those with milder forms of the disease do (Klinnert et al., 2000; MacLean, Perrin, Gortmaker, & Pierre, 1992; Wamboldt et al., 1998). A meta-analysis of behavioral adjustment in children with asthma concluded that, in general, children with asthma do have more behavioral difficulties than their peers, and that these difficulties are more pronounced in the internalizing domain (McQuaid, Kopel, & Nassau, 2001). Disease severity moderates this relationship, such that children with mild illness are not significantly different from healthy peers, but behavioral difficulties are more evident with increasing disease severity (McQuaid, Kopel, & Nassau, 2001).

There is clear evidence that having psychological difficulties puts children with asthma at risk for a problematic disease course. Psychological distress has been associated with poorly controlled asthma marked by problematic nonadherence to treatment regimens (Bender, 2006; Creer, 1993). Early studies in this area indicated that children with asthma who have comorbid behavior problems and/or depressive symptoms tend to have more functional impairment (Gustadt, Gillette, & Mrazek, 1989). Parents and siblings of youths with asthma may also face psychosocial stressors associated with chronic illness management (Barlow & Ellard, 2006). Identifying comorbid behavior problems in patients and families, and initiating appropriate referral for treatment, should be clear priorities for health care providers.

Developmental and Family Implications

A chronic illness such as asthma has the potential to affect the achievement of age-appropriate developmental tasks, such as individuation from parents, socialization outside the family, the establishment of peer relationships, and the formation of a positive self-image. The extent to which asthma exerts influence in these domains is likely to be moderated by disease severity, with children who have more severe and persistent forms of asthma most affected (Fritz & McQuaid, 2000). In addition, the course of asthma may vary across childhood. Although the common notion that many children "outgrow" asthma persists, current conceptualizations propose different asthma course phenotypes—some of which remit in childhood, but many of which fluctuate.

The implementation of skills for effective pediatric asthma management results from a complex set of interactions between family members and other caregivers (Fiese & Everhart, 2006). Children's active participation may vary widely by age, developmental maturity, and attitude toward the illness. Optimally, parents involve children in the disease management process by providing direct guidance, then supervising task performance, and eventually allowing the children to perform the skills independently (Brown, Avery, Mobley, Boccuti, & Golbach, 1996). In the pediatric asthma population, preadolescent children tend to assume responsibility for the tasks of identifying and managing symptoms when they occur. They are less likely to assume responsibility for tasks of preventive management, such as avoiding triggers (McQuaid, Penza-Clyve, et al., 2001). Families often face challenges in optimally distributing responsibilities for asthma management tasks between parents and children, particularly during periods of developmental transition. Some research has demonstrated that adherence may be compromised when parents overestimate the asthma self-management behaviors of adolescents (Walders, Drotar, & Kercsmar, 2000).

Adolescence brings significant challenges with regard to the management of chronic illness, as teenagers may exert their growing independence in ways that can be life-threatening, such as through nonadherence to medication regimens and minimization of acute symptoms. Although all childhood age groups have relatively similar attack prevalence rates, youths ages 11–17 show the highest mortality rates of all the groups, suggesting that this is a period of increased risk (Akinbami & Schoendorf, 2002). Adolescence appears to be a time in which difficulties in adherence to asthma medications can become more pronounced, requiring reinvigored adult supervision of management tasks (Bender, Milgrom, Rand, & Ackerson, 1998; McQuaid, Kopel, Klein, & Fritz, 2003). Specification of developmental expectations for children's self-management of illness, and identification of children at particular risk because of psychological or developmental factors, are key roles for psychologists.

Although much of the existing research assesses how individual- and family-level factors influence asthma outcomes, or how aspects of asthma influence individual and family functioning, most researchers acknowledge that there are multiple, bidirectional influences among these systems (Kaugars, Klinnert, & Bender, 2004; Wamboldt & Wamboldt, 2000). Longitudinal designs provide the most compelling evidence of these reciprocal influences. For example, one recent study evaluated caregiver psychological functioning and infant disease variables for children who were at risk of developing asthma, but had not yet been diagnosed with the disease (Kaugars, Klinnert, Robinson, & Ho, 2008). Caregiver psychological resources and child hospitalizations had significant independent effects on a prospective assessment of parent emotion regulation. More such research is needed to assess how individual, family, and disease factors influence one another longitudinally.

Interdisciplinary Management

Numerous intervention studies have found empirical support for interdisciplinary approaches to asthma management that integrate the expertise of a wide variety of providers, such as physicians, psychologists, nurses, and health educators (Bratton et al., 2001; Evans et al., 1999; Weinstein, Faust, McKee, & Padman, 1992). In addition to establishing criteria for the medical management of asthma, the NIH (2007) guidelines recognize the benefits of an interdisciplinary approach to asthma management under various conditions (such as comorbid psychiatric distress, family problems, or nonadherence) that may jeopardize management of the condition.

Basic Medical Approach

The most recent National Asthma Education and Prevention Program guidelines (NIH, 2007) outline a stepwise approach to managing asthma across the lifespan according to illness severity and level of asthma control. The report highlights four key care components: regular symptom assessment and monitoring; an emphasis on self-management education; efforts to control environmental triggers; and a systematic approach to medication management (NIH, 2007). Depending on the severity and course of the condition, childhood asthma may be medically managed by a primary care pediatrician or may necessitate the involvement of a specialty provider, such as a pulmonologist or an allergist. Pediatric asthma specialists are uniquely qualified to manage challenging asthma cases that require complicated medication management and involve a high risk for morbidity.

In general, practice guidelines recommend a timely response to acute exacerbations at all stages, including preventing disease progression by avoiding asthma triggers and using long-term-control medications (see below) to reduce underlying airway inflammation. A central feature involves a written asthma "action plan." Such a plan typically includes information about medications and dosing. A distinction is made between medications for symptom prevention and those for acute exacerbation. Instruction regarding appropriate health care utilization is included as well (Zemek, Bhogal, & Ducharme, 2008). Collaboration and clear communication between parent and physician also appears instrumental in asthma outcomes (Riekert et al., 2003).

Significant developments in options for the pharmacological management of asthma have been developed and disseminated in recent years. One major change has been the shift from metered-dose inhalers that rely on chlorofluorocarbons (CFCs) to the use of hydrofluoroalkane (HFA), due to the potential harmful environmental effects of CFC-based inhalers. Advantages and challenges to the new drug delivery systems have been described, and some patients may experience a difficult transition to a new medication delivery system (Gustafsson, Taylor, Zanen, & Chrystyn, 2005).

The NIH guidelines (2007) divide the pharmacological management of asthma into two categories: quick-relief/rescue medications and long-term-control medications. Quick-relief medications are used to provide rapid relief of bronchoconstriction found in all forms of asthma; such medications are intended for use on a periodic or as-needed basis. For patients with intermittent asthma that involves infrequent exacerbations, a quick-relief medication, such as a short-acting β_2 agonist (e.g., albuterol) may be the only form of indicated treatment. Systemic corticosteroids (e.g., prednisone) are also considered quick-relief medications, but are generally used to reverse exacerbations when other medications have been ineffective. Excessive reliance on quick-relief medications may indicate that asthma management is insufficient, and that more aggressive treatment (such as additional long-term-control medication) is warranted.

In contrast to quick-relief medications, long-term-control medications are taken on a daily basis to control persistent asthma symptoms. Patients with persistent forms of asthma, marked by underlying inflammation of the airways, generally require both quick-relief and long-term-control medication. Several forms of long-term-control medications are available. Inhaled corticosteroids (e.g., budesonide, fluticasone propionate), which are regarded as effective anti-inflammatory treatments for daily control of symptoms, are commonly prescribed (NIH, 2007). Alternative preventive medications include cromolyn sodium (prescribed in inhaler form) and leukotriene modifiers (e.g., montelukast, prescribed in pill form). In addition, long-acting β_2 agonists may be administered in conjunction with anti-inflammatory medications to provide sustained symptom control. Combinations of medications (e.g., fluticasone propionate and salmeterol) offer a dual delivery of inhaled corticosteroid along with a long-acting β_2 agonist in a single therapeutic dose for patients who require both forms of medication.

Roles of Pediatric Psychologists

Psychologists can provide valuable consultation to health care providers on an outpatient basis, on inpatient units, and through informal consultation. Clinical psychologists will encounter patients with asthma within their general practices, underscoring the importance of asthma awareness for all practitioners. Several roles for pediatric psychologists in facilitating asthma management are emphasized: (1) providing patient, family, and health care provider education; (2) identification and treatment of psychosocial barriers to effective asthma management; and (3) implementation of psychosocial intervention techniques to promote effective family-based asthma management behaviors.

Patient and Family Education

Several types of asthma knowledge deficits, including inaccurate beliefs about the type and use of medications, poor understanding of the etiology and course of asthma, and incorrect beliefs concerning asthma management techniques, have been reported (Clark et al., 1998; Zimmerman, Bonner, Evans, & Mellins, 1999). Numerous educational programs for asthma have been developed. Over the past decade, these programs have been evaluated with increasing methodological rigor. It is now recognized that educational programs emphasizing self-management yield a number of positive effects, including reductions in health care utilization (Bartholomew et al., 2000; DePue et al., 2007) and improved symptom control (Bonner et al., 2002; Clark et al., 2004). Programs that incorporate a focus on behavior change, rather than providing information only, are more likely to yield positive outcomes (Gibson et al., 2002).

Health Care Provider Education

Accomplishing clear patient–provider communication remains a challenge for many families (Modi & Quittner, 2006). Physician-training programs have been developed to improve health care providers' knowledge of asthma treatment guidelines and to enhance their skills in provider–patient interactions (Clark et al., 1998). One example, the Physician Asthma Care Education program, utilizes a structured, interactive curriculum for physician training. Results of a controlled trial indicated many positive outcomes, including higher levels of controller medication prescription in the intervention group, and patient reports of greater frequency of being asked to demonstrate metered-dose inhaler use (Clark et al., 1998). This program has also demonstrated results with patients from low-income backgrounds (Brown, Bratton, Cabana, Kaciroti, & Clark, 2004). Offering health care providers cultural competence training may also improve outcomes. One large study of parents of Medicaid-insured children with asthma found that parents who attended practice sites with policies to promote cultural competence reported being less likely to underuse preventive asthma medications (Lieu et al., 2004).

Identification and Treatment of Psychosocial Barriers to Asthma Management

Various psychosocial stressors have been identified as risk factors for exacerbating asthma morbidity and mortality. For instance, family mental health problems (Weil et al., 1999), limited problem-solving skills (Wade, Holden, Lynn, Mitchell, & Ewart, 2000), and family dysfunction (Strunk, 1987) have been identified as risk factors for morbidity. Medical professionals involved in asthma care may have some expertise in recognizing psychosocial risk factors; however, they frequently do not have the training or the resources to modify psychosocial stressors once these are identified. As a result, collaborative relationships between psychologists and medical staff represent a valuable model for improving asthma outcomes (Walders, Nobile, & Drotar, 2000).

Implementation of Psychosocial Intervention Techniques

In contrast to asthma education efforts that seek to address gaps in asthma knowledge, psychosocial interventions attempt to foster new skills in managing the symptoms and treatments of asthma. The term "asthma self-management" is often used to describe the skills necessary to cope with the treatment demands of asthma and the obligations of patient-directed, rather than physician-facilitated, care (Creer, 2000). In contrast to adult asthma, in which the individual patient is the central figure, self-management in pediatric asthma recognizes the family context of management behaviors. Cooperation among patient, family, and provider in asthma self-management is pivotal in accomplishing optimal outcomes.

Numerous psychosocial interventions for asthma have been described in the published literature and implemented in clinical practice. These include self-management training, problem-solving techniques, family-based interventions, motivational interviewing, and psychophysiological modalities (i.e., relaxation training and biofeedback) (Borrelli, Riekert, Weinstein, & Rathier, 2007; Creer, 2000; Lemanek, Kamps, & Chung, 2001). Psychosocial interventions may be offered to patients singly or in combination, depending on a particular patient's and family's needs. Interventions may be delivered in an inpatient pediatric setting through consultation–liaison work or on an outpatient basis. Psychosocial interventions appear to be particularly effective in maximizing treatment adherence, facilitating cooperation between families and physicians, and delivering asthma education in an optimal manner (Lemanek et al., 2001).

Deficits in problem-solving skills have been identified among families coping with asthma (Wade et al., 2000), resulting in the recommendation to identify and modify ineffective problem-solving strategies (Walders et al., 2006). Interventions that focus on empowering families to optimally manage their children's illness have gained increasing recognition in the literature as tools for successful outcomes (Canino et al., 2008; Warman, Silver, & Wood, 2006). Family-based intervention principles involve encouraging developmentally appropriate distribution of management tasks among family members, promoting a balance between child self-management and parental involvement or supervision, and enhancing asthma awareness among family members (Weinstein et al., 1992).

The recognition of health care disparities among populations affected by asthma has encouraged the development and dissemination of culturally tailored asthma management programs for specific high-risk populations (Weiss, 2007). These efforts have been met with some success. For example, one Web-based, culturally tailored educational program targeting African American urban high school students resulted in decreased symptoms and fewer missed school days for participants compared to controls (Joseph et al., 2007). A family-based program targeted toward Puerto Rican families of children with asthma also demonstrated symptom reduction for participating children compared to a control group (Canino et al., 2008). Given the significance of the health care disparities targeted by these efforts, such programs represent an important priority for future research.

Psychophysiological tools, including relaxation training, progressive/passive muscle relaxation, and biofeedback, have also been evaluated as adjunctive treatments. These interventions attempt to reduce autonomic arousal and emotional distress during an asthma exacerbation (McQuaid & Nassau, 1999). Biofeedback is based on the technique of teaching patients to modify physical symptoms by receiving consistent feedback concerning the exacerbation or reduction of physiological symptoms. Although some forms of biofeedback to modify asthma symptoms are empirically supported, more research is needed to determine whether these strategies effect clinically significant changes (McQuaid & Nassau, 1999). Web-based tools have also shown success as a new modality for delivering educational interventions to patients and families (Joseph et al., 2007; Runge, Lecheler, Horn, Tews, & Schaefer, 2006).

Conclusion

Research and practice in the management of pediatric asthma are at a crossroads. In recent years, spiraling estimates of prevalence and morbidity have engendered coordinated efforts at both national and local levels to diagnose and manage the illness more effectively. Guidelines from national organizations provide recommendations for accurate diagnosis and effective management of the disease (Global Initiative for Asthma [GINA], 2007; NIH, 2007). The pace at which new asthma medications are being developed has been steadily increasing. Despite these advances, asthma remains a critical public health problem with significant morbidity and health care costs. Implementation of the recommendations for asthma management is a difficult task for health care professionals and families—and a significant gap often remains between these recommendations and actual practice. Many families still conceive of asthma as episodic and believe that they are treating asthma effectively by managing the symptoms of the illness, rather than recognizing its chronicity and attempting to prevent future episodes (Callery, Milnes, Verduyn, & Couriel, 2003). Misconceptions about the necessity, nature, and function of asthma medications also persist (Conn, Halterman, Lynch, & Cabana, 2007; Kieckhefer & Spitzer, 1995). Adherence to the medications that are regularly prescribed for children with persistent asthma remains poor, with estimates of adherence rates hovering around 50% (Bender et al., 2000; McQuaid et al., 2003). In order to accomplish reductions in asthma morbidity and improvements in management, research and clinical advances are necessary, and health care policy considerations are relevant. The field of pediatric psychology is uniquely suited to contribute to each of these areas.

Research Directions

Although behavioral research in pediatric asthma has made great strides in recent decades, further empirical work is needed in many areas. Investigations of risk for asthma onset utilizing a biopsychosocial framework can lead to integrated approaches to asthma prevention. Research addressing the complex interactions among stress and emotions, immune function, and asthma exacerbations may lead to new nonpharmacological approaches to asthma control. Further research is needed to explain the gap between physicians' recommendations for asthma management and families' actual implementation of asthma management practices. Research frameworks that identify individual and systems factors supporting adaptive asthma management are necessary and will serve to inform the development of future interventions. Rigorous evaluation of psychosocial interventions through randomized controlled trials will help refine existing programs and promote best-practice guidelines.

Clinical Directions

Psychologists and other mental health professionals can play many roles in working directly with families of children with asthma. Increased collaboration with pediatricians and specialists can facilitate effective asthma care. Specifically, psychologists can help physicians identify family barriers to adherence and can help construct asthma management plans that take family barriers and strengths into account. Individual and family psychological intervention can be critical in preventing mental health problems from complicating treatment adherence or exacerbating physical symptoms, in cases of comorbid psychiatric and medical concerns. Moreover, psychologists can participate in the programming and implementation of educational interventions, emphasizing developmental and family approaches. The interventions provided by psychologists and other mental health professionals can help to "bridge the gap" between health care providers and patients—to assist families in understanding asthma, to help them solve problems related to adherence, and to support them in following their management plan.

Policy Implications

Because of the high prevalence and risks of asthma, along with its disproportionate impact on ethnic minorities, low-income families, and inner-city communities, asthma treatment represents an important public health priority. Through mobilizing communities and health care systems to recognize the complexities of asthma management, psychologists can serve as influential advocates for patients and families. Examples include the many asthma coalitions that have been formed on local levels with mental health representation to promote access to optimal and interdisciplinary asthma care for patients and families.

Pediatric asthma remains a significant health care problem on local, national, and international levels. Research that integrates medical and behavioral aspects of the disease is necessary to increase professional understanding of the illness. Multidisciplinary approaches to clinical care are particularly useful for children with severe asthma and in cases where psychosocial barriers impede asthma care. As clinical issues can serve to inform research agendas, empirical findings should help health care professionals continue to develop effective psychosocial interventions to assist the population of children with asthma. Psychologists are encouraged to evaluate the effectiveness of collaborative care approaches to asthma, in order to document improvements in clinical outcome and cost offset associated with interdisciplinary asthma management. These data are instrumental in securing payment for pediatric psychology services and in promoting the value-added benefit of collaborative care models.

References

Akinbami, L. J., & Schoendorf, K. C. (2002). Trends in childhood asthma: Prevalence, health care utilization, and mortality. *Pediatrics, 110,* 315–322.

Alexander, F. G. (1950). *Psychosomatic medicine: Its principles and applications.* New York: Norton.

Alvarez, G. G., Schulzer, M., Jung, D., & Fitzgerald, J. M. (2005). A systematic review of risk factors associated with near-fatal and fatal asthma. *Canadian Respiratory Journal, 12,* 265–270.

American Academy of Allergy, Asthma and Immunology (AAAAI). (2000). *Allergic disorders: Promoting best practices.* Milwaukee, WI: Author.

American Lung Association. (2007). *Asthma and children fact sheet* [Brochure]. New York: Author.

Austin, J. K., Smith, M. S., Risinger, M. W., & McNelis, A. M. (1994). Childhood epilepsy and asthma: Comparison of quality of life. *Epilepsia, 35,* 608–615.

Barlow, J. H., & Ellard, D. R. (2006). The psychosocial well-being of children with chronic disease, their parents and siblings: An overview of the research evidence base. *Child: Care, Health and Development, 32,* 19–31.

Bartholomew, L. K., Gold, R. S., Parcel, G. S., Czyzewski, D. I., Sockrider, M. M., Fernandez, M., et al. (2000). Watch, Discover, Think, and Act: Evaluation of computer-assisted instruction to improve asthma self-management in inner-city children. *Patient Education and Counseling, 39,* 269–280.

Bender, B. (2006). Risk taking, depression, adherence, and symptom control in adolescents and young adults with asthma. *American Journal of Respiratory and Critical Care Medicine, 173,* 953–957.

Bender, B., Milgrom, H., Rand, C., & Ackerson, L. (1998). Psychological factors associated with medication nonadherence in asthmatic children. *Journal of Asthma, 35,* 347–353.

Bender, B., Wamboldt, F. S., O'Connor, S. L., Rand, C., Szefler, S., Milgrom, H., et al. (2000). Measurement of children's asthma medication adherence by self report, mother report, canister weight, and Doser CT. *Annals of Allergy, Asthma and Immunology, 85,* 416–421.

Bibi, H. S., Feigenbaum, D., Hessen, M., & Shoseyov, D. (2006). Do current treatment protocols adequately prevent airway remodeling in children with mild intermittent asthma? *Respiratory Medicine, 100,* 458–462.

Bloom, B. C., & Cohen, R. A. (2007). *Summary health statistics for U.S. children: National Health Interview Survey, 2006.* Hyattsville, MD: National Center for Health Statistics.

Bonner, S., Zimmerman, B. J., Evans, D., Irigoyen, M., Resnick, D., & Mellins, R. B. (2002). An individualized intervention to improve asthma management among urban Latino and African-American families. *Journal of Asthma, 39,* 167–179.

Borrelli, B., Riekert, K. A., Weinstein, A., & Rathier, L. (2007). Brief motivational interviewing as a clinical strategy to promote asthma medication adherence. *Journal of Allergy and Clinical Immunology, 120,* 1023–1030.

Bratton, D. L., Price, M., Gavin, L., Glenn, K., Brenner, M., Gelfand, E. W., et al. (2001). Impact of a multidisciplinary day program on disease and healthcare costs in children and adolescents with severe asthma: A two-year follow-up study. *Pediatric Pulmonology, 31,* 177–189.

Brown, J. V., Avery, E., Mobley, C., Boccuti, L., & Golbach, T. (1996). Asthma management by preschool children and their families: A developmental framework. *Journal of Asthma, 33,* 299–311.

Brown, R., Bratton, S. L., Cabana, M. D., Kaciroti, N., & Clark, N. M. (2004). Physician asthma education program improves outcomes for children of low-income families. *Chest, 126,* 369–374.

Busse, W. W., & Lemanske, R. F. J. (2001). Advances in immunology: Asthma. *New England Journal of Medicine, 344,* 350–362.

Calhoun, W. J., Sutton, L. B., Emmett, A., & Dorinsky, P. M. (2003). Asthma variability in patients previously treated with beta$_2$-agonists alone. *Journal of Allergy and Clinical Immunology, 112,* 1088–1094.

Callery, P., Milnes, L., Verduyn, C., & Couriel, J. (2003). Qualitative study of young people's and parents' beliefs about childhood asthma. *British Journal of General Practice, 53,* 185–190.

Canino, G., Koinis-Mitchell, D., Ortega, A. N., McQuaid, E. L., Fritz, G. K., & Alegria, M. (2006). Asthma disparities in the prevalence, morbidity, and treatment of Latino children. *Social Science and Medicine, 63,* 2926–2937.

Canino, G., Vila, D., Normand, S. L., Acosta-Perez, E., Ramirez, R., Garcia, P., et al. (2008). Reducing asthma health disparities in poor Puerto Rican children: The effectiveness of a culturally tailored family intervention. *Journal of Allergy and Clinical Immunology, 121,* 665–670.

Centers for Disease Control and Prevention (CDC). (1996). Asthma morbidity and hospitalization among children and young adults—U.S. 1980–1993. *Morbidity and Mortality Weekly Report, 45,* 350–353.

Centers for Disease Control and Prevention (CDC). (2006). Percentage of children aged <18 years with current asthma, by race/ethnicity and sex—United States, 2001–2004. *Morbidity and Mortality Weekly Report, 55,* 185.

Clark, N. M., Brown, R., Joseph, C. L., Anderson, E. W., Liu, M., & Valerio, M. A. (2004). Effects of a comprehensive school-based asthma program on symptoms, parent management, grades, and absenteeism. *Chest, 125,* 1674–1679.

Clark, N. M., Gong, M., Schork, M. A., Evans, D., Roloff, D., Hurwitz, M., et al. (1998). Impact of education on patient outcomes. *Pediatrics, 101,* 831–836.

Conn, K. M., Halterman, J. S., Lynch, K., & Cabana, M. D. (2007). The impact of parents' medication beliefs on asthma management. *Pediatrics, 120,* e521–e526.

Crain, E. F., Kercsmar, C., Weiss, K. B., Mitchell, H., & Lynn, H. (1998). Reported difficulties in access to quality care for children with asthma in the inner city. *Archives of Pediatrics and Adolescent Medicine, 152,* 333–339.

Creer, T. L. (1993). Medication compliance and childhood asthma. In N. A. Krasnegor, L. Epstein, S. B. Johnson, & S. J. Yaffe (Eds.), *Developmental aspects of health compliance behavior* (pp. 303–333). Hillsdale, NJ: Erlbaum.

Creer, T. L. (2000). Self-management and the control of chronic pediatric illness. In D. Drotar (Ed.), *Promoting adherence to medical treatment in chronic illness: Concepts, methods, and interventions* (pp. 95–130). Mahwah, NJ: Erlbaum.

DePue, J. D., McQuaid, E. L., Koinis-Mitchell, D., Camillo, C., Alario, A., & Klein, R. B. (2007). Providence school asthma partnership: School-based asthma program for inner-city families. *Journal of Asthma, 44,* 449–453.

Environmental Protection Agency. (1992). *Respiratory health effects of passive smoking: Lung cancer and other disorders* (Publication No. EPA/600/6-90-006F). Washington, DC: Author.

Evans, R., III, Gergen, P. J., Mitchell, H., Kattan, M., Kercsmar, C., Crain, E., et al. (1999). A randomized clinical trial to reduce asthma morbidity among inner-city children: Results of the National Cooperative Inner-City Asthma Study. *Journal of Pediatrics, 135,* 332–338.

Federico, M. J., & Liu, A. H. (2003). Overcoming childhood asthma disparities of the inner-city poor. *Pediatric Clinics of North American, 50,* 655–675.

Fiese, B. H., & Everhart, R. S. (2006). Medical adherence and childhood chronic illness: Family daily management skills and emotional climate as emerging contributors. *Current Opinion in Pediatrics, 18,* 551–557.

Fritz, G. K., & McQuaid, E. L. (2000). Chronic medical conditions: Impact on development. In A. J. Sameroff, M. Lewis, & S. M. Miller (Eds.), *Handbook of developmental psychopathology* (2nd ed., pp. 277–289). New York: Kluwer Academic/Plenum.

Gibson, P. G., Powell, H., Coughlan, J., Wilson, A. J., Hensley, M. J., Abramson, M., et al. (2002). Limited (information only) patient education programs for adults with asthma. *Cochrane Database of Systematic Reviews,* Issue 2 (Article No. CD001005), DOI: 10.1002/14651858.CD001005.

Global Initiative for Asthma. (2008). *Global strategy for asthma management and prevention.* Retrieved January 29, 2009, from *www.ginasthma.org*

Graham, P. J., Rutter, M. L., Yule, W., & Pless, I. B. (1967). Childhood asthma: A psychosomatic disorder?: Some epidemiological considerations. *British Journal of Preventive and Social Medicine, 21,* 78–85.

Gustadt, L. B., Gillette, J. W., & Mrazek, D. A. (1989). Determinants of school performance in children with chronic asthma. *American Journal of Diseases of Children, 143,* 471–475.

Gustafsson, P., Taylor, A., Zanen, P., & Chrystyn, H. (2005). Can patients use all dry powder inhalers equally well? *International Journal of Clinical Practice, 149,* 13–18.

Hunninghake, G. M., Weiss, S. T., & Celedon, J. C. (2006). Asthma in Hispanics. *American Journal of Respiratory and Critical Care Medicine, 173,* 143–163.

Inkelas, M., Garro, N., McQuaid, E. L., & Ortega, A. N. (2008). Race/ethnicity, language, and asthma care: Findings from a 4-state survey. *Annals of Allergy, Asthma and Immunology, 100,* 120–127.

Isenberg, S. A., Lehrer, P. M., & Hochron, S. (1992). The effects of suggestion and emotional arousal on pulmonary function in asthma: A review and a hypothesis regarding vagal mediation. *Psychosomatic Medicine, 54,* 192–216.

Joseph, C. L., Ownby, D. R., Peterson, E. L., & Johnson, C. C. (2000). Racial differences in physiologic parameters related to asthma among middle-class children. *Chest, 117,* 1336–1344.

Joseph, C. L., Peterson, E., Havstad, S., Johnson, C. C., Hoerauf, S., Stringer, S., et al. (2007). A Web-based, tailored asthma management program for urban African-American high school students. *American Journal of Respiratory and Critical Care Medicine, 175,* 888–895.

Kaugars, A. S., Klinnert, M. D., & Bender, B. G. (2004). Family influences on pediatric asthma. *Journal of Pediatric Psychology, 29,* 475–491.

Kaugars, A. S., Klinnert, M. D., Robinson, J., & Ho, M. (2008). Reciprocal influences in children's and families' adaptation to early childhood wheezing. *Health Psychology, 27,* 258–267.

Kieckhefer, G. M., & Spitzer, A. (1995). School-age children's understanding of the relations between their behavior and their asthma management. *Clinical Nursing Research, 4,* 149–167.

Klinnert, M., & Mrazek, D. A. (1994). Early asthma onset: The interaction between family stressors and adaptive parenting. *Psychiatry, 57,* 51–61.

Klinnert, M. D., McQuaid, E. L., McCormick, D., Adinoff, A. D., & Bryant, N. E. (2000). A multimethod assessment of behavioral and emotional adjustment in children with asthma. *Journal of Pediatric Psychology, 25*, 35–46.

Klinnert, M. D., Nelson, H. S., Price, M. R., Adinoff, A. D., Leung, D. Y., & Mrazek, D. A. (2001). Onset and persistence of childhood asthma: Predictors from infancy. *Pediatrics, 108*, E69.

Kozyrskyj, A. L., Mai, X. M., McGrath, P., Hayglass, K. T., Becker, A. B., & Macneil, B. (2008). Continued exposure to maternal distress in early life is associated with an increased risk of childhood asthma. *American Journal of Respiratory and Critical Care Medicine, 177*, 142–147.

Lemanek, K. L., Kamps, J., & Chung, N. B. (2001). Empirically supported treatments in pediatric psychology: regimen adherence. *Journal of Pediatric Psychology, 26*, 279–282.

Lieu, T. A., Finkelstein, J. A., Lozano, P., Capra, A. M., Chi, F. W., Jensvold, N., et al. (2004). Cultural competence policies and other predictors of asthma care quality for Medicaid-insured children. *Pediatrics, 114*, e102–e110.

Lozano, P., Connell, F. A., & Koepsell, T. D. (1995). Use of health services by African-American children with asthma on Medicaid. *Journal of the American Medical Association, 274*, 469–473.

MacLean, W. E. J., Perrin, J. M., Gortmaker, S., & Pierre, C. B. (1992). Psychological adjustment of children with asthma: Effects of illness severity and recent stressful life events. *Journal of Pediatric Psychology, 17*, 159–171.

Mattes, J., & Karmaus, W. (1999). The use of antibiotics in the first year of life and the development of asthma: Which comes first? *Clinical and Experimental Allergy, 29*, 729–732.

McQuaid, E. L., Fritz, G. K., Nassau, J. H., Mansell, A., Lilly, M. K., & Klein, R. (2000). Stress and airway resistance in children with asthma. *Journal of Psychosomatic Research, 49*, 239–245.

McQuaid, E. L., Kopel, S. J., Klein, R. B., & Fritz, G. K. (2003). Medication adherence in pediatric asthma: Reasoning, responsibility, and behavior. *Journal of Pediatric Psychology, 28*, 323–333.

McQuaid, E. L., Kopel, S. J., & Nassau, J. H. (2001). Behavioral adjustment in children with asthma: A meta-analysis. *Journal of Developmental and Behavioral Pediatrics, 22*, 430–439.

McQuaid, E. L., & Nassau, J. H. (1999). Empirically supported treatments of disease-related symptoms in pediatric psychology: Asthma, diabetes, and cancer. *Journal of Pediatric Psychology, 24*, 306–328.

McQuaid, E. L., Penza-Clyve, S., Nassau, J. H., Fritz, G. K., Klein, R., O'Connor, S., et al. (2001). Sharing family responsibility for asthma management tasks. *Children's Health Care, 30*, 183–199.

Miklich, D. R., Rewey, H. H., Weiss, J. H., & Kolton, S. (1973). A preliminary investigation of psychophysiological responses to stress among different subgroups of asthmatic children. *Journal of Psychosomatic Research, 17*, 1–8.

Miller, B. D., & Wood, B. L. (1994). Psychophysiologic reactivity in asthmatic children: A cholinergically mediated confluence of pathways. *Journal of the American Academy of Child and Adolescent Psychiatry, 33*, 1236–1245.

Miller, G., & Chen, E. (2007). Unfavorable socioeconomic conditions in early life presage expression of proinflammatory phenotype in adolescence. *Psychosomatic Medicine, 69*, 402–409.

Modi, A. C., & Quittner, A. L. (2006). Barriers to treatment adherence for children with cystic fibrosis and asthma: What gets in the way? *Journal of Pediatric Psychology, 31*, 846–858.

Moorman, J. E., Rudd, R. A., Johnson, C. A., King, M., Minor, P., Bailey, C., et al. (2007). National surveillance for asthma—United States, 1980–2004. *Morbidity and Mortality Weekly Report Surveillance Summaries, 56*, 1–54.

Mrazek, D. A., & Klinnert, M. (1991). *Asthma: Psychoneuroimmunologic Considerations* (2nd ed.). San Diego, CA: Academic Press.

Nathan, R. A., Sorkness, C. A., Kosinski, M., Schatz, M., Li, J. T., Marcus, P., et al. (2004). Development of the Asthma Control Test: A survey for assessing asthma control. *Journal of Allergy and Clinical Immunology, 113*, 59–65.

National Institutes of Health (NIH). (2007). *Expert panel report 3: Guidelines for the diagnosis and management of asthma—full report 2007*. Bethesda, MD: Author.

Nelson, D. A., Johnson, C. C., Divine, G. W., Strauchman, C., Joseph, C. L., & Ownby, D. R. (1997). Ethnic differences in the prevalence of asthma in middle class children. *Annals of Allergy, Asthma and Immunology, 78*, 21–26.

Platts-Mills, T. A., Blumenthal, K., Perzanowski, M., & Woodfolk, T. A. (2000). Determinants of clinical allergic disease: The relevance of indoor allergens to the increase in asthma. *American Journal of Respiratory and Critical Care Medicine, 162*, S128–S133.

Riekert, K. A., Butz, A. M., Eggleston, P. A., Huss, K., Winkelstein, M., & Rand, C. S. (2003). Caregiver-physician medication concordance and undertreatment of asthma among inner-city children. *Pediatrics, 111*, e214–e220.

Ritz, T., Dahme, B., Dubois, A. B., Folgering, H., Fritz, G. K., Harver, A., et al. (2002). Guidelines for mechanical lung function measurements in psychophysiology. *Psychophysiology, 39*, 546–567.

Runge, C., Lecheler, J., Horn, M., Tews, J. T., & Schaefer, M. (2006). Outcomes of a Web-based patient education program for asthmatic children and adolescents. *Chest, 129*, 581–593.

Smith, A. D., Cowan, J. O., Brassett, K. P., Herbison, G. P., & Taylor, D. R. (2005). Use of exhaled nitric oxide measurements to guide treatment in chronic asthma. *New England Journal of Medicine, 352*, 2163–2173.

Strunk, R. C. (1987). Asthma deaths in childhood: Identification of patients at risk and intervention. *Journal of Allergy and Clinical Immunology, 80*, 472–477.

Wade, S. L., Holden, G., Lynn, H., Mitchell, H., & Ewart, C. (2000). Cognitive-behavioral predictors of asthma morbidity in inner-city children. *Journal of Developmental and Behavioral Pediatrics, 21*, 340–346.

Walders, N., Drotar, D., & Kercsmar, C. (2000). The allocation of family responsibility for asthma management tasks in African-American adolescents. *Journal of Asthma, 37*, 89–99.

Walders, N., Kercsmar, C., Schluchter, M., Redline, S., Kirchner, H. L., & Drotar, D. (2006). An interdisciplinary intervention for undertreated pediatric asthma. *Chest, 129*, 292–299.

Walders, N., Nobile, C., & Drotar, D. (2000). Promoting adherence to medical treatment in childhood chronic illness: Challenges in a managed care environment. In D. Drotar (Ed.), *Promoting adherence to medical treatment in chronic childhood illness: Concepts, methods, and interventions* (pp. 201–236). Mahwah, NJ: Erlbaum.

Wamboldt, M. Z., Fritz, G. K., Mansell, A., McQuaid, E. L., & Klein, R. B. (1998). Relationship of asthma severity and psychological problems in children. *Journal of the American Academy of Child and Adolescent Psychiatry, 37*, 943–950.

Wamboldt, M. Z., & Wamboldt, F. S. (2000). Role of the family in the onset and outcome of childhood disorders: Selected research findings. *Journal of the American Academy of Child and Adolescent Psychiatry, 39*, 1212–1219.

Warman, K., Silver, E. J., & Wood, P. R. (2006). Asthma risk factor assessment: What are the needs of inner-city families? *Annals of Allergy, Asthma, and Immunology, 97*, S11–S15.

Weil, C. M., Wade, S. L., Bauman, L. J., Lynn, H., Mitchell, H., & Lavigne, J. (1999). The relationship between psychosocial factors and asthma morbidity in inner-city children with asthma. *Pediatrics, 104*, 1274–1280.

Weinstein, A. G., Faust, D. S., McKee, L., & Padman, R. (1992). Outcome of short-term hospitalization for children with severe asthma. *Journal of Allergy and Clinical Immunology, 90*, 66–75.

Weiss, K. B. (2007). Eliminating asthma disparities: A national workshop to set a working agenda. *Chest*, *132*, 753S–756S.

Wood, B. L., Klebba, K. B., & Miller, B. D. (2000). Evolving the biobehavioral family model: The fit of attachment. *Family Process*, *39*, 319–344.

Wood, B. L., Lim, J., Miller, B. D., Cheah, P., Zwetsch, T., Ramesh, S., et al. (2008). Testing the biobehavioral family model in pediatric asthma: Pathways of effect. *Family Process*, *47*, 21–40.

Wright, R., Rodriguez, M., & Cohen, S. (1998). Review of psychosocial stress and asthma: An integrated biopsychosocial approach. *Thorax*, *53*, 1066–1074.

Wright, R. J. (2005). Stress and atopic disorders. *Journal of Allergy and Clinical Immunology*, *116*, 1301–1306.

Zemek, R. L., Bhogal, S. K., & Ducharme, F. M. (2008). Systematic review of randomized controlled trials examining written action plans in children: What is the plan? *Archives of Pediatrics and Adolescent Medicine*, *162*, 157–163.

Zimmerman, B. J., Bonner, S., Evans, D., & Mellins, R. B. (1999). Self-regulating childhood asthma: A developmental model of family change. *Health Education and Behavior*, *26*, 55–71.

CHAPTER 18

Cystic Fibrosis
A Model for Drug Discovery and Patient Care

ALEXANDRA L. QUITTNER
DAVID H. BARKER
KRISTEN K. MARCIEL
MARY E. GRIMLEY

Cystic fibrosis (CF) is the most common fatal genetic disease of European American populations, primarily affecting the lungs, pancreas, and reproductive organs. It is also one of the most complex and difficult-to-treat chronic illnesses of childhood. Median life expectancy has dramatically increased over the past 50 years—from school age in 1955, to about 25 years in 1985, to 37 years in 2006 (Cystic Fibrosis Foundation [CFF], 2008). This increase is due primarily to earlier identification of the disease in infants and toddlers, development of new inhaled medications, and aggressive treatment of lung infections and nutritional deficiencies. Although improvements in lifespan have dramatically altered the outlook for CF, management of the disease requires a substantial investment of time and economic resources by patients and families. The treatment regimen is both complex and time-consuming, requiring patients to spend 2–4 hours per day on a variety of inhaled medications and airway clearance.

CF care provides a unique and innovative model of care. The CFF (*www.cff. org*), established in 1955 (Littlewood, 2007), has been instrumental in simultaneously improving clinical research and patient care. The goals of the CFF include facilitation of basic and clinical research, publication of health outcome data by center to increase accountability, and encouragement of evidence-based medicine by practitioners (Walters & Mehta, 2007). The CFF reviews and accredits 115 CF care centers, requires each center to have a multidisciplinary team, and supports the Therapeutics Development Network to assist in the design and implementation of clinical trials. This model of combining drug discovery with patient care has facilitated basic, clinical, and translational research. Such a model could arguably be applied in other chronic conditions, such as asthma, diabetes, and epilepsy.

The purpose of this chapter is to review the major medical, social, and psychological issues faced by individuals with CF, from infancy through adolescence. First, the basic genetic defect and its sequelae are described; this is followed by a discussion of new, cross-cutting issues in CF, such as the prevalence of CF in minority populations, impact of newborn screening, challenges of adhering to an increasingly complex regimen, and the psychosocial implications of infection control. Finally, relevant medical, behavioral, and psychosocial issues are discussed within a developmental context.

Genetics, Pathophysiology, and Treatments

Clinical symptoms result from incorrect genetic coding of the CF transmembrane conductance regulator (CFTR), which leads to the absence or defective presentation of the CFTR protein (Sharma et al., 2004). This produces a decrease in fluid volume outside the cells and an accumulation of thick, sticky mucus in the lungs and other mucus-secreting organs (e.g., pancreas). A buildup of secretions in the lungs impairs airway clearance and produces an environment that is prone to repeated infections, ultimately leading to respiratory failure and death. The disease process also impedes delivery of pancreatic enzymes to the digestive system. Over time, this dysfunction damages pancreatic tissue and endocrine function, often resulting in CF-related diabetes (Marshall et al., 2005). Finally, 99% of males are sterile due to the blocking of the vas deferens *in utero*, and women face significant challenges to getting pregnant (McMullen et al., 2006).

Because the lungs are unable to clear the thick mucus secretions, which contain a variety of bacteria and other airborne particulates, airway clearance techniques are a standard part of CF care. This process involves inhaling medications that open the airways (e.g., bronchodilators), as well as dornase alpha (which breaks up the by-products of defective proteins) and hypertonic saline (which, along with dornase alpha, thins mucus secretions). These inhaled medications must be coupled with manual airway clearance techniques, which include chest physiotherapy, use of a vest that oscillates the chest wall, or use of positive expiratory pressure physiotherapy or a flutter device. These techniques loosen mucus in the lungs and encourage its removal through productive coughing. This entire process, typically performed twice a day, takes between 40 and 70 minutes.

Despite the rigor of the treatment regimen described above, the lungs eventually become colonized with bacteria, such as *Pseudomonas aeruginosa*, which then become resistant to antibiotics. Prevention or treatment of lung infections (exacerbations) requires an additional 20-minute inhalation of antibiotics, twice per day. If a pulmonary exacerbation persists despite these treatments, patients are prescribed intravenous (IV) antibiotics for 10–14 days. Fighting bacterial infection is a lifelong battle in CF.

CF also affects the digestive system, with a majority of patients born with pancreatic insufficiency. Those who have some pancreatic function typically become pancreatic-insufficient by early adulthood. To address this problem, patients with CF must take orally administered enzymes with every snack and meal. Because malabsorption and elevated resting energy expenditures are problematic in CF, patients must consume 110–200% of the recommended daily allowance of calories (Stallings et al., 2008).

Cross-Cutting Issues

Prevalence in Minority Populations

Although CF was once characterized as a "white" disease, it is more prevalent in minority populations than was once thought. Prevalence rates vary across race and ethnicity. For non-Hispanic white infants, estimates are approximately 1 in 3,500; for Hispanic infants, estimates vary from 1 in 4,000 to 1 in 10,000; for black infants, prevalence varies from 1 in 15,000 to 1 in 20,000. Each year, 1,000 new diagnoses of CF are made in the United States (Centers for Disease Control and Prevention [CDC], 2004). Recently, new diagnoses have been made in adults who present with different genotypes that confer "milder" disease and are associated with longer life expectancy; these patients may have been asymptomatic or misdiagnosed as children. Variations in prevalence rates, particularly for Hispanic infants, are due in part to the ongoing discovery of new CFTR mutations. Diagnostic panels typically include 25–30 of the 1,000 known mutations, potentially underrepresenting those of minority populations. There is also evidence that health outcomes and quality of life are worse in minority populations, but little is known about why these disparities exist (Quittner, Schechter, Rasouliyan, Pasta, & Wagener, 2006).

Infection Control

Due to increased awareness of the precipitous drop in lung function after infection with multiresistant bacteria, new infection control policies were introduced by the CFF in 2001. These guidelines discourage face-to-face interactions among individuals with CF (Saiman & Siegel, 2004). In addition, patients must reside in single rooms while in the hospital and wear face masks; children with CF who attend the same school are segregated; and all CF-specific camps and overnight CF education retreats have been discontinued. Although infection control policies are important for maintaining health, they have increased the sense of stigma and social isolation experienced by patients. However, no studies to date have examined the consequences of these new infection control policies for psychosocial functioning.

Patient-Reported Outcomes

There is growing recognition of the importance of patient-reported outcomes (PROs), such as health-related quality of life (HRQOL), in evaluating the benefits of new medications and treatments (Goss & Quittner, 2007; Quittner, Modi, & Cruz, 2008). The Food and Drug Administration (FDA) has recently issued a guidance that specifies the conceptual and psychometric requirements of PROs that will be utilized in clinical trials, as either primary or secondary outcomes (FDA, 2006). This is an important advance for individuals with chronic conditions, such as CF, because it validates the importance of measuring their perceptions of the benefits of new treatments and may lead to better adherence to chronic therapies. Quittner and colleagues have developed a disease-specific HRQOL measure for CF, the Cystic Fibrosis Questionnaire—Revised (CFQ-R), for children ages 6–13 and their parents, and for adolescents and adults ages 14 and older (Modi & Quittner, 2003; Quittner, Buu, Messer, Modi, & Watrous, 2005). They are currently working on the validation of a downward extension of this measure to preschoolers, ages 3–6 years, using engaging cartoon drawings. This measure may provide insight regarding HRQOL in young children with CF. The reliability and validity of the CFQ-R have been studied extensively, and it has been used in several international trials (Donaldson et al., 2006; Elkins et al., 2006). The CFQ-R was recently utilized as the primary outcome measure in a clinical trial of a new inhaled antibiotic for CF (Retsch-Bogart et al., 2008). This will be the first antibiotic ever approved by the FDA on the basis of a PRO.

Measurement of Adherence

Measuring adherence in CF is particularly challenging because of the complexity of the treatment regimen. Although a full review of adherence measures is beyond the scope of this chapter, relevant issues are discussed below. A more detailed analysis of measurement issues and empirically supported measures is available elsewhere (Quittner, Modi, Lemanek, Ievers-Landis, & Rapoff, 2008). In CF, different measurement approaches are required for different components of the treatment regimen (inhaled vs. oral medications). Electronic monitors are readily available for pills and metered-dose inhalers, but not for other aspects of the treatment regimen, such as airway clearance. Conversely, a daily phone diary instrument has been used successfully in CF to measure adherence to nebulized treatments and airway clearance (Modi et al., 2006; Quittner & Opipari, 1994), but is not ideal for measuring treatments taking less than 5 minutes, such as enzymes or vitamins. Many of these state-of-the-art measures may not be feasible for use in clinical settings (Quittner, Modi, Lemanek, et al., 2008). Electronic monitors are costly, and diary measures are time-intensive. Pharmacy refill histories may be useful if paired with other measures of adherence, but tracking these data is also costly to implement. In sum, there is an urgent need for translational research on the measurement of adherence that could be used in clinical practice. Use of multiple measures, followed by triangulation of these indices, is currently recommended. Smith and Shuchman (2005) also emphasize the importance of working closely with patients and family members to assess their adherence behaviors.

Infancy/Preschool

Medical Issues

Currently, 70% of patients with CF are diagnosed before the age of 1 year (Walters & Mehta, 2007). Diagnosis typically requires documentation of at least one clinical symptom, such as meconium ileus (an obstruction of the bowel), recurrent respiratory infections, or failure to thrive, plus a positive result on a diagnostic test (Walters & Mehta, 2007). Levels of immunoreactive trypsinogen (IRT), an enzyme produced by the pancreas, are commonly used to identify at-risk infants (Southern, 2007). Positive screens based on elevated IRT levels are followed up with genetic testing and/or tests of CFTR dysfunction (nasal potential difference and sweat testing; Walters & Mehta, 2007). Sweat testing, considered the "gold standard," stimulates the skin to sweat and then measures the amount of chloride in sweat found on the arm. This test can be performed as soon as an infant is able to sweat, often as young as 2 weeks of age.

Recent research suggests that early, aggressive care for young children with CF improves long-term outcomes (CDC, 2004). Newborn screening (NBS) is one way to detect CF early and begin treatment before a child presents with significant symptoms. Recently, a majority of states have begun to implement NBS for CF. Preliminary evidence suggests that NBS improves clinical outcomes, such as nutrition (Farrell et al., 1997). An Australian study also found significant improvements in lung function in a group of children diagnosed by NBS versus symptom report (CDC, 2004). These two studies highlight the importance of early interventions. However, additional research on the impact of NBS on families' understanding of and adaptation to CF is needed.

Clinical symptoms are often evident at birth. Respiratory problems are already present in 51% of newborns, and infection with *P. aeruginosa* may occur in early infancy (Walters & Mehta, 2007). Pancreatic abnormalities have also been observed within days of birth (Littlewood, 2007). Approximately 11% of patients with CF are below the 5th percentile for height and weight (Walters & Mehta, 2007), highlighting the importance of early nutritional intervention and enzyme replacement therapy.

Psychosocial Adjustment

Upon receiving a diagnosis of CF, family members enter a period of rapid change as they adjust emotionally and behaviorally to the demands of caring for a child with a chronic illness (Gotz & Gotz, 2000). When the family system begins to stabilize, relationships with the health care team must be established, parents must learn new caregiving tasks, and treatments need to be integrated into daily life. These new tasks and roles build the foundation for how the family will cope with the illness during childhood and adolescence (Rolland, 1988). Thus this period is important for both current and future management of the disease.

Parental Stress and Depression

Adjustment to CF begins with the diagnosis and is marked by significant elevations in caregiver and family stress. Although the diagnosis phase is widely acknowledged as extremely stressful for families, little is known about the processes that lead to increased family stress over the short and long term. In one of the few studies addressing family processes during this phase, Quittner, Opipari, Regoli, Jacobsen, and Eigen (1992) found that mothers often took primary responsibility for their children's treatment regimen. This was in turn associated with increased stress, particularly in relation to the caregiver role, and more symptoms of depression. High rates of depression have also been reported by both mothers and fathers soon after the diagnosis (Glasscoe, Lancaster, Smyth, & Hill, 2007).

Beyond the diagnostic phase, few studies have evaluated the psychological functioning of caregivers. Recently, however, the CFF has funded a large-scale epidemiological study (The International Depression/Anxiety Epidemiological Study of Cystic Fibrosis study; *www.tides-cf.org*), aimed at screening a large representative sample of parents whose children with CF range in age from infancy through age 18. This effort is being coordinated internationally, with screening for depression and anxiety occurring in 17 countries.

Psychosocial Effects of NBS

Studies examining the psychological consequences of NBS for parents have consistently reported clinically elevated levels of psychological distress (i.e., elevated symptoms of depression and anxiety) during the screening process. Results from the Wisconsin research group found that 68% of mothers and 32% of fathers reported elevated symptoms of depression after a positive screen (Tluczek, Koscik, Farrell, & Rock, 2005). At a 6-month follow-up, 17% of mothers and 18% of fathers continued to report depressive symptoms in the clinical range. Elevations in anxiety and parenting stress were also reported. In addition, families reported misunderstandings and confusion following a positive screen (Dillard, Shen, Tluczek, Modaff, & Farrell, 2007). Overall, there is a need for more information and emotional support for families (Tluczek et al., 2006). Even after preliminary genetic counseling, additional interventions may be warranted (McDaniel, Rolland, Feetham, & Miller, 2006).

Family Functioning

Having a child with CF can affect how families function with regard to communication, behavioral control, and division of role responsibilities. Several studies have examined family functioning during mealtimes (Janicke, Mitchell, & Stark, 2005; Mitchell, Powers, Byars, Dickstein, & Stark, 2004). Results of videotaped mealtime interactions have shown that preschoolers with CF evidence more frequent problematic eating behaviors than healthy controls, including whining, crying, delaying eating by talking, refusing to eat, and leaving the table. Parents also engaged in less effective behavioral management of their children during meals, using more physical prompts, commands to eat, coaxing, and spoon feeding (Stark & Powers, 2005). Using multiple-baseline and randomized designs, Stark and colleagues have shown that parent behavior training improves mealtime behavior and results in better nutrition and weight outcomes (Jelalian, Stark, Reynolds, & Seifer, 1998; Stark, Powers, Jelalian, Rape, & Miller, 1994).

Studies examining the effects of a CF diagnosis on family functioning have reported high levels of parental differential treatment. In an early study, parents spent more time with a child with CF than with an older, healthy sibling—a pattern not found in the healthy comparison group (Quittner & Opipari, 1994). Parental differential treatment in the families of children with CF was relatively stable over a follow-up period of 6 months and was found to decrease with age, with significantly less parental differential treatment reported by adolescents. Parental differential treatment may result in psychological and behavioral problems in healthy siblings (Berge & Patterson, 2004). More research is needed for a better understanding of family adjustment to CF.

Adherence

Soon after the diagnosis, parents begin the daunting task of managing the disease. New evidence suggests that parental adjustment may be related to adherence. Using a 3-month longitudinal design, Quittner, Barker, Geller, Butt, and Gondor (2007) found that maternal depression was negatively associated with children's adherence to pancreatic enzymes, which in turn was related to less weight gain in preschool and school-age children.

Children's behavior can also negatively influence treatment adherence. As children become toddlers and preschoolers, treatment refusal often begins. Modi and Quittner (2006) examined the treatment barriers for preschool and school-age children with CF; they found that *both* parents and children cited oppositional behaviors, time management, and ability to swallow pills as key barriers to adherence. Using behavioral principles to teach children to swallow pills at a young age is likely to improve adherence. Future studies should explore effective ways to teach this skill. Behavior management programs that include differential attention, contingency management, shaping, and problem solving appear to be effective for young children (Bernard & Cohen, 2004); however, there is a need for larger, randomized trials.

School Age

Medical Issues

As children get older, they may begin to experience CF-related pain, including abdominal cramping, headaches, and musculoskeletal pain. In one study, children who experienced more CF-related pain also reported worse HRQOL (Palermo, Harrison, & Koh, 2006). To date, no systematic interventions have focused on reducing CF-related pain.

CF also has a substantial impact on sleep. In a recent study, the majority of children with CF (73.9%) reported daytime sleepiness and demonstrated both worse sleep efficiency and less rapid-eye-movement sleep than controls (Naqvi, Sotelo, Murry, & Simakajornboon, 2008). Evidence suggests that inadequate sleep is associated with worse lung function and should be more systematically addressed (Amin, Bean, Burklow, & Jeffries, 2005).

Psychosocial Adjustment

Transition to school brings new challenges for children with CF and their parents. Parents often have to educate school personnel about the disease and make special arrangements at school to facilitate disease management (Quittner, Modi, & Roux, 2004). Berge and Patterson's (2004) review indicated that children with CF, compared to healthy peers, begin to report more internalizing behaviors, particularly depression and anxiety.

During this period, friendships often shift in response to the peers' levels of knowledge and provision of support. Teasing by peers may emerge, as some of the clinical manifestations of CF (e.g., being shorter and thinner, coughing frequently) are now visible. Berlin, Sass, Hobart, Davies, Jandrisevits, and Hains (2005) found that disclosure of the CF diagnosis to peers reduced negative peer evaluations. Disclosure may increase knowledge and acceptance of CF. After disclosure, behaviors that may have seemed abnormal (e.g., eating large portions) may be viewed by others as "normal" in the context of this disease. Appropriate disclosure is likely to influence children's adaptation to the illness and facilitate the establishment of social support from peers, but this has yet to be examined.

Knowledge of Disease Management

Providing developmentally appropriate education and training is needed to increase children's disease-specific knowledge and coping skills. Davis, Quittner, Stack, and Yang (2004) found that children ages 7–17 scored only 57% correct on a basic knowledge measure of CF. A more recent study found similar knowledge scores for children ages 6–12, with the greatest number of errors on questions related to nutrition (e.g., caloric information; Cruz et al., 2007).

Computer-based programs present a cost-effective method for remediating these gaps in knowledge. A Starbright Foundation CD-ROM, titled Fitting CF into Your Life Every Day, is an educational program that teaches children how to cope with such stressors as chronic pain and hospitalizations. Using a waiting-list control group design, Davis and colleagues (2004) found that children who played this CD-ROM demonstrated significant increases in knowledge and generated more competent coping skills. Betterland is an interactive CD-ROM designed to increase knowledge of CF, while providing entertainment for children as they are doing their treatments (Duff, Ball, Wolfe, Blyth, & Brownlee, 2006). These programs represent initial steps in using technology to improve disease-related knowledge and disease management.

Adherence

Disease management becomes more complex as children enter school. Parents are still primarily responsible for their children's treatments, but they must now coordinate care with school personnel. Working with the schools can help ensure that children take their enzymes before lunch and select high-calorie foods at school (Quittner et al., 2004). A recent study at three CF centers in Florida found that 25% of children with CF were not taking their enzymes, suggesting a significant need for improvement (Quittner et al., 2007).

Confusion about prescribed treatment regimens contributes to poor adherence. Ievers and colleagues (1999) found that 12–32% of parents of school-age children with CF did not understand their doctor's prescriptions. More recently, Modi and Quittner (2006) found that parents and physicians disagreed on 17% of the medications prescribed, suggesting that communication problems among providers, parents, and patients constitute one source of the problem. Providing parents with a written, prescribed treatment plan is one basic step CF centers could take to improve communication.

As mentioned earlier, school-age children want to "fit in" and be accepted by their peers. As a result, some children "skip" or refuse treatments to be more similar to their peers (Foster et al., 2001). Children's experiences with their peers are likely to shape their future peer relationships and affect the support they receive from their friends during adolescence. Currently, little is known about how early peer relationships affect treatment adherence in CF.

Children's behavior problems are another significant barrier to adherence in middle childhood (Modi & Quittner, 2006). However, because children's cognitive ability has matured, management strategies other than behavior therapy can be used. For example, Savage and Callery (2005) suggest that parents and children differ in their views of eating, with parents focusing on weight gain and children on energy and feeling healthy.

They recommend that parents acknowledge these differences and begin problem solving with their children.

Adolescence

Medical Issues

During adolescence, patients with CF often experience a decline in lung function, a higher risk of CF-related diabetes (CFRD), delayed puberty, bone disease, and more frequent exacerbations and hospitalizations. Due to damage caused by infection and inflammation, lung function declines approximately 1% each year (Rosenthal, 2007), and these declines may interfere with an adolescent's ability to participate in developmentally appropriate activities (e.g., sports). This decline also varies by gender, with a 3-year survival difference in favor of males (Kulich, Rosenfeld, Goss, & Wilmott, 2003). Gender differences have also been found in HRQOL measures, with females reporting worse HRQOL than males (Gee, Abbott, Conway, Etherington, & Webb, 2003; Quittner et al., 2006).

The prevalence of CFRD increases during adolescence (Elder, Wooldridge, Dolan, & D'Alessio, 2007). CFRD is an additional diagnosis that significantly complicates disease management and is associated with lower lung function (Koch et al., 2001). Treatment for CFRD includes a modified diet and insulin injections. The challenge is to balance the need for increased caloric intake with optimal blood glucose levels. A diet of 35–40% fat, 20% protein, and 40–45% carbohydrate is recommended (White, Morton, Peckham, & Conway, 2004). Because poorly managed CFRD results in a rapid decline in health, annual glucose tolerance tests starting at age 14 are recommended (CFF, 2008).

Nutritional deficiencies lead to delayed puberty and bone disease during adolescence. Adolescents with CF typically do not experience a prepubertal growth spurt and often manifest delayed bone maturation (Bridges, 2007). Delayed bone maturation and malabsorption of fat-soluble vitamins (Vitamins A, D, E, and K) contribute to the development of bone disease. The CFF patient registry data indicates an 8.5% point prevalence of bone disease in patients with CF (CFF, 2008). Better nutritional status may protect against bone disease and osteoporosis (Elkin & Haworth, 2007).

As lung function declines, adolescents experience more pulmonary exacerbations. Treatment of an exacerbation consists of IV antibiotics provided at the hospital or home. Significant improvements in HRQOL were found from pre- to posttreatment with IV antibiotics (Quittner, Stack, Modi, & Davis, 2002); however, IV antibiotics significantly increased the burden of doing treatments and interrupted normal daily activities, such as attending school.

For patients with declining lung function, lung transplantation may be an option. However, pursuit of transplantation is a complex and emotionally difficult decision. Surprisingly, a recent study of adolescents found that lung transplantation did not extend patient survival (Liou, Adler, Cox, & Cahill, 2007). In addition, infections, such as *Burkholderia cepacia* and *Staphylococcus aureus*, were associated with decreased survival. Despite the risks and complications of transplantation, the number of people with CF receiving transplants increased from 5 patients in 1985 to 192 in 2006 (CFF, 2008).

Psychosocial Adjustment

During adolescence, psychosocial adjustment shifts toward increased independence and social development. An adolescent's increased desire for autonomy may result in family conflict and stress. However, family structure and support may also be particularly important during this time of transition to more independence. Szyndler, Towns, van Asperen, and McKay (2005) examined family variables in relation to adolescent psychological functioning. They found that family cohesiveness, expressiveness, and organization were associated with better psychological functioning. In addition, family conflict was associated with worse HRQOL on the CFQ-R. Szyndler and colleagues also suggested that a lack of hope for the future was related to higher levels of psychopathology, but not disease severity. These findings suggest that family conflict negatively influences health outcomes, whereas adaptive family functioning may play a protective role in adolescents' psychosocial adjustment.

Peer support becomes increasingly important during adolescence. For adolescents with CF, the daily management of the disease and lengthy hospital stays decrease contact with healthy peers and limit access to peer support. Graetz, Shute, and Sawyer (2000) conducted one of the few empirical studies addressing social support in this population. Similar to adolescents in other illness groups, adolescents with CF perceived more tangible support from their families and more relational support from their friends. They also found that nonsupportive behaviors, such as nagging or teasing, predicted worse psychological adjustment. In the past, an important source of support was provided by other adolescents with CF. As noted earlier, however, recent infection control policies have prohibited this type of contact, and the effects of this increased isolation are not known. Future studies should focus on peer support and on new technologies (e.g., the Internet, cell phones) that may enable peers with CF to socialize but remain safe.

Because infection control policies make it difficult to conduct group interventions with adolescents, few interventions have been focused on peer relations. One exception is the work of Christian and D'Auria (2006), who conducted group sessions focusing on peer-related issues with adolescents with CF. Each group consisted of four adolescents with CF. Children who tested positive for drug-resistant infections or *B. cepacia* participated in the group via real-time video links in a separate room. Sessions included discussions of strategies to cope with peer relations, explaining CF to peers, dealing with teasing, and keeping up with peers in activities. Adolescents who participated in the support groups reported decreased levels of perceived impact of the illness and loneliness. Again, technology (live videofeeds, the Internet) may provide powerful tools to address peer relations while maintaining infection control guidelines.

Adolescence is also a time of increased awareness of self and body image. In people without CF, adolescence is typically when eating disorders being to emerge. There has been limited research to suggest that some teens with CF may misuse pancreatic enzyme medication to facilitate weight loss (Shearer & Bryon, 2004). Others may engage in maladaptive behaviors, such as overexercising and/or restraining food intake. It is not clear whether these behaviors result from previous eating difficulties (i.e., family conflict associated with eating, gastrointestinal pain, food refusal) or are signs of eating disorder etiology. It is important for researchers and clinicians to distinguish between disease-related and disorder-related eating behaviors, in order to intervene effectively.

Concerns about death and dying emerge at different times for individuals with CF. It may be discussed formally for the first time when adolescents make the transition to adult clinics or when lung transplantation is considered. This discussion often includes advance directives and end-of-life care. Patients may also be anxious about pain management and the possibility of death (Chapman, Landy, Lyon, Haworth, & Bilton, 2005). At this time, a decision about lung transplantation may need to be made. Open and honest communication among the patient, family, and health care team is critical at this time.

Adherence

Adherence during adolescence drops considerably (Zindani, Streetman, Streetman, & Nasr, 2006), and treatment issues become a dominant theme for both teens and parents (DiGirolamo, Quittner, Ackerman, & Stevens, 1997). To understand the difficulties with adherence, it is important to understand the fundamental changes occurring during this time. First, adolescents are spending more time with their friends and receive less supervision from their parents, which may result in more missed treatments (Modi, Marciel, Slater, Drotar, & Quittner, 2008); also, and similar to school-age children, they may stop doing their treatments or stop going to the clinic in order to "be normal" (Badlan, 2006). These changes in family and peer relationships can affect the support provided by friends and family. Social support has been established as an important predictor of treatment adherence in other chronic illness populations (DiMatteo, 2004; Gallant, 2003), but no studies to date have focused on these relationships in CF.

Adolescents also seek greater autonomy and independence from their parents, often leading to conflict about daily treatments (DeLambo, Ievers-Landis, Drotar, & Quittner, 2004). Balancing independence with appropriate supervision is challenging for parents. If they are too restrictive and controlling about the treatment regimen, conflicts are likely to increase among family members, and such struggles decrease appropriate disease management (Fiese & Everhart, 2006; Smith & Wood, 2007). Conversely, if parents shift responsibility too quickly, the adolescents may not have the organizational or treatment-related skills (e.g., cleaning nebulizer) to manage the illness on their own. A recent diary-based study found that the presence of a caregiver during treatment times improved adherence to inhaled medications (Modi et al., 2008).

Emerging Adulthood

As individuals with CF live longer, transfer from pediatric to adult CF centers has become an important issue. The CFF (2008) has encouraged the development of adult CF care centers. Despite the increased availability of care providers who treat adults, approximately 25% of adults with CF receive care from a pediatrician (Anderson, Flume, Hardy, & Gray, 2002). There are distinct and important differences between pediatric and adult centers. Pediatric centers focus on growth and optimal development, whereas adult care centers focus on disease progression and broader lifestyle questions such as fertility, birth control, drug and alcohol use, and transplantation (Brumfield & Lansbury, 2004). One study found that 26% of males first learned about their infertility at age 20 (Fair, Griffiths, & Osman, 2000). Transferring care to a provider who treats adults may assist adolescents and young adults in assuming greater responsibility for management of this disease into emerging adulthood (Schidlow, 2002).

Conclusion

Profound changes in the prognosis, treatment, and lifespan of children and adolescents with CF have occurred over the last 10 years. The unique integration of research and clinical care, utilization of a national registry database, and efforts to improve the quality of care of individuals with CF have been driving forces in this dramatic progress. Despite these advances, such key issues as the impact of NBS, adherence to an increasingly complex regimen, the psychosocial implications of infection control, and the prevalence of depression need to be addressed. Better integration of psychologists into CF clinics would represent an important step in this direction. The shifting landscape of CF and the promise of new medical, psychological, and behavioral treatments are likely to lead to new advances in the decade ahead.

References

Amin, R., Bean, J., Burklow, K., & Jeffries, J. (2005). The relationship between sleep disturbance and pulmonary function in stable pediatric cystic fibrosis patients. *Chest, 128*(3), 1357–1363.

Anderson, D. L., Flume, P. A., Hardy, K. K., & Gray, S. (2002). Transition programs in cystic fibrosis centers: Perceptions of patients. *Pediatric Pulmonology, 33*(5), 327–331.

Badlan, K. (2006). Young people living with cystic fibrosis: An insight into their subjective experience. *Health and Social Care in the Community, 14*(3), 264–270.

Berge, J. M., & Patterson, J. M. (2004). Cystic fibrosis and the family: A review and critique of the literature. *Families, Systems, and Health, 22*(1), 74–100.

Berlin, K. S., Sass, D. A., Hobart Davies, W., Jandrisevits, M. D., & Hains, A. A. (2005). Cystic fibrosis disclosure may minimize risk of negative peer evaluations. *Journal of Cystic Fibrosis, 4*(3), 169–174.

Bernard, R. S., & Cohen, L. L. (2004). Increasing adherence to cystic fibrosis treatment: A systematic review of behavioral techniques. *Pediatric Pulmonology, 37*(1), 8–16.

Bridges, N. (2007). Growth in puberty. In M. Hodson, D. Geddes, & A. Bush (Eds.), *Cystic fibrosis* (3rd ed., pp. 253–260). London: Hodder Arnold.

Brumfield, K., & Lansbury, G. (2004). Experiences of adolescents with cystic fibrosis during their transition from paediatric to adult health care: A qualitative study of young Australian adults. *Disability and Rehabilitation, 26*(4), 223–234.

Centers for Disease Control and Prevention (CDC). (2004). Newborn screening for cystic fibrosis: Evaluation of benefits and risks and recommendations for state newborn screening programs. *Morbidity and Mortality Weekly Report, 53*(RR-13), 1–34.

Chapman, E., Landy, A., Lyon, A., Haworth, C., & Bilton, D. (2005). End of life care for adult cystic fibrosis patients: Facilitating a good enough death. *Journal of Cystic Fibrosis, 4*(4), 249–257.

Christian, B. J., & D'Auria, J. P. (2006). Building life skills for children with cystic fibrosis: Effectiveness of an intervention. *Nursing Research, 55*(5), 300–307.

Cruz, I., Quittner, A. L., McDonald, L., Botteri, M., Barker, D. H., Geller, D., et al. (2007).

Effects of a clinic-based intervention on knowledge and treatment skills for parents and young children with CF [Abstract]. *Journal of Cystic Fibrosis, 6*(S1), 74.

Cystic Fibrosis Foundation (CFF). (2008). *Patient registry 2006 annual report*. Bethesda, MD: Author.

Davis, M. A., Quittner, A. L., Stack, C. M., & Yang, M. C. K. (2004). Controlled evaluation of the Starbright CD-ROM program for children and adolescents with cystic fibrosis. *Journal of Pediatric Psychology, 29*(4), 259–267.

DeLambo, K. E., Ievers-Landis, C. E., Drotar, D., & Quittner, A. L. (2004). Association of observed family relationship quality and problem-solving skills with treatment adherence in older children and adolescents with cystic fibrosis. *Journal of Pediatric Psychology, 29*(5), 343–353.

DiGirolamo, A. M., Quittner, A. L., Ackerman, V., & Stevens, J. (1997). Identification and assessment of ongoing stressors in adolescents with a chronic illness: An application of the behavior-analytic model. *Journal of Clinical Child Psychology, 26*(1), 53–66.

Dillard, J. P., Shen, L., Tluczek, A., Modaff, P., & Farrell, P. M. (2007). The effect of disruptions during counseling on recall of genetic risk information: The case of cystic fibrosis. *Journal of Genetic Counseling, 16*(2), 179–190.

DiMatteo, M. R. (2004). Social support and patient adherence to medical treatment: A meta-analysis. *Health Psychology, 23*(2), 207–218.

Donaldson, S. H., Bennett, W. D., Zeman, K. L., Knowles, M. R., Tarran, R., & Boucher, R. C. (2006). Mucus clearance and lung function in cystic fibrosis with hypertonic saline. *New England Journal of Medicine, 354*(3), 241–250.

Duff, A., Ball, R., Wolfe, S., Blyth, H., & Brownlee, K. (2006). Betterland: An interactive CD-ROM guide for children with cystic fibrosis. *Pediatric Nursing, 18*(7), 30–33.

Elder, D. A., Wooldridge, J. L., Dolan, L. M., & D'Alessio, D. A. (2007). Glucose tolerance, insulin secretion, and insulin sensitivity in children and adolescents with cystic fibrosis and no prior history of diabetes. *Journal of Pediatrics, 151*(6), 653–658.

Elkin, S. L., & Haworth, C. (2007). Cystic-fibrosis-related low bone mineral density. In M. Hodson, D. Geddes, & A. Bush (Eds.), *Cystic fibrosis* (3rd ed., pp. 261–268). London: Hodder Arnold.

Elkins, M. R., Robinson, M., Rose, B. R., Harbour, C., Moriarty, C. P., Marks, G. B., et al. (2006). A controlled trial of long-term inhaled hypertonic saline in patients with cystic fibrosis. *New England Journal of Medicine, 354*(3), 229–240.

Fair, A., Griffiths, K., & Osman, L. M. (2000). Attitudes to fertility issues among adults with cystic fibrosis in Scotland. *Thorax, 55*(8), 672–677.

Farrell, P. M., Kosorok, M. R., Laxova, A., Shen, G., Koscik, R. E., Bruns, W. T., et al. (1997). Nutritional benefits of neonatal screening for cystic fibrosis. *New England Journal of Medicine, 337*(14), 963–969.

Fiese, B. H., & Everhart, R. S. (2006). Medical adherence and childhood chronic illness: Family daily management skills and emotional climate as emerging contributors. *Current Opinion in Pediatrics, 18*(5), 551–557.

Food and Drug Administration (FDA). (2006, February). *Guidance for industry: Patient-reported outcome measures: Use in medical product development to support labeling claims*. Retrieved February 2006 from *www.fda.gov/Cder/Guidance/5460dft.pdf*

Foster, C., Eiser, C., Oades, P., Sheldon, C., Tripp, J., Goldman, P., et al. (2001). Treatment demands and differential treatment of patients with cystic fibrosis and their siblings: Patient, parent and sibling accounts. *Child: Care, Health, and Development, 27*(4), 349–364.

Gallant, M. P. (2003). The influence of social support on chronic illness self-management: A review and directions for research. *Health and Education Behavior, 30*(2), 170–195.

Gee, L., Abbott, J., Conway, S. P., Etherington, C., & Webb, A. K. (2003). Quality of life in cystic fibrosis: The impact of gender, general health perceptions and disease severity. *Journal of Cystic Fibrosis, 2*(4), 206–213.

Glasscoe, C., Lancaster, G. A., Smyth, R. L., & Hill, J. (2007). Parental depression following the early diagnosis of cystic fibrosis: A matched, prospective study. *Journal of Pediatrics, 150*(2), 185–191.

Goss, C. H., & Quittner, A. L. (2007). Patient-reported outcomes in cystic fibrosis. *Proceedings of the American Thoracic Society, 4*(4), 378–386.

Gotz, I., & Gotz, M. (2000). Cystic fibrosis: Psychological issues. *Pediatric Respiratory Reviews, 1*(2), 121–127.

Graetz, B. W., Shute, R. H., & Sawyer, M. G. (2000). An Australian study of adolescents with cystic fibrosis: Perceived supportive and nonsupportive behaviors from families and friends and psychological adjustment. *Journal of Adolescent Health, 26*(1), 64–69.

Ievers, C. E., Brown, R. T., Drotar, D., Caplan, D., Pishevar, B. S., & Lambert, R. G. (1999). Knowledge of physician prescriptions and adherence to treatment among children with cystic fibrosis and their mothers. *Journal of Developmental and Behavioral Pediatrics, 20*(5), 335–343.

Janicke, D. M., Mitchell, M. J., & Stark, L. J. (2005). Family functioning in school-age children with cystic fibrosis: An observational assessment of family interactions in the mealtime environment. *Journal of Pediatric Psychology, 30*(2), 179–186.

Jelalian, E., Stark, L. J., Reynolds, L., & Seifer, R. (1998). Nutrition intervention for weight gain in cystic fibrosis: A meta-analysis. *Journal of Pediatrics, 132*, 486–492.

Koch, C., Cuppens, H., Rainisio, M., Madessani, U., Harms, H. K., Hodson, M. E., et al. (2001). European Epidemiologic Registry of Cystic Fibrosis (ERCF): Comparison of major disease manifestations between patients with different classes of mutations. *Pediatric Pulmonology, 31*(1), 1–12.

Kulich, M., Rosenfeld, M., Goss, C. H., & Wilmott, R. (2003). Improved survival among young patients with cystic fibrosis. *Journal of Pediatrics, 142*(6), 631–636.

Liou, T. G., Adler, F. R., Cox, D. R., & Cahill, B. C. (2007). Lung transplantation and survival in children with cystic fibrosis. *New England Journal of Medicine, 357*(21), 2143–2152.

Littlewood, J. M. (2007). History of cystic fibrosis. In M. Hodson, D. Geddes, & A. Bush (Eds.), *Cystic fibrosis* (3rd ed., pp. 3–19). London: Hodder Arnold.

Marshall, B. C., Butler, S. M., Stoddard, M., Moran, A. M., Liou, T. G., & Morgan, W. J. (2005). Epidemiology of cystic fibrosis-related diabetes. *Journal of Pediatrics, 146*, 681–687.

McDaniel, S. H., Rolland, J. S., Feetham, S., & Miller, S. M. (2006). Psychosocial interventions for patients and families coping with genetic conditions. In S. M. Miller, S. H. McDaniel, J. S. Rolland, & S. L. Feetham (Eds.), *Individuals, families and the new era of genetics: Biopsychosocial perspectives* (pp. 173–196). New York: Norton.

McMullen, A. H., Pasta, D. J., Frederick, P. D., Konstan, M. W., Morgan, W. J., Schechter, M. S., et al. (2006). Impact of pregnancy on women with cystic fibrosis. *Chest, 129*(3), 706–711.

Mitchell, M. J., Powers, S. W., Byars, K. C., Dickstein, S., & Stark, L. J. (2004). Family functioning in young children with cystic fibrosis: Observations of interactions at mealtime. *Journal of Developmental and Behavioral Pediatrics, 25*(5), 335–346.

Modi, A. C., Lim, C. S., Yu, N., Geller, D., Wagner, M. H., & Quittner, A. L. (2006). A multimethod assessment of treatment adherence for children with cystic fibrosis. *Journal of Cystic Fibrosis, 5*(3), 177–185.

Modi, A. C., Marciel, K. K., Slater, S. K., Drotar, D., & Quittner, A. L. (2008). The influence of parental supervision on medical adherence in adolescents with cystic fibrosis: Developmental shifts from pre to late adolescence. *Children's Health Care, 37*(1), 78–92.

Modi, A. C., & Quittner, A. L. (2003). Validation of a disease-specific measure of health-related quality of life for children with cystic fibrosis. *Journal of Pediatric Psychology, 28*(8), 535–546.

Modi, A. C., & Quittner, A. L. (2006). Barriers to treatment adherence for children with cystic fibrosis and asthma: What gets in the way? *Journal of Pediatric Psychology, 31*(8), 846–858.

Naqvi, S. K., Sotelo, C., Murry, L., & Simakajornboon, N. (2008). Sleep architecture in children and adolescents with cystic fibrosis and the association with severity of lung disease. *Sleep and Breathing, 12*(1), 77–83.

Palermo, T. M., Harrison, D., & Koh, J. L. (2006). Effect of disease-related pain on the health-related quality of life of children and adolescents with cystic fibrosis. *Clinical Journal of Pain, 22*(6), 532–537.

Quittner, A. L., Barker, D. H., Geller, D., Butt, S., & Gondor, M. (2007). Effects of maternal depression on electronically monitored enzyme adherence and changes in weight for children with CF [Abstract]. *Journal of Cystic Fibrosis, 6*(Suppl. 1), S77.

Quittner, A. L., Buu, A., Messer, M. A., Modi, A. C., & Watrous, M. (2005). Development and validation of the Cystic Fibrosis Questionnaire in the United States: A health-related quality-of-life measure for cystic fibrosis. *Chest, 128*(4), 2347–2354.

Quittner, A. L., Modi, A. C., & Cruz, I. (2008). Systematic review of health-related quality of life measures for children with respiratory conditions. *Paediatric Respiratory Reviews, 9,* 220–232.

Quittner, A. L., Modi, A. C., Lemanek, K. L., Ievers-Landis, C. E., & Rapoff, M. A. (2007). Evidence-based assessment of adherence to medical treatments in pediatric psychology. *Journal of Pediatric Psychology, 33,* 916–936.

Quittner, A. L., Modi, A. C., & Roux, A. L. (2004). Psychosocial challenges and clinical interventions for children and adolescents with cystic fibrosis: A developmental approach. In R. T. Brown (Ed.), *Handbook of pediatric psychology in school settings* (pp. 333–361). Mahwah, NJ: Erlbaum.

Quittner, A. L., & Opipari, L. C. (1994). Differential treatment of siblings: Interview and diary analyses comparing two family contexts. *Child Development, 65*(3), 800–814.

Quittner, A. L., Opipari, L. C., Regoli, M. J., Jacobsen, J., & Eigen, H. (1992). The impact of caregiving and role strain on family life: Comparisons between mothers of children with cystic fibrosis and matched controls. *Rehabilitation Psychology, 37,* 289–304.

Quittner, A. L., Schechter, M., Rasouliyan, L., Pasta, D., & Wagener, J. (2006). Effects of socioeconomic status, race and ethnicity on quality of life in a national database [Abstract]. *Journal of Cystic Fibrosis, 5*(Suppl. 1), 102.

Quittner, A. L., Stack, C., Modi, A. C., & Davis, M. A. (2002). Evaluation of health-related quality of life before and after antibiotic treatment of a pulmonary exacerbation in children and adolescents with cystic fibrosis [Abstract]. *Pediatric Pulmonology, S24,* 350.

Retsch-Bogart, G. Z., Burns, J. L., Otto, K. L., Liou, T. G., McCoy, K., Oermann, C., et al. (2008). A phase 2 study of aztreonam lysine for inhalation to treat patients with cystic fibrosis and *Pseudomonas aeruginosa* infection. *Pediatric Pulmonology, 43*(1), 47–58.

Rolland, J. (1988). Chronic illness and the family life cycle. In B. Carter & M. McGoldrick (Eds.), *The changing family life cycle: A framework for family therapy* (pp. 433–456). Boston: Allyn & Bacon.

Rosenthal, M. (2007). Physiological monitoring of older children and adults. In M. Hodson, D. Geddes, & A. Bush (Eds.), *Cystic fibrosis* (3rd ed., pp. 345–352). London: Hodder Arnold.

Saiman, L., & Siegel, J. (2004). Infection control in cystic fibrosis. *Clinical Microbiology Reviews, 17*(1), 57–71.

Savage, E., & Callery, P. (2005). Weight and energy: Parents' and children's perspectives on managing cystic fibrosis diet. *Archives of Disease in Childhood, 90*(3), 249–252.

Schidlow, D. V. (2002). Transition in cystic fibrosis: Much ado about nothing? A pediatrician's view. *Pediatric Pulmonology, 33*, 325–326.

Sharma, M., Pampinella, F., Nemes, C., Benharouga, M., So, J., Du, K., et al. (2004). Misfolding diverts CFTR from recycling to degradation: Quality control at early endosomes. *Journal of Cell Biology, 164*, 923–933.

Shearer, J. E., & Bryon, M. (2004). The nature and prevalence of eating disorders and eating disturbance in adolescents with cystic fibrosis. *Journal of the Royal Society of Medicine, 97*(44), 36–42.

Smith, B. A., & Shuchman, M. (2005). Problem of nonadherence in chronically ill adolescents: Strategies for assessment and intervention. *Current Opinion in Pediatrics, 17*(5), 613–618.

Smith, B. A., & Wood, B. L. (2007). Psychological factors affecting disease activity in children and adolescents with cystic fibrosis: Medical adherence as a mediator. *Current Opinion in Pediatrics, 19*(5), 553–558.

Southern, K. W. (2007). The challenge of screening newborn infants for cystic fibrosis. In M. Hodson, D. Geddes, & A. Bush (Eds.), *Cystic fibrosis* (3rd ed., pp. 109–116). London: Hodder Arnold.

Stallings, V. A., Stark, L. J., Robinson, K. A., Feranchak, A. P., Quinton, H., Clinical Practice Guidelines on Growth and Nutrition Subcommittee, et al. (2008). Evidence-based practice recommendations for nutrition-related management of children and adults with cystic fibrosis and pancreatic insufficiency: Results of a systematic review. *Journal of the American Dietetic Association, 108*, 832–839.

Stark, L. J., & Powers, S. W. (2005). Behavioral aspects of nutrition in children with cystic fibrosis. *Current Opinion in Pulmonary Medicine, 11*(6), 539–542.

Stark, L. J., Powers, S. W., Jelalian, E., Rape, R. N., & Miller, D. L. (1994). Modifying problematic mealtime interactions of children with cystic fibrosis and their parents via behavioral parent training. *Journal of Pediatric Psychology, 19*, 751–768.

Szyndler, J. E., Towns, S. J., van Asperen, P. P., & McKay, K. O. (2005). Psychological and family functioning and quality of life in adolescents with cystic fibrosis. *Journal of Cystic Fibrosis, 4*(2), 135–144.

Tluczek, A., Koscik, R., Farrell, P. M., & Rock, M. (2005). Psychosocial risk associated with newborn screening for cystic fibrosis: Parents' experience while awaiting the sweat-test appointment. *Pediatrics, 115*, 1692–1703.

Tluczek, A., Koscik, R., Modaff, P., Pfeil, D., Rock, M., Farrell, P., et al. (2006). Newborn screening for cystic fibrosis: Parents' preferences regarding counseling at the time of infants' sweat test. *Journal of Genetic Counseling, 15*(4), 277–291.

Walters, S., & Mehta, A. (2007). Epidemiology of cystic fibrosis. In M. Hodson, D. Geddes, & A. Bush (Eds.), *Cystic fibrosis* (3rd ed., pp. 21–45). London: Hodder Arnold.

White, H., Morton, A. M., Peckham, D. G., & Conway, S. P. (2004). Dietary intakes in adult patients with cystic fibrosis: Do they achieve guidelines? *Journal of Cystic Fibrosis, 3*(1), 1–7.

Zindani, G. N., Streetman, D. D., Streetman, D. S., & Nasr, S. Z. (2006). Adherence to treatment in children and adolescent patients with cystic fibrosis. *Journal of Adolescent Health, 38*(1), 13–17.

CHAPTER 19

The Psychological Context of Diabetes Mellitus in Youths

TIM WYSOCKI
LISA M. BUCKLOH
PEGGY GRECO

In this chapter, we survey key research findings in three interrelated domains of adaptation of youths and families to diabetes mellitus: (1) the central role of the family in developing and maintaining the complex behavioral repertoire that is crucial to effective diabetes management; (2) the ways in which diabetes management affects, and is affected by, stress, coping, and psychological adjustment of youths and caregivers; and (3) the broader social context in which diabetes management occurs, and the critical importance of effective social supports in promoting effective self-care and coping. Within each domain, we have emphasized studies that have validated measures of these processes and trials of pertinent psychological interventions.

The variants of diabetes mellitus, which may overlap (Ize-Ludlow & Sperling, 2005), include Types 1a and 1b (DM1), Type 2 (DM2), maturity-onset diabetes of youth (MODY), and cystic-fibrosis-related diabetes (CFRD). All involve impaired glucose metabolism due to either insulin deficiency (DM1 and MODY) or insulin resistance (DM2 and CFRD). Since the published psychological research predominantly concerns DM1 and, to a much smaller extent, DM2, this chapter focuses on this existing research.

Treatment of DM1 and MODY includes several daily insulin injections or use of an insulin pump, self-monitoring of blood glucose (SMBG) four to six times daily, regulation of carbohydrate intake, daily exercise, and the prevention or correction of high (hyperglycemia) or low (hypoglycemia) blood glucose levels (Chase, 2006). New continuous glucose monitors may soon enable automatic regulation of insulin delivery via an insulin pump controlled by continuous glucose data (Wood & Laffel, 2007). Management of DM2 differs if a child is in a state of insulin resistance or if the condition has progressed to pancreatic beta cell failure and insulin deficiency. Patients with insulin resistance may be treated with daily oral medications that enhance insulin action and sensitivity. Once DM2 progresses to insulin deficiency, patients are typically started on two or more daily insulin injections and a regimen like that for DM1.

DM1 and DM2 raise long-term risks of heart, kidney, eye, and nerve disease. Major studies (Diabetes Control and Complications Trial Research Group, 1994; U.K. Prospective Diabetes Study Group, 1998) showed that maintaining near-normal hemoglobin A_{1C} (HbA_{1C}) reduces these risks greatly. Current care for DM1 and DM2 strives for near-normal HbA_{1C} (Tamborlane, Gatcomb, Held, & Ahern, 1994) through use of insulin pumps or multiple daily insulin injections, more frequent SMBG, and teaching families to remediate glycemic fluctuations. This requires implementing, monitoring, regulating, and coping with a complex regimen. These demands affect and are affected by many psychological processes. We review the scientific evidence of these interactions, and the assessment and intervention methods that have been tested.

Family Diabetes Management: Knowledge, Skills, and Treatment Adherence

Diabetes Knowledge and Skills

Diabetes knowledge is multifactorial, consisting of basic comprehension of diabetes physiology and management; technical proficiency in insulin administration, SMBG, sick-day management, and dietary regulation; and use of these skills to prevent, detect, and correct glycemic variability. Diabetes knowledge and skills increase with a child's age (Heidgerken et al., 2007), but youths with DM1 and their caregivers are prone to technical errors (Delamater et al., 1988; Johnson, Perwein, & Silverstein, 2000; Schmidt, Klover, Arfken, Delamater, & Hobson, 1992; Weissberg-Benchell et al., 1995). Thus diabetes knowledge and skills should be reevaluated regularly. Parental knowledge may have more impact on the efficacy of diabetes care for young children, whereas teens' knowledge and skills may become more important as parental involvement decreases (La Greca, Follansbee, & Skyler, 1990).

Diabetes knowledge is weakly related to treatment adherence and minimally related to measures of glycemic control (Heidgerken et al., 2007). This weak association should not be surprising, because HbA_{1C} levels are multiply determined by treatment adherence, adequacy of the diabetes regimen, the family's relationship with health care professionals, parent–child communication about diabetes, and the family's diabetes problem-solving skills. Knowledge may be a necessary, but insufficient, condition for effective family management of DM1.

Diabetes subject matter is constantly evolving, and measures of diabetes knowledge may become obsolete quickly. Most previous diabetes knowledge tests measure rote recognition, recall, and comprehension, rather than higher cognitive skills (Wysocki, 2000). A few measures assess diabetes problem-solving skills (Cook, Alkens, Berry, & McNabb, 2001; Heidgerken et al., 2007; Johnson et al., 1982), but these often ask the respondent to select a correct solution from several incorrect solutions, rather than to generate and defend a solution. However, several promising measures have recently been developed. Heidgerken and colleagues (2007) recently reported the psychometric validation of the multiple-choice Diabetes Awareness and Reasoning Test. Internal consistency was .94 for youths and .92 for parents. When demographic variables were controlled for, some subscale scores were significantly associated with HbA_{1C}. To our knowledge, this is the most psychometrically sound measure of diabetes knowledge that is now available for use in pediatric DM1. Wysocki, Iannotti, and colleagues (2008) introduced the Diabetes Problem Solving Interview, a measure of youths' and caregivers' skills in evaluating and proposing solutions to hypothetical glycemic fluctuations. Glycemic control over 9 months was significantly worse among youths whose caregivers had weaker skills on this measure, whereas youths' scores were not predictive of glycemic control. Enhancing caregivers' diabetes problem solving and promoting youths' use of their acquired skills could improve diabetic control.

Diabetes Self-Management and Treatment Adherence

Treatment adherence is a key variable affecting the metabolic status of youths with DM1. Adequate adherence may prevent or delay the long-term complications of DM1 (Diabetes Control and Complications Trial Research Group, 1994). Strict adherence to the diabetes regimen is very difficult, however, and few families or youths succeed at it 100% of the time.

Various adherence measures are available. Patients may rate their adherence to specific regimen components (e.g., La Greca, Swales, Klemp, & Madigan, 1988), record adherence behaviors in a diary, or be interviewed about self-care tasks (Diabetes Research in Children Network Study Group, 2005; Johnson, Silverstein, Rosenbloom, Carter, & Cunningham, 1986). Electronic measures of adherence include computer downloads of memory-stored SMBG data, insulin pump data, or accelerometers to measure physical activity. Like diabetes knowledge tests, adherence measures must evolve as diabetes management changes.

In pediatric diabetes, the "patient" is effectively the family; diabetes management depends heavily on family function. Family communication (Bobrow, AvRuskin, & Siller, 1985), problem solving (Wysocki, Iannotti, et al., 2008), and parental supportive involvement (Anderson, Auslander, Jung, Miller, & Santiago, 1990; Ellis, Podolski, et al., 2007; Wiebe et al., 2005; Wysocki et al., 1996) are key family variables affecting DM1 care.

Interventions Targeting Family Diabetes Management

Many studies of family-focused interventions have targeted treatment adherence, diabetes problem solving, and family diabetes management. Selected studies are summarized below.

Behavioral Contracting and Behavior Modification

Studies have affirmed the efficacy of behavioral contracting (e.g., Carney, Schechter, & Davis, 1983), and behavior modification (e.g., Epstein et al., 1981) as interventions targeting treatment adherence. Such studies confirm that DM1 self-management behavior can be improved with appropriately designed behavioral interventions, and that decreased HbA_{1C} may accompany these treatment effects. For example, Delamater and colleagues (1990) randomly assigned 36 youths newly diagnosed with DM1 to conventional therapy, supportive counseling, or self-management training. The latter was a diabetes-specific behavioral parent training intervention, and it yielded significantly lower HbA_{1C} than conventional therapy over a 2-year follow-up.

Interventions Targeting Family Communication and Problem Solving

Robin and Foster's (1989) behavioral family systems therapy (BFST) has been tested with adolescents with DM1. The first trial improved family communication and conflict resolution (Wysocki et al., 2000) and directly observed family communication (Wysocki et al., 1999), but not treatment adherence or glycemic control. In a second trial, a revised BFST intervention yielded sustained improvements in directly observed family communication (Wysocki, Harris, et al., 2008) and in treatment adherence and glycemic control (Wysocki et al., 2007). Ellis and colleagues have evaluated multisystemic therapy (MST) with urban adolescents in poor glycemic control. MST is an intensive, home-based, problem-focused therapy that seeks to engage the family, school, health care, and peer systems influencing the target behavior(s). MST yields lasting effects on adherence (Ellis et al., 2005; Ellis, Templin, et al., 2007) and health care utilization (Ellis, Naar-King, et al., 2007). The BFST and MST trials suggest that intensive family interventions can yield benefits that may persist over moderately long intervals.

Clinic-Integrated Interventions

Others have evaluated clinic-integrated interventions to promote healthy parent–youth teamwork for diabetes care. Laffel, Brackett, Ho, and Anderson (1998) and Svoren, Butler, Levine, Anderson, and Laffel (2003) compared standard care and a "Care Ambassador" intervention in which families of newly diagnosed children were offered support and assistance in negotiating clinic visits. The "Care Ambassador Plus" group also received psychoeducational modules during clinic visits. The Plus group had significantly less severe hypoglycemia and emergency care over 2 years. For those with baseline HbA_{1C} ≥8.7%, the Plus group achieved significantly lower HbA_{1C} than youths in the other two groups did. The same group also evaluated a family teamwork intervention (Anderson, Brackett, Ho, & Laffel, 1999; Laffel et al., 2003). This significantly improved parental involvement compared to standard care without increasing family conflict. Mean HbA_{1C} in the standard care group increased from 8.2% to 8.7%, whereas that for the intervention group dropped from 8.4% to 8.2% at 1 year. Youths in the intervention group with higher SMBG frequency had significantly lower HbA_{1C} after 1 year.

Stress, Coping, and Psychological Adjustment

Stress and Coping

Psychological stress can affect adolescents' ability to take care of their diabetes by decreasing both metabolic control and adherence. Neuroendocrine responses to stress may directly alter metabolic functioning (e.g., Hanson, Henggeler, & Burghen, 1987). Parental stress may also impede family management of diabetes (e.g., Streisand, Swift, Wickmark, Chen, & Holmes, 2005; Thompson, Auslander, & White, 2001).

Coping style may affect metabolic control. Patients in poor diabetic control tend to use maladaptive ways of coping with stress more often than youths in better control do (Delamater, Kurtz, Bubb, White, & Santiago, 1987; Hanson et al., 1989). Certain coping styles may be related to poorer DM1 outcomes, such as avoidance coping (Grey, Lipman, Cameron, & Thurber, 1997; Reid, Dubow, Carey, & Dura, 1994) or neglecting self-care (Grey et al., 1997). Stress and coping in youths with diabetes can be assessed by using general measures validated with pediatric populations. Blount and colleagues (2008) have provided a comprehensive review of empirically validated assessment measures of stress and coping in pediatric psychology.

Psychological Adjustment

Some studies suggest that youths with DM1 may not differ from the general population in psychological adjustment, especially among younger children (e.g., Helgeson, Snyder, Escobar, Siminerio, & Becker, 2007; Lawrence et al., 2006). But other studies report that having DM1 increases the risk of psychological problems in adolescents, including depression (e.g., Hood et al., 2006; Kovacs, Goldston, Obrosky, & Bonar, 1997), anxiety (Kovacs et al., 1997), and eating disorders (e.g., Jones, Lawson, Daneman, Olmsted, & Rodin, 2000). One review concluded that having DM1 at least doubles the prevalence of depression among youths (Grey, Davidson, Boland, & Tamborlane, 2001). This elevated risk is of significant concern, as psychological problems such as depression have been correlated with poorer glycemic control in youth with DM1 (Hassan, Loar, Anderson, & Heptulla, 2006), and psychological adjustment in adolescents has been linked to glycemic control in early adulthood (e.g., Bryden et al., 2001). A review of this research concluded that anxiety and depression play significant roles in individual adaptation to DM1, but that the relationship to metabolic control is not yet clear (Dantzer, Swendsen, Maurice-Tison, & Salamon, 2003).

Disordered eating and weight control behaviors are special concerns because of both the immediate and long-term impact of these behaviors on glycemic control. In DM1, the rates of eating disorders in preadolescent and adolescent girls (8–30%) are higher than in girls without diabetes (1–4%) (e.g., Colton, Olmsted, Daneman, Rydall, & Rodin, 2004; Jones et al., 2000). These behaviors may include insulin omission, strict dieting, excessive exercise, laxative use, self-induced vomiting, and binge eating (e.g., Colton et al., 2004; Jones et al., 2000), and are more prevalent in girls than in boys (e.g., Bryden et al., 1999). Eating disorders are associated with higher HbA_{1C} and earlier onset of complications (e.g., Rydall, Rodin, Olmsted, Devenyi, & Daneman, 1997).

Children and teens who are overweight are at increased risk for eating disorders, such as binge eating (Stradmeijer, Bosch, Koops, & Seidell, 2000); this is a significant problem that is relevant for youths with DM2, who are usually overweight. Justice (2004) found that adolescents with DM2 with a higher body mass index reported greater body dissatisfaction, and that disordered eating significantly decreased adherence to the daily regimen. Adolescents with DM2 are also at increased risk for psychological adjustment problems that are associated with excess weight, including poor self-esteem and body image, depression, anxiety, and behavioral problems (Kaufman, 2003).

Interventions Targeting Stress, Coping, and Psychological Adjustment in DM1

Several studies have evaluated individual psychological interventions designed to improve coping and stress management, treatment adherence, and treatment of mood and behavioral problems in youths with DM1. See Gage and colleagues (2004) and Wysocki (2006) for reviews, and Winkley, Landau, Eisler, and Ismail (2006) for a meta-analysis of psychological interventions to improve glycemic control in patients with DM1.

Stress Management/Coping Skills Interventions

Studies suggest that stress and anxiety management can reduce stress and, to a lesser extent, improve metabolic control in youths with DM1. Boardway, Delamater, Tomakowsky, and Gutai (1993) reported that a stress management intervention reduced stress but did not improve metabolic control or treatment adherence.

Coping skills training focused on increasing mastery by replacing ineffective coping skills with more constructive behaviors has yielded positive effects for youths with DM1 (e.g., Grey, Boland, Davidson, Li, & Tamborlane, 2000; Grey et al., 2001). These studies demonstrated lasting benefits (1 year) on glycemic control and quality of life. For example, Grey and colleagues (2000) found that adolescents who received coping skills training achieved lower HbA1c, better diabetes self-efficacy, better coping, and less negative impact of DM1 on quality of life.

Cognitive-Behavioral Therapy and Self-Monitoring Interventions

Cognitive-behavioral interventions typically target the identification and modification of negative cognitions to improve problem solving and coping. A multicomponent intervention (Mendez & Belendez, 1997) targeted stress management, social skills, glucose discrimination, problem solving, and self-monitoring with adolescents with DM1 and their parents. This intervention improved adolescents' blood glucose monitoring adherence, diabetes knowledge, and social skills, but did not improve glycemic control. A cognitive-behavioral intervention incorporating problem solving and cognitive restructuring reduced anxiety, anger, and diabetes-related stress in four of six youths (Hains, Davies, Parton, & Silverman, 2001). Five of six youths improved at least one self-care behavior (Silverman, Haines, Davies, & Parton, 2003). Cook, Herold, Edidin, and Briars (2002) reported that a 6-week problem-solving diabetes education program resulted in improved HbA_{1C}, more frequent SMBG, and better problem-solving skills.

Self-monitoring involves active recording of one's diabetes self-management behaviors. Some studies have shown that self-monitoring in youths with DM1 increases treatment adherence (e.g., Kumar, Wentzell, Mikkelsen, Pentland, & Laffel, 2004; Snyder, 1987). Recent advances in technology permit more innovative methods of SMBG. For example, Kumar and colleagues (2004) tested the use of an integrated wireless hand-held modem and diabetes data management software and a wireless-enabled blood glucose monitor, using an integrated motivational game in which participants guessed blood glucose based on prior readings. The researchers found that the game group transmitted significantly more blood glucose results, experienced less hyperglycemia, and increased diabetes knowledge over the 4-week trial, compared to the control group.

Motivational Interviewing and Supportive Therapies

Motivational interviewing (MI) is a flexible, client-centered, directive approach to enhancing motivation for change (Miller & Rollnick, 2002), which can be used to enhance motivation to make changes in treatment adherence in teens with diabetes. MI components include building awareness, generating alternatives, solving problems, making choices, setting goals, and avoiding confrontation (Channon et al., 2007). Channon and colleagues (2007) found that teens with DM1 randomly assigned to MI had significantly lower HbA_{1C} both at the end of the intervention and 12 months later. MI participants also reported improved quality of life, more positive well-being, and differences in personal models of illness. MI has preliminary support for delivery in groups; teens participating in six weekly group sessions of MI and solution-focused therapy showed a 1.5% drop in HbA_{1c} compared to controls 1–3 months after intervention, with some sustained effects 7–12 months later (Viner, Christie, Taylor, & Hey, 2003).

Others have evaluated telephone support interventions with youths with DM1 (Howells et al., 2002; Nunns, King, Smart, & Anderson, 2006). Howells and colleagues (2002) showed that adolescents participating in an intervention using problem solving and social learning principles showed significant improvements in self-efficacy compared to the control group, but there were no effects on HbA_{1c}. These supportive therapies may be of more benefit to children with DM1 if combined with intensive diabetes therapy or other behavioral interventions.

Interventions Targeting Stress, Coping, and Psychological Adjustment in DM2

Studies with psychological components for children with DM2 are ongoing. The National Institutes of Health have funded multicenter diabetes prevention and treatment trials, entitled the Studies to Treat or Prevent Pediatric Type 2 Diabetes, which are testing a multicenter school-based intervention to prevent the onset of DM2 in middle school children. The Treatment Options for Type 2 Diabetes in Adolescents and Youth trial is comparing three treatments for DM2 in the pediatric population (metformin, metformin + rosiglitazone, metformin + lifestyle intervention; Kaufman, 2005). There are also some prevention programs designed to reduce the risk factors associated with DM2. The Bienestar Health Program, which focused on health and education for low-income Hispanic children (Trevino, Hernandez, Yin, Garcia, & Hernandez, 2005), showed improvements in physical fitness for participants compared to controls after an 8-month intervention. Lifestyle interventions, when combined with metformin, have also shown positive effects for children with metabolic syndrome on weight loss (Harden, Cowan, Velasquez-Mieyer, & Patton, 2007) and insulin resistance (Fu et al., 2007).

Social Context of Diabetes

Management of diabetes requires adherence to multiple daily tasks in the home, school, and community. Thus the supportive involvement of family, friends, teachers, and health care professionals is integral to successful diabetes management. Furthermore, there is a need for research that more explicitly investigates cultural and ethnic influences on diabetes management.

Parental Involvement in Diabetes Care

Self-Care Responsibility

Parental involvement in DM1 care has been associated with positive psychological and health outcomes, such as achievement of treatment goals (Grey et al., 2001), decreased family conflict, and improved glycemic control (Anderson et al., 1999). Parental involvement in care should be balanced with a child's level of maturity. Deviation from this balance may have adverse effects; adolescents with excessive self-care autonomy relative to their psychological maturity have worse treatment adherence and more diabetes-related hospitalizations than those whose responsibilities are more developmentally appropriate (Wysocki et al., 1996). Youths who share self-care responsibility with their parents may experience better psychological and health outcomes (Helgeson, Reynolds, Siminerio, Escobar, & Becker, 2008). Parental monitoring of diabetes care may directly improve adherence and indirectly enhance metabolic control (Ellis, Podolski et al., 2007).

Several measures of these processes have been developed. The Diabetes Family Responsibility Questionnaire (Anderson et al., 1990) is a well-validated measure of responsibility for diabetes care. The Parental Monitoring of Diabetes Care Scale (Ellis, Podolski, et al., 2007; Ellis et al., 2008) measures youth and parent reports of parental monitoring of care. Hanna, DiMeglio, and Fortenberry (2007) have pilot-tested adolescent and parent versions of the Perceptions of Adolescents' Assumption of Diabetes Management scales.

Social Support

Positive dimensions of family functioning, such as the provision of social support, are also strongly associated with adaptation to diabetes. Social support from family and friends predicts better self-care (Skinner, John, & Hampson, 2000). Family members are more likely to offer tangible support, such as reminding, assisting, or doing diabetes-related tasks for a child; higher reported levels of family support can yield better adherence for adolescents (La Greca et al., 1995).

There are several measures of diabetes-specific family support. La Greca and colleagues (1995) devised the semistructured Diabetes Social Support Interview to obtain adolescents' perceptions of social support from family and friends. The Diabetes Family Behavior Checklist (Schafer, McCaul, & Glasgow, 1986) measures supportive and nonsupportive family behaviors through a self-report checklist. Higher levels of nonsupportive family behaviors may impede regimen adherence and diabetic control. The Diabetes-Specific Family Behavior Scale (McKelvey et al., 1993) can be used to identify family behaviors in the domains of warmth/caring, guidance/control, and problem solving.

Peer Involvement in Diabetes Care

Peer Pressure

A number of studies have evaluated the influence of friends on DM1 self-management. Adolescents indicate that adherence is more difficult in social and peer contexts (Berlin et al., 2006). Adolescents are more likely than younger children to evidence decreases in adherence in exchange for peer acceptance (Thomas, Peterson, & Goldstein, 1997). Finally, adolescents with DM1 may have more difficulty with social acceptance (e.g., Helgeson et al., 2007), and thus more vulnerability to social pressures that conflict with adequate diabetes self-care.

Social Support

Social support from friends is rated as important by adolescents with diabetes, and peers are a unique source of companionship and emotional support for diabetes care

(La Greca et al., 1995; La Greca, Bearman, & Moore, 2002). Using the Diabetes Social Support Interview, La Greca and colleagues (1995) showed that friend support was most evident for lifestyle aspects of diabetes, such as exercising together or accommodating a meal plan. The relationship between social support and self-care may vary across domains of self-care. Gallant's (2003) review noted a modest positive relationship between social support and self-management, especially for dietary behavior. La Greca and colleagues (2002) also emphasized the important role of friends in disease management for lifestyle aspects of treatment regimens, such as diet and exercise. Hains and colleagues (2007) recently reported that adolescents with negative attributions about friends' reactions to diabetes care were likely to experience more adherence difficulties, more diabetes-related stress, and poorer metabolic control.

Bearman and La Greca (2002) developed the Diabetes Social Support Questionnaire—Friends Version, a self-report form, as another measure of support from friends. This measure demonstrates high internal consistency and has good correspondence with other support measures. Another promising measure is the Diabetes Inventory of Peer Support (Skinner et al., 2000). This self-report questionnaire measures peer support in the areas of diet, exercise, injections, SMBG, and general support. The authors report adequate internal consistency for this measure.

Social Support Interventions

Adolescents' difficulties with regimen demands may not reflect deficient knowledge or problem-solving ability. Thomas and colleagues (1997) suggest a focus on managing peer impressions as a more developmentally appropriate strategy for adolescents with DM1. Hains and colleagues (2007) concur, advocating for cognitive-behavioral interventions to address misattributions of friend and peer reactions. Several of these types of interventions have been evaluated. Greco, Pendley, McDonell, and Reeves (2001) devised a structured short-term group program for integrating friends into adolescents' diabetes management. After intervention, teens and their friends had higher levels of knowledge about diabetes and support, and a higher ratio of peer to family support, while the friends had improved self-perception. Parents also reported improved family functioning and decreased diabetes-related conflict.

In a home-based MST intervention (Pendley et al., 2002), youths ages 8–17 formed a "support network" of friends and adults. The subjects and support teams attended an education and support group session during which a support plan was formed. Three follow-up home visits reinforced utilization of the support team for diabetes management. Adolescents perceived greater diabetes-related support from friends than did school-age children, and friend participation in the intervention was significantly related to metabolic control.

Diabetes Care in Community Settings

School

The American Diabetes Association (2002) has recommended school accommodations, including the training of school personnel in diabetes care and student permission to monitor and treat blood glucose levels in the classroom. A number of interventions have targeted teachers' knowledge of diabetes (e.g., Siminerio & Koerbel, 2000). In one study, 58% of parents reported that their children's school personnel had received diabetes training, and children in these settings had significantly better glycemic control than those in schools with untrained personnel (Wagner, Heapy, James, & Abbott, 2006). This study also showed the positive impact of classmates receiving information about diabetes, and of children having flexibility to perform self-care behaviors in the classroom. Having a diabetes "buddy," the most common strategy reported, may be a cost-effective intervention for improving diabetes care in school (Wagner et al., 2006).

Health Care Settings

There is a lack of research aimed at exploring the variables influencing children's socialization as health care consumers, their internalization of attitudes toward health care delivery and professionals, and their achievement of autonomous relationships with health care providers. Yet every child with DM1 must be prepared to face a lifetime of interactions with health care professionals, and to cultivate a partnership founded on trust and communication. Effective transition of children from pediatric to adult medical services requires a specialized service model, such as the Creating Healthy Futures clinic, a comprehensive transition clinic for adolescents and young adults with special health care needs (Betz & Redcay, 2003).

Reinforcement of clinic recommendations may take inventive forms, such as the Care Ambassador and telephone intervention programs discussed above, or even text messaging to support children and adolescents with diabetes. Franklin, Waller, Pagliari, and Greene (2006) reported a randomized controlled trial of Sweet Talk, a text-messaging system aimed at reinforcing goals set at clinic visits. Positive changes in glycemic control, adherence, and self-efficacy were noted in the Sweet Talk group.

Summary

We have surveyed the major research findings from three lines of diabetes research: family management of diabetes; stress, coping, and psychological adjustment; and the social context of diabetes. This has revealed an impressive array of well-validated and carefully conceived measures of diabetes-specific psychological processes and a wide variety of appropriate interventions that have been tested in randomized controlled trials. Although much attention has been drawn to the roles of psychological variables in family management of diabetes, this research has not had a pervasive practical impact. Few centers have implemented and sustained comprehensive programs of psychological assessment or intervention integrated with the medical care of these children. Achieving effective translation of this research into routine pediatric diabetes care is a substantial challenge for pediatric psychologists—one that will require actions on the levels of multiple complex and interrelated systems. Furthermore, future research and clinical endeavors must consider the broader social, cultural, and ethnic contexts of children with diabetes.

References

American Diabetes Association. (2002). Care of children with diabetes in the school and day care setting. *Diabetes Care, 26,* S131–S135.

Anderson, B. J., Auslander, W. F., Jung, K. C., Miller, J. P., & Santiago, J. V. (1990). Assessing family sharing of diabetes responsibilities. *Journal of Pediatric Psychology, 15,* 477–492.

Anderson, B. J., Brackett, J., Ho, J., & Laffel, L. (1999). An office-based intervention to maintain parent–adolescent teamwork in diabetes management: Impact on parent involvement, family conflict, and subsequent glycemic control. *Diabetes Care, 22,* 713–721.

Bearman, K. J., & La Greca, A. M. (2002). Assessing friend support of adolescents' diabetes care: The Diabetes Social Support Questionnaire—Friends Version. *Journal of Pediatric Psychology, 27,* 417–428.

Berlin, K. S., Davies, W. H., Jastrowski, K. E., Hains, A. A., Patton, E. A., & Alemzadeh, R. (2006). Contextual assessment of problematic situations identified by adolescents using insulin pumps and their parents. *Families, Systems, and Health, 24,* 33–44.

Betz, C. L., & Redcay, G. (2003). Creating healthy futures: An innovative, nurse-managed transition clinic for adolescents and young adults with special health care needs. *Pediatric Nursing, 29,* 25–30.

Blount, R. L., Simons, L. E., Devine, K. A., Jaaniste, T., Cohen, L. L., Chambers, C. T., et al. (2008). Evidence-based assessment of coping and stress in pediatric psychology. *Journal of Pediatric Psychology, 33,* 1021–1045.

Boardway, R. H., Delamater, A. M., Tomakowsky, J., & Gutai, J. P. (1993). Stress management training for adolescents with diabetes. *Journal of Pediatric Psychology, 18,* 29–45.

Bobrow, E. S., AvRuskin, T. W., & Siller, I. (1985). Mother–daughter interactions and adherence to diabetes regimens. *Diabetes Care, 8,* 146–151.

Bryden, K. S., Neil, A., Mayou, R. A., Peveler, R. C., Fairburn, C. G., & Dunger, D. B. (1999). Eating habits, body weight, and insulin misuse: A longitudinal study of teenagers and young adults with Type 1 diabetes. *Diabetes Care, 22,* 1956–1960.

Bryden, K. S., Peveler, R. C., Stein, A., Neil, A., Mayou, R. A., & Dunger, D. B. (2001). Clinical and psychological course of diabetes from adolescence to young adulthood: A longitudinal cohort study. *Diabetes Care, 24,* 1536–1540.

Carney, R. M., Schechter, K., & Davis, T. (1983). Improving adherence to blood glucose monitoring in insulin-dependent diabetic children. *Behavior Therapy, 14,* 247–254.

Channon, S. J., Huws-Thomas, M. V., Rollnick, S., Hood, K., Cannings-John, R. L., Rogers, C., et al. (2007). A multicenter randomized controlled trial of motivational interviewing in teenagers with diabetes. *Diabetes Care, 30,* 1390–1395.

Chase, H. P. (2006). *Understanding diabetes* (11th ed.). Denver, CO: Children's Diabetes Foundation at Denver.

Colton, P., Olmsted, M., Daneman, D., Rydall, A., & Rodin, G. (2004). Disturbed eating behavior and eating disorders in preteen and early teenage girls with Type 1 diabetes. *Diabetes Care, 27,* 1654–1657.

Cook, S., Alkens, J. E., Berry, C. A., & McNabb, W. L. (2001). Development of the Diabetes Problem-Solving Measure for Adolescents. *The Diabetes Educator, 27,* 865–874.

Cook, S., Herold, K., Edidin, D. V., & Briars, R. (2002). Increasing problem solving in adolescents with Type 1 diabetes: The Choices Diabetes Program. *The Diabetes Educator, 28,* 115–123.

Dantzer, C., Swendsen, J., Maurice-Tison, S., & Salamon, R. (2003). Anxiety and depression in juvenile diabetes: A critical review. *Clinical Psychology Review, 23,* 787–800.

Delamater, A. M., Davis, S., Bubb, J., Smith, J., Schmidt, L., White, N. H., et al. (1990). Randomized prospective study of self management training with newly diagnosed diabetic children. *Diabetes Care, 13,* 241–253.

Delamater, A. M., Davis, S., Bubb, J., Smith, J., White, N. H., & Santiago, J. V. (1988). Self monitoring of blood glucose by adolescents with diabetes: Technical skills and utilization of data. *The Diabetes Educator, 15,* 56–61.

Delamater, A. M., Kurtz, S. M., Bubb, J., White, N. H., & Santiago, J. V. (1987). Stress and coping in relation to metabolic control in adolescents with Type 1 diabetes. *Journal of Developmental and Behavioral Pediatrics, 8,* 136–140.

Diabetes Control and Complications Trial Research Group. (1994). Effect of intensive treatment on the development and progression of long term complications in adolescents with insulin-dependent diabetes mellitus. *Journal of Pediatrics, 125,* 177–188.

Diabetes Research in Children Network Study Group. (2005). Diabetes Self Management Profile for flexible insulin regimens: Cross-sectional and longitudinal analysis of psychometric properties in a pediatric sample. *Diabetes Care, 28,* 2034–2035.

Ellis, D. A., Frey, M., Naar-King, S., Templin, T., Cunningham, P., & Cakan, N. (2005). Use of multisystemic therapy to improve regimen adherence among adolescents with Type 1 diabetes in chronic poor metabolic control: A randomized controlled trial. *Diabetes Care, 28,* 1604–1610.

Ellis, D. A., Naar-King, S., Templin, T., Cunningham, P. B., & Frey, M. A. (2007). Improving health outcomes among youth with poorly controlled Type 1 diabetes: The role of treatment fidelity in a randomized clinical trial of multisystemic therapy. *Journal of Family Psychology, 21,* 363–371.

Ellis, D. A., Podolski, C., Frey, M., Naar-King, S., Wang, B., & Moltz, K. (2007). The role of parental monitoring in adolescent health outcomes: Impact of regimen adherence in youth with Type 1 diabetes. *Journal of Pediatric Psychology, 32,* 907–917.

Ellis, D. A., Templin, T., Naar-King, S., Frey, M. A., Cunningham, P. B., Podolski, C. L., et al. (2007). Multisystemic therapy for adolescents with poorly controlled Type 1 diabetes: Stability of treatment effects in a randomized controlled trial. *Journal of Consulting and Clinical Psychology, 75,* 168–174.

Ellis, D. A., Templin, T., Podolski, C., Frey, M., Naar-King, S., & Moltz, K. (2008). The Parental Monitoring of Diabetes Care Scale: Development, reliability, validity of a scale to evaluate parental supervision of adolescent illness management. *Journal of Adolescent Health, 42,* 146–153.

Epstein, L. H., Beck, S., Figueroa, J., Farkas, G., Kazdin, A. E., Daneman, D., et al. (1981). The effects of targeting improvement in urine glucose on metabolic control in children with insulin-dependent diabetes mellitus. *Journal of Applied Behavior Analysis, 14,* 365–375.

Franklin, V. L., Waller, A., Pagliari, C., & Greene, S. A. (2006). A randomized controlled trial of Sweet Talk, a text-messaging system to support young people with diabetes. *Diabetic Medicine, 23,* 1332–1338.

Fu, J. F., Liang, L., Zou, C. C., Hong, F., Wang, C. L., Wang, X. M., et al. (2007). Prevalence of the metabolic syndrome in Zhejiang Chinese obese children and adolescents and the effect of metformin combined with lifestyle intervention. *International Journal of Obesity, 31,* 15–22.

Gage, H., Hampson, S., Skinner, T. C., Hart, J., Storey, L., Foxcroft, D., et al. (2004). Educational and psychosocial programmes for adolescents with diabetes: Approaches, outcomes, and cost-effectiveness. *Patient Education and Counseling, 53,* 333–346.

Greco, P., Pendley, J. S., McDonell, K., & Reeves, G. (2001). A peer group intervention for adolescents with Type 1 diabetes and their best friends. *Journal of Pediatric Psychology, 26,* 485–490.

Grey, M., Boland, E. A., Davidson, M., Li, J., & Tamborlane, W. V. (2000). Coping skills training for youth with diabetes mellitus has long-lasting effects on metabolic control and quality of life. *Journal of Pediatrics, 137,* 107–114.

Grey, M., Davidson, M., Boland, E. A., & Tamborlane, W. V. (2001). Clinical and psychosocial factors associated with achievement of treatment goals in adolescents with diabetes mellitus. *Journal of Adolescent Health, 28,* 377–385.

Grey, M., Lipman, T., Cameron, M. E., & Thurber, F. W. (1997). Coping behaviors at diagnosis and in adjustment one year later in children with diabetes. *Nursing Research, 46,* 312–317.

Hains, A. A., Berlin, K. S., Davies, W. H., Smothers, M. K., Sato, A. F., & Alemzadeh, R. (2007). Attributions of adolescents with Type 1 diabetes related to performing diabetes care around friends and peers: The moderating role of friend support. *Journal of Pediatric Psychology, 32,* 561–570.

Hains, A. A., Davies, W. H., Parton, E., & Silverman, A. H. (2001). A cognitive-behavioral intervention for distressed adolescents with Type 1 diabetes. *Journal of Pediatric Psychology, 26,* 61–66.

Hanna, K. M., DiMeglio, L. A., & Fortenberry, J. D. (2007). Initial testing of scales measuring parents' and adolescents' assumption of diabetes management. *Journal of Pediatric Psychology, 32,* 245–249.

Hanson, C. L., Cigrang, J. A., Harris, M. A., Carle, D. L., Relyea, G., & Burghen, G. (1989). Coping styles in youths with insulin-dependent diabetes mellitus. *Journal of Consulting and Clinical Psychology, 57,* 644–651.

Hanson, C. L., Henggeler, S. W., & Burghen, G. (1987). Model of associations between psychosocial variables and health-outcome measures of adolescents with IDDM. *Diabetes Care, 10,* 752–758.

Harden, K. A., Cowan, P. A., Velasquez-Mieyer, P., & Patton, S. B. (2007). Effects of lifestyle intervention and metformin on weight management and markers of metabolic syndrome in obese adolescents. *Journal of the American Academy of Nurse Practitioners, 19,* 368–377.

Hassan, K., Loar, R., Anderson, B. J., & Heptulla, R. A. (2006). The role of socioeconomic status, depression, quality of life, and glycemic control in Type 1 diabetes mellitus. *Journal of Pediatrics, 149,* 526–531.

Heidgerken, A. D., Merlo, L., Williams, L. B., Lewin, A. B., Gelfand, K., Malasanos, T., et al. (2007). Diabetes Awareness and Reasoning Test: A preliminary analysis of development and psychometrics. *Children's Health Care, 36,* 117–136.

Helgeson, V. S., Reynolds, K. A., Siminerio, L., Escobar, O., & Becker, D. (2008). Parent and adolescent distribution of responsibility for self-care: Links to health outcome. *Journal of Pediatric Psychology, 33,* 497–508.

Helgeson, V. S., Snyder, P. R., Escobar, O., Siminerio, L., & Becker, D. (2007). Comparison of adolescents with and without diabetes on indices of psychosocial functioning for three years. *Journal of Pediatric Psychology, 32,* 794–806.

Hood, K. K., Huestis, S., Maher, A., Butler, D., Volkening, L., & Laffel, L. M. B. (2006). Depressive symptoms in children and adolescents with Type 1 diabetes: Association with diabetes-specific characteristics. *Diabetes Care, 29,* 1389–1391.

Howells, L., Wilson, A. C., Skinner, T. C., Newton, R., Morris, A. D., & Greene, S. A. (2002). A randomized control trial of the effect of negotiated telephone support on glycemic control in young people with Type 1 diabetes. *Diabetic Medicine, 19,* 643–648.

Ize-Ludlow, D., & Sperling, M. A. (2005). The classification of diabetes mellitus: A conceptual framework. *Pediatric Clinics of North America, 52,* 1533–1552.

Johnson, S. B., Perwein, A. R., & Silverstein, J. H. (2000). Response to hypo- and hyperglycemia in adolescents with Type 1 diabetes. *Journal of Pediatric Psychology, 25,* 171–178.

Johnson, S. B., Pollack, R. T., Silverstein, J., Rosenbloom, A., Spillar, R., McCallum, M., et al. (1982). Cognitive and behavioral knowledge about insulin-dependent diabetes among children and parents. *Pediatrics, 69,* 708–713.

Johnson, S. B., Silverstein, J., Rosenbloom, A., Carter, R., & Cunningham, W. (1986). Assessing daily management in childhood diabetes. *Health Psychology, 5,* 545–564.

Jones, J. M., Lawson, M. I., Daneman, D., Olmsted, M. P., & Rodin, G. (2000), Eating disorders in adolescent females with and without Type 1 diabetes: Cross sectional study. *British Medical Journal, 320,* 1563–1566.

Justice, K. A. K. (2004). Eating disorders in adolescents with Type 1 and Type 2 diabetes mellitus: Prevalence and adherence to the regimen. *Dissertation Abstracts International, 64*(12B), 6331B.

Kaufman, F. R. (2003). Type 2 diabetes in children and youth. *Review of Endocrinology and Metabolic Disorders, 4,* 33–42.

Kaufman, F. R. (2005). Type 2 diabetes in children and youth. *Endocrinology and Metabolism Clinics of North America, 34,* 659–676.

Kovacs, M., Goldston, D., Obrosky, D. S., & Bonar, L. K. (1997). Psychiatric disorders in youths with IDDM: Rates and risk factors. *Diabetes Care, 20,* 36–44.

Kumar, V. S., Wentzell, K. J., Mikkelsen, T., Pentland, A., & Laffel, L. (2004). The DAILY (Daily Automated Intensive Log for Youth) trial: A wireless, portable system to improve adherence and glycemic control in youth with diabetes. *Diabetes Technology and Therapeutics, 6,* 445–453.

Laffel, L., Brackett, J., Ho, J., & Anderson, B. J. (1998). Changing the process of diabetes care improves metabolic control and reduces hospitalizations. *Quality Management in Health Care, 6*(4), 53–62.

Laffel, L. M., Vangsness, L., Connell, A., Goebel-Fabri, A., Butler, D., & Anderson, B. J. (2003). Impact of ambulatory, family-focused teamwork intervention on glycemic control in youth with Type 1 diabetes. *Journal of Pediatrics, 142,* 409–416.

La Greca, A. M., Auslander, W. F., Greco, P., Spetter, D., Fisher, E. B., & Santiago, J. V. (1995). I get by with a little help from my family and friends: Adolescents' support for diabetes care. *Journal of Pediatric Psychology, 21,* 449–476.

La Greca, A. M., Bearman, K. J., & Moore, H. (2002). Peer relations of youths with pediatric conditions and health risks: Promoting social support and healthy lifestyles. *Journal of Developmental and Behavioral Pediatrics, 23,* 271–280.

La Greca, A. M., Follansbee, D. M., & Skyler, J. S. (1990). Developmental and behavioral aspects of diabetes management in youngsters. *Children's Health Care, 19,* 132–139.

La Greca, A. M., Swales, T., Klemp, S., & Madigan, S. (1988). Self-care behaviors among adolescents with diabetes. *Proceedings of the Ninth Annual Convention of the Society for Behavioral Medicine,* A42.

Lawrence, J. M., Staniford, D. A., Loots, B., Klingensmith, G. J., Williams, D. E., Ruggiero, A., et al. (2006). Prevalence and correlates of depressed mood among youth with diabetes: The SEARCH for Diabetes in Youth Study. *Pediatrics, 117,* 1348–1358.

McKelvey, J., Waller, D. A., North, A. J., Marks, J. F., Schreiner, B., Travis, L. B., et al. (1993). Reliability and validity of the Diabetes Family Behavior Scale (DFBS). *The Diabetes Educator, 19,* 125–132.

Mendez, F. J., & Belendez, M. (1997). Effects of a behavioral intervention on treatment adherence and stress management in adolescents with IDDM. *Diabetes Care, 24,* 1286–1292.

Miller, W. R., & Rollnick, S. (2002). *Motivational interviewing: Preparing people for change* (2nd ed.). New York: Guilford Press.

Nunns, E., King, B., Smart, C., & Anderson, D. (2006). A randomized controlled trial of telephone calls to young patients with poorly controlled Type 1 diabetes. *Pediatric Diabetes, 7* (5), 254–259.

Pendley, J. S., Kasmen, L. J., Miller, D. L., Donze, J., Swenson, C., & Reeves, G. (2002). Peer and family support in children and adolescents with Type 1 diabetes. *Journal of Pediatric Psychology, 27,* 429–438.

Reid, G. J., Dubow, E. F., Carey, T. C., & Dura, J. R. (1994). Contribution of coping to medical adjustment and treatment responsibility among children and adolescents with diabetes. *Journal of Developmental and Behavioral Pediatrics, 15,* 327–335.

Robin, A. L., & Foster, S. L. (1989). *Negotiating parent–adolescent conflict: A behavioral–family systems approach.* New York: Guilford Press.

Rydall, A. C., Rodin, G. M., Olmsted, M. P., Devenyi, R. G., & Daneman, D. (1997). Disordered eating behavior and microvascular complications in young women with insulin-dependent diabetes mellitus. *New England Journal of Medicine, 336,* 1849–1854.

Schafer, L. C., McCaul, K. D., & Glasgow, R. E. (1986). Supportive and non-supportive family behaviors: Relationships to adherence and metabolic control in persons with Type 1 diabetes. *Diabetes Care, 9,* 179–185.

Schmidt, L. E., Klover, R. V., Arfken, C. L., Delamater, A. M., & Hobson, D. (1992). Compliance with dietary prescriptions in children and adolescents with insulin-dependent diabetes mellitus. *Journal of the American Dietetic Association, 92,* 567–570.

Silverman, A. H., Haines, A. A., Davies, W. H., & Parton, E. (2003). A cognitive-behavioral adherence intervention for adolescents with Type 1 diabetes. *Journal of Clinical Psychology in Medical Settings, 10,* 119–127.

Siminerio, L. M., & Koerbel, G. (2000). A diabetes education program for school personnel. *Practical Diabetes International, 17,* 174–177.

Skinner, T. C., John, M., & Hampson, S. E. (2000). Social support and personal models of diabetes as predictors of self-care and well-being: A longitudinal study of adolescents with diabetes. *Journal of Pediatric Psychology, 25,* 257–267.

Snyder, J. (1987). Behavioral analysis and treatment of poor diabetic self-care and antisocial behavior: A single-subject experimental study. *Behavior Therapy, 18,* 251–263.

Stradmeijer, M., Bosch, J., Koops, W., & Seidell, J. (2000). Family functioning and psychosocial adjustment in overweight youngsters. *International Journal of Eating Disorders, 27,* 110–114.

Streisand, R., Swift, E., Wickmark, T., Chen, R., & Holmes, C. S. (2005). Pediatric parenting stress among parents of children with Type 1 diabetes: The role of self-efficacy, responsibility, and fear. *Journal of Pediatric Psychology, 30,* 513–521.

Svoren, B. M., Butler, D., Levine, B. S., Anderson, B. J., & Laffel, L. (2003). Reducing acute adverse outcomes in youths with Type 1 diabetes: A randomized, controlled trial. *Pediatrics, 112*(4), 914–922.

Tamborlane, W. V., Gatcomb, P., Held, N., & Ahern, J. (1994, September–October) Implications of the DCCT results in treating children and adolescents with diabetes. *Clinical Diabetes,* pp. 115–116.

Thomas, A. M., Peterson, L., & Goldstein, D. (1997). Problem solving and diabetes regimen adherence by children and adolescents with IDDM in social pressure situations: A reflection of normal development. *Journal of Pediatric Psychology, 22,* 541–561.

Thompson, S. J., Auslander, W. F., & White, N. H. (2001). Comparison of single-mother and two-parent families on metabolic control of children with diabetes. *Diabetes Care, 24,* 234–238.

Trevino, R. P., Hernandez, A. E., Yin, Z., Garcia, O. A., & Hernandez, I. (2005). Effect of the Bienestar Health Program on physical fitness in low-income Mexican American children. *Hispanic Journal of Behavioral Sciences, 27,* 120–132.

U.K. Prospective Diabetes Study Group. (1998). Intensive blood glucose control with sulphonylureas or insulin compared with conventional treatment and risk of complications in patients with Type 2 diabetes (UKPDS 33). *Lancet, 352,* 837–853.

Viner, R. M., Christie, D., Taylor, V., & Hey, S. (2003). Motivational/solution-focused intervention improves HbA$_{1c}$ in adolescents with Type 1 diabetes: A pilot study. *Diabetic Medicine, 20,* 739–742.

Wagner, J., Heapy, A., James A., & Abbott, G. (2006). Glycemic control, quality of life, and school experiences among students with diabetes. *Journal of Pediatric Psychology, 31,* 764–769.

Weissberg-Benchell, J., Glasgow, A. M., Tynan, W. D., Wirtz, P., Turek, J., & Ward, J. (1995). Adolescent diabetes management and mismanagement. *Diabetes Care, 18,* 77–82.

Wiebe, D. J., Berg, C. A., Korbel, C., Palmer, D. L., Beveridge, R. M., Upchurch, R., et al. (2005). Children's appraisals of maternal involvement in coping with diabetes: Enhancing our understanding of adherence, metabolic control, and quality of life across adolescence. *Journal of Pediatric Psychology, 30*(2), 167–178.

Winkley, K., Landau, S., Eisler, I., & Ismail, K. (2006). Psychological interventions to improve glycaemic control in patients with Type 1 diabetes: Systematic review and meta-analysis randomized controlled trials. *British Medical Journal, 333*, 65–69.

Wood, J. R., & Laffel, L. M. (2007). Technology and intensive management in youth with Type 1 diabetes: State of the art. *Current Diabetes Reports, 7*, 104–113.

Wysocki, T. (2000). Effective utilization of self-monitored blood glucose data: Cognitive and behavioral prerequisites. In B. Bercu & B. T. Stabler (Eds.), *Symposium on therapeutic outcome of endocrine disorders: Efficacy, innovation and quality of life* (pp. 151–160). New York: Springer-Verlag.

Wysocki, T. (2006). Behavioral assessment and intervention in pediatric diabetes. *Behavior Modification, 30*, 1–21.

Wysocki, T., Harris, M. A., Buckloh, L. M., Mertlich, D., Lochrie, A. S., Mauras, N., et al. (2007). Randomized controlled trial of behavioral family systems therapy for diabetes: Maintenance of effects on diabetes outcomes in adolescents. *Diabetes Care, 30*, 555–560.

Wysocki, T., Harris, M. A., Buckloh, L. M., Mertlich, D., Lochrie, A. S., Taylor, A., et al. (2008). Randomized controlled trial of behavioral family systems therapy for diabetes: Maintenance and generalization of effects on parent–adolescent communication. *Behavior Therapy, 39*, 33–46.

Wysocki, T., Harris, M. A., Greco, P., Bubb, J., Elder, C. L., Harvey, L. M., et al. (2000). Randomized, controlled trial of behavior therapy for families of adolescents with insulin-dependent diabetes mellitus. *Journal of Pediatric Psychology, 25*, 23–33.

Wysocki, T., Iannotti, R., Weissberg-Benchell, J., Hood, K., Laffel, L., Anderson, B. J., et al. (2008). Diabetes problem solving by youths with Type 1 diabetes and their caregivers: Measurement, validation and longitudinal associations with glycemic control. *Journal of Pediatric Psychology, 33*(8), 875–884.

Wysocki, T., Miller, K. M., Greco, P., Harris, M. A., Harvey, L. M., Elder-Danda, C. L., et al. (1999). Behavior therapy for families of adolescents with diabetes: Effects on directly observed family interactions. *Behavior Therapy, 30*, 496–515.

Wysocki, T., Taylor, A., Hough, B. S., Linscheid, T. R., Yeates, K. O., & Naglieri, J. A. (1996). Deviation from developmentally appropriate self-care autonomy: Association with diabetes outcomes. *Diabetes Care, 19*, 119–125.

CHAPTER 20

Sickle Cell Disease

KATHLEEN L. LEMANEK
MARK RANALLI

Sickle cell disease (SCD) is a chronic illness with psychological, social, and physical complications (Barakat, Lash, Lutz, & Nicolaow, 2006). Children and adolescents with SCD are at risk for problems in social-emotional, physical, and school functioning. Previous research on SCD has focused on understanding its pathophysiology and advances in treatment, as well as the neurocognitive functioning of youths with the disease. Within the past 5–10 years, attention has been directed toward pain description and management, neurocognitive functioning of patients who have sustained a stroke or silent infarct, and adolescents' transition to adulthood. Changes in methodology have also been evident with respect to qualitative studies and collaborative projects. This chapter briefly reviews the medical literature on SCD, including prevalence, pathophysiology, clinical manifestations, and approaches to treatment. Studies on the interpersonal, social, and cognitive functioning of youths with SCD are then reviewed. The chapter concludes with recommendations for future research and practice, with attention to integrative and comprehensive care.

Medical Domain

SCD represents a spectrum of inherited disorders of the oxygen-carrying red blood cell protein, hemoglobin (Ballas, 1998). The gene for SCD is found principally in individuals of African ancestry, but this disorder is encountered with increasing frequency in descendants of individuals from Turkey, Greece, southern Mediterranean regions, Saudi Arabia, India, the Caribbean, and Latin America. In the United States, approximately 70,000–100,000 people are affected by SCD (Brawley et al., 2008). The disease occurs in approximately 1 in every 500 African American births and in 1 in every 1,000–1,400 Hispanic American births (National Heart, Lung, and Blood Institute [NHLBI], 1996).

SCD represents a major public health concern. In 2004, there were approximately 113,000 hospitalizations for SCD in the United States, with total hospital costs of $488 million (Steiner & Miller, 2006).

Genetics and Molecular Biology

Normal hemoglobin in humans, called hemoglobin A (HbA), is the major oxygen-carrying protein found in red blood cells. It is composed of two alpha globin and two beta globin chains. The genetic alteration responsible for the most common sickle cell syndromes is a point mutation in the beta globin gene that results in the substitution of valine for glutamic acid at the sixth position of the beta globin (Ingram, 1956). The SCD gene is believed to have persisted in western Africa because of the survival advantage that individuals with "sickle cell trait" experience when infected by malaria (Allison, 1954). Persons with sickle cell trait inherit one normal beta and one sickle beta gene. Approximately 1 in 12 African Americans has sickle cell trait (NHLBI, 1996). Patients with sickle cell trait do not suffer from the spectrum of acute and chronic complications seen in patients with SCD, but under unusual circumstances serious morbidity or mortality can occur. These problems include increased urinary tract infection in women, splenic infarction, and life-threatening results of exercise (e.g., heat stroke, renal failure) or idiopathic sudden death (Serjeant, 1992). Sudden death has usually been seen in athletes or military recruits with the trait, who have become dehydrated after strenuous physical activity.

The most common SCD genotype, also known as sickle cell anemia, is seen in individuals who inherit two sickle beta globin genes (HbSS). Other SCD genotypes occur when other mutant forms of the beta gene are inherited in combination with the sickle beta gene, including HbSC and HbS beta thalassemia. Clinical severity varies within and between genotypes, but the most severe genotype is HbSS. The mean life expectancies of patients with HbSS are 42 years for males and 48 years for females, 25–30 years below expected ages for asymptomatic individuals (Platt et al., 1994). However, the life expectancy for other genotypes, such as HbSC, is similar to that of the general African American population.

Pathophysiology

The sickling process is a multicellular and polygenic phenomenon. Under conditions of hypoxia and acidosis, sickle hemoglobin molecules coalesce with each other into large polymers that damage the erythrocyte membrane, causing the characteristic sickled red blood cell shape (Eaton & Hofrichter, 1990). These rigid and deformed red blood cells are unable to pass through the narrowest blood vessels. A red blood cell "logjam" results, with reduced blood flow to tissues. The resulting oxygen and nutrient starvation, combined with the accumulation of toxic waste products, produces the acute and chronic symptoms seen clinically.

Clinical Manifestations

The variable severity of SCD complications depends on the sickle cell genotype, the influence of other genes, the existence of comorbid illnesses (e.g., asthma or renal disease), knowledge of and adherence to prescribed therapy, and psychosocial factors. After

6 months of age, fetal hemoglobin levels fall and sickle hemoglobin levels rise, with the resulting appearance of clinically evident disease (Ballas, 1998). Early onset of painful events (crises), severe anemia, and high white blood cell count are correlated with later adverse sickle-cell related outcomes (Miller et al., 2001), but the prognostic significance of these hematological variables has been questioned (Quinn et al., 2008).

Pain

Vaso-occlusive crises (VOCs), or recurring episodes of pain, are hallmark clinical features of SCD. Pain episodes differ in intensity, location, and quality, and are categorized as acute (due to blocked blood flow) or chronic (due to damage from repeated pain episodes and tissue ischemia) (Franck, Treadwell, Jacob, & Vichnisky, 2002). Children and adolescents with SCD typically report pain on 7–30% of diary days, with an average duration of 2.5 days and an average pain rating of 5 on a 10-point scale (Dampier, Ely, Brodecki, & O'Neal, 2002; Gil et al., 2000). Pain is described as uncomfortable, achy, and steady; it occurs most often in extremities, the hips, or the abdomen. Events may occur either spontaneously or as a consequence of environmental stress (e.g., exposure to excessive cold or heat), physiological stress (e.g., infection, dehydration), or psychosocial stress (e.g., school exams, peer conflicts) (Ballas, 1998). About 80% of pain episodes are managed at home, but half to two-thirds of hospital admissions in youths are for VOCs (Gil et al., 2000).

Research indicates that both pharmacological and nonpharmacological interventions are used to manage pain at home. Analgesic medication is used on the majority of days with pain (85%) (Dampier et al., 2002), but also is taken on some days without pain by about 15% of adolescents surveyed (Gil et al., 2000). Distracting activities (e.g., sleeping, watching television, talking with others) have been common nonpharmacological interventions utilized to manage pain (Dampier et al., 2002). Parents and caregivers have reported emphasizing efforts either to prevent pain episodes or to stop the pain from worsening by administering medications, applying heat or touch, and giving fluids. Oral analgesics and most nonpharmacological interventions have, however, been rated as only somewhat effective by parents and caregivers (Beyer & Simmons, 2004). Chen, Cole, and Kato (2004) reviewed empirically supported psychosocial interventions for pain and adherence in SCD. Cognitive-behavioral techniques (e.g., calming self-statements, progressive muscle relaxation) were considered probably efficacious for pain. But the efficacy of behavioral techniques and social support interventions for pain or adherence could not be determined, due to the studies' lack of methodological rigor.

Currently, there is no standard treatment implemented in the hospital for more severe pain. Treatment is started with scheduled "bolus" doses of intravenous analgesics, or administration via patient-controlled analgesia units, with rapid transition to oral medications (American Pain Society, 1999). Rehydration with oral or intravenous fluids, rest, and scheduled ambulation are additional components of treatment protocols. Barriers to effective pain management include clinicians' limited knowledge of SCD, inadequate assessment of pain, biases against analgesia use based on ignorance about tolerance, and confusion between physical dependence and addiction (NHLBI, 1996). Sickle cell day hospitals serve as an alternative care delivery system to traditional emergency department care or inpatient hospitalization for management of acute sickle cell complications. (Benjamin et al., 2000). Day hospital management of complications appears to result in shorter length of stays than inpatient care does, and has the potential to provide efficient and timely treatment by professionals specifically trained in the management of acute crises (Benjamin, Swinson, & Nagel, 2000).

Infectious Complications

Poor or absent splenic function seen in SCD prevents the clearance of bacteria, resulting in infections that are rapidly fatal, even if diagnosed properly. The use of daily penicillin prophylaxis, emphasis on routine childhood immunizations (including yearly influenza), and the adoption of aggressive treatment protocols for patients with fever over the past two decades have reduced early death in children with SCD (Gaston et al., 1986).

Pulmonary and Cardiac Complications

As life expectancy in SCD has improved, the impact of added disease activity on organ function is becoming more apparent. Chronic cardiac and pulmonary diseases are replacing infectious complications as the most common causes of death and most frequent reasons for hospitalization (Castro et al., 1994). The catalysts of lung injury in patients with SCD include infection, fat embolism, and bronchoreactive lung disease. Over 50% of patients with SCD have hyperresponsive airways or asthma and may benefit from asthma management (Leong, Dampier, Varlotta, & Allen, 1997). Treatments to control bronchial reactivity seem to exert a beneficial influence in patients with acute pulmonary complications.

The "acute chest syndrome" is the most common reason for mortality in patients with SCD. It is described as chest pain along with respiratory distress, occurs most often as a single episode but may occur as multiple episodes, and is most typical at ages 2–4 years (Castro et al., 1994). High blood pressure in the arteries that supply the lungs is called "pulmonary hypertension" (PHT). As many as 75% of patients with SCD have findings of PHT on autopsy, while 30% have echocardiographic evidence of PHT (Haque et al., 2002). The clinical signs of PHT progress to shortness of breath, exercise intolerance, and lower oxygen levels requiring oxygen supplementation.

Strokes and Other Central Nervous System Complications

Strokes are severe complications of SCD and result from a cumulative interplay among molecular, cellular, and genetic forces. Overt strokes are seen in 9% of patients with SCD before their 14th birthday (Frempong, 1991). The onset is generally abrupt, and they typically occur within the large vessels, commonly involve both cortex and deep white matter, and are associated with greater deficits (Moser et al., 1996).

Silent cerebral infarcts are the most common form of neurological injury in children with SCD, occurring in 22–35% by 14 years of age (Miller et al., 2001). Unlike overt strokes, they occur within small vessels; are generally confined to deep white matter; and involve nonmotor areas of the brain, especially the frontal cortex (Moser et al., 1996). Children with silent infarcts are at increased risk for further overt and silent strokes than are children with SCD (Miller et al., 2001).

Without proper management, in excess of 50–70% of individuals with SCD and stroke experience progression of cerebrovascular injury, or stroke recurrence (Frempong, 1991). Currently, long-term ("chronic") blood transfusion therapy is the most widely accepted treatment for stroke prevention in patients with SCD who have previously experienced strokes. The goal of blood transfusion therapy is to reduce the sickle cell burden to less than 30% of the total hemoglobin content (below that seen in patients with sickle cell trait). Patients should then be free of sickle cell symptomatology, including, presumably, progression of cerebrovascular disease. Indeed, chronic transfusions appear to prevent recurrent strokes in over 80% of patients. Several potential complications are associated with chronic transfusion therapy, including infections (e.g., HIV, hepatitis), the development of antibodies to transfused blood cells, acute and delayed transfusion reactions, and iron overload (Frempong, 1991).

Cognitive and Academic Functioning

Research indicates that individuals with SCD of all ages are at risk for developmental delays, cognitive difficulties, and/or academic deficits. Increased risk status or declines in developmental skills have been found during the first year of life (Hogan et al., 2006) or during the first 3 years of life (Thompson, Gustafson, Bonner, & Ware, 2002). Higher versus lower neurological risks have been identified primarily in language, motor abilities, and executive functions (memory and attention) in toddlers and preschoolers with SCD (Schatz & Roberts, 2007). Deficits on measures of general intelligence, language abilities, visual–motor skills, sequential memory, and attention have been found for children with SCD and overt strokes in previous studies (e.g., Armstrong et al., 1996). Poor school performance has been identified in children with silent infarcts, with 80% showing clinically significant cognitive deficits and 35% demonstrating deficits in academic skills (e.g., Schatz, Brown, Pascual, Hus, & DeBaum, 2001). Declines in global and specific neurocognitive functioning have been found with increasing age in the presence of lower hematocrit levels (percentage of red blood cells in whole blood) (Kral et al., 2006). Whether changes in cognitive functioning represent a stepwise pattern related to distinct structural alterations or a cumulative, gradual decline associated with chronic hypoxia is not known (Kral et al., 2006). Detailed descriptions of neurological and neuropsychological studies, disease-specific models of deficits, and clinical and research implications can be found in reviews by Kral, Brown, and Hynd (2001) and Schatz, Finke, Kellet, and Kramer (2002).

Global deficits and specific deficits in attention, but no differences in academic achievement, have been found when youths with SCD are compared with classmates or siblings (e.g., Noll et al., 2001). However, a large percentage of students with SCD (42%) have reported that disease-related problems pose challenges to participating in school (Peterson, Palermo, Swift, Beebe, & Drotar, 2005), and such students show a higher rate of attainment problems than classmates (31% vs. 14%), which is unexpected based on academic achievement ability (Schatz et al., 2001). The number of individualized education programs (IEPs) also appears less than adequate: Only 70% of youths with identified strokes (Herron, Bacak, King, & DeBaum, 2003), and only 26% with possible learning problems (Peterson et al., 2005), have IEPs. Day and Chismark (2006) have provided detailed recommendations regarding formal presentations to educators that address the effects of SCD on cognitive functioning and academic achievement.

Additional Complications

Skeletal complications are common in patients with SCD; they include weakened bones that fracture easily and degenerative joint disease that causes chronic pain and disability. These complications are probably related to poor nutrition, impaired growth hormone secretion, and delayed puberty (Almeida & Roberts, 2005). With modern management, however, the majority of adolescents achieve full puberty and adult heights within expected norms by 20 years of age (Zemel, Kawchak, Ohene-Frempong, Schall, & Stallings, 2007). Gallbladder disease and renal dysfunction are also common in individuals with SCD, due to high blood flow and chronic sickling within these organs (Kontessis, Mayopoulou-Symvoulidis, Symvoulidis, & Kontopoulou-Griva, 1992). Males may experience prolonged painful erections, due to sickling within the penile tissues that ultimately produces scarring and impotence. In women, amenorrhea and infertility are not uncommon, and pregnancy is accompanied by a substantially increased risk of maternal and fetal complications.

Treatment Approaches

Advances in the understanding of sickle cell pathophysiology, and improvements in early identification and supportive care, have improved patients' quality of life and increased their life expectancy. Whereas pain management has focused largely on symptom control and not on symptom prevention, new treatment approaches show promise as preventive strategies.

Newborn Screening

Early identification of patients with SCD is correlated with better clinical outcomes. This finding, and the fact that prophylactic penicillin markedly reduces the occurrence of bacterial sepsis and death in young patients with SCD, provided the incentive for widespread implementation of neonatal hemoglobinopathy screening (Gaston et al., 1986). As of 2007, all 50 states, Puerto Rico, the U.S. Virgin Islands, and the District of Columbia require universal screening for SCD and other disorders of hemoglobin through heel stick blood spots collected at birth. The primary purpose of screening is to identify infants with SCD and other blood disorders, as well as carriers of such disorders. About 2,000 infants with SCD are identified yearly in the United States through these programs (American Academy of Pediatrics Newborn Screening Taskforce, 2000).

Supportive Care

Hydration, analgesia, and nonsteroidal anti-inflammatory medications are used in the management of the most common SCD complication, pain. Supervised incentive spirometry and early ambulation are recommended to prevent progression of acute pulmonary problems (Bellet, Kalinyak, Rakesh, Elfand, & Rucknagel, 1995). Transfusions are indicated for the management of strokes, pulmonary complications, and chronic pain. Improvements in transfusion technology, including the use of phenotypically similar blood and automated exchange transfusions, reduce the risk of red blood cell antibody formation and potentially fatal iron overload (Rosse et al., 1990).

Novel Agents

Hydroxyurea (HU) is a medication that has numerous beneficial effects on the sickling process, including increasing (protective) fetal hemoglobin levels, improving red blood cell hydration, and interfering with sickle cell adhesion to cells that line blood vessels (Yarbro, 1992). Daily administration of oral HU is the first effective pharmacological intervention documented to provide clinically significant prevention of complications in SCD. The use of HU is related to a reduction in the duration of hospital stays, the frequency of VOC events, and the number of required transfusions (Charache et al., 1995). Longitudinal studies of safety and efficacy are underway in children to determine the long-term benefits and toxicities of HU.

Bone Marrow Transplantation

Bone marrow transplantation (BMT) is currently the only available treatment that offers the prospect of cure for patients with SCD. The goal of a BMT is to replace a patient's defective bone marrow with a donor's normal bone marrow. Morbidity is high and includes infections, infertility, graft versus host disease, and organ complications. However, in the three major studies of BMT for SCD, overall survival was 92–94% (Vermylen et al., 1998). Outcomes for patients with asymptomatic disease appear to be superior to outcomes for those with symptomatic disease (Bernaudin et al., 2007). Marrow from unrelated donors and umbilical cord stem cells are being utilized with increasing frequency for BMT in eligible patients with SCD who have no family donor (Walters et al., 1996).

Psychological Domain

In this section, we examine the intrapersonal and interpersonal adjustment of youths with SCD, the influence of physiological functioning on adjustment, adherence to medical regimen, transition to adult health care, and culturally sensitive practices.

Social-Emotional Functioning

Children and adolescents with SCD are at risk for internalizing symptoms (depression and anxiety), social and peer difficulties, and poorer quality of life (Barakat et al., 2006; Noll et al., 1996; Palermo, Schwartz, Drotar, & McGowan, 2002). Casey, Brown, and Bakeman (2000) have identified impairments in mental abilities or adaptive competencies as general risk factors to psychosocial adjustment. Limited interpersonal, social, and academic opportunities due to illness-related factors (e.g., hospitalizations, VOCs) during critical periods of cognitive, emotional, and social development have been delineated as specific risk factors (Schaeffer et al., 1999).

Active and passive coping strategies used by youths with SCD have been identified as resiliency factors. Examples of active coping strategies include distraction or fantasies to divert attention from pain; examples of passive strategies include rest or sleep and warm baths (Casey et al., 2000; Mitchell et al., 2007). In general, active coping has been associated with decreases in negative thinking, increases in active health management, fewer health care contacts and school absences, and more involvement in daily activities on pain days (Mitchell et al., 2007; Powers, Mitchell, Graumlich, Byars, & Kalinyak, 2002). The specific strategies employed may depend on such factors as developmental level and pain severity, but appear consistent with national recommendations for managing SCD (Casey et al., 2000). Additional risk and resiliency factors have been highlighted in investigations, but there is limited research documenting similarities and differences between youths with and without SCD in these areas.

Demographic variables, such as age and gender, influence psychosocial adjustment (Kell, Kliewer, Erickson, & Ohene-Frempong, 1998). Children with SCD appear more concerned about family and social relationships, while adolescents seem more worried about delayed puberty and physical development, the liability of SCD on family and friends, and death and dying (Schaeffer et al., 1999). Females tend to use more active coping strategies (Casey et al., 2000) and to report a better quality of life than males (Lutz, Barakat, Smith-Whitley, & Ohene-Frempong, 2004). In contrast, males employ denial as a coping strategy to a greater extent (Royal, Headings, Harrell, Ampy, & Hall, 2000) and utilize health care services (e.g., emergency room visits, clinic visits) more often then females (Lutz et al., 2004).

Some gender differences are also evident in peer relationships in youths with SCD. In an earlier study by Noll and colleagues (1996), girls with SCD were rated by their peers as less sociable and less well accepted, and boys were rated as less aggressive than healthy peers. A recent study (Noll, Reiter-Purtill, Vannatta, Gerhardt, & Short, 2007) showed that youths with SCD were selected less often as a best friend but were not less well liked than healthy peers. These nominations may be related to the descriptions of these children by teachers and their peers. Youths with SCD were described by their teachers as more prosocial and less aggressive, and by their peers as less athletic, more ill, and as missing more school.

Family Functioning

Previous research has shown relationships among parent coping, family functioning communication, cohesion), and parent-reported internalizing and externalizing behavior problems in youths with SCD (Brown et al., 2000; Thompson et al., 1999). However, family distress appears to be more related to family conflict and typical child-rearing tasks than to the diagnosis of SCD or its severity (Thompson et al., 2003). The unpredictable nature of the disease and the demands of managing symptoms at home are stressors related to the adjustment of families.

Parents and caregivers of youths with SCD need to be knowledgeable about SCD and its treatment, skilled in recognizing symptoms and implementing treatment plans at home, and persistent in coordinating other family responsibilities and activities (Rao & Kramer, 1993). Both active coping strategies (e.g., information seeking, social support) and passive coping strategies (e.g., prayer) are used by caregivers as they progress through stages of learning about and incorporating SCD into their daily lives (Midence, Fuggle, & Davies, 1993; Northington, 2000). Challenges include the fewer and less effective social contacts and social networks found in mothers of children with SCD (Schuman, Armstrong, Pegelow, & Routh, 1993).

Adaptive family functioning has been associated with active youth coping (Mitchell et al., 2007), but the role of mediating and moderating variables appears critical, according to research by Barakat and colleagues. In one study (Barakat et al., 2007), worse health outcomes were revealed when caregivers reported greater distress in reaction to disease-related stress. Such distress may be affected by caregivers' belief in their ability to manage youths' symptoms at home. In another study (Barakat, Lutz, Nicolaou, & Lash, 2005) higher levels of external locus of control were identified in mothers of children with SCD, but internal locus of control was associated with better family functioning and child self-competence. These authors attribute greater child competence to observing and modeling caregivers' use of problem-solving strategies with respect to medical management of SCD.

Influence of Physiological Functioning on Adjustment

The relationship between disease severity and illness-related stress as measured by medical parameters, including genotype, hemoglobin levels, and SCD-related complications (e.g., pain intensity), has been examined in multiple studies. In general, these studies have not found a relationship between disease variables and adjustment (e.g., Casey et al., 2000); however, the results have varied, depending on the specific outcome variables being examined. For example, the home environment appears more related to cognitive functioning than to disease severity, although level of anemia and temperament may serve as mediators (Schatz & Roberts, 2007). The risk of psychological dysfunction appears more dependent on symptom interference with daily functioning than on disease severity (Barbarin, 1999). The importance of parent and child perceptions of disease severity and illness-related stress as mediators of functioning also may be relevant (Logan, Radcliffe, & Smith-Whitley, 2002; Lutz et al., 2004). For example, Logan and colleagues (2002) found parents' perceptions of illness-related stress to predict routine service use (e.g., clinic visits) and urgent service use (e.g., emergency department visits) in adolescents with SCD.

The relationship between pain severity and various dimensions of adjustment has been studied in recent investigations. Mild pain ratings have been reported for most pain days (95%), and pain appears to interfere with play/sport activities but not with school, social, or home activities in the majority of children and adolescents (80%) (Maikler, Broome, Bailey, & Lea, 2001). However, daily increases in stress and negative mood have been associated with higher daily pain ratings, more health care use, and decreases in school and social activities (Gil et al., 2003). More severe pain ratings have also been related to higher social anxiety in older children and adolescents, in terms of fear of negative evaluation but not social avoidance/distress (Wagner et al., 2004). Overall, adolescents appear to be more adversely affected by the additive stress of a chronic illness that includes pain, which may then limit social activities at a time when peer relationships are more relevant (Wagner et al., 2004).

Adherence

Adherence to pharmacological treatments (e.g., analgesics, oral antibiotics) and non-pharmacological treatments (e.g., hydration) for SCD ranges from 12% for prophylactic penicillin to 96% for HU (Dampier et al., 2002; Witherspoon & Drotar, 2006). The clinical characteristics of SCD and its treatment may generate challenges in investigating adherence assessment and intervention (Barakat, Smith-Whitley, & Ohene-Frempong, 2002). For example, most treatment recommendations are preventive in nature, such as not engaging in excessive physical activity and being well hydrated. Standard treatment recommendations focus on pain and fever management at home and in the hospital, but the specific protocols vary.

Family flexibility in problem solving and use of fewer passive coping strategies appear to promote adherence (Barakat et al., 2002). Better adherence, though, may interfere with physical and social activities, based on an association with poorer quality-of-life ratings (Barakat, Lutz, Smith-Whitley, & Ohene-Frempong, 2005). Adherence is higher for more concrete recommendations, such as follow-up clinic appointments, and less for vague ones, such as maintaining hydration (Baraket, Lutz, Smith-Whitley, et al., 2005). The one study on adherence to prophylactic penicillin revealed forgetting, time constraints, falling asleep, running out of medication, and obtaining refills as common problems (Witherspoon & Drotar, 2006). Forgetting was the primary barrier identified for several treatment components (e.g., pain management, fluids), and caregiver reminders was the main strategy identified as improving adherence, by both caregivers and adolescents assessing multiple components of the SCD treatment regimen (Modi et al., 2009).

Transition to Adult Health Care

Kinney and Ware (1996, p. 1261) have stated that making the transition to adult health care is the "most difficult and potentially traumatic passage faced by adolescents with SCD." This transition usually occurs when adolescents are experiencing other life changes, such as assuming autonomous functioning, separating from their families of origin, and determining their place in society (Baskin et al., 1998; While & Mullen, 2004). These normal developmental tasks may heighten the psychological stress of negotiating the transition into adult health care. The importance of addressing this transition is highlighted by findings of increased disease complications (e.g., organ dysfunction, pain ratings) and medical service utilization in adult patients with SCD (Serjeant, 1992). In a national survey of SCD programs, Telfair and colleagues (Alexander, Allerman-Velez, Loosier, Simmons, & Telfair, 2004) identified the primary concerns of adolescents making the transition to adult centers. These concerns centered on a lack of information related to their transition to adult care, fears of leaving their pediatric care providers, the adult care providers not understanding their needs, and ways to meet adult care providers to identify their needs.

Transition programs not only should attend to specialized health care, but also should assist in educational attainment, life skills, and self-advocacy (Alexander et al., 2004; Baskin et al., 1998). This attention to multiple aspects of care may be related to higher satisfaction scores (i.e., general satisfaction, technical quality, financial aspects) from patients who receive their care from specialized centers versus nonspecialized centers (Aisiku et al., 2007). Unfortunately, few transition programs include topics related to medical management and life skills, and the empirical support for transition programs is lacking (Telfair, Ehiri, Loosier, & Baskin, 2004). In addition, multidisciplinary providers appear not to agree on what constitutes the best practice in regard to transitions (Alexander et al., 2004). Baskin and colleagues (1998) state that transition interventions should be developmentally sensitive and culturally informed, and that they are best implemented within a group setting and with the assistance of mentors who may have SCD or the SCD trait.

Cultural Issues

Guidelines written by the NHLBI (1996) clearly state that families of children with sickle cell disease will participate in health care decision making at all levels and will be satisfied with the services they receive. Parents also report the need for comprehensive health care approaches that meet the physical and psychological needs of patients and families (Mitchell et al., 2007). On the basis of their review, Chen and colleagues (2004) recommended involving extended families in interventions to foster acceptance and implementation. Toward this goal, Schwartz, Radcliffe, and Barakat (2007) found active engagement by adolescents and their families in an investigation of the effects of a culturally sensitive pain management intervention. In addition, the availability of mentors who are demographically similar to patients has been shown to foster racial identity and to reduce the risk for mental health problems (Blechman, 1992).

Several challenges in designing culturally sensitive and comprehensive health care programs are present. First, individuals from ethnic minorities are faced with health care disparities that limit their access to and quality of health care (Baskin et al., 1998). Second, individuals from such minority groups as African Americans have historically been hesitant to seek medical care and may emphasize religious and other cultural practices to manage symptoms (Baskin et al., 1998). Third, the definition of "families" may not be identical across ethnic groups, with nontraditional and single-parent families being heavily represented in studies of youths with SCD (Mitchell et al., 2007). Standard measures of family functioning assessing such constructs as adaptability and cohesiveness may not, therefore, be descriptive of diverse families (Casey et al., 2000). Finally, the differential risk of poverty versus ethnic minority status and/or disease severity needs to be delineated before family-focused, culturally sensitive programs can be designed (Barbarin, 1999; Barbarin, Whitten, Bond, & Conner-Warren, 1999).

Future Directions

This chapter suggests that children and adolescents with SCD are at risk for adjustment difficulties in social-emotional, family, and cognitive functioning. However, the resiliency of youths with SCD is also evident. Several areas of future research are suggested by this review of the literature in SCD. One area pertains to assessment practices that include multiple informants and settings. Barakat and colleagues (e.g., Barakat et al., 2007) advocate using multiple informants (self-report and other report) to understand family functioning related to and separate from disease-related factors. Authors also recommend multidimensional assessment during both the acute phase of the illness and routine care (Noll et al., 2007), and during clinic visits, in day hospitals, and in inpatient settings (Franck et al., 2002). Periodic neuropsychological assessment has been encouraged, to track cumulative and/or discrete structural changes in youths' intellectual and academic performance (Kral et al., 2006). Developmental screenings or testing should also be standard practice, to obtain basic information about the developmental status and early intervention needs of infants, toddlers, and preschool-age children with SCD (Schatz & Roberts, 2007).

Multidisciplinary interventions will be critical in the future and should highlight the individual, the family, and the school. Multiple authors promote the development of family-focused and peer-focused interventions that address communication and problem-solving skills training to manage SCD-related stress, including pain (e.g., Mitchell et al., 2007; Noll et al., 2007). The design and evaluation of educational programs and services for youths with SCD and school personnel should be a priority, due to the paucity of data and subsequent guidelines in this area. As recommended by Chen and colleagues (2004), future research should focus on testing existing interventions rather than on developing new ones, as well as on examining a range of SCD-related outcomes. Data generated from these areas of research can then be translated into clinical practice that not only will minimize the at-risk status of youths with SCD, but will foster optimal social-emotional, family, physical, and academic functioning.

References

Aisiku, I. P., Penberthy, L. T., Smith, W. R., Bovbjerg, V. E., McClish, D. K., & Levenson, J. L. (2007). Patient satisfaction in specialized versus nonspecialized adult sickle cell care centers: The PISCES Study. *Journal of the National Medical Association, 99*, 886–890.

Alexander, L. R., Allerman-Velez, P. L., Loosier, P. S., Simmons, J., & Telfair, J. (2004). Providers' perspectives and beliefs regarding transition to adult care for adolescents with sickle cell disease. *Journal of Health Care for the Poor and Underserved, 15*, 443–461.

Allison, A. C. (1954). Incidence of malarial parasitaemia in African children with and without sickle cell trait. *British Medical Journal, i*, 290–294.

Almeida, A., & Roberts, L. (2005). Bone involvement in sickle cell disease. *British Journal of Haematology, 129*, 482–490.

American Academy of Pediatrics Newborn Screening Taskforce. (2000). Serving the family from birth to the medical home. Newborn screening: A blueprint for the future. *Pediatrics, 106*, 383 – 427.

American Pain Society. (1999). *Guideline for the management of acute and chronic pain in sickle cell disease*. Glenview, IL: Author.

Armstrong, F. D., Thompson, R. J., Wang, W., Zimmerman, R., Pegelow, C. H., Miller, S., et al. (1996). Cognitive functioning and brain magnetic resonance imaging in children with sickle cell disease. *Pediatrics, 97*, 864–870.

Ballas, S. K. (1998). *Sickle cell pain: Progress in pain research and management*. Seattle, WA: International Association for the Study of Pain Press.

Barakat, L. P., Lash, L., Lutz, L. M., & Nicolaow, D. C. (2006). Psychosocial adaptation of children and adolescents with sickle cell disease. In R. T. Brown (Ed.), *Comprehensive handbook of childhood cancer and sickle cell disease: A biopsychosocial approach* (pp. 471–495). New York: Oxford University Press.

Barakat, L. P., Lutz, M., Smith-Whitley, K., & Ohene-Frempong, K. (2005). Is treatment adherence associated with better quality of life in children with sickle cell disease? *Quality of Life Research, 14*, 407–414.

Barakat, L. P., Lutz, M. J., Nicolaou, D. C., & Lash, L. A. (2005). Parental locus of control and family functioning in the quality of life of children with sickle cell disease. *Journal of Clinical Psychology in Medical Settings, 12*, 323–331.

Barakat, L. P., Patterson, C. A., Weinberger, B. S., Simon, K., Gonzalez, E. R., & Dampier, C. (2007). A prospective study of the role of coping and family functioning in health outcomes for adolescents with sickle cell disease. *Journal of Pediatric Hematology and Oncology, 29*, 752–760.

Barakat, L. P., Smith-Whitley, K., & Ohene-Frempong, K. (2002). Treatment adherence in children with sickle cell disease: Disease-related risk and psychosocial resistance factors. *Journal of Clinical Psychology in Medical Settings, 9*, 201–209.

Barbarin, O. (1999). Do parental coping, involvement, religiosity, and racial identity mediate children's psychological adjustment to sickle cell disease? *Journal of Black Psychology, 25*, 391–426.

Barbarin, O., Whitten, C., Bond, S., & Conner-Warren, R. (1999). The social and cultural context of coping with sickle cell disease: III. Stress, coping tasks, and family functioning, and children's adjustment. *Journal of Black Psychology, 25,* 356–377.

Baskin, M. L., Collins, M. H., Brown, F., Griffith, J. R., Samuels, D., Moody, A., et al. (1998). Psychosocial considerations in sickle cell disease (SCD): The transition from adolescence to young adulthood. *Journal of Clinical Psychology in Medical Settings, 5,* 315–341.

Bellet, P., Kalinyak, K. A., Rakesh, S., Elfand, M., & Rucknagel, D. (1995). Incentive spirometry to prevent acute pulmonary complications in sickle cell disease. *New England Journal of Medicine, 333,* 699–703.

Bernaudin, F., Socie, G., Kuentz, M., Chevret, S., Duval, M., Bertrand, Y., et al. (2007). Long-term results of related, myeloablative stem cell transplantation to cure sickle cell disease. *Blood, 110,* 2749–2756.

Benjamin, L. J., Swinson, G. I., & Nagel, R. L. (2000). Sickle cell anemia day hospital: An approach for the management of uncomplicated painful crises. *Blood, 95,* 1130–1137.

Beyer, J. E., & Simmons, L. E. (2004). Home treatment of pain for children and adolescents with sickle cell disease. *Pain Management in Nursing, 5,* 126–135.

Blechman, E. A. (1992). Mentors for high-risk minority youth: From effective communication to bicultural competence. *Journal of Clinical Child Psychology, 21,* 160–169.

Brawley, O. W., Cornelius, L. J., Edwards, L. R., Gamble, V., Green, B., Inturrisi, C., et al. (2008). National Institute of Health Consensus Development Conference statement: Hydroxyurea treatment for sickle cell disease. *Annals of Internal Medicine, 148,* 932–938.

Brown, R. T., Lambert, R., Devine, D., Baldwin, K., Casey, R., Doepke, K., et al. (2000). Risk-resistance adaptation model for caregivers and their children with sickle cell syndromes. *Annals of Behavioral Medicine, 22,* 158–169.

Casey, R., Brown, R. T., & Bakeman, R. (2000). Predicting adjustment in children and adolescents with sickle cell disease: A test of the risk–resistance–adaptation model. *Rehabilitation Psychology, 45,* 155–178.

Castro, O., Brambilla, D. J., Thorington, B., Reindorf, C. A., Scott, R. B., Gillette, P., et al. (1994). The acute chest syndrome in sickle cell disease: Incidence and risk factors in the cooperative study of sickle cell disease. *Blood, 8,* 643–649.

Charache, S., Terrin, M. L., Moore, R. D., Dover, G. J., Barton, F. B., Eckert, S. V., et al. (1995). Effect of hydroxyurea on the frequency of painful crises in sickle cell anemia. *New England Journal of Medicine, 332,* 1317–1322.

Chen, E., Cole, S. W., & Kato, P. M. (2004). A review of empirically supported psychosocial interventions for pain and adherence outcomes in sickle cell disease. *Journal of Pediatric Psychology, 29,* 197–209.

Dampier, C., Ely, B., Brodecki, D., & O'Neal, P. (2002). Characteristics of pain managed at home in children and adolescents with sickle cell disease using diary self-reports. *Journal of Pain, 3,* 461–470.

Day, S., & Chismark, E. (2006). The cognitive and academic impact of sickle cell disease. *Journal of School Nursing, 22,* 330–335.

Eaton, W. A., & Hofrichter, J. (1990). Sickle cell hemoglobin polymerization. *Advances in Protein Chemistry, 40,* 63–79.

Franck, L. S., Treadwell, M., Jacob, E., & Vichnisky, E. (2002). Assessment of sickle cell pain in children and young adults using the Adolescent Pediatric Pain Tool. *Journal of Pain and Symptom Management, 23,* 114–120.

Frempong, K. O. (1991). Stroke in sickle cell disease: Demographic, clinical and therapeutic considerations. *Seminars in Hematology, 28,* 213–219.

Gaston, M. H., Verter, J. I., Woods, G., Pegelow, C., Kelleher, J., Presbury, G., et al. (1986). Prophylaxis with oral penicillin in children with sickle cell anemia: A randomized trial. *New England Journal of Medicine, 314,* 1593–1599.

Gil, K. M., Carson, J. W., Porter, L. S., Ready, J., Valrie, C., Redding-Lallinger, R., et al. (2003).

Daily stress and mood and their association with pain, health-care use, and school activity in adolescents with sickle cell disease. *Journal of Pediatric Psychology*, *28*, 363–373.

Gil, K. M., Porter, L., Ready, J., Workman, E., Sedway, J., & Anthony, K. K. (2000). Pain in children and adolescents with sickle cell disease: An analysis of daily pain diaries. *Children's Health Care*, *29*, 225–241.

Haque, A. K., Gokhale, S., Rampy, B. A., Adegboyega, P., Duarte, A., Saldana, M. J., et al. (2002). Pulmonary hypertension in sickle cell hemoglobinopathy: A clinicopathologic study of 20 cases. *Human Pathology*, *33*, 1037–1043.

Herron, S., Bacak, S. J., King, A., & DeBaum, M. R. (2003). Inadequate recognition of educational resources required for high-risk students with sickle cell disease. *Archives of Pediatrics and Adolescent Medicine*, *157*, 104.

Hogan, A. M., Kirkham, F. J., Prengler, M., Telfer, P., Lane, R., Vargha-Khadem, F., et al. (2006). An exploratory study of physiological correlates of neurodevelopmental delay in infants with sickle cell anemia. *British Journal of Haematology*, *132*, 99–107.

Ingram, V. M. (1956). A specific chemical difference between globins of normal and sickle-cell anemia hemoglobins. *Nature*, *178*, 792–794.

Kell, R. S., Kliewer, W., Erickson, M. T., & Ohene-Frempong, K. (1998). Psychological adjustment of adolescents with sickle cell disease: Relations with demographic, medical, and family competence variables. *Journal of Pediatric Psychology*, *23*, 301–312.

Kinney, T. R., & Ware, R. E. (1996). The adolescent with sickle cell anemia. *Hematology/Oncology Clinics of North America*, *10*, 1255–1264.

Kontessis, P., Mayopoulou-Symvoulidis, D., Symvoulidis, A., & Kontopoulou-Griva, I. (1992). Renal involvement in sickle cell-beta thalassemia. *Nephronology*, *61*, 10–15.

Kral, M. C., Brown, R. T., Connelly, M., Cure, J. K., Besenski, N., Jackson, S. M., et al. (2006). Radiographic predictors of neurocognitive functioning in pediatric sickle cell disease. *Journal of Child Neurology*, *21*, 37–44.

Kral, M. C., Brown, R. T., & Hynd, G. W. (2001). Neuropsychological aspects of pediatric sickle cell disease. *Neuropsychology Review*, *11*, 179–196.

Leong, M. A., Dampier, C., Varlotta, L., & Allen, J. L. (1997). Airway hyperreactivity in children with sickle cell disease. *Journal of Pediatrics*, *131*, 278–283.

Logan, D. E., Radcliffe, J., & Smith-Whitley, K. (2202). Parent factors and adolescent sickle cell disease: Associations with patterns of health service use. *Journal of Pediatric Psychology*, *27*, 475–484.

Lutz, M. J., Barakat, L. P., Smith-Whitley, K., & Ohene-Frempong, K. (2004). Psychological adjustment of children with sickle cell disease: Family functioning and coping. *Rehabilitation Psychology*, *49*, 224–232.

Maikler, V. E., Broome, M. E., Bailey, P., & Lea, G. (2001). Children's and adolescents' use of diaries for sickle cell pain. *Journal of the Society of Pediatric Nursing*, *6*, 161–169.

Midence, K., Fuggle, P., & Davies, S. C. (1993). Psychosocial aspects of sickle cell disease (SCD) in childhood and adolescence: A review. *British Journal of Clinical Psychology*, *11*, 271–280.

Miller, S. T., Macklin, E. A., Pegelow, C. H., Kinney, T. R., Sleeper, L. A., Bello, J. A., et al. (2001). Silent infarction as a risk factor for overt stroke in children with sickle cell anemia: A report from the Cooperative Study of Sickle Cell Disease. *Journal of Pediatrics*, *139*, 385–390.

Mitchell, M. J., Lemanek, K., Palermo, T. M., Crosby, L. E., Nichols, A., & Powers, S. W. (2007). Parent perspectives on pain management, coping, and family functioning in pediatric sickle cell disease. *Clinical Pediatrics*, *46*, 311–319.

Modi, A. C., Crosby, L. E., Guilfoyle, S. M., Lemanek, K. L., Witherspoon, D., & Mitchell, M. J. (2009). Barriers to treatment adherence for pediatric patients with sickle cell disease and their families. *Children's Health Care*, *38*, 107–122.

Moser, F. G., Miller, S. T., Bello, J. A., Pegelow, C. H., Zimmerman, R. A., Wang, W. C., et al. (1996). The spectrum of brain MR abnormalities in sickle cell disease: A report from the cooperative study of sickle cell disease. *American Journal of Neuroradiology, 17,* 965–972.

National Heart, Lung, and Blood Institute (NHLBI). (1996). *Sickle cell anemia* (NIH Publication No. 96-4057). Washington, DC: U.S. Government Printing Office.

Noll, R. B., Reiter-Purtill, J., Vannatta, K., Gerhardt, C. A., & Short, A. (2007). Peer relationships and emotional well-being of children with sickle cell disease. A controlled replication. *Child Neuropsychology, 13,* 173–187.

Noll, R. B., Stith, L., Gartstein, M. A., Ris, M. D., Grueneich, R., Vannatta, K., et al. (2001). Neuropsychological functioning of youths with sickle cell disease: Comparisons with non-chronically ill peers. *Journal of Pediatric Psychology, 26,* 69–78.

Noll, R. B., Vannatta, K., Koontz, K., Kalinyak, K., Bukowski, W. M., & Davies, W. H. (1996). Peer relationships and emotional well-being of youngsters with sickle cell disease. *Child Development, 67,* 423–436.

Northington, L. (2000). Chronic sorrow in caregivers of school age children with sickle cell disease: A grounded theory approach. *Issues in Comprehensive Pediatric Nursing, 23,* 141–154.

Palermo, T. M., Schwartz, L., Drotar, D., & McGowan, K. (2002). Parental report of health-related quality of life in children with sickle cell disease. *Journal of Behavior Medicine, 25,* 269–283.

Peterson, C. C., Palermo, T. M., Swift, E., Beebe, A., & Drotar, D. (2005). Assessment of psychoeducational needs in a clinical sample of children with sickle cell disease. *Children's Health Care, 34,* 133–148.

Platt, O. S., Brambilia, D. J., Rosse, W. F., Milner, P. F., Castro, O., Steinberg, M. H., et al. (1994). Mortality in sickle cell disease: Life expectancy and risk factors for early death. *New England Journal of Medicine, 330,* 1639–1644.

Powers, S. W., Mitchell, M. J., Graumlich, S. E., Byars, K. C., & Kalinyak, K. A. (2002). Longitudinal assessment of pain, coping, and daily functioning in children with sickle cell disease receiving pain management skills training. *Journal of Clinical Psychology in Medical Settings, 9,* 109–119.

Quinn, C. T., Lee, N. J., Shull, E. P., Ahmad, N., Rogers, Z. R., & Buchanan, G. R. (2008). Prediction of adverse outcomes in children with sickle cell anemia: A study of the Dallas newborn cohort. *Blood, 111,* 544–548.

Rao, R., & Kramer, L. (1993). Stress and coping among mothers of infants with a sickle cell condition. *Children's Health Care, 22,* 169–188.

Rosse, W. F., Gallagher, D., Kinney, T. R., Castro, O., Dosik, H., Moohr, J., et al. (1990). Transfusion and alloimmunization in sickle cell disease: The Cooperative Study of Sickle Cell Disease. *Blood, 76,* 1431–1437.

Royal, C. D., Headings, V. E., Harrell, J. P., Ampy, F. R., & Hall, G. W. (2000). Coping strategies in families of children with sickle cell disease. *Ethnicity and Disease, 10,* 237–247.

Schaeffer, J. J., Gil, K. M., Burchinal, M., Kramer, K. D., Nash, K. B., Orringer, E., et al. (1999). Depression, disease severity, and sickle cell anemia. *Journal of Behavioral Medicine, 22,* 115–126.

Schatz, J., Brown, R. T., Pascual, J. M., Hsu, L., & DeBaun, M. R. (2001). Poor school and cognitive functioning with silent cerebral infarction and sickle cell disease. *Neurology, 56,* 1109–1111.

Schatz, J., Finke, R., Kellet, J., & Kramer, J. (2002). Cognitive functioning in children with sickle cell disease: A meta-analysis. *Journal of Pediatric Psychology, 278,* 739–748.

Schatz, J., & Roberts, C. W. (2007). Neurodevelopmental impact of sickle cell disease in early childhood. *Journal of the International Neuropsychological Society, 13,* 933–943.

Schuman, W. B., Armstrong, F. D., Pegelow, C. H., & Routh, D. K. (1993). Enhanced parenting knowledge and skills in mothers of preschool children with sickle cell disease. *Journal of Pediatric Psychology, 18,* 575–591.

Schwartz, L. A., Radcliffe, J., & Barakat, L. P. (2007). The development of a culturally sensitive pediatric pain management intervention of African-American adolescents with sickle cell disease. *Children's Health Care, 36,* 267–283.

Serjeant, G. R. (1992). *Sickle cell disease* (2nd ed.). New York: Oxford University Press.

Steiner, C. A., & Miller, J. L. (2006). *Sickle cell disease patients in U.S. hospitals, 2004* (Statistical Brief No. 21). Rockville, MD: Agency for Healthcare Research and Quality.

Telfair, J., Ehiri, J. E., Loosier, P. S., & Baskin, M. L. (2004). Transition to adult care for adolescents with sickle cell disease: Results of a national survey. *International Journal of Adolescent Medical and Health, 16,* 47–64.

Thompson, R. J., Armstrong, F. D., Kronenberger, W. G., Scott, D., McCabe, M. A., Smith, B., et al. (1999). Family functioning, neurocognitive functioning, and behavior problems in children with sickle cell disease. *Journal of Pediatric Psychology, 24,* 491–498.

Thompson, R. J., Armstrong, F. D., Link, C. L., Pegelow, C. H., Moser, F., & Wang, W. C. (2003). A prospective study of the relationship over time of behavior problems, intellectual functioning, and family functioning in children with sickle cell disease: A report from the Cooperative Study of Sickle Cell Disease. *Journal of Pediatric Psychology, 28,* 59–65.

Thompson, R. J., Gustafson, K. E., Bonner, M. J., & Ware, R. E. (2002). Neurocognitive development of young children with sickle cell disease through three years of age. *Journal of Pediatric Psychology, 27,* 235–244.

Vermylen, C., Cornu, G., Ferster, A., Brichard, B., Ninane, J., Ferrant, A., et al. (1998). Haematopoietic stem cell transplantation for sickle cell anaemia: The first 50 patients transplanted in Belgium. *Bone Marrow Transplant, 22,* 1–6.

Wagner, J. L., Connelly, M., Brown, R. T., Taylor, L., Rittle, C., & Wall-Cloues, B. (2004). Predictors of social anxiety in children and adolescents with sickle cell disease. *Journal of Clinical Psychology in Medical Settings, 11,* 243–252.

Walters, M. C., Patience, M., Leisening, W., Eckman, J. R., Scott, J. P., Mentzer, W. C., et al. (1996). Bone marrow transplantation for sickle cell disease. *New England Journal of Medicine, 335,* 369–376.

While, A. E., & Mullen, J. (2004). Living with sickle cell disease: The perspective of young people. *British Journal of Nursing, 13,* 320–325.

Witherspoon, D., & Drotar, D. (2006). Correlates of adherence to prophylactic penicillin therapy in children with sickle cell disease. *Children's Health Care, 35,* 281–296.

Yarbro, J. W. (1992). Mechanisms of action of hydroxyurea. *Seminars in Oncology, 9,* 1–10.

Zemel, B., Kawchak, D., Ohene-Frempong, K., Schall, J., & Stallings, V. (2007). Effects of delayed pubertal development, nutritional status, and disease severity on longitudinal patterns of growth failure in children with sickle cell disease. *Pediatric Research, 61,* 607–613.

CHAPTER 21

Pediatric Oncology
Progress and Future Challenges

KATHRYN VANNATTA
CHRISTINA G. SALLEY
CYNTHIA A. GERHARDT

Over 12,000 individuals under the age of 20 are diagnosed with cancer each year in the United States (Ries et al., 2006). Although cancer remains the leading cause of death by disease among children, 5-year survival rates now approach 80% overall, and 1 in every 640 young adults is now a survivor of childhood cancer (Lipschitz, Weiner, & Hewitt, 2005). Unfortunately, this progress has been achieved with aggressive medical protocols that create risk for substantial long-term morbidity and threaten quality of life for survivors. Consequently, pediatric psychologists share the challenge of informing and establishing models of care to meet the diverse needs of a growing number of survivors (Rowland, 2005), as well as applying biopsychosocial (Armstrong, 2006) and family ecological (Alderfer & Kazak, 2006) perspectives to the care of children undergoing active treatment. This chapter provides an overview of the short- and long-term impact of pediatric cancer on children and their families, highlighting evidence of both positive and negative outcomes. Particular emphasis is given to the challenges faced by survivors, as well as to models of care and emerging areas of research.

Adjustment of Children and Families during Cancer Treatment

A few decades ago, clinicians and researchers were primarily concerned with the damaging psychological effects of an almost certainly terminal diagnosis on children and their parents (Koocher & O'Malley, 1981), as well as with interventions to improve children's tolerance of treatment that inevitably involved pain, nausea, and conditioned aversions to procedures and settings (Zeltzer, 1994). Despite improvements in survival and supportive medical care, numerous stressors remain that could threaten the adjustment of children with cancer (Sloper, 2000). These include frequent clinic visits and hospitalizations for systemic treatment and invasive procedures, management of side effects (e.g., infection), and monitoring of disease status. Moreover, complicated regimens for medical care at home (e.g., oral medications, intravenous catheter care, and behavioral recommendations to prevent infection) are often met with high rates of nonadherence (Rapoff, McGrath, & Smith, 2006). School attendance and extracurricular activities are often disrupted for children (Katz & Madan-Swain, 2006), while parents struggle with financial and other practical burdens of treatment that may interfere with employment. In addition to all this, parents must master complex medical information (Mack et al., 2007), make treatment decisions (Kodish et al., 2004), manage the flow of information to their ill children (Young, Dixon-Woods, Windridge, & Heney, 2003) and support healthy siblings (Barrera, Fleming, & Fahn, 2004).

Psychologists often serve as consultants or as members of multidisciplinary teams in pediatric oncology. They assist with communication both within families and between families and the medical team, in order to facilitate coping and adjustment as well as treatment decision making. Behavioral interventions for symptom management have been empirically validated and maintain a role in clinical care, despite the growth of pharmacological approaches (e.g., antiemetics and procedural sedation techniques) (Powers, 1999; Tyc, Mulhern, Barclay, Smith, & Bieberich, 1997). Blount and colleagues (Chapter 11, this volume) provide empirically based suggestions for using age-appropriate preparation, imagery, distraction, and other cognitive-behavioral techniques (e.g., modeling and rehearsal) alone or in conjunction with pharmacological techniques to manage pain and distress, such as that experienced during cancer treatment. Although evaluation of interventions to improve adherence has been notably lacking in pediatric oncology, psychologists often collaborate with medical teams to monitor adherence; to identify individual and systemic risk factors for nonadherence; and to implement developmentally appropriate educational, cognitive-behavioral, and family-based intervention strategies that may be extrapolated from work in populations with other chronic illnesses (La Greca & Mackey, Chapter 9, this volume). Caregivers may benefit from assistance with problem-solving skills to manage competing demands or specific challenges. This approach may help caregivers reduce distress earlier in their children's treatment and may particularly benefit single mothers, who may have fewer social resources (Sahler et al., 2005).

Interestingly, most children with cancer do not evidence significant psychopathology (Patenaude & Kupst, 2005), and parents of children treated for cancer may be at greater risk for adverse psychological outcomes than the children themselves (Pai et al., 2007). Levels of child distress may be initially heightened compared to those of healthy children, but these appear to normalize over treatment (Sawyer, Antoniou, Toogood, Rice, & Baghurst, 2000). There is evidence that children with cancer may even demonstrate "better than average" social (Noll et al., 1999) and emotional (Dejong & Fombonne, 2006) functioning—results that this field has been slow to embrace (Phipps, 2005). In contrast, meta-analysis indicates that parents of children with cancer demonstrate mild to moderate distress relative to comparison samples (Pai et al., 2007). Effects appear stronger for mothers than fathers, and for parents of children on versus off treatment. Single mothers, and those with fewer resources, may be at greatest risk for distress and benefit most from assistance (Dolgin et al., 2007). Elevations in posttraumatic stress symptoms have been reported for parents during and after their children's treatment (Kazak et al., 2005). However, such symptoms may also be associated with positive outcomes or growth, such as stronger family relationships (Barakat, Alderfer, & Kazak, 2006). Kazak, Schneider, and Kassam-Adams (Chapter 13, this volume) describe a framework for conceptualizing and addressing traumatic stress at diagnosis, during treatment, and into survivorship.

Future research and models of care face the challenge of identifying risk factors and processes that account for variations in outcomes for children and families affected by cancer. Not all families may need intensive psychosocial services, and tools have been suggested to titrate services according to individual risk profiles (Kazak et al., 2007). Researchers are showing a growing interest in resilience, including work that examines differences in adaptive style (Phipps, 2007), positive affect and optimism (Bisko, Stern, Dillon, Russell, & Laver, 2008), and posttraumatic growth (Barakat et al., 2006). Work is needed that examines family processes as well as individual characteristics contributing to positive outcomes (Barakat, Pulgaron, & Daniel, Chapter 51, this volume). Creativity is needed to conceptualize outcomes beyond the presence or absence of dysfunction, and to integrate novel assessment strategies (e.g., physiological measures, direct observation techniques) with traditional questionnaire approaches.

Late Effects of Cancer Treatment: Neurocognitive, Physical, and Developmental Sequelae

Treatment for pediatric cancer typically requires intensive multiagent chemotherapy and may involve surgical resection or radiation. This treatment creates risk for physical and functional morbidity or "late effects" that emerge after treatment ends (Ness & Gurney, 2007). Some effects, such as impairments in growth, may be manifested during childhood; other late effects, such as cardiac toxicity, may not be apparent until adulthood. Neurological and cognitive late effects of central nervous system (CNS)–directed treatment often emerge after treatment and affect developmental outcomes and adjustment throughout childhood and adulthood (Mulhern & Butler, 2004).

Populations at Risk for Neurocognitive Late Effects

Acute lymphoblastic leukemia (ALL) is the most common form of pediatric cancer, peaking at the age of 4 and accounting for 23% of diagnoses before age 15 (Ries et al., 2006). Survival rates now exceed 80%, as opposed to 50% only 20 years ago. This was accomplished by clinical trials that evaluated doses of craniospinal irradiation (CSI), as well as systemic chemotherapy and intrathecal chemotherapy (i.e., administration of chemotherapy directly into the cerebrospinal fluid via lumbar puncture or spinal tap), to prevent relapse in the CNS (Gaynon, 1995). Neurocognitive declines resulted on these protocols (Cousens, Waters, Said, & Stevens, 1988), and current treatment for ALL reserves CSI for children at higher risk for relapse or CNS involvement. Current protocols, using multiple chemotherapies, are promising but continue to be evaluated for efficacy, as well as preservation of quality of life (Armstrong & Reaman, 2005).

Brain tumors account for 17% of cancer diagnoses and are the most common solid tumors diagnosed before age 20 (Ries et al., 2006). Although brain tumors vary in location, histology, growth patterns, response to treatment, and prognosis, overall survival rates now exceed 65%. Neurodevelopmental risk may result from the tumor mass and perioperative complications, as well as from radiation and chemotherapy directed at the CNS (Ris & Noll, 1994).

Nature and Extent of CNS Late Effects

Pediatric psychologists and neuropsychologists have helped to identify significant consequences of CNS malignancies and CNS-directed treatments, including the nature and timing of sequelae, as well as demographic, diagnostic, and treatment variables associated with increased risk (Mulhern & Butler, 2004). Early studies of neurocognitive outcomes in children with ALL (e.g., Cousens et al., 1988; Stehbens et al., 1991) and brain tumors (Mulhern, Hancock, Fairclough, & Kun, 1992) identified declines in global IQ and academic functioning. Subsequent work focused on specific neuropsychological skills and found that core deficits in attention, working memory, processing speed, executive functions, and fluid abilities led to erosion in broader indicators of cognitive and academic functioning (Campbell et al., 2007; Mulhern & Butler, 2004). A recent meta-analysis by Campbell and colleagues (2007) indicates that moderate deficits ($d = -0.34$ to -0.66) occur for survivors of ALL on measures of attention, information processing, executive functioning, verbal and visual memory, psychomotor and visual–spatial skills, Verbal and Performance IQ, and academic functioning. Longitudinal evaluation indicates that progressive declines represent failures to make age-appropriate gains, rather than a loss of skills or previously acquired knowledge (Palmer et al., 2003).

The neurocognitive impact of cancer treatment is moderated by variations in child characteristics, as well as by variations in treatment (Mulhern & Butler, 2004). Although combinations of whole-brain and focal radiation can complicate evaluation of dose effects (Ris et al., 2005), declines in neurocognitive functioning appear to vary with the dose of whole-brain radiation (Jankovic et al., 1994; Mulhern et al., 1998). Girls (Brown et al., 1998; Waber et al., 1995) and younger children (Mulhern et al., 1998; Reimers et al., 2003) have greater neuropsychological deficits following CNS-directed radiation and chemotherapy. There has been consistent evidence of deficits for children under age 3 (Kaleita, Reaman, MacLean, Sather, & Whitt, 1999), with other studies suggesting deficits for children age 7 and younger (Radcliffe et al., 1992). The interaction of radiation dose and a child's age at the time of treatment may be critical (Fuss, Poljanc, & Hug, 2000; Silber et al., 1992). Fuss and colleagues (2000) concluded that although younger children were vulnerable to varying doses of cranial radiation therapy (CRT), only children over age 6 displayed deficits in Full Scale IQ after high levels of radiation (i.e., 2,400 centigray [cGy]), which exceeds doses in current ALL protocols.

Disease and treatment factors other than radiation may also contribute to neurological and neurocognitive late effects. There are neurotoxic effects of intrathecal, intravenous, and oral chemotherapies such as methotrexate and corticosteroids (Moleski, 2000; Waber et al., 2000), and combinations of chemotherapy and CRT may be more neurotoxic than either alone (Riva et al., 2002; Waber et al., 1995). Substitution of different or higher doses of chemotherapy when CRT is reduced or avoided may lead to comparable deficits in neurocognitive functioning (Moleski, 2000; Mulhern et al., 1998). Neuroimaging has linked postradiation declines in cognitive functioning with diffuse white matter loss or demyelinization (Mulhern et al., 2001). White matter volume is significantly correlated with IQ scores for irradiated patients (Mulhern et al., 1999). Thus a disproportionate loss of normal white matter in frontal lobe, posterior cortical, and subcortical areas may account for disruptions in executive functions in children receiving CRT (Mulhern & Butler, 2004).

Trauma to brain tissue may be associated with an intracranial mass, as well as surgical resection and postoperative complications such as hydrocephalus, infection, and seizures (Chapman et al., 1995). Children who receive only surgical resection for brain tumors also demonstrate deficits in attention, memory, and processing speed (Steinlin et al., 2003). Clear associations between tumor location and neurocognitive and psychosocial functioning have not been demonstrated, perhaps due to challenges in differentiating the effects of tumor location from those of age at onset, growth characteristics, and treatment (Ris & Noll, 1994).

Specific recommendations for ongoing assessment, intervention, and advocacy related to neurocognitive risk in survivors have been published by the Children's Oncology Group (Nathan et al., 2007). Pharmacological and rehabilitative approaches have been employed to target neurocognitive deficits (Butler & Mulhern, 2005). Butler and colleagues (2008) evaluated a multicomponent cognitive remediation program to improve sustained attention and attentional control, in which repetitive computerized training, training in metacognitive strategies, and cognitive-behavioral skills were used to promote adaptive coping with cognitive dysfunction. Interestingly, this intervention called for teachers and parents to encourage generalization of these skills, thus combining ecological and patient-centered approaches. Significant intervention effects were found on performance measures of academic achievement and on parent ratings, but not objective measures, of attention. Computerized training targeting the deficits in phonetic skills that are thought to underlie reading impairments is also being evaluated and could be a future direction for intervention (Palmer, Reddick, & Gaijar, 2007). Further development of these approaches, and demonstration of their effectiveness when disseminated in broader practice, will be challenges for the future.

Interrelation of Neurocognitive Late Effects and Social, Emotional, and Behavioral Functioning

Risk and resilience models of child development and developmental psychopathology emphasize the interdependence of biological, cognitive, emotional, and social development within individuals and across development (Cicchetti & Cohen, 2006). Unfortunately, only limited research has examined the processes by which medical risk factors and neurocognitive late effects shape developmental outcomes. Children with ALL represent a significant proportion of samples that have demonstrated resilient outcomes during and shortly after treatment (e.g., Noll et al., 1999). However, a large epidemiological study suggested that adolescent survivors of ALL and brain tumors may be at increased risk for symptoms of depression and anxiety, inattention, and social difficulties, relative to siblings and to adolescents treated for other types of cancer (Schultz et al., 2007). CRT, with or without intrathecal methotrexate, was predictive of these outcomes—a pattern congruent with some (Hill et al., 1998; Vannatta, Gerhardt, Wells, & Noll, 2007), but not all (Noll et al., 1997), studies. It is interesting that the latter study did not include children who received the higher doses of CRT (2,400 vs. 1,800 cGy) common to early protocols. In addition, Vannatta and colleagues (2007) found associations between the intensity of CNS treatment and social functioning only for children who were treated at a young age.

Psychosocial difficulties have been increasingly documented for children following treatment for brain tumors (Fuemmeler, Elkin, & Mullins, 2002). Internalizing problems have been described from multiple sources, but more so from the perspective of parents than of children themselves (Carpentieri et al., 2003; Poggi et al., 2005; Ribi et al., 2005). This could reflect a repressive adaptive style (Phipps, 2007) or difficulty in obtaining valid self-reports from children with cognitive difficulties (Tao & Parsons, 2005). Social withdrawal, isolation, and reduced participation in social activities have been frequently described by brain tumor survivors, as well as by their parents, teachers, and classmates (Aarsen et al., 2006; Poggi et al., 2005; Schultz et al., 2007). Children treated for brain tumors are more likely to be bullied or victimized by peers and to have difficulty establishing or maintaining friendships (Vance, Eiser, & Horne, 2004; Vannatta, Gartstein, Short, & Noll, 1998). These difficulties may be greater following CRT and/or CNS-directed chemotherapy (Holmquist & Scott, 2002; Ribi et al., 2005; Schultz et al., 2007), but problems also remain for children who only receive surgical resection (Aarsen et al., 2006).

The consequences of cancer and of cancer treatment that involves the CNS are likely to extend well past childhood. Survivors of pediatric brain tumors are less likely to be employed in adulthood (de Boer, Verbeek, & van Dijk, 2006), perhaps reflecting the continuation of CNS late effects and prior deficits in academic achievement and progress (Brown et al., 1998; Langeveld et al., 2003; Mitby et al., 2003). Adult survivors of pediatric brain tumors are also more likely to be single, particularly if they are males (Frobisher, Lancashire, Winter, Jenkinson, & Hawkins, 2007; Langeveld et al., 2003), which could reflect deficits in social competence or in establishment of economic independence. Finally, adults who received CRT during treatment for pediatric cancer appear to represent a subset of survivors at risk for persistent impairments in quality of life (Langeveld, Stam, Grootenhuis, & Last, 2002).

Research examining mechanisms that account for links between neurocognitive late effects and more distal psychosocial and developmental outcomes has been quite limited. Correlations have been reported among broad indicators of intellectual functioning, verbal memory, learning deficits, and social withdrawal (Holmquist & Scott, 2002; Poggi et al., 2005), but this work has been exploratory and not based on theoretical models of how core neurocognitive deficits influence social and emotional adaptation. Models of social information processing recognize that attention, executive functions, and emotion regulation play a key role in the execution of social problem solving (Yeates et al., 2007). There is some evidence that pediatric brain tumor survivors have social problem-solving deficits (Lewis, Morris, Morris, & Foster, 2000) and demonstrate biases in their recognition of nonverbal emotional cues (Bonner, Hardy, Willard, & Hutchinson, 2008)—a skill that has been associated with peer acceptance (Nowicki & Duke, 1994). Campbell and colleagues (2007) have suggested that neurocognitive late effects may influence subsequent emotional and behavioral functioning via alterations in coping strategies that are dependent on higher-order executive functions (Compas, 2006). Data with a small sample of adolescents treated for ALL showed evidence of covariation among measures of memory and cognitive flexibility, coping, and emotional–behavioral functioning. Further investigation of this model is warranted, particularly with youths at heightened risk for neurocognitive late effects.

Finally, further investigations of family functioning in relation to neurocognitive late effects are needed (Peterson & Drotar, 2006). Family resources and processes may moderate the impact of cancer treatment on these outcomes or the extent to which neurocognitive late effects alter psychosocial outcomes (Carlson-Green, Morris, & Krawiecki, 1995). In addition, morbidity experienced by survivors may create elevated demands on families that could disrupt parent and family functioning (Foley, Barakat, Herman-Liu, Radcliffe, & Molloy, 2000).

Health Challenges Associated with Survivorship

Survivors of pediatric cancer are at marked risk for physical late effects, including organ damage, functional impairments, and secondary malignancies that may require primary treatment and could affect quality of life (Ness & Gurney, 2007). Data suggest that two-thirds of adult survivors of pediatric cancer have at least one such late effect, a third report two or more, and a quarter report a severe or life-threatening condition (Oeffinger et al., 2006). These can include cardiovascular, endocrine, orthopedic, neurological, sensory–motor, respiratory, renal, or reproductive impairments that can range from mild to severe. Variations in growth and body mass index are evident for survivors, with elevated risk of obesity for some (e.g., survivors of ALL who are female or receive high levels of CRT) and short stature and underweight for others (e.g., brain tumor survivors who received adjuvant therapies) (Gurney et al., 2008; Meacham et al., 2005; Oeffinger et al., 2003). Secondary malignancies may occur, particularly skin cancer or brain, bone, testicular, and breast tumors within prior fields of radiation therapy (Yeazel et al., 2004). These late effects contribute to a mortality rate among survivors that is nearly 11 times higher than that of the general U.S. population (Mertens et al., 2001). Health challenges among survivors emerge over time after treatment completion and may not become evident until adulthood. Consequently, behavioral factors that attenuate or exacerbate risk for health problems have become a focus of interest for clinicians and researchers. Attention is particularly warranted for patterns of health behaviors that may become established during adolescence (Tercyak & Tyc, 2006).

Much of our knowledge about the physical late effects of treatment for pediatric cancer has been obtained through epidemiological studies of older adolescent and adult survivors. The Childhood Cancer Survivorship Study has assessed the relative risk of diverse health outcomes in a sample of over 14,000 survivors and 3,000 siblings (Robison et al., 2002). Sufficient numbers of participants have allowed assessment of outcomes as a function of diagnostic and treatment risk factors, but reliance on self-report questionnaires and phone interviews has provided limited detail about processes of interest. Additional approaches are needed to identify behavioral practices that may moderate risk over time and contribute to the development of secondary prevention strategies. Prospective evaluation is needed of theoretically based individual factors (e.g., health beliefs and readiness) and contextual factors (e.g., family, peer, and community) evident during childhood and adolescence that are associated with health behaviors, as well as with intermediate and distal health outcomes (Ford & Ostroff, 2006; Tercyak et al., 2004). Factors that influence health screening behaviors (e.g., self-exams and medical follow-up), reductions in health risk behaviors (e.g., tobacco, alcohol, and drug use), and promotion of positive health behaviors (e.g., sunscreen usage, physical activity) are all warranted. As children progress through adolescence and into adulthood, they assume increasing autonomy for their health and health care practices, and early phases of survivorship may represent "teachable moments" for health promotion (Rowland, 2005).

Lifelong surveillance is recommended for early detection of secondary malignancies and severe late effects (Landier et al., 2004); however, by the time survivors are responsible for their own health care decisions, cancer screening self-exams (Yeazel et al., 2004) and medical follow-up (Oeffinger et al., 2004) fall short of recommendations. Although involvement in some risk-taking and health-compromising behaviors, such as experimentation with alcohol and tobacco, is normative during adolescence (Centers for Disease Control and Prevention, 2008), such actions may have heightened consequences for youths at risk for pulmonary, cardiac, or liver disease (Ford & Ostroff, 2006). Specific health risk behaviors, such as use of tobacco, alcohol, and illegal substances; unsafe sexual practices; and sun exposure without sunscreen may be equally or slightly less prevalent in survivors than in the general population (Clarke & Eiser, 2007). Individuals who engage in one risk behavior may be more likely to engage in others, further threatening their health (Butterfield et al., 2004). Data suggest that adolescent survivors do perceive heightened health vulnerability (Tyc, Hudson, & Hinds, 1999); however, perceived vulnerability has been inconsistently associated with teens' reported health behaviors and intent to engage in future risk behaviors (Tyc, Hadley, & Crockett, 2001; Tyc et al., 2005).

Interest has grown in promotion of health behaviors, such as physical activity and healthy nutrition. Survivors may be at risk for being either overweight or underweight, depending on specific disease and treatment risk factors (Meacham et al., 2005). Suboptimal bone mineral density, body composition, and muscle strength may all be additional risks, particularly among survivors of ALL or those who received radiation for brain tumors (Ness et al., 2007). Reduced physical activity and quality of life may be linked to these health risks (Odame et al., 2006). Research suggests that adolescent cancer survivors are as likely as, but not more likely than, the general population to engage in health-promoting behaviors (e.g., exercise, diet, sleep, seat belt use) (Mulhern et al., 1995). Perceived barriers to specific health behaviors such as exercise and a low-fat diet may reflect general factors (e.g., poor weather, influence of friends, being too busy) rather than health-related factors (e.g., being too tired) (Arroyave et al., 2008).

Education about medical history and future health risks has been a cornerstone of models for long-term care (Hudson et al., 2004); however, deficits in knowledge are widespread among survivors. Kadan-Lottick and colleagues (2002) found that nearly 30% of 635 survivors over the age of 18 could not accurately report their diagnosis, and many were unaware of specific treatments they had received. Improved knowledge and appreciation of vulnerability may result from interventions, but such awareness does not necessarily translate into changes in health behaviors (Clarke & Eiser, 2007). Research is only beginning to consider theoretically based cognitive and behavioral factors, such as decision-making skills, health beliefs, and readiness, that may influence risk taking and health promotion (Emmons et al., 2003; Tercyak et al., 2004; Yeazel et al., 2004). This is expected to be an active area of research and program development in the years to come. Despite the need for lifelong follow-up for survivors of pediatric cancer, current practice falls short of this ideal. Numerous resources and guidelines are being developed to help survivors and providers tailor follow-up care that is specific to risk exposure (Oeffinger & Hudson, 2004); these include a detailed online resource (*www.survivorshipguidelines.org*) by the Children's Oncology Group. A great deal of work and multidisciplinary collaboration is needed to determine the best way to ensure utilization of resources.

In summary, rapid evolution in the field of oncology has led to new challenges and opportunities for pediatric psychologists. At this time, it appears as though the majority of children with cancer will demonstrate resilience during and after treatment; however, subgroups at risk for neurocognitive late effects may be at greater risk for social and developmental deficits. Survivors may need assistance in mastering and acting on knowledge of their specific health risks and health care needs. Pediatric psychologists can, and no doubt will, continue to make significant contributions to clinical services, research, and public policy regarding these challenges.

References

Aarsen, F. K., Paquier, P. F., Reddingius, R. E., Streng, I. C., Arts, W. F., Evera-Preesman, M., et al. (2006). Functional outcome after low-grade astrocytoma treatment in childhood. *Cancer, 106*, 396–402.

Alderfer, M. A., & Kazak, A. E. (2006). Family issues when a child is on treatment for cancer. In R. T. Brown (Ed.), *Comprehensive handbook of childhood cancer and sickle cell disease: A biopsychosocial approach* (pp. 53–74). New York: Oxford University Press.

Armstrong, F. D. (2006). Cancer and blood disorders in childhood: Biopsychosocial-developmental issues in assessment and treatment. In R. T. Brown (Ed.), *Comprehensive handbook of childhood cancer and sickle cell disease: A biopsychosocial approach* (pp. 17–32). New York: Oxford University Press.

Armstrong, F. D., & Reaman, G. H. (2005). Psychological research in childhood cancer: The Children's Oncology Group perspective. *Journal of Pediatric Psychology, 30*, 89–97.

Arroyave, W. D., Clipp, E., Miller, P. E., Jones, L. W., Ward, D. S., Bonner, M. J., et al. (2008). Childhood cancer survivors' perceived barriers to improving exercise and dietary behaviors. *Oncology Nursing Forum, 35*, 121–130.

Barakat, L. P., Alderfer, M. A., & Kazak, A. E. (2006). Posttraumatic growth in adolescent survivors of cancer and their mothers and fathers. *Journal of Pediatric Psychology, 31*, 413–419.

Barrera, M., Fleming, C., & Fahn, F. (2004). Social support and related factors associated with psychological adjustment of siblings of children with cancer. *Child: Care, Health, and Development, 30*, 103–111.

Bisko, M. J., Stern, J., Dillon, R., Russell, E. C., & Laver, J. (2008). Happiness and time perspective as potential mediators of quality of life and depression in adolescent cancer. *Pediatric Blood and Cancer, 50*, 613–619.

Bonner, M. J., Hardy, K. K., Willard, V. W., & Hutchinson, K. C. (2008). Brief report: Psychosocial functioning of fathers as primary caregivers of pediatric oncology patients. *Journal of Pediatric Psychology, 32*, 851–856.

Brown, R. T., Madan-Swain, A., Walco, G. A., Cherrick, I., Ievers, C. E., Conte, P. M., et al. (1998). Cognitive and academic late effects among children previously treated for acute lymphocytic leukemia receiving chemotherapy as CNS prophylaxis. *Journal of Pediatric Psychology, 23*, 333–340.

Butler, R. W., Copeland, D. R., Fairclough, D. L., Mulhern, R. K., Katz, E. R., Kazak, A. E., et al. (2008). A multicenter, randomized clinical trial of a cognitive remediation program for childhood survivors of pediatric malignancy. *Journal of Consulting and Clinical Psychology, 76*, 367–378.

Butler, R. W., & Mulhern, R. K. (2005). Neurocognitive interventions for children and adolescents surviving cancer. *Journal of Pediatric Psychology, 30*, 65–78.

Butterfield, R. M., Park, E. R., Puleo, E., Mertens, A., Gritz, E. R., Li, F. P., et al. (2004). Multiple risk behaviors among smokers in the Childhood Cancer Survivors Study Cohort. *Psycho-Oncology, 13*, 619–629.

Campbell, L. K., Scaduto, M., Sharp, W., Dufton, L., Van Slyke, D., Whitlock, J. A., et al. (2007). A meta-analysis of the neurocognitive sequelae of treatment for childhood acute lymphocytic leukemia. *Pediatric Blood and Cancer, 49*, 65–73.

Carlson-Green, B., Morris, R. D., & Krawiecki, N. (1995). Family and illness predictors of outcome in pediatric brain tumors. *Journal of Pediatric Psychology, 20*, 769–784.

Carpentieri, S. C., Meyer, E. A., Delaney, B. L., Victoria, M. L., Gannon, B. K., Doyle, J. M., et al. (2003). Psychosocial and behavioral functioning among pediatric brain tumor survivors. *Journal of Neuro-Oncology, 63*, 279–287.

Centers for Disease Control and Prevention. (2008). Youth risk behavior surveillance: United States 2007. Surveillance summaries. *Morbidity and Mortality Weekly Report, 57*(SS-4).

Chapman, C. A., Waber, D. P., Bernstein, J. H., Pomeroy, S. L., LaVally, B., Sallen, S. E., et al. (1995). Neurobehavioral and neurologic outcome in long-term survivors of posterior fossa brain tumors: Role of age and perioperative factors. *Journal of Child Neurology, 10*, 209–212.

Cicchetti, D., & Cohen, D. J. (Eds.). (2006). *Developmental psychopathology: Vol. 1. Theory and method* (2nd ed.). Hoboken, NJ: Wiley.

Clarke, S. A., & Eiser, C. (2007). Health behaviours in childhood cancer survivors: A systematic review. *European Journal of Cancer, 43*, 1373–1384.

Compas, B. E. (2006). Psychobiological processes of stress and coping: Implications for resilience in children and adolescents—comments on the papers of Romeo & McEwen and Fisher et al. *Annals of the New York Academy of Sciences, 1094*, 226–234.

Cousens, P., Waters, B., Said, J., & Stevens, M. (1988). Cognitive effects of cranial irradiation in leukaemia: A survey and meta-analysis. *Journal of Child Psychology and Psychiatry, 29*, 839–852.

de Boer, A. G., Verbeek, J. H., & van Dijk, F. J. (2006). Adult survivors of childhood cancer and unemployment: A meta-analysis. *Cancer, 107*, 1–11.

Dejong, M., & Fombonne, E. (2006). Depression in paediatric cancer: An overview. *Psycho-Oncology, 15*, 553–566.

Dolgin, M. J., Phipps, S., Fairclough, D. L., Sahler, O. J. Z., Askins, M., Noll, R. B., et al. (2007). Trajectories of adjustment in mothers of children with newly diagnosed cancer: A natural history investigation. *Journal of Pediatric Psychology, 32*, 771–782.

Emmons, K. M., Butterfield, R. M., Puleo, E., Park, E. R., Mertens, A., Gritz, E. R., et al. (2003). Smoking among participants in the childhood cancer survivors cohort: The Partnership for Health Study. *Journal of Clinical Oncology, 21*, 189–196.

Foley, B., Barakat, L. P., Herman-Liu, A., Radcliffe, J., & Molloy, P. (2000). The impact of childhood hypothalamic/chiasmatic brain tumors on child adjustment and family functioning. *Children's Health Care, 29*, 209–223.

Ford, J. S., & Ostroff, J. S. (2006). Health behaviors of childhood cancer survivors: What we've learned. *Journal of Clinical Psychology in Medical Settings, 13*, 151–167.

Frobisher, C., Lancashire, E. R., Winter, D. L., Jenkinson, H. C., & Hawkins, M. M. (2007). Long-term population-based marriage rates among adult survivors of childhood cancer in Britain. *International Journal of Cancer, 121*, 846–855.

Fuemmeler, B. F., Elkin, T. D., & Mullins, L. L. (2002). Survivors of childhood brain tumors: Behavioral, emotional, and social adjustment. *Clinical Psychology Review, 22*, 547–586.

Fuss, M., Poljanc, K., & Hug, E. B. (2000). Full Scale IQ (FSIQ) changes in children treated with whole brain and partial brain irradiation: A review and analysis. *Strahlenther Onkologia*, *176*, 573–581.

Gaynon, P. S. (1995). Acute leukemia in children. *Current Opinion in Hematology*, *2*, 240–246.

Gurney, J. G., Ness, K. K., Stovall, M., Wolden, S., Punyko, J. A., Neglia, J. P., et al. (2008). Final height and body mass index among adult survivors of childhood brain cancer: Childhood Cancer Survivor Study. *Journal of Clinical Endocrinology and Metabolism*, *88*, 4731–4739.

Hill, J. M., Kornblith, A. B., Jones, D., Freeman, A., Holland, J. F., Glicksman, A. S., et al. (1998). A comparative study of the long term psychosocial functioning of childhood acute lymphoblastic leukemia survivors treated by intrathecal methotrexate with or without cranial radiation. *Cancer*, *82*, 208–218.

Holmquist, L. A., & Scott, J. (2002). Treatment, age, and time-related predictors of behavioral outcome in pediatric brain tumor survivors. *Journal of Clinical Psychology in Medical Settings*, *9*, 315–321.

Hudson, M. M., Hester, A., Sweeney, T., Kippenbrock, S., Majcina, R., Vear, S., et al. (2004). A model of care for childhood cancer survivors that facilitates research. *Journal of Pediatric Oncology Nursing*, *21*, 170–174.

Jankovic, M., Brouwers, P., Valsecchi, M. G., Van Veldhuizen, A., Huisman, J., Kamphuis, R., et al. (1994). Association of 1800 cGy cranial irradiation with intellectual function in children with acute lymphoblastic leukaemia. ISPACC: International Study Group on Psychosocial Aspects of Childhood Cancer. *Lancet*, *344*, 224–227.

Kadan-Lottick, N. S., Robison, L. L., Gurney, J. G., Neglia, J. P., Yasui, Y., Hayashi, R., et al. (2002). Childhood cancer survivors' knowledge about their past diagnosis and treatment: Childhood Cancer Survivor Study. *Journal of the American Medical Association*, *287*, 1832–1839.

Kaleita, T. A., Reaman, G. H., MacLean, W. E., Sather, H. N., & Whitt, J. K. (1999). Neurodevelopmental outcome of infants with acute lymphoblastic leukemia: A Children's Cancer Group report. *Cancer*, *85*, 1859–1865.

Katz, E. R., & Madan-Swain, A. (2006). Maximizing school, academic, and social outcomes in children and adolescents with cancer. In R. T. Brown (Ed.), *Comprehensive handbook of childhood cancer and sickle cell disease: A biopsychosocial approach* (pp. 313–338). New York: Oxford University Press.

Kazak, A. E., Rourke, M. T., Alderfer, M. A., Pai, A., Reilly, A. F., & Meadows, A. T. (2007). Evidence-based assessment, intervention and psychosocial care in pediatric oncology: A blueprint for comprehensive services across treatment. *Journal of Pediatric Psychology*, *32*, 1099–1110.

Kazak, A. E., Simms, S., Alderfer, M. A., Rourke, M. T., Crump, T., McClure, K., et al. (2005). Feasibility and preliminary outcomes from a pilot study of a brief psychological intervention for families of children newly diagnosed with cancer. *Journal of Pediatric Psychology*, *30*, 644–655.

Kodish, E., Eder, M., Noll, R. B., Ruccione, K., Lange, B., Angiolillo, A., et al. (2004). Communication of randomization in childhood leukemia trials. *Journal of the American Medical Association*, *291*, 470–475.

Koocher, G. P., & O'Malley, J. E. (1981). *The Damocles syndrome: Psychological consequences of surviving childhood cancer*. New York: McGraw-Hill.

Landier, W., Bhatia, S., Eshelman, D. A., Forte, K. J., Sweeney, T., Hester, A. L., et al. (2004). Development of risk-based guidelines for pediatric cancer survivors: The Children's Oncology Group long-term follow-up guidelines from the Children's Oncology Group Late Effects Committee and Nursing Discipline. *Journal of Clinical Oncology*, *22*, 4979–4990.

Langeveld, N. E., Stam, H., Grootenhuis, M. A., & Last, B. F. (2002). Quality of life in young adult survivors of childhood cancer. *Supportive Care in Cancer, 10,* 579–600.

Langeveld, N. E., Ubbink, M. C., Last, B. F., Grootenhuis, M. A., Voute, P. A., & De Haan, R. J. (2003). Educational achievement, employment and living situation in long-term young adult survivors of childhood cancer in the Netherlands. *Psycho-Oncology, 12,* 213–225.

Lewis, J., Morris, M., Morris, R. N. K., & Foster, M. A. (2000). Social problem solving in children with acquired brain injuries. *Journal of Head Trauma Rehabilitation, 15,* 930–942.

Lipschitz, S., Weiner, J. V., & Hewitt, M. E. (2005). *Childhood cancer survivorship: Improving care and quality of life.* Washington, DC: National Academies Press.

Mack, J. W., Cook, E. F., Wolfe, J., Grier, H. E., Cleary, P. D., & Weeks, J. C. (2007). Understanding of prognosis among parents of children with cancer: Parental optimism and the parent–physician interaction. *Journal of Clinical Oncology, 25,* 1357–1362.

Meacham, L. R., Gurney, J. G., Mertens, A. C., Ness, K. K., Sklar, C. A., Robison, L. L., et al. (2005). Body mass index in long-term adult survivors of childhood cancer: A report of the Childhood Cancer Survivor Study. *Cancer, 103,* 1730–1739.

Mertens, A., Yasui, Y., Neglia, J., Potter, J., Nesbit, M., Ruccione, K., et al. (2001). Late mortality experience in five-year survivors of childhood cancer. *Journal of Clinical Oncology, 19,* 3163–3172.

Mitby, P. A., Robison, L. L., Whitton, J. A., Zevon, M. A., Gibbs, I. C., Tersak, J. M., et al. (2003). Utilization of special education services and educational attainment among long-term survivors of childhood cancer: A report from the Childhood Cancer Survivor Study. *Cancer, 97,* 1115–1126.

Moleski, M. (2000). Neuropsychological, neuroanatomical, and neurophysiological consequences of CNS chemotherapy for acute lymphoblastic leukemia. *Archives of Clinical Neuropsychology, 15,* 603–630.

Mulhern, R. K., & Butler, R. W. (2004). Neurocognitive sequelae of childhood cancers and their treatment. *Pediatric Rehabilitation, 7,* 1–14.

Mulhern, R. K., Hancock, J., Fairclough, D., & Kun, L. (1992). Neuropsychological status of children treated for brain tumors: A critical review and integrative analysis. *Medical Pediatric Oncology, 20,* 181–191.

Mulhern, R. K., Kepner, J. L., Thomas, P. R., Armstrong, F. D., Friedman, H. S., & Kun, L. E. (1998). Neuropsychologic functioning of survivors of childhood medulloblastoma randomized to receive conventional or reduced-dose craniospinal irradiation: A Pediatric Oncology Group study. *Journal of Clinical Oncology, 16,* 1723–1728.

Mulhern, R. K., Palmer, S. L., Reddick, W. E., Glass, J. O., Kun, L. E., Taylor, J., et al. (2001). Risks of young age for selected neurocognitive deficits in medulloblastoma are associated with white matter loss. *Journal of Clinical Oncology, 19,* 472–479.

Mulhern, R. K., Reddick, W., Palmer, S. L., Glass, J. O., Elkin, T. D., Kun, L. E., et al. (1999). Neurocognitive deficits in medulloblastoma survivors and white matter loss. *Annals of Neurology, 46,* 834–841.

Mulhern, R. K., Tyc, V. L., Phipps, S., Crom, D., Barclay, D., Greenwald, C., et al. (1995). Health-related behaviors of survivors of childhood cancer. *Medical Pediatric Oncology, 25,* 159–165.

Nathan, P. C., Patel, S. K., Dilley, K., Goldsby, R., Harvey, J., Jacobsen, C., et al. (2007). Guidelines for identification of, advocacy for, and intervention in neurocognitive problems in survivors of childhood cancer: A report from the Children's Oncology Group. *Archives of Pediatrics and Adolescent Medicine, 161,* 798–806.

Ness, K. K., Baker, K. S., Dengel, D. R., Youngren, N., Sibley, S., Mertens, A. C., et al. (2007). Body composition, muscle strength deficits and mobility limitations in adult survivors of childhood acute lymphoblastic leukemia. *Pediatric Blood and Cancer, 49,* 975–981.

Ness, K. K., & Gurney, J. G. (2007). Adverse late effects of childhood cancer and its treatment on health and performance. *Annual Review of Public Health, 28,* 279–302.

Noll, R. B., Gartstein, M. A., Vannatta, K., Correll, J., Bukowski, W. M., & Davies, W. H. (1999). Social, emotional, and behavioral functioning of children with cancer. *Pediatrics, 103,* 71–78.

Noll, R. B., MacLean, W. E., Jr., Whitt, J. K., Kaleita, T. A., Stehbens, J. A., Waskerwitz, M. J., et al. (1997). Behavioral adjustment and social functioning of long-term survivors of childhood leukemia: Parent and teacher reports. *Journal of Pediatric Psychology, 22,* 827–841.

Nowicki, S., & Duke, M. (1994). Individual differences in the nonverbal communications of affect: The Diagnostic Analysis of Nonverbal Accuracy Scale. *Journal of Nonverbal Behavior, 18,* 9–35.

Odame, I., Duckworth, J., Talsma, D., Beaumont, L., Furlong, W., Webber, C., et al. (2006). Osteopenia, physical activity and health-related quality of life in survivors of brain tumors treated in childhood. *Pediatric Blood and Cancer, 46,* 357–362.

Oeffinger, K. C., & Hudson, M. M. (2004). Long-term complications following childhood and adolescent cancer: Foundations for providing risk-based health care for survivors. *CA: A Cancer Journal for Clinicians, 54,* 208–236.

Oeffinger, K. C., Mertens, A. C., Hudson, M. M., Gurney, J. G., Casillas, J., Chen, H., et al. (2004). Health care of young adult survivors of childhood cancer: A report from the Childhood Cancer Survivor Study. *Annals of Family Medicine, 2,* 61–70.

Oeffinger, K. C., Mertens, A. C., Sklar, C. A., Kawashima, T., Hudson, M. M., Meadows, A. T., et al. (2006). Chronic health conditions in adult survivors of childhood cancer. *New England Journal of Medicine, 355,* 1572–1582.

Oeffinger, K. C., Mertens, A. C., Sklar, C. A., Yasui, Y., Fears, T., Stovall, M., et al. (2003). Obesity in adult survivors of childhood acute lymphoblastic leukemia: A report from the Childhood Cancer Survivor Study. *Journal of Clinical Oncology, 21,* 1359–1365.

Pai, A. L. H., Greenley, R. N., Lewandowski, A., Drotar, D., Youngstrom, E., & Peterson, C. C. (2007). A meta-analytic review of the influence of pediatric cancer on parent and family functioning. *Journal of Family Psychology, 21,* 407–415.

Palmer, S. L., Gajjar, A., Reddick, W. E., Glass, J. O., Kun, L. E., Wu, S., et al. (2003). Predicting intellectual outcome among children treated with 35–40 Gy craniospinal irradiation for medulloblastoma. *Neuropsychology, 17,* 548–555.

Palmer, S. L., Reddick, W. E., & Gajjar, A. (2007). Understanding the cognitive impact on children who are treated for medulloblastoma. *Journal of Pediatric Psychology, 32,* 1040–1049.

Patenaude, A. F., & Kupst, M. J. (2005). Psychosocial functioning in pediatric cancer. *Journal of Pediatric Psychology, 30,* 9–27.

Peterson, C. C., & Drotar, D. (2006). Family impact of neurodevelopmental late effects in survivors of pediatric cancer: Review of research, clinical evidence, and future directions. *Clinical Child Psychology and Psychiatry, 11,* 349–366.

Phipps, S. (2005). Commentary: Contexts and challenges in pediatric psychosocial oncology research: Chasing moving targets and embracing "good news" outcomes. *Journal of Pediatric Psychology, 30,* 41–45.

Phipps, S. (2007). Adaptive style in children with cancer: Implications for a positive psychology approach. *Journal of Pediatric Psychology, 32,* 1055–1066.

Poggi, G., Liscio, M., Galbiati, S., Adduci, A., Massimino, M., Gandola, L., et al. (2005). Brain tumors in children and adolescents: Cognitive and psychological disorders at different ages. *Psycho-Oncology, 14,* 386–395.

Powers, S. (1999). Empirically supported treatments in pediatric psychology: Procedure-related pain. *Journal of Pediatric Psychology, 24,* 131–145.

Radcliffe, J., Packer, R. J., Atkins, T. E., Bunin, G. R., Schut, L., Goldwein, J. W., et al. (1992). Three- and four-year cognitive outcome in children with noncortical brain tumors treated with whole-brain radiotherapy. *Annals of Neurology, 32,* 551–554.

Rapoff, M. A., McGrath, A. M., & Smith, S. D. (2006). Adherence to treatment demands. In R. T. Brown (Ed.), *Comprehensive handbook of childhood cancer and sickle cell disease: A biopsychosocial approach* (pp. 138–169). New York: Oxford University Press.

Reimers, T. S., Ehrenfels, S., Mortensen, E. L., Schmiegelow, M., Sonderkaer, S., Carstensen, H., et al. (2003). Cognitive deficits in long-term survivors of childhood brain tumors: Identification of predictive factors. *Medical Pediatric Oncology, 40,* 26–34.

Ribi, K., Relly, C., Landolt, M. A., Alber, F. D., Boltshauser, E., & Grotzer, M. A. (2005). Outcome of medulloblastoma in children: Long-term complications and quality of life. *Neuropediatrics, 36,* 357–365.

Ries, L. A. G., Melbert, D., Krapcho, M., Stinchcomb, D. G., Howlader, N., Horner, M. J., et al. (Eds.). (2006). *SEER cancer statistics review, 1975–2005.* Bethesda, MD: National Cancer Institute.

Ris, M. D., & Noll, R. B. (1994). Long-term neurobehavioral outcome in pediatric brain-tumor patients: Review and methodological critique. *Journal of Clinical and Experimental Neuropsychology, 16,* 21–42.

Ris, M. D., Ryan, P., Lamba, M., Brenemen, J., Cecil, K., Succop, P., et al. (2005). An improved methodology for modeling neurobehavioral late-effects of radiotherapy in pediatric brain tumors. *Pediatric Blood and Cancer, 44,* 487–493.

Riva, D., Giorgi, C., Nichelli, F., Bulgheroni, S., Massimino, M., Cefalo, G., et al. (2002). Intrathecal methotrexate affects cognitive function in children with medulloblastoma. *Neurology, 59,* 48–53.

Robison, L. L., Mertens, A. C., Boice, J. D., Breslow, N. E., Donaldson, S. S., Green, D. M., et al. (2002). Study design and cohort characteristics of the Childhood Cancer Survivor Study: A multi-institutional collaborative project. *Medical and Pediatric Oncology, 38,* 229–239.

Rowland, J. H. (2005). Foreword: Looking beyond cure: Pediatric cancer as a model. *Journal of Pediatric Psychology, 30,* 1–3.

Sahler, O. J., Fairclough, D. L., Phipps, S., Mulhern, R. K., Dolgin, M. J., Noll, R. B., et al. (2005). Using problem solving skills training to reduce negative affectivity in mothers of children with newly diagnosed cancer: Report of a multisite randomized trial. *Journal of Consulting and Clinical Psychology, 73,* 272–283.

Sawyer, M., Antoniou, G., Toogood, I., Rice, M., & Baghurst, P. (2000). Childhood cancer: A 4-year prospective study of the psychological adjustment of children and parents. *Journal of Pediatric Hematology/Oncology, 22,* 214–220.

Schultz, K. A. P., Ness, K. K., Whitton, J., Recklitis, C., Zebrack, B., Robison, L. L., et al. (2007). Behavioral and social outcomes in adolescent survivors of childhood cancer: A report from the Childhood Cancer Survivor Study. *Journal of Clinical Oncology, 25,* 3649–3656.

Silber, J. H., Radcliffe, J., Peckham, V., Perilongo, G., Kishnani, P., Fridman, M., et al. (1992). Whole-brain irradiation and decline in intelligence: The influence of dose and age on IQ score. *Journal of Clinical Oncology, 10,* 1390–1396.

Sloper, P. (2000). Predictors of distress in parents of children with cancer: A prospective study. *Journal of Pediatric Psychology, 25,* 79–91.

Stehbens, J. A., Kaleita, T. A., Noll, R. B., MacLean, W. E., Jr., O'Brien, R. T., Waskerwitz, M. J., et al. (1991). CNS prophylaxis of childhood leukemia: What are the long-term neurological, neuropsychological, and behavioral effects? *Neuropsychology Review, 2,* 147–177.

Steinlin, M., Imfeld, S., Zulauf, P., Boltshauser, E., Lovblad, K. O., Ridolfi Luthy, A., et al. (2003). Neuropsychological long-term sequelae after posterior fossa tumour resection during childhood. *Brain, 126,* 1998–2008.

Tao, M. L., & Parsons, S. K. (2005). Quality-of-life assessment in pediatric brain tumor patients and survivors: Lessons learned and challenges to face. *Journal of Clinical Oncology, 23,* 5424–5426.

Tercyak, K. P., Nicolas, M., Councill, T., Prahlad, S., Taylor, K. L., & Shad, A. T. (2004). Brief report: Health beliefs among survivors of childhood cancer. *Journal of Pediatric Psychology, 29,* 397–402.

Tercyak, K. P., & Tyc, V. L. (2006). Opportunities and challenges in the prevention and control of cancer and other chronic diseases: Children's diet and nutrition and weight and physical activity. *Journal of Pediatric Psychology, 31,* 750–763.

Tyc, V. L., Hadley, W., & Crockett, G. (2001). Prediction of health behaviors in pediatric cancer survivors. *Medical and Pediatric Oncology, 37,* 42–46.

Tyc, V. L., Hudson, M. M., & Hinds, P. (1999). Health promotion intervention for adolescent cancer survivors. *Cognitive and Behavioral Practice, 6,* 128–136.

Tyc, V. L., Lensing, S., Rai, S. N., Klosky, J. L., Stewart, D. B., & Gattuso, J. (2005). Predicting perceived vulnerability to tobacco-related health risks and future intentions to use tobacco among pediatric cancer survivors. *Patient Education and Counseling, 62,* 198–204.

Tyc, V. L., Mulhern, R. K., Barclay, D. R., Smith, B. F., & Bieberich, A. A. (1997). Variables associated with anticipatory nausea and vomiting in pediatric cancer patients receiving ondansetron antiemetic therapy. *Journal of Pediatric Psychology, 22,* 45–58.

Vance, Y. H., Eiser, C., & Horne, B. (2004). Parents' views of the impact of childhood brain tumours and treatment on young people's social and family functioning. *Clinical Child Psychology and Psychiatry, 9,* 271–288.

Vannatta, K., Gartstein, M. A., Short, A., & Noll, R. B. (1998). A controlled study of peer relationships of children surviving brain tumors: Teacher, peer, and self ratings. *Journal of Pediatric Psychology, 23,* 279–287.

Vannatta, K., Gerhardt, C. A., Wells, R. J., & Noll, R. B. (2007). Intensity of CNS treatment for pediatric cancer: Prediction of social outcomes in survivors. *Pediatric Blood and Cancer, 49,* 716–722.

Waber, D. P., Carpentieri, S. C., Klar, N., Silverman, L. B., Schwenn, M., Hurwitz, C. A., et al. (2000). Cognitive sequelae in children treated for acute lymphoblastic leukemia with dexamethasone or prednisone. *Journal of Pediatric Hematology/Oncology, 22,* 206–213.

Waber, D. P., Tarbell, N. J., Fairclough, D., Atmore, K., Castro, R., Isquith, P., et al. (1995). Cognitive sequelae of treatment in childhood acute lymphoblastic leukemia: Cranial radiation requires an accomplice. *Journal of Clinical Oncology, 13,* 2490–2496.

Yeates, K. O., Bigler, E. D., Dennis, M., Gerhardt, C. A., Rubin, K. H., Stancin, T., et al. (2007). Social outcomes in childhood brain disorder: A heuristic integration of social neuroscience and developmental psychology. *Psychological Bulletin, 133,* 535–556.

Yeazel, M. W., Oeffinger, K. C., Gurney, J. G., Mertens, A. C., Hudson, M. M., Emmons, K. M., et al. (2004). The cancer screening practices of adult survivors of childhood cancer: A report from the Childhood Cancer Survivor Study. *Cancer, 100,* 631–640.

Young, B., Dixon-Woods, M., Windridge, K. C., & Heney, D. (2003). Managing communication with young people who have a potentially life threatening chronic illness: Qualitative study of patients and parents. *British Medical Journal, 326,* 305.

Zeltzer, L. (1994). Pain and symptom management. In D. J. Bearison & R. K. Mulhern (Eds.), *Pediatric psychooncology: Psychological perspectives on children with cancer* (pp. 61–83). New York: Oxford University Press.

CHAPTER 22

Pediatric Traumatic Brain Injury and Spinal Cord Injury

SHARI L. WADE
NICOLAY CHERTKOFF WALZ
GLENDALIZ BOSQUES

This chapter provides an overview of the medical, cognitive, and psychosocial consequences of traumatic brain injury (TBI) and spinal cord injury (SCI). These central nervous system (CNS) conditions share the characteristics of a sudden, traumatic onset of a life-altering condition in a previously healthy child or adolescent, and an uncertain (and often extended) course of recovery. However, they differ with respect to the relative effects on cognitive-behavioral versus physical functioning, as well as the attendant caregiving demands. In addition, although TBI affects children of all ages, with peaks in early childhood and adolescence, SCI primarily affects teenagers. This chapter focuses on the assessment and treatment issues associated with these conditions, as well as promising approaches for intervention.

Traumatic Brain Injury

Epidemiology

TBI is a brain insult acquired as the result of an external mechanical force. TBI is a subset of acquired brain injury but does not include acquired insults sustained from nontraumatic causes, such as anoxia or tumors. It is the most common cause of death and long-term disability for children under 15 years of age, with nearly half a million children in this age range suffering a TBI every year. About 90% of pediatric TBI is considered mild (Glasgow Coma Scale [GCS] scores in the 13–15 range, typically without neuroimaging evidence of brain injury), with children treated and released from the emergency department. Thus most children with TBI survive; however, traumatic injuries are the leading cause of death among children, with about 50% involving brain injuries. Mortality rates are highest in infancy. Falls are the leading cause of TBI, with rates highest among children ages 0–4 and older adults. Child abuse as a cause of TBI is most common among infants (about 25%). Among children ages 0–2, boys are more likely than girls, and non–European American children are more likely than European American children, to incur inflicted TBI (Keenan et al., 2003). The rates of TBI related to motor vehicle traffic accidents and to assault are highest among adolescents. Overall, TBI occurs about 1.5 times as often among males as among females (Keenan & Bratton, 2006; Langlois, Rutland-Brown, & Thomas, 2006).

Neuropathology and Pathophysiology

The pathophysiology of TBI is usually discussed in terms of "primary" and "secondary" effects. Primary effects are the effects of the trauma itself, such as skull fractures, contusions, and hemorrhages. These primary injuries most commonly occur as results of the biochemical forces of acceleration–deceleration. Rotational movement can produce focal contusions (bruises), as well as diffuse axonal injury. Focal injury is most common in the frontal and anterior temporal areas, whereas shear strain injury occurs most commonly at the white–gray matter boundaries. Secondary effects occur subsequent to the trauma and include brain swelling, cerebral edema, elevated intracranial pressure, hypoxia, mass lesions, and seizures. Research advances in the neurochemical mechanisms of pediatric TBI suggest a number of changes in cerebral metabolism that affect the developing brain over an extended period of time, such as excessive production of free radicals and excessive production of excitatory amino acids (Beers, Berger, & Adelson, 2007).

Outcomes

Medical Complications

Possible acute medical complications of TBI include seizures, hydrocephalus, and intracranial infections arising from penetrating injuries (National Institute of Neurological Disorders and Stroke [NINDS], 2002). Pain, particularly headache, is a common acute and long-term consequence of TBI. Acute postconcussive symptoms may include dizziness, vertigo, and sleep difficulties. Children may also experience coordination difficulties and unsteady gait. Other senses, such as vision, hearing, and taste, may be affected; results may include difficulty recognizing or processing what is being seen, ringing or rushing sounds in the ears (tinnitus), and odd tastes or smells (NINDS, 2002). TBI can also result in endocrine changes, including the early onset of puberty (Behan, Phillips, Thompson, & Agha, 2008). Despite the range of medical complications, behavioral changes remain a primary concern for families.

Neurobehavioral and Psychosocial Consequences

A more comprehensive review of the neuropsychological consequences of pediatric TBI is presented by Yeates (2000), and this is supplemented by sources cited below. The pediatric psychologist should be aware that moderate to severe TBI in children is typically associated with significant cognitive morbidity. The extensive literature shows that TBI can produce short- and long-term deficits in many domains, including orientation to person, place, and time; intellectual functioning; academic skills; language skills; nonverbal skills; attention, memory, and other executive functions (EFs); and adaptive behavioral competence (e.g., Ewing-Cobbs et al., 2004; Levin & Hanten, 2005; Taylor et al., 2002; Yeates, Taylor, Wade, et al., 2002). Children with TBI often display characteristics similar to those of children with attention-deficit/hyperactivity disorder (ADHD) or learning disorders, such as concentration problems, memory deficits, and uneven academic performance. Most important from the perspective of assessment and intervention is that cognitive consequences for a given child can be highly variable, with deficits in some domains or settings and intact abilities in others (Ylvisaker et al., 2001). Although cognitive deficits show improvement over time, there is also evidence that some problems may not emerge or become evident until higher-level skills are required (Anderson et al., 2006). Thus children with TBI are sometimes described as "growing into" their deficits, making it important to follow children with more severe injuries over time.

In recent years, deficits in EFs, discourse, and language pragmatics have been identified as common consequences of pediatric TBI that adversely affect both academic and social functioning (Chapman et al., 2006; Dennis, Purvis, Barnes, Wilkinson, & Winner, 2001; Levin & Hanten, 2005). EFs include a constellation of core metacognitive abilities, such as attentional control, working memory, and problem solving, that enable individuals to organize and regulate their behavior successfully. Deficits in these skills may not be apparent on traditional intelligence or achievement testing, but may contribute to classroom failure following TBI. Similarly, children with TBI may have difficulties abstracting meaning from both written and spoken language, despite normal performance on tests of language abilities (Chapman et al., 2006). This discrepancy between capacity as assessed in structured testing situations and performance in everyday settings presents challenges for psychologists involved in assessment and treatment planning (Ylvisaker et al., 2001). As such, observation in classroom or community settings may provide a valuable complement to traditional office-based assessments.

Behavioral and psychiatric problems are also frequent outcomes of moderate to severe TBI, with longer-term follow-up suggesting that behavioral and personality changes represent the most persistent consequences of TBI in children (Bloom et al., 2001; Max et al., 1997). It is often difficult to truly estimate the effects of TBI on a child's behavior, because children with behavior or learning problems are more likely to sustain traumatic injuries (Goldstrohm & Arffa, 2005). Children with preinjury behavior problems may also be more likely to develop diagnosable disorders after their injuries. Behavioral problems often fail to resolve despite some recovery of cognitive functions. Initial improvements in behavior may be most evident in children with severe TBI, but persistent or even worsening symptoms may also characterize these children. In general, postinjury behavior is not strongly related to children's cognitive skills (e.g., Schwartz et al., 2003; Taylor et al., 2002; Yeates, Taylor, Wade, et al., 2002). More severe injuries, less advantaged family environments, and younger age at injury are predictive of poorer outcomes (e.g., Anderson et al., 2006; Stancin et al., 2002; Taylor et al., 1999, 2002). However, research on predictors of behavioral recovery is complex, and clinicians should be aware that there is substantial variation in outcome at the individual level.

Research on the development of psychiatric disorders suggests that in the 2 years following injury, a new psychiatric disorder (e.g., emotional disorders, disinhibited states, conduct disorder) develops in 10–21% of children with mild TBI, and in 62–71% of children with severe TBI (Max et al., 1997; Schwartz et al., 2003). These new psychiatric disorders cut across diagnoses and often involve personality changes marked by increased impulsivity and affective lability (Max et al., 2000). Anxiety symptoms are also common (Vasa et al., 2002). Although there have been fewer investigations of social outcomes, recent studies have identified specific problems with social information-processing skills and social competence, including fewer friendships (Janusz, Kirkwood, Yeates, & Taylor, 2002; Prigatano & Gupta, 2006; Yeates et al., 2004). Taken together, these findings suggest that social participation and quality of life may be adversely affected for many children with TBI (Stancin et al., 2002).

Family Burden and Distress

TBI creates significant stress for parents and families that may persist for many years following severe injuries (Rivara et al., 1996; Wade et al., 2002; Wade, Taylor, et al., 2006). TBI has also been linked to high levels of psychological symptoms and distress in family members (Wade, Taylor, Drotar, Stancin, & Yeates, 1998). Although a significant portion of parents experience burden and distress, many families adapt successfully to the increased demands of the injury. Such factors as socioeconomic status, ethnicity, preinjury family resources and stresses, and initial response to the injury appear to moderate the injury's impact on caregivers, placing some families at greater risk for long-term difficulties (Rivara et al., 1996; Wade et al., 2001, 2004; Yeates, Taylor, Woodrome, et al., 2002). Specifically, families with poorer preinjury functioning, social environments characterized by high levels of stresses and inadequate resources, and maladaptive coping strategies evidence poorer adaptation over time. Careful assessment of family resources and stresses should enable pediatric psychologists to identify families who may benefit from more intensive intervention.

Assessment

TBI severity is usually assessed by the Glasgow Coma Scale (GCS), a 15-point scale that incorporates specific assessment of eye opening, motor response, and verbal response. Typically, scores of 13–15 are indicative of mild injury; scores of 9–12 represent moderate injury; and scores of 8 or less reflect severe injury (Teasdale & Jennett, 1974). GCS scores are less reliable and sensitive in younger children (Foreman et al., 2007). Other indicators of severity, such as duration of impaired unconsciousness, length of posttraumatic amnesia, and neuroimaging findings, can be helpful in understanding neurobehavioral outcomes. Advances in understanding the neuropathology and pathophysiology of pediatric TBI have been facilitated by increasingly sophisticated technology. Techniques such as susceptibility-weighted imaging, magnetic resonance spectroscopy, diffusion-weighted imaging, and diffusion tensor imaging appear to be particularly sensitive to the diffuse axonal injury of TBI and can now be used to better characterize the nature of the initial injury, the underlying mechanisms, and the evolution of the injury. An improved understanding of the developing brain's neurochemical and pathophysiological response to TBI has the potential to lead to the development of novel interventions and to improve prediction of outcomes (e.g., Ashwal, Holshouser, & Tong, 2006;

Berger, Adelson, Richichi, & Kochanek, 2006; Robertson, Soane, Siegel, & Fiskum, 2006).

A pediatric psychologist is most likely to be involved in cases of moderate to severe TBI, where children and/or family members are having difficulty adjusting to the physical and/or neurobehavioral sequelae of TBI. Thus we refer the reader to recent, comprehensive reviews of outcomes and management of mild TBI (Kirkwood et al., 2007; McCrea, 2008; Yeates & Taylor, 2005). In most cases of moderate to severe TBI, a comprehensive neuropsychological evaluation is warranted to elucidate any neurobehavioral deficits and to assist with reentry into the school and community. Office-based assessments should be integrated with parent and teacher reports as well as direct observation, to provide an ecologically valid assessment of a child's strengths and weaknesses (Ylvisaker et al., 2001). Assessments of child and family adjustment are also recommended, because posttraumatic stress symptoms and poor family adaptation may complicate the child's recovery.

Intervention

Recent review articles outline existing interventions for pediatric TBI (Laatsch et al., 2007; Ylvisaker et al., 2007). Although the nature of an intervention depends to some extent on the target problem (e.g., memory vs. anger), randomized clinical trials (RCTs) are rare. Treatment approaches can be divided into psychoeducation/information; cognitive remediation and orthotics; behavioral approaches; family-centered treatments/positive behavioral supports; and medication. In the acute and chronic phases, TBI can result in injury-related neurological changes that may be also amenable to existing behavioral interventions for such conditions as sleep problems and headaches (Beebe et al., 2007; Kirkwood et al., 2007).

Educational and Informational Interventions

Surveys suggest that additional information about recovery following TBI is a prominent family need. Findings from an RCT in children with mild TBI indicated that informational pamphlets may significantly reduce behavioral symptoms in the initial postinjury months (Ponsford et al., 2001). However, an investigation with parents of severely injured children found education to be inferior to stress management strategies in reducing parental distress (Singer et al., 1994). In addition, an informational intervention directed at children with TBI was unsuccessful in ameliorating self-awareness deficits (Beardmore, Tate, & Liddle, 1999). Thus educational approaches directed at parents and/or children with TBI are unlikely to be sufficient when the children are experiencing marked cognitive or behavioral consequences.

Cognitive Remediation and Compensatory Approaches

Cognitive remediation approaches include strategies for improving attention, memory, and other EFs (see Limond & Leeke, 2005, for a review). Although evidence is limited, recent studies from Sweden (Van't Hooft et al., 2005) suggest that a structured approach to retraining specific elements of attention and memory may contribute to improved neuropsychological functioning. Compensatory strategies and devices, such as pagers, personal digital assistants, and talking watches, may also be used to address ongoing difficulties with memory, planning, and organization skills in older children (Wilson, Emslie, Quirk, & Evans, 2001). Pediatric psychologists may play a role in helping children to identify compensatory strategies (including devices) to enable them to reduce the effects of EF deficits on school performance and everyday functioning (Catroppa & Anderson, 2006).

Behavioral and Cognitive-Behavioral Approaches to Interventions

Recent reviews (Laatsch et al., 2007; Ylvisaker et al., 2007) indicate that most published reports of treatments to improve behavioral functioning following TBI involve single- or multiple-case-design studies of operant behavioral conditioning and token economies to reduce disruptive or aggressive behaviors. Evidence suggests that such programs are successful in reducing problem behaviors in severely injured children. However, concerns have been raised that traditional behavioral approaches may not generalize across settings or behaviors, in part due to the inability of children with frontal lobe injuries to benefit and learn from the consequences.

Although investigations of cognitive-behavioral interventions are less numerous, they suggest that providing training in such metacognitive strategies as self-monitoring (Selznick & Savage, 2000), self-regulation, and self-reinforcement (Suzman, Morris, Morris, & Milan, 1997) may be effective in improving self-awareness and problem-solving skills. However, small sample sizes and the absence of comparison groups limit the generalizability of these findings.

Positive Behavioral Supports and Family-Centered Interventions

In response to the limitations of traditional behavioral treatment paradigms, Ylvisaker, Jacobs, and Feeney (2003) developed an intervention model incorporating positive behavioral supports and antecedent behavior control to improve on-task behaviors/task completion and to reduce aggressive and disruptive behaviors. Their approach engages a child's parents and/or teachers in identifying and addressing environmental antecedents to problem behaviors, and in providing appropriate supports and scaffolding to the child to ensure successful task completion. Principles include negotiating with the child to make tasks interesting, meaningful, and doable; providing frequent support and feedback early and then fading these over time; and structuring the environment to maximize successes. Although limited to multiple, well-designed single-case studies, the growing evidence base for positive behavioral supports suggests that they can provide an effective approach for addressing behavioral issues in the school and home.

Family problem solving (FPS), a treatment integrating TBI education with training in problem solving, communication skills, and positive behavioral supports, has shown promise in reducing internalizing symptoms following TBI in school-age children (Wade, Michaud, & Brown, 2006). As the use of positive behavioral supports does, FPS involves collaborative problem solving among child, family, and therapist to address family-identified concerns. An online version of FPS, integrating Web-based didactic sessions with synchronous video conferences to assist families in implementing the problem-solving process to achieve family goals was shown to reduce parental depression, anxiety, and distress relative to an Internet resource control treatment (Wade, Carey, & Wolfe,

2006a). Improvements in child functioning were also demonstrated, with greater effects among older and economically disadvantaged children (Wade, Carey, & Wolfe, 2006b). These RCTs suggest that cognitive-behavioral approaches with demonstrated efficacy for other conditions (D'Zurilla & Nezu, 1999) may be also beneficial following TBI.

Medications and Other Treatment Approaches

Because TBI results in secondary psychiatric disorders, most notably ADHD, treatments that have proven efficacious for these other conditions may also be successful in the treatment of TBI (see Barkley, 2002, and Daly, Cohen, Carpenter, & Brown, Chapter 36, this volume, for descriptions of treatments for ADHD). Several small RCTs suggest that psychostimulant medications used in the treatment of ADHD may also be effective in reducing attention and behavioral problems following pediatric TBI (Beers, Skold, Dixon, & Adelson, 2005; Jin & Schachar, 2004; Mahalick et al., 1998). However, because the efficacy of behavioral treatments for ADHD has not been documented in populations with brain injuries, it is unclear what adaptations might be necessary.

Although further research is necessary to establish evidence-based recommendations, increasing numbers of promising interventions are at the pediatric psychologist's disposal. Importantly, both the cognitive and behavioral consequences of pediatric TBI appear to be responsive to behavioral interventions.

School Reentry and Intervention

The return to school following a TBI can be challenging for both the student and the school, as confusion, concentration/memory difficulties, and fatigue are typically greatest during the initial weeks following the injury. Because TBI is relatively uncommon, teachers and counselors may be unfamiliar with its common cognitive and behavioral consequences. Intraindividual variability in abilities can prove particularly challenging for teachers, who may misattribute uneven performance to low motivation or behavioral difficulties. Thus pediatric psychologists can play an important role in facilitating the hospital-to-school transition by educating classroom personnel as well as peers (see DePompei, Blosser, Savage, & Lash, 1999). The positive behavioral supports described previously, as well as self-monitoring strategies, have been used successfully in classroom settings to reduce behavior problems and increase work completion (Selznick & Savage, 2000; Ylvisaker et al., 2003). Because cognitive deficits may emerge over time with increasing academic or organizational demands, psychologists can also facilitate transitions from one academic setting to another (Ylvisaker et al., 2001).

Spinal Cord Injury

Epidemiology

Although less common than TBI, SCI is a devastating event for the injured child as well as his or her family members. According to recent epidemiological evidence (Vitale, Goss, Matsumoto, & Roye, 2006), approximately 2 children per 100,000 are admitted to hospitals in the United States for treatment of SCI. Males are three times more likely to sustain SCI than females, especially during adolescence. Motor vehicle crashes are the most common causes of SCI in youths (56%), and the majority involved in these incidents did not wear seat belts (67%) and/or were intoxicated with alcohol or drugs (30%). Other causes of SCI include falls (14%), gunshot wounds (9%), and sports injuries (7%). Although having SCI as a result of trauma is uncommon in children, some groups may be at higher risk: African American children have a higher rate of this type of injury than other ethnic and racial groups, followed by Native Americans, Hispanics, and Asians (Vitale et al., 2006). The nature and etiology of SCI also vary as a function of a child's age: Infants may sustain SCI as a result of birth trauma or abuse, whereas adolescents are most likely to be injured in motor vehicle crashes.

As a result of advances in medicine and technology, increasing numbers of children are surviving previously fatal injuries. Although a GCS score of 3 has been reported as a negative predictor for survival following SCI (40% mortality rate), 99% of patients who have a GSC score of 4 or greater survive (Vitale et al., 2006). With high survival rates, there will be an increasing number of adults with childhood-onset SCI. As a survivor faces the problems that follow a life-altering event such as SCI, a pediatric psychologist can play a valuable role in helping the child and family to understand and address the long-term psychosocial implications, as well as the complex interdisciplinary medical management needs.

Neuropathology and Pathophysiology

Like TBI, SCI is discussed in terms of primary and secondary effects. The primary effects are typically initiated when fractured or dislocated vertebrae bruise or tear spinal cord tissue, causing bleeding and damage to axons and cell membranes (NINDS, 2003). However, younger children may sustain bruising or ischemic injury to the spinal cord in the absence of fracture or dislocation (Boyd & Perrin, 1992). Due to swelling, the spinal cord fills the spinal canal, cutting off blood flow and oxygen to spinal cord tissue. Secondary biochemical effects resulting in neuronal death, axonal demyelinization, and inflammation contribute to more extensive damage.

Because a SCI affects the neurological input and output beneath the level of the lesion, it is associated with varying degrees of loss of sensation and motor function. The American Spinal Injury Association has developed an Impairment Scale to classify the extent of remaining motor and sensory functioning. Injuries are classified as "complete" or "incomplete," depending on whether any sensory or motor function is preserved below the level of the injury (NINDS, 2003).

Outcomes

Medical Complications

The loss of sensory and motor function arising from SCI contributes to a range of medical complications, including pressure ulcers, deep vein thrombosis, and pulmonary embolisms. The latter are a common cause of morbidity and mortality following SCI if not properly managed (Consortium for Spinal Cord Medicine, 2000; DeVivo, Black, & Stover, 1993). In addition to loss of ambulation, if the injury is high enough, the child no longer has diaphragm control and will therefore require a mechanical ventilator for respiratory management. For patients with cervical or higher thoracic injuries, autonomic dysreflexia is a life-threatening potential medical complication of SCI (Karlsson, 1999). Due to an imbalance of the peripheral nervous system and the CNS, dysreflexia results in elevated blood pressure, slowed heart rate, headaches, and profuse sweating and flushing above the level of injury.

In addition, patients with SCI often develop bladder and bowel incontinence, commonly referred to as "neurogenic bladder and bowel" (Beneveto & Sipski, 2002). In order to manage these complications, most patients are required to perform intermittent catheterizations on a consistent basis to empty the bladder and avoid urinary tract infections, and to follow a bowel program with stool softeners and suppositories to prevent chronic constipation, impaction, and incontinence episodes. Incontinence can be a source of embarrassment for older children and adolescents, and its successful management necessitates considerable adherence on their part.

Other chronic medical problems that may arise include frequent pneumonias, chronic pressure ulcers, spasticity, neurogenic erectile dysfunction, osteoporosis, high cholesterol, and obesity. Muscle spasticity can lead to pain or physical discomfort (NINDS, 2003). Given the chronic (and in some cases life-threatening) medical complications associated with pediatric SCI, it is particularly important to consider a child's and family's psychosocial needs.

Psychosocial and Behavioral Consequences

Prospective investigations of short- and long-term psychological consequences of pediatric SCI are lacking. However, existing studies and clinical reports suggest that the acute emotional impact of SCI can be profound: SCI can result in feelings of shock, anger, denial, anxiety, grief, and depression, especially among adolescents. Psychologists may be called in during inpatient rehabilitation to assess depressive symptoms and potential suicidal ideation, and to address denial and nonadherence with rehabilitative recommendations. Given that SCI is most frequently caused by vehicular crashes and violence, posttraumatic stress disorder (PTSD) is also common, affecting 25% or more of pediatric survivors (Boyer, Knolls, Kafkalas, Tollen, & Swartz, 2000). When compared to the general population, patients with childhood-onset SCI have equivalent educational attainment, but lower levels of community participation, employment, income, independent living, and marriage (Anderson, Krajci, & Vogel, 2002).

Various demographic, medical, and behavioral characteristics have been identified as predictors of more positive medical and psychosocial outcomes, including younger onset of injury, higher educational level, greater functional independence, fewer medical complications, and higher levels of participation in everyday activities (Massagli, 2000; Tasiemski, Kennedy, Gardner, & Taylor, 2005). Family functioning is also predictive of functional independence, with children from higher-functioning families achieving greater functional independence (Boyer, Hitelman, Knolls, & Kafkalas, 2003). Moreover, posttraumatic stress symptoms mediate the association between family functioning and functional independence, suggesting that poor family functioning may influence a child's adjustment through increased symptoms of PTSD.

Despite poorer outcomes than those of their peers, patients with childhood-onset SCI have better outcomes than individuals with adult-onset injuries do. Sustaining an injury at a younger age may enable these individuals to adapt successfully to their changed circumstances by developing educational and/or professional career goals despite their disability (Molnar & Alexander, 1999). In addition, the level of the injury and the associated degree of sensory and motor dysfunction are not predictive of quality of life or satisfaction, suggesting that factors other than the degree of physical impairment may be the most salient determinants of long-term functioning (Anderson, Vogel, Betz, & Willis, 2004). Similarly, for patients with long-term dependence on a mechanical ventilator, life satisfaction has been shown to be unrelated to the years of ventilator assistance. However, it may be more important to evaluate the social environment of individuals using ventilators, including caregivers and available support, because these factors relate directly to their quality of life as adults (Nelson, Dixon, & Warschausky, 2004).

Family Burden and Distress

Given the demands for medical and physical care and the risks of medical complications associated with SCI, it is not surprising that caregivers experience elevated levels of depressive symptoms and clinical depression (Dreer, Elliot, Shewchuk, Berry, & Rivara, 2007). In addition, parents of children with SCI report high rates of PTSD (Boyer et al., 2000). In the adult SCI literature, such factors as caregiver problem solving and support have been shown to influence adjustment (Dreer et al., 2007). Because parental and child psychological adjustment are closely linked (Boyer et al., 2000), facilitating parent/family functioning may also improve child adaptation.

Approaches to Community Reentry and Intervention

Since community reintegration, advanced education, and functional independence have been associated with higher life satisfaction and better quality of life (Anderson et al., 2002, 2004), proactive psychological interventions can focus on increasing community participation levels. It is also essential to discuss adulthood transition issues early in the course of adjustment to pediatric SCI, with the goals of increasing functional independence and mobility, as well as social interaction and community integration skills. Children with SCI need to be provided with the necessary tools for decision making, including community integration and participation at every developmental stage. Activities that can facilitate skill development and integration include specialized camps, adaptive sports, school activities, sleepovers, and exercise programs, among others (Molnar & Alexander, 1999).

Behavioral and Cognitive-Behavioral Approaches

Although empirical evidence is lacking, standard cognitive-behavioral treatments for depression and PTSD should also be effective in reducing these symptoms following pediatric SCI (Boyer et al., 2000). In addition, standard behavioral approaches may be used to address adherence to treatment regimens (Gorski, Slifer, Townsend, Kelly-Suttka, & Amari, 2005). Established pain management protocols may be adapted to address discomfort arising from spasticity.

Family-Centered Approaches

Family-centered treatments may be helpful in reducing caregiver burden and improving family functioning. Family therapy may also be useful in addressing parental overprotectiveness, thereby helping parents give older children and adolescents exposure to normative experiences such as chores and volunteer or part-time jobs, in order to help form educational and professional goals. Moreover, as patients develop necessary cognitive and physical skills, psychologists can help them assume the responsibility for self-care and prevention of medical complications, such as pressure ulcers, urinary tract infections, and respiratory complications.

Developmental Transitions

Sexuality, relationships, and marriage pose significant concerns for survivors of childhood SCI and may not be adequately addressed by medical providers. However, research suggests that being able to have meaningful relationships is essential to greater life satisfaction (Anderson et al., 2002). Hence psychological treatment for adolescents and young adults may also focus on such matters as sexual functioning, birth control methods and fertility, and employment.

Conclusions and Future Directions

TBI and SCI are both caused by traumatic, and in some cases violent, events in previously healthy children. Thus they both require considerable adaptation on the part of the injured individuals and their families, and contribute to both acute and longer-term child and caregiver distress, depression, and PTSD. Similarly, for both conditions, social-environmental characteristics such as family functioning and resources can have as much or more influence on long-term adaptation as injury severity or level can. Accordingly, clinicians treating both TBI and SCI must understand recovery in the broader contexts of family, school, and community. As for other pediatric conditions discussed in this volume, successful psychological intervention is likely to involve coordination with other medical and rehabilitation professionals. However, TBI, unlike SCI, may have profound effects on subsequent learning, EFs, behavioral organization, and self-awareness (Trahan, Pepin, & Hopps, 2006). As a result, TBI poses more significant challenges in many respects for parents, teachers, and clinicians.

Considerable research remains to be done to establish evidence-based treatments for children with TBI and SCI. For example, the field knows little about the generalizability and maintenance of treatment gains, what treatments work best for which families and for children at which ages, the efficacy of school reentry programs and school-based rehabilitation programs, or the applicability of rehabilitation methods that have been drawn from adult models. However, a growing literature highlights several promising approaches for treating behavioral and family issues following TBI. For SCI that is not comorbid with TBI, established treatments for the target diagnosis or symptom (e.g., cognitive-behavioral treatment for PTSD or depression) are likely to be appropriate. However, psychologists assessing and treating children who have sustained both TBI and SCI must take into account neuropsychological deficits arising from the TBI when developing and implementing treatment plans. Treatment of both conditions also necessitates communication with school personnel, as well as education and advocacy when academic and social needs are not being met. Effective treatment also requires the acknowledgment that these injuries occur in the context of a child's or adolescent's development, and thus that the effects may be lifelong, evolving, and evident in various areas of functioning.

The future holds the potential for considerable changes in the evaluation and treatment of both conditions. Improvements in neuroimaging may allow clinicians to more precisely identify and target neural changes arising from TBI. Identification of genes (e.g., apolipoprotein E4) associated with neurological vulnerability may enable clinicians to identify children at greatest risk for long-term consequences (see Alexander et al., 2007). Research on the use of functional electrical stimulation to trigger movements in limbs that have lost sensory and motor input may allow individuals to regain motor function after SCI. Although use of these devices is currently limited, bioengineering research should contribute to advances in the ease of implantation and their ability to stimulate natural-looking movements. Pediatric psychologists can play an important role in helping patients and their families understand the implications and limitations of these technological advances, while supporting adaptation and growth. In fact, as research on outcomes of pediatric TBI and SCI continues, and as more evidence-based interventions are developed to improve child and family outcomes, pediatric psychologists will have much more information and many more interventions to offer injured children and their families.

References

Alexander, S., Kerr, M. E., Kim, Y., Kamboh, M. I., Beers, S. R., & Conley, Y. P. (2007). Apolipoprotein E4 allele presence and functional outcome after severe traumatic brain injury. *Journal of Neurotrauma, 24,* 790–797.

Anderson, C. J., Krajci, K. A., & Vogel, L. C. (2002). Life satisfaction in adults with pediatric-onset spinal cord injuries. *Journal of Spinal Cord Medicine, 25,* 184–190.

Anderson, C. J., Vogel, L. C., Betz, R. R., & Willis, K. M. (2004). Overview of adult outcomes in pediatric-onset spinal cord injuries: Implications for transition to adulthood. *Journal of Spinal Cord Medicine, 27,* S98–S106.

Anderson, V. A., Catroppa, C., Dudgeon, P., Morse, S. A., Haritou, F., & Rosenfeld, J. V. (2006). Understanding predictors of functional recovery and outcome 30 months following early childhood head injury. *Neuropsychology, 20,* 42–57.

Ashwal, S., Holshouser, B. A., & Tong, K. A. (2006). Use of advanced neuroimaging techniques in the evaluation of pediatric traumatic brain injury. *Developmental Neuroscience, 28,* 309–326.

Barkley, R. A. (2002). Psychosocial treatments for attention deficit hyperactivity disorder. *Journal of Clinical Psychiatry, 63,* S36–S43.

Beardmore, S., Tate, R., & Liddle, B. (1999). Does information and feedback improve children's knowledge and awareness of deficits after traumatic brain injury? *Neuropsychological Rehabilitation, 9,* 45–62.

Beebe, D. W., Krivitzky, L., Wells, C. T., Wade, S. L., Taylor, H. G., & Yeates, K. O. (2007). Brief report: Parental report of sleep behaviors following moderate of severe pediatric traumatic brain injury. *Journal of Pediatric Psychology, 32,* 845–850.

Beers, S. R., Berger, R. P., & Adelson, P. D. (2007). Neurocognitive outcome and serum biomarkers in inflicted versus non-inflicted traumatic brain injury in young children. *Journal of Neurotrauma, 24,* 97–105.

Beers, S. R., Skold, A., Dixon, C. E., & Adelson, P. E. (2005). Neurobehavioral effects of amantadine after pediatric traumatic brain injury. *Journal of Head Trauma Rehabilitation, 20,* 450–463.

Behan, L. A., Phillips, J., Thompson, C. J., & Agha, A. (2008). Neuroendocrine disorders after traumatic brain injury. *Journal of Neurology, Neurosurgery and Psychiatry, 79,* 753–759.

Beneveto, B. T., & Sipski, M. L. (2002). Neurogenic bladder, neurogenic bowel, and sexual dysfunction in people with spinal cord injury. *Physical Therapy, 82,* 601–612.

Berger, R. P., Adelson, P. D., Richichi, R., & Kochanek, P. M. (2006). Serum biomarkers after traumatic and hypoxemic brain injuries: Insight into the biochemical response of the pediatric brain to inflicted brain injury. *Developmental Neuroscience, 28,* 327–335.

Bloom, D. R., Levin, H. S., Ewing-Cobbs, L., Saunders, A. E., Song, J., Fletcher, J. N., et al. (2001). Lifetime and novel psychiatric disorders after pediatric traumatic brain injury. *Journal of the American Academy of Child and Adolescent Psychiatry, 40,* 572–579.

Boyd, J., & Perrin, J. C. S. (1992). Spinal cord injury. In E. Molnar (Ed.), *Pediatric rehabilitation* (2nd ed., pp. 336–362). Baltimore: Williams & Wilkins.

Boyer, B. A., Hitelman, J. S., Knolls, M. L., & Kafkalas, C. M. (2003). Posttraumatic stress and family functioning in pediatric spinal cord injuries: Moderation or mediation? *American Journal of Family Therapy, 31,* 23–37.

Boyer, B. A., Knolls, M. L., Kafkalas, C. M., Tollen, L. G., & Swartz, M. (2000). Prevalence and relationships of posttraumatic stress in families experiencing pediatric spinal cord injury. *Rehabilitation Psychology, 45,* 339–355.

Catroppa, C., & Anderson, V. (2006). Planning, problem-solving and organizational abilities in children following TBI: Intervention techniques. *Pediatric Rehabilitation, 9,* 89–97.

Chapman, S. B., Gamino, J. F., Cook, L. G., Hanten, G., Li, X., & Levin, H. S. (2006). Impaired discourse gist and working memory in children after brain injury. *Brain and Language, 78,* 178–188.

Consortium for Spinal Cord Medicine. (2000). *Pressure ulcer prevention and treatment following spinal cord injury.* Washington, DC: Paralyzed Veterans of America.

Dennis, M., Purvis, K., Barnes, M. A., Wilkinson, M., & Winner, E. (2001). Understanding of literal truth, ironic criticism, and deceptive praise following childhood head injury. *Brain and Language, 78,* 1–16.

DePompei, R., Blosser, J., Savage, R., & Lash, M. (1999). *Back to school after a moderate to severe brain injury.* Wake Forest, NC: Lash & Associates.

DeVivo, M. J., Black, K. J., Stover, S. L. (1993). Causes of death during the first 12 years after spinal cord injury. *Archives of Physical Medicine and Rehabilitation, 74,* 248–254.

Dreer, L. E., Elliot, T. R., Shewchuk, R., Berry, J. W., & Rivara, P. (2007). Family caregivers of persons with spinal cord injury: Predicting caregivers at risk for probable depression. *Rehabilitation Psychology, 52,* 351–357.

D'Zurilla, T. J., & Nezu, A. M. (1999). *Problem-solving therapy: A social competence approach to clinical intervention* (2nd ed.). New York: Springer.

Ewing-Cobbs, L., Barnes, M., Fletcher, J. M., Levin, H. S., Swank, P. R., & Song, J. (2004). Modeling of longitudinal academic achievement scores after pediatric traumatic brain injury. *Developmental Neuropsychology, 25,* 107–133.

Foreman, B. P., Caesar, R. R., Parks, J., Madden, C., Gentilello, L. M., Shafi, S., et al. (2007). Usefulness of the Abbreviated Injury Score and the Injury Severity Score in comparison to the Glasgow Coma Scale in predicting outcome after traumatic brain injury. *Journal of Trauma, 62,* 946–950.

Goldstrohm, S. L., & Arffa, S. (2005). Preschool children with mild to moderate traumatic brain injury: An exploration of immediate and post-acute morbidity. *Archives of Clinical Neuropsychology, 20,* 675–695.

Gorski, H. A., Slifer, K. J., Townsend, V., Kelly-Suttka, J., & Amari, A. (2005). Behavioural treatment of non-compliance in adolescents with newly acquired spinal cord injuries. *Pediatric Rehabilitation, 8,* 187–198.

Janusz, J. A., Kirkwood, M. W., Yeates, K. O., & Taylor, H. G. (2002). Social problem-solving skills in children with traumatic brain injury: Long-term outcomes and prediction of social competence. *Child Neuropsychology, 8,* 179–194.

Jin, C., & Schachar, R. (2004). Methylphenidate treatment of attention-deficit/hyperactivity disorder secondary to traumatic brain injury: A critical appraisal of treatment studies. *CNS Spectrums, 9,* 217–226.

Karlsson, A. K. (1999). Autonomic dysreflexia. *Spinal Cord, 37,* 383–391.

Keenan, H. T., & Bratton, S. L. (2006). Epidemiology and outcomes of pediatric traumatic brain injury. *Developmental Neuroscience, 28,* 256–263.

Keenan, H. T., Runyan, D. K., Marshall, S. W., Nocera, M. A., Merten, D. F., & Sinai, S. H. (2003). A population-based study of inflicted traumatic brain injury in young children. *Journal of the American Medical Association, 290,* 621–626.

Kirkwood, M. W., Yeates, K. O., Taylor, H. G., Randolph, C., McCrea, M., & Anderson, V. A. (2007). Management of pediatric mild traumatic brain injury: A neuropsychological review from injury through recovery. *The Clinical Neuropsychologist,* 1–32.

Laatsch, L., Harrington, D., Hotz, G., Marcantuono, J., Mozzoni, M. P., Walsh, V., et al. (2007). An evidence-based review of cognitive and behavioral rehabilitation treatment studies in children with acquired brain injury. *Journal of Head Trauma Rehabilitation, 22,* 248–256.

Langlois, J. A., Rutland-Brown, W., & Thomas, K. E. (2006). *Traumatic brain injury in the United States: Emergency department visits, hospitalizations, and deaths.* Atlanta, GA: Centers for Disease Control and Prevention, National Center for Injury Prevention and Control.

Levin, H. S., & Hanten, G. (2005). Executive functions after traumatic brain injury in children. *Pediatric Neurology, 33,* 79–93.

Limond, J., & Leeke, R. (2005). Practitioner review: Cognitive rehabilitation for children with acquired brain injury. *Journal of Child Psychology and Psychiatry, 46,* 339–352.

Mahalick, D. M., Carmel, P. W., Greenberg, J. P., Molofsky, W., Brown, J. A., Heary, R. F., et al. (1998). Psychopharmocologic treatment of acquired attention disorders in children with brain injury. *Pediatric Neurosurgery, 29,* 121–126.

Massagli, T. L. (2000). Medical and rehabilitation issues in the care of children with spinal cord injury. *Physical Medicine and Rehabilitation Clinics of North America, 11,* 169–181.

Max, J. E., Koele, S. L., Castillo, C. C., Lindgren, S. D., Arndt, S., Bokura, H., et al. (2000). Personality change disorder in children and adolescents following traumatic brain injury. *Journal of the International Neuropsychological Society, 6,* 279–289.

Max, J. E., Robin, D. A., Lindgren, S. D., Smith, W. L., Sato, Y., Mattheis, P. J., et al. (1997). Traumatic brain injury in children and adolescents: Psychiatric disorders at two years. *Journal of the American Academy of Child and Adolescent Psychiatry, 36,* 1278–1285.

McCrea, M. A. (2008). *Mild traumatic brain injury and postconcussion syndrome: The new evidence base for diagnosis and treatment.* New York: Oxford University Press.

Molnar, G. E., & Alexander, M. A. (1999). *Pediatric rehabilitation.* Philadelphia: Hanley & Belfus.

National Institute of Neurological Disorders and Stroke (NINDS). (2002). *Traumatic brain injury: Hope through research* (NIH Publication No. 02-2478). Bethesda, MD: National Institutes of Health.

National Institute of Neurological Disorders and Stroke (NINDS). (2003). *Spinal cord injury:*

Hope through research (NIH Publication No. 03-160). Bethesda, MD: National Institutes of Health.

Nelson, V. S., Dixon, P. J., & Warschausky, S. A. (2004). Long-term outcome of children with high tetraplegia and ventilator dependence. *Journal of Spinal Cord Medicine, 27,* S93–S97.

Ponsford, J., Willmott, C., Rothwell, A., Cameron, P., Ayton, G., Nelms, R., et al. (2001). Impact of early intervention after mild traumatic brain injury in children. *Pediatrics, 108,* 1297–1303.

Prigatano, G. P., & Gupta, S. (2006). Friends after traumatic brain injury in children. *Journal of Head Trauma Rehabilitation, 21,* 505–513.

Rivara, J. B., Jaffe, K. M., Polissar, N. L., Fay, G. C., Liao, S., & Martin, K. M. (1996). Predictors of family functioning and change 3 years after traumatic brain injury in children. *Archives of Physical Medicine and Rehabilitation, 77,* 754–764.

Robertson, C. L., Soane, L., Siegel, Z. T., & Fiskum, G. (2006). The potential role of mitochondira in pediatric traumatic brain injury. *Developmental Neuroscience, 28,* 432–446.

Schwartz, L., Taylor, H. G., Drotar, D., Yeates, K. O., Wade, S. L., & Stancin, T. (2003). Long-term behavior problems after pediatric traumatic brain injury: Prevalence, predictors, and correlates. *Journal of Pediatric Psychology, 28,* 251–264.

Selznick, L., & Savage, R. C. (2000). Using self-monitoring procedures to increase on-task behavior with three adolescent boys with brain injury. *Behavioral Interventions, 15,* 243–260.

Singer, G. H. S., Glang, A., Nixon, C., Cooley, E., Kerns, K. A., Williams, D., et al. (1994). A comparison of two psychosocial interventions for parents of children with acquired brain injury: An exploratory study. *Journal of Head Trauma Rehabilitation, 9,* 38–49.

Stancin, T., Drotar, D., Taylor, H. G., Yeates, K. O., Wade, S. L., & Minich, N. M. (2002). Health-related quality of life of children and adolescents following traumatic brain injury. *Pediatrics, 109,* e34.

Suzman, K. B., Morris, R. D., Morris, M. K., & Milan, M. A. (1997). Cognitive-behavioral remediation of problem-solving deficits in children with acquired brain injury. *Journal of Behavior Therapy and Experimental Psychiatry, 28,* 203–212.

Tasiemski, T., Kennedy, P., Gardner, B. P., & Taylor, N. (2005). The association of sports and physical recreation with life satisfaction in a community sample of people with spinal cord injuries. *NeuroRehabilitation, 20,* 253–265.

Taylor, H. G., Yeates, K. O., Wade, S. L., Drotar, D., Klein, S. K., & Stancin, T. (1999). Influences on first-year recovery from traumatic brain injury in children. *Neuropsychology, 13,* 76–89.

Taylor, H. G., Yeates, K. O., Wade, S. L., Drotar, D., Stancin, T., & Minich, N. (2002). A prospective study of short- and long-term outcomes after traumatic brain injury in children: Behavior and achievement. *Neuropsychology, 16,* 15–27.

Teasdale, G., & Jennett, B. (1974). Assessment of coma and impaired consciousness: A practical scale. *Lancet, ii,* 81–84.

Trahan, E., Pepin, M., & Hopps, S. (2006). Impaired awareness of deficits and treatment adherence among people with traumatic brain injury or spinal cord injury. *Journal of Head Trauma Rehabilitation, 21,* 226–235.

Van't Hooft, I., Andersson, K., Bergman, B., Sejersen, T., Von Wendt, L., & Bartfai, A. (2005). Beneficial effect from a cognitive training programme on children with acquired brain injuries demonstrated in a controlled study. *Brain Injury, 19,* 511–518.

Vasa, R. A., Gerring, J. P., Grados, M., Slomine, B., Cristensen, J. R., Rsing, W., et al. (2002). Anxiety after severe pediatric closed head injury. *Journal of the American Academy of Child and Adolescent Psychiatry, 41,* 148–156.

Vitale, M. G., Goss, J. M., Matsumoto, H., & Roye, D. P., Jr. (2006). Epidemiology of pediatric spinal cord injury in the United States: Years 1997 and 2000. *Journal of Pediatric Orthopedics, 26,* 745–749.

Wade, S. L., Borawski, E. A., Taylor, H. G., Drotar, D., Yeates, K. O., & Stancin, T. (2001). The relationship of caregiver coping to family outcomes during the initial year following pediatric traumatic injury. *Journal of Consulting and Clinical Psychology, 69*, 406–415.

Wade, S. L., Carey, J., & Wolfe, C. R. (2006a). The efficacy of an online cognitive-behavioral, family intervention in improving child behavior and social competence following pediatric brain injury. *Rehabilitation Psychology, 51*, 179–189.

Wade, S. L., Carey, J., & Wolfe, C. R. (2006b). The efficacy of an online family intervention to reduce parental distress following pediatric brain injury. *Journal of Consulting and Clinical Psychology, 74*, 445–454.

Wade, S. L., Michaud, L., & Brown, T. M. (2006). Putting the Pieces Together: Preliminary efficacy of a family problem-solving intervention for children with traumatic brain injury. *Journal of Head Trauma Rehabilitation, 21*, 50–60.

Wade, S. L., Taylor, H. G., Drotar, D., Stancin, T., & Yeates, K. O. (1998). Family burden and adaptation following traumatic brain injury (TBI) in children. *Pediatrics, 102*, 110–116.

Wade, S. L., Taylor, H. G., Drotar, D., Stancin, T., Yeates, K. O., & Minich, N. M. (2002). A prospective study of long-term caregiver and family adaptation following brain injury in children. *Journal of Head Trauma Rehabilitation, 17*, 96–111.

Wade, S. L., Taylor, H. G., Drotar, D., Yeates, K. O., Stancin, T., & Minich, N. M. (2004). Interpersonal stressors and resources as predictors of caregiver adaptation following pediatric traumatic injury. *Journal of Consulting and Clinical Psychology, 72*, 776–784.

Wade, S. L., Taylor, H. G., Yeates, K. O., Drotar, D., Stancin, T., Minich, N. M., et al. (2006). Long-term family adaptation following pediatric brain injury. *Journal of Pediatric Psychology, 31*, 1072–1083.

Wilson, B. A., Emslie, H. C., Quirk, K., & Evans, J. J. (2001). Reducing everyday memory and planning problems by means of a paging system: A randomized control crossover study. *Journal of Neurology, Neurosurgery and Psychiatry, 70*, 477–482.

Yeates, K. O. (2000). Pediatric closed head injury. In K. O. Yeates, M. D. Ris, & H. G. Taylor (Eds.), *Pediatric neuropsychology: Research, theory, and practice* (pp. 92–116). New York: Guilford Press.

Yeates, K. O., Swift, K., Taylor, H. G., Wade, S. L., Drotar, D., Stancin, T., et al. (2004). Short- and long-term social outcomes following pediatric traumatic brain injury. *Journal of the International Neuropsychological Society, 10*, 412–426.

Yeates, K. O., & Taylor, H. G. (2005). Neurobehavioral outcomes of mild head injury in children and adolescents. *Pediatric Rehabilitation, 8*, 5–16.

Yeates, K. O., Taylor, H. G., Wade, S. L., Drotar, D., Stancin, T., & Minich, N. (2002). A prospective study of short- and long-term neuropsychological outcomes after traumatic brain injury in children. *Neuropsychology, 16*, 514–523.

Yeates, K. O., Taylor, H. G., Woodrome, S. E., Wade, S. L., Stancin, T., & Drotar, D. (2002). Race as a moderator of parent and family outcomes following pediatric traumatic brain injury. *Journal of Pediatric Psychology, 27*, 393–404.

Ylvisaker, M., Jacobs, H. E., & Feeney, T. (2003). Positive supports for people who experience behavioral and cognitive disability after brain injury: A review. *Journal of Head Trauma Rehabilitation, 18*, 7–32.

Ylvisaker, M., Todis, B., Glang, A., Urbanczyk, B., Franklin, C., DePompei, R., et al. (2001). Educating students with TBI: Themes and recommendations. *Journal of Head Trauma Rehabilitation, 16*, 76–93.

Ylvisaker, M., Turkstra, L., Coehlo, C., Yorkston, K., Kennedy, M., Sohlerg, M. M., et al. (2007). Behavioral interventions for children and adults with behavioural disorders after TBI: A systematic review of the evidence. *Brain Injury, 21*, 769–805.

CHAPTER 23

Central Nervous System Disorders
Epilepsy and Spina Bifida as Exemplars

KATHLEEN K. M. DEIDRICK
MAUREEN O. GRISSOM
JANET E. FARMER

The term "neurodevelopmental disorders" applies to central nervous system (CNS) impairments that can or do interfere with children's adaptive functioning and participation in age-appropriate activities (e.g., recreational, academic, or household activities) (Mudrick, 2002). Neurodevelopmental disorders can be categorized by the period of time in which CNS impairment originated: prenatal, perinatal, and postnatal periods (see Table 23.1) (Luckasson et al., 2002). Although prevalence rates for CNS disorders can be difficult to ascertain, the 1994–1995 National Health Interview Survey—Disability Supplement for Children indicated that 1.9% of children had neurodevelopmental disorders (e.g., neurosensory problems, mental retardation, autism, genetic disorders) (Msall et al., 2003). Of the children who received special education services, 17% were identified with neurodevelopmental disorders. Children with these disorders are vulnerable to the same risks to psychological adjustment as children with other medical disorders (e.g., distress and pain related to medical procedures, multiple hospitalizations that reduce time in school and with peers, other difficulties). In addition, children with neurodevelopmental disorders are at increased risk for cognitive deficits and related school, behavioral, and emotional difficulties, making them more likely to come to the attention of pediatric psychologists (Farmer & Deidrick, 2006). The purpose of this chapter is to provide an overview of issues relevant to pediatric psychologists working with children who have neurodevelopmental disorders, and to offer information on assessment and treatment approaches in these populations. The chapter begins with a brief review of a framework for understanding neurodevelopmental disorders. It then describes two such conditions, epilepsy and spina bifida (SB), and provides guidelines for assessment and intervention in these populations.

350

TABLE 23.1. Common Causes of Neurodevelopmental Disabilities

Prenatal	Perinatal	Postnatal

• Genetic/metabolic disorders
  o Chromosome abnormalities
  o Fragile X syndrome
  o Down syndrome
  o Phenylketonuria
  o Hypothyroidism
  o Autism
• Disruption of normal brain development
  o Spina bifida
  o Hydrocephalus
  o Cerebral palsy
• Hearing impairment
• Environmental causes
  o Fetal alcohol exposure
  o Irradiation during pregnancy
	• Intrauterine disorders
	  o Chronic placental insufficiency
	• Neonatal disorders
	  o Prematurity and associated early medical risks, such as:
	    ▪ Periventricular hemorrhage and leukomalacia
	    ▪ Retinopathy
	    ▪ Respiratory distress syndrome
	• Human immunodeficiency virus
		• Traumatic brain injury
		• Spinal cord injury
		• Infections
		  o Encephalitis
		  o Meningitis
		• Demyelinating and neurodegenerative disorders
		• Seizure disorders
		• Chronic illnesses with central nervous system effects
		  o Sickle cell anemia
		  o Acute lymphocytic leukemia
		  o End-stage renal disease
		  o Diabetes
		• Lead poisoning
		• Malnutrition

Note. From Luckasson et al. (2002). Copyright 2002 by the American Association on Mental Retardation. Adapted by permission.

A Framework for Understanding Neurodevelopmental Disorders

The *International Classification of Functioning, Disability and Health for Children and Youth* (ICF-CY) is a recently developed multifactorial method of describing and categorizing outcomes for young people, including those with neurodevelopmental concerns (World Health Organization, 2007). This classification system provides a strategy for coding children's health in multiple domains, including any relevant health conditions, their impact on physical structures and function, and the resulting effect on activities and participation in the community (see Figure 23.1). This system also takes into account contextual factors that can influence outcomes, such as stages of development and a child's environment. Careful description of such concerns through the ICF-CY provides a framework for understanding child functioning and may help clinicians, educators, and parents develop a proactive plan for each child's health and educational needs. This chapter utilizes the following ICF-CY categories to discuss our two exemplars of neurodevelopmental disorders: body functions and structures (physical, cognitive, and emotional and behavioral); child activities; participation; and environmental factors.

An Overview of Neurodevelopmental Disorders: Two Exemplars

Epilepsy and SB are neurodevelopmental conditions resulting in a variety of associated medical and cognitive-developmental concerns. Although many conditions could have been chosen, epilepsy and SB are targeted because this choice allows us to cover the

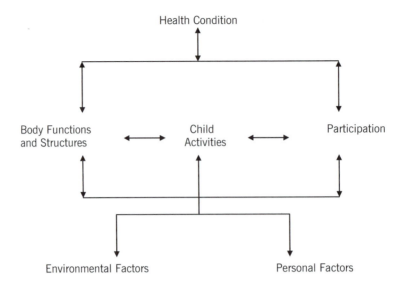

FIGURE 23.1. Conceptual model of factors that influence child outcome, based on the *International Classification of Functioning, Disability and Health for Children and Youth* (World Health Organization, 2007). From Farmer and Deidrick (2006). Copyright 2006 by The Guilford Press. Reprinted by permission.

complex impairments that can co-occur in children with neurodevelopmental disorders. Epilepsy is a relatively common condition that pediatric psychologists are likely to encounter in their practice, and it is a prototypical example of a neurodevelopmental condition that can be "invisible" to others. SB provides a contrasting example in which mobility difficulties may also be present. Children with these conditions vary considerably in their presentation, with notable differences in severity and comorbid conditions even among children with the same medical diagnosis.

Epilepsy

Body Functions and Structures

Physical Functioning. "Seizures" are atypical electrical discharges in the brain that may cause a variety of effects, including loss of consciousness, loss of muscle tone or increased muscle tone, and automatisms. Some seizures may have an identifiable cause (i.e., can be localized to a specific area of the brain or related to a particular event or neurological condition, such as a head injury), whereas others may not. In the case of more than one seizure that is not caused by a particular event or insult, a diagnosis of epilepsy is made (Hauser & Beghi, 2008). According to the Epilepsy Foundation of America (2002), approximately 1% of U.S. children under the age of 20 years are diagnosed with epilepsy. Seizures are categorized according to their type of onset (generalized vs. partial), as well as their effects (e.g., absence seizures with staring, tonic seizures with stiffening of muscles, atonic seizures with loss of muscle tone) (Friedman & Sharieff, 2006). Seizure onset is categorized as partial (involving a single area of the brain, though it may progress to other areas during the course of the seizures) or generalized (involving both hemispheres of the brain and a loss of consciousness). For a detailed review of the various seizure types, the reader is referred to Blackburn, Zelko, and Shurtleff (2007).

Medical interventions varying in terms of effectiveness and invasiveness are available for the treatment of epilepsy. In the past two to three decades, there has been an increase in the availability of antiepileptic drugs (AEDs), which are chosen according to seizure type. AEDs have been found to control seizures in 80–90% of children with absence epilepsy, juvenile myoclonic epilepsy, and new-onset partial seizures (Garofalo, 2007). In the remaining group of children, various treatments are considered, including surgical intervention in children with identified tumors, malformations, or localized regions of seizure activity. The vagus nerve stimulator is another treatment that has been found to result in reduced seizure frequency and severity, as well as improved quality of life in some children (Lundgren, Amark, Blennow, Stromblad, & Wallstedt, 1998). Some research suggests efficacy for certain diets (e.g., a ketogenic diet) in reducing seizures as much as 84%. There is still only limited support for this approach, based on studies with small sample sizes (Remahl, Dahlin, & Amark, 2008). The mechanism underlying the low-carbohydrate ketogenic diet is not well understood, but it is thought to be related to alterations in neurotransmitters due to the changes in metabolism caused by the diet (Hartman, Gasior, Vining, & Rogawski, 2007).

Cognitive Functioning. The overall intellectual functioning of children with epilepsy is generally within the average range, although there is a greater likelihood of impairment related to generalized seizure type, earlier onset, and seizure intractability (LaJoie & Moshe, 2004; Nolan et al., 2004) or the presence of significant neurological abnormalities (Williams, 2003). Particularly when seizures are not well controlled, children with epilepsy are at greater risk for difficulties in the areas of attention, memory (Nolan et al., 2004), and processing speed (Aldenkamp et al., 2000). Children and adolescents with epilepsy receive special education services at higher rates and are at risk for academic underachievement (Berg et al., 2005). A recent study found that nearly half of all children with epilepsy (N = 164 children and adolescents with several seizure types; the study excluded individuals with mental retardation, head injury, or other chronic physical or medical conditions) exceeded the cutoff for a learning disability (one standard deviation IQ–achievement discrepancy) in one or more academic domains, with such discrepancies being most common in the area of writing (Fastenau, Jianzhao, Dunn, & Austin, 2008). Consequently, screening for learning disabilities is an important consideration for any child identified with epilepsy. The most effective approach to minimizing cognitive difficulties is through control of the seizures, which unfortunately is not always an attainable goal (Berg et al., 2001). In addition to the effects of seizures themselves, medications used to treat epilepsy and concomitant difficulties can contribute to cognitive difficulties.

Emotional and Behavioral Functioning. Children with epilepsy are at increased risk for psychopathology, such as depressive symptoms (Wagner & Smith, 2006). Specifically, children with epilepsy are nearly five times more likely to experience psychopathology than children in the general population, and more than twice as likely as children with non-CNS-related chronic conditions (Austin & Caplan, 2007). Other factors that could contribute to the presence or absence of psychopathology include AEDs, individual and family adaptation to epilepsy, and underlying neurological dysfunction that may be related to both seizures and behavioral difficulties (Austin et al., 2001). There are also numerous demographic factors to consider (e.g., gender, age of onset, seizure characteristics), and methodological differences make it difficult to understand the impact of these variables on outcome. Age of onset has been more strongly related to IQ and language difficulties than to behavioral problems, although cognitive and language deficits can contribute to behavior problems (Austin & Caplan, 2007). An increase in behavioral difficulties has been found to be associated with higher levels of family stress, lower parental educational status, lower levels of extended family support, and poorer maternal mental health (Austin & Caplan, 2007). The reader is referred to Austin and Caplan (2007) for more information on behavior problems in children with epilepsy.

Activities and Participation

As noted above, children with epilepsy are also at risk for academic problems (Bailet & Turk, 2000). Factors that may contribute to academic difficulties include attention and memory difficulties, the side effects of AEDs, possible underlying neurological abnormalities, and psychological/behavioral issues (MacLeod & Austin, 2003). Children with epilepsy have been found to have poorer social skills than their healthy siblings (Tse, Hamiwka, Sherman, & Wirrell, 2007). Finally, the development of independence during adolescence may be affected by such issues as difficulty in obtaining a driver's license (Epilepsy Foundation of America, 2002).

Environmental Factors

In addition to the potential effects of epilepsy on children's functioning and activities, such children are affected by family factors and more distal environmental factors, such as societal reactions and health care–related issues. Reviews of the literature on families of children with epilepsy (Rodenburg, Meijer, Dekovic, & Aldenkamp, 2005) have found that these families report higher levels of stress than do control families of children with other conditions, such as asthma. Parents of children with epilepsy have been found to be more overprotective of their children; however, this finding has not been linked to emotional and behavioral problems in the children. It has been hypothesized that due to the unique issues faced by these parent–child dyads, such as medical compliance and the need to supervise the children's activities, overprotectiveness may be largely adaptive (Hodes, Garralda, Rose, & Schwartz, 1999). Other aspects of the parent–child relationship, such as psychological control (e.g., intrusive and manipulative parenting strategies, such as creating feelings of guilt) exerted by parents, have been found to be problematic and related to depression and anxiety (Rodenburg et al., 2005).

The social stigma related to epilepsy has been associated with depression, low self-esteem, and anxiety and negativity (MacLeod & Austin, 2003), particularly in adolescents (Dunn, 2003). A commonly cited finding is that at the time of the onset of seizures, parents feel that they lack knowledge about their child's condition (Shore, Perkins, & Austin, 2008). Seizures may generate anxiety on the part of the public, and parents may worry about stigma for their child as well as future consequences (Chapieski et al., 2005). Parental attitudes, however, have been found to become more positive across time, with an initial period of high stress at the onset of seizures followed by better adjustment (Rodenburg et al., 2005).

Several issues have been noted to impede the timely identification and treatment of epilepsy; these include parents' neglecting to seek treatment or not recognizing symptoms, and health care professionals' failing to recognize seizures and in some cases initiating inappropriate treatment (Buelow & Shore, 2006). Although quantitative studies of this topic were not available in the extant literature, these issues were identified via a qualitative study (Buelow & Shore, 2006) in which approximately as many parents reported problems in the diagnostic process as reported satisfaction with the process of diagnosis. Also affecting children and adults with seizures are barriers to seeking or complying with medical treatment. A survey study of neurologists revealed low income, lack of health insurance, transportation, social stigma, and misconceptions (e.g., of epilepsy as a mental illness) as some of the major obstacles (Hawley et al., 2007).

Spina Bifida

Body Functions and Structures

Physical Functioning. SB occurs when the neural tube does not fuse properly in early pregnancy, resulting in malformations of the spinal cord and cerebral cortex (Mitchell et al., 2004). The most common form of SB is myelomeningocele, in which the meninges and spinal nerves are not contained in the spinal cord and protrude from the open vertebrae. This condition results in weakness or paralysis of the lower extremities, as well as problems with bowel and bladder control. Children with myelomeningocele frequently exhibit malformations of the cerebral cortex, including malformation of subcortical midline brain structures (e.g., midbrain and corpus callosum). Arnold–Chiari II malformations are common; these consist of structural abnormalities of the cerebellum in which brain tissue herniates through the base of the skull, due to insufficient room in the skull cavity. Blockage of cerebrospinal fluid (CSF) in the third and forth ventricles often results in the buildup of excessive CSF in the ventricles (hydrocephalus), requiring the placement of a shunt to divert the CSF. Secondary CNS insults due to multiple shunt revisions, shunt infections, or seizures are also common (Dennis, Landry, Barnes, & Fletcher, 2006). Prevalence rates for SB without anencephaly vary across country of origin and race, with one recent study estimating a prevalence rate of 3.74 per 10,000 in the United States (Canfield et al., 2006; Mitchell, 2005).

Children with SB experience multiple medical treatments, beginning with surgery to close the lesion either prenatally or immediately after birth. Placement of a shunt to divert CSF from the ventricles to the abdominal cavity often occurs in the neonatal period. Children are followed closely so that neurologists can monitor shunt functioning and perform revisions of the shunt as needed. During early school age, children learn to manage their own bowel programs and perform intermittent catheterization to prevent bladder infections and protect the kidneys (Edwards, Borzyskowski, Cox, & Badcock, 2004). Children and families must also learn regimens for skin care (e.g., prevention of pressure sores due to braces or poor positioning in wheelchairs) and for maintaining function through physical therapy. Ongoing monitoring by physicians is also needed to prevent and treat secondary orthopedic and physical health issues (e.g., scoliosis, obesity) (Simeonsson, McMillen, & Huntington, 2002).

Cognitive Functioning. Children with SB present with typically intact overall intellectual functioning (low-average range), basic language skills, and single-word reading skills. However, these skills often mask subtle weaknesses in visual–spatial and visual–motor skills and in higher-level language (Dennis et al., 2006; Ewing-Cobbs, Barnes, & Fletcher, 2003). Some researchers suggest that at least a subset of these children exhibit a nonverbal learning disorder pattern (Yeates, Loss, Colvin, & Enrile, 2003). Burgeoning research indicates difficulties with attention and other aspects of executive functioning (e.g., initiation, organization, self-monitoring) among children with SB and hydrocephalus (Mahone, Zabel, Levey, Verda, & Kinsman, 2002; Rose & Holmbeck, 2007). Although echoic and implicit memory (e.g., memory for routines) may be intact, difficulties with learning, long-term memory, and retrieval of previously stored memories may be present. A current model of cognitive functioning in SB suggests that this profile originates from basic processing deficits in the posterior attention systems (orienting) and in the areas of timing and motor movement (Dennis et al., 2006).

Emotional and Behavioral Functioning. The research on psychological adjustment in SB is mixed, but recent studies suggest increased risk for adjustment and psychiatric problems. Early studies suggested a general tendency toward internalizing symptoms (e.g., withdrawal, somatic symptoms) and depression for children with SB (Appleton et al., 1997). However, other studies indicate that children with SB may also be at increased risk for externalizing behavior problems. For example, a 1998 study examining parent-reported psychiatric symptoms among 54 children and adolescents with SB reported that 43% of these youths met screening criteria on a parent questionnaire for at least one disorder, and that 13% met criteria for more than one disorder (Ammerman et al., 1998). The most common disorders for which children met screening cutoff criteria were attention-deficit hyperactivity disorder (33%), other behavior disorders (15%), and anxiety disorders (21%). In addition, some literature suggests potential difficulties in adjusting to the condition, including poor knowledge of critical disease-related information (e.g., reasons for intermittent catheterization, signs of shunt malfunction) (Greenley, Coakley, Holmbeck, Jandasek, & Wills, 2006) and poor adherence to bowel, skin care, and catheterization regimens (Holmbeck et al., 1998).

Activities and Participation

Academically, children with SB exhibit intact basic reading skills (particularly at younger ages when word decoding is emphasized), in contrast to weaker comprehension skills. Difficulties with mathematics and specific learning disabilities in math are common (Barnes et al., 2006). These weaknesses are consistent with the cognitive profile described above, including deficits in visual–spatial processing and in problem solving and planning. Children with SB, therefore, generally receive poorer grades than healthy children and are less likely to be seen as academically capable, particularly when the effects of SB are combined with the impact of low socioeconomic status (Holmbeck et al., 2003). Children may be more dependent upon adults, showing decreased responsibility for household tasks and less ability to make independent decisions (Holmbeck et al., 2003). These children are described as less involved in extracurricular physical and social activities and more reluctant to initiate social interactions (Holmbeck et al., 2003); these characteristics contribute to their having smaller groups of friends and fewer reciprocal friendships (Cunningham, Thomas, & Warschausky, 2007). Social information-processing weaknesses and other weaknesses in social skills may also be present and are closely tied to cognitive deficits (Warschausky, Argento, Hurvitz, & Berg, 2003).

Environmental Factors

Recent reviews and meta-analyses examining family functioning in children with SB suggest that families typically show a pattern of resilience, with positive adaptation to the task of raising a child with a neurodevelopmental disorder (Holmbeck, Greenley, Coakley, Greco, & Hagstrom, 2006; Vermaes, Gerris, & Janssens, 2007). These reviews suggest that marriages typically remain stable and that relationships between family members are generally positive. However, a subset of parents display high levels of stress (19–56% of mothers and 25–28% of fathers), including stressful interactions with their affected children and doubts about their own parenting abilities (Vermaes, Janssens, Bosman, & Gerris, 2005). Parents who are single, are older, are members of a minority group, lack financial or social resources, and have poorer coping skills may be particularly vulnerable to high levels of stress. In addition, some aspects of parenting appear to be influenced. Mothers of children with SB may show a pattern of overprotection, greater use of psychological control, and an authoritarian style, particularly if their children exhibit weaker cognitive skills. Maternal overprotection may be associated with less autonomous decision-making skill, and may be related to depression and behavior problems, for children with SB as well as for healthy children (Holmbeck et al., 2002).

Psychological Assessment and Treatment

Because children with neurodevelopmental disorders, such as SB and epilepsy, are at increased risk of emotional and behavioral disturbance, pediatric psychologists are likely to encounter these populations. Psychologists will quickly discover that the core approaches and skills used in other medical and mental health populations also apply to children with neurodevelopmental disorders. Many of the factors that promote well-being in children with neurodevelopmental disorders are universally beneficial. For example, the literature suggests that parent well-being (e.g., parent stress, psychopathology, marital relationship) and child characteristics (e.g., intrinsic motivation, cognitive ability, coping skills, behavior) are as strongly related to adjustment in children with SB as in typically developing children (Coakley, Holmbeck, & Bryant, 2006).

However, the cognitive characteristics that are unique to children with neurodevelopmental disorders require a subtle shift in perspective and awareness. Assessment and treatment for children with neurodevelopmental disorders and their families should be based on principles gathered from the pediatric rehabilitation literature, including (1) capitalizing on child and family strengths to enhance functional outcome; (2) centering interventions within a child's natural environment and daily routines; (3) using a team approach to address the child's diverse needs; (4) acknowledging the interaction of child development and neurodevelopment with the disease or injury process; and (5) understanding and addressing the relationship between cognitive abilities and psychological functioning through remediational, compensatory, and supportive strategies (Farmer, Kanne, & Grissom, in press). Below, we review the aspects of inpatient and outpatient treatment that may be different for children with neurodevelopment disorders than for children with non-neurological physical health concerns.

Inpatient Assessment and Treatment

Children with neurodevelopmental disorders present at inpatient hospitals for treatment related to their neurodevelopmental condition (e.g., treatment of shunt malfunction in SB), as well as for typical childhood illnesses. Overall, children with neurodevelopmental concerns such as SB may be more likely to present for hospitalization than healthy children, due to disease-specific health vulnerabilities (Ouyang, Grosse, Armour, & Waitzman, 2007). Psychology consultations may be requested for a variety of reasons (e.g., poor adherence to medical treatments, behavior problems, pain management concerns). Although a consulting psychologist's approach is likely to be similar regardless of the presence or absence of CNS dysfunction, the orientation and focus may differ slightly.

Kazak, Simms, and Rourke (2002) provide a model for family-focused consultations in pediatric populations that is consistent with rehabilitation principles and can easily be adapted to populations with CNS disorders. This approach emphasizes family competence and reframes behaviors that are problematic for medical teams as attempts to cope with stressors. For children with neurodevelopmental disorders, who sometimes do not have the communication skills necessary to get their needs met in a socially appropriate manner, this orientation is particularly important. A psychologist responds to a consultation request by clarifying the referral question and assembling a collaborative team (or therapeutic triad) that includes the child, a family member, and a member of the medical team (e.g., physician, physical or occupational therapist, nurse). The team collaborates to help the family use preexisting coping skills to calm distress, promote positive relationships between the family and medical team member, and manage the specific conflict that prompted the consultation (Kazak et al., 2002). For example, in a child with SB who presents with an acute illness and refusal to eat, the team will work to identify the child's preexisting strengths, reinforcement history, and preferences. Using this information, the team can help the child to communicate more effectively and develop a simple behavior system to promote eating (e.g., ignoring refusal behaviors and providing high levels of social attention to eating behaviors).

During the information-gathering portion of the consultation, the consulting psychologist can rely on the ICF-CY as a framework for identifying broad areas that should be targeted. Cognitive screening is conducted (1) to clarify the role that cognitive weaknesses may play in the problem leading to the consultation request, and (2) to identify strengths that the family and medical team can use to promote positive adaptation for the child. Depending on the consultation question, a variety of assessment strategies may be appropriate, including informal strategies (e.g., obtaining cognitive functioning history from the parents, reviewing educational records, observing the child's cognitive processing during an interview), brief cognitive screenings, and formal, targeted cognitive evaluations. Brief neuropsychological screening batteries, such as those described by Baron (2004), may be helpful in getting a more comprehensive understanding of child functioning across domains and may serve as a preliminary step to more comprehensive outpatient evaluation.

Specialized assessment in the area of pain may also be warranted, as children can experience both acute pain related to medical procedures and chronic, life-limiting pain related to primary disease symptoms (Berrin et al., 2007; Oddson, Clancy, & McGrath, 2006). Pain may be underrecognized and undertreated among children with neurodevelopmental disorders, due to their higher frequency of exposure to painful procedures, communication deficits, and atypical facial and body responses to pain, as well as an underlying bias that undervalues the experiences of children with cognitive disabilities (Hadden & von Baeyer, 2005). Psychologists may adapt common self-report pain assessment scales (e.g., enlarging and/or simplifying the scales, allowing simple pointing responses, or providing training in the use of the scales), and/or may use measures that have been developed for children who have communication problems (Breau, McGrath, Camfield, & Finley, 2002; Hadden & von Baeyer, 2005).

Outpatient Assessment and Treatment

Specialized outpatient treatments for children with neurodevelopmental disorders are rapidly emerging in the literature. Two recently published edited volumes are devoted to emerging treatment approaches in this population (Farmer, Donders, & Warschausky, 2006; Hunter & Donders, 2007). In addition to the general principles of rehabilitation that guide this work, this literature reflects a shift in treatment approach to address cognitive deficits and their impact on child functioning. Treatment approaches include direct services to remediate, or assist children in compensating for, cognitive deficits; positive behavior support approaches, which structure the environment to promote success; family supports to teach specific skills or assist with care coordination; and modifications of cognitive-behavioral therapies.

Cognitive Remediation and Compensatory Strategies

Many children with neurodevelopmental disorders are eligible for comprehensive early intervention services through the educational system. Such services (typically in-home or center-based treatments) may include physical, occupational, and speech/language therapies, as well as specialized instruction. The types of services available and the criteria for qualification for services vary widely across states. Familiarity with local services and regulations will be very useful to pediatric psychologists (National Early Childhood Technical Assistance Center, 2008). The utility of comprehensive early intervention programs in preventing secondary impairments in children with known neurodevelopmental risks has been examined. In one example, the Infant Health and Development Program targeted children who were born at low birthweights, and provided family supports and an enriched day care experience. This program showed promise in preventing the cognitive, academic, functional, health, and behavioral consequences of low birthweight (Gross, Spiker, & Haynes, 1997).

In addition to preventive developmental programs, psychologists may attempt to remediate the consequences of neurodevelopmental disorders directly, through providing cognitive rehabilitation or assisting children in generating compensatory strategies. In order to choose the correct strategy, a psychologist must complete a comprehensive neuropsychological evaluation that describes a child's strengths and weaknesses in a variety of domains, including intellectual and academic functioning; adaptive skills; language; visual–spatial and visual–motor skills; and memory, attention, and other aspects of executive functioning. These findings can be used to develop individualized recommendations to improve the child's functioning. A few cognitive rehabilitation programs that directly involve a child in "mental exercises" designed to strengthen basic skills have received support in the literature (Butler et al., 2008). In addition, specialized instruction programs have been adopted for working with children with neurodevelopmental concerns (e.g., Direct Instruction for children with Traumatic Brain Injuries; Glang, Singer, Cooley, & Tish, 1992). Provision of individualized compensatory strategies based on neuropsychological test findings can also be very helpful (e.g., extended time for processing, simplification of visual information).

Positive Behavior Supports

Traditional behavior modification strategies are helpful for working with children who have neurodevelopmental disorders (Warschausky, Kewman, & Kay, 1999). Misbehavior in children with such disorders can develop as the result of the same factors that predispose typically developing children to misbehave, such as inconsistent or inappropriate discipline and monitoring. However, misbehavior can also develop as a result of inability to communicate, difficulty understanding or processing language, poor memory, frustration due to inappropriate task demands, or difficulty learning from experience. Therefore, positive behavior support approaches, which involve skill-building strategies and antecedent controls, are gathering support for use in these populations (Bambara, Dunlap, & Schwartz, 2004; Feeney & Ylvisaker, 2003).

Family Supports

Various family support interventions have been described that include one or a combination of the following components: assisting families in coordinating care, psychoeducation, family therapy, and informal supports. Because the system of care for children with neurodevelopmental disorders is fragmented, a family may benefit from coordination of care and creation of a "medical home" for a child (Farmer & Drewel, 2006). Psychoeducation to increase the caregiver's knowledge of the child's illness, its cognitive impact, and strategies for behavior management and educational support may also be useful, as families often report needs for more information about their children's condition (Farmer, Marien, Clark, Sherman, & Selva, 2004). Although traditional family therapy approaches have not been thoroughly studied in these populations, promising pilot studies are emerging (Glueckauf et al., 2002). Although the research on less formal supports is unclear, respite care (skilled caregiving for short periods of time to allow family members a break), parent-to-parent supports (e.g., support groups, parent-matching programs) (Hastings & Beck, 2004), and sibling supports (Lobato & Kao, 2005) are often recommended.

Psychotherapeutic Approaches

Direct psychotherapy services to children with CNS disorders are largely uninvestigated, with a few notable exceptions. The "gold standard" cognitive-behavioral treatment programs used to treat children with mental health concerns in the absence of neurological insults may have limitations in these populations, due to these programs' inherent demands for higher-level language, metacognitive skills, and abstraction. However, there are some promising pilot programs for social skills training in children with SB and cerebral palsy (King et al., 1997) and children with brain tumors (Die-Trill et al., 1996). Initial investigations using modified cognitive-behavioral treatments in children with Asperger's disorder, who frequently exhibit higher-level language and executive functioning deficits, are promising (Sofronoff, Attwood, & Hinton, 2005). Stress innoculation training has been used in treatment for children with cognitive disorders resulting from cancer, and may be useful in children with other neurodevelopmental disorders (Butler & Mulhern, 2005).

Conclusions

In conclusion, the ICF-CY and the burgeoning literature on neurodevelopmental disorders provide useful information for psychologists working with children who have such disorders and their families. The basic psychological skills possessed by most practitioners will address many of the concerns observed in these populations. However, the most promising interventions incorporate assessment and intervention strategies that are based on rehabilitation principles and take cognitive weaknesses into account. Although information on interventions is scattered across literatures in multiple disciplines (psychology, medicine, nursing, education, occupational and speech/language therapy, social work), a set of promising approaches is developing. In the future, researchers should continue to explore the impact of biological, cognitive, psychological, and psychosocial factors on outcomes for children with neurodevelopmental disorders. Transition to adulthood should also be a focus of future research efforts, as this period is commonly described as a time of uncertainty and difficulty for persons with neurodevelopmental disorders, and empirically supported interventions to promote transition are not plentiful. Finally, continued efforts to determine whether standard cognitive-behavioral and family treatments are appropriate in this population, what modifications to standard treatments are needed, and where innovation is needed are encouraged.

References

Aldenkamp, A., van Bronswijk, K., Braken, M., Diepman, L. A., Verwey, L. E., & van den Wittenboer, G. (2000). A clinical comparative study evaluating the effect of epilepsy versus ADHD on timed cognitive tasks in children. *Child Neuropsychology, 6*, 209–217.

Ammerman, R. T., Kane, V. R., Slomka, G. T., Reigel, D. H., Franzen, M. D., & Gadow, K. D. (1998). Psychiatric symptomatology and family functioning in children and adolescents with spina bifida. *Journal of Clinical Psychology in Medical Settings, 5*, 449–465.

Appleton, P. L., Ellis, N. C., Minchom, P. E., Lawson, V., Boll, V., & Jones, P. (1997). Depressive symptoms and self-concept in young people with spina bifida. *Journal of Pediatric Psychology, 22*, 707–722.

Austin, J. K., & Caplan, R. (2007). Behavioral and psychiatric comorbidities in pediatric epilepsy: Toward an integrative model. *Epilepsia, 48*, 1639–1651.

Austin, J. K., Harezlak, J., Dunn, D. W., Huster, G. A., Rose, D. F., & Ambrosius, W. T. (2001). Behavior problems in children before first recognized seizures. *Pediatrics, 107*, 115–122.

Bailet, L. L., & Turk, W. R. (2000). The impact of childhood epilepsy on neurocognitive and behavioral performance: A prospective longitudinal study. *Epilepsia, 41*, 426–431.

Bambara, L. M., Dunlap, G., & Schwartz, I. S. (Eds.). (2004). *Positive behavior support: Criti-*

cal articles on improving practice for individuals with severe disabilities. Austin, TX: PRO-ED and TASH.

Barnes, M. A., Wilkinson, M., Khemani, E., Boudesquie, A., Dennis, M., Fletcher, J. M., et al. (2006). Arithmetic processing in children with spina bifida: Calculation accuracy, strategy use, and fact retrieval fluency. *Journal of Learning Disabilities, 39*, 174–187.

Baron, I. S. (2004). *Neuropsychological evaluation of the child*. New York: Oxford University Press.

Berg, A. T., Shinnar, S., Levy, S., Testa, F., Smith-Rapaport, S., & Beckerman, B. (2001). Early development of intractable epilepsy in children: A prospective study. *Neurology, 56*, 1445–1452.

Berg, A. T., Smith, S. N., Frobish, D., Levy, S. R., Testa, F. M., Beckerman, B., et al. (2005). Special education needs of children with newly diagnosed epilepsy. *Developmental Medicine and Child Neurology, 47*, 749–753.

Berrin, S. J., Malcarne, V. L., Varni, J. W., Burwinkle, T. M., Sherman, S. A., Artavia, K., et al. (2007). Pain, fatigue, and school functioning in children with cerebral palsy: A path-analytic model. *Journal of Pediatric Psychology, 32*, 330–337.

Blackburn, L. B., Zelko, F., & Shurtleff, H. (2007). Seizure disorders. In S. J. Hunter & J. Donders (Eds.), *Pediatric neuropsychological intervention* (pp. 133–150). Cambridge, UK: Cambridge University Press.

Breau, L. M., McGrath, P. J., Camfield, C. S., & Finley, G. (2002). Psychometric properties of the Non-Communicating Children's Pain Checklist—Revised. *Pain, 99*, 349–357.

Buelow, J. M., & Shore, C. P. (2006). Childhood epilepsy: Failures along the path to diagnosis and treatment. *Epilepsy and Behavior, 9*, 440–447.

Butler, R. W., Copeland, D. R., Fairclough, D. L., Mulhern, R. K., Katz, E. R., Kazak, A. E., et al. (2008). A multicenter, randomized clinical trial of a cognitive remediation program for childhood survivors of a pediatric malignancy. *Journal of Consulting and Clinical Psychology, 76*, 367–378.

Butler, R. W., & Mulhern, R. K. (2005). Neurocognitive interventions for children and adolescents surviving cancer. *Journal of Pediatric Psychology, 30*, 65–78.

Canfield, M. A., Honein, M. A., Yuskiv, N., Xing, J., Mai, C. T., Collins, J. S., et al. (2006). National estimates and race/ethnic-specific variation of selected birth defects in the United States, 1999–2001. *Birth Defects Research, 76*, 747–756.

Chapieski, L., Brewer, V., Evankovich, K., Culhane-Shelburne, K., Zelman, K., & Alexander, A. (2005). Adaptive functioning in children with seizures: Impact of maternal anxiety about epilepsy. *Epilepsy and Behavior, 7*, 246–252.

Coakley, R. M., Holmbeck, G. N., & Bryant, F. B. (2006). Constructing a prospective model of psychosocial adaptation in young adolescents with spina bifida: An application of optimal data analysis. *Journal of Pediatric Psychology, 31*, 1084–1099.

Cunningham, S. D., Thomas, P. D., & Warschausky, S. (2007). Gender differences in peer relations of children with neurodevelopmental conditions. *Rehabilitation Psychology, 52*, 331–337.

Dennis, M., Landry, S. H., Barnes, M., & Fletcher, J. M. (2006). A model of neurocognitive function in spina bifida over the life span. *Journal of the International Neuropsychological Society, 12*, 285–296.

Die-Trill, M., Bromberg, J., LaVally, B., Portales, L. A., Sanfeliz, A., & Patenaude, A. (1996). Development of social skills in boys with brain tumors: A group approach. *Journal of Psychosocial Oncology, 14*, 23–41.

Dunn, D. W. (2003). Neuropsychiatric aspects of epilepsy in children. *Epilepsy and Behavior, 4*, 101–106.

Edwards, M., Borzyskowski, M., Cox, A., & Badcock, J. (2004). Neuropathic bladder and intermittent catheterization: Social and psychological impact on children and adolescents. *Developmental Medicine and Child Neurology, 46*, 168–177.

Epilepsy Foundation of America. (2002). *Answer place: Epilepsy and seizure statistics*. Retrieved February 1, 2008, from *www.epilepsyfoundation.org*

Ewing-Cobbs, L., Barnes, M. A., & Fletcher, J. M. (2003). Early brain injury in children: Development and reorganization of cognitive function. *Developmental Neuropsychology, 24,* 669–704.

Farmer, J. E., & Deidrick, K. K. (2006). Introduction to childhood disability. In J. E. Farmer, J. Donders, & S. Warschausky (Eds.), *Treating neurodevelopmental disabilities: Clinical research and practice* (pp. 3–20). New York: Guilford Press.

Farmer, J. E., Donders, J., & Warschausky, S. (Eds.). (2006). *Treating neurodevelopmental disabilities: Clinical research and practice*. New York: Guilford Press.

Farmer, J. E., & Drewel, E. H. (2006). Systems interventions for comprehensive care. In J. E. Farmer, J. Donders, & S. Warschausky (Eds.), *Treating neurodevelopmental disabilities: Clinical research and practice* (pp. 269–288). New York: Guilford Press.

Farmer, J. E., Kanne, S. M., & Grissom, M. O. (in press). Pediatric neuropsychology. In R. J. Frank & T. R. Elliott (Eds.), *Handbook of rehabilitation psychology*. New York: Guilford Press.

Farmer, J. E., Marien, W. E., Clark, M. J., Sherman, A., & Selva, T. J. (2004). Primary care supports for children with chronic health conditions: Identifying and predicting unmet family needs. *Journal of Pediatric Psychology, 29,* 355–367.

Fastenau, P. S., Jianzhao, S., Dunn, D. W., & Austin, J. K. (2008). Academic underachievement among children with epilepsy: Proportion exceeding psychometric criteria for learning disability and associated risk factors. *Journal of Learning Disabilities, 41,* 195–207.

Feeney, T. J., & Ylvisaker, M. (2003). Context-sensitive behavioral supports for young children with TBI: Short-term effects and long-term outcome. *Journal of Head Trauma Rehabilitation, 18,* 33–51.

Friedman, M. J., & Sharieff, G. Q. (2006). Seizures in children. *Pediatric Clinics of North America, 53,* 257–277.

Garofalo, E. (2007). Clinical development of antiepileptic drugs for children. *Neurotherapeutics, 4,* 70–74.

Glang, A., Singer, G., Cooley, E., & Tish, N. (1992). Tailoring direct instruction techniques for use with elementary students with brain injury. *Journal of Head Trauma Rehabilitation, 7,* 93–108.

Glueckauf, R. L., Fritz, S. P., Ecklund-Johnson, E. P., Liss, H. J., Dages, P., & Carney, P. (2002). Videoconferencing-based family counseling for rural teenagers with epilepsy: Phase 1 findings. *Rehabilitation Psychology, 47,* 49–72.

Greenley, R. N., Coakley, R. M., Holmbeck, G. N., Jandasek, B., & Wills, K. (2006). Condition-related knowledge among children with spina bifida: Longitudinal changes and predictors. *Journal of Pediatric Psychology, 31,* 828–839.

Gross, R. T., Spiker, D., & Haynes, C. W. (1997). *Helping low birth weight, premature babies: The Infant Health and Development Program*. Stanford, CA: Stanford University Press.

Hadden, K. L., & von Baeyer, C. L. (2005). Global and specific behavioral measures of pain in children with cerebral palsy. *Clinical Journal of Pain, 21,* 140–146.

Hartman, A. L., Gasior, M., Vining, E. P., & Rogawski, M. A. (2007). The neuropharmacology of the ketogenic diet. *Pediatric Neurology, 36,* 281–292.

Hastings, R. P., & Beck, A. (2004). Practitioner review: Stress intervention for parents of children with intellectual disabilities. *Journal of Child Psychology and Psychiatry, 45,* 1338–1349.

Hauser, W. A., & Beghi, E. (2008). First seizure definitions and worldwide incidence and mortality. *Epilepsia, 49,* 8–12.

Hawley, S. R., Paschal, A. M., Ablah, E., St. Romain, T., Liow, K., & Molgaard, C. A. (2007). Initial perspectives from Midwestern neurologists: Epilepsy patients' barriers and motivators for seeking treatment. *Epilepsia, 48,* 1920–1925.

Hodes, M., Garralda, M. E., Rose, G., & Schwartz, R. (1999). Maternal expressed emotion and adjustment in children with epilepsy. *Journal of Child Psychology and Psychiatry, 40,* 1083–1093.

Holmbeck, G. N., Belvedere, M. C., Christensen, M., Czerwinski, A. M., Hommeyer, J. S., Johnson, S. Z., et al. (1998). Assessment of adherence with multiple informants in pre-adolescents with spina bifida: Initial development of a multidimensional, multitask parent-report questionnaire. *Journal of Personality Assessment, 70,* 427–440.

Holmbeck, G. N., Greenley, R. N., Coakley, R. M., Greco, J., & Hagstrom, J. (2006). Family functioning in children and adolescents with spina bifida: An evidence-based review of research and interventions. *Journal of Developmental and Behavioral Pediatrics, 27,* 249–277.

Holmbeck, G. N., Johnson, S. Z., Wills, K. E., McKernon, W., Rose, B., Erklin, S., et al. (2002). Observed and perceived parental overprotection in relation to psychosocial adjustment in preadolescents with a physical disability: The mediational role of behavioral autonomy. *Journal of Consulting and Clinical Psychology, 70,* 96–110.

Holmbeck, G. N., Westhoven, V. C., Phillips, W. S., Bowers, R., Gruse, C., Nikolopoulos, T., et al. (2003). A multimethod, multi-informant, and multidimensional perspective on psychosocial adjustment in preadolescents with spina bifida. *Journal of Consulting and Clinical Psychology, 71,* 782–796.

Hunter, S., & Donders, J. (Eds.). (2007). *Pediatric neuropsychological intervention.* Cambridge, UK: Cambridge University Press.

Kazak, A. E., Simms, S., & Rourke, M. T. (2002). Family systems practice in pediatric psychology. *Journal of Pediatric Psychology, 27,* 133–143.

King, G. A., Specht, J. A., Schultz, I., Warr-Leeper, G., Redekop, W., & Risebrough, N. (1997). Social skills training for withdrawn unpopular children with physical disabilities: A preliminary evaluation. *Rehabilitation Psychology, 42,* 47–60.

LaJoie, J., & Moshe, S. L. (2004). Effects of seizures and their treatment on fetal brain. *Epilepsia, 45*(Suppl. 8), 48–52.

Lobato, D. J., & Kao, B. T. (2005). Brief report: Family-based group intervention for young siblings of children with chronic illness and developmental disability. *Journal of Pediatric Psychology, 30,* 678–682.

Luckasson, R., Borthwick-Duffy, S., Buntinx, W. H. E., Coulter, D. L., Craig, E. M., Reeve, A., et al. (2002). *Mental retardation: Definition, classification, and systems of supports* (10th ed.). Washington, DC: American Association on Mental Retardation.

Lundgren, J., Amark, P., Blennow, G., Stromblad, L. G., & Wallstedt, L. (1998). Vagus nerve stimulation in 16 children with refractory epilepsy. *Epilepsia, 39,* 809–813.

MacLeod, J. S., & Austin, J. K. (2003). Stigma in the lives of adolescents with epilepsy: A review of the literature. *Epilepsy and Behavior, 4,* 112–117.

Mahone, E., Zabel, T., Levey, E., Verda, M., & Kinsman, S. (2002). Parent and self-report ratings of executive function in adolescents with myelomeningocele and hydrocephalus. *Child Neuropsychology, 8,* 258–270.

Mitchell, L. E. (2005). Epidemiology of neural tube defects. *American Journal of Medical Genetics: Part C. Seminars in Medical Genetics, 135,* 88–94.

Mitchell, L. E., Adzick, N. S., Melchionne, J., Pasquariello, P. S., Sutton, L. N., Whitehead, A. S., et al. (2004). Spina bifida. *Lancet, 364,* 1885–1895.

Msall, M. E., Avery, R. C., Tremont, M. R., Lima, J. C., Rogers, M. L., & Hogan, D. P. (2003). Functional disability and school activity limitations in 41,300 school-age children: Relationship to medical impairments. *Pediatrics, 111,* 548–553.

Mudrick, N. R. (2002). The prevalence of disability among children: Paradigms and estimates. *Physical Medicine and Rehabilitation Clinics of North America, 13,* 775–792.

National Early Childhood Technical Assistance Center. (2008). *State Part C Coordinators.* Retrieved September 25, 2008, from *www.nectac.org/contact/ptccoord.asp*

Nolan, M. A., Redoblado, M. A., Lah, S., Sabaz, M., Lawson, J. A., Cunningham, A. M., et al. (2004). Memory function in childhood epilepsy syndromes. *Journal of Paediatrics and Child Health, 40,* 20–27.

Oddson, B. E., Clancy, C. A., & McGrath, P. J. (2006). The role of pain in reduced quality of life and depressive symptomology in children with spina bifida. *Clinical Journal of Pain, 22,* 784–789.

Ouyang, L., Grosse, S. D., Armour, B. S., & Waitzman, N. J. (2007). Health care expenditures of children and adults with spina bifida in a privately insured U.S. population. *Birth Defects Research, 79,* 552–558.

Remahl, S., Dahlin, M. G., & Amark, P. E. (2008). Influence of the ketogenic diet on 24-hour electroencephalogram in children with epilepsy. *Pediatric Neurology, 38,* 38–43.

Rodenburg, R., Meijer, A. M., Dekovic, M., & Aldenkamp, A. P. (2005). Family factors and psychopathology in children with epilepsy: A literature review. *Epilepsy and Behavior, 6,* 488–503.

Rose, B. M., & Holmbeck, G. N. (2007). Attention and executive functions in adolescents with spina bifida. *Journal of Pediatric Psychology, 32,* 983–994.

Shore, C. P., Perkins, S. M., & Austin, J. K. (2008). The Seizures and Epilepsy Education (SEE) program for families of children with epilepsy: A preliminary study. *Epilepsy and Behavior, 12,* 157–164.

Simeonsson, R. J., McMillen, J. S., & Huntington, G. S. (2002). Secondary conditions in children with disabilities: Spina bifida as a case example. *Mental Retardation and Developmental Disabilities Research Reviews, 8,* 198–205.

Sofronoff, K., Attwood, T., & Hinton, S. (2005). A randomised controlled trial of a CBT intervention for anxiety in children with Asperger syndrome. *Journal of Child Psychology and Psychiatry, 46,* 1152–1160.

Tse, E., Hamiwka, L., Sherman, E. M. S., & Wirrell, E. (2007). Social skills problems in children with epilepsy: Prevalence, nature and predictors. *Epilepsy and Behavior, 11,* 499–505.

Vermaes, I. P., Gerris, J. R., & Janssens, J. M. (2007). Parents' social adjustment in families of children with spina bifida: A theory-driven review. *Journal of Pediatric Psychology, 32,* 1214–1226.

Vermaes, I. P., Janssens, J. M., Bosman, A. M., & Gerris, J. R. (2005). Parents' psychological adjustment in families of children with spina bifida: A meta-analysis. *BMC Pediatrics, 5,* 32.

Wagner, J. L., & Smith, G. (2006). Psychosocial intervention in pediatric epilepsy: A critique of the literature. *Epilepsy and Behavior, 8,* 39–49.

Warschausky, S., Argento, A. G., Hurvitz, E., & Berg, M. (2003). Neuropsychological status and social problem solving in children with congenital or acquired brain dysfunction. *Rehabilitation Psychology, 48,* 250–254.

Warschausky, S., Kewman, D., & Kay, J. (1999). Empirically supported psychological and behavioral therapies in pediatric rehabilitation of TBI. *Journal of Head Trauma Rehabilitation, 14,* 373–383.

Williams, J. (2003). Learning and behavior in children with epilepsy. *Epilepsy and Behavior, 4,* 107–111.

World Health Organization. (2007). *International classification of functioning, disability and health for children and youth.* Geneva: Author.

Yeates, K. O., Loss, N., Colvin, A. N., & Enrile, B. G. (2003). Do children with myelomeningocele and hydrocephalus display nonverbal learning disabilities?: An empirical approach to classification. *Journal of the International Neuropsychological Society, 9,* 653–662.

CHAPTER 24

Medical and Psychosocial Aspects
of Juvenile Rheumatoid Arthritis

MICHAEL A. RAPOFF
CAROL B. LINDSLEY
CYNTHIA KARLSON

Pediatric rheumatic diseases are chronic multisystem disorders that involve acute and chronic tissue inflammation of the musculoskeletal system, blood vessels, and skin. Juvenile rheumatoid arthritis is the most common type of childhood arthritis and a major cause of short- and long-term disability among chronic pediatric diseases (Cassidy & Petty, 2005). The term "juvenile rheumatoid arthritis" (hereafter abbreviated as JRA) is used here because the criteria for this diagnosis (American College of Rheumatology) were the inclusion criteria for almost all of the studies cited in this chapter. The newer classification schema, "juvenile idiopathic arthritis," has broader inclusion criteria, including children with psoriatic arthritis, enthesitis-associated arthritis, and an undifferentiated group. Children with chronic arthritis and their families must adhere to complex daily medical regimens, and must cope with pain and the psychosocial impact of living with a chronic disease. This chapter reviews the medical and psychosocial aspects of JRA, including adherence to medical regimens, chronic pain, and psychosocial adjustment and coping. Clinical and research implications are reviewed at the end of each section.

Medical Aspects

The etiology of JRA is not known, although variables thought to be important in the pathophysiology of the disease include genetic predisposition, unknown environmental triggers, and immune reactivity. The hallmark of the disease is synovitis (inflammation of the synovial membrane of a joint). There are three subtypes of JRA; the categorization is made according to the symptomatology that occurs over the first 6 months of disease (Cassidy & Petty, 2005).

Systemic-Onset JRA

The systemic-onset subtype affects approximately 10% of children with JRA and is defined by the presence of a characteristic rash or high cyclic fevers, along with joint symptoms, either arthritis or arthralgias. Children with systemic-onset JRA frequently show other manifestations, such as lymphadenopathy (inflammation of lymph nodes), hepatosplenomegaly (enlargement of the liver and spleen), pericarditis (inflammation of the pericardium or sac enclosing the heart), serositis (inflammation of a serous membrane), and marked laboratory abnormalities. The systemic symptoms will generally subside over the first few months of disease as the joint symptoms persist and often progress. Children with systemic-onset JRA are frequently admitted to the hospital to establish a firm diagnosis and begin therapy. Most children will respond to appropriate therapy. However, this subtype remains the most difficult to treat, and up to 25% of children with it have a poor prognosis with continually active and poorly responsive disease. The severest involvement is generally in the hands, hips, and neck, so both mobility and dexterity are at risk.

Polyarticular JRA

The polyarticular subtype occurs in about 40% of children with JRA and is defined as involvement of more than four joints. Usually these include hands, wrists, hips, knees, ankles, and neck. If the disease begins at an early age, there may be involvement of the mandibular growth centers, which leads to facial asymmetry and creates a potential for long-term temporomandibular joint problems. About 25% of these children have a positive rheumatoid factor test, which is a marker for more severe disease.

Pauciarticular (Oligoarticular) JRA

The pauciarticular (or oligoarticular) subtype occurs in 40–50% of children with JRA and is defined as involvement of four or fewer joints, with the joints most frequently involved being the knees or ankles. There are two subgroups of these patients: (1) young girls who test positive for antinuclear antibody and have a high risk for eye involvement (uveitis); and (2) older boys who have a long-term risk for developing involvement of the axial skeleton, hips, and back. The diagnosis is made with the demonstration of persistent arthritis in one or more joints for a minimum of 6 weeks and with the exclusion of other diagnoses. Early, accurate diagnosis is critical to achieving optimal outcome in these children.

Medical Treatment

Once the diagnosis of JRA is established, most children require regular therapy. The specific therapy used depends on the age of the child and the severity of the arthritis. Nonsteroidal anti-inflammatory drugs (NSAIDs) are the standard first-line therapy. Well-established drugs (such as naproxen or ibuprofen) are used in young children, and longer-acting, once-a-day drugs (such as nambutome, piroxicam, or the newer cyclooxygenase-2 inhibitor celicoxib) are often used in older children and adolescents.

Most children with pauciarticular disease respond to NSAIDs, but intra-articular corticosteroids may be needed for unresponsive joints, and occasionally second-line agents (e.g., sulfasalazaine) are added. In polyarticular disease, NSAIDs are the initial therapy; second-line agents or disease-modifying antirheumatic drugs (DMARDs), such as hydroxychloroquine, sulfasalazaine, or methotrexate, are added for poorly responsive or unresponsive disease after weeks to months. Low-dose short-term corticosteroid therapy may be used as "bridge therapy" to control symptoms during a transitional period, as DMARDs take weeks to months to be effective. In systemic disease, DMARDs (hydroxychloroquine or methotrexate) may be added early in the disease course, and daily corticosteroids may be required for pericarditis or unresponsive disease. Children with eye involvement are generally treated with corticosteroid eye drops and dilating agents. The activity of the eye disease does not usually fluctuate with that of the joint disease. Every effort is made to avoid long-term corticosteroid therapy in children because of the serious effects of toxicity, including growth retardation, iatrogenic Cushing disease, osteoporosis, fractures, obesity, and hypertension. Patients with persistent, severe polyarticular or systemic disease who do not respond to methotrexate therapy are candidates for biological agents such as antitumor necrosis factor drugs (e.g., enteracept).

In addition to drug therapy, children with JRA must be carefully monitored for growth abnormalities, nutrition, vision, and school and social functioning, as well as psychological and emotional health. Therapeutic exercise programs with professional supervision may be needed to maximize joint motion and minimize muscle atrophy. Overall, the disease outcomes have markedly improved over the past two decades, and most children with JRA who have early diagnosis and receive appropriate treatment will have minimal joint deformity and can lead active, normal lives.

Adherence to Medical Regimens

Children with JRA and their parents are usually asked to adhere consistently and over a long period of time to a variety of therapeutic regimens, most notably medications, therapeutic exercises, and splinting of joints. Many of these regimens may have delayed beneficial effects and in the short term may cause unwanted side effects, such as gastrointestinal irritation and pain. The need for consistent adherence over a long period of time, delayed beneficial effects, and negative side effects have all been factors predicting greater adherence problems in pediatric chronic diseases (Rapoff, 1999).

Adherence Rates to Regimens for JRA

Relatively few studies have specifically addressed adherence to regimens for JRA. Adherence to NSAIDs varies depending on the measure used, with higher rates (83–95%) by parent or child report or pill counts (April, Feldman, Platt, & Duffy, 2006; Feldman et al., 2007; Kvien & Reimers, 1983), and lower rates (45–70%) by serum assay or electronic monitoring (Litt & Cuskey, 1981; Litt, Cuskey, & Rosenberg, 1982; Rapoff, Belmont, Lindsley, & Olson, 2005). They also vary depending on the cutoff point used to classify patients as adherent or nonadherent. Using the convention of classifying patients as nonadherent if they took <80% of doses (Rapoff, 1999), Brewer, Giannini, Kuzmina, and Alekseev (1986) found nonadherence rates of 11–14% for active and placebo medications, whereas Rapoff and colleagues (2005) found that 48% of newly diagnosed patients with JRA were nonadherent. There is also consistent evidence that adherence is lower to therapeutic exercise regimens than to medications, by parent or patient report (April et al., 2006; Feldman et al., 2007; Hayford & Ross, 1988; Rapoff, Lindsley, & Christophersen, 1985). A few studies have targeted improvements in adherence to regimens (primarily medications) for JRA.

Adherence Intervention Studies

Two studies have examined the efficacy of parent-managed token reinforcement programs in altering adherence to regimens for JRA. The first study (Rapoff, Lindsley, & Christophersen, 1984) focused on improving adherence to medications, splint wearing, and prone lying (to prevent hip contractures) for a 7-year-old female with severe systemic-onset JRA. Introduction of a token system increased adherence from 59 to 95% for medications, from 0 to 77% for splint wearing, and from 0 to 71% for prone lying. At the 10-week follow-up (with the token system withdrawn), adherence to medications, splint wearing, and prone lying averaged 90%, 91%, and 80%, respectively. The second study (Rapoff, Purviance, & Lindsley, 1988b) tested the efficacy of a token system program in improving adherence to medications for a 14-year-old male with polyarticular JRA. Medication adherence increased from an average of 44% during baseline to an average of 97% at 9-month follow-up. In the second study, improvements were also seen in clinical outcomes (e.g., number of active joints).

Although the above-described studies showed that token systems can be effective in improving adherence, they are labor-intensive for families and require well-trained personnel to implement and monitor. One study (Rapoff, Purviance, & Lindsley, 1988a) evaluated less complex behavioral strategies (self-monitoring and positive verbal feedback) combined with educational strategies. This study involved three female patients with JRA, ages 3, 10, and 13 years. Adherence increased from an average of 38% and 54% for the youngest two patients at baseline to an average of 97% and 92% during the intervention, respectively. Adherence increased only slightly (from 44 to 49%) for the 13-year-old, who had less parental supervision of her regimen. Adherence decreased for all three patients at 4-month follow-up (means ranged from 24 to 89%).

The success of interventions with limited numbers of patients who were persistently nonadherent led our group to conducted a randomized controlled trial for newly diagnosed patients with JRA that evaluated a clinic-based, nurse-administered educational and behavioral intervention to promote adherence and prevent nonadherence to nonsteroidal medications (Rapoff et al., 2002). Thirty-four participants (mean age = 8.44 years) were randomly assigned to the experimental or (attention placebo) control groups. Patients and parents in the experimental group were given information about adherence improvement strategies (prompting, monitoring, positive reinforcement, and discipline techniques; Rapoff, 1998). The control group received only educational information about JRA and its treatments. At 52-week follow-up, the experimental group showed significantly better overall average adherence than the control group (77.7% vs. 56.9%)—and, as predicted, the trend in adherence levels significantly dropped over time in the control group, but not in the experimental group. There were, however, no significant postintervention group differences on disease activity and functional status measures, perhaps due to "floor effects" (e.g., 68% of experimental participants and 67% of controls had quiescent or mild disease at baseline).

A unique randomized clinical trial focused on preventing osteoporosis in children with JRA (mean age 6 years) by increasing calcium intake (Stark et al., 2005). Children assigned to the behavioral intervention group, who received nutritional education and behavior modification, achieved a significantly greater increase in dietary calcium intake compared to the group receiving an enhanced standard care control (i.e., education on JRA only). In addition, and of clinical significance, 92% of children in the intervention group achieved the treatment goal of 1,500 mg of calcium per day, compared to 17% of children in the control group. The above-mentioned studies suggest that behavioral strategies combined with education is the most effective way to improve adherence to regimens for JRA and to prevent deterioration in adherence over time in newly diagnosed patients.

Clinical and Research Implications

Based on his adherence intervention research, Rapoff (2000) has suggested a three-tiered approach to minimizing nonadherence: "primary," "secondary," and "tertiary" prevention. Primary prevention efforts would be most relevant for those patients who have not yet exhibited clinically significant nonadherence—possibly those recently diagnosed or those who are able to sustain adequate adherence over time. Interventions at this level would involve educational approaches (e.g., stressing the importance of adherence), organizational strategies (e.g., simplifying regimens), and relatively simple behavioral strategies (e.g., monitoring of regimen adherence by providers or parents). Secondary prevention might be most applicable to those patients for whom clinically significant nonadherence has been identified early in the disease course or has yet to compromise their health and well-being. Interventions at this level might include more frequent monitoring of regimen adherence by parents and patients, specific and consistent positive social reinforcement for adherence, and general discipline strategies (e.g., time out for younger children). Tertiary prevention efforts would apply to patients with an ongoing pattern of clinically significant nonadherence. Strategies at this level might include token system programs, contingency contracting, self-management training (e.g., problem solving to anticipate and manage obstacles to adherence), and possibly psychotherapy. Whereas pediatric psychologists could train primary health care providers and nurses to implement primary- and secondary-level interventions, pediatric psychologists would be responsible for implementing strategies at the tertiary level, due to the demanding and technical nature of these strategies.

Pain

Chronic pain is a primary clinical manifestation of JRA (Anthony & Schanberg, 2003; Cassidy & Petty, 2005). Although some children with JRA (14% in one study) report no pain (Sherry, Bohnsack, Salmonson, Wallace, & Mellins, 1990), the majority of children report mild to moderate levels of pain intensity (Gragg et al., 1996; Hagglund, Schopp,

Alberts, Cassidy, & Frank, 1995; Ilowite, Walco, & Pochaczevsky, 1992; Thompson, Varni, & Hanson, 1987; Varni, Rapoff, et al., 1996a). In addition, about 25–30% report pain intensities in the moderate to severe range (Ross, Lavigne, Hayford, Dyer, & Pachman, 1989; Schanberg, Lefebvre, Keefe, Kredich, & Gil, 1997). In one study, 82% of children with JRA reported a mean pain duration of 4.3 hours per day (range = 30 minutes to 24 hours; Benestad, Vinje, Veierød, & Vandvik, 1996).

A daily dairy study over a 2-month period found that children with JRA reported having mild to moderate pain an average of 73% of days, and 31% reported pain in the severe range (Schanberg, Anthony, Gil, & Maurin, 2003). Also, a long-term follow-up study from the Mayo Clinic found that adults who had been diagnosed with JRA reported significantly greater pain, fatigue, and disability than to gender-matched healthy adults did (Peterson, Mason, Nelson, O'Fallon, & Gabriel, 1997). Higher levels of pain have also been linked to reductions in quality of life for children with rheumatic diseases (Dhanani, Quenneville, Perron, Abdolell, & Feldman, 2002; Sawyer et al., 2004). Thus pain is a significant problem for some children with JRA, is associated with greater disability, and can persist into adulthood.

Biobehavioral Model of Pain

Beginning with the introduction of the gate control theory of pain (Melzack & Wall, 1965), researchers have gravitated to a biobehavioral model of pain that focuses on the unique and interactive components of nociceptive activity, emotions, cognitions, and behavior in the experience of pain (Rapoff & Lindsley, 2000).

Nociception

Physiological, anatomical, and chemical properties of the nervous system contribute to the perception of pain. Nociceptive afferents (nerve fibers) in the joint are located in the joint capsule and ligaments, bone, periosteum, articular fat pads, and perivascular sites, and respond to noxious mechanical, thermal, and chemical stimulation (Randich, 1993). The enhanced pain associated with arthritis is probably due to the response of joint afferent fibers to mechanical and heat stimulation present during inflammation and to chemical mediators of joint inflammation, such as prostaglandins (Meyer, Campbell, & Raja, 1994). Studies of experimentally induced pain found reduced pain threshold in inflamed and noninflamed joints of children with active arthritis, and, to a lesser degree, in the joints of children in remission (Hogeweg et al., 1995; Hogeweg, Kuis, Oostendorp, & Helders, 1995; Thastum, Zachariae, Schøler, Bjerring, & Herlin, 1997). The persistence of lowered pain threshold, even after nociceptive input to the joint might be expected to cease, suggests a role for long-lasting structural and functional changes— that is, "neuroplastic alterations" due to "central sensitization" (Coderre & Katz, 1997; Kuis, Heijnen, Hogeweg, Sinnema, & Helders, 1997).

Emotions

Pain is an emotional as well as a sensory experience (Banks & Kerns, 1996; Chapman, 2001). There is strong correlational support for the link between negative emotions, particularly anxiety and depression, and increased pain intensity and interference in the lives of children with JRA (Gragg et al., 1996; Hagglund et al., 1995; Hoff, Palermo, Schluchter, Zebracki, & Drotar, 2006; Ross et al., 1993; Schanberg et al., 2003; Thompson et al., 1987; Varni, Rapoff, et al., 1996a, 1996b). Also, daily stressful events and negative mood have been linked to increased pain, stiffness, and fatigue in children with JRA (Schanberg et al., 2000). Although causality studies examining the link between emotional distress and pain have yet to be conducted, emotional distress and pain may share common etiological factors, are reciprocally linked, and can occur concurrently (Banks & Kerns, 1996; Gamsa, 1990). For example, increased anxiety can induce muscle tension, thereby directly inducing or exacerbating musculoskeletal pain, or increased pain can induce anxiety about future prognosis or interference with life activities.

Cognitions

A third variable is concerned with how people attend to and think about the experience of pain. The focus in the pain literature has been on maladaptive rather than adaptive thinking. Cognitive processing of pain can be maladaptive in at least two ways: (1) People can fail to attend to information or fail to generate self-talk that might be helpful in coping with pain; or (2) people can engage in dysfunctional thinking that leads to maladaptive coping and greater pain (such as wishful or catastrophic thinking). Catastrophizing may be the most "toxic" type of dysfunctional thinking related to pain and seems to include three components: (1) rumination (preoccupation with pain-related thoughts); (2) magnification (exaggeration of the threat value of pain); and (3) helplessness (adopting a helpless orientation to coping with pain) (Sullivan, Bishop, & Pivik, 1995).

Several studies have investigated cognitive coping strategies in children with JRA. Studies in Denmark have found that catastrophizing is associated with higher pain intensity during a cold-pressor paradigm (Thastum, Zachariae, Schøler, & Herlin, 1998) and over an extended 3-week period (Thastum, Herlin, & Zachariae, 2005). Reid, Gilbert, and McGrath (1998) found that "emotion-focused avoidance" coping (catastrophizing and expressing negative emotions) was associated with greater pain intensity, pain duration, and anxiety. Varni, Waldron, and colleagues (1996) found that "cognitive self-instruction" (primarily wishful thinking) was related to greater emotional distress, and that "cognitive refocusing" (engaging in activities as a distraction from pain) was related to less pain intensity and emotional distress. Another study (Schanberg et al., 1997) found that "pain control and rational thinking" (controlling and decreasing pain while avoiding catastrophizing) predicted lower pain intensity.

Behavior

When children are in pain, they exhibit a wide variety of pain behaviors, such as limping, grimacing, crying, resting, or asking for medication. These pain behaviors and how others respond to them can be either adaptive or maladaptive for a child experiencing pain. Some pain behaviors, such as guarding and malpositioning of affected joints, may be maladaptive for children with JRA (Cassidy & Petty, 2005). Caregivers' responses to children's pain-related behaviors may also be maladaptive, such as when parents allow children to avoid attending school, resulting in low academic performance and missed opportunities for social interactions. Conversely, if children engage in "well" behaviors (e.g., positive coping strategies) and parents reinforce adaptive behaviors, children would be expected to experience less pain and disability from pain. For instance, one study found that children with JRA who reported resting more and withdrawing from activities showed higher levels of pain and emotional distress (Varni, Waldron, et al., 1996). Another study found that children with JRA who engaged in "approach" coping (including talking to a friend or family member about how they felt) showed less functional disability (Reid et al., 1998).

Clinical and Research Implications

A biobehavioral model of pain would suggest a number of treatment options (Rapoff & Lindsley, 2000). Early and aggressive pharmacological treatment of JRA could lead to enhanced pain relief and function, in both the short term and the long term, via a reduction in peripheral and central sensitization mechanisms. Psychological interventions that reduce negative emotional states and teach cognitive restructuring could directly or indirectly reduce pain intensity and pain interference. In addition, imagery techniques (e.g., vividly imagining a relaxing place or experience) combined with relaxation exercises are often helpful in diverting attention from pain, thereby reducing pain.

There is a need for well-controlled, multisite pain intervention trials for children with JRA. Studies to date have been promising, but have involved small samples and no control or alternative-treatment comparison groups (Lavigne, Ross, Berry, Hayford, & Pachman, 1992; Walco, Varni, & Ilowite, 1992). Investigators should also consider using electronic pain diaries (e-diaries) rather than paper diaries, as e-diaries are well accepted by children and adolescents with arthritis, and result in fewer errors and omissions than paper diaries do (Palermo, Valenzuela, & Stork, 2004; Stinson et al., 2006).

Psychosocial Adjustment and Coping

A substantial body of research exists on the psychosocial adjustment and coping of children and adolescents with JRA (for other reviews, see Bradley, 1985; Lavigne & Faier-Routman, 1992; Quirk & Young, 1990; Turkel & Pao, 2007). Overall, studies evaluating the psychosocial adjustment of children with JRA report mixed findings. Early studies suggested increased psychosocial problems; however, these studies often involved small sample sizes, hospitalized children, and the use of nonstandardized measures (Cleveland, Reitman, & Brewer, 1965; Rimon, Belmaker, & Ebstein, 1977). More recent studies tend to include larger samples, standardized measures, a specific theoretical perspective, and more sophisticated statistical approaches. Yet researchers still find a mixed picture of adjustment and coping in children with JRA. Recent studies have also expanded their focus to include the parents and siblings of children and adolescents with JRA.

Social and Emotional Adjustment

Many studies have found no significant psychosocial deficits in children with JRA, compared with normative or healthy controls. Kellerman, Zeltzer, Ellenberg, Dash, and Rigler (1980) assessed 168 chronically ill adolescents (30 with rheumatic disease) and 349 healthy controls, and found no significant differences between healthy and ill adolescents or between illness subgroups on measures of anxiety or self-esteem. In a case–control study, Noll and colleagues (2000) compared children with JRA to control classmates and found no significant differences on any measure of social and emotional functioning. Huygen, Kuis, and Sinnema (2000) conducted a study of 47 Dutch patients with JRA, 52 healthy peers, and their parents. Results indicated that self-esteem, perceived competence, body image, social competence, social support, and psychopathology were equivalent across groups, despite the facts that the children with JRA had less ability to participate in sports, less frequent opportunities to play with friends, and lower perceived athletic competence.

Several other studies have found significant differences between the psychosocial functioning of children with JRA and healthy control children. Mullick, Nahar, and Haq (2005) compared 40 children with JRA to 40 age- and sex-matched healthy children and found that the children with JRA were significantly more likely to have a depressive disorder (15.0%) than the healthy controls (0%). In a 1-year prospective study that examined quality of life in children with JRA, Sawyer and colleagues (2004) found that children with arthritis reported significantly lower quality of life than previously reported by healthy children in the general community. In a meta-analytic review, LeBovidge, Lavigne, Donenberg, and Miller (2003) concluded that children with juvenile arthritis display an increased overall risk for adjustment problems and internalizing (anxious and depressive) symptoms, but no increased risk for lowered self-concept or externalizing problems. Thus it appears that children with JRA do nearly as well as their healthy peers, but that they are at increased risk for anxiety and depressive disorders.

School Adjustment

An early epidemiological study indicated that chronically ill children were significantly delayed in school achievement when compared with their peers, possibly because of their increased school absences (Pless & Roughmann, 1971). Other early studies addressing school absence found that children with JRA tended to be absent significantly more often than their healthy peers (Fowler, Johnson, & Atkinson, 1985). However, Sturge, Garralda, Boissin, Dore, and Woo (1997) found the mean school attendance rate to be 92%. Children with more severe JRA were significantly more likely to miss school.

More recent studies have examined not only school attendance, but adjustment within the school setting, along with peer support. Schanberg and colleagues (2003) found that 56% of children with JRA reduced their school activities at least once during a 2-month period when they experienced increased disease activity (increased pain, stiffness, and fatigue). Higher classmate support was found to predict fewer adjustment problems and fewer depressive symptoms (von Weiss et al., 2002), whereas peer rejection was associated with increased adjustment problems and increased depressive symptoms (Sandstrom & Schanberg, 2004). Fortunately, children with JRA generally report sufficient peer support from friends and boyfriends or girlfriends (Kyngäs, 2004).

Long-Term Psychosocial Adjustment

Miller, Spitz, Simpson, and Williams (1982) conducted a follow-up study of 121 individuals with JRA who had reached at least the age of 18 years and found that most of them were working, attending school full time, or a combination of the two. The authors also compared 50 patients with their siblings and found no significant differences on any demographic or psychosocial variables. However, Peterson and colleagues (1997) conducted a 25-year follow-up study of 44 individuals diagnosed with JRA (mean age = 33.5 years) and found that these individuals had significantly lower functional status, more physical disability, higher unemployment, and less ability to exercise than matched controls. Therefore, it is possible that children with JRA function fairly typically through the age of dependence (when they typically live with their families), but tend to have more difficulty as they progress through life.

Packham, Hall, and Pimm (2002) conducted a long-term follow-up of 246 adults diagnosed with JRA (mean age = 35.4 years) and compared results to general population norms. Results indicated that adults with JRA experienced higher levels of anxiety (31.6%) than the general population (18%), but similar or lower levels of depression (5.2% current, 21.1% past) than the general population (12% current, 20% past). Those individuals with systemic-onset JRA had higher levels of anxiety and depression, whereas those with oligoarticular JRA had lower levels of anxiety and depression. Furthermore, depression was more common when JRA onset was between 6 and 12 years of age, and anxiety was more common in the late-onset group (over 12 years of age).

Adjustment in Parents and Siblings of Children with JRA

Parental distress, family cohesion, and cognitive appraisals of JRA are important factors in child and family adjustment (Helgeson, Janicki, Lerner, & Barbarin, 2003; Wagner et al., 2003). Families of children with JRA report multiple illness-related stressors, such as school difficulties, fears for the children's future, problems managing treatment regimens, and financial burdens (Degotardi, Revenson, & Ilowite, 1999). However, the majority of families appear to be fairly well adjusted, reporting high levels of family cohesion and expressiveness and low levels of family conflict. Reid, McGrath, and Lang (2005) examined parent–child interactions among children with juvenile fibromyalgia, children with JRA, and healthy controls during a pain-inducing exercise task. Controlling for pain, they found no significant differences across groups on parent–child interactions.

Despite an overall positive picture, increased family burden and increased parental distress has been found in families of children with JRA. Henoch, Batson, and Baum (1978) compared a sample of children with JRA to control children and found that families of children with JRA were significantly more likely to have unmarried parents due to divorce, separation, or death, and were more likely to experience adoption in their families, than the control sample. In a study of maternal functioning, Manuel (2001) found that mothers of children with JRA reported significantly higher levels of emotional distress than normative groups of mothers. Although they do so to a lesser extent than mothers, fathers of children with JRA also report higher levels of emotional distress (McNeill, 2004) and a large number of concerns over their children's illness (Hovey, 2005).

Regarding siblings, Daniels, Miller, Billings, and Moos (1986) compared 72 children with a rheumatic disease (58 with JRA) and their siblings with 60 demographically matched siblings of healthy children on measures of psychological functioning and family functioning. Results indicated no differences between groups on any measures, with siblings of children with JRA and siblings of healthy children functioning equally well. Thus research indicates that JRA may have little effect on siblings, but probably contributes to increased stress for mothers and fathers.

Clinical and Research Implications

The bulk of the empirical evidence suggests that children and adolescents with JRA do not appear to be at greater risk of developing clinically significant adjustment problems. However, it is possible that this risk has been underestimated, due to underreporting of psychosocial difficulties or fluctuations in psychosocial functioning concomitant with fluctuations in disease severity (which may not be captured in cross-sectional studies). Children who experience more severe disease appear to be at greater risk for adjustment problems. Alternatively, family cohesion appears to be a protective factor in both child and parent adjustment. More longitudinal studies are needed to assess psychosocial adjustment and coping among children with JRA, coupled with well-timed psychosocial interventions for those deemed to be at risk. Studies on adjustment and coping should also include measures of adaptive or protective factors specific to children with JRA, such as the parent and child arthritis self-efficacy scales developed by Barlow, Shaw, and Wright (2000, 2001).

References

Anthony, K. K., & Schanberg, L. E. (2003). Pain in children with arthritis: A review of the current literature. *Arthritis Care and Research, 49,* 272–279.

April, K. T., Feldman, D. E., Platt, R. W., & Duffy, C. M. (2006). Comparison between children with juvenile idiopathic arthritis and their parents concerning perceived treatment adherence. *Arthritis Care and Research, 55,* 558–563.

Banks, S. M., & Kerns, R. D. (1996). Explaining high rates of depression in chronic pain: A diathesis–stress framework. *Psychological Bulletin, 119,* 95–110.

Barlow, J. H., Shaw, K. L., & Wright, C. C. (2000). Development and preliminary validation of a self-efficacy measure for use among parents of children with juvenile idiopathic arthritis. *Arthritis Care and Research, 13,* 227–236.

Barlow, J. H., Shaw, K. L., & Wright, C. C. (2001). Development and preliminary validation of a children's arthritis self-efficacy scale. *Arthritis Care and Research, 45,* 159–166.

Benestad, B., Vinje, O., Veierød, M. B., & Vandvik, I. H. (1996). Quantitative and qualitative assessments of pain in children with juvenile chronic arthritis based on the Norwegian version of the Pediatric Pain Questionnaire. *Scandinavian Journal of Rheumatology, 25,* 293–299.

Bradley, L. A. (1985). Psychological aspects of arthritis. *Bulletin on the Rheumatic Diseases, 35,* 1–12.

Brewer, E. J., Giannini, E. H., Kuzmina, N., & Alekseev, L. (1986). Penicillamine and hydroxychloroquine in the treatment of severe juvenile rheumatoid arthritis. *New England Journal of Medicine, 314,* 1269–1276.

Cassidy, J. T., & Petty, R. E. (2005). *Textbook of pediatric rheumatology* (5th ed.). Philadelphia: Saunders.

Chapman, C. R. (2001). The psychophysiology of pain. In J. D. Loser (Ed.), *Bonica's management of pain* (3rd ed., pp. 461–477). Philadelphia: Lippincott Williams & Wilkins.

Cleveland, S. E., Reitman, E. E., & Brewer, E. J. (1965). Psychological factors in juvenile rheumatoid arthritis. *Arthritis and Rheumatism, 8,* 1152–1158.

Coderre, T. J., & Katz, J. (1997). Peripheral and central hyperexcitability: Differential signs and symptoms in persistent pain. *Behavioral and Brain Sciences, 20,* 404–419.

Daniels, D., Miller, J. J., Billings, A. G., & Moos, R. H. (1986). Psychosocial functioning of siblings of children with rheumatic disease. *Journal of Pediatrics, 109,* 379–383.

Degotardi, P. J., Revenson, T. A., & Ilowite, N. T. (1999). Family-level coping in juvenile rheumatoid arthritis: Assessing the utility of a quantitative family interview. *Arthritis Care and Research, 12,* 314–324.

Dhanani, S., Quenneville, J., Perron, M., Abdolell, M., & Feldman, B. M. (2002). Minimal difference in pain associated with change in quality of life in children with rheumatic disease. *Arthritis Care and Research, 47,* 501–505.

Feldman, D. E., De Civita, M., Dobkin, P. L., Malleson, P., Meshefedjian, G., & Duffy, C. (2007). Perceived adherence to prescribed treatment in juvenile idiopathic arthritis over a one-year period. *Arthritis Care and Research, 57,* 226–233.

Fowler, M. G., Johnson, M. P., & Atkinson, S. S. (1985). School achievement and absence in children with chronic health conditions. *Journal of Pediatrics, 106,* 683–687.

Gamsa, A. (1990). Is emotional disturbance a precipitator or a consequence of chronic pain? *Pain, 42,* 183–195.

Gragg, R. A., Rapoff, M. A., Danovsky, M. B., Lindsley, C. B., Varni, J. W., Waldron, S. A., et al. (1996). Assessing chronic musculoskeletal pain associated with rheumatic disease: Further validation of the Pediatric Pain Questionnaire. *Journal of Pediatric Psychology, 21,* 237–250.

Hagglund, K. J., Schopp, L. M., Alberts, K. R., Cassidy, J. T., & Frank, R. G. (1995). Predicting pain among children with juvenile rheumatoid arthritis. *Arthritis Care and Research, 8,* 36–42.

Hayford, J. R., & Ross, C. K. (1988). Medical compliance in juvenile rheumatoid arthritis: Problems and perspectives. *Arthritis Care and Research, 1,* 190–197.

Helgeson, V. S., Janicki, D., Lerner, J., & Barbarin, O. (2003). Brief report: Adjustment to juvenile rheumatoid arthritis: A family systems perspective. *Journal of Pediatric Psychology, 28,* 347–353.

Henoch, M. J., Batson, J. W., & Baum, J. (1978). Psychosocial factors in juvenile rheumatoid arthritis. *Arthritis and Rheumatism, 21,* 229–233.

Hoff, A. L., Palermo, T. M., Schluchter, M., Zebracki, K., & Drotar, D. (2006). Longitudinal relationships of depressive symptoms to pain intensity and functional disability among children with disease-related pain. *Journal of Pediatric Psychology, 31,* 1046–1056.

Hogeweg, J. A., Huygen, A. C., De Jong-De Vos Van Steenwijk, C., Bernards, A. T., Oostendorp, R. A., & Helders, P. J. (1995). The pain threshold in juvenile chronic arthritis. *British Journal of Rheumatology, 34,* 61–67.

Hogeweg, J. A., Kuis, W., Oostendorp, R. A. B., & Helders, P. J. M. (1995). General and segmental reduced pain thresholds in juvenile chronic arthritis. *Pain, 62,* 11–17.

Hovey, J. K. (2005). Fathers' parenting chronically ill children: Concerns and coping strategies. *Issues in Comprehensive Pediatric Nursing, 28,* 83–95.

Huygen, A. C. J., Kuis, W., & Sinnema, G. (2000). Psychological, behavioral, and social adjustment in children and adolescents with juvenile chronic arthritis. *Annals of Rheumatic Disease, 59,* 276–282.

Ilowite, N. T., Walco, G. A., & Pochaczevsky, R. (1992). Assessment of pain in patients with juvenile rheumatoid arthritis: Relation between pain intensity and degree of joint inflammation. *Annals of the Rheumatic Diseases, 51,* 343–346.

Kellerman, J., Zeltzer, L., Ellenberg, L., Dash, J., & Rigler, D. (1980). Psychological effects of illness in adolescence: I. Anxiety, self-esteem, and perception of control. *Journal of Pediatrics, 97,* 126–131.

Kuis, W., Heijnen, C. J., Hogeweg, J. A., Sinnema, G., & Helders, P. J. M. (1997). How painful is juvenile chronic arthritis? *Archives of Disease in Childhood, 77,* 451–453.

Kvien, T. K., & Reimers, S. (1983). Drug handling and patient compliance in an outpatient paediatric trial. *Journal of Clinical and Hospital Pharmacy, 8,* 251–257.

Kyngäs, H. (2004). Support network of adolescents with chronic disease: Adolescents' perspective. *Nursing and Health Sciences, 6,* 287–293.

Lavigne, J. V., & Faier-Routman, J. (1992). Psychological adjustment to pediatric physical disorders: A meta-analytic review. *Journal of Pediatric Psychology, 17,* 133–157.

Lavigne, J. V., Ross, C. K., Berry, S. L., Hayford, J. R., & Pachman, L. M (1992). Evaluation of a psychological treatment package for treating pain in juvenile rheumatoid arthritis. *Arthritis Care and Research, 5,* 101–110.

LeBovidge, J. S., Lavigne, J. V., Donenberg, G. R., & Miller, M. L. (2003). Psychological adjustment of children and adolescents with chronic arthritis: A meta-analytic review. *Journal of Pediatric Psychology, 28,* 29–39.

Litt, I. F., & Cuskey, W. R. (1981). Compliance with salicylate therapy in adolescents with juvenile rheumatoid arthritis. *American Journal of Diseases of Children, 135,* 434–436.

Litt, I. F., Cuskey, W. R., & Rosenberg, A. (1982). Role of self-esteem and autonomy in determining medication compliance among adolescents with juvenile rheumatoid arthritis. *Pediatrics, 69,* 15–17.

Manuel, J. C. (2001). Risk and resistance factors in the adaptation in mothers of children with juvenile rheumatoid arthritis. *Journal of Pediatric Psychology, 26,* 237–246.

McNeill, T. (2004). Fathers' experience of parenting a child with juvenile rheumatoid arthritis. *Qualitative Health Research, 14,* 526–545.

Melzack, R., & Wall, P. D. (1965). Pain and mechanisms: A new theory. *Science, 150,* 971–979.

Meyer, R. A., Campbell, J. N., & Raja, S. N. (1994). Peripheral neural mechanisms of nociception. In P. D. Wall & R. Melzack (Eds.), *Textbook of pain* (3rd ed., pp. 13–44). Edinburgh, UK: Churchill Livingstone.

Miller, J. J., Spitz, P. W., Simpson, U., & Williams, G. F. (1982). The social functioning of young adults who had arthritis in childhood. *Journal of Pediatrics, 100,* 378–382.

Mullick, M. S., Nahar, J. S., & Haq, S. A. (2005). Psychiatric morbidity, stressors, impact, and burden in juvenile idiopathic arthritis. *Journal of Health, Population and Nutrition, 23,* 142–149.

Noll, R. B., Kozlowski, K., Gerhardt, C., Vannatta, K., Taylor, J., & Passo, M. (2000). Social, emotional, and behavioral functioning of children with juvenile rheumatoid arthritis. *Arthritis and Rheumatism, 43,* 1387–1396.

Packham, J. C., Hall, M. A., & Pimm, T. J. (2002). Long-term follow-up of 246 adults with juvenile idiopathic arthritis: Predictive factors for mood and pain. *Rheumatology, 41,* 1444–1449.

Palermo, T. M., Valenzuela, D., & Stork, P. P. (2004). A randomized trial of electronic versus paper pain diaries in children: Impact on compliance, accuracy, and acceptability. *Pain, 107,* 213–219.

Peterson, L. S., Mason, T., Nelson, A. M., O'Fallon, W. M., & Gabriel, S. E. (1997). Psychosocial outcomes and health status of adults who have had juvenile rheumatoid arthritis. *Arthritis and Rheumatism, 40,* 2235–2240.

Pless, K. B., & Roughmann, K. J. (1971). Chronic illness and its consequences: Observations based on three epidemiologic surveys. *Journal of Pediatrics, 79,* 351–359.

Quirk, M. E., & Young, M. H. (1990). The impact of JRA on children, adolescents, and their families: Current research and implications for future studies. *Arthritis Care and Research, 3,* 36–43.

Randich, A. (1993). Neural substrates of pain and analgesia. *Arthritis Care and Research, 6,* 171–177.

Rapoff, M. A. (1998). *Helping children follow their medical treatment program: Guidelines for parents of children with rheumatic diseases.* (Available from the author, University of Kansas Medical Center, Department of Pediatrics, 3901 Rainbow Boulevard, Kansas City, KS 66160-7330)

Rapoff, M. A. (1999). *Adherence to pediatric medical regimens.* New York: Kluwer Academic/ Plenum Press.

Rapoff, M. A. (2000). Facilitating adherence to medical regimens for pediatric rheumatic diseases: Primary, secondary, and tertiary prevention. In D. Drotar (Ed.), *Promoting adherence to medical treatment in chronic childhood illness: Concepts, methods, and interventions* (pp. 329–345). Mahwah, NJ: Erlbaum.

Rapoff, M. A., Belmont, J., Lindsley, C., Olson, N., Morris, J., & Padur, J. (2002). Prevention of nonadherence to nonsteroidal anti-inflammatory medications for newly diagnosed patients with juvenile rheumatoid arthritis. *Health Psychology, 21,* 620–623.

Rapoff, M. A., Belmont, J. M., Lindsley, C. B., & Olson, N. Y. (2005). Electronically monitored adherence to medications by newly diagnosed patients with juvenile rheumatoid arthritis. *Arthritis Care and Research, 53,* 905–910.

Rapoff, M. A., & Lindsley, C. B. (2000). The pain puzzle: A visual and conceptual metaphor for understanding and treating pain in pediatric rheumatic disease. *Journal of Rheumatology, 58*(Suppl.), 29–33.

Rapoff, M. A., Lindsley, C. B., & Christophersen, E. R. (1984). Improving compliance with medical regimens: Case study with juvenile rheumatoid arthritis. *Archives of Physical Medicine and Rehabilitation, 65,* 267–269.

Rapoff, M. A., Lindsley, C. B., & Christophersen, E. R. (1985). Parent perceptions of problems experienced by their children in complying with treatments for juvenile rheumatoid arthritis. *Archives of Physical Medicine and Rehabilitation, 66,* 427–430.

Rapoff, M. A., Purviance, M. R., & Lindsley, C. B. (1988a). Educational and behavioral strategies for improving medication compliance in juvenile rheumatoid arthritis. *Archives of Physical Medicine and Rehabilitation, 69,* 439–441.

Rapoff, M. A., Purviance, M. R., & Lindsley, C. B. (1988b). Improving medication compliance for juvenile rheumatoid arthritis and its effect on clinical outcome: A single-subject analysis. *Arthritis Care and Research, 1,* 12–16.

Reid, G. J., Gilbert, C. A., & McGrath, P. J. (1998). The Pain Coping Questionnaire: Preliminary validation. *Pain, 76,* 83–96.

Reid, G. J., McGrath, P. J., & Lang, B. A. (2005). Parent–child interactions among children with juvenile fibromyalgia, arthritis, and healthy controls. *Pain, 113,* 201–210.

Rimon, R., Belmaker, R. H., & Ebstein, R. (1977). Psychosomatic aspects of juvenile rheumatoid arthritis. *Scandinavian Journal of Rheumatology, 6,* 1–10.

Ross, C. K., Lavigne, J. V., Hayford, J. R., Berry, S. L., Sinacore, J. M., & Pachman, L. M. (1993). Psychological factors affecting reported pain in juvenile rheumatoid arthritis. *Journal of Pediatric Psychology, 18,* 561–573.

Ross, C. K., Lavigne, J. V., Hayford, J. R., Dyer, A. R., & Pachman, L. M. (1989). Validity of reported pain as a measure of clinical state in juvenile rheumatoid arthritis. *Annals of the Rheumatic Diseases, 48,* 817–819.

Sandstrom, M. J., & Schanberg, L. E. (2004). Brief report: Peer rejection, social behavior, and psychological adjustment in children with juvenile rheumatic disease. *Journal of Pediatric Psychology, 29,* 29–34.

Sawyer, M. G., Whitham, J. N., Roberton, D. M., Taplin, J. E., Varni, J. W., & Baghurst, P. A. (2004). The relationship between health-related quality of life, pain and coping strategies in juvenile idiopathic arthritis. *Rheumatology, 43,* 325–330.

Schanberg, L. E., Anthony, K. K., Gil, K. M., & Maurin, E. C. (2003). Daily pain and symptoms in children with polyarticular arthritis. *Arthritis and Rheumatism, 48,* 1390–1397.

Schanberg, L. E., Lefebvre, J. C., Keefe, F. J., Kredich, D. W., & Gil, K. M. (1997). Pain coping and the pain experience in children with juvenile chronic arthritis. *Pain, 73,* 181–189.

Schanberg, L. E., Sandstrom, M. J., Starr, K., Gil, K. M., Lefebvre, J. C., Keefe, F. J., et al.

(2000). The relationship of daily mood and stressful events to symptoms in juvenile rheumatic disease. *Arthritis Care and Research*, 13, 33–41.

Sherry, D. D., Bohnsack, J., Salmonson, K., Wallace, C. A., & Mellins, E. (1990). Painless juvenile rheumatoid arthritis. *Journal of Pediatrics*, 116, 921–923.

Stark, L. J., Janicke, D. M., McGrath, A. M., Mackner, L. M., Hommel, K. A., & Lovell, D. (2005). Prevention of osteoporosis: A randomized clinical trial to increase calcium intake in children with juvenile rheumatoid arthritis. *Journal of Pediatric Psychology*, 30, 377–386.

Stinson, J. N., Petroz, G. C., Tait, G., Feldman, B. M., Streiner, D., McGrath, P. J., et al. (2006). e-Ouch: Usability testing of an electronic chronic pain diary for adolescents with arthritis. *Clinical Journal of Pain*, 22, 295–305.

Sturge, C., Garralda, M. E., Boissin, M., Dore, C. J., & Woo, P. (1997). School attendance and juvenile chronic arthritis. *British Journal of Rheumatology*, 36, 1218–1223.

Sullivan, M. J. L., Bishop, S. R., & Pivik, J. (1995). The Pain Catastrophizing Scale: Development and validation. *Psychological Assessment*, 7, 524–532.

Thastum, M., Herlin, T., & Zachariae, R. (2005). Relationship of pain-coping strategies and pain-specific beliefs to pain experience in children with juvenile idiopathic arthritis. *Arthritis Care and Research*, 53, 178–184.

Thastum, M., Zachariae, R., Schøler, M., Bjerring, P., & Herlin, T. (1997). Cold pressor pain: Comparing responses of juvenile arthritis patients and their parents. *Scandinavian Journal of Rheumatology*, 26, 272–279.

Thastum, M., Zachariae, R., Schøler, M., & Herlin, T. (1998). A Danish adaptation of the Pain Coping Questionnaire for children: Preliminary data concerning reliability and validity. *Acta Paediatrica*, 88, 132–138.

Thompson, K. L., Varni, J. W., & Hanson, V. (1987). Comprehensive assessment of pain in juvenile rheumatoid arthritis: An empirical model. *Journal of Pediatric Psychology*, 12, 241–255.

Turkel, S., & Pao, M. (2007). Late consequences of chronic pediatric illness. *Psychiatric Clinics of North America*, 30, 819–835.

Varni, J. W., Rapoff, M. A., Waldron, S. A., Gragg, R. A., Bernstein, B. H., & Lindsley, C. B. (1996a). Chronic pain and emotional distress in children and adolescents. *Journal of Developmental and Behavioral Pediatrics*, 17, 154–161.

Varni, J. W., Rapoff, M. A., Waldron, S. A., Gragg, R. A., Bernstein, B. H., & Lindsley, C. B. (1996b). Effects of perceived stress on pediatric chronic pain. *Journal of Behavioral Medicine*, 19, 515–528.

Varni, J. W., Waldron, S. A., Gragg, R. A., Rapoff, M. A., Bernstein, B. H., Lindsley, C. B., et al. (1996). Development of the Waldron/Varni Pediatric Pain Coping Inventory. *Pain*, 67, 141–150.

von Weiss, R. T., Rapoff, M. A., Varni, J. W., Lindsley, C. B., Olson, N. Y., Madson, K. L., et al. (2002). Daily hassles and social support as predictors of adjustment in children with pediatric rheumatic disease. *Journal of Pediatric Psychology*, 27, 155–165.

Wagner, J. L., Chaney, J. M., Hommel, K. A., Page, M. C., Mullins, L. L., White, M. M., et al. (2003). The influence of parental distress on child depressive symptoms in juvenile rheumatoid diseases: The moderating effect of illness intrusiveness. *Journal of Pediatric Psychology*, 28, 453–462.

Walco, G. A., Varni, J. W., & Ilowite, N. T. (1992). Cognitive behavioral pain management in children with juvenile rheumatoid arthritis. *Pediatrics*, 89, 1075–1079.

CHAPTER 25

Cardiovascular Disease

ALAN M. DELAMATER
JASON F. JENT

Cardiovascular disease in children includes congenital heart disease (CHD), acquired heart disease, arrhythmias, and systemic hypertension. Surgical advances have allowed many children with cardiovascular disease to live relatively normal lives. The increased longevity of pediatric cardiac patients, along with the child and family stress associated with diagnosis, treatment, and ongoing management, has inspired many studies to evaluate the psychological and cognitive effects of cardiovascular disease in children (particularly CHD). In this chapter, the various types of pediatric cardiac disease and their medical management are briefly described, followed by sections reviewing the effects of cardiac disease on psychological functioning.

Pediatric Cardiac Disorders

Congenital Heart Disease

CHD includes a variety of disorders involving structural defects to the heart or the coronary blood vessels that occur during fetal development. The etiology in most cases is not known, but it is presumed to be due to a combination of genetic predisposition, chromosomal abnormalities, and environmental factors. The prevalence of CHD is between 5 and 8 in 1,000 live births (Bernstein, 2004), and most cases are diagnosed prenatally. CHD is grouped into two subtypes: acyanotic (e.g., ventricular septal defects, atrial septal–atrial ventricular canal defects and patent ductus arteriosis, coarctation of the aorta, and valvular lesions) and cyanotic (e.g., cardiomyopathy, hypoplastic left heart syndrome, pulmonary atresia, tetralogy of Fallot, tricuspid artesia, and transposition of the great arteries) (Bernstein, 2004). Acyanotic CHD is the more common type of CHD and involves holes in the walls of the heart chambers, the effect of which is to shunt fully oxygenated blood away from the body and back into the lungs. Cyanotic CHD is characterized by lesions that result in an obstruction to normal blood flow; this process results in reduced oxygenation of the blood, or cyanosis. Many patients with mild CHD require little or no treatment, as the heart defect corrects itself over time or results in little or no functional impairment. However, some patients with moderate to severe CHD may need significant medical intervention (e.g., cardiac surgery, heart transplantation).

Acquired Heart Disease and Arrhythmias

Acquired heart disease in childhood also includes a variety of disorders, generally resulting from bacterial and/or viral infections that damage the heart. These disorders include infective endocarditis, cardiomyopathy, rheumatic heart disease, diseases of the myocardium and pericardium, and coronary artery disease secondary to Kawasaki syndrome (Bernstein, 2004).

Childhood cardiac rhythm disturbances or arrhythmias can result from CHD (both acyanotic and cyanotic subtypes), acquired heart diseases, or acquired systemic disorders. The main risk associated with an arrhythmia is severe tachycardia (fast heart rate) or bradycardia (slow heart rate), resulting in decreased cardiac output; severe untreated arrhythmia may lead to sudden death.

Cognitive and Behavioral Functioning

Numerous studies have examined the cognitive development and behavioral functioning of children with CHD. The results of these studies are mixed with regard to the negative impact of CHD on children's functioning. However, a number of factors (e.g., type of CHD, disease severity, preoperative factors, surgery type, surgery support mechanisms, postoperative factors, and family dynamics) appear to moderate the effects of CHD on children's cognitive and behavioral functioning.

Cognitive and Behavioral Functioning Prior to Cardiac Surgery

Research has suggested that infants with CHD who require cardiovascular surgery are at increased risk for problematic parent–infant interactions and adverse neurodevelopmental outcomes. In particular, infants and toddlers with CHD have been found to be less active, rhythmic, and responsive to parents' cues, and more withdrawn and intense in negative emotional reactions (Goldberg, Morris, Simmons, Fowler, & Levinson, 1990; Lobo, 1992; Marino & Lipshitz, 1991).

There has also been an increased emphasis in recent research to examine how genetic factors and preoperative functioning may affect neurodevelopmental outcomes in children with CHD. In patients with CHD with preexisting genetic syndromes (e.g., Turner syndrome, Down syndrome), the apolipoprotein ε2 allele and/or deletion 22q11.2 have been associated with adverse neurodevelopmental outcomes (Atallah et al., 2007; Gaynor et al., 2007; Zeltser et al., 2008). Research has also shown that newborns with CHD requiring cardiovascular surgery often exhibit preexisting brain abnormalities, such as white matter injury, stroke, intraventricular hemorrhage, abnormal brain metabolism, and microcephaly (Limperopoulos et al., 1999, 2002; Miller et al. 2007). A number of factors occurring immediately prior to surgery, including acidosis, hypoxia, cerebral oxygen saturation, and seizure activity, have been linked to adverse neurodevelopmental outcomes in children with CHD (Hovels-Gurich et al., 2002; Mahle et al., 2000; Toet et al., 2005).

Operative Factors

With an increasing number of standardized corrective surgeries and treatments of CHD, more research has been dedicated to evaluating the effects of specific types of surgery (e.g., arterial switch operation, heart transplantation) on neurodevelopmental outcomes. Of particular interest are the effects of life support techniques used during cardiac surgery on neurodevelopmental outcomes.

Life Support Mechanisms during and after Cardiac Surgery

Deep hypothermic circulatory arrest (DHCA) and cardiopulmonary bypass (CPB) are both life support techniques used during cardiovascular surgery with children with CHD. During DHCA, the body and blood are cooled and cardiac arrest is induced, to allow surgeons to have adequate exposure to correct complex lesions. CPB mechanically circulates blood and oxygen throughout the body, bypassing the heart and lungs with a heart–lung machine.

A series of studies evaluated the effects of DHCA and CPB on children with transposition of the great arteries. In a large randomized clinical trial, children were randomly assigned to undergo predominantly either DHCA or low-flow CPB during the arterial switch operation. Early follow-up studies demonstrated a higher prevalence of motor skill, expressive language, and neurological problems in children who received DHCA than in children who received CPB (Bellinger et al., 1995; Bellinger, Rappaport, Wypij, Wernovsky, & Newburger, 1997). In a follow-up study of these children at 8 years of age, children in the DHCA group achieved significantly worse scores on measures of fine motor dexterity of the nondominant hand, apraxia of speech, visual–motor tracking, and phonological awareness than children in the CPB group (Bellinger et al., 2003). However, children in the CPB group displayed worse functioning in impulsivity and reaction time, and were rated by teachers as displaying more difficult behaviors, than children in the DHCA group. It was noted that both groups displayed behavioral functioning within normal limits.

Cardiac arrest time during surgery also appears to affect outcomes in children with CHD. That is, multiple studies have suggested that increased cardiac arrest time during surgery is related to subsequent neurodevelopmental impairment in children with CHD (Hovels-Gurich et al., 2001; Massaro, El-dib, Glass, & Aly, 2008; Oates, Simpson, Turnbull, & Cartmill, 1995; Wray, 2006).

Another type of life support mechanism, extracorporeal membrane oxygenation (ECMO), is a surgical procedure involving cardiopulmonary bypass of blood via cannulation of the right common carotid artery and right internal jugular vein. ECMO is a temporary life-saving technique for the most severely ill children, but carries with it a number of risks to neurological functioning, including intraventricular hemorrhage. ECMO is considered a standard therapy for neonatal respiratory failure that is unresponsive to other interventions. Some research has suggested an increased prevalence (approximately 25%) of abnormal neurodevelopmental outcomes in children with CHD who receive ECMO (Hamrick et al., 2003). In one study, young children who received ECMO after cardiac surgery displayed significantly more impairment than cardiac and healthy control groups on measures of abstract reasoning, lateralized motor functioning (left hand), visual memory, and visual–spatial constructive skills (Tindall, Rothermel, Delamater, Pinsky, & Klein, 1999).

Heart Transplantation

Several studies examined the cognitive development and psychological adjustment of children before and after heart transplantation, and found that some patients may be at risk for cognitive and psychosocial problems following transplantation (Todaro, Fennell, Sears, Rodrigue, & Roche, 2000). In a study designed to examine preoperative functioning in children awaiting heart transplantation, children with CHD and cardiomyopathy displayed developmental quotients within the average range (Wray & Radley-Smith, 2004b). With regard to postoperative functioning, most children who received heart transplants displayed cognitive development within normal limits, but there appears to be an increased prevalence of developmental delays and motor skill problems within this population (Fleisher et al., 2002; Freier et al., 2004). The degree to which cognitive status is affected by transplantation itself, or by factors related to the medical conditions that necessitated transplant, is currently unknown.

A number of studies have also examined the emotional and behavioral functioning of children awaiting heart transplants and those who have received heart transplants. Specifically, children awaiting heart transplants have increased prevalence of depression, psychosocial difficulties, and/or other psychiatric disorders (Serrano-Ikkos, Lask, Whitehead, Rees, & Graham, 1999; Wray & Radley-Smith, 2004a). In addition, children who receive heart transplants are more likely to have increased problems with social functioning at school, peer relationships, participation in sports and activities, and depression (Wray, Long, Radley-Smith, & Yacoub, 2001; Wray & Radley-Smith, 2006). Such children also were more likely to be experiencing difficulties in reading and arithmetic 5 years after transplant (Wray et al., 2001).

Postoperative Factors

Given the risk of brain injury during cardiac surgery, there has been an increased emphasis on monitoring and evaluating neurological functioning in the days following surgery. A study using magnetic resonance imaging found that preoperative brain injuries in newborns with CHD persisted postoperatively and/or that new brain injuries were identified (Miller et al., 2007). Similar, a neurobehavioral study found that developmental disabilities were predicted by postoperative brain injuries (Limperopoulos et al., 2002). Postoperative seizures appear to occur in between 11 and 20% of children who receive cardiac surgery, but their effects on long-term neurodevelopmental outcomes remain unclear (Bellinger et al., 1995; Gaynor et al., 2006; Newburger, et al., 1993). The presence of postoperative cardiocirculatory insufficiency has been associated with increases in internalizing, externalizing, and attention problems in children with transposition of the great arteries (Hovels-Gurich et al., 2002). In addition, postoperative length of stay in the hospital has been shown to be related to worse cognitive functioning at 8-year follow-up, even after sociodemographic variables, perioperative factors, and perfusion events were controlled for (Newburger et al., 2003).

Long-Term Effects of Cardiovascular Surgery

Research examining the long-term effects of CHD on children who have undergone cardiovascular surgery is mixed. Several methodological factors (e.g., small sample sizes; no comparison groups; failure to account for preoperative, perioperative, and postoperative factors) have likely contributed to the inconsistent evidence regarding the effects of CHD on cognitive and behavioral functioning. In an attempt to better understand the existing literature on the effects of CHD, a meta-analysis of 25 CHD studies was conducted to systematically evaluate the cognitive and behavioral functioning in children with CHD who have undergone cardiovascular surgery (Karsdrop, Everaerd, Kindt, & Mulder, 2007). The meta-analysis included peer-reviewed articles published between 1980 and 2005, 2- to 19-year-old patients with CHD, and measures of cognitive and behavioral functioning. Overall, it was determined that the presence of CHD per se was not associated with cognitive deficits. However, youths with more severe CHD demonstrated lower overall cognitive functioning than did those with less severe CHD (Karsdrop et al., 2007). In particular, children with hypoplastic left heart syndrome or transposition of the great arteries displayed lower cognitive functioning relative to study control groups and normative data. Specifically, these children experienced more difficulties with perceptual organizational abilities. Children with other types of CHD, including atrium septum defect, ventricular septum defect, and tetralogy of Fallot, displayed cognitive functioning within the average range.

The meta-analysis also systematically evaluated research (11 studies) that used the Child Behavior Checklist to examine the effects of CHD on behavioral functioning. Results indicated that only older patients with CHD (>10 years old) were perceived by their parents as having more overall, internalizing, and externalizing problems than control groups. Unlike the cognitive outcomes, the behavioral outcomes were not related to disease severity in children and adolescents with CHD. The generalizability of the meta-analysis is limited in that measures of cognitive functioning, family functioning, and quality of life for very young children (<2 years old) were not included.

Other, more recent research has been specifically devoted to gaining a better understanding of the neurodevelopmental functioning of children with tetralogy of Fallot who have undergone surgery. In a series of studies where such children were compared to children with acyanotic CHD conditions and/or healthy controls, the children with tetralogy of Fallot performed significantly worse on measures of language, attention, executive functioning, academic performance, visual–spatial skills, and sensorimotor functioning (Hovels-Gurich, Konrad, Skorzenski, Herpertz-Dahlmann, et al., 2007; Hovels-Gurich, Konrad, Skorzenski, Minkenberg, et al., 2007; Miatton, De Wolf, Francois, Thiery, & Vingerhoets, 2007b).

Gross and fine motor skills appear to be another area of concern for children with CHD who have undergone cardiovascular surgery. Several studies have shown that these children are at increased risk for gross and fine motor delays that remain relatively stable over time (Brosig, Mussatto, Kuhn, & Tweddell, 2007a; Holm, Fredriksen, Fosdahl, Olstad, & Vollestad, 2007; Majnemer et al., 2006; McGusker et al., 2007).

Despite increasing awareness of the higher prevalence of neurodevelopmental deficits in children with severe CHD, less empirical attention has been given to how these deficits affect academic performance. The limited research in this areas has suggested that children with surgically corrected CHD are viewed as having significantly lower academic achievement, more school problems in general, and a higher rate of repeating a grade, compared to healthy controls (Mahle et al., 2000; Miatton, De Wolf, Francois, Thiery, & Vingerhoets, 2007a).

Family Factors

The presence of specific parental factors appears to moderate the effects of CHD on children's behavioral outcomes. That is, children with CHD whose parents are identified as exhibiting poor parental control skills, high maternal worry, insecure maternal attachment, and/or increased maternal psychopathology are at risk for poorer behavioral adjustment (Berant, Mikulincer, & Shaver, 2008; McGusker et al., 2007).

Other studies have explored parenting stress and parenting style of parents of children with CHD. Although some literature suggests that approximately 20% of parents of children with CHD report clinically significant parenting stress, other research has found no differences in parenting stress between parents of children with CHD and healthy control parents (Brosig, Mussatto, Kuhn, & Tweddell, 2007b; DeMaso et al., 1991; Uzark & Jones, 2003; Visconti, Saudino, Rappaport, Newburger, & Bellinger, 2002). However, similar to other populations, parents who reported significant parenting stress viewed their children with CHD as exhibiting more behavior problems (Uzark & Jones, 2003; Visconti et al., 2002).

Quality of Life

As success with cardiac surgery continues to increase, greater emphasis has been given to self-concept and quality of life in children with CHD. Particular attention has been given to the effects of CHD on children's and adolescents' health-related quality of life. Some research indicates that children and adolescents with CHD have a quality of life similar to that of healthy controls (Brosig et al., 2007b; Culbert et al., 2003; Hovels-Gurich, Konrad, Skorzenski, Minkenberg, et al., 2007; Mahle et al., 2000). In contrast, other studies have shown that youths with CHD report significantly lower quality of life relative to healthy peers (Krol et al., 2003; Mussatto & Tweddell, 2005). Specifically, patients with cyanotic heart disease and/or complex CHD who have received palliative surgery appear to be at increased risk for perceived physical limitations and decreased exercise tolerance (Casey, Sykes, Craig, Power, & Mulholland, 1996; Chen, Li, & Wang, 2005; Kamphuis et al., 2002). In an attempt to explore what factors might explain these different findings, Cohen, Mansoor, Langut, and Lorber (2007) evaluated health-related quality of life, depression, self-esteem, and perceived heart disease severity in adolescents with acquired heart disease or CHD and healthy adolescents. Findings revealed that depressive symptoms and perceived disease severity mediated the relationship between an objective measure of disease severity (i.e., based on medical record review) and health-related quality of life.

Quality of life has also been examined in children with arrhythmias, with most children reporting their health to be excellent or good. Children who had received previous surgery for their cardiac condition reported increased worries regarding their arrhythmias. Greater frequency of daily medications was associated with more worries about their arrhythmias and greater impact of the arrhythmias on their lives (Schneider, Delamater, Geith, Young, & Wolff, 2001).

Summary and Implications for Future Research

Overall, the effects of CHD on children's cognitive and behavioral functioning are mixed and are partially explained by a number of moderating variables (e.g., genetic syndromes, preoperative factors, life support mechanism, disease severity). However, it is difficult to draw firm conclusions about the effect of different moderator variables on cognitive and behavioral functioning, because many of these variables are closely related. For example, it is difficult to separate the effect of disease severity and number of operations, because children with more severe CHD may need more surgeries.

Research findings suggest that children with CHD who require corrective surgery have a high prevalence of preoperative brain injuries and brain abnormalities. Furthermore, the presence of genetic abnormalities or syndromes, preoperative cyanosis, or preoperative seizure activity in children with CHD has been linked to adverse neurodevelopmental outcomes. After heart transplantation, children's cognitive development appears to proceed normally, but these children appear to be at increased risk for depression, social skill problems, motor skill deficits, and learning difficulties. Children who receive CPB during cardiac surgery generally display better neurodevelopmental outcomes than children who receive predominantly DHCA during surgery. Children treated with ECMO after cardiac surgery appear to experience higher cognitive impairment and lateralized deficits of functions performed by the right hemisphere.

Overall, the presence of CHD in children per se is not associated with cognitive deficits and/or behavioral problems. However, youths with more severe CHD (specifically, hypoplastic left heart syndrome and transposition of the great arteries) demonstrate lower levels of cognitive functioning than youths with less severe CHD do. More recent evidence has indicated that children with CHD are at significant risk for gross and fine motor delays, as well as lower academic achievement.

The research literature on behavioral and emotional functioning suggests that infants with CHD are viewed as having more difficult temperamental characteristics and are less responsive to cues for feeding. Older children and adolescents (>10 years old) with CHD demonstrate more overall, internalizing, and externalizing behavior problems than controls. Family factors appear to play a role in children's behavioral functioning: Ineffective parenting, insecure maternal attachment, parenting stress, and increased maternal psychopathology have been identified as risk factors for adverse behavioral outcomes. Research findings are mixed regarding health-related quality of life in children and adolescents with CHD. Increased disease severity and depressive symptoms appear to be related to lower ratings of quality of life in children with CHD or arrhythmias.

The research literature on CHD is limited by several methodological problems. Study samples are usually small, raising concerns about sampling bias. When sociodemographic characteristics of the sample are reported, in most cases the sample is predominantly white and in the middle range of socioeconomic status. In addition, samples are often heterogeneous with regard to type of cardiac defect. Several studies have not used control groups, relying instead on comparisons with test norms. Many studies also fail to account for preoperative, operative, and postoperative factors.

Few controlled studies have been reported with respect to the developmental outcomes of children undergoing transplantation. Further studies with larger samples are needed to more precisely determine the nature and characteristics of longer-term neurodevelopmental outcomes in these children. A significant number of such children may have learning difficulties, and there is some evidence of increased depression and lower social competence among school-age children. This issue remains important for future studies.

Despite the increased risk for cognitive, emotional, and behavioral difficulties in children with CHD, very little research on interventions or academic placement has been conducted. Pediatric psychologists can make significant contributions by designing and evaluating specifically tailored interventions for parental stress, child depression, and social difficulties in families of children with CHD. Academic achievement in children with CHD also needs to be further explored, to gain a better understanding of the need for potential academic and occupational accommodations. In addition, counseling regarding potential academic difficulties and reasonable expectations for age-appropriate activities (including participation in sports) may be useful, particularly for school-age children with more severe disease. These children should have comprehensive psychoeducational evaluations and individual educational plans made as needed to facilitate optimal academic performance.

With regard to children with acquired heart disease, little systematic research has been reported. This area needs more attention from pediatric psychologists. Research studies should particularly target adherence to prophylactic drug regimens, as this is a significant clinical issue related to morbidity of children and clinical decisions regarding transplantation.

References

Atallah, J., Joffe, A. R., Robertson, C. M., Leonard, N., Blakeley, P. M., Nettel-Aguirre, A., et al. (2007). Two-year general and neurodevelopmental outcome after neonatal complex cardiac surgery in patients with deletion 22q11.2: A comparative study. *Journal of Thoracic and Cardiovascular Surgery, 134,* 772–779.

Bellinger, D. C., Jonas, R. A., Rappaport, L. A., Wypij, D., Wernovsky, G., Kuban, K., et al. (1995). Developmental and neurologic status of children after heart surgery with hypothermic circulatory arrest or low-flow cardiopulmonary bypass. *New England Journal of Medicine, 332,* 549–555.

Bellinger, D. C., Rappaport, L. A., Wypij, D., Wernovsky, G., & Newburger, J. W. (1997). Patterns of developmental dysfunction after surgery during infancy to correct transposition of the great arteries. *Journal of Developmental and Behavioral Pediatrics, 18,* 75–83.

Bellinger, D. C., Wypij, D., duPlessis, A. J., Rappaport, L. A., Jonas, R. A., Wernovsky, G., et al. (2003). Neurodevelopmental status at eight years in children with dextro-transposition of the great arteries: The Boston Circulatory Arrest Trial. *Journal of Thoracic and Cardiovascular Surgery, 126,* 1385–1396.

Berant, E., Mikulincer, M., & Shaver, P. R. (2008). Mothers' attachment style, their mental health, and their children's emotional vulnerabilities: A 7-year study of children with congenital heart disease. *Journal of Personality, 76,* 31–65.

Bernstein, D. (2004). The cardiovascular system. In R. E. Behrman, R. M. Kliegman, & H. B. Jenson (Eds.), *Nelson textbook of pediatrics* (17th ed., pp. 1475–1598). Philadelphia: Saunders.

Brosig, C. L., Mussatto, K. A., Kuhn, E. M., & Tweddell, J. S. (2007a). Neurodevelopmental outcome in preschool survivors of complex congenital heart disease: Implications for clinical practice. *Journal of Pediatric Health Care, 21,* 3–12.

Brosig, C. L., Mussatto, K. A., Kuhn, E. M., & Tweddell, J. S. (2007b). Psychosocial outcomes for preschool children and families after surgery for complex congenital heart disease. *Pediatric Cardiology, 28,* 255–262.

Casey, R. A., Sykes, D. H., Craig, B., Power, R., & Mulholland, H. C. (1996). Behavioral adjustment of children with surgically palliated complex congenital heart disease. *Journal of Pediatric Psychology, 21,* 335–352.

Chen, C., Li, C., & Wang, J. (2005). Self-concept: Comparison between school-aged children with congenital heart disease and normal school-aged children. *Journal of Clinical Nursing, 14,* 394–402.

Cohen, M., Mansoor, D., Langut, H., & Lorber, A. (2007). Quality of life, depressed mood, and self-esteem in adolescents with heart disease. *Psychosomatic Medicine, 69,* 313–318.

Culbert, E. L., Ashburn, D. A., Cullen-Dean, G., Joseph, J. A., Williams, W. G., Blackstone, E. H., et al. (2003). Quality of life of children after repair of transposition of the great arteries. *Circulation, 108,* 857–862.

DeMaso, D. R., Campis, L. K., Wypij, D., Bertram, S., Lipshitz, M., & Freed, M. (1991). The impact of maternal perceptions and medical severity on the adjustment of children with congenital heart disease. *Journal of Pediatric Psychology, 16,* 137–149.

Fleisher, B. E., Baum, D., Brudos, G., Burge, M., Carson, E., Constantinou, J., et al. (2002). Infant heart transplantation at Stanford: Growth and neurodevelopmental outcome. *Pediatrics, 109,* 1–7.

Freier, M. C., Babikian, T., Pivonka, J., Aaen, T. B., Gardner, J. M., Baum, M., et al. (2004). A longitudinal perspective on neurodevelopmental outcome after infant cardiac transplantation. *Journal of Heart and Lung Transplantation, 23,* 857–864.

Gaynor, J. W., Jarvik, G. P., Bernbaum, J., Gerdes, M., Wernovsky, G., Burnham, J., et al. (2006). The relationship of postoperative electographic seizures to neurodevelopmental outcome at 1 year of age after neonatal and infant cardiac surgery. *Journal of Thoracic and Cardiovascular Surgery, 131,* 181–189.

Gaynor, J. W., Wernovsky, G., Jarvik, G. P., Bernbaum, J., Gerdes, M., Zackai, E., et al. (2007). Patient characteristics are important determinants of neurodevelopmental outcome at one year of age after neonatal and infant cardiac surgery. *Journal of Thoracic and Cardiovascular Surgery, 133,* 1344–1353.

Goldberg, S., Morris, P., Simmons, R. J., Fowler, R. S., & Levinson, H. (1990). Chronic illness in infancy and parenting stress: A comparison of three groups of parents. *Journal of Pediatric Psychology, 15,* 347–358.

Hamrick, S. E., Gremmels, D. B., Keet, C. A., Leonard, C. H., Connell, J. K., Hawgood, S., et al. (2003). Neurodevelopmental outcome of infants supported with extracorporeal membrane oxygenation after cardiac surgery. *Pediatrics, 111,* 671–675.

Holm, I., Fredriksen, P. M., Fosdahl, M. A., Olstad, M., & Vollestad, N. (2007). Impaired motor competence in school-aged children with complex congenital heart disease. *Archives of Pediatrics and Adolescent Medicine, 161,* 945–950.

Hovels-Gurich, H. H., Konrad, K., Skorzenski, D., Herpertz-Dahlmann, B., Messmer, B. J., & Seghaye, M. (2007). Attentional dysfunction in children after corrective cardiac surgery in infancy. *Annals of Thoracic Surgery, 83,* 1425–1430.

Hovels-Gurich, H. H., Konrad, K., Skorzenski, D., Minkenberg, R., Herpertz-Dahlmann, B., Messmer, B. J., et al. (2007). Long-term behavior and quality of life after corrective cardiac surgery in infancy for tetralogy of Fallot or ventricular septal defect. *Pediatric Cardiology*, *28*, 346–354.

Hovels-Gurich, H. H., Seghaye, M., Schnitker, R., Wiesner, M., Huber, W., Minkenberg, R., et al. (2002). Long-term neurodevelopmental outcomes in school-aged children after neonatal arterial switch operation. *Journal of Thoracic and Cardiovascular Surgery*, *124*, 448–458.

Hovels-Gurich, H. H., Seghaye, M., Sigler, M., Kotlarek, F., Bartl, A., Neuser, J., et al. (2001). Neurodevelopmental outcome related to cerebral risk factors in children after neonatal arterial switch operation. *Annals of Thoracic Surgery*, *71*, 881–888.

Kamphuis, M., Ottencamp, J., Vliegen, H. W., Vogels, T., Zwinderman, K. H., Kamphuis, R. P., et al. (2002). Health related quality of life of health status in adult survivors with previously operated complex congenital heart disease. *Heart*, *87*, 356–362.

Karsdrop, P. A., Everaerd, W., Kindt, M., & Mulder, B. J. (2007). Psychological and cognitive functioning in children and adolescents with congenital heart disease: A meta-analysis. *Journal of Pediatric Psychology*, *32*, 527–541.

Krol, Y., Grootenhuis, M. A., Destree-Vonk, A., Lubbers, L. J., Koopman, H. M., & Last, B. F. (2003). Health related quality of life in children with congenital heart disease. *Psychology and Health*, *18*, 251–260.

Limperopoulos, C., Majnemer, A., Shevell, M., Rosenblatt, B., Rohlicek, C., & Tchervenkov, C. (1999). Neurologic status of newborns with congenital heart defects before open heart surgery. *Pediatrics*, *103*, 402–408.

Limperopoulos, C., Majnemer, A., Shevell, M. I., Rohlicek, C., Rosenblatt, B., Tchervenkov, C., et al. (2002). Predictors of developmental disabilities after open heart surgery in young children with congenital heart defects. *Journal of Pediatrics*, *142*, 51–58.

Lobo, M. (1992). Parent–infant interaction during feeding when the infant has congenital heart disease. *Journal of Pediatric Nursing*, *7*, 97–105.

Mahle, W. T., Clancy, R. R., Moss, E. M., Gerdes, M., Jobes, D. R., & Wernovsky, G. (2000). Neurodevelopmental outcome and lifestyle assessment in school-aged and adolescent children with hypolastic left heart syndrome. *Pediatrics*, *105*, 1082–1089.

Majnemer, A., Limperopoulos, C., Shevell, M., Rosenblatt, B., Rohlicek, C., & Tchervenkov, C. (2006). Long-term neuromotor outcome at school entry of infants with congenital heart defects requiring open-heart surgery. *Journal of Pediatrics*, *148*, 72–77.

Marino, B. L., & Lipshitz, M. (1991). Temperament in infants and toddlers with cardiac disease. *Pediatric Nursing*, *17*, 445–448.

Massaro, A. N., El-dib, M., Glass, P., & Aly, H. (2008). Factors associated with adverse neurodevelopmental outcomes in infants with congenital heart disease. *Brain Development*, *30*, 437–446.

McGusker, C. G., Doherty, N. N., Molloy, B., Casey, F., Rooney, N., Mulholland, C., et al. (2007). Determinants of neuropsychological and behavioral outcomes in early childhood survivors of congenital heart disease. *Archives of Disease in Childhood*, *92*, 137–141.

Miatton, M., De Wolf, D., Francois, K., Thiery, E., & Vingerhoets, G. (2007a). Behavior and self-perception in children with a surgically corrected congenital heart disease. *Journal of Developmental and Behavioral Pediatrics*, *28*, 294–301.

Miatton, M., De Wolf, D., Francois, K., Thiery, E., & Vingerhoets, G. (2007b). Intellectual, neuropsychological, and behavioral functioning in children with tetralogy of Fallot. *Journal of Thoracic and Cardiovascular Surgery*, *133*, 449–455.

Miller, S. P., McQuillen, P. S., Hamrick, S., Xu, D., Glidden, D. V., Charlton, N., et al. (2007). Abnormal brain development in newborns with congenital heart disease. *New England Journal of Medicine*, *357*, 1928–1938.

Mussatto, K., & Tweddell, J. (2005). Quality of life following surgery for congenital cardiac malformations in neonates and infants. *Cardiology in the Young*, *15*(Suppl. 1), 174–178.

Newburger, J. W., Jonas, R. A., Wernovsky, G., Wypij, D., Hickey, P. R., Karl, C. K., et al. (1993).

Comparison of the perioperative neurologic effects of hypothermic circulatory arrest versus low-flow cardiopulmonary by-pass in infant heart surgery. *New England Journal of Medicine, 329,* 1057–1064.

Newburger, J. W., Wypij, D., Bellinger, D. C., du Plessis, A. J., Kuban, K. C., Rappaport, L. A., et al. (2003). Length of stay after infant cardiac surgery is related to cognitive outcome at age 8 years. *Journal of Pediatrics, 143,* 67–73.

Oates, R. K., Simpson, J. M., Turnbull, J. A., & Cartmill, T. B. (1995). The relationship between intelligence and duration of circulatory arrest with deep hypothermia. *Journal of Thoracic and Cardiovascular Surgery, 110,* 786–792

Schneider, K., Delamater, A., Geith, T., Young, M., & Wolff, G. (2001). Quality of life in children with cardiac arrhythmia. *Annals of Behavioral Medicine, 23*(Suppl.), S180.

Serrano-Ikkos, E., Lask, B., Whitehead, B., Rees, P., & Graham, P. (1999). Heart or heart–lung transplantation: Psychosocial outcome. *Pediatric Transplantation, 3,* 301–308.

Tindall, S., Rothermel, R., Delamater, A. M., Pinsky, W., & Klein, M. (1999). Neuropsychological abilities of children with cardiac disease treated with extracorporeal membrane oxygenation. *Developmental Neuropsychology, 16,* 101–115.

Todaro, J. F., Fennell, E. B., Sears, S. F., Rodrigue, J. R., & Roche, A. K. (2000). Cognitive and psychological outcomes in pediatric heart transplantation. *Journal of Pediatric Psychology, 25,* 567–576.

Toet, M. C., Flinterman, A., Laar, I., Vries, J. W., Bennink, G. B., Uiterwaal, C. S., et al. (2005). Cerebral oxygen saturation and brain electrical activity before, during, and up to 36 h after arterial switch procedure in neonates without pre-existing brain damage: Its relationship to neurodevelopmental outcomes. *Experimental Brain Research, 165,* 343–350.

Uzark, K., & Jones, K. (2003). Parenting stress and children with heart disease. *Journal of Pediatric Health Care, 17,* 163–168.

Visconti, K. J., Saudino, K. J., Rappaport, L. A., Newburger, J. W., & Bellinger, D. C. (2002). Influence of parental stress and social support on the behavioral adjustment of children with transposition of the great arteries. *Journal of Developmental and Behavioral Pediatrics, 23,* 314–321.

Wray, J. (2006). Intellectual development of infants, children, and adolescents with congenital heart disease. *Developmental Science, 9,* 368–378.

Wray, J., Long, T., Radley-Smith, R., & Yacoub, M. (2001). Returning to school after heart or heart–lung transplantation: How well do children adjust? *Transplantation, 72,* 100–106.

Wray, J., & Radley-Smith, R. (2004a). Depression in pediatric patients before and 1 year after heart or heart–lung transplantation. *Journal of Heart and Lung Transplantation, 23,* 1103–1110.

Wray, J., & Radley-Smith, R. (2004b). Developmental and behavioral status of infants and young children awaiting heart or heart–lung transplantation. *Pediatrics, 113,* 488–495.

Wray, J., & Radley-Smith, R. (2006). Longitudinal assessment of psychological functioning in children after heart or heart–lung transplantation. *Journal of Heart and Lung Transplantation, 25,* 345–352.

Zeltser, I., Jarvik, G. P., Bernbaum, J., Wernovsky, G., Nord, A. S., Gerdes, M., et al. (2008). Genetic factors are important determinants of neurodevelopmental outcome after repair of tetralogy of Fallot. *Journal of Thoracic and Cardiovascular Surgery, 135,* 91–97.

CHAPTER 26

Pediatric Organ Transplantation

JAMES R. RODRIGUE
NATALIYA ZELIKOVSKY

Transplantation of the kidney, heart, liver, lung, and small intestine is now performed at pediatric medical centers worldwide. In the United States alone, there have been more than 20,000 pediatric transplants performed in the past decade (*www.unos.org*). Pediatric transplant outcomes and the management of young transplant patients have improved over time. In most instances, survival is as good as, or better than, that seen in adults (Sweet et al., 2006). Other outcomes, including physical growth, cognitive development, neurological functioning, academic performance, quality of life, and the psychological adaptation of children and families, are increasingly topics of investigation within pediatric transplant programs and represent excellent collaborative research opportunities for pediatric psychologists. Fortunately, the number of children and adolescents awaiting organ transplantation has leveled off since 2001, with nearly 2,000 on the U.S. waiting list at the end of 2007. Waiting times are generally less for children than for adults, in large part because children are given priority on the transplant waiting list.

Clinical Issues

Organ transplantation is a process that, for most children and their families, begins with the diagnosis of a serious illness that leads to intensive, prolonged medical and pharmacological interventions and multiple hospitalizations. After months or years of dealing with the rigors and demands of chronic illness and its treatment, referral for transplant evaluation inevitably leads to both excitement and anxiety—excitement about the prospect of living disease-free, and anxiety about the uncertainty of waiting for a suitable organ. For many children, an organ is eventually procured, and renewed hope for long-term survival follows transplant surgery. Unfortunately, the dynamic process does not end there, as transplant recipients must consume a cocktail of medications on a daily basis (usually for life) and navigate successfully through an assortment of complications that are part of the posttransplant experience. Such complications may include graft rejection, infections, hospital readmissions, various toxicities, and other systemic problems (Magee, Krishnan, Benfield, Hsu, & Shneider, 2008).

Although the point of entry may vary across centers, pediatric psychologists working in large medical centers are often consulted to provide clinical services to children and families at various points along the transplant spectrum. Psychological evaluations are often conducted to identify psychological, developmental, and behavioral health strengths and liabilities as they relate to the transplant process, and to determine a child's baseline level of functioning along these various dimensions. Clinical interviews and some formal testing may serve as the basis for these evaluations (Maloney, Clay, & Robinson, 2004; Rodrigue, Gonzalez-Peralta, & Langham, 2004; Streisand & Tercyak, 2001). More recently, there has been an effort to develop and validate specific tools to guide clinicians' assessment of pediatric transplant candidates (Fung & Shaw, 2008). For some children and their families, psychological interventions are necessary to optimize the children's transplant candidacy and to increase the likelihood of positive health outcomes, both before and after transplantation. This includes interventions to reduce risks of nonadherence, attenuate family stress, facilitate reintegration into school and/or other activities, and improve overall quality of life.

Organ Donation

The single most pressing issue confronting the field of transplantation is the severe organ shortage. The scarcity of donor organs is especially acute for children, since organ size matters for liver, heart, and lung transplantation, and there are not many size-matched deaths in younger children. The widening gap between the number of people awaiting transplantation and the number of donated organs, and the best ways to reverse this trend, have been topics of considerable dialogue and debate among health professionals, bioethicists, and health policy experts (Childress & Liverman, 2006).

There are two ways in which organs become available for transplantation: through deceased or live donation. In the case of deceased donation, a family has consented to donate the organs of a loved one who has suffered a traumatic injury or medical event, and has been declared brain-dead. There are many important factors that play a role in how family members decide whether to donate organs under such intensely traumatic circumstances (e.g., Rodrigue, Cornell, & Howard, 2006, 2008; Siminoff, Gordon, Hewlett, & Arnold, 2001). Some of these factors include knowledge of the deceased's donation intentions, any previous discussion about organ donation that has occurred within the family, the quality of the interactions with hospital staff and organ requestors, and previous attitudes toward organ donation. Increasingly, psychologists are working collaboratively with organ procurement organizations to provide educational programs on grief and bereavement, the impact of traumatic injury and brain death on families, and how best to approach families when requesting consent for organ donation.

Children may also receive organs from living donors. Healthy individuals can now donate a kidney (the remaining kidney enlarges and assumes the function of the one donated), a liver segment (which regenerates in days), a portion of the pancreas, or a lobe of the lung (which does not regenerate). Living donor transplants may have some advantages over deceased donor transplants, depending on the specific organ type. These advantages may include better graft and/or patient survival rates, preemption of more costly and debilitating medical or surgical interventions while a patient is awaiting deceased donor transplantation, and improved quality of life for the recipient. Despite these possible advantages, living donation poses risks to otherwise healthy individuals, with greater risks associated with certain donation types (liver) over others (kidney). Possible risks include physical pain and discomfort; wound infections; bleeding; psychological trauma; the development of hypertension, proteinuria, or progressive organ failure; and death (Ghobrial et al., 2008; Hartmann, Fauchald, Westlie, Brekke, & Holdaas, 2003). Overall, however, the quality of life and psychological outcomes have been quite favorable for living donors (Switzer, Dew, & Twillman, 2000). Because parents make up a large percentage of those who opt to donate an organ to their children, pediatric psychologists consulting with transplant programs may be asked to play an active role in providing evaluation services throughout the living donation process. The Consensus Statement on the Live Organ Donor (Live Organ Donor Consensus Group, 2000) strongly emphasizes the need for careful psychosocial evaluation of the prospective donor—with a focus on examining the donor's psychological stability, competence, and ability to provide informed consent, as well as on determining whether the donation decision is being made freely and without coercion (Olbrisch, Benedict, Haller, & Levenson, 2001).

Adherence to Medical Regimens

Prior to transplantation, most children and adolescents have dealt with a complex regimen of medications, surgery, frequent laboratory tests, clinic appointments, dietary restrictions or supplements, and activity limitations. Organ transplantation offers a chance at improved quality of life and better long-term medical prognosis. In order to optimize graft survival however, patients must commit themselves to lifelong immunosuppressant medications designed to prevent the occurrence of both acute and chronic rejection episodes. Poor adherence contributes to acute rejection episodes, graft loss, lower quality of life, higher health care utilization, and ethical dilemmas regarding retransplantation (Cleemput, Kesteloot, & De Geest, 2002).

Despite the serious implications for clinical outcomes, nonadherence is a common problem among pediatric patients and particularly among adolescents. The prevalence of nonadherence ranges from 9 to 75% (Dobbels, Van Damme-Lombaert, Vanhaecke, & De Geest, 2005; Fredericks et al., 2008), depending on the conceptualization, methodology, and measurement strategies used. The biological and psychological developmental changes that occur during adolescence place teens at a higher risk of nonadherence and poor outcome than other age groups (Berquist et al., 2008). Nonadherence may not become evident for a couple of years, as adolescents tend to do well with their medication regimen initially, but show more signs of nonadherence over time (Berquist et al., 2008). Indeed, adolescents have the best 1-year graft survival of any age group, but the long-term transplant outcomes in adolescents are disappointing, most often because of poor adherence.

As in the assessment of most pediatric illnesses, various subjective and objective methods (e.g., self-report, collateral ratings by health care providers, blood serum levels, pharmacy refills, electronic monitoring) are used with pediatric transplant patients to assess adherence with the immunosuppression regimens. No singular method has strong diagnostic value in predicting clinical outcomes, so a multimethod approach in which a composite adherence score can be calculated may be optimal. Several measures have been developed recently that quantify nonadherence and identify specific barriers to care in the transplant population; these include the Medical Adherence Measure (Zelikovsky, Schast, Palmer, & Meyers, 2008) and the Adolescent and Parent Medication Barriers Survey (Simons & Blount, 2007). Regardless of the methods used, several aspects of nonadherence should be evaluated, including overall versus partial nonadherence (inconsistent taking), problems with all versus some of the medications, and complete absence (missed) versus timing (off-schedule dosing).

Risk factors for nonadherence have been grouped into socioeconomic, patient-related, condition-related, treatment-related, and health care system factors (for a review, see Dobbels et al., 2005). Behavioral and emotional problems, psychiatric and abuse history, and posttraumatic stress have been implicated as predictors of nonadherence (Maikranz, Steele, Dreyer, Startman, & Bovaird, 2007; Penkower et al., 2003; Shemesh et al., 2007). In addition, nonadherence may be associated with lower health-related quality of life, with deficits in school functioning, limitations in emotional/behavioral and physical functioning, poorer mental health, and lower general health perceptions (Fredericks, Lopez, Magee, Shieck, & Opipari-Arrigan, 2007; Fredericks et al., 2008). High parent stress, low parental involvement, and strained parent–child interactions have also been associated with poor medication adherence (Gerson, Furth, Neu, & Fivush, 2004); however, but specific relational factors, including family cohesion, conflict, and communication, have not yet been fully explored. Finally, medical regimens that require lifestyle changes, have cosmetic side effects, interrupt social activities, require more self-care responsibility, and have more perceived barriers are most difficult for teenagers (Annunziato et al., 2007; Wray, Waters, Radley-Smith, & Sensky, 2006; Zelikovsky et al., 2008).

There is preliminary evidence that nonadherence patterns may vary as a function of race. For instance, Tucker and colleagues (2001) found that medication regimen factors (e.g., pill size, complexity) and self-efficacy may be more predictive of nonadherence among African American patients, while "forgetting" may be more common among European American patients. African American transplant recipients were also more adherent with transplant medications if they had dialysis prior to transplant (vs. preemptive transplant) and if they received a deceased donor (vs. live, related donor) transplant (Fennell, Tucker, & Pedersen, 2001). These race findings should be interpreted cautiously, as they may be confounded by other variables, including education level, health literacy, family income, and family size. Clearly, there is a need to examine unique predictors of adherence among racially and ethnically diverse transplant patients, as well as to examine the influence of these other contextual factors on adherence.

Although more progress has been made recently in delineating the psychosocial factors affecting adherence in pediatric transplantation, the risk factors are still not well understood. Most of the psychosocial variables (e.g., depression, social support) have been explored in very few studies, using different methodologies and measurement tools; all this makes it difficult to draw consistent and generalizable conclusions. Developmental transitions (adolescence, transition to adult centers) when the risks for adherence problems are heightened deserve additional attention. Furthermore, we must begin to move beyond retrospective or cross-sectional designs and toward multisite longitudinal protocols. In this way, researchers can pool intellectual and practical resources to increase sample sizes, examine adherence patterns across the different organ groups, and allow for more optimal geographical representation.

Long-Term Psychosocial Adaptation

As pediatric transplant survival rates improve, researchers have increasingly focused on describing the impact of transplantation on quality of life and psychological functioning. Most pediatric transplant recipients experience improved quality of life (Cole et al., 2004; Sundaram, Landgraf, Neighbors, Cohn, & Alonso, 2007), although there may be some problems with long-term adaptation (Bucuvalas et al., 2003; Fredericks et al., 2007). Similarly, psychological outcomes are positive for most recipients, although about 25% of patients experience clinically significant emotional and behavioral adjustment issues (DeMaso, Douglas Kelley, Bastardi, O'Brien, & Blume, 2004; Todaro, Fennell, Sears, Rodrigue, & Roche, 2000; Wray & Radley-Smith, 2007; Wu, Aylward, Steele, Maikrantz, & Dreyer, 2008). It is important, however, to consider the many differences across studies in measurement strategies, sample sociodemographic characteristics, time since transplant, and medical factors. Moreover, most quality-of-life research in pediatric transplantation has focused on survivors of liver and kidney transplants, with comparatively fewer studies focused on the long-term outcomes after heart or lung transplantation.

The neurocognitive functioning of children who undergo transplantation has received relatively sparse empirical attention, despite the fact that most diseases leading to the need for transplantation have known cognitive ramifications. In addition to disease type and severity, the long-term neurocognitive status of children may be affected by medication side effects, age at the time of organ failure, multiple surgeries and lengthy hospitalizations, and missed educational opportunities due to illness (Brosig, Hintermeyer, Zlotocha, Behrens, & Mao, 2006; Brouhard et al., 2000; Kennard et al., 1999). For some, transplantation may precipitate recovery of neurocognitive functions, including sustained attention, mental processing/decision speed, visuospatial abilities, and memory (Mendley & Zelko, 1999; Qvist et al., 2002), although there may be some age-based limits to recovery (Freier et al., 2004; Wray & Radley-Smith, 2005). More longitudinal research is needed to better understand the long-term developmental and neurocognitive late effects of end-stage disease and changes in functioning after organ transplant. Such research may now be facilitated by the recent requirement by the United Network for Organ Sharing (*www.unos.org*) that pediatric transplant centers document the cognitive and motor development for each transplant recipient at 6 months and then annually for up to 5 years after transplant, with continued follow-up assessments until age 25, if possible. Although the policy allows programs to estimate the recipient's deficits (e.g., "probable," "questionable"), we recommend that transplant programs use standardized measures to document functioning and to assist in specifying deficits for intervention.

An additional area of psychosocial functioning that requires further study is the impact of pediatric transplantation on family systems. Preliminary studies show heightened stress and depressive symptoms for some parents, and possible changes in family dynamics (Rodrigue et al., 1997; Simons, Ingerski, & Janicke, 2007; Tarbell & Kosmach, 1998; Zelikovsky, Schast, & Jean-Francois, 2007). Because mothers and fathers (or other caretakers) experience the stress of caring for an ill child differently and rely on different coping strategies, all primary caretakers need to be included in psychosocial evaluations (Simons et al., 2007; Zelikovsky et al., 2007). Although there is no empirically defined schedule for optimal clinical care, we recommend a psychological screening of each child and family at 6-month intervals during the pretransplant waiting period and in the first 2 years after transplant surgery, as well as annual evaluations in all subsequent years. Focusing on quality of life, developmental progress, cognitive functioning, academic achievement, behavioral and psychological adaptation, adherence behaviors, and family functioning during these evaluations would provide much-needed information about the effects of transplantation (and its associated medical demands), as well as opportunities for immediate intervention to prevent poor health outcomes. In addition, close collaboration with schoolteachers, school nurses, and administrators is imperative to ensure successful integration of the child into the academic and social milieu.

Transition to Adult Care

Because transplant recipients receive ongoing care for life, and long-term survival is now a reality for many, the pediatric-to-adult care transition has assumed greater importance in recent years. Transition to adult health care systems consists of two components: first, a transfer of health care responsibilities from the caregivers to the patients, and then the actual transfer from a children's hospital to an adult health care setting (Annunziato et al., 2007). We have found that it is critical for the transition to occur gradually over time; for the process to occur as a collaborative effort among the patient, family, and health care team; and for the transition to occur at a developmentally appropriate time. Emerging research emphasizes the need to develop a coordinated transitional plan, as medical outcomes can be compromised if the transition is not handled effectively (Annunziato et al., 2007; Watson, 2000). Moreover, changes in insurance coverage (and its associated implications) further highlight the importance of this transition and its timing. For instance, Medicare coverage currently ends 3–4 years after transplant or whenever a minor child reaches adulthood, which may affect out-of-pocket expenses, adherence behaviors, and health outcomes (Willoughby et al., 2007).

Some centers have developed protocols to assess adolescents' emotional and developmental readiness for transition from pediatric-to-adult care, and to assist them and their parents with this often intimidating and emotionally difficult process. Although the actual transfer of care usually occurs when a person is between 18 and 21 years of age, we conceptualize the transition process as beginning in early adolescence. For instance, we recommend a gradual transition of medical responsibility from parents to adolescents: The adolescent begins to see the health care provider without the parents, with the corresponding expectation that the adolescent will increase his or her level of knowledge about illness, transplantation, and long-term recovery. The psychosocial evaluation at this time might focus on regimen knowledge and adherence; ability to summarize one's own medical history; independent decision-making skills and responsibility in illness management; academic and career goals; risk-taking behaviors that can have an impact on transplant outcomes; psychological adjustment and coping; and availability of peer mentoring and family support.

An emerging area of clinical investigation is the impact of pediatric-to-adult care transitions on transplant outcomes—graft and patient survival, quality of life, adherence, and psychological functioning. As programs are developed to assist in the transition process, pediatric psychologists are best positioned to evaluate the effectiveness of these intervention strategies in preparing adolescents emotionally and practically for increased medical responsibility. To date, we are aware of only one study that has examined the impact of the transition process on adolescent transplant recipients (Annunziato et al., 2008). Findings from this study (which showed poorer adherence rates to immunosuppression medications after the transition) underscore the vulnerability of this period for adolescents and young adults, as well as the need to develop a coordinated approach to facilitating the transition effectively.

Research Agenda

The pace of psychological research on pediatric transplantation lags far behind that focused on adult transplantation (Engle, 2001). Until recently, research in this area has been limited largely to single-site retrospective studies with small sample sizes. Intervention research is virtually nonexistent. What is needed now is a clear research agenda for pediatric psychologists with interests in transplantation.

In light of the critical organ shortage, one of the most significant ways in which psychologists can advance the field of pediatric transplantation is by identifying the most effective strategies for increasing deceased organ donation. The Division of Transplantation in the Health Resources and Services Administration has an excellent research grants program (*www.organdonor.gov*) designed to facilitate behavioral and psychological studies on organ donation. Psychologists have a unique opportunity to lend scientific expertise to help increase the likelihood that adolescents will consider registering to be organ donors. Moreover, psychologists have expertise in the cognitive decision-making processes underlying donation decisions, and they can help to develop effective models for approaching grieving parents upon the traumatic death of their child.

Health care professionals in pediatric transplantation now recognize the importance of measuring clinical outcomes that extend beyond survival. Relevant outcomes for children have been discussed throughout this chapter and include those at the individual (developmental, cognitive, affective, quality of life), family (family stress, caregiver burden, sibling adjustment), school (academic functioning, peer relations), and health care system (transition from pediatric to adult medicine) levels. With longer survival times, it is imperative that psychologists systematically assess these clinical outcomes beyond the first few years after transplantation and into early adulthood. Longitudinal studies from the pretransplant evaluation through 10 or 15 years after transplant surgery would permit the disentangling of effects due to disease from those due to transplant surgery and the posttransplant regimen. Such research also would provide valuable insight into the full range of benefits associated with pediatric transplantation. Multisite collaborations must be forged to obtain adequate and statistically meaningful sample sizes, since most transplant programs handle very few pediatric cases per year, and there is considerable heterogeneity in these samples.

Finally, there is also a need for pediatric psychology researchers to demonstrate how psychological interventions can affect the range of health outcomes both before and after transplantation. Interventions promoting physical and mental health (e.g., higher quality of life, psychological adaptation, effective school reintegration), preventing negative health outcomes (e.g., organ rejection and death from nonadherence, posttraumatic stress, family conflict), and highlighting medical cost offsets (e.g., lower health care costs, staff time savings, less utilization of health care resources) are desperately needed. The human, financial, and societal costs associated with nonadherence following transplantation are substantial. Consequently, the development, implementation, and evaluation of services designed to promote posttransplant adherence among adolescents in particular would represent a major advance in this field.

Summary and Conclusions

In summary, pediatric transplantation offers children a chance at life extension and improved quality of life, and affords many exciting opportunities for psychologists. The field is riddled with clinical, ethical, and scientific issues that potentially affect the physical and mental well-being of children and families. As the number of children who are affected by transplantation increases, so too does the expectation that pediatric psychologists will continue to play a vital role as integral members of transplant teams. Moreover, pediatric psychologists may be called on to assess the psychological strengths and liabilities of pediatric transplant candidates and their families; to design, implement, and evaluate interventions to reduce behavioral health liabilities and to promote positive adaptation; and to conduct behavioral health research. Pediatric psychologists may also be asked to educate other health professionals and health policy experts about behavioral health issues and their relevance to pediatric transplantation. Several pediatric psychologists have already made substantial contributions to advancing our understanding of the psychological and behavioral health concomitants of organ transplantation, and we should continue to build on and expand their efforts. In this chapter, we have attempted to highlight some of the emerging issues that warrant our attention and consideration as clinicians, scientists, and educators. We have no doubt that the horizons of pediatric transplantation will continue to expand over the next several years. Pediatric psychologists must be ready to embrace these challenges and to participate actively in the interdisciplinary dialogue that characterizes this field.

Acknowledgments

Support for the preparation of this chapter was provided in part by grants from the National Institutes of Health (Nos. DK079665 and DK077322) and the Health Resources and Services Administration (No. HS08576) to James R. Rodrigue.

References

Annunziato, R. A., Emre, S., Shneider, B. L., Barton, C., Dugan, C. A., & Shemesh, E. (2007). Adherence and medical outcomes in pediatric liver transplant recipients who transition to adult services. *Pediatric Transplantation, 11,* 608–614.

Annunziato, R. A., Emre, S., Shneider, B. L., Dugan, C. A., Aytaman, Y., McKay, M. M., et al. (2008). Transitioning health care responsibility from caregivers to patient: A pilot study aiming to facilitate medication adherence during this process. *Pediatric Transplantation, 12,* 309–315.

Berquist, R. K., Berquist, W. E., Esquivel, C. O., Cox, K. L., Wayman, K. I., & Litt, I. F. (2008). Non-adherence to post-transplant care: Prevalence, risk factors and outcomes in adolescent liver transplant recipients. *Pediatric Transplantation, 12,* 194–200.

Brosig, C., Hintermeyer, M., Zlotocha, J., Behrens, D., & Mao, J. (2006). An exploratory study of the cognitive, academic, and behavioral functioning of pediatric cardiothoracic transplant recipients. *Progress in Transplantation, 16,* 38–45.

Brouhard, B. H., Donaldson, L. A., Lawry, K. W., McGowan, K. R. B., Drotar, D., Davis, I., et al. (2000). Cognitive functioning in children on dialysis and post-transplantation. *Pediatric Transplantation, 4,* 261–267.

Bucuvalas, J. C., Britto, M., Krug, S., Ryckman, F. C., Atherton, H., Alonso, M. P., et al. (2003). Health related quality of life in pediatric liver transplant recipients: A single-center study. *Liver Transplantation, 9,* 62–71.

Childress, J. F., & Liverman, C. T. (Eds.). (2006). *Organ donation: Opportunities for action.* Washington, DC: National Academies Press.

Cleemput, I., Kesteloot, K., & De Geest, S. (2002). A review of the literature on the economics of noncompliance: Room for methodological improvement. *Health Policy, 59,* 65–94.

Cole, C. R., Bucuvalas, J. C., Hornung, R. W., Krug, S., Ryckman, F. C., Atherton, H., et al. (2004). Impact of liver transplantation on HRQOL in children less than 5 years old. *Pediatric Transplantation, 8,* 222–227.

DeMaso, D. R., Douglas Kelley, S., Bastardi, H., O'Brien, P., & Blume, E. D. (2004). The longitudinal impact of psychological functioning, medical severity, and family functioning in pediatric heart transplantation. *Journal of Heart and Lung Transplantation, 23,* 473–480.

Dobbels, F., Van Damme-Lombaert, R., Vanhaecke, J., & De Geest, S. (2005). Growing pains: Non-adherence with the immunosuppressive regimen in adolescent transplant recipients. *Pediatric Transplantation, 9,* 381–390.

Engle, D. (2001). Psychosocial aspects of the organ transplant experience: What has been established and what we need for the future. *Journal of Clinical Psychology, 57,* 521–549.

Fennell, R. S., Tucker, C., & Pedersen, T. (2001). Demographic and medical predictors of medication compliance among ethnically different pediatric renal transplant patients. *Pediatric Transplantation, 5,* 343–348.

Fredericks, E. M., Lopez, M. J., Magee, J. C., Shieck, V., & Opipari-Arrigan, L. (2007). Psychological functioning, nonadherence and health outcomes after pediatric liver transplantation. *American Journal of Transplantation, 7,* 1974–1983.

Fredericks, E. M., Magee, J. C., Opipari-Arrigan, L., Shieck, V., Well, A., & Lopez, M. J. (2008). Adherence and health-related quality of life in adolescent liver transplant recipients. *Pediatric Transplantation, 12,* 289–299.

Freier, M. C., Babikian, T., Pivonka, J., Burley Aaen, T., Gardner, J. M., Baum, M., et al. (2004). A longitudinal perspective on neurodevelopmental outcome after infant cardiac transplantation. *Journal of Heart and Lung Transplantation, 23,* 857–864.

Fung, E., & Shaw, R. J. (2008). Pediatric Transplant Rating Instrument: A scale for the pretransplant psychiatric evaluation of pediatric organ transplant recipients. *Pediatric Transplantation, 12,* 57–66.

Gerson, A. C., Furth, S. L., Neu, A. M., & Fivush, B. A. (2004). Assessing associations between medication adherence and potentially modifiable psychosocial variables in pediatric kidney transplant recipients and their families. *Pediatric Transplantation, 8,* 543–550.

Ghobrial, R. M., Freise, C. E., Trotter, J. F., Tong, L., Ojo, A. O., Fair, J. H., et al. (2008). Donor morbidity after living donation for liver transplantation. *Gastroenterology, 135,* 468–476.

Hartmann, A., Fauchald, P., Westlie, L., Brekke, I. B., & Holdaas, H. (2003). The risk of living kidney donation. *Nephrology Dialysis and Transplantation, 18,* 871–873.

Kennard, B. D., Stewart, S. M., Phelan-McAuliffe, D., Waller, D. A., Bannister, M., Fioravani,

V., et al. (1999). Academic outcome in long-term survivors of pediatric liver transplantation. *Journal of Developmental and Behavioral Pediatrics, 20,* 17–23.

Live Organ Donor Consensus Group. (2000). Consensus statement on the live organ donor. *Journal of the American Medical Association, 284,* 2919–2926.

Magee, J. C., Krishnan, S. M., Benfield, M. R., Hsu, D. T., & Shneider, B. L. (2008). Pediatric transplantation in the United States, 1997–2006. *American Journal of Transplantation, 8,* 935–945.

Maikranz, J. M., Steele, R. G., Dreyer, M. L., Startman, A. C., & Bovaird, J. A. (2007). The relationship of hope and illness-related uncertainty to emotional adjustment and adherence among pediatric renal and liver recipients. *Journal of Pediatric Psychology, 32,* 571–581.

Maloney, R., Clay, D. L., & Robinson, J. (2004). Sociocultural issues in pediatric transplantation: A conceptual model. *Journal of Pediatric Psychology, 30,* 235–246.

Mendley, S. R., & Zelko, F. A. (1999). Improvement in specific aspects of neurocognitive performance in children after renal transplantation. *Kidney International, 56,* 318–323.

Olbrisch, M. E., Benedict, S. M., Haller, D. L., & Levenson, J. L. (2001). Psychosocial assessment of living organ donors: Clinical and ethical considerations. *Progress in Transplantation, 11,* 40–49.

Penkower, L., Dew, M. A., Ellis, D., Sereika, S. M., Kitutu, J. M., & Shapiro, R. (2003). Psychological distress and adherence to the medical regimen among adolescent renal transplant recipients. *American Journal of Transplantation, 3,* 1418–1425.

Qvist, E., Pihko, H., Fagerudd, P., Valanne, L., Lamminranta, S., Karikoski, J., et al. (2002). Neurodevelopmental outcomes in high-risk patients after renal transplantation in early childhood. *Pediatric Transplantation, 6,* 53–62.

Rodrigue, J. R., Cornell, D. L., & Howard, R. J. (2006). The organ donation experience: A comparison of donor and non-donor families. *American Journal of Transplantation, 6,* 190–198.

Rodrigue, J. R., Cornell, D. L., & Howard, R. J. (2008). Pediatric organ donation: What factors most influence parents' donation decisions? *Pediatric Critical Care Medicine, 9,* 180–185.

Rodrigue, J. R., Gonzalez-Peralta, R., & Langham, M. (2004). Solid organ transplantation. In R. T. Brown (Ed.), *Handbook of pediatric psychology in school settings* (pp. 679–699). Mahwah, NJ: Erlbaum.

Rodrigue, J. R., MacNaughton, K., Hoffmann, R. G., Graham-Pole, J., Andres, J. M., Novak, D. A., et al. (1997). Transplantation in children: A longitudinal assessment of mothers' stress, coping, and perceptions of family functioning. *Psychosomatics, 38,* 478–486.

Shemesh, E., Annunziato, R. A., Yehuda, R., Shneider, B. L., Newcorn, J. H., Hutson, C., et al. (2007). Childhood abuse, non-adherence, and medical outcome in pediatric liver transplant recipients. *Journal of American Academy of Child and Adolescent Psychiatry, 46,* 1280–1289.

Siminoff, L. A., Gordon, N., Hewlett, J., & Arnold, R. M. (2001). Factors influencing families' consent for donation of solid organs for transplantation. *Journal of the American Medical Association, 286,* 71–77.

Simons, L., & Blount, R. L. (2007). Identifying barriers to medication adherence in adolescent transplant recipients. *Journal of Pediatric Psychology, 32,* 831–844.

Simons, L., Ingerski, L. M., & Janicke, D. M. (2007). Social support, coping, and psychological distress in mothers and fathers of pediatric transplant candidates: A pilot study. *Pediatric Transplantation, 11,* 781–787.

Streisand, R. M., & Tercyak, K. P. (2001). Evaluating the pediatric transplant patient: General considerations. In J. R. Rodrigue (Ed.), *Biopsychosocial perspectives on transplantation* (pp. 71–92). New York: Kluwer Academic/Plenum Press.

Sundaram, S. S., Landgraf, J. M., Neighbors, K., Cohn, R. A., & Alonso, E. M. (2007). Adolescent health-related quality of life following liver and kidney transplantation. *American Journal of Transplantation, 7*, 982–989.

Sweet, S. C., Wong, H. H., Webber, S. A., Horslen, S., Guidinger, M. K., Fine, R. N., et al. (2006). The 2005 SRTR report on the state of transplantation: Pediatric transplantation in the United States, 1995–2004. *American Journal of Transplantation, 6*, 1132–1152.

Switzer, G. E., Dew, M. A., & Twillman, R. K. (2000). Psychosocial issues in living organ donation. In P. T. Trzepacz & A. F. DiMartini (Eds.), *The transplant patient: Biological, psychiatric, and ethical issues in organ transplantation* (pp. 42–66). New York: Cambridge University Press.

Tarbell, S. E., & Kosmach, B. (1998). Parental psychosocial outcomes in pediatric liver and/or intestinal transplantation: Pretransplantation and the early postoperative period. *Liver Transplantation and Surgery, 4*, 378–387.

Todaro, J. F., Fennell, E. B., Sears, S. F., Rodrigue, J. R., & Roche, A. K. (2000). A review of cognitive and psychological outcomes in pediatric heart transplant recipients. *Journal of Pediatric Psychology, 25*, 567–576.

Tucker, C. M., Pedersen, S., Herman, K. C., Fennell, R. S., Bowling, B., Pedersen, T., et al. (2001). Self-regulation predictors of medication adherence among ethnically different patients with renal transplants. *Journal of Pediatric Psychology, 26*, 455–464.

Watson, A. R. (2000). Non-compliance and transfer from pediatric to adult transplant unit. *Pediatric Nephrology, 14*, 469–472.

Willoughby, L. M., Fukami, S., Bunnapradist, S., Gavard, J. A., Lentine, K. L., Hardinger, K. L., et al. (2007). Health insurance considerations for adolescent transplant recipients as they transition to adulthood. *Pediatric Transplantation, 11*, 127–131.

Wray, J., & Radley-Smith, R. (2005). Beyond the first year after pediatric heart or heart–lung transplantation: Changes in cognitive function and behaviour. *Pediatric Transplantation, 9*, 170–177.

Wray, J., & Radley-Smith, R. (2007). Prospective psychological evaluation of pediatric heart and heart–lung recipients. *Journal of Pediatric Psychology, 32*, 217–222.

Wray, J., Waters, S., Radley-Smith, R., & Sensky, T. (2006). Adherence in adolescents and young adults following heart or heart–lung transplantation. *Pediatric Transplantation, 10*, 694–700.

Wu, Y. P., Aylward, B. S., Steele, R. G., Maikrantz, J. M., & Dreyer, M. L. (2008). Psychosocial functioning of pediatric renal and liver transplant recipients. *Pediatric Transplantation, 2*, 582–587.

Zelikovsky, N., Schast, A. P., & Jean-Francois, D. (2007). Parent stress and coping: Waiting for a child to receive a kidney transplant. *Clinical Psychology in Medical Settings, 14*, 320–329.

Zelikovsky, N., Schast, A. P., Palmer, J., & Meyers, K. E. C. (2008). Perceived barriers to adherence in pediatric kidney transplant candidates. *Pediatric Transplantation, 12*, 300–308.

CHAPTER 27

Abdominal Pain–Related Gastrointestinal Disorders

Irritable Bowel Syndrome and Inflammatory Bowel Disease

GERARD A. BANEZ
CARIN L. CUNNINGHAM

Irritable Bowel Syndrome

Irritable bowel syndrome (IBS) is a functional gastrointestinal disorder (FGID) characterized by chronic or recurrent abdominal pain/discomfort, together with altered bowel function (urgency, altered stool consistency, altered stool frequency, incomplete evacuation, and bloating/distention). These symptoms stem from problems in bowel functioning and are not explained by identifiable structural or biochemical abnormalities. The most commonly used symptom-based criteria for IBS are the Rome III criteria (Rasquin et al., 2006). These criteria require that the primary IBS symptoms be present at least once/week for at least 2 months. The abdominal pain or discomfort is associated with two or more of the following at least 25% of the time: It is (1) improved with defecation, (2) associated with a change in frequency of stool, and/or (3) associated with a change in form (appearance) of stool. No inflammatory, anatomic, metabolic, or neoplastic process explains the three symptoms.

Within the Rome III classification, IBS is categorized as one subtype of abdominal pain–related FGID. Others include functional dyspepsia, abdominal migraine, childhood functional abdominal pain, and childhood functional abdominal pain syndrome. The extent to which the etiologies of these disorders differ is not clear. Symptoms of altered bowel function (i.e., diarrhea, constipation) distinguish IBS from the other abdominal pain–related FGIDs. When appropriate, the Rome III criteria classify IBS as either "diarrhea-predominant" or "constipation-predominant" on the basis of the predominant bowel habit. For some individuals, diarrhea and constipation alternate. IBS has been conceptualized by some investigators as a later-stage manifestation of the recurrent nonorganic abdominal pain seen in childhood. Walker, Guite, Duke, Barnard, and Greene (1998) reported that 5 years after their initial evaluation, female patients with recurrent abdominal pain were more likely than controls to meet criteria for IBS. Howell, Poulton, and Talley (2005) found that IBS at age 26 years was significantly more common among individuals with a history of childhood abdominal pain between ages 7 and 9 years than among those with no such history.

Causes/Conceptualization

The cause of IBS has not been definitively established. Multiple factors are thought to contribute; these include physiological factors, such as abnormal motility (increased or irregular movement of the gut) and enhanced visceral sensitivity, as well as psychosocial factors, such as stress and emotions. The etiology and course of IBS are increasingly conceptualized from a biopsychosocial perspective (Drossman, 1998): The patient's IBS symptoms and daily functioning are presumed to involve multiple factors (e.g., genetic predisposition, environmental factors, motility, sensation, life stress, psychological status, coping, social support) and their interactions along the central nervous system–enteric nervous system or "brain–gut" axis.

In IBS, the nerve endings in the bowel lining are thought to be hypersensitive. Symptoms of abdominal pain and discomfort appear to be the results of increased sensitivity to distension of the gastrointestinal tract by gas or fecal material, and a tendency for the bowel to be overly reactive to eating, stress, emotional arousal, or gaseous distension. For example, Faure and Wieckowska (2007) demonstrated that children with IBS sensed rectal pain at a lower pressure threshold, compared with controls and children with functional dyspepsia. Alterations in bowel habits are probably related to alterations in autonomic regulation of gut motility (e.g., more pronounced bowel contractions cause the feces to move through the colon quickly, not allowing sufficient time for water reabsorption and resulting in loose, watery stools).

The role of stress and other psychosocial factors (e.g., anxiety, depression, social learning) is multifaceted. Although psychosocial stressors do not cause IBS, they can clearly exacerbate a patient's gastrointestinal symptoms (Bennett, Tennant, Piesse, Badcock, & Kellow, 1998). Major and daily stressors, including events related to family illness, also affect the patient's symptom experience, efforts to cope, and eventual clinical outcome (Levy et al., 2004; Walker, Garber, Smith, Van Slyke, & Lewis Claar, 2001). Although children with recurrent abdominal pain and IBS have been found to score higher on measures of anxiety-related and depressive symptoms (Campo et al., 2004; Hodges, Kline, Barbero, & Woodruff, 1985), these symptoms may be the results rather than the causes of pain in at least some patients. The ways in which family members respond to their children's IBS may also have an important role in the development and course of symptoms. Specifically, positive consequences (e.g., excusing a child from having to do the dishes or allowing the child to stay home from school) may serve to reinforce and maintain pain behaviors and associated functional disability (Walker, 1999).

The abdominal pain, altered bowel habits, and psychological factors associated with IBS can contribute significantly to a negative quality of life (Hahn, Yan, & Strassels, 1999). Patients with IBS have rated their quality of life as lower than the norm and comparable to that of patients with inflammatory bowel disease (IBD) (Pace et al., 2003). IBS is the second most common cause (after the common cold) of work and school absenteeism. According to a recent survey (International Foundation for Functional Gastrointestinal Disorders, 2002), IBS symptoms caused missed leisure activities even more than absenteeism at work or school. Missed leisure activities were reported as occurring among over two-thirds of the respondents (68%), with 5% reporting missing such occasions more than 50 times in a 3-month period. For children and adolescents with IBS, missed school, peer activities, and sports/extracurricular activities are not uncommon when symptoms are severe. In a multisite study, Varni and his colleagues (2006) found that pediatric patients with IBS demonstrated significantly lower physical, emotional, social, and school functioning than healthy children did. Their impairment in health-related quality of life (HRQOL) was comparable to that of patients with organic gastrointestinal disorders.

Prevalence

IBS is common in children and adolescents. In a population-based study of 507 suburban middle and high school students (Hyams, Burke, Davis, Rzepski, & Andrulonis, 1996), 6% of the middle school students and 14% of the high school students reported symptoms consistent with a diagnosis of IBS. The likelihood of seeing a physician was four times greater in those students whose pain affected their activities. In a medical practice–based study (Hyams et al., 1995), IBS symptoms were present in the majority of 227 children and adolescents presenting to a pediatric gastroenterology clinic with recurrent abdominal pain. Of the 171 patients whose symptoms were deemed functional, 117 manifested the IBS symptoms of lower abdominal pain, cramping, and increased flatus.

IBS is generally regarded as a chronic relapsing condition (Collins, 2001). In most patients, the presence and severity of IBS symptoms fluctuate over time. Though some reports suggest that 80% of patients are symptom-free at 5 years, other studies contradict this finding (Svendsen, Munck, & Anderson, 1985). One possible explanation is that IBS symptoms do not disappear altogether, but that patients may tend to respond to different sites and types of abdominal pain at different times (American Digestive Health Foundation, 2001). The dominance of abdominal pain, coexisting psychological difficulties, and/or multiple abdominal surgeries (e.g., cholecystectomy, appendectomy, hysterectomy) are factors associated with poor prognosis (Collins, 2001).

Clinical Evaluation

A history of abdominal pain and disordered defecation that meets the Rome III diagnostic criteria, along with a normal medical history and physical exam, support the diagnosis of IBS (Rasquin et al., 2006). A nutritional history can be useful to assess for the intake of caffeine, fructose, sorbitol, and other substances that might contribute to pain, bloating, or diarrhea. Some patients require diagnostic testing (e.g., sigmoidoscopy, colonoscopy, barium enema) to exclude other medical conditions, but such evaluation is not necessary for the majority of patients. In fact, superfluous testing may create additional anxiety and lead to unnecessary costs and risks. Limited laboratory screening may include complete blood count, erythrocyte sedimentation rate, stool studies, and breath hydrogen testing. If a patient has IBS, the results of these tests will be essentially negative. The presence of "red flag" warning signs (e.g., presence of blood in the stool, involuntary weight loss, deceleration of linear growth, significant vomiting, chronic severe diarrhea) warrants more medical evaluation. In the absence of this evidence, the degree of functional impairment, parental concerns, and the physician's fear of a missed diagnosis influence the extent of evaluation (Hyams, 1999). The differential diagnosis of IBS requires consideration of the following categories of disease conditions: (1) dietary factors; (2) infection, bacterial or parasitic; (3) some form of IBD (see discussion below); (4) mental health difficulties; (5) malabsorptive disorders; and (6) miscellaneous disease conditions, including endometriosis, Zollinger–Ellison syndrome, and other endocrine tumors, and HIV-related diseases. It is important to note that IBS may coexist with some of these conditions, such as an IBD. When this occurs, treatment of the coexisting conditions will be critical.

Our psychosocial assessment includes a pain and IBS symptom history, review of diagnostic criteria, and evaluation of social-emotional contributors. Particular attention is given to psychological and social factors that precipitate or maintain IBS symptoms and poor levels of functioning. We utilize a number of checklists and questionnaires to gather relevant clinical data, including but not limited to measures of stress (Compas, Davis, Forsythe, & Wagner, 1987), coping (Walker, Smith, Garber, & Van Slyke, 1997), emotional and behavioral problems (Achenbach, 1991), functional disability (Walker & Greene, 1991), and parental responses to pain/gastrointestinal symptoms (Van Slyke & Walker, 2006). A daily log of the frequency and severity of a child's primary IBS symptoms (e.g., abdominal pain, diarrhea, distention) provides a method of ongoing behavioral assessment. Entries for each IBS episode are helpful for establishing the frequency and pattern of symptoms.

Treatment

To date, no cure for IBS has been found. Current treatment approaches are aimed at providing effective reassurance and symptom relief, modifying symptom perceptions, and developing effective management strategies. A confident diagnosis, confirmation, and explanation of the pain experience, and even reassurance by itself, can be therapeutic (Hyams, 2000). Drossman and Thompson (1992) have recommended a graduated, multicomponent treatment approach to IBS. In their approach, the amount and types of treatment are based on the severity of the IBS. For patients with mild IBS symptoms and no significant functional disability, education about IBS, reassurance of its nonserious nature, and dietary changes are indicated. Behavioral treatments (e.g., relaxation therapy, hypnosis, and biofeedback) and certain medications for symptom relief may be considered for patients with moderate to severe IBS and disruptions in daily activities.

To our knowledge, there have been few randomized controlled trials examining IBS treatments for children and adolescents. Despite the absence of empirical support, intervention strategies used with adults are often used with pediatric populations. Huertas-Ceballos, Logan, Bennett, and Macarthur (2008a, 2008b, 2009) recently completed an informative series of Cochrane reviews of psychosocial, pharmacological, and dietary interventions for recurrent abdominal pain and IBS in childhood. Their review of psychosocial interventions (Huertas-Ceballos et al., 2008c) identified five randomized trials that examined interventions broadly based on cognitive-behavioral therapy (CBT) (e.g., contingency management training for parents, instruction to the child on progressive muscle relaxation, diaphragmatic breathing, cognitive coping). The five studies reported statistically significant improvements in pain, leading the authors to recommend consideration of CBT for some children with recurrent abdominal pain, including

IBS. These findings are consistent with reviews written by Janicke and Finney (1999) and Weydert, Ball, and Davis (2003), who also documented empirical support for CBT in the treatment of childhood recurrent abdominal pain. Also relevant to IBS in some children is the growing evidence base for psychological or behavioral treatments for toileting difficulties (e.g., Cox, Sutphen, Borowitz, Kovatchev, & Ling, 1998; Stark et al., 1997). For patients whose IBS includes constipation, documentation of stool passage, scheduled sits, rewards for compliance with medication and sitting times, and anorectal biofeedback may be beneficial.

Reviews of pharmacological and dietary interventions for childhood recurrent abdominal pain and IBS have not provided much support for these approaches. Huertas-Ceballos and colleagues (2008a) identified three pharmacological trials that met their inclusion criteria and found only weak evidence of benefit. The medications evaluated in these trials included pizotifen, peppermint oil, and famotidine. The authors concluded that there is little reason for their use outside clinical trials. A review of dietary interventions (Huertas-Ceballos et al., 2009) included seven trials and provided no evidence that fiber supplementation, lactose-free diets, or lactose bacillus supplementation are effective in the management of children with recurrent abdominal pain.

Suggested CBT Approach

In our practice, we typically collaborate with pediatric gastroenterologists and dietitians on an interdisciplinary treatment approach for IBS. In terms of psychological treatment, we utilize a CBT approach that targets misinformation about IBS, chronic overarousal, and inability to manage stress and anxiety effectively (Neff & Blanchard, 1987). Treatment typically includes some, if not all, of the following: (1) information and education about IBS, (2) pain behavior management training for parents, (3) relaxation training, (4) skin temperature biofeedback, and (5) stress management training. Although many patients benefit from attention to each of these areas, some patients do best with a more focused approach that emphasizes their particular areas of need over others. As warranted, specific training in toileting skills is offered. For example, a patient with constipation-predominant IBS may be instructed to sit on the toilet for 10 minutes after every meal and to practice external anal sphincter strengthening exercises to prevent overflow incontinence.

IBS, Pain-Associated Disability Syndrome, and Interdisciplinary Rehabilitation

Some child and adolescent patients with IBS experience significant functional impairment. They do not attend school, interact with peers, and/or participate in sports, extracurricular activities, and other personal/family events. Bursch (1999, p. 8.2) coined the term "pain-associated disability syndrome" (PADS) to describe the severe manifestation of this presentation. She defined PADS as "a downward spiral of increasing pain-associated disability, lasting at least 3 months, for which symptom-focused strategies have not led to an acceptable resolution." For severely affected patients with IBS and PADS, an interdisciplinary rehabilitation approach provides an understandable and useful model of care. A rehabilitation approach blends pediatric subspecialty care, behavioral health, and rehabilitation therapies, such as physical and occupational therapies. Pain is accepted as a symptom that may or may not be eradicated. The focus of the approach is on independent functioning (rather than pain), improved coping, and increased self-efficacy. Preliminary outcomes for a combined inpatient–day hospital interdisciplinary rehabilitation program for children and adolescents with various chronic pain disorders, including IBS, and associated disability suggest promise for this approach (Banez et al., 2008). At the conclusion of treatment, patients reported a 36% improvement in pain severity and a 50% improvement in physical functioning. One month after the program, they reported a 46% improvement in social functioning and a 50% improvement in pain-specific anxiety.

Inflammatory Bowel Disease

IBD, a chronic, relapsing condition of digestive tract inflammation in which periods of active disease alternate with periods of disease control, includes three separate diagnostic categories: Crohn disease (CD), ulcerative colitis (UC), and indeterminate colitis (IC). In CD, inflammation occurs at any point in the digestive tract from the mouth to the skin surrounding the anus, and there is mucosal inflammation. In UC, the inflammation is restricted to the large colon and is confined to the inner lining of the large intestine mucosal wall. A diagnosis of IC is given until the disease has progressed and a differentiation can be made (Rice & Chuang, 1999). In 2005, an algorithm standardizing the diagnosis/classification of pediatric IBD was created to aid in differentiating childhood CD from UC, thereby reducing variability among practitioners (European Society of Pediatric Gastroenterology, Hepatology, and Nutrition, IBD Working Group, 2005).

Symptoms of IBD vary in frequency and severity. Symptoms of CD and UC include diarrhea, rectal bleeding, rectal urgency, abdominal cramps, weight loss, fatigue, and fever. Children diagnosed with UC report worse symptoms and complications than adults with UC do (Griffiths et al., 1999). In youths, the range of symptoms and presenting signs of IBD are broad and often subtle, and diagnosis can be difficult. The mean delay for the diagnosis of CD in children is between 7 and 11 months, in UC between 5 and 8 months, and in IC 14 months (Mamula, Markowitz, & Baldassano, 2003).

The management of pediatric IBD can include pharmacological, nutritional, and surgical interventions. Treatment goals include controlling the inflammatory process, maintaining adequate nutrition to promote growth, and facilitating participation in age-appropriate activities (Baldassano & Piccoli, 1999). Surgery is necessary when medication cannot control the symptoms or when there is an intestinal obstruction or other complications. More than a third of pediatric patients with IBD will require surgery within 20 years of diagnosis (Langholz, Munkholm, Krasilinikoff, & Binder, 1998).

Prevalence

IBD is diagnosed during childhood or adolescence in 25–30% of patients (Cuffari & Darbari, 2002). Current epidemiological studies of IBD report that approximately 1.1 million people in the United States have IBD (Loftus et al., 2007), over 100,000 of whom are children and adolescents (Carvalho & Hyams, 2007). Kugathasan and colleagues (2003) found a twofold predominance in pediatric CD prevalence relative to UC, and a significantly higher rate of CD in boys than in girls. The number of patients diagnosed with IC has been increasing (Cuffari & Darbari, 2002), accounting for approximately 15% of the cases that present as colitis (King, 2003).

Prognosis

The disease course of IBD is unpredictable. For children with CD, 40–50% relapse in the first year after remission, and only 1% never relapse after diagnosis and initial therapy (Ballinger, 2000). 70% of children diagnosed with UC enter remission within 3 months following initial therapy, and approximately 50% remain in remission over the next year. Colectomy (i.e., removal of the colon) is curative for UC and is required within 5 years in up to 26% of children presenting with severe disease, compared with 10% of those with mild disease. There is a markedly increased risk of cancer for patients with long-standing colonic CD or long-standing UC (Hyams, 2000).

Causes/Conceptualization

The exact etiology of IBD is unknown. Current research proposes a multifactorial cause: The pathogenesis of IBD proceeds from a genetic predisposition (susceptible host) coupled with specific triggers (bacteria and viruses) that interact with the body's immune system and trigger the disease (Kim & Ferry, 2004). A person who has a relative with IBD has a 10–15% greater than average risk of developing IBD (Achkar, 2007). Two genes have been identified in the regulation of immunity and inflammation in IBD: NOD2 (Cuffari & Dubbari, 2002) and the IL23R gene (Duerr et al., 2006). Existing data do not support diet or psychological factors as causes of IBD (Bremner & Beattie, 2002).

Psychological Factors

Issues unique to pediatric IBD include delay in diagnosis; unpredictability of the course of illness; unknown etiology of illness; embarrassment about "bathroom-related" symptoms (e.g., rectal urgency, frequent need to use the bathroom), leading to school avoidance; and symptoms of growth retardation and delayed puberty, which may affect the development of autonomy. Difficulties associated with IBD medications include side effects of corticosteroids (e.g., cushingoid features, weight gain, mood swings, striae) and increased risk of cancer with use of infliximab (Banez & Cunningham, 2003).

Depressive and Anxiety Symptoms

Rates of depressive and anxiety disorders in children and adolescents with IBD vary, with estimated prevalence rates of 25–60% among those with long-standing illness (Burke et al., 1989b; Engstrom & Lindquist, 1991) and 14–28% among those who have been recently diagnosed (Burke, Neigut, Kochosis, Chandra, & Sauer, 1994). Rates of internalizing symptoms among youths with IBD have been found to be higher than among youths with cystic fibrosis (Burke et al., 1989b) or healthy comparison groups (Engstrom, 1999; Mackner, Crandall, & Szigethy, 2006), but are comparable to youth with chronic headaches or diabetes (Engstrom, 1991). Gold, Issenman, Roberts, and Watt (2000) reported lower rates of depressive symptoms in a sample of youths with

IBD than in a matched sample of youths with other FGIDs. This study's results, however, are equivocal due to small sample sizes, lack of reliability checks for diagnoses, and cross-sectional designs. Studies utilizing larger samples report a lower prevalence of psychiatric disorders (Mackner & Crandall, 2006). Szigethy, Levy-Warren, and Whitoon (2004) found that later age of diagnosis was associated with greater depressive symptoms; however, overall age was not significantly associated with depressive symptoms. Factors associated with depressive symptoms among youths with IBD include later age of diagnosis, greater parental depression, greater frequency of stressful life events, lower family cohesion, and higher family conflict (Burke et al., 1994; Szigethy et al., 2004).

Social and School Functioning

Social skills development may be adversely affected in youths with a diagnosis of IBD. Mackner and Crandall (2006) found that more parents of children with IBD reported clinically significant problems in social competence than parents of healthy children did (22% vs. 2%). Similarly, Moody, Eaden, and Mayberry (1999) found that patients with IBD had problems interacting with peers and a decrease in sports-related activities. The timing of diagnosis has been associated with decreased social functioning: More patients diagnosed with IBD during adolescence had significantly low social competence scores than those diagnosed in childhood (35% vs. 5%) (Mackner & Crandall, 2005a).

School-related concerns have also been documented among youths with IBD. Ferguson, Sedgwick, and Drummond (1994) found that young adults with juvenile-onset IBD reported increased school absences, interference with exams, and problems in pursuing higher education. Mayberry (1999) reported that 66% of patients ages 6–17 years had problems with school attendance, leading to academic underachievement; in another study, children with CD missed more school and participated in fewer peer-related activities (Akobeng, Mirajkar, et al., 1999).

Health-Related Quality of Life

Initial HRQOL studies, limited by small sample sizes and the use of nonvalidated instruments, documented that 31–50% of children with IBD have limitations in social functioning, concerns about weight gain, flareups in their condition, and school absenteeism (Akobeng, Mirajkar, et al., 1999; Griffiths et al., 1999; Rabbett et al., 1996). More recent HRQOL studies addressing these methodological issues have provided mixed results. Cunningham, Drotar, Palermo, McGowan, and Arendt (2007) found that children and adolescents reported worse HRQOL than physically healthy children in one domain: general health. Loonen, Grootenhuis, Last, Koopman, and Derkx (2002) found no significant differences in generic HRQOL between younger children with IBD and a healthy control group. Adolescents with IBD, however, reported a significantly lower HRQOL in four domains: motor functioning, bodily complaints, autonomy, and negative emotion (Loonen et al., 2002). Another study reported that boys with IBD had significantly lower HRQOL than healthy peers had (De Boer, Grootenhuis, Derkx, & Last, 2005). Otley and colleagues (2002) conducted a prospective study using the IMPACT questionnaire, a disease-specific measure of HRQOL, and found significant improvement in HRQOL during the first year following diagnosis. Patients with increasing disease severity reported worse HRQOL.

Youths with more frequent symptoms and greater steroidal side effects have been found to exhibit greater limitations in HRQOL (Cunningham et al., 2007). Higher self-esteem (DeBoer et al., 2005) and use of predictive coping strategies (van der Zaag-Loonen, Grootenhuis, Last, & Derkx, 2004) have been shown to be associated with higher HRQOL, whereas male gender and older age have been associated with lower HRQOL (DeBoer et al., 2005; Otley et al., 2002).

Adherence

Adherence to IBD treatment is challenging, since medications need to be taken continuously to maintain remission, the relapse rate is high, and the side effects of medications often affect physical appearance. For youths with IBD, nonadherence with the medical treatment regimen may increase the risk of colorectal cancer and need for health care utilization (Achkar, 2007). Hommel, Davis, and Baldassano (2008) reported high rates of adherence (93–97%) based on patient self-report. In contrast, Mackner and Crandall (2005b) utilized a structured interview to assess oral medication adherence among 50 preadolescents and adolescents with IBD, and found that only 38% of parents and 48% of children reported perfect adherence to IBD medications. Similarly, Oliva-Hemker, Abadom, Cuffari, and Thompson (2007) reported 34–50% adherence rates based on pharmacy refill records, with rates varying according to medication. Hommel and colleagues found lower adherence rates (52–63%) via pill counts, depending on the medication. Factors such as less optimal coping strategies and lower patient-perceived HRQOL have been associated with lower levels of adherence (Hommel et al., 2008; Mackner & Crandall, 2005b).

Family Functioning

Parents of adolescents with IBD have reported worries regarding their children's medication (including negative side effects), school absenteeism, and future plans (Akobeng, Miller, et al., 1999; Rabbett et al., 1996). Caregivers reported that they experienced more emotional worry, greater impact on their personal time, a decrease in social activities, and changes in financial resources, compared to caregivers of healthy same-age children (Cunningham et al., 2007; Engstrom, 1992). Greenley and Cunningham (2009) reported that greater youth disease activity and poorer youth HRQOL were predictive of lower parent quality of life.

Difficulties with family and parent functioning have been shown to be associated with more severe disease, more bowel movements, increased pain, youth fatigue, and a greater number of behavioral and emotional symptoms (Burke, Kocoshis, Chandra, Whiteway, & Sauer, 1990; Greenley & Cunningham, 2009; Tojek, Lumley, Corlis, Ondersma, & Tolia, 2002). Siblings of patients with IBD have reported concerns about their parents keeping them uninformed about the illness, their ill sibling being teased at school, and their sibling needing to be hospitalized (Akobeng, Miller, et al., 1999).

Clinical Evaluation

Assessment measures specific to IBD in youths are lacking, with the exception of one measure for HRQOL, the IMPACT questionnaire mentioned above (Otley et al., 2002).

Anecdotally, we have found that clinical assessment of the following issues may facilitate youths' adjustment to IBD (Banez & Cunningham, 2003).

Knowledge of IBD

Assessment of a youth's and parent's knowledge of IBD beginning at the time of diagnosis is an "ongoing process," identifying areas where education is warranted. Helpful assessment questions include these: What is the youth's/parent's understanding of IBD and its causes? Do the family members understand the treatment regimen and medication side effects? What are their biggest fears about IBD?

Psychological Functioning

Since no IBD disease-specific measures exist, we recommend evidence-based measures that have already been used in pediatric IBD research (Holmbeck, Li, Schurman, Friedman, & Coakley, 2002), such as the Children's Depression Inventory (Kovacs, 1985) and the Children's Global Assessment Scale (Shaffer et al., 1983). Patient and family interviews also yield important information.

Social and School Functioning

Assessment of social and school functioning should include such questions as these: Are the child's friends aware of his or her IBD? Does having IBD interfere with socializing with peers? Are there activity limitations due to IBD? Has a Section 504 plan been established to help with special needs (e.g., bathroom privileges, need to take medicine during the day or to rest between classes) and to address the academic sequelae of missed school days?

Youth HRQOL

Assessment of HRQOL includes attention to general domains as well as disease-specific HRQOL. The Child Health Questionnaire (Landgraf, Abetz, & Ware, 1996) and the TNO-AZL Preschool Children Quality of Life questionnaire (Verrips, Vogels, den Ouden, Paneth, & Verloove-Vanhorick, 2000) are well-established assessment methods previously used in samples with IBD. Disease-specific measures are useful in identifying which IBD symptoms or treatments influence youths' well-being. The IMPACT is a disease-specific HRQOL instrument that is valid and reliable (Otley et al. 2002), with four factor-analytically supported domains: general well-being and symptoms, emotional functioning, social interactions, and body image (Perrin et al., 2008).

Family Functioning

Identification of the family's support system, the presence of financial pressures, insurance concerns, and other family members with a diagnosis of IBD is helpful. Evidence-based assessment of parental functioning (Alderfer et al., 2008), with attention to levels of psychological distress, parent quality of life, and parent coping skills, is important. Attention to sibling adjustment is also warranted. We have found that the following information is useful: Do siblings understand what IBD is? Are they afraid that they will "get" IBD? Are they functioning well in their daily activities? Are they jealous of the extra attention that their ill sibling receives?

Adherence

Assessment of adherence should include (1) multiple methods, (2) electronic data when available, (3) assessment of barriers to adherence, and (4) assessment of patient and family knowledge (Quittner, Modi, Lemanek, Ievers-Landis, & Rapoff, 2008). One parent–adolescent report interview of adherence to IBD medication has reported moderate correlations between parents' and youths' reports of adherence (Mackner & Crandall, 2005b).

Treatment

Pediatric psychologists adhering to an evidence-based practice model can play an important role in maximizing the adjustment of youths with IBD. The treatment literature on psychosocial interventions for youths with IBD is anecdotal, with the exception of an evidence-based treatment for depression (which used a manual-based CBT approach) in adolescents with IBD. Results indicated that the use of this treatment, the Primary and Secondary Control Enhancement Training Program, may be an efficacious intervention for subdromal depression in adolescents with IBD (Szigethy, Kenney, Carpenter, & Hardy, 2007). There are no evidence-based treatments specific for anxiety, social functioning, or school functioning in IBD; nor are there evidence-based treatments to improve parent, family, or sibling functioning in pediatric IBD. Anecdotal reports suggest that psychosocial treatment is helpful at strategic points: at diagnosis, at recurrence, and in regard to treatment-related issues (Cunningham & Banez, 2006).

Data do not support the benefits of psychotherapy, behavioral techniques, complementary therapies, or psychotropic medications for the long-term medical course of IBD in youths. No published studies exist on enhancing adherence in pediatric IBD. Anecdotally, the following strategies have been successful: written treatment plans, visual reminders, visibly storing pills, cell phone reminders, and formulating medication plans in advance. We also offer these general suggestions for clinical care of youths with IBD:

1. Be familiar with the medical aspects of IBD, including presenting symptoms, diagnostic procedures, treatment modalities, and medication side effects.

2. Introduce psychosocial services at diagnosis, since an approach that includes education, anticipatory guidance, and a multidisciplinary team approach can set a model for treatment.

3. Clarify the patient's or family members' misconceptions regarding the etiology, treatment, and prognosis of IBD, and provide information on an ongoing basis (Day, Whitten, & Bohane, 2005).

4. Normalize patient and familial reactions to dealing with IBD. Knowing that fears about bathroom issues or medication side effects are common for patients with IBD may help to decrease anxiety.

5. Facilitate the transition to adult care, to help adolescents prepare to assume responsibility for their medical care and learn how to access care and support systems

(see Desir & Seidman, 2003). An effective transition may result in improved compliance with therapy, and effective planning of long-range needs can address the need for benefits to cover issues of continuing health insurance, life insurance, and disability (Mamula et al., 2003). Hait, Arnold, and Fishman (2006) offer a timeline to facilitate this transition process.

References

Achenbach, T. M. (1991). *Manual for the Child Behavior Checklist/4–18 and 1991 Profile*. Burlington: University of Vermont, Department of Psychiatry.

Achkar, T. (2007). *New vistas in inflammatory bowel disease*. Paper presented at the Crohn's and Colitis Foundation of Northeast Ohio Education Seminar, Independence, OH.

Akobeng, A., Miller, V., Firth, D., Suresh-Babu, M. V., Mir, P., & Thomas, A. G. (1999). Quality of life of parents and siblings of children with inflammatory bowel disease. *Journal of Pediatric Gastroenterology and Nutrition, 28*, S40–S42.

Akobeng, A. K., Mirajkar, B., Suresh-Babu, M. V., Firth, D., Miller, D., Mir, P., et al. (1999). Quality of life in children with Crohn's disease: A pilot study. *Journal of Pediatric Gastroenterology and Nutrition, 28*, S37–S39.

Alderfer, M. A., Fiese, B. H., Gold, J., Cutuli, J., Holmbeck, G. N., Goldbeck, L., et al. (2008). Evidence-based assessment in pediatric psychology: Family measures. *Journal of Pediatric Psychology, 33*, 1046–1061.

American Digestive Health Foundation. (2001). *Irritable bowel syndrome: Part 1: Nosology, epidemiology, and pathophysiology*. Bethesda, MD: Author.

Baldassano, R. N., & Piccoli, D. A. (1999). Inflammatory bowel disease in pediatric and adolescent patients. *Gastroenterology Clinics of North America, 28*, 445–458.

Ballinger, A. B. (2000). Epidemiology, natural history and prognosis of inflammatory bowel disease. In D. Ramptain (Ed.), *Inflammatory bowel disease* (pp. 59–70). London: Martin Dunitz.

Banez, G. A., Buchannan, K., Kenagy, D., Frantsuzov, J., Hall, J., Hashkes, P., et al. (2008, April). *Chronic pain in adolescents: Preliminary evaluation of an interdisciplinary pain rehabilitation program (research in progress)*. Paper presented at the National Conference on Child Health Psychology, Miami, FL.

Banez, G. A., & Cunningham, C. (2003). Pediatric gastrointestinal disorders: Recurrent abdominal pain, inflammatory bowel disease, and rumination disorder/cyclic vomiting. In M. C. Roberts (Ed.), *Handbook of pediatric psychology* (3rd ed., pp. 462–480). New York: Guilford Press.

Bennett, E. J., Tennant, C. C., Piesse, C., Badcock, C.-A., & Kellow, J. E. (1998). Level of chronic life stress predicts clinical outcome in irritable bowel syndrome. *Gut, 43*, 256–261.

Bremner, A. R., & Beattie, R. M. (2002). Theory of Crohn's disease in childhood. *Expert Opinions in Pharmacology, 3*(7), 809–825.

Burke, P., Kocoshis, S. A., Chandra, R., Whiteway, M., & Sauer, J. (1990). Determinants of depression in recent onset pediatric inflammatory bowel disease. *Journal of American Academy of Child and Adolescent Psychiatry, 29*, 608–610.

Burke, P., Meyer, V., Kocoshis, S., Orenstein, D., & Sauer, J. (1989). Obsessive–compulsive symptoms in childhood inflammatory bowel disease and cystic fibrosis. *Journal of the American Academy of Child and Adolescent Psychiatry, 4*, 525–527.

Burke, P., Meyer, V., Kocoshis, S., Orenstein, D. M., Chandra, R., Nord, D. J., et al. (1989). Depression and anxiety in pediatric inflammatory bowel disease and cystic fibrosis. *Journal of the American Academy of Child and Adolescent Psychiatry, 28*, 948–951.

Burke, P. M., Neigut, D., Kocoshis, S., Chandra, R., & Sauer, J. (1994). Correlates of depression in new onset pediatric inflammatory bowel disease. *Child Psychiatry and Human Development*, 24(4), 275–283.

Bursch, B. (1999). Pain-associated disability syndrome. In P. E. Hyman (Ed.), *Pediatric functional gastrointestinal disorders* (pp. 8.1–8.14). New York: Academic Professional Information Services.

Campo, J. V., Ehmann, M., Altman, S., Lucas, A., Birmaher, B., DiLorenzo, C., et al. (2004). Recurrent abdominal pain, anxiety, and depression in primary care. *Pediatrics*, 113, 817–824.

Carvalho, R., & Hyams, J. S. (2007). Diagnosis and management of inflammatory bowel disease in children. *Seminars in Pediatric Surgery*, 16(3), 164–171.

Collins, S. M. (2001). Natural history and prognosis. In R. Stockbrugger & F. Pace (Eds.), *The irritable bowel syndrome manual* (pp. 81–86). London: Mosby-Wolfe.

Compas, B. E., Davis, G. E., Forsythe, C. J., & Wagner, B. M. (1987). Assessment of major and daily life events during adolescence: The Adolescent Perceived Events Scale. *Journal of Consulting and Clinical Psychology*, 55, 534–541.

Cox, D. J., Sutphen, J., Borowitz, S., Kovatchev, B., & Ling, W. (1998). Contributions of behavior therapy and biofeedback to laxative therapy in the treatment of pediatric encopresis. *Annals of Behavioral Medicine*, 20, 70–76.

Cuffari, C., & Darbari, A. (2002). Inflammatory bowel disease in the pediatric and adolescent patient. *Gastroenterology Clinics of North America*, 31, 275–291.

Cunningham, C., & Banez, G. A. (2006). *Pediatric gastrointestinal disorders: Biopsychosocial assessment and treatment*. New York: Springer.

Cunningham, C., Drotar, D., Palermo, T., McGowan, K., & Arendt, R. (2007). Health related quality of life in children and adolescents with inflammatory bowel disease. *Children's Health Care*, 36, 29–43.

Day, A. S., Whitten, K. E., & Bohane, T. D. (2005). Childhood inflammatory bowel disease: Parental concerns and expectations. *World Journal of Gastroenterology*, 11(7), 1028–1031.

De Boer, M. A., Grootenhuis, M., Derkx, B., & Last, B. (2005). Health-related quality of life and psychosocial functioning of adolescents with inflammatory bowel disease. *Inflammatory Bowel Diseases*, 11, 400–406.

Desir, B., & Seidman, E. G. (2003). Transitioning the pediatric IBD patient to adult care. *Best Practice and Research: Clinical Gastroenterology*, 17(2), 197–212.

Drossman, D. A. (1998). Presidential address: Gastrointestinal illness and the biopsychosocial model. *Psychosomatic Medicine*, 60, 258–267.

Drossman, D. A., & Thompson, G. (1992). The irritable bowel syndrome: Review and a graduated multicomponent approach. *Annals of Internal Medicine*, 116, 1009–1016.

Duerr, R. H., Taylor, K. D., Brant, S. R., Rioux, J. D., Silverberg, M. S., Daly, M. J., et al. (2006). A genome-wide association study identifies IL23R as an inflammatory bowel disease gene. *Science*, 314, 1403–1405.

Engstrom, I. (1991). Parental distress and social interaction in families with children with inflammatory bowel disease. *Journal of the American Academy of Child and Adolescent Psychiatry*, 30, 904–912.

Engstrom, I. (1992). Mental health and psychological functioning in children and adolescents with inflammatory bowel disease: A comparison with children having other chronic illnesses and with healthy children. *Journal of Child Psychology and Psychiatry*, 33, 563–582.

Engstrom, I. (1999). Inflammatory bowel disease in children and adolescents: Mental health and family functioning. *Journal of Pediatric Gastroenterology and Nutrition*, 28, S28–S33.

Engstrom, I., & Lindquist, B. L. (1991). Inflammatory bowel disease in children and adolescents: A somatic and psychiatric investigation. *Acta Paediatrica Scandinavica*, *80*(6–7), 640–647.

European Society of Gastroenterology, Hepatology, and Nutrition, IBD Working Group. (2005). Inflammatory bowel disease in children and adolescents: Recommendations for diagnosis— the Porto criteria. *Journal of Pediatric Gastroenterology and Nutrition*, *1*(1), 1–7.

Faure, C., & Wieckowska, A. (2007). Somatic referral of visceral sensations and rectal sensory threshold for pain in children with functional gastrointestinal disorders. *Journal of Pediatrics*, *150*, 66–71.

Ferguson, A., Sedgwick, D. M., & Drummond, J. (1994). Morbidity of juvenile-onset inflammatory bowel disease: Effects on education and employment in early adult life. *Gut*, *35*, 665–668.

Gold, N., Issenman, R., Roberts, J., & Watt, S. (2000). An alternate view of children with inflammatory bowel disease and functional gastrointestinal complaints. *Inflammatory Bowel Disease*, *6*, 1–7.

Greenley, R. N., & Cunningham, C. (2009). Parent quality of life in the context of pediatric inflammatory bowel disease. *Journal of Pediatric Psychology*, *34*(2), 129–136.

Griffiths, A. M., Nicholas, D., Smith, C., Munk, M., Stephens, D., Durno, C., et al. (1999). Development of a quality of life index for pediatric inflammatory bowel disease: Dealing with differences related to age and IBD type. *Journal of Pediatric Gastroenterology and Nutrition*, *28*, S46–S52.

Hahn, B. A., Yan, S., & Strassels, S. (1999). Impact of irritable bowel syndrome on quality of life and resource use in the United States and United Kingdom. *Digestion*, *60*, 77–81.

Hait, E., Arnold, J. H., & Fishman, L. N. (2006). Educate, communicate, anticipate: Practical recommendations for transitioning adolescents with IBD to adult health care. *Inflammatory Bowel Diseases*, *12*, 170–173.

Hodges, K., Kline, J. J., Barbero, G., & Woodruff, C. (1985). Anxiety in children with recurrent abdominal pain and in their parents. *Psychosomatics*, *26*, 859–866.

Holmbeck, G. N., Li, S. T., Schurman, J. V., Friedman, D., & Coakley, R. M. (2002). Collecting and managing multisource and multimethod data in studies of pediatric populations. *Journal of Pediatric Psychology*, *27*, 5–18.

Hommel, K., Davis, C. M., & Baldassano, R. N. (2008). Medication adherence and quality of life in pediatric inflammatory bowel disease. *Journal of Pediatric Psychology*, *33*, 867–874.

Howell, S., Poulton, R., & Talley, N. J. (2005). The natural history of childhood abdominal pain and its association with adult irritable bowel syndrome: Birth-cohort study. *American Journal of Gastroenterology*, *100*, 2071–2078.

Huertas-Ceballos, A., Logan, S., Bennett, C., & Macarthur, C. (2008a). Pharmacological interventions for recurrent abdominal pain (RAP) and irritable bowel syndrome (IBS) in childhood. *Cochrane Database of Systematic Reviews*, Issue 1 (Article No. CD003017), DOI: 10.1002/14651858.CD003017.pub2.

Huertas-Ceballos, A., Logan, S., Bennett, C., & Macarthur, C. (2008b). Psychosocial interventions for recurrent abdominal pain (RAP) and irritable bowel syndrome (IBS) in childhood. *Cochrane Database of Systematic Reviews* Issue 1 (Article No. CD003014), DOI: 10.1002/14651858.CD003014.pub2.

Huertas-Ceballos, A., Logan, S., Bennett, C., & Macarthur, C. (2009). Dietary interventions for recurrent abdominal pain (RAP) and irritable bowel syndrome (IBS) in childhood. *Cochrane Database of Systematic Reviews*, Issue 1 (Article No. CD003019), DOI: 10.1002/14651858.CD003019.pub3.

Hyams, J. S. (1999). Chronic and recurrent abdominal pain. In P. E. Hyman (Ed.), *Pediatric functional gastrointestinal disorders* (pp. 7.1–7.21). New York: Academic Professional Information Services.

Hyams, J. S. (2000). Inflammatory bowel disease. *Pediatrics in Review*, *21*(9), 291–295.

Hyams, J. S., Burke, G., Davis, P. M., Rzepski, B., & Andrulonis, P. A. (1996). Abdominal pain and irritable bowel syndrome in adolescents: A community-based study. *Journal of Pediatrics, 129,* 220–226.

Hyams, J. S., Treem, W. R., Justinich, C. J., Davis, P., Shoup, M., & Burke, G. (1995). Characterization of symptoms in children with recurrent abdominal pain: Resemblance to irritable bowel syndrome. *Journal of Pediatric Gastroenterology and Nutrition, 20,* 209–214.

International Foundation for Functional Gastrointestinal Disorders. (2002). *IBS in the Real World Survey: Summary findings.* Milwaukee, WI: Author.

Janicke, D. M., & Finney, J. W. (1999). Empirically supported treatments in pediatric psychology: Recurrent abdominal pain. *Journal of Pediatric Psychology, 24,* 115–127.

Kim, S. C., & Ferry, G. D. (2004). Inflammatory bowel disease in pediatric and adolescent patients: Clinical, therapeutic and psychosocial considerations. *Gastroenterology, 126,* 1550–1560.

King, R. A. (2003). Pediatric inflammatory bowel disease. *Child and Adolescent Psychiatric Clinics of North America, 12,* 967–995.

Kovacs, M. (1985). Children's Depression Inventory (CDI). *Psychopharmacology Bulletin, 21,* 995–998.

Kugathasan, S., Judd, R. H., Hoffmann, R. G., Helkenen, J., Telega, G., Khan, F., et al. (2003). Epidemiologic and clinical characteristics of children with newly diagnosed inflammatory bowel disease in Wisconsin: A statewide population-based study. *Journal of Pediatrics, 143,* 525–531.

Landgraf, J. M., Abetz, L., & Ware, J. E. (1996). *The CHQ user's manual.* Boston: Health Institute, New England Medical Center.

Langholz, E., Munkholm, P., Krasilinikoff, P. A., & Binder, V. (1998). Inflammatory bowel diseases in children. *Ugeskrift for Laeger, 160,* 5648–5464.

Levy, R. L., Whitehead, W. E., Walker, L. S., Von Korff, M., Feld, A. D., Garner, M., et al. (2004). Increased somatic complaints and health-care utilization in children: Effects of parent IBS status and parent response to gastrointestinal symptoms. *American Journal of Gastroenterology, 99,* 2442–2451.

Loftus, C. G., Loftus, E. V., Jr., Harmsen, W. S., Zinsmeister, A. R., Tremaine, W. J., Melton, L. J., III, et al. (2007). Update on the incidence and prevalence of Crohn's disease and ulcerative colitis in Olmsted County, Minnesota, 1940–2000. *Inflammatory Bowel Diseases, 3,* 254–261.

Loonen, H. J., Derkx, B. H. F., Koopman, H. M., & Heymans, H. S. A. (2002). Are parents able to rate the symptoms and quality of life of their offspring with IBD? *Inflammatory Bowel Diseases, 8,* 270–276.

Loonen, H. J., Grootenhuis, M. A., Last, B. P., Koopman, H. M., & Derkx, H. H. F. (2002). Quality of life in pediatric inflammatory bowel disease measured by a generic and a disease specific questionnaire. *Acta Paediatrica, 91,* 347–354.

Mackner, L. M., & Crandall, W. V. (2005a). Long-term psychosocial outcomes reported by children and adolescents with inflammatory bowel disease. *American Journal of Gastroenterology, 100,* 1386–1392.

Mackner, L. M., & Crandall, W. V. (2005b). Oral medication adherence in pediatric inflammatory bowel disease. *Inflammatory Bowel Diseases, 11,* 1006–1012.

Mackner, L. M., & Crandall, W. V. (2006). Psychological factors affecting pediatric inflammatory bowel disease. *Current Opinion in Pediatrics, 19,* 548–552.

Mackner, L. M., Crandall, W. V., & Szigethy, E. M. (2006). Brief report: Psychosocial functioning in pediatric inflammatory bowel disease. *Inflammatory Bowel Disease, 12,* 239–244.

Mamula, P., Markowitz, J. E., & Baldassano, R. N. (2003). Inflammatory bowel disease in early childhood and adolescence: Special considerations. *Gastroenterology Clinics of North America, 32,* 967–995.

Mayberry, J. F. (1999). Impact of inflammatory bowel disease on educational achievements and work prospects. *Journal of Pediatric Gastroenterology and Nutrition, 28,* S34–S36.

Moody, G., Eaden, J., & Mayberry, J. F. (1999). Social implications of childhood Crohn's disease. *Journal of Pediatric Gastroenterology and Nutrition, 28,* S43–S45.

Neff, D. F., & Blanchard, E. B. (1987). A multi-component treatment for irritable bowel syndrome. *Behaviour Therapy, 18,* 70–83.

Oliva-Hemker, M. M., Abadom, V., Cuffari, C., & Thompson, R. E. (2007). Nonadherence with thiopurine immunomodulator and mesalamine medications in children with Crohn disease. *Journal of Pediatric Gastroenterology and Nutrition, 44,* 180–184.

Otley, A., Smith, C., Nicholas, D., Munk, M., Avolio, J., Sherman, P. M., et al. (2002).The IMPACT questionnaire: A valid measure of health-related quality of life in pediatric inflammatory bowel disease. *Journal of Pediatric Gastroenterology and Nutrition, 35,* 557–563.

Pace, F., Molteni, P., Bollani, S., Sarzi-Puttini, P., Stockbrugger, R., Bianchi Porro, G., et al. (2003). Inflammatory bowel disease versus irritable bowel syndrome Quality-of-life in children with Crohn's disease. *Journal of Pediatric Gastroenterology and Nutrition, 5,* 528–533.

Perrin, J. M., Kuhlthau, K., Chughtai, A., Romm, D., Kirschner, B. S., Ferry, G. D., et al. (2008). Measuring quality of life in pediatric patients with inflammatory bowel disease: Psychometric and clinical characteristics. *Journal of Pediatric Gastroenterology and Nutrition, 46,* 164–171.

Quittner, A. L., Modi, A. C., Lemanek, K. L., Ievers-Landis, C. E., & Rapoff, M. (2008). Evidence-based assessment of adherence to medical treatments in pediatric psychology. *Journal of Pediatric Psychology, 33,* 916–936.

Rabbett, H., Elbadri, A., Thwaites, R., Northover, H., Dady, I., & Firth, D. (1996). Quality-of-life in children with Crohn's disease. *Journal of Pediatric Gastroenterology and Nutrition, 5,* 528–533.

Rasquin, A., Di Lorenzo, C., Forbes, D., Guiraldes, E., Hyams, J. S., Staiano, A., et al. (2006). Childhood functional gastrointestinal disorders: Child/adolescent. *Gastroenterology, 130,* 1527–1537.

Rice, H. E., & Chuang, E. (1999). Current management of pediatric inflammatory bowel disease. *Seminars in Pediatric Surgery, 8,* 221–228.

Shaffer, D., Gould, M. S., Brasic, J., Ambrosini, P., Fisher, P., Bird, H., et al. (1983). A Children's Global Assessment Scale. *Archives of General Psychiatry, 40,* 1228–1231.

Stark, L. J., Opirari, L. C., Donaldson, D. L., Danovsky, M. B., Rasile, D. A., & DelSanto, A. F. (1997). Evaluation of a standard protocol for retentive encopresis. *Journal of Pediatric Psychology, 22,* 619–633.

Svendsen, J. H., Munck, L. K., & Andersen, J. R. (1985). Irritable bowel syndrome prognosis and diagnostic safety: A 5-year follow-up study. *Scandinavian Journal of Gastroenterology, 20,* 415–418.

Szigethy, E., Kenney, E., Carpenter, J., & Hardy, D. M. (2007). Cognitive-behavioral therapy for adolescents with inflammatory bowel disease and subsyndromal depression. *Journal of the American Academy of Child and Adolescent Psychiatry, 46*(10), 1290–1298.

Szigethy, E., Levy-Warren, A., & Whitoon, S. (2004). Depressive symptoms and inflammatory bowel disease in children and adolescents: A cross sectional study. *Journal of Pediatric Gastroenterology and Nutrition, 39,* 395–403.

Tojek, T. M., Lumley, M. A., Corlis, M., Ondersma, S., & Tolia, V. (2002). Maternal correlates of health status in adolescents with inflammatory bowel disease. *Journal of Psychosomatic Research, 52,* 173–179.

van der Zaag-Loonen, H. J., Grootenhuis, M. A., Last, B. P., & Derkx, H. H. F. (2004). Coping strategies and quality of life of adolescents with inflammatory bowel disease. *Quality of Life Research, 13,* 1011–1019.

Van Slyke, D. A., & Walker, L. S. (2006). Mothers' responses to children's pain. *Clinical Journal of Pain, 22*(4), 387–391.

Varni, J. W., Lane, M. M., Burwinkle, T. M., Fontaine, E. N., Youssef, N. N., Schwimmer, J. B., et al. (2006). Health-related quality of life in pediatric patients with irritable bowel syndrome. *Journal of Developmental and Behavioral Pediatrics, 27*(6), 451–458.

Verrips, G. H., Vogels, A. G., den Ouden, A. L., Paneth, N., & Verloove-Vanhorick, S. P. (2000). Measuring health-related quality of life in adolescents: Agreement between raters and between methods of administration. *Child: Care, Health, and Development, 26*(6), 457–469.

Walker, L. S. (1999). The evolution of research on recurrent abdominal pain: History, assumptions, and a conceptual model. In P. J. McGrath & G. A. Finley (Eds.), *Chronic and recurrent pain in children and adolescents* (pp. 141–172). Seattle, WA: International Association for the Study of Pain Press.

Walker, L. S., Garber, J., Smith, C. A., Van Slyke, D. A., & Lewis Claar, R. (2001). The relation of daily stressors to somatic and emotional symptoms in children with and without recurrent abdominal pain. *Journal of Consulting and Clinical Psychology, 69*, 85–91.

Walker, L. S., & Greene, J. W. (1991). The Functional Disability Inventory: Measuring a neglected dimension of child health status. *Journal of Pediatric Psychology, 16*, 39–58.

Walker, L. S., Guite, J. W., Duke, M., Barnard, J. A., & Greene, J. W. (1998). Recurrent abdominal pain: A potential precursor of irritable bowel syndrome in adolescents and young adults. *Journal of Pediatrics, 132*, 1010–1015.

Walker, L. S., Smith, C. A., Garber, J., & Van Slyke, D. A. (1997). Development and validation of the Pain Response Inventory for Children. *Psychological Assessment, 9*, 392–405.

Weydert, J. A., Ball, T. M., & Davis, M. F. (2003). Systematic review of treatments for recurrent abdominal pain. *Pediatrics, 111*, e1–e11.

CHAPTER 28

Pediatric Burns

KENNETH J. TARNOWSKI
RONALD T. BROWN

Burns are among the most devastating types of injuries, are often life-threatening, and pose significant acute and chronic biopsychosocial challenges to patients and their families. Indeed, burns are among the most resource-intensive (in terms of hospitalization time, cost, and staff resources) forms of trauma sustained by children (Lukish et al., 2001), and they share characteristics of acute medical disorders as well as those associated with chronic illnesses (e.g., short- and long-term medical and psychosocial challenges) (Tarnowski, 1994). This chapter provides an overview of the epidemiology and nature of burn injuries, as well as biopsychosocial considerations during the acute and rehabilitation phases.

Epidemiology

Annually, approximately 1.5–2.0 million individuals sustain burn injuries in the United States. It is estimated that 70,000–100,000 of these individuals have injuries that require hospitalization. Of the patients that require hospitalization, approximately one-half are under 18 years of age (Pruitt, Goodwin, & Mason, 2002). Burn injuries remain the fifth most common cause of injury-related mortality (Centers for Disease Control and Prevention, 2008).

Burns may occur as a result of exposure to chemicals, radiation, flames, electrical current, or scalding liquids. Most burns are not severe and do not result in hospitalization. The ways in which children sustain burn injuries vary as a function of age and developmental capabilities. For example, as toddlers refine their motor capabilities, they are at increased risk of injuries from spills and hot household tap water. Toddlers also have a high rate of contact burns due to touching hot objects (e.g., stoves, heaters).

School-age children often sustain injuries in experimental play with matches and light-ers, while adolescents are often injured outside the home in the context of risk-taking activities involving fireworks and liquid flammables. More males than females sustain burn injuries, and this gender discrepancy increases as a function of age. It is also well known that cigarettes are a leading cause of house fires and are responsible for approxi-mately 35% of fatal residential fires in the United States (McLoughlin & McGuire, 1990). Finally, child abuse in the form of intentional burn injury accounts for an esti-mated 10–20% of pediatric burns (Joffe, 2000).

Medical Considerations

Classification of Burn Injuries

Burns are typically described in terms of depth and total body surface area (TBSA). TBSA is calculated through the use of special charts called "burn diagrams" that graph-ically depict dorsal and ventral views of the body, divided into smaller discrete areas of known percentage of TBSA. Heat intensity and duration of contact determine the extent and depth of skin injury.

Burn injuries that are restricted to the epidermis are first-degree burns. The skin is red and painful to touch, but the epidermis is intact, and there is an absence of blis-ters. First-degree burns are typically not included in the calculation of TBSA, given that these injuries do not markedly influence care provision or outcome. Second-degree burns involve the dermis and are also referred to as partial-thickness burns. Burns of this extent can vary widely in appearance, from those at the periphery of an injury site that are red with the inclusion of blisters, to those that are deeper with a white appearance but less painful presentation due to the damaged peripheral nerve endings. Full-thickness (third-degree) burns are the most extensive injuries, involving multiple skin layers and possible destruction of subcutaneous tissue and peripheral nerve fibers, These injuries have a leathery appearance and are painless due to the destruction of nerve endings (Passaretti & Billmire, 2003). Occasionally, one sees references to fourth-degree burns, involving destruction of tendons, nerves, muscle, and bone; however, this terminology is used infrequently and is usually invoked in the context of deep electrical burns (Reed & Pomerantz, 2005).

Treatment Overview

The following information is based on the succinct overview of the medical and sur-gical aspects of pediatric burn care provided by Reed and Pomerantz (2005). Emer-gency treatment at the scene of injury involves removing the heat source and ensuring an unobstructed airway. Cardiopulmonary resuscitation may be required. Following admission, bronchoscopy may be required to fully assess the airway, and intubation is commonly required. Burns cause intravascular fluid diffusion, and intravenous provision of isotonic saline is needed to rectify homeostatic imbalance. Cardiac, gastrointestinal, and pulmonary status; temperature; and fluid titration are closely monitored. Partial-thickness burns are commonly treated with antibiotic ointments, and wound dressings are changed once or twice daily. Full-thickness burns are treated with silver sulfadiazine or mafeninide acetate preparations. Alternatively, synthetic occlusive dressings, human allograft, or pigskin can be used until epithelization occurs. Infection needs to be closely monitored and treated aggressively. Eschar (dead tissue) needs to be surgically removed, and necrotic tissue needs to be debrided. Autografting is conducted in stages due to the limited availability of donor material. Pressure dressings and garments are used to minimize scarring. Multiple reconstructive surgeries for scar revision may be conducted over a period of years. Advances in cultured dermatological materials hold promise for refinements in the care of patients with severe burns.

Psychosocial Considerations

Premorbid Risk Factors

Clearly, the development of strategies to prevent pediatric burn injuries is dependent upon the identification of relevant risk-related variables. Although child risk may be potentiated by such factors as parental smoking, failure to adjust hot water heaters, and the like, we have limited understanding of how specific child developmental variables (e.g., emerging motoric capabilities) interact with parental and family psychosocial variables (e.g., socioeconomic status, decreased vigilance associated with parental psychopathology such as depression) in relation to injury risk (Tarnowski, 1994). Furthermore, we have very little information on how premorbid parental and family psychopathology influences the psychological sequelae of severe burn injury (Noronha & Faust, 2007). In sum, much work remains to be done on identification of specific utilitarian and psychological risk variables related to pediatric burn injury, as well as on how such variables are related to the long-term psychosocial fate of pediatric burn victims (Tarnowski & Simonian, 2003).

Issues during the Acute Phase

Major areas of concern during the acute phase include mental status, nutritional intake, body image disturbances, self-excoriation, posttraumatic symptoms, treatment adherence, pain management, and issues associated with child and family adaptation to the recovery process (Sarwer et al., 2006). These issues are described below.

Mental Status

Following burn injury, there are frequently central nervous system dysfunctions resulting from anoxic and hypoxic conditions (e.g., carbon monoxide inhalation), medications, or sleep deprivation. Moreover, individuals who are severely burned frequently suffer from metabolic complications and infections that often produce altered mental status (Reed & Pomerantz, 2005). The management of such disoriented states often includes correction of electrolyte imbalances resulting from fluid loss following injury. Psychological approaches to enhance orientation may include the use of visual aids for the purpose of orienting the individual to time of day (e.g., clocks, the use of windows) and date (e.g., calendars) (Sarwer et al., 2006). In addition, assigning a child to the same staff members over the course of several days assists in orienting the child to time and place.

Nutritional Intake

Ensuring adequate caloric intake is a common problem on pediatric burn units, and staff members frequently seek consultation from a pediatric psychologist. Behavioral approaches to improve nutrition, including contingency management, may be used to increase caloric and fluid intake and to reduce the need for tube and intravenous feedings. The physical task of eating often proves to be a formidable challenge due to structural impairments, and occupational therapists often can be helpful with adaptive devices that promote the transition to self-sufficiency.

Disturbances in Body Image

Burns often lead to disfigurement, which may negatively influence children's sense of competence as well as their relationships with peers, particularly in adolescence (Passaretti & Billmire, 2003; Sarwer et al., 2006; Saxe et al., 2005). Saxe and colleagues (2005) have demonstrated that body image is associated with symptoms of acute stress disorder in children, and that this association is mediated by the size of the burn. Thus children who have sustained severe burn injuries are at particular risk for loss of identity, reduced sense of physical competence, and social stigmatization (Rawlins, Khan, Shenton, & Sharpe, 2007; Stoddard, 2002). It is noteworthy that adjustment difficulties and problems with peer relationships increase following the acute phase of injury, when children are discharged from the hospital and are away from the support of hospital staff (Passaretti & Billmire, 2003; Sarwer et al., 2006). It is not surprising that these adjustment difficulties are especially salient for adolescents (Landolt, Grubenmann, & Meuli, 2002), and ongoing monitoring of adjustment and adaptation is especially important over the course of the burn injury and after discharge from the hospital (Meyer et al., 2007; Passaretti & Billmire, 2003). Social skills training may be of benefit in managing taunting from peers and in negotiating reactions from strangers (Blakeney et al., 2005).

Self-Excoriation

Following the healing of burned skin tissue, there is frequently intense itching (Lukish et al., 2001). Such excoriation can compromise wound healing, and behavioral techniques including response interruption and distraction have frequently proved efficacious for younger children (Sarwer et al., 2006).

Posttraumatic Stress Disorder

Over the past several years, a compelling literature has shown that children who have survived chronic or acute diseases frequently suffer from posttraumatic stress disorder (PTSD). Many youths who have survived burns have endured additional traumatic experiences, including accidents. For this reason, it is no surprise that burn survivors often exhibit trauma symptoms in both the acute and rehabilitative phases of recovery (Stoddard & Saxe, 2001; Stoddard et al., 2006). Meyer, Robert, Murphy, and Blakeney (2000) have argued that determining how behavioral problems are related to posttrauma sequelae and the preburn environment will be important in developing intervention programs for these children. Over the years, there has been a great deal of progress in recognizing and managing PTSD, and pediatric psychologists have become especially vigilant in recognizing these symptoms in children who have survived serious trauma (see Kazak, Schneider, & Kassam-Adams, Chapter 13, this volume). Stoddard and colleagues (2006) have provided important data to suggest that even preschool children who have been burned also demonstrate symptoms of PTSD.

Adherence to Treatment Demands

Numerous treatments and procedures are required during the acute phase of a burn injury; these include physical and occupational therapy, use of pressure garments, and various medication regimens. Adherence to prescribed procedures may become a major issue following hospitalization. Empirically supported interventions for improving adherence in pediatric burn patients are lacking, but techniques that have been demonstrated to be efficacious in managing the adherence of children and their families to treatments for other pediatric conditions may be of value (see La Greca & Mackey, Chapter 9, this volume).

Pain Management

Children and adolescents frequently experience significant pain during the acute phase of a burn injury, due to the burn itself as well as the necessary procedures for the care of the injury (e.g., dressing changes, debridement) (Ratcliff et al., 2006). Appropriate management of pain during the acute phase following the burn injury is important in diminishing later symptoms associated with anxiety and PTSD (Stoddard & Saxe, 2001). For example, one study provided important findings that higher doses of pain analgesia during the acute phase of hospitalization were associated with fewer symptoms of PTSD 6 months after the burn injury (Stoddard & Saxe, 2001).

The pediatric psychologist has an array of assessment techniques available to evaluate pain, including self-report rating scales, physiological assessments, and various coding techniques documenting pain behavior (for a review, see Cohen et al., 2008). Details on effective psychological pain management methods for children are summarized by Blount and colleagues (Chapter 11, this volume). Pharmacotherapies are also widely used in the management of pain for children who have sustained burn injuries. These include nonsteroidal anti-inflammatory drugs, as well as morphine and synthetic opioids that are delivered by numerous venues (including patient-controlled analgesia; regional blocks; and intravenous, intramuscular, and oral routes) (Ratcliff et al., 2006). The use of benzodiazepines (e.g., diazepam [Valium]) has received support when used as an adjunct to pain analgesia (Stoddard, Martyn, & Sheridan, 1997). Finally, the use of other pharmacotherapies, including the stimulants and tricyclic antidepressants, has been demonstrated to diminish the need for higher doses of traditional pain analgesia (Ratcliff et al., 2006).

It has been demonstrated that ongoing pharmacological management of acute pain in general, and timely management of pain for various procedures (including dressing changes) in particular, have been associated with an individual's increase in the sense of control over these aversive procedures, and even in reductions in the rates of postoperative morbidity and health utilization patterns (e.g., number of days hospitalized) (Saxe et al., 2001). Nonetheless, despite the benefits of pharmacological management of pain, ongoing assessment of adverse effects and toxicities associated with various pharmaco-therapies is of utmost importance.

Child and Familial Adjustment Issues

There is frequently a positive association between behavioral disturbances and children's exposure to aversive procedures. Given the myriad aversive procedures that must be endured by children who have sustained burn injuries, behavioral disturbances are frequently encountered on pediatric burn units. Such painful procedures as debridement and hydrotherapy may be perceived by children as random and promote a form of learned helplessness. For this reason, it is important that the hospital environment be both predictive and consistent, and that children and adolescents be empowered with maximum control. They should be given choices pertaining to times of hydrotherapy and dressing changes, and allow children to remove dressings and splints themselves whenever this is feasible and possible (Stoddard & Saxe, 2001).

Familial variables that have been demonstrated to be predictive of good adjustment following a significant stressor or chronic illness include cohesiveness, effective communication skills within the family system, social support networks, and skills in conflict resolution among family members. These characteristics have been found to assist children in regulating affect and trusting others, such as medical staff members (Stoddard & Saxe, 2001). In addition, families that have financial resources available and that support an active or engaged style of coping rather than a passive or disengaged style of coping (e.g., avoidance, denial) often have children who fare better during the postburn adjustment phase. Premorbid adjustment and time since the injury have been noted to be generally stable and viable predictors of adjustment and adaptation to the burn injury (Landolt et al., 2002). Landolt and colleagues (2002) have also provided important data to suggest that compromised familial relationships are associated with poor psychological adjustment among survivors of burn injuries. Because adaptation to burn injuries in children is highly related to family functioning, it is important for the pediatric psychologist to address the needs and concerns of all family members during the course of hospitalization. Family therapy may be a viable approach in managing other chronic diseases, and these approaches should be investigated through controlled clinical trials to examine the efficacy of family systems therapy for children who have been burned and their families.

Rehabilitation Issues

During the rehabilitation phase, children are required to adhere to specific self-care practices, including physical therapy and the wearing of pressure garments. Often multiple hospitalizations are necessary for the purpose of reconstructive surgeries. During this period, children and their families often must come to terms with the children's loss of functional capacity and permanent disfigurement. There are frequently a number of familial stressors, and, as in other chronic illnesses, the children must negotiate the difficulties associated with school reentry.

Long-Term Psychological Adaptation

For children who have sustained burn injuries, the clinical literature has documented difficulties of self-esteem, body image, and peer relationships; altered academic and career trajectories; coping with disfigurement and societal reactions; and increased family stressors (for reviews, see Noronha & Faust, 2007; Sarwer et al., 2006; Stoddard & Saxe, 2001). Consistent with the acute phase of injury, symptoms of PTSD are often present; problems with mood and symptoms of internalizing and externalizing adjustment difficulties may also be seen (Stoddard & Saxe, 2001). However, contrary to the expectation that the majority of children will suffer poor long-term psychosocial outcomes because of the devastating nature of burn injuries, the literature generally suggests that most children are able to negotiate the recovery process successfully (Tarnowski, 1994).

Clearly, adaptation to burn injuries is especially complex and is predicted by a number of variables, including premorbid functioning, behavioral risk factors, and child and family resource variables. Noronha and Faust (2007) examined those variables that had the greatest impact on psychological adjustment following burn injuries for children, adolescents, and young adults. Findings of this meta-analysis of the extant literature (13 studies) revealed that location of the injury, parental adjustment, and children's premorbid functioning were most strongly associated with postmorbid psychological adjustment and adaptation. It is likely that risk and resource variables may differentially combine to predict outcome, as in other chronic illnesses. Such a model for pediatric burns has been provided by Tarnowski and Simonian (2003).

Conclusions

Burns are relatively common pediatric injuries that are classified in terms of depth, location, and TBSA. Severe burn injuries are associated with a host of serious biopsychosocial challenges. Although the treatment of these injuries is among the most resource-intensive and psychologically taxing of any form of treatment for human injury, recent medical, surgical, and psychological advances have markedly improved the survival rate and outcomes for children with burn injuries. Consultation with pediatric burn victims and their families requires significant treatment breadth and versatility, as many of the commonly encountered problems (e.g., mental status, nutritional intake, body image disturbance, adherence, family issues, pain management) will require the use of treatments that have largely been developed/refined with other pediatric populations. Often these empirically supported treatments will need to be adapted and tailored to the unique challenges of youths with devastating burns. Frequently one will witness the practical, if not the theoretical, limits of such interventions because of the protracted and severe biopsychosocial stressors that are unique to pediatric burns.

Studies examining the intermediate to long-term psychosocial sequelae of pediatric burns have improved methodological rigor (e.g., use of psychometrically sound measures, structured interview data), and there is emerging evidence in support of the role of premorbid child and family psychopathology in mediating long-term outcomes. Recent studies (Landolt et al., 2002; Rosenberg et al., 2006) have assessed quality of life for pediatric burn survivors, but these data are preliminary, and future work is required to address conflicting findings. Although progress has been made in the prevention of burn injuries, much work remains to significantly reduce the mortality and biopsychosocial morbidity associated with these injuries.

Acknowledgments

We would like to thank the anonymous reviewers for their helpful input, and Charity Barone for her kind assistance in the preparation of this chapter.

References

Blakeney, P., Thomas, C., Holzer, C. E., Rose, M., Berniger, F., & Meyer, W. J. (2005). Efficacy of a short-term, intensive social skills training program for burned adolescents. *Journal of Burn Care Rehabilitation, 26,* 546–555.

Centers for Disease Control and Prevention, National Center for Injury Prevention and Control. (2008). *Fire deaths and injuries: Fact sheet.* Retrieved March 15, 2009, from *www/cdc.gov/ncipc/factsheets/fire.htm*

Cohen, L. L., Lemanek, K., Blount, R. L., Dahlquist, L. M., Lim, C. S., Palermo, T. M., et al. (2008). Evidence-based assessment of pediatric pain. *Journal of Pediatric Psychology, 33,* 939–955.

Joffe, M. D. (2000). Burns. In G. R. Fleisher & S. Ludwig (Eds.), *Textbook of pediatric emergency medicine* (4th ed., pp. 1427–1434). Philadelphia: Lippincott Williams & Wilkins.

Landolt, M. A., Grubenmann, S., & Meuli, M. (2002). Family impact greatest: Predictors of quality of life and psychological adjustment in pediatric burn survivors. *Journal of Trauma Injury, Infection, and Critical Care, 53,* 1146–1151.

Lukish, J. R., Eichelberger, M. R., Newman, K. D., Pao, M., Nobuhara, K., Keating, M., et al. (2001). The use of a bioactive skin substitute decreases length of stay for pediatric burn patients. *Journal of Pediatric Surgery, 36,* 1118–1121.

McLoughlin, E., & McGuire, A. (1990). The causes, cost, and prevention of childhood burn injuries. *American Journal of Diseases of Children, 144,* 677–683.

Meyer, W. J., Blakeney, P., Thomas, C. R., Russell, W., Robert, R. S., & Holzer, C. E. (2007). Prevalence of major psychiatric illness in young adults who were burned as children. *Psychosomatic Medicine, 69,* 377–382.

Meyer, W. J., Robert, R., Murphy, L., & Blakeney, P. E. (2000). Evaluating the psychosocial adjustment of 2- and 3-year-old pediatric burn survivors. *Journal of Burn Care and Rehabilitation, 21,* 179–184.

Noronha, D., & Faust, J. (2007). Identifying the variables impacting post-burn psychological adjustment: A meta-analysis. *Journal of Pediatric Psychology, 32,* 380–391.

Passaretti, D., & Billmire, D. A. (2003). Management of pediatric burns. *Journal of Craniofacial Surgery, 14,* 713–718.

Pruitt, B. A., Goodwin, C. W., & Mason, A. D. (2002). Epidemiological, demographic, and outcome characteristics of burn injury. In D. Herndon (Ed.), *Total burn care* (2nd ed., pp. 16–30). Philadelphia: Saunders.

Ratcliff, S. L., Brown, A., Rosenberg, L., Rosenberg, M., Robert, R., & Cuervo, L. J. (2006). The effectiveness of a pain and anxiety protocol to treat the acute pediatric burn patient. *Burns, 32,* 554–562.

Rawlins, J. M., Khan, A. A., Shenton, A. F., & Sharpe, D. T. (2007). Epidemiology and outcome analysis of 208 children with burns attending an emergency department. *Pediatric Emergency Care, 23,* 289–293.

Reed, J. L., & Pomerantz, W. J. (2005). Emergency management of pediatric burns. *Pediatric Emergency Care, 21*, 118–129.

Rosenberg, M., Blakeney, P., Robert, R., Thomas, C., Holzer, C., & Meyer, W. (2006). Quality of life of young adults who survived pediatric burns. *Journal of Burn Care and Research, 27*, 773–778.

Sarwer, D. B., Pruzinsky, T., Cash, T. F., Goldwyn, R. M., Persing, J. A., & Whitaker, L. A. (2006). *Psychological aspects of reconstructive and cosmetic plastic surgery: Clinical, empirical and ethical perspectives.* Philadelphia: Lippincott Williams & Wilkins.

Saxe, G., Stoddard, F., Chawla, N., Lopez, C. G., Hall, E., Sheridan, et al. (2005). Risk factors for acute stress disorder in children with burns. *Journal of Trauma and Dissociation, 6*, 37–49.

Saxe, G., Stoddard, E., Courtney, D., Cunningham, K., Chawla, N., Sheridan, R., et al. (2001). Relationship between acute morphine and the course of PTSD in children with burns. *Journal of the American Academy of Child and Adolescent Psychiatry, 40*, 915–921.

Stoddard, E. J., Martyn, J., & Sheridan, R. (1997). Psychiatric issues in pain of burn injury. *Current Review of Pain, 1*, 130–136.

Stoddard, F. J. (2002). Care of infants, children and adolescents with burn injuries. In M. Lewis (Ed.), *Child and adolescent psychiatry: A comprehensive textbook* (3rd ed., pp. 1188–1208). Philadelphia: Lippincott Williams & Wilkins.

Stoddard, F. J., Ronfeldt, H., Kagan, J., Drake, J. E., Snidman, N., Murphy, J. M., et al. (2006). Young burned children: The course of acute stress and physiological and behavioral responses. *American Journal of Psychiatry, 163*, 1084–1090.

Stoddard, F. J., & Saxe, G. (2001). Ten-year research review of physical injuries. *Journal of the American Academy of Child and Adolescent Psychiatry, 40*, 1128–1145.

Tarnowski, K. J. (1994). *Behavioral aspects of pediatric burns.* New York: Plenum Press.

Tarnowski, K. J., & Simonian, S. J. (2003). Psychological aspects of catastrophic pediatric injury: Considerations in traumatic burn and head injuries. In K. Anchor, J. E. Shmerling, & J. M. Anchor (Eds.), *The handbook of catastrophic injury* (pp. 200–212). Dubuque, IA: Kendall/Hunt.

CHAPTER 29

Feeding and Vomiting Problems in Pediatric Populations

ALAN H. SILVERMAN
SALLY TARBELL

Children with feeding, growth, and vomiting problems are commonly seen by primary care doctors for management of these difficulties. Given the complexity of these disorders, interdisciplinary treatment approaches are optimal. This chapter reviews literature pertinent to prevalence, etiology, assessment, diagnosis, and treatment of these disorders, with an emphasis on an interdisciplinary biobehavioral approach to care.

Feeding Problems

Feeding a child is one of the most fundamental caregiving tasks of parenting. Unfortunately, feeding problems are common (Linscheid, Budd, & Rasnake, 1995), often adversely affecting childhood nutrition and family relationships (Hagekull & Dahl, 1987; Lindberg, Bohlin, Hagekull, & Thunstrome, 1994; Singer, Song, Hill, & Jaffe, 1990). Feeding problems are often identified in the first 2–3 years of life when a child does not progress from one feeding stage to the next. Problems may include (but are not limited to) food refusal, disruptive mealtime behavior, rigid food preferences, suboptimal growth, and failure to master feeding skills consistent with the child's developmental level. Approximately half to two-thirds of children with feeding disorders present with mixed etiologies that include behavioral, physiological, and developmental factors (Budd et al., 1992; Rommel, De Meyer, Feenstra, & Veereman-Wauters, 2003).

Prevalence

Feeding problems occur in 25–45% of children in the general population (Bentovim, 1970; Forsyth, Leventhal, & McCarthy, 1985). Generally, younger children have more feeding problems than older children. Although some children's feeding habits improve as they age, the general trend is for early feeding problems to persist (Babbitt, Hoch, & Coe, 1994; Dahl & Sundelin, 1992). Some research suggests that untreated feeding problems may predict eating disorders in adolescence and adulthood (Marchi & Cohen, 1990).

The primary concern of caregivers and clinicians is the child's nutritional status. Inadequate caloric intake manifests itself as undernutrition with "failure to thrive" (a condition in which children have suboptimal weight gain followed by a deceleration in linear growth). One survey found that 10–20% of children in the United States are undernourished, and that these children account for 1–5% of pediatric hospital admissions (Bithoney & Rathbun, 1983). If malnutrition ensues (weight less than 80% of the ideal body weight for height), adverse effects on cognitive development (Drotar & Sturm, 1988; Galler, Ramsey, Solimano, Lowell, & Mason, 1983), and emotional regulation (Polan et al., 1990; Wolke, Skuse, & Mathisen, 1989) may result.

Etiology

A variety of problems may affect an infant's or child's ability or desire to eat. These include medical or physical disorders, developmental delays, caregiver–child interactive problems, caregiver competence, and societal problems such as food scarcity or poverty.

Medical or Physical Disorders

Acute medical conditions (e.g., gastroenteritis, strep infection) may cause decreased appetite, fatigue, nausea, and abdominal pain. Fortunately, these conditions tend to have transient effects on nutritional status. However, chronic conditions (e.g., cleft lip and palate, trisomy 21), are of greater concern, as they can lead to nutritional compromise (Kirby & Noel, 2007; Needlman, Adair, & Bresnahan, 1998). Furthermore, some medications have side effects (e.g., diarrhea, constipation, nausea, vomiting, anorexia, dyspepsia, and abdominal pain) that can contribute to feeding problems (Needlman et al., 1998). Conditions that require nasal or gastric tube feeding frequently disrupt a child's association of oral feeding with satiation of hunger (Blackman & Nelson, 1985, 1987; Geertsma, Hyams, Pelletier, & Reiter, 1985). In some instances, feeding safety concerns stemming from aspiration prohibit oral feeding during sensitive periods, resulting in disrupted oral–motor skill development (Field, Garland, & Williams, 2003).

Developmental Disability

Feeding disorders are prevalent in developmentally disabled populations, with approximately one-third affected (Gouge & Ekvall, 1975). As many as 80% of children with severe or profound mental retardation have a feeding disorder (Manikam & Perman, 2000; Perske, Clifton, McLean, & Stein, 1977). These high prevalence rates are likely due to delayed development of, or deficiencies in, the oral–motor skills and fine motor skills required for independent feeding. The prevalence rates of feeding problems due to medical and developmental problems are expected to rise as the survival rate of children with developmental disabilities increases.

Sensory Processing

Some theorists posit that sensory processing problems (Morris & Klein, 1987), due to neurological abnormalities (Walter, 1994), contribute to or cause feeding problems. To date, however, there is scant research supporting the validity of sensory diagnoses and the efficacy of sensory treatments. It is also unclear whether "sensory therapies" actually use well-validated desensitization techniques (Fishbein et al., 2006; Gibbons, Williams, & Riegel, 2007). In spite of limited empirical support, sensory integration treatments are widely used for pediatric feeding disorders.

Social and Environmental Factors

Feeding is an interactive process. In a normally developing child, feeding success depends on the caregiver's ability to create an environment that facilitates the child's ability to attend to cues of hunger and satiety. Caregiver overcontrol of meals (Birch & Marlin, 1982; Johnson & Birch, 1994) and caregiver concerns about child health, weight, and food consumption (Crist et al., 1994) can disrupt self-regulation of food intake and increase behavioral problems. Likewise, childhood feeding problems are associated with high levels of parenting stress (Babbitt et al., 1994; Crist et al., 1994; Garro, Thurman, Kerwin, & Ducette, 2005; Powers et al., 2002). Caregiver physical and mental health problems, knowledge of medical and nutritional conditions, family financial difficulties, and cultural expectations for feeding also influence feeding problems. These environmental variables have not been systematically studied, but warrant attention in both diagnosis and treatment of feeding problems.

In conclusion, most feeding problems have multiple etiologies. Therapists and researchers alike are advised to consider medical, developmental, social, and environmental factors in the diagnosis, treatment, and study of these conditions.

Assessment

Assessment should clarify a family's treatment objectives, identify components of the feeding problem, and determine whether the family's objectives are appropriate and achievable. Typically, assessment consists of a medical record review, caregiver-completed questionnaires, a clinical interview, and observation of the child during feeding. Interdisciplinary assessments, including those completed by a physician, speech and language pathologist and/or occupational therapist, dietitian, and pediatric psychologist, are particularly well suited to achieving the goals listed above.

Medical Records and Questionnaires

Assessment of a child's medical, developmental, and environmental status can be obtained in part by questionnaires. Feeding questionnaires have been developed to assess the severity of behavioral problems occurring during meals (Archer, Rosenbaum, & Streiner, 1991; Davies et al., 2006), the feeding relationship (Davies, Ackerman, Davies, Vannatta, & Noll, 2007; Johnson & Birch, 1994; Musher-Eizenman & Holub, 2007), and feeding skills (Crist et al., 1994). Parents may also be asked to report on their own psychosocial functioning; such instruments as the Symptom Checklist-90—Revised (Derogatis, 1983) and the Parenting Stress Index (Abidin, 1995) may be useful in gauging caregiver factors that affect feeding behaviors. Although questionnaires can be useful for extracting clinically relevant information, they are not substitutes for a clinical interview.

Clinical Interview

The clinical interview is used to clarify the family's concerns and to obtain information for making a diagnosis and developing treatment strategies. Interdisciplinary interviews are especially beneficial, as each team member benefits from questions asked by others during feeding assessments. Interviews focus on the child's medical and developmental history, feeding milestones, family mealtimes and daily routines, onset and nature of the specific feeding problems, and previous attempts at interventions. Questions regarding cultural meal practices can provide important information regarding the family's mealtime expectations; perceptions of feeding problems; and desire to engage in medical, behavioral, and/or other therapeutic interventions. The psychologist also assesses the family's mental health history and current family stressors.

Mealtime Observation

An observation of child and caregiver interaction during a meal is central to a feeding assessment (Linscheid, Budd, & Rasnake, 2003). The goal of the observation is to determine whether the parent–child interaction is reinforcing the feeding problem (e.g., the parent is coaxing the child to eat). Typically, feeding observations are done *in vivo* with a simulated meal. Ideally, a meal is simulated when the child would be expected to be hungry (e.g., after 2 hours of fasting), with the interdisciplinary team observing behind a one-way mirror or via closed-circuit television to minimize the effects of direct observation on the feeding interactions. Preferred and nonpreferred foods are presented, and the psychologist records specific behaviors (e.g., bites accepted, refusal frequency and severity). To facilitate the observation, some objective observation rating scales have been developed to assess caregiver–child interactions. These include the Mother–Infant/Toddler Feeding Scale (Chatoor, 1986), the Dyadic Interaction Nomenclature for Eating (Stark et al., 1997), and the Mealtime Observation Schedule (Sanders, Patel, Le Grice, & Shepherd, 1993).

Behavioral Treatment

Considerable evidence supports the use of behavioral approaches in the treatment of feeding disorders (Babbitt et al., 1994; Kerwin, 1999; Linscheid, 2006). Consequently, behavioral treatment strategies are used in outpatient, day treatment, and inpatient care settings. Treatment goals typically consist of (1) decreasing behavioral problems at meals; (2) decreasing parent stress at meals; (3) increasing pleasurable parent–child interactions at meals; (4) increasing oral intake or variety of oral intake; (4) advancing texture (e.g., moving from pureed and smooth foods to chewable solids); and (5) increasing meal structure and routine (Fischer & Silverman, 2007). Behavioral treatment includes implementation of a feeding schedule, appetite manipulation, behavior management, and parent training. Ongoing consultation with other specialists (especially a dietitian and a speech pathologist) is often needed to monitor the safety of the treatment plan, which can at times result in transient weight loss, or unmask oral–motor or swallowing deficits.

Feeding Environment

A consistent feeding environment is perhaps the most basic and easily implemented of the behavioral interventions. Naturalistic observations (Drotar, Eckerle, Satola, Pallotta, & Wyatt, 1990; Mathisen, Skuse, Wolke, & Reilly, 1989) and common clinical practices support the creation of a predictable feeding environment (e.g., all meals in the dining room), use of secure seating for the child (e.g., a highchair or booster seat with a strap), and creation of a mealtime environment free from distractions (e.g., elimination of television and toys). Ideally, the meal is prepared before the child comes to the table, reducing distraction from non-food-related stimuli. During mealtimes, food and beverage should be placed in front of the child, regardless of the child's interest in eating. Sitting at the table, in turn, allows for ongoing exposure to foods and beverages and gives family members the opportunity to model appropriate feeding behaviors. All of these interventions are intended to create an environment that reduces ambiguity about the tasks associated with feeding, to enhance the caregiver's control over the feeding interaction.

Feeding Schedule and Appetite Manipulation

Children who eat on a fixed schedule without "grazing" between scheduled meals generally consume more calories than do same-age peers without these restrictions. Mealtimes that are too short (Mathisen et al., 1989) or too long (Linscheid et al., 1995) are associated with increased frequency and severity of feeding problems. Once children learn that meals are only offered at specific times and that food selection is left to caregivers, they are no longer reinforced for maintaining food refusal. Creating a predictable feeding schedule facilitates promotion of appetite, motivating children to reach specific feeding goals (Linscheid, 2006). It also allows children to experience the natural consequences of hunger after a low-volume or "failed" meal, and teaches them to be responsive to internal cues of hunger and satiety. Caregivers are often surprised to learn that restricting access to foods has this benefit.

Some medications have been used to induce hunger (e.g., cyproheptadine) or to reduce anxiety that may cause a child to ignore hunger cues (e.g., clonidine), but few data are available on the efficacy of these interventions. The children who benefit most from appetite stimulants are those with suboptimal nutrition who have intact oral skills but are unresponsive to internal hunger cues.

Prior to implementing appetite manipulation, the clinician should assess (1) medical conditions that prohibit periods of fasting; (2) the child's hunger drive; (3) the child's developmental and oral–motor skills, to ensure that foods presented are commensurate with the child's feeding abilities; and (4) the caregiver's acceptance of appetite manipulation, so as not to cause undue stress on the family. Given the medical and nutritional concerns that can arise with this treatment strategy, it should be conducted in consultation with a dietitian and pediatrician.

Behavior Management

Behavioral strategies can be used to promote eating new foods, advance acceptance of foods with different textures, increase caloric intake, decrease dependence on milk or supplemental feedings, and reduce negative feeding behaviors. The essential elements of behavior management are (1) identifying the targeted behavior for change; (2) selecting techniques to increase or decrease behaviors congruent with feeding goals; and (3) developing a treatment plan that consistently pairs a contingency (positive or negative) with the targeted behavior. Strategies to increase behaviors include use of positive and negative reinforcement, as well as discrimination training. Extinction, satiation, punishment, and desensitization are used to reduce behavior. Typically, these strategies are used in combination to create the strongest treatment effects in the shortest time. For comprehensive reviews, see Linscheid (2006) and Kedesdy and Budd (1998).

Parent Training

Parents learn interventions from providers and implement these recommendations in the home environment. Parents are educated about how adaptive and maladaptive behaviors develop and become reinforced, how to assess antecedents and consequences as they affect behavior, and how to use basic behavioral interventions to effect change. Parent training often includes (1) the provision of written information, including descriptions of intervention techniques to be used; (2) therapist modeling intervention techniques during a simulated meal; (3) *in vivo* coaching, directly with the child in the room or through remote coaching (e.g., behind a one-way mirror) to refine parent skills; and (4) review of video-recorded feeding in the natural environments in which the child eats.

Treatment Setting

Feeding problems are typically treated in outpatient settings by individual practitioners. Some outpatient clinics have interdisciplinary care models, but these programs are generally housed within large children's hospitals that have resources for comprehensive clinics. Outpatient settings are typically more accessible to families and may be advantageous when interdisciplinary care is not essential. Outpatient treatment may be best suited to treatments that primarily involve parent training. When a feeding disorder is severe or complex, intensive treatment (day treatment or inpatient care) is warranted. Intensive treatment facilities have several advantages over outpatient settings, including (1) greater environmental control; (2) greater intensity of treatment; (3) accelerated learning by increased contact with caregivers; and (4) daily medical and nutritional monitoring, thus providing clinicians with more treatment options (e.g., appetite manipulation, swallow induction). Intensive feeding programs are designed to allow a high frequency of interactions with a behavior therapist and frequent assessment by other interdisciplinary team members (e.g., a physician, nutritionist, speech and language therapist, occupational therapist). When a child is dependent on supplemental tube feeding, appetite manipulation can be used safely to create hunger and to help the child experience satiation of hunger through oral feeding. Under these conditions, the child must be monitored closely for nutrient and fluid intake. Reductions in supplemental tube feeding without appropriate supervision and without the behavioral component of the intervention are unlikely to be successful and can be associated with medical risk due to ketosis, which inhibits appetite (Johnstone, Horgan, Murison, Bremner, & Lobley, 2008). Disadvantages of inpatient care include high cost, disruption of family life during treatment, and the scarcity of treatment programs.

Feeding Problems: Summary

Feeding problems are commonly encountered in children and can have substantial negative consequences for child development and family dynamics. Increasingly, health care professionals are recognizing the complex contributions of anatomic, physiological, developmental, and behavioral factors in the development of feeding problems. Behavioral treatment of feeding disorders in children is well established and empirically supported. Applied in an interdisciplinary clinic, behavioral treatments address the multiple etiologies of feeding problems in young children.

Vomiting Disorders and Rumination

Functional vomiting disorders and rumination are characterized by chronic and/or recurrent gastrointestinal symptoms for which no medical cause has been identified (Rasquin et al., 2006). The current diagnostic standard for functional gastrointestinal disorders, the Rome III criteria, provide for better recognition of these disorders and help guide research to improve treatment of these conditions in children (Hyman et al., 2006; Rasquin et al., 2006). However, the application of these criteria in clinical practice is sometimes difficult, as children often present with symptoms that either overlap classified disorders or are not easily classified by these criteria (Caplan, Walker, & Rasquin, 2006).

Cyclic vomiting syndrome (CVS) is the only pediatric vomiting disorder identified in Rome III. Although functional vomiting and chronic idiopathic nausea are included in Rome III as diagnoses of functional gastrointestinal disorders in adults, they also occur in the pediatric population, so they are briefly reviewed as well.

Cyclic Vomiting Syndrome

CVS is characterized by recurring, severe, stereotypic vomiting/retching episodes, lasting from hours to days, with periods of normal health between episodes (Li, 2000). CVS is diagnosed only after other serious medical conditions that may mimic its symptomatology (e.g., intestinal malrotation, increased intracranial pressure, hydronephrosis, metabolic disorders) have been excluded (Li, 2000). Although CVS is the most well described and researched of the functional vomiting disorders, it is still poorly recognized by pediatric professionals, with children having symptoms for an average of 2.6 years before being correctly diagnosed with CVS (Li, 2000). Pediatric population-based studies report a prevalence rate of approximately 2% (Abu-Arafeh & Russell, 1995; Ertekin, Selimoglu, & Altnkaynak, 2006). The median age of onset is 4.8 years, with a slight predominance of girls over boys (Li & Misiewicz, 2003). The presentation of CVS remains stable across development, with the exception that the duration of CVS episodes increases progressively with age (Prakash, Staiano, Rothbaum, & Clouse, 2001). Clinical reports of children with CVS indicate that it lasts approximately 2–5 years and typically resolves between 9 and 14 years of age; however, CVS can also begin in adolescence or adulthood (Li, 2000).

Vomiting episodes are stereotypic for a majority of children (Li & Balint, 2000). Prodromal symptoms may appear before the vomiting, including loss of appetite, nausea, pallor, lethargy, social withdrawal, and irritability (Li & Misiewicz, 2003). Onset of the vomiting attack commonly occurs in the early morning hours or upon awakening, with high-intensity vomiting accompanied by symptoms of unrelenting nausea, retching, and severe abdominal pain (Li & Misiewicz, 2003). Notably, the vomiting does not relieve symptoms of nausea and abdominal discomfort, as is typically the case with gastroenteritis or influenza. Associated signs and symptoms can include fever, diarrhea, light and sound sensitivity, abdominal pain, vertigo, headache, and excess salivation (Li, 2000; Li & Misiewicz, 2003). Episodes occur with an average frequency of every 2–4 weeks (Li & Misiewicz, 2003).

A majority (82%) of children with CVS have a subtype considered to be a migraine variant, based on similarities in symptoms (e.g., pallor, nausea, abdominal pain, vomiting), as well as their clinical response to antimigraine therapies and a positive family history of migraine (Li & Misiewicz, 2003; Stickler, 2005). As is the case with migraine headache, families frequently report "triggers" for the attacks, including infections (31%) and psychological stress (47%)—especially excitement or "positive stress," such as birthdays, holidays, and special events (Li & Misiewicz, 2003), as well as negative stressors, such as school or family problems, sleep changes, and missed meals (Li & Balint, 2000). Episodes tend to improve in the summer, perhaps because of fewer school related stressors and infections (Li & Misiewicz, 2003). It is estimated that 28% of children with CVS will develop migraines by the time they reach the age of 18 years (Li & Misiewicz, 2003). Other distinct CVS subtypes include disorders of energy metabolism with an earlier onset of CVS (i.e., ≤ 1 year of age) (Boles, Powers, & Adams, 2006); menstrual-related episodes (Li & Misiewicz, 2003); the Sato subtype, which is characterized by profound lethargy and hypertension, and is associated with the most prolonged (6 days) and intense episodes (92 emeses/episode) (Li, 2000); and timed or calendar-based CVS, wherein attacks reliably occur after a specific number of days (Li, 2000).

Etiology/Pathophysiology

Although the pathogenesis of CVS is unknown, several theories have been advanced to account for this disorder. Given that CVS is heterogeneous in its manifestations, it is unlikely that one theory will account for all variations of this vomiting disorder. Taché and Li have hypothesized that a perturbation of the hypothalamic–pituitary–adrenal axis—in particular, an increase in corticotropin-releasing hormone—acts as a possible mediator of the vomiting attack (Sunku, Kagawalla, & Li, 2003; Taché, 1999). Measurements of stress hormones taken during CVS episodes offer preliminary support for this hypothesis (Marcus et al., 2006). Autonomic abnormalities have also been identified in children with CVS. Chelimsky and Chelimsky (2007) found abnormal sympathetic function and postural hypotension in a small sample of children with CVS. To, Issenman, and Kamath (1999) assessed heart rate variability in children with CVS and found enhanced sympathetic and diminished parasympathetic modulation of the heart. It is noteworthy that autonomic abnormalities are also associated with migraine headaches (Mosek, Novak, & Opfer-Gehrking, 1999; Sanya, Brown, & von Wilmowsky, 2005).

Mitochondrial disorders, which are maternally inherited conditions that affect cellular energy production, have been found in children with cyclic vomiting, including both those with and those without significant medical and developmental comorbidities (Boles et al., 2006). These disorders of energy metabolism are likely to account for the findings that some children with CVS are heat-intolerant, have difficulties sustaining athletic activities, and tend to "graze" (because they require food at shorter intervals to sustain their activities). These children also are more likely to have a CVS episode during fasting, or when they need to step up energy production, as occurs with illness and exercise.

Medical Treatment

There have been no randomized clinical trials for the medical management of CVS, and thus the information on treatment is based on clinical reports. Medical interventions can significantly improve CVS symptoms, including both the duration and frequency of episodes, but it is not uncommon for a child or adolescent to have CVS attacks intermittently. Medical management includes preventive, abortive, and palliative strategies. For children with one or more episodes per month, or those with long episodes (≥5 days), a preventive strategy is typically used, given the morbidity associated with these episodes. Medications including tricyclic antidepressants, cyproheptadine, beta blockers, oral contraceptives, and antiseizure medications have been used successfully to prevent CVS attacks, particularly those with migraine variants (Pareek, Fleisher, & Abell, 2007). When episodes are infrequent, an abortive approach is typically taken: The child receives antimigraine medications, antiemetics, sedatives, analgesics, and/or intravenous fluids as needed to abort or shorten the attack, or for symptom relief. Children who have calendar-based episodes have been less responsive to these approaches. Generally, the sooner medical intervention is offered in the setting of an acute attack, the better chance there is of symptom control. For those who cannot be managed on an outpatient basis, emergency room visits or hospital admission is indicated to restore electrolyte imbalances, provide intravenous hydration, and relieve symptoms. Complications of CVS include dehydration, electrolyte imbalances, esophagitis, Mallory–Weiss tears, and dental decay (Catto-Smith & Ranuh, 2003).

Psychosocial Factors

Family and School Impact. There is considerable morbidity associated with CVS, for both the affected child and the family as a whole. Children miss nearly 5 weeks of school per year due to CVS (mean = 24 days) (Li & Misiewicz, 2003), compromising not only their education but also their social and recreational activities. Parents attending to their sick child both at home and during hospitalization must spend time away from their other children, miss days of work, and in some cases lose or quit their jobs due to multiple absences related to caring for their sick child. Helpful information for the family can be obtained from the Cyclic Vomiting Syndrome Association, a support organization developed by families of children with CVS (*www.cvsaonline.org*).

The lack of recognition of this disorder by both health care and educational professionals can make educational supports difficult to obtain. An individualized education program, and particularly a Section 504 plan, can provide educational accommodations for children and adolescents whose CVS symptoms interfere with school attendance. Modest educational adjustments can have a significant impact for children with CVS. For example, schools have modified the schedules of students with CVS so that core courses occur later in the day, with electives or study periods in the morning, given the prevalence of the early morning onset of CVS symptoms. Schools also need to be informed that the children are not suffering from a contagious illness such as gastroenteritis or flu, to allow for school attendance once CVS symptoms have resolved.

Psychiatric Comorbidity. Preliminary data suggest that CVS is associated with internalizing psychiatric disorders. Using parent reports on the Child Behavior Checklist (Achenbach, 1991), Forbes, Withers, Silburn and McKelvey (1999) found that children with CVS had significantly higher Total Problem scores than age- and gender-matched controls. These researchers also found that scores for the Internalizing, Somatic Complaints, and Anxious/Depressed scales were more likely to fall in the clinical range for children with CVS. Tarbell and Li (2008) evaluated the prevalence of psychiatric symptoms in children and adolescents with CVS and their parents, using psychiatric symptom reports completed by parents, as well as adolescent self-reports. They found a high prevalence of internalizing disorders, especially anxiety symptoms, in these children and adolescents. Thirty-five percent of mothers also endorsed anxiety disorders in themselves. These preliminary data suggest that children and adolescents with CVS be screened for psychiatric disorders.

Behavioral Treatments

Published descriptions of psychological treatment of CVS are limited to a few case reports. Treatments have included interventions delivered on inpatient psychiatry services, as well as dynamically oriented outpatient family and individual therapy, including play therapy (Fennig & Fennig, 1999; Magagna, 1995; Reinhart, Evans, & McFadden, 1977). The intensity of the services described in these reports may not be necessary to achieve improvement in the psychological and vomiting symptoms for a majority of children. The association between CVS and migraine provides an opportunity to apply well-developed, empirically supported treatments shown to be effective for pediatric migraine to CVS. Behavioral treatments for migraine in children include biofeedback-assisted relaxation therapy to lower physical arousal (e.g., hand warming); cognitive therapy directed toward identification of headache triggers and maladaptive cognitions; and training in coping skills to modify how a child responds to stress (Penzien, Rains, & Andrasik, 2002). Studies reporting the successful use of behavioral treatments (including hypnotherapy, biofeedback, guided imagery, and cognitive-behavioral therapy) for other functional gastrointestinal complaints, such as irritable bowel syndrome and functional abdominal pain in children and adolescents (Blanchard & Scharff, 2002; Humphreys & Gevirtz, 2000; Vlieger, Menko-Frankenhuis, Wolfcamp, Tromp, & Benninga, 2007; Youssef et al., 2004), also may offer promise for children with CVS. Empirically supported behavioral treatments for management of comorbid anxiety and depression (Compton et al., 2004), as well as medication consultation, should be considered as well for children and adolescents with CVS who have comorbid psychiatric disorders.

Changes in functional status and quality of life associated with treatment can be evaluated with measures developed to assess functional status in children with migraine, such as the PedsMIDAS (Hershey et al., 2001), or a more general assessment of quality of life, such as the PedsQL™ (Varni, Seid, Knight, Uzark, & Szer, 2002). Any reductions in the frequency or intensity of the vomiting episodes and associated psychiatric comorbidity should also be noted. To date, there are no adequately validated inventories for the assessment of nausea, vomiting, and retching in children and adolescents. Scales that have been developed use Likert and visual analogue scale ratings for children (and, in some cases, parents) to report on nausea, vomiting, and retching associated with chemotherapy or anesthesia, which may have limited applicability to CVS (Baker & Ellett, 2006).

Functional Vomiting

The criteria for the diagnosis of functional vomiting include one or more episodes of vomiting per week; absence of an eating disorder, rumination, or major *Diagnostic and Statistical Manual of Mental Disorders*, fourth edition (DSM-IV) psychiatric disorder; and absence of self-induced vomiting, central nervous system or metabolic disorders, or chronic marijuana use. These criteria need to be fulfilled for the last 3 months, with symptom onset at least 6 months before diagnosis (Tack et al., 2006). These children and adolescents present with intermittent vomiting that can occur with sufficient frequency to affect their own and their families' activities. Typically children will describe vomiting only once per incident, with the vomiting occurring prior to or during exciting or stressful events such as competitive athletic meets, performances, vacations, and holidays. Impairment is significantly less than that described for CVS; however, these children can be sent home from school or miss activities, due to concerns about infectious illness. There is sparse literature on this condition in children, and our own clinical experience with these youths is that there are often comorbid anxiety symptoms that do not meet criteria for DSM-IV-TR diagnosis. Clinically, these children have responded to cognitive and behavioral interventions focused on lowering arousal during times of anticipated stress (cognitive restructuring, biofeedback-assisted relaxation training). No treatment literature exists for the behavioral management of this condition in children, and there is no evidence that medications are particularly useful for this condition.

Chronic Idiopathic Nausea

The diagnosis of chronic idiopathic nausea includes the presence of bothersome nausea, occurring at least several times per week, not typically associated with vomiting, in the absence of medical abnormalities that would explain the nausea (e.g., peptic ulcer disease, gastritis, celiac disease, delayed gastric emptying, Type 1 diabetes). These criteria need to be fulfilled for the past 3 months, with symptom onset at least 6 months before diagnosis (Tack et al., 2006). This disorder has been noted particularly in adolescent females, who describe severe nausea upon awakening that typically remits by midday. The nausea is of sufficient intensity to interfere with daily activities, including school. Again, no treatment literature to date is directed to the management of this functional disorder, but given the significant functional impairment associated with these symptoms, this disorder is included here to facilitate its recognition by pediatric psychologists.

Rumination

Rumination involves the repeated regurgitation of gastric contents into the mouth, which are either rechewed and reswallowed or expectorated (Hyman et al., 2006). Exclusionary criteria are that the symptoms do not respond to treatment for gastroesophageal reflux disease or anticholinergic medications; do not occur during sleep; and are not accompanied by signs of nausea, distress, or pain. For diagnosis in an infant, the onset of the symptoms occurs between 3 and 8 months, and the symptoms are not responsive to hand restraint, formula changes, gavage, or gastrostomy feedings. In addition, the symptoms are absent when the infant is interacting with others and must be present for at least 3 months (Hyman et al., 2006). In an adolescent, the symptoms should occur soon after meals, with no retching and no evidence of a medical condition that explains the symptoms. These criteria need to be fulfilled at least once per week for at least 2 months before diagnosis (Rasquin et al., 2006). Eating disorders such as bulimia nervosa also need to be ruled out (Eckern, Stevens, & Mitchell, 1999). There is currently no medical treatment for rumination. Surgery (Nissen fundoplication) has been used in a few adult cases with mixed results (Oelschlager, Chan, Eubanks, Pope, & Pellegrini, 2002). Morbidity due to persistent rumination includes weight loss, malnutrition, dental erosions, electrolyte abnormalities, and functional disability (Chial, Camilleri, Williams, Litzinger, & Perrault, 2003).

Rumination is reported to be most common in infants and in children with pervasive developmental disorders and mental retardation (Malcolm, Thumshirn, Camilleri, & Williams, 1997). Psychosocial problems, such as caretaker neglect or lack of stimulation, are considered to be predisposing factors in infants and those with developmental disabilities. However, Lavigne, Burns, and Cotter (1981) described a population of infants with rumination who were developmentally normal and had healthy parent–child interactions. These infants responded to an intervention that included punishment (scolding), time out from positive social reinforcement, and differential reinforcement of nonruminative behaviors. Although there have been no clinical trials of the behavioral treatment of rumination, case studies detail a variety of effective behavioral interventions, including providing starchy food following meals (Thibadeau, Blew, Reedy, & Liuiselli, 1999), food satiation (Clauser & Scibak, 1990), noncontingent high-frequency feeding immediately following meals (Thibadeau et al., 1999), oral hygiene (Singh, Manning, & Angell, 1982), and cognitive-behavioral therapy and biofeedback (Chial et al., 2003).

Recently, there have been several reports on the prevalence and management of rumination in cognitively normal adolescents and adults. A review by Chial and colleagues (2003) reported that the diagnosis of rumination in children and adolescents is often delayed, resulting in significant morbidity, with 72.7% (32/44) missing school secondary to rumination and 46% (35/76) being hospitalized for treatment or complications associated with rumination. Habit reversal, such as diaphragmatic breathing as a competing response for rumination, has been found to be effective for management of rumination in several case reports (Chitkara, Van Tilburg, Whitehead, & Talley, 2006; Malcolm et al., 1997).

Vomiting Disorders and Rumination: Summary

In summary, there is much potential for the pediatric psychologist to contribute to the management children with vomiting disorders and rumination; however, psychological treatment needs to follow a thorough medical evaluation to rule out nonbehavioral factors contributing to these disorders. The limited data available on psychological management of these conditions provide an opportunity for pediatric psychologists to develop and test new behavioral interventions that can contribute to the care of children with these underrecognized disorders, which have a significant impact on quality of life for the children and their families.

References

Abidin, R. (1995). *Parenting Stress Index—Short Form*. Odessa, FL: Psychological Assessment Resources.

Abu-Arafeh, I., & Russell, G. (1995). Cyclical vomiting syndrome in children: A population based study. *Journal of Pediatric Gastroenterology and Nutrition, 21*, 454–458.

Achenbach, T. M. (1991). *Manual for the Child Behavior Checklist/4–18 and 1991 Profile*. Burlington: University of Vermont, Department of Psychiatry.

Archer, L. A., Rosenbaum, P. L., & Streiner, D. L. (1991). The Children's Eating Behavior Inventory: Reliability and validity results. *Journal of Pediatric Psychology, 16*, 629–642.

Babbitt, R. L., Hoch, T. A., & Coe, D. A. (1994). Behavioral feeding disorders. In D. N. Tuchman & R. S. Walters (Eds.), *Disorders of feeding and swallowing in infants and children* (pp. 77–95). San Diego, CA: Singular.

Baker, P. D., & Ellett, M. L. (2006). Measuring nausea and vomiting in adolescents. *Gastroenterology Nursing, 30*, 18–28.

Bentovim, A. (1970). The clinical approach to feeding disorders of childhood. *Journal of Psychosomatic Research, 14*, 267–276.

Birch, L. L., & Marlin, D. W. (1982). I don't like it; I never tried it: Effects of exposure on two-year-old children's food preferences. *Appetite, 3*, 353–360.

Bithoney, W. G., & Rathbun, J. M. (1983). Failure to thrive. In M. Levine, W. Carey, A. Crocker, & R. Gross (Eds.), *Developmental-behavioral pediatrics* (pp. 557–572). Philadelphia: Saunders.

Blackman, J. A., & Nelson, C. L. A. (1985). Reinstituting oral feedings in children fed by gastrostomy tube. *Clinical Pediatrics, 24*, 434–438.

Blackman, J. A., & Nelson, C. L. A. (1987). Rapid introduction of oral feedings to tube-fed patients. *Journal of Developmental and Behavioral Pediatrics, 8*, 63–67.

Blanchard, E. B., & Scharff, L. (2002). Psychosocial aspects of assessment and treatment of irritable bowel syndrome in adults and recurrent abdominal pain in children. *Journal of Consulting and Clinical Psychology, 70*, 725–738.

Boles, R. G., Powers, A. L. R., & Adams, K. (2006). Cyclic vomiting syndrome plus. *Journal of Child Neurology, 21*, 182–188.

Budd, K. S., McGraw, T. E., Farbisz, R., Murphy, T. B., Hawkins, D., Heilman, N., et al. (1992). Psychosocial concomitants of children's feeding disorders. *Journal of Pediatric Psychology, 17*, 81–94.

Caplan, A., Walker, L., & Rasquin, A. J. (2006). Validation of the pediatric Rome III criteria for functional gastrointestinal disorders using the questionnaire on pediatric gastrointestinal symptoms. *Pediatric Gastroenterology and Nutrition, 41*, 305–316.

Catto-Smith, A. G., & Ranuh, R. (2003). Abdominal migraine and cyclical vomiting. *Seminars in Pediatric Surgery, 12*, 254–258.

Chatoor, I. (1986). *Mother–Infant/Toddler Feeding Scale*. Unpublished manuscript, Children's National Medical Center, Washington, DC.

Chelimsky, T. C., & Chelimsky, G. C. (2007). Autonomic abnormalities in cyclic vomiting syndrome. *Journal of Pediatric Gastroenterology and Nutrition, 44*, 326–300.

Chial, H. J., Camilleri, M., Williams, D. E., Litzinger, K., & Perrault, J. (2003). Rumination syndrome in children and adolescents: Diagnosis, treatment, and prognosis. *Pediatrics, 111*, 158–162.

Chitkara, D. K., Van Tilburg, M., Whitehead, W. E., & Talley, N. J. (2006). Teaching diaphragmatic breathing for rumination syndrome. *American Journal of Gastroenterology, 101,* 2449–2452.

Clauser, B., & Scibak, J. W. (1990). Direct and generalized effects of food satiation in reducing rumination. *Research in Developmental Disabilities, 11,* 23–36.

Compton, S. N., Marsh, J. S., Bent, D., Albano, A. M., Weersing, R., & Curry, J. (2004). Cognitive-behavioral psychotherapy for anxiety and depressive disorders in children and adolescents: An evidence-based review. *Journal of the American Academy of Child and Adolescent Psychiatry, 43,* 930–959.

Crist, W., McDonnel, P., Beck, M., Gillespie, C. T., Barrett, P., & Mathews, J. (1994). Behavior at mealtimes and the young child with cystic fibrosis. *Journal of Developmental and Behavioral Pediatrics, 15,* 279–286.

Dahl, M., & Sundelin, C. (1992). Feeding problems in an affluent society: Follow-up at four years of age in children with early refusal to eat. *Acta Paediatrica, 81,* 575–579.

Davies, W. H., Ackerman, L. K., Davies, C. M., Vannatta, K., & Noll, R. B. (2007). About Your Child's Eating: Factor structure and psychometric properties of a feeding relationship measure. *Eating Behaviors, 8,* 457–463.

Davies, W. H., Satter, E., Berlin, K. S., Sato, A. F., Silverman, A. H., Fischer, E. A., et al. (2006). Reconceptualizing feeding and feeding disorders in interpersonal context: The case for a relational disorder. *Journal of Family Psychology, 20,* 409–417.

Derogatis, L. R. (1983). *SCL-90-R: Administration, scoring and interpretation manual.* Towson, MD: Clinical Psychometric Research.

Drotar, D., Eckerle, D., Satola, J., Pallotta, J., & Wyatt, B. (1990). Maternal interactional behavior with nonorganic failure-to-thrive infants: A case comparison study. *Child Abuse and Neglect, 14,* 41–51.

Drotar, D., & Sturm, L. (1988). Prediction of intellectual development in young children with early histories of failure to thrive. *Journal of Pediatric Psychology, 13,* 281–295.

Eckern, M., Stevens, W., & Mitchell, J. (1999). The relationship between rumination and eating disorders. *International Journal of Eating Disorders, 26,* 414–419.

Ertekin, V., Selimoglu, M. A., & Altnkaynak, S. (2006). Prevalence of cyclic vomiting syndrome in a sample of Turkish school children in an urban area. *Journal of Clinical Gastroenterology, 40,* 896–898.

Fennig, S., & Fennig, S. (1999). Cyclic vomiting syndrome: Role of a psychiatric inpatient unit in a general children's hospital. *Journal of Pediatric Gastroenterology and Nutrition, 29,* 207–210.

Field, D., Garland, M., & Williams, K. (2003). Correlates of specific childhood feeding problems. *Journal of Paediatrics and Child Health, 39,* 299–304.

Fischer, E. A., & Silverman, A. H. (2007). Behavioral conceptualization, assessment, and treatment of pediatric feeding disorders. *Seminars in Speech and Language, 28,* 223–231.

Fishbein, M., Cox, S., Swenny, C., Mogren, C., Walbert, L., & Fraker, C. (2006). Food chaining: A systematic approach for the treatment of children with feeding aversion. *Nutrition in Clinical Practice, 21,* 182–184.

Forbes, D., Withers, G., Silburn, S., & McKelvey, R. (1999). Psychological and social characteristics and precipitants of vomiting in children with cyclic vomiting syndrome. *Digestive Diseases and Sciences, 44,* 19S–22S.

Forsyth, B. W. C., Leventhal, J. M., & McCarthy, P. L. (1985). Mothers' perceptions of problems of feeding and crying behaviors: A prospective study. *American Journal of Diseases of Children, 139,* 269–272.

Galler, J. R., Ramsey, F., Solimano, G., Lowell, W. E., & Mason, E. (1983). The influence of early malnutrition on subsequent behavioral development: I. Degree of impairment in intellectual performance. *Journal of the American Academy of Child Psychiatry, 22,* 8–15.

Garro, A., Thurman, S. K., Kerwin, M. E., & Ducette, J. P. (2005). Parent/caregiver stress during pediatric hospitalization for chronic feeding problems. *Journal of Pediatric Nursing*, *20*, 268–275.

Geertsma, M. A., Hyams, J. S., Pelletier, J. M., & Reiter, S. (1985). Feeding resistance after parenteral hyperalimentation. *American Journal of Diseases of Children*, *139*, 255–256.

Gibbons, B. G., Williams, K. E., & Riegel, K. E. (2007). Reducing tube feeds and tongue thrust: Combining an oral–motor and behavioral approach to feeding. *American Journal of Occupational Therapy*, *61*, 384–391.

Gouge, A. L., & Ekvall, S. W. (1975). Diets of handicapped children: Physical, psychological, and socioeconomic correlations. *American Journal of Mental Deficiency*, *80*, 149–157.

Hagekull, B., & Dahl, M. (1987). Infants with and without feeding difficulties: Maternal experiences. *International Journal of Eating Disorders*, *6*, 83–98.

Hershey, A. D., Powers, S. W., Vockell, A.-L. B., LeCates, S., Kabbouche, M. A., & Maynard, M. K. (2001). PedMIDAS: Development of a questionnaire to assess disability of migraines in children. *Neurology*, *57*, 2034–2039.

Humphreys, P. A., & Gevirtz, R. N. (2000). Treatment of recurrent abdominal pain: Components analysis of four treatment protocols. *Journal of Pediatric Gastroenterology and Nutrition*, *31*, 47–51.

Hyman, P. E., Milla, P. J., Benninga, M. A., Davidson, G. P., Fleisher, D. F., & Taminiau, J. (2006). Childhood functional gastrointestinal disorders: Neonate/toddler. *Gastroenterology*, *130*, 1519–1526.

Johnson, S. L., & Birch, L. L. (1994). Parents' and children's adiposity and eating style. *Pediatrics*, *94*, 653–661.

Johnstone, A. M., Horgan, G. W., Murison, S. D., Bremner, D. M., & Lobley, G. E. (2008). Effects of a high-protein ketogenic diet on hunger, appetite, and weight loss in obese men feeding ad libitum. *American Journal of Clinical Nutrition*, *87*, 44–55.

Kedesdy, J. H., & Budd, K. S. (1998). Environmental interventions in feeding: An overview. In J. H. Kedesdy & K. S. Budd (Eds.), *Childhood feeding disorders: Biobehavioral assessment and intervention* (pp. 115–157). Baltimore: Brookes.

Kerwin, M. E. (1999). Empirically supported treatments in pediatric psychology: Severe feeding problems. *Journal of Pediatric Psychology*, *24*(3), 193–214.

Kirby, M., & Noel, R. J. (2007). Nutrition and gastrointestinal track assessment and management of children with dysphagia. *Seminars in Speech and Language*, *28*(3), 180–189.

Lavigne, J. V., Burns, W. J., & Cotter, P. D. (1981). Rumination in infancy: Recent behavioral approaches. *International Journal of Eating Disorders*, *1*, 70–82.

Li, B. U. K. (2000). Cyclic vomiting syndrome and abdominal migraine. *International Seminars in Pediatric Gastroenterology and Nutrition*, *9*, 1–9.

Li, B. U. K., & Balint, J. P. (2000). Cyclic vomiting syndrome: Evolution of our understanding of a brain–gut disorder. *Advances in Pediatrics*, *47*, 117–160.

Li, B. U. K., & Misiewicz, L. (2003). Cyclic vomiting syndrome: A brain–gut disorder. *Gastroenterology Clinics of North America*, *32*, 997–1019.

Lindberg, L., Bohlin, G., Hagekull, B., & Thunstrome, M. (1994). Early food refusal: Infant and family characteristics. *Infant Mental Health Journal*, *15*, 262–277.

Linscheid, T. J. (2006). Behavioral treatments for pediatric feeding disorders. *Behavior Modification*, *30*, 6–23.

Linscheid, T. R., Budd, K. S., & Rasnake, L. K. (1995). Pediatric feeding disorders. In M. C. Roberts (Ed.), *Handbook of pediatric psychology* (2nd ed., pp. 501–515). New York: Guilford Press.

Linscheid, T. J., Budd, K. S., & Rasnake, L. K. (2003). Pediatric feeding problems. In M. C. Roberts (Ed.), *Handbook of pediatric psychology* (3rd ed., pp. 481–498.). New York: Guilford Press.

Magagna, J. (1995). Psychophysiologic treatment of cyclic vomiting. *Journal of Pediatric Gastroenterology and Nutrition, 21*(Suppl. 1), S31–S36.

Malcolm, A., Thumshirn, M. B., Camilleri, M., & Williams, D. E. (1997). Rumination syndrome. *Mayo Clinic Proceedings, 72,* 646–652.

Manikam, R., & Perman, J. A. (2000). Pediatric feeding disorders. *Journal of Clinical Gastroenterology, 30,* 34–46.

Marchi, M., & Cohen, P. (1990). Early childhood eating behaviors and adolescent eating disorders. *Journal of the American Academy of Child and Adolescent Psychiatry, 29,* 112–117.

Marcus, S. B., Agiabe-Williams, M., Grigoriadis, D. E., Taché, Y., Zimmerman, D., & Li, B U. K. (2006). Corticotropin-releasing factor (CRF) levels are elevated during episodes of cyclic vomiting syndrome. *Gastroenterology, 130*(4, Suppl. 2), A-4, Abstract 24.

Mathisen, B., Skuse, D., Wolke, D., & Reilly, S. (1989). Oral–motor dysfunction and failure to thrive among inner-city infants. *Developmental Medicine and Child Neurology, 31,* 293–302.

Morris, S. E., & Klein, M. D. (1987). *Pre-feeding skills: A comprehensive resource for feeding development.* Tucson, AZ: Therapy Skill Builders.

Mosek, A., Novak, V., & Opfer-Gehrking, T. L. (1999). Autonomic dysfunction in migraineurs. *Headache, 39,* 108–117.

Musher-Eizenman, D., & Holub, S. (2007). Comprehensive Feeding Practices Questionnaire: Validation of a new measure of parental feeding practices. *Journal of Pediatric Psychology, 32*(8), 960–972.

Needlman, B., Adair, R. H., & Bresnahan, K. (1998). Biological factors in feeding and growth. In J. H. Kedesdy & K. S. Budd (Eds.), *Childhood feeding disorders: Biobehavioral assessment and intervention* (pp. 33–77). Baltimore: Brookes.

Oelschlager, B. K., Chan, M. M., Eubanks, T. R., Pope, C. E., II, & Pellegrini, C. A. (2002). Effective treatment of rumination with Nissen fundoplication. *Journal of Gastrointestinal Surgery, 6,* 638–644.

Pareek, N., Fleisher, D. R., & Abell, T. A. (2007). Cyclic vomiting syndrome: What a gastroenterologist needs to know. *American Journal of Gastroenterology, 102,* 2832–2840.

Penzien, D. B., Rains, J. C., & Andrasik, F. (2002). Behavioral treatment of recurrent headache: Three decades of experience and empiricism. *Applied Psychophysiology and Biofeedback, 27,* 163–181.

Perske, R., Clifton, A., McLean, B. M., & Stein, J. E. (Eds.). (1977). *Mealtimes for severely and profoundly handicapped persons: New concepts and attitudes.* Baltimore: University Park Press.

Polan, H. J., Leon, A., Kaplan, M. D., Kessler, D. B., Stern, D. N., & Ward, M. J. (1990). Disturbances of affect expression in failure-to-thrive. *Journal of the American Academy of Child and Adolescent Psychiatry, 30,* 897–903.

Powers, S. W., Byars, K. C., Mitchell, M. J., Patton, S. R., Standiford, D. A., & Dolan, L. M. (2002). Parent report of mealtime behavior and parenting stress in young children with Type 1 diabetes and in healthy control subjects. *Diabetes Care, 25,* 313–318.

Prakash, C., Staiano, A., Rothbaum, R. J., & Clouse, R. E. (2001). Similarities in cyclic vomiting syndrome across age groups. *American Journal of Gastroenterology, 96,* 684–688.

Rasquin, A., Di Lorenzo, C., Forbes, D., Guiraldes, E., Hyams, J. S., Staiano, A., et al. (2006). Childhood functional gastrointestinal disorders: Child/adolescent. *Gastroenterology, 130,* 1527–1537.

Reinhart, J. B., Evans, S. L., & McFadden, D. L. (1977). Cyclic vomiting in children: Seen through the psychiatrist's eye. *Pediatrics, 59,* 371–377.

Rommel, N., De Meyer, A. M., Feenstra, L., & Veereman-Wauters, G. (2003). The complexity of feeding problems in 700 infants and young children presenting to a tertiary care institution. *Journal of Pediatric Gastroenterology and Nutrition, 37,* 75–84.

Sanders, M. R., Patel, R. K., Le Grice, B., & Shepherd, R. W. (1993). Children with persistent feeding difficulties: An observational analysis of the feeding interactions of problem and non-problem eaters. *Health Psychology, 12,* 64–73.

Sanya, E. O., Brown, C. M., & von Wilmowsky, C. (2005). Impairment of parasympathetic baroflex responses in migraine patients. *Acta Neurologica Scandinavica, 111,* 102–107.

Singer, L. T., Song, L. Y., Hill, B. P., & Jaffe, A. C. (1990). Stress and depression in mothers of failure-to-thrive children. *Journal of Pediatric Psychology, 15*(6), 711–720.

Singh, N. N., Manning, P. J., & Angell, M. J. (1982). Effects of an oral hygiene punishment procedure on chronic rumination and collateral behaviors in monozygous twins. *Journal of Applied Behavior Analysis, 15,* 309–314.

Stark, L. J., Mulvihill, M. M., Jelalian, E., Bowen, A. M., Powers, S. W., Tao, S., et al. (1997). Descriptive analysis of eating behavior in school-age children with cystic fibrosis and healthy control children. *Pediatrics, 99,* 665–671.

Stickler, G. B. (2005). Relationship between cyclic vomiting syndrome and migraine. *Clinical Pediatrics, 44,* 505–508.

Sunku, B., Kagawalla, A., & Li, B. U. K. (2003). *Is Sato's subtype of cyclic vomiting syndrome more severe?* Paper presented at the meeting of the North American Society of Pediatric Gastroenterology, Hepatology and Nutrition, Montréal.

Taché, Y. (1999). Cyclic vomiting syndrome: The corticotropin-releasing factor hypothesis. *Digestive Diseases and Sciences, 44*(Suppl.), 79S–86S.

Tack, J., Talley, N. J., Camilleri, M., Holtmann, G., Hu, P., Malagelada, J.-R., et al. (2006). Functional gastroduodenal disorders. *Gastroenterology, 130,* 1466–1479.

Tarbell, S., & Li, B. U. K. (2008). Psychiatric symptoms in children and adolescents with cyclic vomiting syndrome and their parents. *Headache, 48,* 259–266.

Thibadeau, S., Blew, P., Reedy, P., & Liuiselli, J. K. (1999). Access to white bread as an intervention for chronic ruminative vomiting. *Journal of Behavior Therapy and Experimental Psychiatry, 30,* 137–144.

To, J., Issenman, R. M., & Kamath, M. V. (1999). Evaluation of neurocardiac signals in pediatric patients with cyclic vomiting syndrome through power spectral analysis of heart rate variability. *Journal of Pediatrics, 135,* 363–366.

Varni, J. W., Seid, M., Knight, T., Uzark, K., & Szer, I. (2002). The PedsQL 4.0 Generic Core scales: Sensitivity, responsiveness, and impact on clinical decision-making. *Journal of Behavioral Medicine, 25,* 175–193.

Vlieger, A. M., Menko-Frankenhuis, C., Wolfcamp, S. C. S., Tromp, E., & Benninga, M. A. (2007). Hypnotherapy for children with functional abdominal pain or irritable bowel syndrome: A randomized controlled trial. *Gastroenterology, 133,* 1430–1436.

Walter, R. S. (1994). Issues surrounding the development of feeding and swallowing. In D. N. Tuchman & R. S. Walters (Eds.), *Disorders of feeding and swallowing in infants and children: Pathophysiology, diagnosis, and treatment* (pp. 421–433). San Diego, CA: Singular.

Wolke, D., Skuse, D., & Mathisen, B. (1989). Behavioral style in failure-to-thrive infants: A preliminary communication. *Journal of Pediatric Psychology, 15,* 237–254.

Youssef, N. N., Rosh, J. R., Loughran, M., Schuckalo, S. G., Cotter, A. N., Verga, B. G., et al. (2004). Treatment of functional abdominal pain in childhood with cognitive behavioral strategies. *Journal of Pediatric Gastroenterology and Nutrition, 39,* 192–196.

CHAPTER 30

Pediatric Obesity

ELISSA JELALIAN
CHANTELLE N. HART

Pediatric obesity has increased dramatically over the past 30 years, and adult obesity is considered a leading cause of preventable deaths. Data from the National Health and Nutrition Examination Survey (NHANES) indicate that 16.3% of U.S. children 2–19 years old are obese (body mass index [BMI] ≥ 95th percentile for age and gender; Ogden, Carroll, & Flegal, 2008). Rates of obesity in children vary by age, gender, and ethnicity, with older children and ethnic minority children at increased risk. Data from the NHANES indicate that 17.6% of adolescents (12–19 years old), 20.7% of non-Hispanic African American children, and 20.9% of Mexican American children are obese (Ogden et al., 2008). Although these recent estimates suggest that rates of obesity in children may be flattening, they nevertheless mark a threefold increase in obesity over the last three decades. Moreover, overweight youths have become heavier (Jolliffe, 2004). Given the dramatic increase in prevalence, pediatric overweight and obesity have become common concerns for families and health care providers, and provide a unique opportunity for involvement of pediatric psychologists.

Definitions of Overweight and Obesity

"Obesity" is generally defined as excess body fat or adiposity in comparison to overall body weight when considered in relation to a given weight standard (Flegal, Tabak, & Ogden, 2006). Because measures of body fatness are more challenging to obtain, BMI, which is a measure of weight adjusted for height (kilograms/meters^2), is commonly used (Barlow, 2007; Flegal et al., 2006). Although absolute BMI values can be used to define obesity in adulthood, BMI fluctuates with age and varies by gender in children.

As a result, BMI percentile scores for a given age and gender are calculated to determine obesity status in children. Children with a BMI at or above the 85th percentile for their age and gender, but less than the 95th percentile, are now considered "overweight"; those with BMI values at or above the 95th percentile are considered "obese" (Barlow, 2007). Formerly, these cutoffs were defined as "at risk for overweight" and "overweight," respectively. The recent changes in terminology were recommended by an expert committee to parallel adult definitions of obesity more closely, decrease the confusion associated with the category "at risk for overweight," and more accurately describe the excess adiposity associated with each category (Barlow, 2007). However, because many earlier studies have used "overweight" and "obese" interchangeably, we do the same in this chapter.

Health Consequences

Pediatric obesity negatively affects a number of systems within the body, including the cardiovascular, metabolic, pulmonary, gastrointestinal, and skeletal systems (Daniels, 2006; Daniels et al., 2005). Specifically, children and adolescents who are obese exhibit increased rates of impaired glucose tolerance and insulin resistance, and are at increased risk for development of the metabolic syndrome (Daniels et al., 2005). Furthermore, pediatric obesity is believed to be the leading cause of Type 2 diabetes; it is also associated with risk factors associated with cardiovascular disease, including high diastolic and systolic blood pressure, left ventricular hypertrophy, and atherosclerosis (Daniels, 2006; Freedman, Dietz, Srinivasan, & Berenson, 1999). Moreover, pediatric obesity is associated with asthma and obstructive sleep apnea, as well as nonalcoholic fatty liver disease—a condition previously believed to occur only in adulthood (Daniels, 2006).

In addition, pediatric obesity in childhood and adolescence is associated with obesity in adulthood (Singh, Mulder, Twisk, van Mechelen, & Chinapaw, 2008; Whitaker, Wright, Pepe, Seidel, & Dietz, 1997), which is more difficult to treat and is associated with increased morbidity and mortality (Bray, 2004; Hill & Trowbridge, 1998). Risk of obesity in adulthood increases with increased child age, and preadolescents' weight status is a stronger predictor of adult overweight status than parental weight (Whitaker et al., 1997). Thus pediatric obesity is a serious condition associated with both concurrent and future disease risk.

Psychosocial Correlates

Being overweight during childhood and adolescence is potentially associated with a number of negative emotional correlates. We provide an overview of the areas of psychosocial functioning that have been evaluated in overweight and obese pediatric samples. The reader is referred to reviews by Wardle and Cooke (2005) and Zeller and Modi (2008) for more in-depth coverage of the topic. During the last 5 years, considerable attention has been paid to the impact of obesity on health-related quality of life (HRQOL), including domains of physical, social, emotional, and academic functioning. Overweight children and adolescents consistently describe impairments in daily functioning similar to those of children with cancer, and significantly greater than those of normal-weight healthy controls (Schwimmer, Burwinkle, & Varni, 2003). Furthermore, subsequent research has documented a relationship between degree of overweight and HRQOL (Williams, Wake, Hesketh, Maher, & Waters, 2005). Taken together, findings highlight the negative effects on quality of life experienced by these children.

A second area that has received considerable attention is the relationship between weight status and self-concept, typically defined as perceived competence across a number of specific domains. Although findings have been mixed in studies with school-age children, there is a suggested inverse relationship between BMI and self-concept in both cross-sectional and prospective studies with adolescents (French, Story, & Perry, 1995). Across both children and adolescents, there appears to be a stronger relationship between obesity and self-worth related to physical appearance or body image. Fairly consistent findings of decreased physical self-worth and higher body dissatisfaction have been documented in overweight children and adolescents relative to normal-weight peers (Wardle & Cooke, 2005). In a recent study of adolescent girls 14–17 years of age, girls who were overweight or at risk of overweight reported higher levels of body dissatisfaction and made more negative attributions regarding their appearance than normal-weight peers did (Thompson et al., 2007). Although these discrepancies in self-worth are significant, it is important to note that children who are overweight typically do not endorse clinically significant low levels of self-worth.

Recent studies have extended beyond evaluation of self-concept to consider symptoms of depression and anxiety as well. Limited research has been conducted regarding the association between obesity and anxiety, with mixed results (Tanofsky-Kraff et al., 2004; Zeller, Saelens, Roehrig, Kirk, & Daniels, 2004); more attention has been paid to the association between obesity and depressive symptoms. Data from the National Longitudinal Study of Adolescent Health (Add Health) indicate comparable rates of depressive symptoms in overweight and nonoverweight adolescents, with approximately 9% of depressed adolescents categorized as obese (Goodman & Whitaker, 2002). In contrast, a second large-scale survey of adolescents (Project EAT; Crow, Eisenberg, Story, & Neumark-Sztainer, 2006), relying on different criteria, reported that 25% of overweight boys and 41% of overweight girls were in the top quartile with regard to a measure of depressive symptoms. Generally, rates of co-occurrence reported from studies of adolescents seeking weight control treatment tend to be higher than those reported in epidemiological studies. For example, approximately one-third of a small treatment-seeking sample of adolescents met criteria for major depressive disorder (Erermis et al., 2004). However, in a subsequent study of treatment-seeking youths, approximately 11% of the sample met criteria for clinically significant depressive symptoms as measured by the Children's Depression Inventory (Zeller & Modi, 2006)—a percentage comparable to the population base rates. Differences in the prevalence rates of depressive symptoms in overweight samples probably result from inconsistent measurement strategies and criteria for determining clinical significance.

The social functioning of overweight youths is a topic that has received considerable attention. Studies of treatment-seeking children have found global deficits in parents' ratings of their social competence compared to that of normal-weight controls (Braet, Mervielde, & Vandereycken, 1997) and community samples (Banis et al., 1988; Wallander & Varni, 1989). Estimates of the prevalence of social problems in children who are overweight and present for treatment vary, ranging from 11% (Epstein, Wisniewski, & Weng, 1994) to 45% of boys and 28% of girls with elevated scores on the Social Problems subscale of the Child Behavior Checklist (CBCL) (Epstein, Myers, & Anderson, 1996).

Subsequent studies have examined difficulties in specific dimensions of social functioning. With regard to peer relationships, a higher rate of overt victimization (i.e., physical) was reported by obese boys, and a higher rate of relational victimization (i.e., damage to friendships) by obese girls, relative to average-weight peers (Pearce, Boergers, & Prinstein, 2002). Similarly, obese adolescents were both victims and perpetrators of verbal bullying in interactions with peers (Janssen, Craig, Boyce, & Pickett, 2004). A significant percentage of adolescents with BMI greater than or equal to the 95th percentile endorsed weight-related teasing by peers and family members (Neumark-Sztainer et al., 2002). Furthermore, data from the Add Health Study indicate that obese adolescents are less likely than normal-weight teens to be nominated by peers as friends (Strauss & Pollack, 2003).

Recent investigations have moved beyond simple characterization of overweight populations to description of factors that help explicate the heterogeneity in psychosocial outcomes within this population. Several studies have demonstrated the negative qualities attributed to overweight children in hypothetical situations—for example, "ugly," "sad," and "lazy" (Bell & Morgan, 2000; Latner & Stunkard, 2003)—and many others have documented a relationship between weight-based teasing and psychosocial outcomes. For example, in a sample of overweight African American children, weight-related teasing was negatively related to both appearance and global self-worth (Young-Hyman, Schlundt, Herman-Wenderoth, & Bozylinski, 2003). Similarly, weight-based teasing by peers and parental criticism of weight predicted lower self-concept in a sample of overweight children (Davison & Birch, 2002). A recent review provides an excellent summary of the psychosocial and physical consequences associated with weight stigma and weight-based teasing (Puhl & Latner, 2007).

A second construct that has been related to psychosocial outcomes among overweight youths is that of body satisfaction/shape concern. For example, overweight adolescents categorized as "high-risk" on the basis of weight/shape concern were found to have higher levels of anxiety, depression, and stress, as well as more impaired social functioning (Celio Doyle, Le Grange, Goldschmidt, & Wilfley, 2007). Of interest, body satisfaction has also been related longitudinally to weight status such that among adolescent girls with BMI at or above the 85th percentile, higher body satisfaction at initial evaluation was associated with smaller BMI increase 5 years later (van den Berg & Neumark-Sztainer, 2007).

In summary, empirical findings suggest that overweight children and adolescents are not systematically at risk for increased psychological distress; they suggest the importance of potential mediators of psychological distress, including weight-related teasing and stigma, and body satisfaction. Practical implications of these findings include the importance of assessing dimensions of social and emotional functioning in children and adolescents presenting for weight loss treatment. Conversely, it may be important to evaluate weight-related concerns in overweight youths presenting with emotional or behavioral problems, to determine the extent to which weight concerns contribute to psychological difficulties.

Influences on Obesity: An Ecological Perspective

An ecological model of diet, physical activity, and obesity has been proposed to understand how multiple influences affect body weight (National Heart, Lung, and Blood Institute, 2004). These include individual-level variables such as genetic and psychological factors, as well as environmental influences ranging from family factors to the policies and incentives of the society at large. We first review the larger societal context in which pediatric obesity develops, to provide a framework for understanding the current obesity epidemic. We then review the relative influences of both genetic and more proximal environmental influences on pediatric obesity risk.

Changes in the Larger Cultural Environment Associated with Obesity Risk

In recent decades, U.S. society has become increasingly sedentary, less physically active, and more likely to consume diets rich in calories and fat and deficient in nutrient-dense foods. It has been estimated that children spend more than 25% of their waking hours in front of televisions (Robinson, 2001). Furthermore, data from the Youth Risk Behavior Surveillance show that almost 25% of adolescents spend 3 or more hours in front of computers daily (for non-school-related activities), and that approximately 35% watch television for 3 or more hours per day (Eaton et al., 2008). Data indicate that children who watch more television are at increased risk for obesity (e.g., Dowda, Ainsworth, Addy, Saunders, & Riner, 2001; Dubois, Farmer, Girard, & Peterson, 2008; O'Brien et al., 2007), probably due to the influence of television viewing on children's food intake. For example, one study found that increased television viewing was associated with fewer fruits and vegetables consumed, increased consumption of sugar-sweetened beverages, and increased overall caloric intake (Miller, Taveras, Rifas-Shiman, & Gillman, 2008). Although findings regarding television and obesity risk are consistent, research linking obesity with other sedentary behaviors (such as video games and computer usage) is limited (Spear et al., 2007). Further research is needed to tease apart the potential role of these additional sedentary behaviors in the current obesity epidemic.

Coinciding with increased sedentary behavior is reduction in frequency of physical activity (Dollman, Norton, & Norton, 2005). For example, between 55 and 66% of adolescents do not meet the current recommendation of 60 minutes per day of moderate to vigorous physical activity (Eaton et al., 2008; Sanchez et al., 2007). A number of studies show that physical activity is associated with decreased BMI in children and adolescents. For example, one large prospective study of children 10–15 years old showed that a 1-year increase in physical activity was associated with a decrease in relative BMI in girls and overweight boys (Berkey, Rockett, Gillman, & Colditz, 2003). Participation in athletics or organized exercise programs may also provide protection against obesity in children and adolescents (Dowda et al., 2001).

The quality of children's and adolescents' diets has steadily declined over the past 20–30 years (Jahns, Siega-Riz, & Popkin, 2001), with many children not meeting current dietary recommendations (Briefel & Johnson, 2004; Kant, 2003; Sanchez et al., 2007). Data show that most adolescents (i.e., >85%) do not eat five or more servings of fruits and vegetables daily (Sanchez et al., 2007). In contrast, almost one-third of daily energy intake for children and adolescents comes from snack foods, such as desserts, salty snacks, and sweeteners/sweetened drinks (Kant, 2003). These declines in dietary quality mirror changes in societal eating patterns. Within the past two to three decades, there has been an increased reliance on meals prepared outside the home (French, Story, & Jeffery, 2001), and a "supersizing" of meals at restaurants, at fast-food establishments, and within the home environment (Nielsen & Popkin, 2003). Estimates suggest that Americans spend almost half of their food budget on meals consumed outside the home (Lin, Franzao, & Guthrie, 1999), with one study indicating that 40% of children's meals come from sources other than home (Murphy, 2000). Given the increase in calories associated with meals eaten in restaurants and fast-food establishments when compared to the same foods prepared at home (French et al., 2001), it is not surprising that the quality of children's and adolescent's diets has decreased.

In summary, a number of societal factors have tipped the scales toward obesity risk in children and adolescents. In addition to these broader societal influences on eating and activity habits, research has uncovered both genetic and more proximal environmental factors associated with the development of obesity, which are reviewed below.

Genetic Influences on Obesity Risk

Twin and adoption studies suggest that measures of body size and composition, such as height, weight, waist circumference, and percentage of body fat, are heritable traits (Schousboe et al., 2004), with estimations of the contribution of genes to variations in obesity status ranging between 40 and 70% (Farooqi, 2005). With the completion of the Human Genome Project and the International HapMap, our understanding of the role of genetics in the development of obesity is rapidly unfolding. One exciting discovery is the identification of the fat mass and obesity-associated (FTO) gene, which has been associated with increased BMI and obesity in a number of studies (Loos & Bouchard, 2008). Although heritability clearly influences risk for obesity, it is widely believed that genes and the environment interact to determine obesity status.

Family Influences on Pediatric Obesity

The home environment and parents, in particular, play an important role in children's eating and activity behaviors and weight status. Parental weight is correlated with children's weight and is often one of the most important predictors of children's BMI status (Agras, Hammer, McNicholas, & Kraemer, 2004; Dowda et al., 2001). Although, as noted above, this is in part due to genetic factors, familial correlations in weight also reflect the shared environment, highlighting the influence that specific parenting practices may have on children's eating/activity behaviors and weight status.

The structure of the home environment is an important determinant of eating and activity behaviors. Availability of food items and of physical versus sedentary activities is associated with food intake and time spent being active, respectively (Atkinson, Sallis, Saelens, Cain, & Black, 2005; Spurrier, Magarey, Golley, Curnow, & Sawyer, 2008). For example, Spurrier and colleagues (2008) found that among preschool-age children, the amount of outdoor play equipment available at home was associated with the amount of time spent in outdoor play. Furthermore, the presence of a computer game station was associated with increased time spent in sedentary activities. Finally, increased availability of fruits, vegetables, and sweetened beverages was associated with increased intake of each food group, respectively (Spurrier et al., 2008). Additional studies confirm the important role of stimulus control (i.e., availability of food items and activities) in children's engagement in eating and activity behaviors (Atkinson et al., 2005; Hanson, Neumark-Sztainer, Eisenberg, Story, & Wall, 2005).

Beyond making healthy foods and activities accessible to their children, parents play an important role in children's obesity risk through establishment of familial eating patterns and rules. Particularly with younger children, parents decide where to eat, how meals will be prepared, and what types and how much food to present to children. A number of studies have shown that presentation of larger portions is associated with increased food intake, even in children as young as 5 years old (Rolls, Engell, & Birch, 2000). Furthermore, where and with whom children eat may affect dietary intake and weight status. Eating in front of the television is associated with increased caloric intake (Wiecha et al., 2006). Conversely, sitting down for a family dinner may provide some protection against obesity. Studies regarding the effects of family meals have shown mixed results, with increased intake of nutrient-dense foods (Gillman et al., 2000) and decreased risk of being or becoming overweight (Sen, 2006) found in two studies, and another prospective study failing to find a relationship between family dinners and weight status (Taveras et al., 2005). Finally, food restriction is consistently associated with higher BMI (Clark, Goyder, Bissell, Blank, & Peters, 2007), possibly due to the increased attention that is drawn to restricted food items when they are limited (Fisher & Birch, 1999).

Additional parenting behaviors associated with obesity risk include modeling and the use of an authoritative parenting style. Children learn about appropriate eating behaviors through both experience and observation (Savage, Fisher, & Birch, 2007); thus parental modeling of eating behaviors can play an important role in determining food intake. Although there is limited research on parental modeling, one study found that in middle-school children, those who perceived their parents modeling fruit and vegetable consumption were more likely to eat fruits and vegetables themselves (Young, Fors, & Hayes, 2004). Furthermore, a recent meta-analysis showed a moderate relationship between parental modeling of physical activity and child engagement in physical activity (Pugliese & Tinsley, 2007). In addition to modeling, research has shown that parenting style may be associated with children's obesity risk: Positive parenting approaches, such as an authoritative style (Rhee, Lumeng, Appugliese, Kaciroti, & Bradley, 2006; Wake, Nicholson, Hardy, & Smith, 2007) and use of positive reinforcement (Arredondo et al., 2006), may have protective effects on obesity risk. Specifically, use of positive reinforcement (e.g., parent report of praise when child ate a healthy snack or engaged in physical activity) was associated with increased intake of healthier foods such as fruits and vegetables, decreased intake of sweetened beverages and snacks, and increased physical activity in a sample of Latino/Latina children (Arredondo et al., 2006). A recent review concludes that although there is clearly a relationship between parenting practices and child weight status, there is minimal research regarding pathways, with a potential bidirectional relationship between parenting and child eating behaviors (Ventura & Birch, 2008).

Additional Influences on Eating, Activity, and Obesity

There are a number of additional influences on obesity risk, including organizational factors, the physical environment, and policies and incentives (National Heart, Lung, and Blood Institute, 2004). Of particular interest in recent years is the adoption of policies to promote healthier eating and activity environments within school settings (see just below). Furthermore, the built environment, including neighborhood walkability and recreational infrastructure, has been shown to be an important predictor of physical activity (e.g., Davison & Lawson, 2006).

Prevention and Intervention Efforts

Efforts to regulate weight in children and adolescents range from primary prevention, typically targeting large groups of children, to tertiary interventions focused on individual overweight children and their families. We review intervention and prevention efforts separately, as these involve fairly distinct strategies and are targeted at different populations.

School-Based Prevention Programs and Policy Initiatives

The broadest-level strategies to prevent development or progression of obesity are policy changes, which may be implemented at the school district, state, or national level. Targets for school-based policies include the school nutrition environment, education related to nutrition and physical activity, BMI-reporting requirements, and development of safe school routes, with the majority of legislation related to school nutrition standards and vending machines (Boehmer, Brownson, Haire-Joshu, & Dreisinger, 2007). During the last several years, there has been a notable increase in implementation of policies to improve school food and activity environments (Boehmer et al., 2007). We provide a brief overview of school-based prevention programs, and refer the reader to Brown and Summerbell (2009) for more detailed information.

Historically, prevention programs included multicomponent interventions with educational curricula, behavior change strategies, and manipulation of the school nutrition or physical activity environment (French et al., 2001). A recent review of school-based interventions concludes that combined diet and physical activity interventions may be effective in preventing pediatric obesity, with 45% of reviewed studies on combined interventions demonstrating significant BMI decreases in intervention groups relative to controls (Brown & Summerbell, 2009). Of note, key intervention components (e.g., dance vs. other physical activity, single vs. multiple targets) could not be determined from the review. Although some interventions were developed specifically for children from particular ethnic or racial backgrounds (e.g., Pathways, GEMs), programs that included heterogeneous samples did not typically report findings by ethnicity (Brown & Summerbell, 2009).

Lifestyle Interventions for Treatment of Pediatric Obesity

Prevention programs and policy initiatives are population-based efforts geared toward children and adolescents regardless of weight status, whereas targeted interventions focus on children who are at increased risk or who are already overweight or obese. Very few interventions have identified and targeted children who are at increased risk for obesity. One such intervention targeted families with normal-weight children but at least one obese parent, and evaluated the relative utility of two messages: one to increase healthy foods, and one to decrease unhealthy foods. Parents whose families were instructed to increase fruit and vegetable consumption showed greater decreases in percent overweight than parents whose families were instructed to decrease high-fat and high-sugar foods (Epstein, Gordy, et al., 2001). Additional research needs to be conducted to determine the long-term efficacy of interventions that promote healthy practices without specifically targeting restriction of less healthy behaviors.

Several comprehensive reviews have addressed the efficacy of lifestyle intervention for treatment of pediatric obesity (e.g., Jelalian & Saelens, 1999; Oude Luttikhuis et al., 2009), and a recent paper provides a quantitative analysis of pediatric obesity treatments (e.g., Wilfley, Tibbs, et al., 2007). We provide here a summary of intervention strategies and supporting evidence, and refer the reader to the references noted above for more detailed reviews.

Lifestyle interventions for children and adolescents who are overweight are typically delivered in a group setting and incorporate several common components. These include dietary restriction, physical activity prescription, behavior modification components (such as self-monitoring of diet and physical activity), stimulus control strategies, and contingency management, as well as varying levels of parent involvement. There is considerable empirical support documenting the efficacy of comprehensive behavioral weight management interventions with school-age children (8–12 years), with decreases in overweight ranging from approximately 5 to 20% observed immediately following the interventions (Jelalian & Saelens, 1999). A recent meta-analysis found that lifestyle interventions demonstrated significant effects in decreasing pediatric obesity when compared to waiting-list/no-treatment controls or education-only comparison groups (Wilfley, Tibbs, et al., 2007).

Randomized behavioral weight control trials exclusively targeting adolescents demonstrate variable findings (Jelalian et al., 2008). A recent review concludes that despite multiple methodological limitations, comprehensive interventions involving behavioral strategies combined with attention to diet and physical activity show promise in decreasing adolescent obesity (Tsiros, Sinn, Coates, Howe, & Buckley, 2008). One randomized trial combining group-based behavioral treatment with one of two activity interventions (peer-enhanced adventure therapy or supervised aerobic exercise) demonstrated an average reduction of 1.75 BMI units across conditions (Jelalian, Mehlenbeck, Lloyd-Richardson, Birmaher, & Wing, 2006).

Relatively few pediatric obesity interventions have been conducted with children and adolescents from diverse ethnic and racial backgrounds. In a study of African American adolescent girls conducted by Wadden and colleagues (1990), no significant differences in outcome were observed, regardless of whether parents were seen together with adolescents, in separate groups, or not included in treatment. A second randomized trial with African American adolescent girls (Resnicow, Taylor, Baskin, & McCarty, 2005) compared a high-intensity intervention (weekly behavioral sessions, messages via two-way pager, and phone calls) to a moderate-intensity intervention (six psychoeducational sessions) and found no significant differences between groups at 6 months, with the moderate-intensity group demonstrating a slight increase and the high-intensity group a slight decrease in BMI. An Internet-based intervention for African American girls and their parents led to greater reduction in body fat and weight than an education-only control did (White et al., 2004). Finally, in a recent randomized controlled trial with

overweight Mexican American youths, intensive intervention delivered in a school setting resulted in greater decreases in z BMI than a self-help condition did (Johnston et
al., 2007).

Another area that has received minimal attention is maintenance of weight loss.
Although some studies provide long-term follow-up of participants in weight control
interventions (Epstein, McCurley, Wing, & Valoski, 1990; Epstein, Valoski, Wing, &
McCurley, 1994), investigation of specific strategies for maintenance of weight loss has
been virtually nonexistent (Wilfley, Stein, et al., 2007). In contrast, developing effective weight maintenance strategies has become a critical topic for adult weight control
research (Perri & Corsica, 2002). In the one published study evaluating the efficacy
of different weight maintenance approaches, children who were randomly assigned to
either behavioral skills maintenance or social facilitation maintenance demonstrated
greater weight loss maintenance than those assigned to the control condition did (Wilfley, Stein, et al., 2007).

Improvements in Psychosocial Outcomes Secondary to Lifestyle Interventions

The effectiveness of pediatric weight control interventions is typically judged with reference to changes in weight status of participants. Secondarily, improvements in psychosocial functioning have also been reported. In particular, behavioral weight control interventions have been associated with improvements in self-concept (French et
al., 1995; Jelalian et al., 2006), reduction in eating disorder symptomatology (Braet &
Van Winckel, 2000), and fewer behavior problems as measured by the CBCL (Epstein,
Paluch, Saelens, Ernst, & Wilfley, 2001).

Intensive Weight Control Interventions

Given the increased prevalence of obesity in children and adolescents, intensive interventions—such as very-low-calorie diets or protein-sparing modified fasts, behavioral
treatment offered in residential or camp settings, pharmacotherapy, and bariatric surgery—have become viable treatment options with severely obese adolescents. Treatments provided in residential and inpatient settings show some promise as effective
strategies for weight loss (e.g., Barton, Walker, Lambert, Gately, & Hill, 2004). Pharmacotherapy (e.g., the use of sibutramine and orlistat) also shows some promise when
used alone or in combination with behavioral interventions (Berkowitz et al., 2006;
Godoy-Matos et al., 2005). However, more research is needed to ensure that pharmacotherapy is a safe and effective alternative for treatment of pediatric obesity (Han
& Yanovski, 2008). Finally, bariatric surgery, though still uncommon, has been performed with increased frequency on severely obese adolescents during the last several
years (Tsai, Inge, & Burd, 2007). It has been recommended that bariatric surgery be
used with caution: More conservative selection criteria should be used for adolescents
than for adults—that is, BMI ≥ 40 kg/m^2 in combination with medical comorbidity
(Inge, Zeller, Garcia, & Daniels, 2004)—and such surgery should not be performed
at all in children (i.e., <13 years) who do not have the decisional capacity for serious
interventions (Inge et al., 2004). A review of bariatric surgery approaches is provided
by Inge, Zeller, Lawson, and Daniels (2005), and detailed consideration of intensive
therapies is provided by Han and Yanovski (2008).

Future Directions

Given the current status of obesity prevention and intervention efforts, several directions for future research studies and clinical initiatives are suggested. There are a number of exciting areas for future research, including recognizing the role of perinatal factors in obesity risk, understanding the dynamic interaction of genetic and environmental risk factors, and investigating applications of technology to enhance adherence to behavioral weight control strategies. We focus discussion on three specific areas where pediatric psychologists, in particular, are well positioned to advance our understanding of obesity prevention and intervention efforts.

Primary Care Settings

Recent expert committee recommendations note the importance of developing interventions for prevention and treatment of pediatric obesity in primary care settings (Barlow, 2007). Primary care providers are on the front line for providing health care for children, and are therefore in an advantageous position to offer services for preventing obesity (Story et al., 2002). They have the stature and the authority to make lifestyle recommendations, and have great access to the population at large, with the average U.S. child making two to three office visits per year to a pediatrician (Manson, Skerrett, Greenland, & VanItallie, 2004). Although few interventions have been conducted in primary care settings, results from these studies suggest that primary care settings may provide a unique opportunity to influence a large segment of the population (Saelens et al., 2002). Primary care is also a setting in which pediatric psychologists may be effective in both coordinating clinical care and collaborating on research initiatives.

Translational Research

A second area focuses on translation of research from efficacy trials to effectiveness and dissemination studies. Existing interventions tend to target a small number of participants in well-controlled environments. An example of extension to an applied setting is provided by delivery of an intervention based on the "Traffic Light Diet" in a clinic setting, with promising results (Johnston & Steele, 2007). Another key area is the translation of research in the behavioral, social, and basic sciences to the area of obesity prevention and intervention. Pediatric psychologists have expertise with established interventions targeting other chronic conditions, as well as with such key constructs as adherence, making them uniquely qualified to contribute to this objective.

Treatment of Comorbid Conditions

A final area in need of additional research is better understanding of the role of comorbid conditions in the development and treatment of pediatric obesity. The reader is referred to Zametkin, Jacobs, and Parrish (2008) for a comprehensive review of this topic. To date, studies show that although subgroups of children who are obese may be at increased risk of psychiatric disorders, in general children who are obese do not exhibit higher rates of these conditions (Zametkin et al., 2008). Nevertheless, a number of children with psychiatric disorders are obese or experience weight gain as a result of psychopharmacological treatment of their disorders. It is therefore of particular importance to develop interventions to treat pediatric obesity and comorbid psychiatric disturbance. One potential approach may be physical activity, which has benefits for treatment of both psychiatric concerns and excess weight.

Summary and Conclusions

There has been a dramatic increase in pediatric obesity during the last three decades. Obesity places children and adolescents at increased risk for both concurrent and future negative health and psychosocial outcomes. Several studies have documented the efficacy of lifestyle interventions in the treatment of pediatric obesity, and limited evidence supports the efficacy of multicomponent interventions for prevention of obesity. Recent policy initiatives targeting improvements in the school nutrition and activity environments may provide important progress in this area. Relatively minimal attention has been given to establishing interventions in pediatric settings, conducting effectiveness studies in practical settings, and developing combined treatments for obesity and psychological concerns, all of which are important areas for clinical initiatives and future research.

References

Agras, W. S., Hammer, L. D., McNicholas, F., & Kraemer, H. C. (2004). Risk factors for childhood overweight: A prospective study from birth to 9.5 years. *Journal of Pediatrics*, *145*, 20–25.

Arredondo, E. M., Elder, J. P., Ayala, G. X., Campbell, N., Baquero, B., & Duerksen, S. (2006). Is parenting style related to children's healthy eating and physical activity in Latino families? *Health Education Research*, *21*, 862–871.

Atkinson, J. L., Sallis, J. F., Saelens, B. E., Cain, K. L., & Black, J. B. (2005). The association of neighborhood design and recreational environments with physical activity. *American Journal of Health Promotion*, *19*, 304–309.

Banis, H. T., Varni, J. W., Wallander, J. L., Korsch, B. M., Jay, S. M., Adler, R., et al. (1988). Psychological and social adjustment of obese children and their families. *Child Care Health Development*, *14*, 157–173.

Barlow, S. E. (2007). Expert committee recommendations regarding the prevention, assessment, and treatment of child and adolescent overweight and obesity: Summary report. *Pediatrics*, *120*(Suppl. 4), S164–S192.

Barton, S. B., Walker, L. L., Lambert, G., Gately, P. J., & Hill, A. J. (2004). Cognitive change in obese adolescents losing weight. *Obesity Research*, *12*, 313–319.

Bell, S. K., & Morgan, S. B. (2000). Children's attitudes and behavioral intentions toward a peer presented as obese: Does a medical explanation for the obesity make a difference? *Journal of Pediatric Psychology*, *25*, 137–145.

Berkey, C. S., Rockett, H. R., Gillman, M. W., & Colditz, G. A. (2003). One-year changes in activity and in inactivity among 10- to 15-year-old boys and girls: Relationship to change in body mass index. *Pediatrics*, *111*, 836–843.

Berkowitz, R. I., Fujioka, K., Daniels, S. R., Hoppin, A. G., Owen, S., Perry, A. C., et al. (2006). Effects of sibutramine in obese adolescents: A randomized trial. *Annals of Internal Medicine*, *145*, 81–90.

Boehmer, T. K., Brownson, R. C., Haire-Joshu, D., & Dreisinger, M. L. (2007). Patterns of childhood obesity prevention legislation in the United States. *Preventing Chronic Disease*, 4(3). Available at *www.cdc.gov/ped/issues/2007/jul/06_0082.htm*

Braet, C., Mervielde, I., & Vandereycken, W. (1997). Psychological aspects of childhood obesity: A controlled study in a clinical and nonclinical sample. *Journal of Pediatric Psychology*, 22, 59–71.

Braet, C., & Van Winckel, M. (2000). Long-term follow-up of cognitive behavioral treatment program for obese children. *Behavior Therapy*, 31, 55–74.

Bray, G. A. (2004). Medical consequences of obesity. *Journal of Endocrinology and Metabolism*, 89, 2583–2589.

Briefel, R. R., & Johnson, C. L. (2004). Secular trends in dietary intake in the United States. *Annual Review of Nutrition*, 24, 401–431.

Brown, T., & Summerbell, C. (2009). Systematic review of school-based interventions that focus on changing dietary intake and physical activity levels to prevent childhood obesity: An update to the obesity guidance produced by the National Institute for Health and Clinical Excellence. *Obesity Reviews*, 10, 110–141.

Clark, H. R., Goyder, E., Bissell, P., Blank, L., & Peters, J. (2007). How do parents' child-feeding behaviours influence child weight?: Implications for childhood obesity policy. *Journal of Public Health*, 29, 132–141.

Crow, S., Eisenberg, M. E., Story, M., & Neumark-Sztainer, D. (2006). Psychosocial and behavioral correlates of dieting among overweight and non-overweight adolescents. *Journal of Adolescent Health*, 38, 569–574.

Daniels, S. R. (2006). The consequences of childhood overweight and obesity. *The Future of Children*, 16, 47–67.

Daniels, S. R., Arnett, D. K., Eckel, R. H., Gidding, S. S., Hayman, L. L., Kumanyika, S., et al. (2005). Overweight in children and adolescents: Pathophysiology, consequences, prevention, and treatment. *Circulation*, 111, 1999–2012.

Davison, K. K., & Birch, L. L. (2002). Processes linking weight status and self-concept among girls from ages 5 to 7 years. *Developmental Psychology*, 38, 735–748.

Davison, K. K., & Lawson, C. T. (2006). Do attributes in the physical environment influence children's physical activity?: A review of the literature. *International Journal of Behavioral Nutrition and Physical Activity*, 3, 19.

Dollman, J., Norton, K., & Norton, L. (2005). Evidence for secular trends in children's physical activity behaviour. *British Journal of Sports Medicine*, 39, 892–897.

Dowda, M., Ainsworth, B. E., Addy, C. L., Saunders, R., & Riner, W. (2001). Environmental influences, physical activity, and weight status in 8- to 16-year-olds. *Archives of Pediatrics and Adolescent Medicine*, 155, 711–717.

Doyle, A. C., Le Grange, D., Goldschmidt, A., & Wilfley, D. E. (2007). Psychosocial and physical impairment in overweight adolescents at high risk for eating disorders. *Obesity*, 15, 145–154.

Dubois, L., Farmer, A., Girard, M., & Peterson, K. (2008). Social factors and television use during meals and snacks is associated with higher BMI among pre-school children. *Public Health Nutrition*, 12, 1–13.

Eaton, D. K., Kann, L., Kinchen, S., Shanklin, S., Ross, J., Hawkins, J., et al. (2008). Youth Risk Behavior Surveillance—United States, 2007. *Morbidity and Mortality Weekly Report Surveillance Summaries*, 57, 1–131.

Epstein, L. H., Gordy, C. C., Raynor, H. A., Beddome, M., Kilanowski, C. K., & Paluch, R. (2001). Increasing fruit and vegetable intake and decreasing fat and sugar intake in families at risk for childhood obesity. *Obesity Research*, 9, 171–178.

Epstein, L. H., McCurley, J., Wing, R. R., & Valoski, A. (1990). Five-year follow-up of family-based behavioral treatments for childhood obesity. *Journal of Consulting and Clinical Psychology, 58*, 661–664.

Epstein, L. H., Myers, M. D., & Anderson, K. (1996). The association of maternal psychopathology and family socioeconomic status with psychological problems in obese children. *Obesity Research, 4*, 65–74.

Epstein, L. H., Paluch, R. A., Saelens, B. E., Ernst, M. M., & Wilfley, D. E. (2001). Changes in eating disorder symptoms with pediatric obesity treatment. *Journal of Pediatrics, 139*, 58–65.

Epstein, L. H., Valoski, A., Wing, R. R., & McCurley, J. (1994). Ten-year outcomes of behavioral family-based treatment for childhood obesity. *Health Psychology, 13*, 373–383.

Epstein, L. H., Wisniewski, L., & Weng, R. (1994). Child and parent psychological problems influence child weight control. *Obesity Research, 2*, 509–515.

Erermis, S., Cetin, N., Tamar, M., Bukusoglu, N., Akdeniz, F., & Goksen, D. (2004). Is obesity a risk factor for psychopathology among adolescents? *Pediatrics International, 46*, 296–301.

Farooqi, I. S. (2005). Genetic and hereditary aspects of childhood obesity. *Best Practice and Research: Clinical Endocrinology and Metabolism, 19*, 359–374.

Fisher, J. O., & Birch, L. L. (1999). Restricting access to palatable foods affects children's behavioral response, food selection, and intake. *American Journal of Clinical Nutrition, 69*, 1264–1272.

Flegal, K. M., Tabak, C. J., & Ogden, C. L. (2006). Overweight in children: Definitions and interpretation. *Health Education Research, 21*, 755–760.

Freedman, D. S., Dietz, W. H., Srinivasan, S. R., & Berenson, G. S. (1999). The relation of overweight to cardiovascular risk factors among children and adolescents: The Bogalusa Heart Study. *Pediatrics, 103*, 1175–1182.

French, S. A., Story, M., & Jeffery, R. W. (2001). Environmental influences on eating and physical activity. *Annual Review of Public Health, 22*, 309–335.

French, S. A., Story, M., & Perry, C. L. (1995). Self-esteem and obesity in children and adolescents: A literature review. *Obesity Research, 3*, 479–490.

Gillman, M. W., Rifas-Shiman, S. L., Frazier, A. L., Rockett, H. R., Camargo, C. A., Jr., Field, A. E., et al. (2000). Family dinner and diet quality among older children and adolescents. *Archives of Family Medicine, 9*, 235–240.

Godoy-Matos, A., Carraro, L., Vieira, A., Oliveira, J., Guedes, E. P., Mattos, L., et al. (2005). Treatment of obese adolescents with sibutramine: A randomized, double-blind, controlled study. *Journal of Clinical Endocrinology and Metabolism, 90*, 1460–1465.

Goodman, E., & Whitaker, R. C. (2002). A prospective study of the role of depression in the development and persistence of adolescent obesity. *Pediatrics, 110*, 497–504.

Han, J. C., & Yanovski, J. A. (2008). Intensive therapies for the treatment of pediatric obesity. In E. Jelalian & R. G. Steele (Eds.), *Handbook of childhood and adolescent obesity* (pp. 241–260). New York: Springer.

Hanson, N. I., Neumark-Sztainer, D., Eisenberg, M. E., Story, M., & Wall, M. (2005). Associations between parental report of the home food environment and adolescent intakes of fruits, vegetables and dairy foods. *Public Health Nutrition, 8*, 77–85.

Hill, J. O., & Trowbridge, F. L. (1998). Childhood obesity: Future directions and research priorities. *Pediatrics, 101*, 570–574.

Inge, T. H., Zeller, M., Garcia, V. F., & Daniels, S. R. (2004). Surgical approach to adolescent obesity. *Adolescent Medicine Clinics, 15*, 429–453.

Inge, T. H., Zeller, M. H., Lawson, M. L., & Daniels, S. R. (2005). A critical appraisal of evidence supporting a bariatric surgical approach to weight management for adolescents. *Journal of Pediatrics, 147*, 10–19.

Jahns, L., Siega-Riz, A. M., & Popkin, B. M. (2001). The increasing prevalence of snacking among US children from 1977 to 1996. *Journal of Pediatrics, 138*, 493–498.

Janssen, I., Craig, W. M., Boyce, W. F., & Pickett, W. (2004). Associations between overweight and obesity with bullying behaviors in school-aged children. *Pediatrics, 113*, 1187–1194.

Jelalian, E., Hart, C. N., Mehlenbeck, R. S., Lloyd-Richardson, E. E., Kaplan, J. D., Flynn-O'Brien, K. T., et al. (2008). Predictors of attrition and weight loss in an adolescent weight control program. *Obesity, 16*, 1318–1323.

Jelalian, E., Mehlenbeck, R., Lloyd-Richardson, E. E., Birmaher, V., & Wing, R. R. (2006). 'Adventure therapy' combined with cognitive-behavioral treatment for overweight adolescents. *International Journal of Obesity, 30*, 31–39.

Jelalian, E., & Saelens, B. E. (1999). Empirically supported treatments in pediatric psychology: Pediatric obesity. *Journal of Pediatric Psychology, 24*, 223–248.

Johnston, C. A., & Steele, R. G. (2007). Treatment of pediatric overweight: An examination of feasibility and effectiveness in an applied clinical setting. *Journal of Pediatric Psychology, 32*, 106–110.

Johnston, C. A., Tyler, C., McFarlin, B. K., Poston, W. S., Haddock, C. K., Reeves, R., et al. (2007). Weight loss in overweight Mexican American children: A randomized, controlled trial. *Pediatrics, 120*, e1450–e1457.

Jolliffe, D. (2004). Continuous and robust measures of the obesity epidemic. *Demography, 41*, 303–314.

Kant, A. K. (2003). Reported consumption of low-nutrient-density foods by American children and adolescents: Nutritional and health correlates, NHANES III, 1988 to 1994. *Archives of Pediatrics and Adolescent Medicine, 157*, 789–796.

Latner, J. D., & Stunkard, A. J. (2003). Getting worse: The stigmatization of obese children. *Obesity Research, 11*, 452–456.

Lin, B. H., Franzao, E., & Guthrie, J. (1999). *Away-from-home foods increasingly important to quality of American diet* (Agricultural Information Bulletin No. 749). Washington, DC: U.S. Department of Agriculture.

Loos, R. J., & Bouchard, C. (2008). FTO: The first gene contributing to common forms of human obesity. *Obesity Reviews, 9*, 246–250.

Manson, J. E., Skerrett, P. J., Greenland, P., & VanItallie, T. B. (2004). The escalating pandemics of obesity and sedentary lifestyle: A call to action for clinicians. *Archives of Internal Medicine, 164*, 249–258.

Miller, S. A., Taveras, E. M., Rifas-Shiman, S. L., & Gillman, M. W. (2008). Association between television viewing and poor diet quality in young children. *International Journal of Pediatric Obesity, 3*, 168–176.

Murphy, J. (2000). *The super-sizing of America: Are fast food chains to blame for the nation's obesity?* Retrieved January 21, 2002, from *www.speakout.com*

National Heart, Lung, and Blood Institute. (2004, August). *Predictors of Obesity, Weight Gain, Diet, and Physical Activity Workshop*. Workshop presented by the National Heart, Lung, and Blood Institute, Bethesda, MD.

Neumark-Sztainer, D., Falkner, N., Story, M., Perry, C., Hannan, P. J., & Mulert, S. (2002). Weight-teasing among adolescents: Correlations with weight status and disordered eating behaviors. *International Journal of Obesity, 26*, 123–131.

Nielsen, S. J., & Popkin, B. M. (2003). Patterns and trends in food portion sizes, 1977–1998. *Journal of the American Medical Association, 289*, 450–453.

O'Brien, M., Nader, P. R., Houts, R. M., Bradley, R., Friedman, S. L., Belsky, J., et al. (2007). The ecology of childhood overweight: A 12-year longitudinal analysis. *International Journal of Pediatric Obesity, 31*, 1469–1478.

Ogden, C. L., Carroll, M. D., & Flegal, K. M. (2008). High body mass index for age among US children and adolescents, 2003–2006. *Journal of the American Medical Association, 299,* 2401–2405.

Oude Luttikhuis, H., Baur, L., Jansen, H., Shrewsbury, V. A., O'Malley, C., Stolk, R. P., et al. (2009). Interventions for treating obesity in children. *Cochrane Database of Systematic Reviews,* Issue I (Article No. CD001872), DOI: 10.1002/14651858.CD001872.pub2.

Pearce, M. J., Boergers, J., & Prinstein, M. J. (2002). Adolescent obesity, overt and relational peer victimization, and romantic relationships. *Obesity Research, 10,* 386–393.

Perri, M. G., & Corsica, J. A. (2002). Improving the maintenance of weight loss in behavioral treatment of obesity. In T. A. Wadden & A. J. Stunkard (Eds.), *Handbook of obesity treatment* (pp. 357–379). New York: Guilford Press.

Pugliese, J., & Tinsley, B. (2007). Parental socialization of child and adolescent physical activity: A meta-analysis. *Journal of Family Psychology, 21,* 331–343.

Puhl, R. M., & Latner, J. D. (2007). Stigma, obesity, and the health of the nation's children. *Psychological Bulletin, 133,* 557–580.

Resnicow, K., Taylor, R., Baskin, M., & McCarty, F. (2005). Results of Go Girls: A weight control program for overweight African-American adolescent females. *Obesity Research, 13,* 1739–1748.

Rhee, K. E., Lumeng, J. C., Appugliese, D. P., Kaciroti, N., & Bradley, R. H. (2006). Parenting styles and overweight status in first grade. *Pediatrics, 117,* 2047–2054.

Robinson, T. N. (2001). Television viewing and childhood obesity. *Pediatric Clinics of North America, 48,* 1017–1025.

Rolls, B. J., Engell, D., & Birch, L. L. (2000). Serving portion size influences 5-year-old but not 3-year-old children's food intakes. *Journal of the American Dietetic Association, 100,* 232–234.

Saelens, B. E., Sallis, J. F., Wilfley, D. E., Patrick, K., Cella, J. A., & Buchta, R. (2002). Behavioral weight control for overweight adolescents initiated in primary care. *Obesity Research, 10,* 22–32.

Sanchez, A., Norman, G. J., Sallis, J. F., Calfas, K. J., Cella, J., & Patrick, K. (2007). Patterns and correlates of physical activity and nutrition behaviors in adolescents. *American Journal of Preventive Medicine, 32,* 124–130.

Savage, J. S., Fisher, J. O., & Birch, L. L. (2007). Parental influence on eating behavior: Conception to adolescence. *Journal of Law, Medicine, and Ethics, 35,* 22–34.

Schousboe, K., Visscher, P. M., Erbas, B., Kyvik, K. O., Hopper, J. L., Henriksen, J. E., et al. (2004). Twin study of genetic and environmental influences on adult body size, shape, and composition. *International Journal of Obesity, 28,* 39–48.

Schwimmer, J. B., Burwinkle, T. M., & Varni, J. W. (2003). Health-related quality of life of severely obese children and adolescents. *Journal of the American Medical Association, 289,* 1813–1819.

Sen, B. (2006). Frequency of family dinner and adolescent body weight status: Evidence from the National Longitudinal Survey of Youth, 1997. *Obesity, 14,* 2266–2276.

Singh, A. S., Mulder, C., Twisk, J. W., van Mechelen, W., & Chinapaw, M. J. (2008). Tracking of childhood overweight into adulthood: A systematic review of the literature. *Obesity Reviews, 9,* 474–488.

Spear, B. A., Barlow, S. E., Ervin, C., Ludwig, D. S., Saelens, B. E., Schetzina, K. E., et al. (2007). Recommendations for treatment of child and adolescent overweight and obesity. *Pediatrics, 120*(Suppl. 4), S254–S288.

Spurrier, N. J., Magarey, A. A., Golley, R., Curnow, F., & Sawyer, M. G. (2008). Relationships between the home environment and physical activity and dietary patterns of preschool children: A cross-sectional study. *International Journal of Behavioral Nutrition and Physical Activity, 5,* 31.

Story, M. T., Neumark-Stzainer, D. R., Sherwood, N. E., Holt, K., Sofka, D., Trowbridge, F. L., et al. (2002). Management of child and adolescent obesity: Attitudes, barriers, skills, and training needs among health care professionals. *Pediatrics, 110,* 210–214.

Strauss, R. S., & Pollack, H. A. (2003). Social marginalization of overweight children. *Archives of Pediatrics and Adolescent Medicine, 157,* 746–752.

Tanofsky-Kraff, M., Yanovski, S. Z., Wilfley, D. E., Marmarosh, C., Morgan, C. M., & Yanovski, J. A. (2004). Eating-disordered behaviors, body fat, and psychopathology in overweight and normal-weight children. *Journal of Consulting and Clinical Psychology, 72,* 53–61.

Taveras, E. M., Rifas-Shiman, S. L., Berkey, C. S., Rockett, H. R., Field, A. E., Frazier, A. L., et al. (2005). Family dinner and adolescent overweight. *Obesity Research, 13,* 900–906.

Thompson, J. K., Shroff, H., Herbozo, S., Cafri, G., Rodriguez, J., & Rodriguez, M. (2007). Relations among multiple peer influences, body dissatisfaction, eating disturbance, and self-esteem: A comparison of average weight, at risk of overweight, and overweight adolescent girls. *Journal of Pediatric Psychology, 32,* 24–29.

Tsai, W. S., Inge, T. H., & Burd, R. S. (2007). Bariatric surgery in adolescents: Recent national trends in use and in-hospital outcome. *Archives of Pediatrics and Adolescent Medicine, 161,* 217–221.

Tsiros, M. D., Sinn, N., Coates, A. M., Howe, P. R., & Buckley, J. D. (2008). Treatment of adolescent overweight and obesity. *European Journal of Pediatrics, 167,* 9–16.

van den Berg, P., & Neumark-Sztainer, D. (2007). Fat 'n happy 5 years later: Is it bad for overweight girls to like their bodies? *Journal of Adolescent Health, 41,* 415–417.

Ventura, A. K., & Birch, L. L. (2008). Does parenting affect children's eating and weight status? *International Journal of Behavioral Nutrition and Physical Activity, 5,* 15.

Wadden, T. A., Stunkard, A. J., Rich, L., Rubin, C. J., Sweidel, G., & McKinney, S. (1990). Obesity in black adolescent girls: A controlled clinical trial of treatment by diet, behavior modification, and parental support. *Pediatrics, 85,* 345–352.

Wake, M., Nicholson, J. M., Hardy, P., & Smith, K. (2007). Preschooler obesity and parenting styles of mothers and fathers: Australian national population study. *Pediatrics, 120,* e1520–e1527.

Wallander, J. L., & Varni, J. W. (1989). Social support and adjustment in chronically ill and handicapped children. *American Journal of Community Psychology, 17,* 185–201.

Wardle, J., & Cooke, L. (2005). The impact of obesity on psychological well-being. *Best Practice and Research: Clinical Endocrinology and Metabolism, 19,* 421–440.

Whitaker, R. C., Wright, J. A., Pepe, M. S., Seidel, K. D., & Dietz, W. H. (1997). Predicting obesity in young adulthood from childhood and parental obesity. *New England Journal of Medicine, 337,* 869–873.

White, M. A., Martin, P. D., Newton, R. L., Walden, H. M., York-Crowe, E. E., Gordon, S. T., et al. (2004). Mediators of weight loss in a family-based intervention presented over the Internet. *Obesity Research, 12,* 1050–1059.

Wiecha, J. L., Peterson, K. E., Ludwig, D. S., Kim, J., Sobol, A., & Gortmaker, S. L. (2006). When children eat what they watch: Impact of television viewing on dietary intake in youth. *Archives of Pediatrics and Adolescent Medicine, 160,* 436–442.

Wilfley, D. E., Stein, R. I., Saelens, B. E., Mockus, D. S., Matt, G. E., Hayden-Wade, H. A., et al. (2007). Efficacy of maintenance treatment approaches for childhood overweight: A randomized controlled trial. *Journal of the American Medical Association, 298,* 1661–1673.

Wilfley, D. E., Tibbs, T. L., Van Buren, D. J., Reach, K. P., Walker, M. S., & Epstein, L. H. (2007). Lifestyle interventions in the treatment of childhood overweight: A meta-analytic review of randomized controlled trials. *Health Psychology, 26,* 521–532.

Williams, J., Wake, M., Hesketh, K., Maher, E., & Waters, E. (2005). Health-related quality of life of overweight and obese children. *Journal of the American Medical Association, 293,* 70–76.

Young, E. M., Fors, S. W., & Hayes, D. M. (2004). Associations between perceived parent behaviors and middle school student fruit and vegetable consumption. *Journal of Nutrition Education and Behavior, 36,* 2–8.

Young-Hyman, D., Schlundt, D. G., Herman-Wenderoth, L., & Bozylinski, K. (2003). Obesity, appearance, and psychosocial adaptation in young African American children. *Journal of Pediatric Psychology, 28,* 463–472.

Zametkin, A., Jacobs, A., & Parrish, J. (2008). Treatment of children and adolescents with obesity and comorbid psychiatric conditions. In E. Jelalian & R. G. Steele (Eds.), *Handbook of childhood and adolescent obesity* (pp. 425–444). New York: Springer.

Zeller, M. H., & Modi, A. C. (2006). Predictors of health-related quality of life in obese youth. *Obesity, 14,* 122–130.

Zeller, M. H., & Modi, A. C. (2008). Psychosocial factors related to obesity in children and adolescents. In E. Jelalian & R. G. Steele (Eds.), *Handbook of childhood and adolescent obesity* (pp. 25–42). New York: Springer.

Zeller, M. H., Saelens, B. E., Roehrig, H., Kirk, S., & Daniels, S. R. (2004). Psychological adjustment of obese youth presenting for weight management treatment. *Obesity Research, 12,* 1576–1586.

CHAPTER 31

Eating Disorders

ANGELA CELIO DOYLE
DANIEL LE GRANGE

Eating disorders most typically begin during adolescence (Flament, Ledoux, Jeammet, Choquet, & Simon, 1995; Lucas, Beard, O'Fallon, & Kurland, 1991) and have been diagnosed in children as young as 7 years old (Bostic, Muriel, Hack, Weinstein, & Herzog, 1997), making it essential for mental health professionals working with youths to be familiar with the assessment, diagnosis, and treatment of eating problems. Despite this, the development, maintenance, and treatment of eating disorders have been especially understudied among children and adolescents (Steiner & Lock, 1998). In this chapter, we first provide an overview of the diagnostic categories of eating disorders, with the accompanying age-related considerations pertaining to diagnosis. The prevalence, comorbidities, course, and prognosis associated with pediatric eating disorders are also described. A multifaceted evaluation for eating disorders is essential and, as such, is delineated in this chapter for use by clinicians. Finally, empirically supported treatments for pediatric eating disorders are reviewed.

Diagnostic Categories

The *Diagnostic and Statistical Manual of Mental Disorders*, fourth edition, text revision (DSM-IV-TR; American Psychiatric Association, 2000) provides three diagnoses for eating disorders: anorexia nervosa (AN), bulimia nervosa (BN), and eating disorder not otherwise specified (EDNOS). Binge-eating disorder (BED) is described as a criteria set needing further study in the DSM-IV-TR and is presently best captured diagnostically as EDNOS.

The DSM-IV-TR defines AN as a refusal to maintain weight or lack of weight gain at a time of growth at 85% of expected weight for height (ideal body weight, or IBW). This is accompanied by an intense fear of gaining weight or becoming fat, despite a low body weight. Individuals with AN also experience a disturbance in the way they perceive their body shape or weight, assign undue influence to body shape or weight in their self-evaluation, or deny the seriousness of their low body weight. Finally, in postmenarchal females, a diagnosis of AN is only made when menstrual cycles are absent for 3 consecutive months (amenorrhea). Note that a woman is considered to be amenorrheic if her periods only occur while she is using hormones (e.g., through oral contraceptives). Two subtypes further describe AN: the "restricting type," in which the individual purely restricts his or her caloric intake; and the "binge-eating/purging type," which is characterized by regular binge-eating and purging behaviors (i.e., self-induced vomiting or the misuse of laxatives or diuretics) while also possessing a low body weight.

BN is characterized by a pattern of binge eating coupled with inappropriate compensatory methods intended to prevent weight gain, as well as overvaluation of body weight and shape (American Psychiatric Association, 2000). Binge eating is defined as consuming an objectively large amount of food (e.g., more than what most people would eat during a discrete period of time under similar circumstances), accompanied by a feeling of loss of control. Compensatory behaviors can include self-induced vomiting, misuse of laxatives, misuse of diuretics, excessive exercise, and fasting. To meet criteria for BN, binge eating and compensatory behaviors must occur at least twice per week over a 3-month period. Two subtypes further describe BN: the "purging type" and the "nonpurging type." The purging type of BN is marked by purging behaviors (see above), and the nonpurging type is marked by compensatory behaviors such as excessive exercise or fasting. Body weight in individuals with BN tends to be in the normal range. For those who concurrently meet BN and AN diagnostic criteria (i.e., low weight with high frequency of binge eating and purging), a diagnosis of AN is given.

The diagnosis of EDNOS captures several common variations on AN and BN, BED, and more rare disordered eating presentations (e.g., chewing and spitting out large quantities of food). For instance, EDNOS would be diagnosed when a female meets all criteria for AN except that she has a regular menstrual cycle. In addition, EDNOS would be diagnosed when all of the criteria for BN are met, but the duration of illness has been less than 3 months or the frequency of binge eating/purging is less than two times per week. Although EDNOS was originally conceived of as a category for exceptions to more common presentations, the diagnosis of EDNOS is particularly prevalent in children and adolescents. In fact, when the strict criteria provided by the DSM-IV-TR are followed, the majority of all adolescents with eating disorders are considered to have EDNOS. In a recent study examining comparative diagnoses of eating disorders in adolescents, 59.1% of 281 consecutive referrals to an eating disorders program met criteria for EDNOS, while 20.3% were diagnosed with AN and 20.6% were diagnosed with BN (Eddy, Celio Doyle, Hoste, Herzog, & Le Grange, 2008). The adolescents categorized as having EDNOS ranged in presentation from subthreshold AN to BED, limiting the usefulness of the EDNOS diagnosis for purposes of concisely communicating relevant symptoms and guiding treatment recommendations. Furthermore, a comparison of children and adolescents presenting for eating disorder treatment found that younger patients (i.e., <13 years old) are more likely to be diagnosed with EDNOS (rather than AN or BN) than their older adolescent counterparts (Peebles, Wilson, & Lock, 2006). This suggests that the current classification scheme for eating disorders, which was developed on the basis of adult psychopathology, may not adequately describe or sensitively represent eating psychopathology among younger people.

A multidisciplinary Workgroup for Classification of Eating Disorders in Children and Adolescents (WCEDCA) was recently formed to evaluate the shortcomings of the current classification schemes for diagnosing eating disorders in children and adolescents, and this group has suggested several important adjustments to and cautions regarding the current criteria (Bravender et al., 2007). In regard to AN, a primary criterion is low weight, defined as at or below 85% IBW or a body mass index (BMI) of 17.5 kg/m^2. Weight-to-height ratios like BMI, or other weight cutoffs, can be problematic to interpret in younger populations. In children and adolescents, for whom continuous growth is expected, the WCEDCA highlights the importance of using slowed or halted growth due to malnutrition and several data points plotted on a growth chart over time, rather than a single point in time, in determining pathological weight status. Another criterion for the diagnosis of AN that can be problematic because of developmental considerations is amenorrhea. Menstrual cycles early in adolescence can take some time to establish a regular pattern, making it difficult to determine whether three consecutive periods have been missed. Some adolescents will have delayed menarche due to malnutrition (i.e., primary amenorrhea), and boys with AN do not have a parallel criterion in terms of sexual development. Two notable differences in the clinical presentation of AN among children and adolescents compared with adults are a lack of verbally articulated body dissatisfaction and non-weight-related motivation for their restrictive behaviors. Many children and younger adolescents do not report body image distortion and express a desire to "be healthy" rather than to lose weight, unlike older adolescents or adults with AN (Lock & Le Grange, 2006).

In regard to BN, the DSM-IV-TR criteria may not reflect a consideration of developmental factors in the eating-disordered psychopathology of younger adolescents, for whom regular, sustained patterns of binge eating and purging may not be firmly established yet. Specifically, to meet criteria for BN, bingeing and purging must occur an average of twice a week for 3 months. Unlike older individuals with more chronic symptoms of BN, adolescents may demonstrate more vacillation in their symptom frequency, experiencing brief periods of high-frequency behaviors followed by an absence of symptoms. Yet children and adolescents with more inconsistent binge–purge behaviors report comparable levels of general psychopathology and may represent the early form of what will later become a chronic and sustained pattern of pathological behavior (Le Grange, Loeb, Van Orman, & Jellar, 2004). Developmentally sensitive adaptations to the DSM for eating disorders have not yet been made.

Epidemiology

AN most commonly begins during adolescence, with a point prevalence rate of 0.48% in adolescent females (Lucas et al., 1991). Rates of AN are lower in boys, with a

19:2 female-to-male ratio in adults (Hoek, 1993), but some investigators have identified increased referral rates for males with eating disorders (Braun, Sunday, Huang, & Halmi, 1999). The peak age of onset is estimated to be between 14 and 18 years (American Psychiatric Association, 2000), but AN has been diagnosed in children as young as 7 years old (Bostic et al., 1997). Although AN affects individuals of all racial/ethnic backgrounds, it is more commonly found in European American, Hispanic, and Asian American females than in African American females, and is most prevalent in industrialized societies (American Psychiatric Association, 2000). In terms of prognosis, adolescent-onset AN tends to be associated with better outcome than either prepubertal or adult-onset AN; prepubertal AN may be associated with a more severe psychiatric profile (Russell, 1985).

Research on the course and outcome of AN in adults suggests considerable variability, with fewer than half of surviving patients achieving full recovery, one-third showing improvements but continuing to experience symptoms, and one-fifth remaining chronically ill (Steinhausen, 2002). Research on treatment outcome of AN in adolescents appears to be more favorable. Approximately 75% of adolescents in a 6-month intensive inpatient program achieved full recovery over longitudinal follow-up, with a median recovery time of 5 years (Strober, Freeman, & Morrell, 1997). Substantial improvement and recovery is also seen through outpatient treatment over short- and long-term follow-ups as well (Le Grange & Lock, 2005).

Regarding BN, estimates show that 1–5% of adolescent girls in the United States meet full criteria (American Academy of Pediatrics, 2003) and that one-fifth of adolescents with BN are male (Steiner & Lock, 1998). BN in premenarchal youths is relatively rare (Kent, Lacey, & McClusky, 1992), and BN is more likely to be diagnosed in adolescents between the ages of 13 and 20 years old than in children less than 13 years old (Peebles et al., 2006). The peak age of onset is estimated to be between 15.7 and 18.1 years (Fairburn, Cooper, Doll, Norman, & O'Connor, 2000; Herzog, Keller, Sacks, Yeh, & Lavori, 1992). Although BN typically begins in adolescence, the disorder may not be identified and treatment may not be sought until years later, due to the secretiveness and shame frequently accompanying BN. BN affects individuals of all socioeconomic and racial/ethnic groups, but may be less common among African Americans (Striegel-Moore et al., 2003). Multiple studies have demonstrated that a shorter duration of BN predicts good outcome in treatment (e.g., Keel & Mitchell, 1997; Reas, Schoemaker, Zipfel, & Williamson, 2001). In a longitudinal study following adolescents with full-syndrome eating disorders over 17 years, the authors found that untreated BN predicted a 20-fold (younger adolescents) to 35-fold (older adolescents) increase in the risk for BN in adulthood (Kotler, Cohen, Davies, Pine, & Walsh, 2001), highlighting the significance of BN in adolescents and the need to intervene early.

Treatment outcome in adult BN is moderately successful, with approximately 50% reaching full recovery (Keel & Mitchell, 1997). In short-term outcome studies of adolescents with BN, cognitive-behavioral and family-based treatments reveal significant reductions in eating disorder symptoms and initial binge–purge abstinence rates in between 40 and 60% of these adolescents (Le Grange, Crosby, Rathouz, & Leventhal, 2007; Lock, 2005; Schapman-Williams, Lock, & Couturier, 2006; Schmidt et al., 2007).

Psychiatric and Medical Comorbidity

Both psychiatric and medical comorbidity are commonly found in adolescents with eating disorders. In a recent study of 86 adolescents with AN participating in a treatment trial, 24% reported a mood disorder and 14% reported an anxiety disorder (Lock, Agras, Bryson, & Kraemer, 2005). In a study of 80 adolescents with BN or subthreshold BN, 62.5% of the sample had a comorbid diagnosis (Fischer & Le Grange, 2007); the majority of these presented with a major mood disorder, and 25% had previously attempted suicide or harmed themselves. AN and BN confer risk for developing other eating disorders as well. Although the diagnosis of personality disorders may not be appropriate in children and adolescents, certain patterns of personality styles have been associated with AN and BN: Adolescents with AN tend to exhibit more avoidant, inhibited, and constricted personality traits, whereas adolescents with bulimic symptoms tend to demonstrate affective lability and undercontrolled behaviors and emotions (Steiner & Lock, 1998; Thompson-Brenner, Eddy, Satir, Boisseau, & Westen, 2008).

Medical sequelae of both AN and BN are significant, and medical problems are highly likely in youths with EDNOS as well. Low weight and amenorrhea are hallmark criteria of AN, and numerous medical consequences are related to these conditions. Malnutrition is accompanied by lowered body temperature, hypotension, structural brain abnormalities, cardiac dysfunction, and gastrointestinal difficulties. Changes in skin/hair texture and growth can occur, such as the development of lanugo (fine, downy hair on the body), dry skin, hair loss, and brittle hair and nails. Osteopenia and osteoporosis are often found to result from low weight and can persist even following weight gain (Misra & Klibanski, 2006). Acute medical problems include bradycardia (very slow heart rate), hypothermia (very low body temperature), and dehydration, which may become life-threatening (Fisher et al., 1995). The medical consequences of AN are particularly pronounced in childhood and adolescence, when physical development can be stunted and otherwise compromised. Medical signs of malnutrition may take time to be identified by a physician, in part due to the body's natural resiliency; that is, common signs of starvation may not initially be detected, and an early lack of these signs should not invite complacency. Among adults, standard mortality rates for AN are elevated, with some estimates indicating an almost 18-fold increase in mortality compared with that in the general population (Steinhausen, 2002). Approximately half of the deaths in individuals with AN are due to suicide (Keel et al., 2003). Following weight restoration, psychological and social impairment may persist, but vocational or academic functioning is more likely to remain high (Deter & Herzog, 1994).

Medical complications occurring in individuals with BN are largely related to binge–purge behaviors and include low potassium (hypokalemia), esophageal tears, gastric disturbances, dehydration, and severe changes in blood pressure or heart rate when standing or sitting (orthostasis), which may require intermittent hospitalization. Among individuals with BN, as many as one-quarter may require hospitalization due to medical reasons (Golden et al., 2003). Mortality rates are not elevated in adolescents with BN, although any of the above-described medical comorbidities could result in death.

Etiology and Risks for Pediatric Eating Disorders

A developmental psychopathological perspective of eating disorders postulates that a "perfect storm" of biological, familial/individual, and sociocultural forces may converge to precipitate the development of an eating disorder (Steiner et al., 2003). Genetic research has yielded increasing evidence for the familial clustering of eating disorders and related attitudes (Kendler et al., 1995), and current research is underway to add to our understanding of genetic variants that put individuals at risk for eating disorders (Kaye et al., 2008). It is believed that 50% of the risk for AN is attributable to additive genetic factors. Furthermore, biological influences in the development of eating disorders have been implicated through studies of serotonergic activity in cortical and limbic systems, and through brain imaging studies showing altered activity in different regions of the brain (Frank et al., 2007). However, in several areas of this research, it remains unclear whether these neurobiological differences are premorbid risk factors or secondary effects of disordered eating and starvation.

Hypotheses regarding family characteristics as risk factors for the development of eating disorders have been postulated. For instance, seminal work by Minuchin, Rosman, and Baker (1978) hypothesized that families of patients with eating disorders are characterized by being overly enmeshed, conflict-avoidant, and inflexible. A more recent theory suggested that insecure attachment (i.e., dismissive attachment styles) may contribute to risk for an eating disorder (Ward et al., 2001). Some research suggests that families of individuals with BN are more chaotic, conflicted, and critical, whereas families of individuals with AN are more controlling and organized (Humphrey, 1987). However, these family characteristics have not yet been demonstrated to be definitive or specific risk factors for the development of eating disorders.

Weight/shape concerns and dieting behaviors are considered to be specific and highly potent risk factors for the development of eating disorders (Jacobi, Hayward, de Zwaan, Kraemer, & Agras, 2004). Adolescence is generally characterized by an increased focus on bodily appearance, due to a greater emphasis on sexual attractiveness, social acceptance, and the ability to undertake actions related to these issues—all of which are likely to increase the risk of an eating disorder. In a survey study of almost 5,000 adolescents, 57% of girls and 33% of boys reported using unhealthy methods in attempts to lose weight (e.g., fasting, skipping meals) (Neumark-Sztainer, Story, Hannan, Perry, & Irving, 2002). In addition, early onset of puberty in girls and sexual abuse, as well as difficult transitions (e.g., new school, parent divorce), have been hypothesized to play a role in the etiology of eating disorders. However, only a small percentage of youths who have these experiences go on to develop true eating disorder psychopathology, suggesting other influences in the development of these disorders.

The mass media are often described as playing an important environmental role in the development of eating disorders, particularly due to the "thin ideal" that is promoted (McCabe, Ricciardelli, & Finemore, 2001). It has been argued that the internalization of the thin ideal makes young females more vulnerable to the development of disordered eating behaviors and attitudes (Ohring, Graber, & Brooks-Gunn, 2001), while an increased emphasis on muscularity and lower body fat leads to increased shape/weight concerns and eating disorders in males (Leit, Pope, & Gray, 2001). Although the precise developmental pathways of eating disorders remain unknown, these disorders are probably influenced by a complex combination of biological, psychological, and sociocultural factors.

Evaluation

The evaluation of eating disorders in youths is multifaceted. It is essential to meet with both an adolescent and his or her caregiver(s) to obtain a more complete picture of current eating disturbance and a historical account of other psychiatric problems, as well as aspects of healthy psychosocial development.

Interview with Adolescent

The evaluation should begin by meeting with the adolescent alone to demonstrate respect for his or her developing identity. Although the adolescent may present as defensive or hostile, it is important that the assessor convey a warm, supportive atmosphere and ask open-ended questions to obtain a good understanding of the adolescent and his or her family. A comprehensive evaluation will entail a history of weight loss efforts, including calorie restriction (e.g., limiting fat intake, limiting fluid consumption, fasting/skipping meals), exercise patterns, avoidance of eating, secretive eating, hoarding of food, binge eating, self-induced vomiting, misuse of laxatives and diuretics for weight control purposes, use of stimulants/diet pills, and (for clients with Type 1 diabetes) misuse of insulin for appetite suppression. Inquiring about potential triggers for the onset of the dieting behavior will provide a context for later case conceptualization. Some potential triggers include recent transitions or other stressors (e.g., academic problems, friendship/romantic relationship breakups, parental divorce), exposure to weight-related criticism or teasing, onset of menses, dating experiences, stressful family environment, and exposure to dieting within the adolescent's social circle or family. Finally, it is important to carefully assess current pretreatment levels of dietary restriction, binge eating, compensatory behaviors, severity of weight/shape concerns, and preoccupation with eating, as these will be targets in treatment.

Interview with Parents

After the interview with the adolescent, parents (or the caregivers) should be interviewed without the adolescent present to gain a complete picture of the client's psychopathology. Youths with the restricting subtype of AN or EDNOS may have a tendency to underreport symptomatology (Couturier, Lock, Forsberg, Vanderheyden, & Yen, 2007). Some adolescents and children may minimize their symptoms unconsciously due to a distorted perception of their behaviors/attitudes, while others may purposely deny or underreport symptoms to evade treatment. Some parents are apprehensive about the evaluation and treatment experience because they feel shame or guilt regarding their child's problems. For this reason, it is again important to convey supportiveness and warmth when asking about parents' observations of their child.

Parents should be asked more generally about their child's physical and social development (e.g., performance in school, relationships with family members, peer relationships), as well as any history of psychiatric illness in immediate and extended family members. Information obtained from the parents can be compared to the adolescent's interview in order to explore similarities and differences; together, the two interviews provide a more comprehensive history of the development and maintenance of the eating disorder.

Psychometric Assessments

Clinical assessment can be improved through the use of standardized interview and self-report questionnaires. These allow for comparison with normative data and can be used to monitor progress during treatment. The following are a few of the many assessments specifically evaluating the cognitive, attitudinal, and behavioral components of eating disorders in youths.

The Eating Disorder Examination (EDE; Cooper & Fairburn, 1987) is a standardized investigator-based interview that measures the severity of specific eating disorder psychopathology. The EDE also generates operational eating disorder diagnoses. With the exception of the diagnostic items, it is exclusively concerned with the preceding 4 weeks. It assesses both the frequency of key behaviors (e.g., various forms of overeating and purging), and the severity of psychopathology as characterized by four subscales: Dietary Restraint, Eating Concern, Shape Concern, and Weight Concern. The psychometric properties of the EDE are good (e.g., Rizvi, Peterson, Crow, & Agras, 2000), and it has been used in many treatment studies. Adolescents as young as age 12 are able to understand and respond to the interview (Binford, Le Grange, & Jellar, 2005). A child version of the EDE with preliminary psychometric support (Watkins, Frampton, Lask, & Bryant-Waugh, 2005) has been developed for use with younger children, who may have difficulty understanding the more complicated constructs.

The EDE–Questionnaire (EDE-Q; Fairburn & Beglin, 1994) is a self-report version of the EDE and demonstrates good psychometric properties (Peterson et al., 2007). Among adolescents, there is good correspondence between the EDE interview and the EDE-Q (Binford et al., 2005).

Other self-report measures include the Eating Disorder Inventory, for which normative data are available down to age 14 years (Shore & Porter, 1990); the Eating Attitudes Test, which has a version for school-age children (Maloney, McQuire, & Daniels, 1988); and the Kids Eating Disorders Survey, which is applicable for children up to middle school age (Childress, Brewerton, Hodges, & Jarrell, 1993).

General Psychopathology

In addition to assessing specific psychopathology of eating disorders, the evaluator needs to assess for the presence of psychiatric comorbidities (anxiety, depression, substance use, and other disorders). It is not unusual for clients to report difficulties with feelings of depression, anxiety, obsessionality, and delusional beliefs. However, it is important to understand how disturbances in these domains may sometimes be attributable to the eating disorder itself. For instance, reports of anxiety or obsessiveness may focus exclusively on eating and weight loss behaviors; in this example, the eating disorder is the primary and root problem. Thorough attention to discriminating these symptoms from other psychiatric disorders is important.

Medical Examination

Because eating disorders are so likely to have medical sequelae, it is essential to obtain a medical evaluation from a physician who has experience working with eating disorders. A complete physical exam to check for signs of malnutrition (e.g., dehydration, lanugo), as well as effects of purging (e.g., tooth erosion, electrolyte imbalance), helps to assess the severity of the illness. Furthermore, it is important to rule out other possible organic reasons for weight loss, including thyroid disease, celiac disease, or cancers.

Treatment

Comprehensive psychiatric and medical care using a team approach is urged for the treatment of eating disorders (Commission on Adolescent Eating Disorders, 2005). The severity of the eating disorder typically dictates the level of care selected; however, the availability of resources and third-party coverage may play a major role in treatment selection. Inpatient hospitalization in a psychiatric unit that specializes in eating disorders and residential treatments may be warranted for severe and persistent cases of AN and BN—for example, when comorbidities are present that require close medical or psychiatric monitoring (Golden et al., 2003). This more intensive level of care may also be warranted when an individual has been unresponsive to multiple outpatient treatment attempts. However, in most cases where medical stability has been established, outpatient psychotherapy with or without psychopharmacology is a prudent first step.

Anorexia Nervosa

Psychotherapy

Although AN has been recognized by the medical community for over 125 years, research on the psychological treatment of AN is very limited. There are relatively few published outpatient controlled psychotherapy trials for AN across age groups, and their findings are limited by small sample sizes and variable outcome measures, making it difficult to draw more general conclusions (Bulik, Berkman, Brownley, Sedway, & Lohr, 2007). Five randomized controlled trials (RCTs) have focused on adolescents with AN (Eisler et al., 2000; Le Grange, Eisler, Dare, & Russell, 1992; Lock et al., 2005; Robin et al., 1999; Russell, Szmukler, Dare & Eisler, 1987), and additional research on these same approaches has included case series and pilot studies (Le Grange, Binford, & Loeb, 2005; Loeb et al., 2007). Both family-based treatment (FBT) and individual psychotherapy for adolescent AN have garnered empirical support. However, FBT currently appears to demonstrate superior outcomes to individual psychotherapy.

FBT for adolescent AN was devised by Dare and Eisler (1997) at the Maudsley Hospital in London, and it incorporates elements of Minuchin's and others' earlier family-based work. FBT is also referred to as the "Maudsley approach," due to the location of its development and early trials. FBT is one of the only treatments for adolescent AN with consistent empirical support (National Collaborating Centre for Mental Health,

2004). In one trial, approximately two-thirds of adolescent patients treated with FBT for AN were recovered at the end of FBT, while 75–90% were fully weight-recovered at 5-year follow-up (Eisler et al., 1997). Similar improvements in terms of psychological factors were also noted for these patients.

The primary aims of FBT are to assist parents in restoring their afflicted child to physical health and returning him or her to normal adolescent development unencumbered by the eating disorder. FBT is agnostic as to the etiology of the disorder, and family members are assured that they are not the causes of the eating disorder, to alleviate guilt and motivate action. FBT is problem-focused, and the principal strategy consists of behavioral change directed by unified parents. FBT also aims to externalize and separate the AN pathology from the affected adolescent, to promote parental action and encourage adolescent cooperation. There are three phases that span 6–12 months of treatment (approximately 15–24 sessions). Parents play an active and positive role in order to help restore their child's weight to levels expected for their adolescent's age and height (Phase 1); hand the control over eating back to the adolescent (Phase 2); and encourage normal adolescent development through an in-depth discussion of these crucial developmental issues as they pertain to their child (Phase 3). A manual for FBT as it has been implemented in almost all of the Maudsley studies is available to clinicians (Lock, Le Grange, Agras, & Dare, 2001), as well as a parent handbook that can assist and guide parents through treatment (Lock & Le Grange, 2005).

Individual therapy may also be efficacious for adolescent AN, although there is less persuasive evidence available. Individual treatment is hypothesized to support autonomy and independence, promote self-development and confidence, and provide an opportunity for the adolescent to comment on problems and issues without parental involvement (e.g., dating, substance experimentation, the patient's evaluations of the parents). In a study comparing ego-oriented individual therapy with a family treatment based on FBT, the family treatment restored weight and menses more quickly than the individual treatment, and there were no group differences on such psychological variables as eating attitudes, depression, and self-reported eating-related family conflict (Robin et al., 1999). Due to a small study sample ($N = 37$), conclusions based on these findings should be drawn with caution. It is important to note that in practice, family treatments are often combined with individual therapy (Lock, 2002), and that in cases of highly critical parents, FBT for AN can be administered in "separate" sessions (i.e., parents can be seen apart from their adolescent) (Le Grange et al., 1992).

Psychopharmacology

Psychopharmacology in the treatment of AN in adolescents is relatively unexplored. Low-dose neuroleptics may be used to address severe obsessional thinking and anxiety, but to date have only been studied in case reports and open-label trials (Mehler-Wex, Romanos, Kirchheiner, & Schulze, 2008). Specifically, newer antipsychotic agents (e.g., olanzapine) at doses of 5 mg/day or more yields decreased anxiety about eating, improved sleep, and decreased rumination about food and body concerns (Dennis, Le Grange, & Bremer, 2006). Currently, a double-blind RCT of olanzapine is underway in Ontario, Canada (Spettigue et al., 2008).

Bulimia Nervosa

Psychotherapy

There have been close to 50 RCTs studying treatments for BN in adults (Shapiro et al., 2007), pointing to cognitive-behavioral therapy (CBT), interpersonal psychotherapy, and the adjunctive use of selective serotonin reuptake inhibitors as effective treatments. In comparison, only two RCTs have been published for adolescent BN (Le Grange et al., 2007; Schmidt et al., 2007), despite the fact that BN typically begins in adolescence.

Given the relative success of CBT with adults, CBT may be an effective approach for adolescents (Le Grange & Schmidt, 2005) and has been evaluated in a case series with promising results (rate of abstinence from bulimic behaviors = 56%; Lock, 2005). In addition, an RCT evaluating a CBT guided self-care condition demonstrated positive results in abstinence from bingeing and purging at posttreatment (20%) and 6-month follow-up (40%; Schmidt et al., 2007). In CBT for adolescents, parent involvement is expected, although the degree of involvement that is needed is unspecified.

The model of CBT for BN assumes that the maintenance of the disorder is centered on dysfunctional thoughts, attitudes, and behaviors regarding body shape and weight (Fairburn, Marcus, & Wilson, 1993). Concerns about weight and shape, along with low self-esteem, result in attempts at dietary restriction. The pattern of restrictive eating results in psychological and physiological deprivation, which potentiates the likelihood of binge eating, especially in the presence of negative affect. Compensatory behaviors are used to lessen the individual's fear of weight gain following a binge, and the pernicious cycle of dietary restriction, binge eating, and purging continues.

A second promising treatment that has been tested with adolescents is FBT for BN (FBT-BN). Similar to FBT for AN, FBT-BN is agnostic about the causes of the disorder and assumes that adolescent development is negatively affected by secrecy, shame, and dysfunctional eating patterns characteristic of BN. FBT-BN follows the same three stages of treatment as in FBT for AN; however, several important differences between the two forms of FBT exist. First, in FBT-BN treatment is not focused on weight restoration, but rather on the regulation of eating patterns and the elimination of bingeing–purging. Second, the treatment of BN is more collaborative between parents and the affected adolescent. Finally, adolescents with BN may be more likely to have psychiatric comorbidity than those with AN, which is an additional factor that often arises in treatment. These competing issues are dealt with as clinically necessary, but a focus on the eating disorder is persistently maintained when possible. Many adolescents respond well to parental involvement in meal planning and assisting with efforts to decrease binge-eating and purging episodes, once the therapist succeeds in assuring them that the parental involvement is supportive rather than critical. At the same time, family involvement helps the therapist to highlight for the parents the medical and psychological problems associated with BN, and to elicit their support in helping their child.

FBT-BN has been evaluated in adolescents in two case series (Dodge, Hodes, Eisler, & Dare, 1995; Le Grange, Lock, & Dymek, 2003) and one RCT (Le Grange et al., 2007), for which a treatment manual was developed (Le Grange & Lock, 2007). In this RCT, FBT-BN was compared with a nonspecific individual supportive psychotherapy. FBT-BN yielded a greater proportion of adolescents who were abstinent from bingeing–purging at posttreatment (39% vs. 17.9%; $p < .05$) and at 6-month follow-up (29.3% vs. 10.3%; $p = .05$). Also, greater reductions on all measures of eating pathology were demonstrated for FBT-BN. A variation of FBT-BN was used in Schmidt and colleague's RCT (2007; described above) and compared favorably to CBT guided self-care at 6-month follow-up (family therapy = 41% abstinent).

Psychopharmacology

The use of psychopharmacological interventions in adolescents with BN has only been studied in one open-label medication trial (Kotler, Devlin, Davies, & Walsh, 2003). In this promising study, 8 weeks of fluoxetine (60 mg/day) was well tolerated in conjunction with supportive psychotherapy, yielding improvement rates of approximately 70%. Additional double-blind RCT studies are needed to evaluate psychopharmacology in adolescents with BN.

Current Needs and Future Directions

Additional clinical trials studying treatments for pediatric eating disorders are greatly needed. To date, there have only been seven RCTs of psychotherapy for AN and BN in adolescents. There is early evidence from these few trials that involving parents in treatment may be helpful, particularly through FBT (i.e., the Maudsley approach), and that guided CBT may be useful for older adolescents with BN. Pharmacological interventions in youths could also be useful, but have been largely unexplored. Due to the extensive physical and psychological sequelae of eating disorders, early identification and intervention are needed. Physicians, teachers, and parents should be educated as to the early warning signs of eating disorders in youths. In addition, practitioners should be well equipped to provide aggressive and targeted treatments to reduce symptoms as quickly as possible.

References

American Academy of Pediatrics. (2003). Policy statement: Identifying and treating eating disorders. *Pediatrics, 111,* 204–211.

American Psychiatric Association. (2000). *Diagnostic and statistical manual of mental disorders* (4th ed., text rev.). Washington, DC: Author.

Binford, R. B., Le Grange, D., & Jellar, C. C. (2005). Eating Disorders Examination versus Eating Disorders Examination—Questionnaire in adolescents with full and partial-syndrome bulimia nervosa and anorexia nervosa. *International Journal of Eating Disorders, 37,* 44–49.

Bostic, J. Q., Muriel, A. C., Hack, S., Weinstein, S., & Herzog, D. (1997). Anorexia nervosa in a 7-year-old girl. *Journal of Developmental and Behavioral Pediatrics, 18,* 331–333.

Braun, D., Sunday, S., Huang, A., & Halmi, C. A. (1999). More males seek treatment for eating disorders. *International Journal of Eating Disorders, 25,* 415–424.

Bravender, T., Bryant-Waugh, R., Herzog D., Katzman, D., Kreipe, R. D., Lask, B., et al. (2007). Workgroup for Classification of Eating Disorders in Children and Adolescents: Classification of child and adolescent eating disturbances. *International Journal of Eating Disorders, 40*(Suppl.), S117–S122.

Bulik, C. M., Berkman, N. A., Brownley, K. A., Sedway, J. A., & Lohr, K. N. (2007). Anorexia nervosa treatment: A systematic review of randomized controlled trials. *International Journal of Eating Disorders, 40,* 310–320.

Childress, A., Brewerton, T., Hodges, E., & Jarrell, M. (1993). The Kids Eating Disorder Survey (KEDS): A study of middle school students. *Journal of the American Academy of Child and Adolescent Psychiatry, 32,* 843–850.

Commission on Adolescent Eating Disorders. (2005). Treatment of eating disorders. In D. L. Evans, E. B. Foa, R. E. Gur, H. Hendin, C. P. O'Brien, M. E. P. Seligman, et al. (Eds.), *Treating and preventing adolescent mental health disorders: What we know and what we don't know—a research agenda for improving the mental health of our youth* (pp. 283–301). Oxford, UK: Oxford University Press.

Cooper, Z., & Fairburn, C. (1987). The Eating Disorder Examination: A semi-structured interview for the assessment of the specific psychopathology of eating disorders. *International Journal of Eating Disorders, 6,* 1–8.

Couturier, J., Lock, J., Forsberg, S., Vanderheyden, D., & Yen, H. L. (2007). The addition of a parent and clinician component to the Eating Disorder Examination for children and adolescents. *International Journal of Eating Disorders, 40,* 472–475.

Dare, C., & Eisler, I. (1997). Family therapy for anorexia nervosa. In D. M. Garner & P. Garfinkel (Eds.), *Handbook of treatment for eating disorders* (pp. 307–324). New York: Guilford Press.

Dennis, K., Le Grange, D., & Bremer, J. (2006). Olanzapine use in adolescent anorexia nervosa. *Eating and Weight Disorders, 11,* e53–e56.

Deter, H. C., & Herzog, W. (1994). Anorexia nervosa in a long-term perspective: Results of the Heidelberg–Mannheim Study. *Psychosomatic Medicine, 56,* 20–27.

Dodge, E., Hodes, M., Eisler, I., & Dare, C. (1995). Family therapy for bulimia nervosa in adolescents: An exploratory study. *Journal of Family Therapy, 17,* 59–77.

Eddy, K. T., Celio Doyle, A., Hoste, R., Herzog, D. B., & Le Grange, D. (2008). Eating disorder not otherwise specified in adolescents. *Journal of the American Academy of Child and Adolescent Psychiatry, 47,* 156–164.

Eisler, I., Dare, C., Hodes, M., Russell, G., Dodge, E., & Le Grange, D. (2000). Family therapy for adolescent anorexia nervosa: The results of a controlled comparison of two family interventions. *Journal of Child Psychology and Psychiatry, 41,* 727–736.

Eisler, I., Dare, C., Russell, G. F. M., Szmukler, G. I., Le Grange, D., & Dodge, E. (1997). Family and individual therapy in anorexia nervosa: A five-year follow-up. *Archives of General Psychiatry, 54,* 1025–1030.

Fairburn, C., & Beglin, S. (1994). Assessment of eating disorders: Interview or self-report questionnaire? *International Journal of Eating Disorders, 16,* 363–370.

Fairburn, C. G., Cooper, Z., Doll, H. A., Norman, P., & O'Connor, M. (2000). The natural course of bulimia nervosa and binge eating disorder in young women. *Archives of General Psychiatry, 57,* 659–665.

Fairburn, C. G., Marcus, M. D., & Wilson, G. T. (1993). Cognitive-behavioral therapy for binge eating and bulimia nervosa: A comprehensive treatment manual. In C. G. Fairburn & G. T. Wilson (Eds.), *Binge eating: Nature, assessment, and treatment* (pp. 361–404). New York: Guilford Press.

Fischer, S., & Le Grange, D. (2007). Co-morbidity and high-risk behaviors in treatment seeking adolescents with bulimia nervosa. *International Journal of Eating Disorders, 40,* 751–753.

Fisher, M., Golden, N., Katzman, D., Kreipe, R., Rees, J., Schebendach, J., et al. (1995). Eating disorders in adolescents: A background paper. *Journal of Adolescent Health, 16,* 420–437.

Flament, M., Ledoux, S., Jeammet, P., Choquet, M., & Simon, Y. (1995). A population study of bulimia nervosa and subclinical eating disorders in adolescence. In H. Steinhausen (Ed.),

Eating disorders in adolescence: Anorexia and bulimia nervosa (pp. 21–36). New York: Brunner/Mazel.

Frank, G. K., Bailer, U. F., Meltzer, C. C., Price, J. C., Mathis, C. A., Wagner, A., et al. (2007). Regional cerebral blood flow after recovery from anorexia or bulimia nervosa. *International Journal of Eating Disorders, 40,* 488–492.

Golden, N. H., Katzman, D. K., Kreipe, R. E., Stevens, S. L., Sawyer, S. M., Rees, J., et al. (2003). Eating disorders in adolescents: Position paper of the Society for Adolescent Medicine. *Journal of Adolescent Health, 33,* 496–503.

Herzog, D. B., Keller, M. B., Sacks, N. R., Yeh, C. J., & Lavori, P. W. (1992). Psychiatric comorbidity in treatment-seeking anorexics and bulimics. *Journal of the American Academy of Child and Adolescent Psychiatry, 31,* 810–818.

Hoek, H. (1993). Review of epidemiological studies of eating disorders. *International Review of Psychiatry, 5,* 61–74.

Humphrey, L. (1987). Comparison of bulimic–anorexic and nondistressed families using structural analysis of behavior. *Journal of the American Academy of Child and Adolescent Psychiatry, 26,* 248–255.

Jacobi, C., Hayward, C., de Zwaan, M., Kraemer, H. C., & Agras, W. S. (2004). Coming to terms with risk factors for eating disorders: Application of risk terminology and suggestions for a general taxonomy. *Psychological Bulletin, 130,* 19–65.

Kaye, W. H., Bulik, C. M., Plotnicov, K., Thornton, L., Devlin, B., Fichter, M. M., et al. (2008). The genetics of anorexia nervosa collaborative study: Methods and sample description. *International Journal of Eating Disorders, 41,* 289–300.

Keel, P. K., Dorer, D. J., Eddy, K. T., Franko, D., Charatan, D. L., & Herzog, D. B. (2003). Predictors of mortality in eating disorders. *Archives of General Psychiatry, 60,* 179–183.

Keel, P. K., & Mitchell, J. E. (1997). Outcome in bulimia nervosa. *American Journal of Psychiatry, 154,* 313–321.

Kendler, K. S., Walters, E. E., Neale, M. C., Kessler, R. C., Heath, A. C., & Eaves, L. J. (1995). The structure of genetic and environmental risk factors for six major psychiatric disorders in women. *Archives of General Psychiatry, 52,* 374–383.

Kent, A., Lacey, H., & McClusky, S. E. (1992). Pre-menarchal bulimia nervosa. *Journal of Psychosomatic Research, 36,* 205–210.

Kotler, L. A., Cohen, P., Davies, M., Pine, D. S., & Walsh, B. T. (2001). Longitudinal relationships between childhood, adolescent, and adult eating disorders. *Journal of the American Academy of Child and Adolescent Psychiatry, 40,* 1434–1440.

Kotler, L. A., Devlin, M. J., Davies, M., & Walsh, B. T. (2003). An open trial of fluoxetine for adolescents with bulimia nervosa. *Journal of Child and Adolescent Psychopharmacology, 13,* 329–335.

Le Grange, D., Binford, R., & Loeb, K. L. (2005). Manualized family-based treatment for anorexia nervosa: A case series. *Journal of the American Academy of Child and Adolescent Psychiatry, 44,* 41–46.

Le Grange, D., Crosby, R. D., Rathouz, P. J., & Leventhal, B. L. (2007). A randomized controlled comparison of family-based treatment and supportive psychotherapy for adolescent bulimia nervosa. *Archives of General Psychiatry, 64,* 1049–1056.

Le Grange, D., Eisler, I., Dare, C., & Russell, G. (1992). Evaluation of family treatments in adolescent anorexia nervosa: A pilot study. *International Journal of Eating Disorders, 12,* 347–357.

Le Grange, D., & Lock, J. (2005). The dearth of psychological treatment studies for anorexia nervosa. *International Journal of Eating Disorders, 37,* 79–91.

Le Grange, D., & Lock, J. (2007). *Treating bulimia in adolescents: A family-based approach.* New York: Guilford Press.

Le Grange, D., Lock, J., & Dymek, M. (2003). Family-based therapy for adolescents with bulimia nervosa. *American Journal of Psychotherapy, 57*, 237–251.

Le Grange, D., Loeb, K. L., Van Orman, S., & Jellar, C. C. (2004). Bulimia nervosa in adolescents: A disorder in evolution? *Archives of Pediatrics and Adolescent Medicine, 58*, 478–482.

Le Grange, D., & Schmidt, U. (2005). The treatment of adolescents with bulimia nervosa. *Journal of Mental Health, 14*, 587–597.

Leit, R., Pope, H. G., & Gray, J. (2001). Cultural expectations of muscularity in men: The evolution of Playgirl centerfolds. *International Journal of Eating Disorders, 29*, 90–93.

Lock, J. (2002). Treating adolescents with eating disorders in the family context: Empirical and theoretical considerations. *Child and Adolescent Psychiatric Clinics of North America, 11*, 331–342.

Lock, J. (2005). Adjusting cognitive behavior therapy for adolescents with bulimia nervosa: Results of a case series. *American Journal of Psychotherapy, 59*, 267–281.

Lock, J., Agras, W. S., Bryson, S., & Kraemer, H. (2005). A comparison of short- and long-term family therapy for adolescent anorexia nervosa. *Journal of the American Academy of Child and Adolescent Psychiatry, 44*, 632–639.

Lock, J., & Le Grange, D. (2005). *Help your teenager beat an eating disorder.* New York: Guilford Press.

Lock, J., & Le Grange, D. (2006). Eating disorders. In D. A. Wolfe & E. J. Mash (Eds.), *Behavioral and emotional disorders in adolescents: Nature, assessment, and treatment* (pp. 485–504). New York: Guilford Press.

Lock, J., Le Grange, D., Agras, W. S., & Dare, C. (2001). *Treatment manual for anorexia nervosa: A family-based approach.* New York: Guilford Press.

Loeb, K. L., Walsh, B. T., Lock, J., Le Grange, D., Jones, J., Marcus, S., et al. (2007). Open trial of family-based treatment for adolescent anorexia nervosa: Evidence of successful dissemination. *Journal of the American Academy of Child and Adolescent Psychiatry, 46*, 792–800.

Lucas, A. R., Beard, C. M., O'Fallon, W. M., & Kurland, L. T. (1991). 50-year trends in the incidence of anorexia nervosa in Rochester, Minn: A population-based study. *American Journal of Psychiatry, 148*, 917–929.

Maloney, M., McQuire, J., & Daniels, S. (1988). The reliability testing of a children's version of the Eating Attitudes Test. *Journal of the American Academy of Child and Adolescent Psychiatry, 27*, 541–543.

McCabe, M., Ricciardelli, L., & Finemore, J. (2001). The role of puberty, media and popularity with peers on strategies to increase weight, decrease weight and increase muscle tone among adolescent boys and girls. *Journal of Psychosomatic Research, 52*, 145–153.

Mehler-Wex, C., Romanos, M., Kirchheiner, J., & Schulze, U. M. (2008). Atypical antipsychotics in severe anorexia nervosa in children and adolescents: Review and case reports. *European Eating Disorders Review, 6*, 100–108.

Minuchin, S., Rosman, B., & Baker, I. (1978). *Psychosomatic families: Anorexia nervosa in context.* Cambridge, MA: Harvard University Press.

Misra, M., & Klibanski, A. (2006). Anorexia nervosa and osteoporosis. *Reviews in Endocrine and Metabolic Disorders, 7*, 91–99.

National Collaborating Centre for Mental Health. (2004). *Eating disorders: Core interventions in the treatment and management of anorexia nervosa, bulimia nervosa and related eating disorders.* London: British Psychological Society/Gaskell, UK.

Neumark-Sztainer, D. M., Story, M., Hannan, P. J., Perry, C. L., & Irving, L. M. (2002). Weight-related concerns and behaviors among overweight and nonoverweight adolescents: Implications for preventing weight-related disorders. *Archives of Pediatrics and Adolescent Medicine, 156*, 171–178.

Ohring, R., Graber, J., & Brooks-Gunn, J. (2001). Girls' recurrent and concurrent body dis-satisfaction: Correlates and consequences over 8 years. *International Journal of Eating Disorders, 31,* 404–415.

Peebles, R., Wilson, J., & Lock, J. (2006). How do children and adolescents with eating disorders differ at presentation? *Journal of Adolescent Health, 39,* 800–805.

Peterson, C., Crosby, R., Wonderlich, S., Joiner, T., Crow, S., Mitchell, J., et al. (2007). Psychometric properties of the Eating Disorder Examination—Questionnaire: Factor structure and internal consistency. *International Journal of Eating Disorders, 40,* 386–389.

Reas, D. L., Schoemaker, C., Zipfel, S., & Williamson, D. A. (2001). Prognostic value of duration of illness and early intervention in bulimia nervosa: A systematic review of the outcome literature. *International Journal of Eating Disorders, 30,* 1–10.

Rizvi, S., Peterson, C., Crow, S., & Agras, W. (2000). Test–retest reliability of the Eating Disorder Examination. *International Journal of Eating Disorders, 28,* 311–316.

Robin, A., Siegal, P., Moye, A., Gilroy, M., Dennis, A., & Sikand, A. (1999). A controlled comparison of family versus individual therapy for adolescents with anorexia nervosa. *Journal of the American Academy of Child and Adolescent Psychiatry, 38,* 1482–1489.

Russell, G. F. M. (1985). Premenarchal anorexia nervosa and its sequelae. *Journal of Psychiatric Research, 19,* 363–369.

Russell, G. F. M., Szmukler, G. I., Dare, C., & Eisler, I. (1987). An evaluation of family therapy in anorexia and bulimia nervosa. *Archives of General Psychiatry, 44,* 1047–1056.

Schapman-Williams, A. M., Lock, J., & Couturier, J. (2006). Cognitive-behavioral therapy for adolescents with binge eating syndromes: A case series. *International Journal of Eating Disorders, 39,* 252–255.

Schmidt, U., Lee, S., Beecham, J., Perkins, S., Treasure, J., Yim, I., et al. (2007). A randomized controlled trial of family therapy and cognitive behavior therapy guided self-care for adolescents with bulimia nervosa and related disorders. *American Journal of Psychiatry, 164,* 591–598.

Shapiro, J. R., Berkman, N. D., Brownley, K. A., Sedway, J. A., Lohr, K. N., & Bulik, C. M. (2007). Bulimia nervosa treatment: A systematic review of randomized controlled trials. *International Journal of Eating Disorders, 40,* 321–336.

Shore, R., & Porter, J. (1990). Normative and reliability data for 11–18 year olds on the Eating Disorder Inventory. *International Journal of Eating Disorders, 9,* 201–207.

Spettigue, W., Buchholz, A., Henderson, K., Feder, S., Moher, D., Kourad, K., et al. (2008). Evaluation of the efficacy and safety of olanzapine as an adjunctive treatment for anorexia nervosa in adolescent females: A randomized, double-blind, placebo-controlled trial. *BMC Pediatrics, 8,* 4.

Steiner, H., Kwan, W., Shaffer, T. G., Walker, S., Miller, S., Sagar, A., et al. (2003). Risk and protective factors for juvenile eating disorders. *European Child and Adolescent Psychiatry, 12*(Suppl. 1), 38–46.

Steiner, H., & Lock, J. (1998). Anorexia nervosa and bulimia nervosa in children and adolescents: A review of the past 10 years. *Journal of the American Academy of Child and Adolescent Psychiatry, 37,* 352–359.

Steinhausen, H. C. (2002). The outcome of anorexia nervosa in the 20th century. *American Journal of Psychiatry, 159,* 1284–1293.

Striegel-Moore, R., Dohm, F., Kraemer, H., Taylor, C. B., Daniels, S., Crawford, P., et al. (2003). Eating disorders in white and black women. *American Journal of Psychiatry, 160,* 1326–1331.

Strober, M., Freeman, R., & Morrell, W. (1997). The long-term course of severe anorexia nervosa in adolescents: Survival analysis of recovery, relapse, and outcome predictors over 10–15 years in a prospective study. *International Journal of Eating Disorders, 22,* 339–360.

Thompson-Brenner, H., Eddy, K. T., Satir, D., Boisseau, C., & Westen, D. (2008). Personality subtypes in adolescents with eating disorders: Validation of a classification approach. *Journal of Child Psychology and Psychiatry*, *49*, 170–180.

Ward, A., Ramsey, R., Turnbull, S. J., Steele, M., Steele, H., & Treasure, J. L. (2001). Attachment in anorexia nervosa: A transgenerational perspective. *British Journal of Medical Psychology*, *74*, 497–505.

Watkins, B., Frampton, I., Lask, B., & Bryant-Waugh, R. (2005). Reliability and validity of the child version of the Eating Disorder Examination: A preliminary investigation. *International Journal of Eating Disorders*, *38*, 183–187.

CHAPTER 32

Elimination Disorders

Enuresis and Encopresis

LAURA K. CAMPBELL
DANIEL J. COX
STEPHEN M. BOROWITZ

The mastery of bowel and bladder control is a major developmental milestone, influenced by neurocognitive and physiological maturation, temperamental characteristics, and parental and cultural expectations for toilet training. As a general guideline, continence for stool is expected by age 4 and continence for urine by age 5. In the United States, toilet training for both typically occurs by a child's third year of life (Brazelton et al., 1999). Delays in reaching or disruptions after achieving this milestone are sources of significant stress and embarrassment for children and their families. In this chapter, we provide an overview of the biopsychosocial issues associated with the functional elimination disorders, enuresis and encopresis, and we briefly review empirically supported treatments for each disorder.

Enuresis

The *Diagnostic and Statistical Manual of Mental Disorders*, fourth edition, text revision (DSM-IV-TR; American Psychiatric Association, 2000) defines enuresis as the repeated voiding of urine into the bed or clothing in children with a chronological and developmental age of at least 5 years. The behavior may be involuntary or intentional; must occur at a rate of twice a week for at least 3 months or result in clinically significant distress or functional impairment; and cannot be caused by a substance or a general medical condition. The DSM-IV-TR also specifies three subtypes of enuresis: nocturnal only, diurnal only, and nocturnal and diurnal.

Enuresis and subclinical bedwetting are very common conditions in children. Prevalence rates vary broadly (Butler, Golding, Northstone, & ALSPAC Study Team,

2005), with overall estimates of approximately 10% of school-age children (Jarvelin, Vikevainen-Tervonen, Moilanen, & Huttunen, 1988). Enuresis is more than twice as likely in boys as in girls (Butler et al., 2005). Prevalence rates decline steadily with age, with approximately 1% experiencing bedwetting into adolescence (Feehan, McGee, Stanton, & Silva, 1990).

Biological Factors: The Pathophysiology of Enuresis

Nocturnal enuresis is a physiologically normal voiding of urine occurring only during sleep without daytime urinary incontinence (van Gool, Nieuwenhuis, ten Doeschate, Messer, & de Jong, 1999). In most children, nocturnal enuresis results from a maturational delay in the ability to recognize the sensation of a full bladder while asleep. Children who experience nightly wetting accidents may also experience a reduction in bladder capacity overnight, leaving them unable to hold all the urine produced while sleeping (Yeung et al., 2002). They may also produce a large amount of urine, due to insufficient production of the antidiuretic hormone vasopressin (Devitt et al., 1999). Nocturnal enuresis has a strong genetic component, and approximately 77% of children with the condition have a first-degree relative with a history of enuresis (Bartolozzi, Boldrini, Salmeri, & Vitali, 1991; see von Gontard, Schaumburg, Hollmann, Eiberg, & Rittig, 2001, for a review). Only 2–3% of nocturnal enuresis cases have identifiable organic causes of nocturnal enuresis (e.g., neurological disorders; Schmitt, 1997). Although it is commonly believed that bedwetting occurs in children who are heavy sleepers, little scientific evidence supports this theory (Neveus, Stenberg, Lackgren, Tuvemo, & Hetta, 1999).

Approximately 5–10% of children with nocturnal enuresis also experience dysfunctional daytime urination, including increased urgency and frequency (Schmitt, 1997). Urinary urgency is typically caused by muscle spasms of the bladder wall (i.e., detrusor muscle) and small bladder capacity, though urinary tract infections and constipation may also be responsible (Schmitt, 1997). Constipation occurs in up to 36.1% of children with enuresis (McGrath, Caldwell, & Jones, 2007). Although it is considered rare, detrusor–sphincter discoordination and paradoxical contraction of the urethral sphincter—conditions that result in incomplete voiding due to muscle contractions during urination—can also cause daytime urinary incontinence (Norgaard, van Gool, Hjalmas, Djurhuus, & Hellstrom, 1998).

Psychosocial Factors

As mentioned above, nocturnal enuresis and daytime wetting caused by bladder dysfunction are involuntary experiences and as such are not thought to be caused by psychological issues. However, emotional and behavioral problems may develop as consequences of the disorder, due to the social stigma of having wetting accidents. Enuresis is a major source of stress and embarrassment for both children and their parents.

The literature on psychological problems in children with enuresis has yielded mixed results. Some studies report no increase in psychological problems (e.g., Friman, Handwerk, Swearer, McGinnis, & Warzak, 1998; Hirasing, van Leerdam, Bolk-Bennink, & Bosch, 1997), and others indicate higher rates of clinically significant emotional and behavioral problems, including internalizing, externalizing, and attention problems (Joinson, Heron, Emond, & Butler, 2007). Children with diurnal enuresis may exhibit significantly more parent-reported externalizing problems, diagnosable psychiatric conditions, and encopresis than children with nocturnal enuresis only (Zink, Freitag, & von Gontard, 2008).

Many cases of diurnal enuresis are caused by postponement of voiding or withholding of urine. This behavior typically occurs when a child is intensely engaged in another activity (e.g., playing, watching television, homework) and ignores the urge to urinate. Children who postpone voiding have been found to exhibit significantly higher rates of attention problems, oppositional behavior problems, withdrawn behavior, stool withholding, and encopresis, compared to normative data, children with nocturnal enuresis only, and children with urge incontinence only (Lettgen et al., 2002; Zink et al., 2008). Treatment for comorbid emotional and behavioral disorders—including attention-deficit/hyperactivity disorder, which could interfere with attention to bladder distension cues, treatment adherence, and outcome—is imperative.

Treatment

Although enuresis has a high rate of spontaneous remission by late childhood, intervention to promote rapid resolution minimizes its psychosocial impact on a child and family. However, it should be noted that before treatment for enuresis is initiated in a mental health clinic, children should be referred to their pediatrician to rule out organic causes of urinary incontinence (e.g., urinary tract infection).

Medical Interventions

As we discuss in the next section, the urine alarm is the most effective treatment method for most cases of nocturnal enuresis (Mellon & McGrath, 2000). However, the medication desmopressin acetate (DDAVP), a synthetic analogue of the hormone vasopressin, is also useful in the treatment of nocturnal enuresis. DDAVP is an antidiuretic, which decreases urine production and concentrates urine. Children usually respond relatively quickly to the medication, making it an ideal option for sleepovers/overnight events, as well as for children at risk for parental punishment after bedwetting episodes (Butler, 2004). Although DDAVP is effective during treatment, bedwetting typically resumes upon its discontinuation, limiting its utility for long-term treatment (see Glazener & Evans, 2002, and Houts, Berman, & Abramson, 1994, for reviews). Combining DDAVP with the urine alarm may boost the success rate of the urine alarm conditioning process in children who overproduce urine and are at risk for dropping out of treatment (Mellon & McGrath, 2000). The tricyclic antidepressant imipramine can also be used to treat nocturnal enuresis; however, the relapse rate is high (as with DDAVP), and the medication can cause significant side effects in children (Riddle et al., 1991). Therefore, it tends to be reserved for children who have not responded to standard treatment (Gepertz & Neveus, 2004).

Behavioral Interventions

As Mellon and McGrath (2000) have pointed out in their review, nocturnal enuresis is unique in that the research literature clearly supports one specific behavioral intervention for the successful treatment of the disorder: the urine alarm. This treatment approach, which employs an alarm that is activated by moisture sensors worn on night garments or placed on the mattress, is deemed efficacious and superior to other forms of therapy, including medications (Mellon & McGrath, 2000). Combined therapies for nocturnal enuresis pairing urine alarms with other behavioral strategies or medications may also be effective, though it is unclear whether these treatment components have an additive effect on treatment outcome. Two multicomponent treatment protocols combining the urine alarm with other behavioral interventions, such as overlearning and positive reinforcement, are dry-bed training (Azrin, Sneed, & Foxx, 1974) and full-spectrum home training (Houts & Leibert, 1984). For a comprehensive review of empirically supported treatments of nocturnal enuresis, please refer to Mellon and McGrath (2000).

Although the behavioral treatment of nocturnal enuresis is well established and empirically supported, no large studies or clinical trials currently exist on treatment for diurnal or combined enuresis. Behavioral strategies employed in our clinic and in various published case studies for children with daytime wetting, particularly those who postpone voiding, include positive reinforcement for appropriate toileting and independent responding to internal cues to urinate, decreased fluid intake, scheduled toilet sitting, overlearning, and cleanliness training. In children with urge incontinence or bladder dysfunction, strengthening of pelvic floor muscles by stopping urinary flow midstream and basing urination on brief time intervals (rather than urges) can also be helpful in preventing urinary accidents while children are attempting to reach a bathroom.

Encopresis

The DSM-IV-TR (American Psychiatric Association, 2000) defines encopresis as the repeated passage of feces into inappropriate places (e.g., clothing or floor) in children with a chronological and developmental age of at least 4 years. The behavior may be involuntary or intentional, must occur at a rate of one event a month for at least 3 months, and cannot be caused by a substance or a general medical condition. The DSM-IV-TR also requires that constipation and overflow incontinence be indicated as present or absent. More than 80% of children with encopresis have a history of constipation or large, hard, painful bowel movements that are difficult to pass (Benninga, Buller, & Heymans, Tytgat, & Taminiau, 1994; Johanson & Lafferty, 1996; Levine, 1975; Loening-Baucke, 1993; Molnar, Taitz, Urwin, & Wales, 1983), with most developing constipation before age 3 (Partin, Hamill, Fischel, & Partin, 1992). Although encopresis is a functional disorder with no organic etiology, in most cases medical intervention is needed to alleviate chronic constipation (i.e., fewer than three stools per week).

Encopresis is common in school-age children, accounting for approximately 3% of general pediatric outpatient visits (Loening-Baucke, 1993), 25% of visits to pediatric gastroenterology clinics (Taitz, Wales, Urwin, & Molnar, 1986), and over 3% of psychiatric referrals (Levine, 1975). Few epidemiological studies of encopresis have been conducted, but estimates of its prevalence range from 1 to 7.5% of elementary school-age children (Doleys, Schwartz, & Ciminero, 1981; Loening-Baucke, 1996). In clinical/epidemiological studies, males are four to six times more likely to develop encopresis than females (Levine, 1975).

Biological Factors: The Pathophysiology of Encopresis

Chronic constipation often results from stool-withholding behavior due to painful defecation, but it may also occur in response to specific toilet-related fears, aversion to public/unfamiliar bathrooms, or dietary changes, or even without any apparent cause (Benninga, Voskuijl, & Taminiau, 2004; Borowitz et al., 2003; Iacono et al., 1998; Luxem, Christophersen, Purvis, & Baer, 1997). As stool is chronically retained, it becomes harder, larger, and more difficult to evacuate, causing abdominal and/or perianal pain with defecation. Loss of appetite, early satiety, nausea, and vomiting may also result. With chronic constipation, the walls of the rectum stretch to accommodate large amounts of retained stool (i.e., acquired megacolon), causing reduced rectal tone and lessened urge to defecate. Overflow incontinence occurs when new, soft stool leaks around the mass of retained stool and into a child's underwear or pull-up diaper. Soiling typically occurs during the day, though it may occur while the child is asleep at night if the child has a severe fecal impaction (Di Lorenzo & Benninga, 2004).

More than 50% of children with constipation and encopresis exhibit abnormal defecation dynamics, including paradoxical constriction of the external anal sphincter (EAS; van der Plas et al., 1996). Paradoxical constriction occurs when a child involuntarily contracts the EAS while attempting to push out stool, leading to unproductive straining. This process often develops in conjunction with stool withholding. Approximately 30% of children with encopresis also experience enuresis, due at least in part to pressure on the bladder caused by fecal impaction (Levine, 1975; O'Regan & Yazbeck, 1985). Children with encopresis, especially females, may be at increased risk for urinary tract infections, because soiling accidents may introduce fecal bacteria into the urethra.

Psychosocial Factors

The role of psychological factors in the development and maintenance of encopresis is controversial. Although encopresis may be associated with emotional distress and behavioral problems in some children, psychopathology is no longer thought to be a primary cause of the disorder. That being said, a small subset of children with encopresis have co-occurring behavioral issues and developmental delays severe enough to interfere with optimal treatment adherence (Cox, Morris, Borowitz, & Sutphen, 2002; Joinson, Heron, Butler, von Gontard, & ALSPAC Study Team, 2006).

While many cases of encopresis can be effectively managed with brief, symptom-focused medical and behavioral therapy, children with comorbid behavioral disorders often require more comprehensive intervention. As compared to healthy children without a history of defecation problems, children with encopresis are significantly more likely to exhibit behavioral problems, including attention problems, disruptive behaviors, anxiety, and poorer academic and social competency (Cox et al., 2002; Joinson et al., 2006). Children with constipation are also perceived by their parents as being more stubborn (i.e., disobedient, defiant, and resistant to following instructions) than are children without constipation (Burket et al., 2006).

It has long been thought that encopresis may be an indicator of sexual abuse. However, as Mellon, Whiteside, and Friedrich (2006) point out, most studies examining the association of sexual abuse and encopresis fail to include control groups, making it impossible to determine how the prevalence of sexual abuse in children with encopresis compares with that of the general population. One study by Mellon and colleagues found comparable rates of fecal soiling in children who had been sexually abused (10.3%) and children with externalizing behavior problems and no sexual abuse history (10.5%).

It is important to note that chronic fecal soiling can produce psychosocial consequences within a family, in peer relationships, and within a patient. Parents sometimes have a history of blaming or punishing the patient for accidents and develop significant guilt once they understand the physiological causes of encopresis. Peers frequently develop stereotypes about affected children, often labeling them as "dirty" or "stinky," and therefore reject them. Even after the soiling has resolved, these labels may persist. Affected children may respond to parent or peer rejection with hostility or poor self-esteem, or may respond to persistent soiling with learned helplessness.

Treatment

Treatment success rates vary considerably, depending on the type and combination of interventions used, the study methods employed, and how improvement is defined (see Brazzelli & Griffiths, 2007, and McGrath, Mellon, & Murphy, 2000, for reviews). In brief, combining medical treatment and behavioral strategies is the standard of care for treating encopresis. Biofeedback has also been used to treat encopresis. Each of these treatment components is described separately below. However, it should be noted that before treatment for encopresis is initiated in a mental health clinic, children should be referred to their pediatrician to rule out organic causes of constipation and/or fecal incontinence (e.g., Hirschsprung disease, neurological disorders). Also, essential parts of any treatment protocol for encopresis are demystification of the disorder and thorough psychoeducation regarding the condition and its treatment.

Medical Interventions

In children with constipation and encopresis, treatment usually begins with disimpaction of the colon through some form of "cleanout" procedure with high-dose laxatives or a series of enemas. Although enemas produce faster, more predictable results, they are more invasive and often perceived as aversive by children and their parents. Polyethylene glycol (PEG 3350), an orally administered laxative, is frequently used in high doses to perform an "oral cleanout" and may be preferred over enemas. However, a major disadvantage to oral cleanout procedures is that they cause diarrhea and necessitate frequent trips to the toilet over as long as 2–3 days. Consequently, oral cleanouts are often postponed until weekends or holidays to avoid school absence. Next, daily maintenance laxative therapy to prevent recurrence of constipation is initiated. Nearly any laxative (e.g., PEG 3350, lactulose) can be used for maintenance therapy in sufficient doses. Laxatives containing senna (e.g., Ex-Lax), which act as a mild colonic irritant and thereby strengthen the urge to defecate, are also useful in maintenance therapy. The review paper by Benninga and colleagues (2004) includes a table of frequently used laxatives, along with common dosages and side effects. It is essential to establish daily bowel movements to allow the colon to decompress and resume normal tone, as well as to increase the child's sensitivity to rectal distension and facilitate more efficient rectal evacuation. Laxative regimens and adjustments should be always performed in consultation with a pediatrician or a pediatric gastroenterologist.

Dietary recommendations—such as increasing the dietary fiber with fruits, vegetables, whole grains, and/or a fiber supplement; increasing fluid intake; eliminating dairy products; and consuming probiotics—are frequently recommended as adjuncts to encopresis treatment. However, the efficacy of such dietary changes in encopresis has not been established, as no randomized clinical trials have been published.

Behavioral Interventions

Behavioral protocols should be used in conjunction with medical interventions in children with constipation and encopresis, but may be used alone in children with nonretentive encopresis. Behavioral interventions for encopresis typically focus on (1) appropriate and immediate response to rectal distension/urge to defecate with trips to the toilet; (2) resolution of toilet avoidance/fear; (3) appropriate toilet-sitting and defecation dynamics; (4) having the child spend sufficient time on the toilet to promote complete evacuation; and (5) implementing a toilet-sitting schedule 10–30 minutes after breakfast and supper. Appropriate defecation dynamics training through instruction and modeling is a particularly important aspect of treatment and is emphasized in the comprehensive behavioral approach known as "enhanced toilet training" (ETT; Cox, Sutphen, Ling, Quillian, & Borowitz, 1996) and its Internet-based version (*www.ucanpooptoo.com*; for a description of both ETT and the Internet version, please refer to Ritterband et al., 2003). Behavioral interventions in combination with laxatives have been shown to be more effective than either treatment alone (Borowitz, Cox, Sutphen, & Kovatchev, 2002; Brazzelli & Griffiths, 2007).

Biofeedback

EAS biofeedback is used in attempt to correct abnormal defecation dynamics in children with encopresis. Biofeedback teaches a child to reverse the learned behavior of paradoxical constriction by relaxing the EAS during straining. Although this intervention makes theoretical sense, a recent meta-analysis concluded that in the treatment of children suffering from encopresis, in general EAS-exhibiting biofeedback therapy does not provide any additional benefit to the combination of medical and behavioral therapy (i.e., laxative therapy, toilet training, and dietary changes) (Brazzelli & Griffiths, 2007; Cox et al., 1996). Nevertheless, biofeedback may be helpful for selected patients exhibiting prolonged, effortful, and unproductive straining who have not responded to medical and behavioral interventions.

Summary

The elimination disorders, enuresis and encopresis, are biopsychosocial disorders; as such, the various physiological, behavioral, family, peer, and environmental factors must be addressed in the diagnosis and treatment of these conditions. In most children, enuresis and encopresis do not signify serious psychopathology. Nevertheless, the embarrassment and stress these disorders cause for children and families necessitate swift and appropriate treatment to prevent emotional sequelae and peer rejection. Fortunately, the majority of children with elimination disorders respond favorably to the empirically supported behavioral and medical interventions available.

References

American Psychiatric Association. (2000). *Diagnostic and statistical manual of mental disorders* (4th ed., text rev.). Washington, DC: Author.

Azrin, N. H., Sneed, T. J., & Foxx, R. M. (1974). Dry-bed training: Rapid elimination of childhood enuresis. *Behaviour Research and Therapy, 12,* 147–156.

Bartolozzi, G., Boldrini, A., Salmeri, A., & Vitali, E. (1991). Evaluation and treatment of the enuretic child: Eight years experience. *Medical and Surgical Pediatrics, 13,* 389–393.

Benninga, M. A., Buller, H. A., Heymans, H. S., Tytgat, G. N., & Taminiau, J. A. (1994). Is encopresis always the result of constipation? *Archives of Disease in Childhood, 71,* 186–193.

Benninga, M. A., Voskuijl, W. P., & Taminiau, J. A. J. M. (2004). Invited review: Childhood constipation: Is there new light in the tunnel? *Journal of Pediatric Gastroenterology and Nutrition, 39,* 448–464.

Borowitz, S., Cox, D. J., Sutphen, J., & Kovatchev, B. (2002). Treatment of childhood encopresis: A randomized trial comparing three protocols. *Journal of Pediatric Gastroenterology and Nutrition, 34,* 378–384.

Borowitz, S. M., Cox, D. J., Tam, A., Ritterband, L., Sutphen, J., & Penberthy, J. K. (2003). Precipitants of constipation during early childhood. *Journal of the American Board of Family Practice, 16,* 213–218.

Brazelton, T. B., Christopherson, E. R., Frauman, A. C., Gorski, P. A., Poole, J. M., Stadtler, A. C., et al. (1999). Instruction, timeliness, and medical influences affecting toilet training. *Pediatrics, 103,* 1353–1358.

Brazzelli, M., & Griffiths, P. (2006). Behavioural and cognitive interventions with or without other treatments for the management of faecal incontinence in children. *Cochrane Database of Systematic Reviews,* Issue 2 (Article No. CD002240), DOI: 10.1002/14651858. CD002240.pub3.

Burket, R. C., Cox, D. J., Tam, A. P., Ritterband, L., Borowitz, S., Sutphen, J., et al. (2006). Does stubbornness have a role in pediatric constipation? *Journal of Developmental and Behavioral Pediatrics, 27,* 106–111.

Butler, R. J. (2004). Childhood nocturnal enuresis: Developing a conceptual framework. *Clinical Psychology Review, 24,* 909–931.

Butler, R. J., Golding, J., Northstone, K., & ALSPAC Study Team. (2005). Nocturnal enuresis at 7.5 years old: Prevalence and analysis of clinical signs. *British Journal of Urology International, 96,* 404–410.

Cox, D. J., Morris, J. B. J., Borowitz, S. M., & Sutphen, J. L. (2002). Psychological differences between children with and without chronic encopresis. *Journal of Pediatric Psychology, 27,* 585–591.

Cox, D. J., Sutphen, J., Ling, W., Quillian, W., & Borowitz, S. (1996). Additive benefits of laxative, toilet training, and biofeedback therapies in the treatment of pediatric encopresis. *Journal of Pediatric Psychology, 21,* 659–670.

Devitt, H., Holland, P., Butler, R., Redfern, E., Hiley, E., & Roberts, G. (1999). Plasma vasopressin and response to treatment in primary nocturnal enuresis. *Archives of Disease in Childhood, 80,* 448–451.

Di Lorenzo, C., & Benninga, M. A. (2004). Pathophysiology of pediatric fecal incontinence. *Gastroenterology, 126,* S33–S40.

Doleys, D. M., Schwartz, M. S., & Ciminero, A. R. (1981). Elimination problems: Enuresis and encopresis. In E. J. Mash & L. G. Terdal (Eds.), *Behavioral assessment of childhood disorders* (pp. 679–710). New York: Guilford Press.

fFeehan, M., McGee, R., Stanton, W., & Silva, P. A. (1990). A 6 year follow up of childhood enuresis: Prevalence in adolescence and consequences for mental health. *Journal of Pediatrics and Child Health, 26,* 75–79.

Friman, P. C., Handwerk, M. L., Swearer, S. M., McGinnis, C., & Warzak, W. J. (1998). Do children with primary nocturnal enuresis have clinically significant behavior problems? *Archives of Pediatrics and Adolescent Medicine, 152,* 537–539.

Gepertz, S., & Neveus, T. (2004). Imipramine for therapy resistant enuresis: A retrospective evaluation. *Journal of Urology, 171,* 2607–2610.

Glazener, C. M. A., & Evans, J. H. C. (2002). Desmopressin for nocturnal enuresis in children. *Cochrane Database of Systematic Reviews,* Issue 3 (Article No. CD002112), DOI: 10.1002/14651858.CD002112.

Hirasing, R. A., van Leerdam, F. J., Bolk-Bennink, L. B., & Bosch, J. D. (1997). Bedwetting and behavioral and/or emotional problems. *Acta Paediatrica, 86,* 1131–1134.

Houts, A. C., Berman, J. S., & Abramson, H. (1994). Effectiveness of psychological and pharmacological treatments for nocturnal enuresis. *Journal of Consulting and Clinical Psychology, 62,* 737–745.

Houts, A. C., & Leibert, R. M. (1984). *Bedwetting: A guide for parents and children.* Springfield, IL: Thomas.

Iacono, G., Cavataio, F., Montalto, G., Florena, A., Tumminello, M., Soresi, M., et al. (1998). Intolerance of cow's milk and chronic constipation in children. *New England Journal of Medicine, 339,* 1100–1104.

Jarvelin, M. R., Vikevainen-Tervonen, L., Moilanen, I., & Huttunen, N. P. (1988). Enuresis in seven-year-old children. *Acta Paediatrica Scandinavia, 77,* 148–153.

Johanson, J. F., & Lafferty, J. (1996). Epidemiology of fecal incontinence: The silent affliction. *American Journal of Gastroenterology, 91,* 33–36.

Joinson, C., Heron, J., Butler, U., von Gontard, A., & ALSPAC Study Team. (2006). Psychological differences between children with and without soiling problems. *Pediatrics, 117,* 1575–1584.

Joinson, C., Heron, J., Emond, A., & Butler, R. (2007). Psychological problems in children with bedwetting and combined (day and night) wetting: A UK population-based study. *Journal of Pediatric Psychology, 32,* 605–616.

Lettgen, B., von Gontard, A., Olbing, H., Heiken-Lowenau, C., Gaebel, E., & Schmitz, I. (2002). Urge incontinence and voiding postponement in childhood: Somatic and psychosocial factors. *Acta Paediatrica, 91,* 978–984.

Levine, M. D. (1975). Children with encopresis: A descriptive analysis. *Pediatrics, 56,* 412–416.

Loening-Baucke, V. (1993). Chronic constipation in children. *Gastroenterology, 105,* 1557–1564.

Loening-Baucke, V. (1996). Encopresis and soiling. *Pediatric Clinics of North America, 43,* 279–298.

Luxem, M. C., Christophersen, E. R., Purvis, P. C., & Baer, D. M. (1997). Behavioral–medical treatment of pediatric toileting refusal. *Journal of Developmental and Behavioral Pediatrics, 18,* 34–41.

McGrath, K. H., Caldwell, P. H. Y., & Jones, M. P. (2007). The frequency of constipation in children with nocturnal enuresis: A comparison with parental reporting. *Journal of Pediatrics and Child Health, 44,* 19–27.

McGrath, M., Mellon, M., & Murphy, L. (2000). Empirically supported treatments in pediatric psychology: Constipation and encopresis. *Journal of Pediatric Psychology, 25,* 225–254.

Mellon, M. W., & McGrath, M. L. (2000). Empirically supported treatments in pediatric psychology: Nocturnal enuresis. *Journal of Pediatric Psychology, 25*, 194–214.

Mellon, M. W., Whiteside, S. P., & Friedrich, W. N. (2006). The relevance of fecal soiling as an indicator of child sexual abuse: A preliminary analysis. *Journal of Developmental and Behavioral Pediatrics, 27*, 25–32.

Molnar, D., Taitz, L. S., Urwin, O. M., & Wales, J. K. H. (1983). Anorectal manometry results in defecation disorders. *Archives of Disease in Childhood, 58*, 257–261.

Neveus, T., Stenberg, A., Lackgren, G., Tuvemo, T., & Hetta, J. (1999). Sleep of children with enuresis: A polysomnographic study. *Pediatrics, 103*, 1193–1197.

Norgaard, J. P., van Gool, J. D., Hjalmas, K., Djurhuus, J. C., & Hellstrom, A. L. (1998). Standardization and definitions in lower urinary tract dysfunction in children. *British Journal of Urology, 81*, 1–16.

O'Regan, S., & Yazbeck, S. (1985). Obstipation: A cause of enuresis, urinary tract infection and vesicouretral reflux in children. *Medical Hypotheses, 17*, 409–413.

Partin, J. C., Hamill, S. K., Fischel, J. E., & Partin, J. S. (1992). Painful defecation and fecal soiling in children. *Pediatrics, 89*, 1007–1009.

Riddle, M. A., Nelson, J. C., Kleinman, C. S., Rasmusson, A., Leckman, J. F., & King, R. A. (1991). Sudden death in children receiving Norpramin: A review of three reported cases and a commentary. *Journal of the American Academy of Child and Adolescent Psychiatry, 30*, 104–108.

Ritterband, L. M., Cox, D. J., Walker, L. S., Kovatchev, B., McKnight, L., Patel, K., et al. (2003). An Internet intervention as adjunctive therapy for pediatric encopresis. *Journal of Consulting and Clinical Psychology, 71*, 910–917.

Schmitt, B. D. (1997). Nocturnal enuresis. *Pediatrics in Review, 18*, 183–190.

Taitz, L. S., Wales, J. K. H., Urwin, O. M., & Molnar, D. (1986). Factors associated with outcome in management of defecation disorders. *Archives of Disease in Childhood, 61*, 472–477.

van der Plas, R. N., Benninga, M. A., Buller, H. A., Bossyut, P. M., Akkermans, L. M., Redekop, W. K., et al. (1996). Biofeedback training in treatment of childhood constipation: A randomized controlled study. *Lancet, 348*, 776–780.

van Gool, J. D., Nieuwenhuis, E., ten Doeschate, I. O., Messer, T. P., & de Jong, T. P. (1999). Subtypes in monosymptomatic nocturnal enuresis: II. *Scandinavian Journal of Urology and Nephrology*, Suppl. 202, 8–11.

von Gontard, A., Schaumburg, H., Hollmann, E., Eiberg, H., & Rittig, S. (2001). The genetics of enuresis. *Journal of Urology, 166*, 2438–2443.

Yeung, C. K., Sit, F. K., To, L. K., Chiu, H. N., Sihoe, J. D., Lee, E., et al. (2002). Reduction in nocturnal functional bladder capacity is a common factor in the pathogenesis of refractory enuresis. *British Journal of Urology, 90*, 302–307.

Zink, S., Freitag, C. M., & von Gontard, A. (2008). Behavioral comorbidity differs in subtypes of enuresis and urinary incontinence, *Journal of Urology, 179*, 295–298.

CHAPTER 33

Pediatric Sleep

LISA J. MELTZER
JODI A. MINDELL

Sleep is a universal phenomenon. Across development, children and adolescents spend an average of 40% of their day sleeping (Mindell & Owens, 2003). When children and adolescents do not obtain sufficient sleep, there are numerous consequences, affecting growth, development, cognitive functioning, performance, health, mood, and family functioning. Sleep problems are common even in healthy, typically developing children, with 25–40% experiencing some type of sleep problem (Owens, 2005b). Furthermore, disrupted sleep can often be associated with physical or psychiatric illness. This chapter reviews normal sleep during development, evaluation for sleep problems, common pediatric sleep disorders, and special issues related to sleep in children and adolescents with medical or psychiatric issues.

Normal Sleep in Children and Adolescents

The amount and timing of sleep change over the developmental lifespan, especially for children and adolescents. It is important for all clinicians to consider how much sleep a child needs versus how much he or she is currently obtaining. Insufficient sleep can contribute to poor emotion regulation, negative mood, increased behavior problems, and a decrease in coping skills (Mindell & Owens, 2003). In addition, insufficient sleep will manifest itself differently across the age span (e.g., toddlers become more overactive, while adolescents become more moody or lethargic). Although recent studies have shown variability in how much sleep children and adolescents need (Iglowstein, Jenni, Molinari, & Largo, 2003), the following guidelines are appropriate for most youths.

Newborns (0–3 Months)

In a 24-hour period, most newborns will sleep 10–18 hours, although premature infants may sleep longer. Newborns will sleep in short periods (typically 45 minutes to 3 hours), with no differentiation between night and day. It is important to ensure that parents are following safe sleep practices, especially putting their infant to sleep on his or her back to reduce the risk of sudden infant death syndrome.

Infants (3–12 Months)

At about 3 months of age, most infants will begin to sleep longer stretches at night (8–10 hours), with two to three naps per day (for a total of 3–4 hours of daytime sleep). Between 3 and 6 months of age, sleep begins to consolidate, and most healthy infants no longer need night feedings by 6 months. The majority of infants are able to "sleep through the night" by 9 months of age (Goodlin-Jones, Burnham, Gaylor, & Anders, 2001; Sadeh, Mindell, Luedtke, & Wiegand, 2009). In addition, most 6-month-olds take a nap twice a day, although some continue to take three naps a day until 9 or 10 months. Between 9 and 12 months, developmental milestones (e.g., crawling, walking) have been shown to be related to disrupted sleep for several nights to several weeks before and after each milestone is achieved (Scher & Cohen, 2005).

All infants have multiple arousals during the night. "Signalers" will let their parents know they are awake, while "self-soothers" will return to sleep independently. To help infants develop self-soothing sleep skills, parents should be encouraged to put infants to bed "drowsy but awake." Infants who are rocked or nursed to sleep at bedtime will likely require this same association to help them return to sleep after a normal nighttime arousal.

Toddlers (12 Months–3 Years)

Toddlers in the United States sleep on average 9–10 hours at night with an additional 1–3 hours during the day (Mindell, Meltzer, Carskadon, & Chervin, 2009; National Sleep Foundation, 2004). Between 12 and 18 months, most toddlers will make the transition from two daytime naps to one. Some 25–30% of toddlers experience sleep problems, with many related to bedtime struggles and night wakings (Owens, 2005b). A consistent bedtime routine is essential to facilitate sleep. Because many toddlers have not yet developed the cognitive reasoning skills or the behavioral control to follow instructions related to staying in bed, most toddlers should be kept in a crib until approximately 3 years of age.

Preschoolers (3–5 Years)

Preschoolers sleep approximately 9–10 hours at night (Mindell et al., 2009; National Sleep Foundation, 2004), although it is expected that they need approximately 11–12 hours. The primary change in sleep during the preschool years is the cessation of daytime naps, although 25% of 5-year-olds continue to nap. Sleep problems are common in this age group, and are often related to the development of language, cognitive reasoning, imagination, and limit testing. In combination, these factors can result in bedtime struggles over a child's multiple requests for attention (e.g., one more kiss, one more story), nighttime fears, and resisting going to bed if his or her parents are still awake. Finally, obstructive sleep apnea (OSA) and partial-arousal parasomnias (see "Pediatric Sleep Disorders," below) peak in this age group. Contrary to the popular belief that children will outgrow sleep problems, if not addressed, these sleep problems can become chronic (Kataria, Swanson, & Trevathan, 1987).

School-Age Children (5–12 Years)

For many years, school-age children were considered "golden sleepers" with one 10- to 12-hour sleep period at night, little daytime sleepiness, and few sleep problems. However, studies and surveys have shown that school-age children average 9.5 hours of sleep, and that one-third develop or continue to have sleep problems (Mindell et al., 2009; National Sleep Foundation, 2004; Owens, Spirito, McGuinn, & Nobile, 2000; Sadeh, Raviv, & Gruber, 2000). Anxiety is a common factor contributing to delayed sleep onset or prolonged night wakings in this age group. Furthermore, OSA and poor sleep habits can contribute to sleep difficulties and daytime sleepiness. Sleep problems in school-age children can negatively affect attention, behavior, learning, memory, and mood (Sadeh, Gruber, & Raviv, 2002, 2003).

Adolescents (13–18 Years)

Studies have shown that adolescents need about 9 hours of sleep, and that some benefit from a short afternoon nap (~45 minutes) (Carskadon, Wolfson, Acebo, Tzischinsky, & Seifer, 1998). In addition, these studies have shown that with puberty adolescents experience a shift in their circadian rhythm (internal clock), with sleep onset physiologically delayed for approximately 2 hours. On average, however, adolescents only get 7–7.5 hours of sleep nightly (National Sleep Foundation, 2006). With late bedtimes and early wake times for school, the majority of adolescents experience chronic partial sleep deprivation, resulting in significant daytime sleepiness. The consequences of this regular sleep loss in teens include problems with learning and attention, poor emotion regulation, and an increased risk of injuries and "drowsy driving" crashes (Dahl & Lewin, 2002; National Sleep Foundation, 2006). Along with early school start times, several other environmental factors may contribute to adolescent sleep deprivation; these include after-school jobs, extracurricular activities, academic demands, and technology (e.g., Internet, television, text messaging) (see Moore & Meltzer, 2008, for a review).

Evaluation of Sleep Problems

Sleep History

Although parents are the primary reporters of sleep problems in young children, it is important to interview school-age children and adolescents directly, as parents may not be aware of sleep disruptions. Furthermore, though sleep mostly occurs at night, information about a child's day can also provide information about sleep problems. A comprehensive sleep history should include multiple components:

- *Bedtime.* Along with the actual time a child goes to bed (including weekdays, weekends, school holidays, and the summer), questions should also focus on the bedtime routine; whether there is any bedtime resistance, and how parents respond to these behaviors; uncomfortable sensations in the legs (see below); the amount of time it takes the child to fall asleep (sleep onset latency); and whether the child requires any sleep onset association (e.g., bottle, parental presence, television turned on) to fall asleep.
- *Sleep environment.* It is important to find out where a child falls asleep (own room, parents' bedroom, living room), as well as information about the room conditions. Bedrooms ideally should be cool, dark, quiet, and technology-free (no computer or television).
- *During the night.* Information about what happens while the child is sleeping includes the timing, frequency, and duration of night wakings (and parental response); symptoms of sleep-disordered breathing (e.g., snoring, pauses in breathing, gasping); presence of parasomnias (sleepwalking, sleep terrors) and periodic limb movements; and whether the child has seizures or enuresis.
- *Daytime.* Questions about the child's daytime should focus on what time the child wakes in the morning (weekdays and weekends), whether it is difficult to wake the child, the timing and duration of naps, caffeine use, daytime behavior problems, and daytime sleepiness.

Additional Measures of Sleep Problems

To complement the clinical interview, sleep diaries, questionnaires, actigraphy, and polysomnography (PSG) can be used to help with the diagnosis and treatment of sleep disorders. Sleep diaries are daily records of sleep patterns, including bedtime, sleep onset latency, night wakings, morning wake time, and naps. Two weeks of sleep diaries typically provide sufficient information for clinical purposes. A number of questionnaires are available to assess sleep patterns and daytime sleepiness. The most common questionnaires to assess sleep patterns include the Brief Infant Sleep Questionnaire for ages 0–3 (Sadeh, 2004), the Children's Sleep Habit Questionnaire for school-age children (Owens, Spirito, & McGuinn, 2000), and the Sleep Habits Survey for adolescents (Wolfson & Carskadon, 1998). For daytime sleepiness, two scales have been validated in children and adolescents: the Cleveland Adolescent Sleepiness Questionnaire (Spilsbury, Drotar, Rosen, & Redline, 2007) and the Pediatric Daytime Sleepiness Scale (Drake et al., 2003).

An actigraph is a watch-sized activity monitor worn on the wrist (or ankle in infants), differentiating between sleep and wake periods. These devices have been found to provide accurate estimates of sleep patterns for an extended period of time (e.g., 1–2 weeks); their use can supplement the clinical interview, or can provide additional information for families who may be poor historians. PSG is an overnight sleep study used to examine sleep stages, breathing quality, periodic limb movements, and arousals during sleep. PSG is considered the "gold standard" for the diagnosis of OSA. For patients with excessive daytime sleepiness who have a sufficient amount of sleep and no underlying sleep disrupters, a multiple sleep latency test (MSLT) can be conducted during the day. An MSLT consists of four naps spaced 2 hours apart, providing objective information about daytime sleepiness. PSG and MSLT are primarily conducted in the lab; both involve a modified electroencephalogram (EEG), as well as monitors of respiratory effort, ventilation, airflow, heart rate, respiratory rate, oxygen saturation, body movements, snoring, and muscle tone.

Pediatric Sleep Disorders

Not only are pediatric sleep disorders common, but they can become chronic if left untreated. Sleep disorders vary in their presentation and treatment recommendations, with similar symptoms representative of different disorders (e.g., sleeplessness, daytime sleepiness). Furthermore, there is often a comorbid presentation of physiological sleep disorders (e.g., OSA) and behavioral sleep issues (e.g., poor sleep habits).

Behavioral Insomnia of Childhood

Behavioral insomnia of childhood (BIC) is the most common behavioral sleep disorder experienced by infants and young children, with patients presenting with complaints of bedtime problems and frequent night wakings (ICSD-2; American Academy of Sleep Medicine [AASM], 2005). There are three types of BIC. The sleep onset association type (BIC-SOA) most commonly presents as frequent night wakings, and is reported in 10–30% of infants and toddlers. A sleep onset association is a condition required for a child to fall asleep at bedtime and return to sleep following normal nighttime arousals. Children who have BIC-SOA have developed negative sleep onset associations that require another person or situation beyond their immediate control in order to fall asleep (e.g., nursing, rocking, being driven in the car). The limit-setting type of BIC (BIC-LS) presents most often as complaints of bedtime problems, particularly bedtime stalling or resistance. BIC-LS is seen in 10–30% of toddlers and preschoolers, as this is the age where it is developmentally normal to test the limits, and in 15% of 4- to 10-year-old children. BIC-LS often involves multiple requests for attention at bedtime (e.g., one more story or drink of water) or having tantrums at bedtime, including refusing to go to bed. If parents set consistent limits, these behaviors will typically disappear. However, if limits are not present or are set inconsistently, children will continue to engage in these negative behaviors at bedtime, resulting in delayed sleep onset. Once asleep, children with BIC-LS typically have few night wakings, but may appear sleepy during the day because of shortened total sleep time. The combined type of BIC occurs when there are inconsistent or no limits set at bedtime, and the child is then unable to fall asleep without the presence of a negative sleep onset association (e.g., a parent lying next to the child). Children with the combined type will present with both bedtime problems and frequent night wakings.

Treatment for BIC includes a number of behavioral interventions that have shown to be highly efficacious, producing durable changes (Mindell et al., 2006). These treatment approaches include standard extinction, graduated extinction, positive routines, and parent education (Morgenthaler et al., 2006). The key components to treatment include (1) setting a consistent, age-appropriate bedtime; (2) having a short, consistent bedtime routine that progresses toward and ends in the child's sleeping environment; and (3) teaching the child to fall asleep independently. Although standard extinction (or "cry it out") can produce lasting changes in as few as 3 days, most parents are unable to tolerate their child's prolonged crying, and prefer instead to use a graduated extinction approach (France, 1994; Rickert & Johnson, 1988). This treatment involves the use of parental "checks" on the child, often at increasingly longer intervals. For example, these intervals can increase in length in one night (2 minutes, 4 minutes, 6 minutes) or over several nights (first night, 2 minutes; second night, 5 minutes). If they are able to check on their child during sleep training, parents are more likely to be adherent to treatment (Mindell et al., 2006). The combination of efficacy and parental acceptance/adherence makes graduated extinction the most clinically appropriate treatment option, and it is commonly recommended by popular parenting books (Ferber, 2006; Mindell, 2005).

Insomnia

Insomnia is a complaint of difficulty initiating or maintaining sleep. It is a complex problem because it can be a disorder, as well as either a symptom or an outcome of another disorder. Because some children do not perceive their sleep disruptions as problematic, the complaint of insomnia will often come from parents. As a disorder, insomnia results primarily from a combination of maladaptive sleep behaviors (e.g., poor sleep habits) and negative cognitions (thoughts and beliefs about sleep). Insomnia can also be a symptom of many psychiatric disorders (e.g., anxiety, depression), as well as a consequence of both psychiatric and medical disorders (e.g., resulting from pain, medication).

Although several pharmacological agents are used to treat insomnia in adults, the Food and Drug Administration has not yet approved medications to treat insomnia in children. Cognitive-behavioral treatment for insomnia has been shown to be highly effective in the treatment of insomnia for adults (Edinger & Means, 2005), and is expected to be an appropriate treatment approach for some children and adolescents. This approach consists of a combination of behavioral interventions (e.g., restricting the amount of time a patient spends in bed, controlling stimulus in the sleep environment) and cognitive reframing (targeting maladaptive beliefs about sleep). Institution of good sleep habits is also important, including maintaining a regular sleep–wake schedule, following a consistent bedtime routine, and avoiding caffeine and other stimulating activities (e.g., television viewing at bedtime).

Circadian Rhythm Disorder, Delayed Sleep Phase Type

Circadian rhythm disorder, delayed sleep phase type or delayed sleep phase syndrome (DSPS), is seen primarily in adolescents, although it also can be diagnosed in children. The presenting complaint for DSPS is difficulty falling asleep before the early hours of the morning, combined with difficulty waking for school and daytime sleepiness. The diagnostic criteria for DSPS includes a sleep onset time more than 2 hours after the desired sleep onset time, causing significant daytime impairment (ICSD-2; AASM, 2005). Typically, adolescents with DSPS are unable to fall asleep before 2:00–4:00 A.M. Once they are asleep, the quality and staging of their sleep are normal, although they get insufficient sleep if they have to wake for school. A distinguishing feature between DSPS and insomnia is that an adolescent with DSPS will have no problem falling asleep at the delayed hour, while a patient with insomnia will have difficulty falling asleep regardless of his or her bedtime. Treatment for DSPS typically involves chronotherapy, or a gradual shift in the patient's sleep schedule. The reader is referred to Wyatt (2004) and

Morgenthaler and colleagues (2007) for more details. For treatment to be successful, adolescents must be highly motivated to maintain a consistent sleep schedule 7 nights a week. Bright light therapy and melatonin have also been recommended as adjuncts to chronotherapy (Morgenthaler et al., 2007); however, the safety and efficacy of melatonin in children and adolescents are not yet well understood.

Partial-Arousal Parasomnias

Partial-arousal parasomnias are a spectrum of arousal disorders that include confusional arousals, sleep terrors, and sleepwalking. Parasomnias occur during the transition from slow-wave sleep to lighter sleep, rapid eye movement (REM) sleep, or a brief arousal, resulting in patients appearing to be awake, even though they are asleep. Common features of parasomnias include (1) the timing of the events (typically the first third of the night, when slow-wave sleep is the predominant sleep stage); (2) the appearance of being awake, although a patient will be nonresponsive to a parent or other person; (3) the length of the events (typically 5–15 minutes), ending suddenly with a rapid return to sleep; and (4) retrograde amnesia, with the child or adolescent having no memory of the event the following morning (ICSD-2; AASM, 2005). Parasomnias occur regularly in approximately 3% of children, with 15–40% of children sleepwalking on at least one occasion (Mindell & Owens, 2003). Most children outgrow sleep terrors in adolescence, whereas sleepwalking is more likely to continue for 5–10 years (Mindell & Owens, 2003).

The most common trigger for parasomnias is insufficient sleep (including sleep deprivation and OSA) or changes to sleep routines (e.g., illness, vacation, change to schedule). There appears to be a strong genetic component, with 80–90% of patients having an identifiable first-degree relative with a history of parasomnias (Mindell & Owens, 2003). Treatment includes increasing sleep time (as little as 30 minutes per night can be sufficient); maintaining safety (e.g., putting a bell on a child's door to alert family members that the child is sleepwalking); providing reassurance that these events do not indicate underlying psychopathology; and instructing parents not to wake the patient, as this can prolong the duration of the parasomnia event (Mindell & Owens, 2003).

Obstructive Sleep Apnea

The prevalence of OSA is estimated at 1–3% (Katz & Marcus, 2005). In young children, the most common causes of OSA are enlarged tonsils and adenoids, which result in airway obstruction during sleep. Overnight PSG is considered the gold standard for diagnosing OSA; as such, children with loud, regular snoring and daytime sleepiness (which may be manifested as hyperactivity) should be referred for PSG. Untreated OSA can result in excessive daytime sleepiness, delayed growth, hyperactivity, and inattention. The removal of the tonsils and adenoids is curative for approximately 70% of patients (Katz & Marcus, 2005).

OSA can also be caused by a crowded airway due to craniofacial anomalies, a large tongue or low palate (as seen in children with Down syndrome), hypotonia, or obesity. For these children, a primary treatment approach may be positive airway pressure (PAP). Although PAP is a highly effective treatment when used (forcing the airway to remain open during sleep), many children are unable to tolerate the discomfort of the mask or air pressure, resulting in poor adherence for at least 30% of children (Marcus et al., 2006; Uong, Epperson, Bathon, & Jeffe, 2007). While the lack of adherence to PAP has only begun to receive attention in the literature, the use of desensitization has been suggested as one promising intervention to improve adherence rates (Marcus et al., 2006).

Narcolepsy

Narcolepsy is a disorder that presents as excessive daytime sleepiness. Prevalence rates in children and adolescents are unknown, although retrospective studies of adults with narcolepsy suggest that 34% experienced narcolepsy symptoms before the age of 15 (Challamel et al., 1994). Along with excessive daytime sleepiness, symptoms of narcolepsy include cataplexy (a weakening of muscle tone following a strong emotion), sleep paralysis, and hypnogogic/hypnopompic hallucinations at sleep onset/offset (ICSD-2; AASM, 2005). Narcolepsy is diagnosed by overnight PSG (to rule out other sleep disorders), followed by a multiple sleep latency test (MSLT). Treatment for narcolepsy includes the use of stimulant medications, regular sleep–wake schedules, and scheduled daytime naps.

Restless-Legs Syndrome/Periodic Limb Movement Disorder

Restless-legs syndrome (RLS) is a clinical diagnosis with these features: (1) A patient reports uncomfortable sensation in the legs (e.g., creepy-crawly, tingling, soda bubbles, ants crawling); (2) the discomfort is relieved with movement; and (3) the sensations have a circadian component, worsening in the evening and during the night (ICSD-2; AASM, 2005). In children and adolescents, the most common cause of RLS is low ferritin, with treatment focusing on supplemental iron. Population estimates of RLS are 5–15%, but the prevalence in children and adolescents is unknown (Mindell & Owens, 2003).

Periodic limb movement disorder (PLMD) is a disorder of movement during sleep, resulting in fragmented sleep, multiple arousals, and daytime sleepiness. PLMD is diagnosed by overnight PSG, and RLS and PLMD are often comorbid conditions. Rates of PLMD in children are unknown. The treatment for PLMD can include iron and other supplements, sleep hygiene, and dopaminergic medications (Standards of Practice Committee of the AASM, 2004).

Sleep-Related Rhythmic Movement Disorder

Rhythmic movement disorder presents as a repetitive movement (e.g., head banging, body rocking) that is present at sleep onset. Youths with rhythmic movement disorder will require this movement both at bedtime and following normal nighttime arousals (similar to a sleep onset association). Rhythmic movement disorder is common in very young children, with approximately 60% of infants having at least one rhythmic behavior; fewer than half of these behaviors continue at age 18 months, and most resolve by age 4, although some children continue the behaviors into adolescence and even adulthood (ICSD-2; AASM, 2005). Approximately 3–15% of children are believed to have significant head banging. Treatment approaches include safety (tightening screws and bolts on the crib or bed, installing guard rails), behavioral management (avoiding rein-forcement of the behavior, dampening the noise, increasing sleep), and the treatment of underlying sleep disrupters (e.g., OSA, ear infections) (Mindell & Owens, 2003). In severe cases for older children and adolescents, a short trial of a mild benzodiazepine (e.g., 2–3 weeks) may lead to long-term cessation. For others, this medication may be used on a short-term basis for special events (e.g., sleepovers with friends, overnight camp).

Medical and Psychiatric Issues and Sleep

Although sleep problems are common for all children, sleep disturbances are even more likely to occur with comorbid medical illnesses or psychiatric disorders (Palermo & Owens, 2008). Much remains to be learned about the relationship of sleep and these disorders, but recent studies have begun to document the frequency and consequences of sleep disruptions in children with chronic physical or mental illness and their families.

Medical Issues

Pain

There is a bidirectional relationship between sleep and pain, with pain increasing the frequency of sleep disruptions, and poor or insufficient sleep increasing pain severity (Lewin & Dahl, 1999). Sleep disturbances have been reported in children with juvenile rheumatoid arthritis (Bloom et al., 2002; Ward et al., 2008), adolescents with muscu-loskeletal pain (Meltzer, Mindell, & Logan, 2005; Tsai et al., 2008), and youths with migraine headaches (Aaltonen, Hamalainen, & Hoppu, 2000; Miller, Palermo, Powers, Scher, & Hershey, 2003) and sickle cell disease (Valrie, Gil, Redding-Lallinger, & Dae-schner, 2007). Across studies, patients report more sleep disruptions, with a relationship between sleep and pain.

Asthma

Studies using both objective measures (PSG and actigraphy) and subjective measures of sleep (sleep diaries) have found that children with asthma have more night wak-ings and poorer sleep quality than healthy controls (Sadeh, Horowitz, Wolach-Benodis, & Wolach, 1998; Stores, Ellis, Wiggs, Crawford, & Thomson, 1998). Several conse-quences of these sleep disturbances have been found, including asthma exacerbation (Strunk, Sternberg, Bacharier, & Szefler, 2002), poorer daytime functioning (mood, concentration, and memory) (Stores et al., 1998), and more missed days of school for children (Diette et al., 2000).

Traumatic Brain Injury

For children and adolescents with mild to moderate traumatic brain injuries, there have been mixed findings in the literature about the prevalence and persistence of sleep prob-lems. One study of almost 700 youths found that sleep problems were present at 1 and 4 months after injury, but had resolved by 10 months (Hooper et al., 2004). Two actigraphy studies of adolescents with mild traumatic brain injuries found greater sleep disturbances than in noninjured controls (Kaufman et al., 2001; Pillar et al., 2003), but a third study found no differences on actigraphy (Milroy, Dorris, & McMillan, 2008). Clearly, more research in this area is needed.

Hospitalization

Sleep disruptions during hospitalization are commonly accepted. However, given that sleep is related to health and healing, sleep during hospitalization has begun to receive more attention in recent years. Early studies reported that 25% of hospitalized young children (3–8 years) had delayed sleep onset and multiple night wakings (Hagemann, 1981; White, Williams, Alexander, Powell-Cope, & Conlon, 1990). Since these studies were conducted, it has become commonplace in the United States and Canada for parents either to "room in" with their children or to be provided with nearby sleeping accommodations (Stremler, Wong, & Parshuram, 2008). Still, recent studies of sleep patterns in hospitalized youths have also found significant sleep disruptions, particularly for younger children (Meltzer, Davis, & Mindell, 2008), children with cancer (Hinds et al., 2007), and children with sickle cell disease (Jacob et al., 2006).

Injury

An underreported consequence of insufficient sleep in children is unintentional injury. Several studies have found increased rates of injuries as a result of sleep deprivation in young children (Owens, Fernando, & McGuinn, 2005). In a study of a nationally representative sample followed longitudinally, even mild sleep loss was found to predict increased risk of injuries after a number of external covariates (e.g., maternal depression, socioeconomic status, externalizing behaviors) were controlled for (Schwebel & Brezausek, 2008). In adolescents, risk-taking behaviors have also been related to poor sleep (O'Brien & Mindell, 2005).

Other Illnesses

Several other illnesses have also recently received increased attention in their relation to sleep. These include eczema (Chamlin et al., 2005; Moore, David, Murray, Child, & Arkwright, 2006), HIV (Franck et al., 1999), cystic fibrosis (Amin, Bean, Burklow, & Jeffries, 2005), cancer (Sanford et al., 2008), and epilepsy (Batista & Nunes, 2007; Becker, Fennell, & Carney, 2003).

Disrupted Caregiver Sleep

Sleep disruptions in children with chronic illnesses can have a significant impact on their parents/caregivers, as parents are frequently required to provide medical care during the night. Disrupted caregiver sleep can have consequences for the entire family. Readers are referred to a recent review of 19 studies documenting disrupted sleep for parents of children with chronic illnesses (Meltzer & Moore, 2008).

Psychiatric Issues

Attention-Deficit/Hyperactivity Disorder

Sleep problems are commonly reported in children with attention-deficit/hyperactivity disorder (ADHD), including difficulties falling asleep, prolonged or frequent night wakings, and early morning awakening. Studies have shown that sleep patterns and sleep quality are more disrupted for children with ADHD than for healthy controls (Golan, Shahar, Ravid, & Pillar, 2004; Gruber, Sadeh, & Raviv, 2000). Interestingly, inconsistencies between parental reports of sleep disturbances and objective measures of sleep disturbances have been found (Corkum, Tannock, Moldofsky, Hogg-Johnson, & Humphries, 2001). Furthermore, a number of children with ADHD may have undiagnosed underlying sleep disrupters, including OSA, RLS, and PLMD.

Similar to the bidirectional relationship of sleep and pain, a "conundrum" about the relationship between sleep and daytime functioning in children with ADHD has been discussed (Owens, 2005a). Namely, the fact that children with ADHD have more sleep disturbances may in part be attributable to the same arousal mechanism as the one involved in the ADHD (Corkum, Moldofsky, Hogg-Johnson, Humphries, & Tannock, 1999; Tirosh, Sadeh, Munvez, & Lavie, 1993). Conversely, insufficient or disrupted sleep can contribute to an increase in ADHD symptoms. Studies also indicate that medication for ADHD can disrupt sleep (Corkum, Panton, Ironside, Macpherson, & Williams, 2007), although newer medications may lead to fewer sleep disruptions (Sangal et al., 2006).

Autism Spectrum Disorders

Overall 44 to 83% of children with autism spectrum disorders have been reported to have sleep disruptions, including prolonged sleep onset latency, multiple or prolonged night wakings, or early morning awakenings (Wiggs & Stores, 2004). Although the cause of sleep problems in this group has yet to be determined, suggested etiologies include poor stimulation regulation, abnormal melatonin production, brain pathology, anxiety, and/or abnormal sleep EEG (Richdale, 1999; Wasdell et al., 2008). As in children with ADHD, there have been inconsistent findings when sleep is measured by parent report versus objective measures of sleep (Hering, Epstein, Elroy, Iancu, & Zelnik, 1999). Questions also remain about the impact of these sleep disruptions on the children's daytime behavior (including stereotypic symptoms of autism and related disorders), as well as on parents' sleep and daytime functioning (Meltzer, 2008; Schreck, Mulick, & Smith, 2004).

Depression

The prevalence of sleep problems in children and adolescents with depression is between 66 and 90% (Ivanenko, Crabtree, & Gozal, 2005). The relationship between sleep and depression is complex and often bidirectional (Chorney, Detweiler, Morris, & Kuhn, 2007). That is, sleep disturbances (i.e., insomnia and hypersomnia) are reported as symptoms of depression in children and adolescents (Liu et al., 2007), in addition to exacerbating the other symptoms of depression (Breslau, Roth, Rosenthal, & Andreski,

1996). It has been suggested that sleep disruptions may be prodromal symptoms of depression, with two studies demonstrating that children and adolescents with sleep disturbances are at an increased risk for developing later depression (Breslau et al., 1996; Johnson, Chilcoat, & Breslau, 2000).

Treatment for sleep problems in youths with depression typically requires a multimodal approach, due to the complex interplay of these disorders (Ivanenko et al., 2005). The first step includes the behavioral treatment for insomnia described earlier, including a consistent sleep–wake schedule, relaxation skills, and cognitive restructuring. The medications children and adolescents take for their depression also need to be considered, as some antidepressants can cause either insomnia or hypersomnia (Ivanenko et al., 2005).

Anxiety

Sleep disturbances and anxiety are also highly associated; again, sleep problems are both symptoms of and functional impairments that result from anxiety disorders (Chorney et al., 2007). A recent study found that 88% of youths with anxiety disorders had at least one sleep-related problem (Alfano, Ginsburg, & Kingery, 2007); other studies have reported that 42–66% of children with generalized anxiety disorder have sleep disturbances (Kendall & Pimentel, 2003; Masi et al., 2004). Children who are anxious during the day may have difficulties initiating sleep due to worries or fears, and the resulting shortened sleep can exacerbate their symptoms of anxiety. Traumatic events, life stressors, and other underlying causes of anxiety may also contribute to excessive arousal, hypervigilance, and fears at bedtime when youths are expected to fall asleep in a dark room, often alone (Sadeh, 1996). A multimodal approach is also required for the treatment of sleep disturbances in children with anxiety disorders—concurrently addressing the underlying cause of the children's anxiety, while reinforcing good sleep habits, positive reinforcement for desired behaviors, and graduated extinction to help the children learn to fall asleep independently.

Summary

Sleep problems in children and adolescents are common and represent a wide range of disorders. It is essential for all pediatric psychologists to understand normal sleep across the developmental span and to inquire about sleep. When doing so is appropriate, youths should be referred to a pediatric sleep center for the evaluation of underlying sleep disrupters (e.g., snoring, OSA, PLMD). In addition, there is a complex and bidirectional relationship between sleep and a number of physical and psychiatric illnesses. Pediatric psychologists need to recognize both how an illness or disorder can result in sleep problems, and how sleep disturbances can exacerbate an illness or disorder. Finally, there are many behavioral interventions that are highly efficacious for the treatment of behaviorally based sleep disorders. Overall, pediatric psychologists are uniquely positioned to identify and provide treatment for sleep issues in children and adolescents.

References

Aaltonen, K., Hamalainen, M. L., & Hoppu, K. (2000). Migraine attacks and sleep in children. *Cephalalgia, 20*, 580–584.

Alfano, C. A., Ginsburg, G. S., & Kingery, J. N. (2007). Sleep-related problems among children and adolescents with anxiety disorders. *Journal of the American Academy of Child and Adolescent Psychiatry, 46*, 224–232.

American Academy of Sleep Medicine (AASM). (2005). *International classification of sleep disorders: Diagnostic and coding manual* (2nd ed.). Westchester, IL: American Academy of Sleep Medicine.

Amin, R., Bean, J., Burklow, K., & Jeffries, J. (2005). The relationship between sleep disturbance and pulmonary function in stable pediatric cystic fibrosis patients. *Chest, 128*, 1357–1363.

Batista, B. H. B., & Nunes, M. L. (2007). Evaluation of sleep habits in children with epilepsy. *Epilepsy and Behavior, 11*, 60–64.

Becker, D. A., Fennell, E. B., & Carney, P. R. (2003). Sleep disturbance in children with epilepsy. *Epilepsy and Behavior, 4*, 651–658.

Bloom, B. J., Owens, J. A., McGuinn, M., Nobile, C., Schaeffer, L., & Alario, A. J. (2002). Sleep and its relationship to pain, dysfunction, and disease activity in juvenile rheumatoid arthritis. *Journal of Rheumatology, 29*, 169–173.

Breslau, N., Roth, T., Rosenthal, L., & Andreski, P. (1996). Sleep disturbance and psychiatric disorders: A longitudinal epidemiological study of young adults. *Biological Psychiatry, 39*, 411–418.

Carskadon, M. A., Wolfson, A. R., Acebo, C., Tzischinsky, O., & Seifer, R. (1998). Adolescent sleep patterns, circadian timing, and sleepiness at a transition to early school days. *Sleep, 21*, 871–881.

Challamel, M. J., Mazzola, M. E., Nevsimalova, S., Cannard, C., Louis, J., & Revol, M. (1994). Narcolepsy in children. *Sleep, 17*, S17–S20.

Chamlin, S. L., Mattson, C. L., Frieden, I. J., Williams, M. L., Mancini, A. J., Cella, D., et al. (2005). The price of pruritus: Sleep disturbance and cosleeping in atopic dermatitis. *Archives of Pediatrics and Adolescent Medicine, 159*, 745–750.

Chorney, D. B., Detweiler, M. F., Morris, T. L., & Kuhn, B. R. (2008). The interplay of sleep disturbance, anxiety, and depression in children. *Journal of Pediatric Psychology, 33*, 339–348.

Corkum, P., Moldofsky, H., Hogg-Johnson, S., Humphries, T., & Tannock, R. (1999). Sleep problems in children with attention-deficit/hyperactivity disorder: Impact of subtype, comorbidity, and stimulant medication. *Journal of the American Academy of Child and Adolescent Psychiatry, 38*, 1285–1293.

Corkum, P., Panton, R., Ironside, S., Macpherson, M., & Williams, T. (2008). Acute impact of immediate release methylphenidate administered three times a day on sleep in children with attention-deficit/hyperactivity disorder. *Journal of Pediatric Psychology, 33*, 368–379.

Corkum, P., Tannock, R., Moldofsky, H., Hogg-Johnson, S., & Humphries, T. (2001). Actigraphy and parental ratings of sleep in children with attention-deficit/hyperactivity disorder (ADHD). *Sleep, 24*, 303–312.

Dahl, R. E., & Lewin, D. S. (2002). Pathways to adolescent health: Sleep regulation and behavior. *Journal of Adolescent Health, 31*, 175–184.

Diette, G. B., Markson, L., Skinner, E. A., Nguyen, T. T., Gatt-Bergstrom, P., & Wu, A. W. (2000). Nocturnal asthma in children affects school attendance, school performance, and parents' work attendance. *Archives of Pediatrics and Adolescent Medicine, 154*, 923–928.

Drake, C., Nickel, C., Buruvalie, E., Roth, T., Jefferson, C., & Badia, P. (2003). The Pediatric

Daytime Sleepiness Scale (PDSS): Sleep habits and school outcomes in middle-school children. *Sleep, 26,* 455–458.

Edinger, J. D., & Means, M. K. (2005). Cognitive-behavioral therapy for primary insomnia. *Clinical Psychology Review, 25,* 539–558.

Ferber, R. (2006). *Solve your child's sleep problems.* New York: Fireside.

France, K. G. (1994). Handling parents' concerns regarding the behavioural treatment of infant sleep disturbance. *Behaviour Change, 11,* 101–109.

Franck, L. S., Johnson, L. M., Lee, K., Hepner, C., Lambert, L., Passeri, M., et al. (1999). Sleep disturbances in children with human immunodeficiency virus infection. *Pediatrics, 104,* e62.

Golan, N., Shahar, E., Ravid, S., & Pillar, G. (2004). Sleep disorders and daytime sleepiness in children with attention-deficit/hyperactivity disorder. *Sleep, 27,* 261–266.

Goodlin-Jones, B. L., Burnham, M. M., Gaylor, E. E., & Anders, T. F. (2001). Night waking, sleep–wake organization, and self-soothing in the first year of life. *Journal of Developmental and Behavioral Pediatrics, 22,* 226–233.

Gruber, R., Sadeh, A., & Raviv, A. (2000). Instability of sleep patterns in children with attention-deficit/hyperactivity disorder. *Journal of the American Academy of Child and Adolescent Psychiatry, 39,* 495–501.

Hagemann, V. (1981). Night sleep of children in a hospital: Part I. Sleep duration. *Maternal–Child Nursing Journal, 10,* 1–13.

Hering, E., Epstein, R., Elroy, S., Iancu, D. R., & Zelnik, N. (1999). Sleep patterns in autistic children. *Journal of Autism and Developmental Disorders, 29,* 143–147.

Hinds, P. S., Hockenberry, M., Rai, S. N., Zhang, L., Razzouk, B. I., McCarthy, K., et al. (2007). Nocturnal awakenings, sleep environment interruptions, and fatigue in hospitalized children with cancer. *Oncology Nursing Forum, 34,* 393–402.

Hooper, S. R., Alexander, J., Moore, D., Sasser, H. C., Laurent, S., King, J., et al. (2004). Caregiver reports of common symptoms in children following a traumatic brain injury. *NeuroRehabilitation, 19,* 175–189.

Iglowstein, I., Jenni, O. G., Molinari, L., & Largo, R. H. (2003). Sleep duration from infancy to adolescence: Reference values and generational trends. *Pediatrics, 111,* 302–307.

Ivanenko, A., Crabtree, V. M., & Gozal, D. (2005). Sleep and depression in children and adolescents. *Sleep Medicine Reviews, 9,* 115–129.

Jacob, E., Miaskowski, C., Savedra, M., Beyer, J. E., Treadwell, M., & Styles, L. (2006). Changes in sleep, food intake, and activity levels during acute painful episodes in children with sickle cell disease. *Journal of Pediatric Nursing, 21,* 23–34.

Johnson, E. O., Chilcoat, H. D., & Breslau, N. (2000). Trouble sleeping and anxiety/depression in childhood. *Psychiatry Research, 94,* 93–102.

Kataria, S., Swanson, M. S., & Trevathan, G. E. (1987). Persistence of sleep disturbances in preschool children. *Behavioral Pediatrics, 110,* 642–646.

Katz, E. S., & Marcus, C. L. (2005). Diagnosis of obstructive sleep apnea syndrome in infants and children. In S. H. Sheldon, R. Ferber, & M. H. Kryger (Eds.), *Principles and practice of pediatric sleep medicine* (4th ed., pp. 197–210). Philadelphia: Elsevier/Saunders.

Kaufman, Y., Tzischinsky, O., Epstein, R., Etzioni, A., Lavie, P., & Pillar, G. (2001). Long-term sleep disturbances in adolescents after minor head injury. *Pediatric Neurology, 24,* 129–134.

Kendall, P. C., & Pimentel, S. S. (2003). On the physiological symptom constellation in youth with generalized anxiety disorder (GAD). *Journal of Anxiety Disorders, 17,* 211–221.

Lewin, D. S., & Dahl, R. E. (1999). Importance of sleep in the management of pediatric pain. *Journal of Developmental and Behavioral Pediatrics, 20,* 244–252.

Liu, X., Buysse, D. J., Gentzler, A. L., Kiss, E., Mayer, L., Kapornai, K., et al. (2007). Insomnia and hypersomnia associated with depressive phenomenology and comorbidity in childhood depression. *Sleep, 30*, 83–90.

Marcus, C. L., Rosen, G., Ward, S. L., Halbower, A. C., Sterni, L., Lutz, J., et al. (2006). Adherence to and effectiveness of positive airway pressure therapy in children with obstructive sleep apnea. *Pediatrics, 117*, e442–e451.

Masi, G., Millepiedi, S., Mucci, M., Poli, P., Bertini, N., & Milantoni, L. (2004). Generalized anxiety disorder in referred children and adolescents. *Journal of the American Academy of Child and Adolescent Psychiatry, 43*, 752–760.

Meltzer, L. J. (2008). Brief report: Sleep in parents of children with autism spectrum disorders. *Journal of Pediatric Psychology, 33*, 380–386.

Meltzer, L. J., Davis, K. A., & Mindell, J. A. (2008). Sleep in hospitalized pediatric patients and their parents. *Sleep, 31*, A89.

Meltzer, L. J., Mindell, J. A., & Logan, D. E. (2005). Sleep patterns in adolescent females with chronic musculoskeletal pain. *Behavioral Sleep Medicine, 3*, 305–314.

Meltzer, L. J., & Moore, M. (2008). Sleep disruptions in parents of children and adolescents with chronic illnesses: Prevalence, causes, and consequences. *Journal of Pediatric Psychology, 33*, 279–291.

Miller, V. A., Palermo, T. M., Powers, S. W., Scher, M. S., & Hershey, A. D. (2003). Migraine headaches and sleep disturbances in children. *Headache, 43*, 362–368.

Milroy, G., Dorris, L., & McMillan, T. M. (2008). Brief report: Sleep disturbances following mild traumatic brain injury in childhood. *Journal of Pediatric Psychology, 33*, 242–247.

Mindell, J. A. (2005). *Sleeping through the night: How infants, toddlers, and their parents can get a good night's sleep* (rev. ed.). New York: HarperCollins.

Mindell, J. A., Kuhn, B. R., Lewin, D. S., Meltzer, L. J., Sadeh, A., & Owens, J. A. (2006). Behavioral treatment of bedtime problems and night wakings in infants and young children. *Sleep, 29*, 1263–1276.

Mindell, J. A., Meltzer, L. J., Carskadon, M. A., & Chervin, R. (2009). Developmental aspects of sleep hygiene: Findings from the 2004 National Sleep Foundation *Sleep in America Poll*. *Sleep Medicine*.

Mindell, J. A., & Owens, J. A. (2003). *A clinical guide to pediatric sleep: Diagnosis and management of sleep problems*. Philadelphia: Lippincott Williams & Wilkins.

Moore, K., David, T. J., Murray, C. S., Child, F., & Arkwright, P. D. (2006). Effect of childhood eczema and asthma on parental sleep and well-being: A prospective comparative study. *British Journal of Dermatology, 154*, 514–518.

Moore, M., & Meltzer, L. J. (2008). The sleepy adolescent: Causes and consequences of sleepiness in teens. *Paediatric Respiratory Reviews, 9*, 114–120.

Morgenthaler, T. I., Lee-Chiong, T., Alessi, C., Friedman, L., Aurora, R. N., Boehlecke, B., et al. (2007). Practice parameters for the clinical evaluation and treatment of circadian rhythm sleep disorders: An American Academy of Sleep Medicine report. *Sleep, 30*, 1445–1459.

Morgenthaler, T. I., Owens, J., Alessi, C., Boehlecke, B., Brown, T. M., Coleman, J., et al. (2006). Practice parameters for behavioral treatment of bedtime problems and night wakings in infants and young children: An American Academy of Sleep Medicine report. *Sleep, 29*, 1277–1281.

National Sleep Foundation. (2004). Sleep in America poll. Retrieved May 11, 2007, from *www.sleepfoundation.org/site/c.huIXKjM0IxF/b.2419041/k.1302/2004SleepinAmericaPoll.htm*

National Sleep Foundation. (2006). Sleep in America poll. Retrieved March 31, 2006, from *www.sleepfoundation.org/site/c.huIXKjM0IxF/b.2419037/k.1466/2006SleepinAmericaPoll.htm*

O'Brien, E. M. & Mindell, J. A. (2005). Sleep and risk-taking behavior in adolescents. *Behavioral Sleep Medicine, 3*, 113–133.

Owens, J. A. (2005a). The ADHD and sleep conundrum: A review. *Journal of Developmental and Behavioral Pediatrics, 26,* 312–322.

Owens, J. A. (2005b). Epidemiology of sleep disorders during childhood. In S. H. Sheldon, R. Ferber, & M. H. Kryger (Eds.), *Principles and practices of pediatric sleep medicine* (4th ed., pp. 27–33). Philadelphia: Elsevier/Saunders.

Owens, J. A., Fernando, S., & McGuinn, M. (2005). Sleep disturbance and injury risk in young children. *Behavioral Sleep Medicine, 3,* 18–31.

Owens, J. A., Spirito, A., & McGuinn, M. (2000). The Children's Sleep Habits Questionnaire (CSHQ): Psychometric properties of a survey instrument for school-aged children. *Sleep, 23,* 1043–1051.

Owens, J. A., Spirito, A., McGuinn, M., & Nobile, C. (2000). Sleep habits and sleep disturbance in elementary school-aged children. *Journal of Developmental and Behavioral Pediatrics, 21,* 27–36.

Palermo, T. M., & Owens, J. (2008). Introduction to the special issue: Sleep in pediatric medical populations. *Journal of Pediatric Psychology, 33,* 227–231.

Pillar, G., Averbooch, E., Katz, N., Peled, N., Kaufman, Y., & Shahar, E. (2003). Prevalence and risk of sleep disturbances in adolescents after minor head injury. *Pediatric Neurology, 29,* 131–135.

Richdale, A. L. (1999). Sleep problems in autism: Prevalence, cause, and intervention. *Developmental Medicine and Child Neurology, 41,* 60–66.

Rickert, V. I., & Johnson, C. M. (1988). Reducing nocturnal awakening and crying episodes in infants and young children: A comparison between scheduled awakenings and systematic ignoring. *Pediatrics, 81,* 203–212.

Sadeh, A. (1996). Stress, trauma and sleep in children. *Child and Adolescent Psychiatric Clinics of North America, 5,* 685–700.

Sadeh, A. (2004). A brief screening questionnaire for infant sleep problems: Validation and findings for an Internet sample. *Pediatrics, 113,* 570–577.

Sadeh, A., Gruber, R., & Raviv, A. (2002). Sleep, neurobehavioral functioning, and behavior problems in school-age children. *Child Development, 73,* 405–417.

Sadeh, A., Gruber, R., & Raviv, A. (2003). The effects of sleep restriction and extension on school-age children: What a difference an hour makes. *Child Development, 74,* 444–455.

Sadeh, A., Horowitz, I., Wolach-Benodis, L., & Wolach, B. (1998). Sleep and pulmonary function in children with well-controlled, stable asthma. *Sleep, 21,* 379–384.

Sadeh, A., Mindell, J. A., Luedtke, K., & Wiegand, B. (2009). Sleep and sleep ecology in the first three years. *Journal of Sleep Research, 18,* 60–73.

Sadeh, A., Raviv, A., & Gruber, R. (2000). Sleep patterns and sleep disruptions in school-age children. *Developmental Psychology, 36,* 291–301.

Sanford, S. D., Okuma, J. O., Pan, J., Srivastava, D. K., West, N., Farr, L., et al. (2008). Gender differences in sleep, fatigue, and daytime activity in a pediatric oncology sample receiving dexamethasone. *Journal of Pediatric Psychology, 33,* 298–306.

Sangal, R. B., Owens, J., Allen, A. J., Sutton, V., Schuh, K., & Kelsey, D. (2006). Effects of atomoxetine and methylphenidate on sleep in children with ADHD. *Sleep, 29,* 1573–1585.

Scher, A., & Cohen, D. (2005). Locomotion and nightwaking. *Child: Care, Health, and Development, 31,* 685–691.

Schreck, K. A., Mulick, J. A., & Smith, A. F. (2004). Sleep problems as possible predictors of intensified symptoms of autism. *Research in Developmental Disabilities, 25,* 57–66.

Schwebel, D. C., & Brezausek, C. M. (2008). Nocturnal awakenings and pediatric injury risk. *Journal of Pediatric Psychology, 33,* 323–332.

Spilsbury, J. C., Drotar, D., Rosen, C. L., & Redline, S. (2007). The Cleveland Adolescent Sleepiness Questionnaire: A new measure to assess excessive daytime sleepiness in adolescents. *Journal of Clinical Sleep Medicine, 3,* 603–612.

Standards of Practice Committee of the American Academy of Sleep Medicine (AASM). (2004). Practice parameters for the dopaminergic treatment of restless legs syndrome and periodic limb movement disorder. *Sleep, 27,* 557–559.

Stores, G., Ellis, A. J., Wiggs, L., Crawford, C., & Thomson, A. (1998). Sleep and psychological disturbance in nocturnal asthma. *Archives of Disease in Childhood, 78,* 413–419.

Stremler, R., Wong, L., & Parshuram, C. (2008). Practices and provisions for parents sleeping overnight with a hospitalized child. *Journal of Pediatric Psychology, 33,* 292–297.

Strunk, R. C., Sternberg, A. L., Bacharier, L. B., & Szefler, S. J. (2002). Nocturnal awakening caused by asthma in children with mild-to-moderate asthma in the childhood asthma management program. *Journal of Allergy and Clinical Immunology, 110,* 395–403.

Tirosh, E., Sadeh, A., Munvez, R., & Lavie, P. (1993). Effects of methylphenidate on sleep in children with attention-deficit hyperactivity disorder. *American Journal of Diseases of Children, 147,* 1313–1315.

Tsai, S. Y., Labyak, S. E., Richardson, L. P., Lentz, M. J., Brandt, P. A., Ward, T. M., et al. (2008). Brief report: Actigraphic sleep and daytime naps in adolescent girls with chronic musculoskeletal pain. *Journal of Pediatric Psychology, 33,* 307–311.

Uong, E. C., Epperson, M., Bathon, S. A., & Jeffe, D. B. (2007). Adherence to nasal positive airway pressure therapy among school-aged children and adolescents with obstructive sleep apnea syndrome. *Pediatrics, 120,* e1203–e1211.

Valrie, C. R., Gil, K. M., Redding-Lallinger, R., & Daeschner, C. (2007). The influence of pain and stress on sleep in children with sickle cell disease. *Children's Health Care, 36,* 335–353.

Ward, T. M., Brandt, P., Archbold, K., Lentz, M., Ringold, S., Wallace, C. A., et al. (2008). Polysomnography and self-reported sleep, pain, fatigue, and anxiety in children with active and inactive juvenile rheumatoid arthritis. *Journal of Pediatric Psychology, 33,* 232–241.

Wasdell, M. B., Jan, J. E., Bomben, M. M., Freeman, R. D., Rietveld, W. J., Tai, J., et al. (2008). A randomized, placebo-controlled trial of controlled release melatonin treatment of delayed sleep phase syndrome and impaired sleep maintenance in children with neurodevelopmental disabilities. *Journal of Pineal Research, 44,* 57–64.

White, M. A., Williams, P. D., Alexander, D. J., Powell-Cope, G. M., & Conlon, M. (1990). Sleep onset latency and distress in hospitalized children. *Nursing Research, 39,* 134–139.

Wiggs, L., & Stores, G. (2004). Sleep patterns and sleep disorders in children with autistic spectrum disorders: Insights using parent report and actigraphy. *Developmental Medicine and Child Neurology, 46,* 372–380.

Wolfson, A. R., & Carskadon, M. A. (1998). Sleep schedules and daytime functioning in adolescents. *Child Development, 69,* 875–887.

Wyatt, J. K. (2004). Delayed sleep phase syndrome: Pathophysiology and treatment options. *Sleep, 27,* 1195–1203.

CHAPTER 34

Autism Spectrum Disorders and Developmental Disabilities

JONATHAN M. CAMPBELL
MATTHEW J. SEGALL
AILA K. DOMMESTRUP

W̲e present a brief overview of defining characteristics, proposed etiological mechanisms, diagnosis and assessment, treatment, and outcomes for individuals with autism spectrum disorders (ASDs) and intellectual disability (ID). We selectively introduce recent research and identify comprehensive resources to guide assessment and intervention practice. Our discussion of developmental disabilities focuses primarily on ID as opposed to the larger group of children with developmental disabilities. We use the term "ID," as opposed to "mental retardation," to reflect the change in terminology being adopted within the field.

Autism Spectrum Disorders

Leo Kanner (1943) identified the defining features of autism in his description of 11 children who showed a unique cluster of social, communicative, and behavioral symptoms differentiating them from other children. Autism and related disorders are characterized by pervasive impairments in several areas of development: reciprocal social interaction; communication; and unusual behaviors, interests, and/or repetitive activities. These symptoms usually are observed early in development and persist across the lifespan. Social impairments, such as a lack of social responsiveness or initiation of social interaction, represent the hallmark features of ASDs and are often present early in development. Although repetitive behaviors and restrictive interests constitute important components of the symptom picture, individuals with ASDs may be best understood as exhibiting pervasive social communication disorders. Additional examples of symptomatology are presented in the discussion below of specific diagnostic standards.

Diagnostic Standards and Epidemiology

For clinical purposes, the most widely used diagnostic criteria for autism and related disorders are those appearing in the *Diagnostic and Statistical Manual of Mental Disorders*, fourth edition, text revision (DSM-IV-TR; American Psychiatric Association, 2000), which identifies four subtypes of pervasive developmental disorders (PDDs): autistic disorder (autism), Asperger's disorder (AD), Rett's disorder (Rett's), and childhood disintegrative disorder (CDD). Individuals who show social impairment and associated symptoms of autism, but fail to meet diagnostic criteria for another PDD, are diagnosed with PDD not otherwise specified (PDD-NOS). Regardless of diagnosis, all children with PDDs show severe impairments emerging in early childhood, typically in communication and social interactions, and deviating from overall developmental level. The DSM-IV-TR classification system assumes a diagnostic hierarchy, whereby certain disorders take precedence over others in terms of differential diagnosis. For example, CDD and Rett's take precedence over autism and AD, which in turn take precedence over PDD-NOS (American Psychiatric Association, 2000). Although CDD and Rett's are officially listed as PDD diagnoses, the majority of our chapter focuses on autism, AD, and PDD-NOS; for the purposes of our chapter, we use the term "ASDs" to refer to these disorders.

Autistic Disorder

Consistent with many of Kanner's (1943) initial ideas about autism, the DSM-IV-TR describes three clusters of symptoms, often known as the "autistic triad," that must be present early in development for diagnosis. DSM-IV-TR criteria require a minimum of six symptoms from three areas for diagnosis. Highlighting the core social deficits that define autism, at least two symptoms of qualitative impairment in social interaction are required, such as failure to develop peer relationships appropriate to developmental level and lack of shared enjoyment. At least one symptom indicating qualitative impairment in communication is required, such as delays in development of spoken language or stereotyped and repetitive use of language. At least one symptom indicating restricted, repetitive, and stereotyped patterns of behavior, interests, and/or activities (abbreviated hereafter as RRB) is also required. For the RRB criterion to be satisfied, a child may show an all-encompassing preoccupation that is abnormal in *intensity*, such as a developmentally appropriate interest in a topic (e.g., Thomas the Tank Engine) that is pursued to the exclusion of other interests. The RRB criterion may also be satisfied by an interest that is abnormal in *focus*, such as an obsessive interest in deep-fat fryers. Finally, the RRB criterion may be satisfied if a child engages in stereotyped and repetitive motor mannerisms (e.g., hand flapping). For diagnosis, delays or dysfunction must be present prior to 36 months of age.

Asperger's Disorder

According to the DSM-IV-TR, the two essential features of AD are identical to two of those for autism: (1) qualitative impairments in social interaction, and (2) restricted and stereotyped patterns of behavior. For a DSM-IV-TR diagnosis of AD, children must show *no* significant delays in (1) general language functioning, (2) self-help skills, (3) adaptive behavior (with the exception of social interaction), or (4) cognitive development (American Psychiatric Association, 2000). Significant delays are only generally defined in the DSM-IV-TR, however. For example, age-appropriate language functioning is defined as the use of single words by the age of 2 years and communicative phrases by age 3 years. In the DSM-IV-TR, AD is differentiated from autism in that individuals with AD do not present with early cognitive or language delays. In addition, the DSM-IV-TR guides the differential diagnosis of AD versus autism as follows. The RRB criterion for AD is described as taking the form of an "all-encompassing pursuit" (American Psychiatric Association, 2000, p. 82); in autism, stereotypic behavior, preoccupation with parts of objects, and/or distress at changes in routines or rituals are usually also present. In addition, individuals with AD are described as interested in social interaction, but take a verbose, one-sided, and insensitive approach to such interaction; by contrast, self-isolation is often characteristic of autism.

The Disintegrative Disorders: CDD and Rett's

CDD is characterized by at least 2 years of normal development followed by a period of severe regression across multiple areas of functioning (American Psychiatric Association, 2000). The 2-year period of normal development must be marked by age-appropriate communication, social relatedness, play, and adaptive behavior. After typical development, clinically significant losses in acquired skills must take place prior to the age of 10 and occur in at least two of five areas (e.g., language). Diagnosis of CDD also requires abnormal functioning in two of three domains of the autistic triad. CDD is reported to be very rare and is typically associated with functioning in the range of severe to profound ID. Medical causes for deterioration (e.g., head injury) must be ruled out before a diagnosis of CDD can be made. Rett's is a disorder known to be caused by mutations on the MECP2 gene on the X chromosome. Rett's is also characterized by developmental deterioration; in this case, a brief period of normal development is followed by a significant loss of previously acquired skills, purposeful hand movements, severe psychomotor retardation, and deceleration of head growth (American Psychiatric Association, 2000). Rett's is identified as a PDD due to loss of social interaction, communication delays, and stereotypic movements. Rett's is associated with severe ID, and until recently had been documented only in females.

Pervasive Developmental Disorder Not Otherwise Specified

A diagnosis of PDD-NOS is rendered in the presence of severe and pervasive impairment in reciprocal social interaction *and either* verbal or nonverbal communication *or* stereotyped behavior, interests, or activities (American Psychiatric Association, 2000, p. 84). Children with PDD-NOS do not meet formal diagnostic criteria for any of the previously described PDD diagnoses, or for schizophrenia, schizotypal personality disorder, or avoidant personality disorder. Individuals with PDD-NOS are characterized by heterogeneity above and beyond that already observed within the other PDD groups. Less is known about individuals diagnosed with PDD-NOS than about those with other PDD diagnoses; however, limited data suggest that social and communication deficits are usually less severe and prognosis is generally better in this group than in individuals with autistic disorder (Towbin, 2005).

Prevalence rates for ASDs (i.e., autism, AD, and PDD-NOS) are in the range of 6–7 per 1,000 children. Fombonne (2005) reported prevalence rates of 2.6 per 10,000 for AD, 13 per 10,000 for autism, and 21 per 10,000 for PDD-NOS. The Centers for Disease Control and Prevention (CDC, 2007) reported a mean prevalence rate of 6.6 per 1,000 children for autism, AD, and PDD-NOS, or roughly 1 of every 152 children. Males are more frequently diagnosed with ASDs, at a ratio of 3.7:1 (CDC, 2007).

Heterogeneity across the ASDs

As may be apparent in the description of the varied symptoms associated with ASDs, individuals with ASDs differ widely from one another, such as degree of interest in social interaction and presence or absence of speech. This heterogeneity is perhaps best captured within the domain of intellectual functioning, which can extend from ID to superior cognitive ability. Persons with ASDs also frequently demonstrate a remarkable range of intraindividual variability. For example, children with ASDs can show a remarkable combination of well-preserved or age-appropriate abilities in the presence of severe disability. Discrepancies between areas of functioning are best exemplified by "savant" abilities, which are infrequent combinations of memory, calendar calculation, or musical talents in the presence of profound ID.

Comorbid Conditions

Children with ASDs often present with comorbid neurocognitive, affective, or medical disorders. ID frequently co-occurs with autism, with traditionally reported estimates in the range of 70–80%. Edelson (2006), however, argued that the high rates of ID were due to re-reporting of early flawed data. As classification has begun to include higher-functioning individuals, such as those with AD, historical data most certainly overestimate the presence of ID. Children with ASDs frequently show problems with various aspects of attention and executive functioning, such as sustaining attention and organizing academic tasks. Medical disorders frequently reported for children with autism include epilepsy (20–30%); neurocutaneous syndromes, such as tuberous sclerosis and neurofibromatosis (1–4%); and chromosomal disorders, such as fragile X syndrome (FXS; 1–8.1%) (Fombonne, 2005). Internalizing disorders also co-occur with ASDs, with estimates up to 56% for depressive or anxiety disorders (Howlin, 2005).

Etiological Considerations

There is little doubt that ASDs are associated with neurobiological dysfunction; however, the exact nature of the dysfunction is unresolved. Due to the heterogeneity observed for individuals with ASDs and the absence of universal findings with respect to etiology, some experts have concluded that there is no single cause of autism (Happé, Ronald, & Plomin, 2006).

Genetic Findings

A long-standing literature highlights genetic liability as a risk factor for the presence of an ASD, because autism concordance rates increase as a result of greater genetic similarity. For example, autism concordance rates for dizygotic (i.e., fraternal) twins hover around 5%, while autism concordance rates for monozygotic twins increase to 60% (Rutter, 2005). Autism concordance rates also increase as the case definition expands, such that the concordance rates for monozygotic twins increase to 90% for social and communicative symptoms related to ASDs, such as social aloofness and circumscribed interests (Rutter, 2005). Genetic causes are clearly identified in about 5–10% of individuals with autism.

Neurocognitive Theories

Researchers have attempted to account for autistic symptomatology via basic neurocognitive deficits, such as impaired attention/executive functioning and weak central coherence, among others. Ozonoff, South, and Provencal (2005) documented consistent executive functioning impairments for individuals with ASDs. Executive functioning appears related to social-cognitive tasks, such as joint attention (e.g., sharing experience), social attribution, and social reasoning tasks, and there is some suggestion that executive functioning impairment may be associated with RRB symptoms. Interestingly, problems with social attribution, such as assigning social meaning to ambiguous stimuli as measured in the social attribution task, has been associated with hypoactivation of the medial prefrontal cortex—a brain area associated with executive functions (Castelli, Frith, Happé, & Frith, 2002).

Happé (2005) has reviewed evidence related to the "weak central coherence" theory of autism. This theory ascribes symptoms of autism to problems with central coherence (i.e., the tendency to process information in context for higher-level meaning, such as conceptual understanding). As such, weak central coherence as a cognitive style has been invoked to explain obsessive interests (i.e., heightened focus on details), aspects of cognitive test performance (e.g., better memory for details versus general ideas), and savant skills infrequently seen in autism. As yet, clear connections between weak central coherence and neurobiological findings have not been established; however, premature brain growth and arrest, discussed below, may lend support to this theory of autism.

The fact that individuals with ASDs often demonstrate deficits in multiple domains of cognitive functioning, as opposed to a single "core" deficit, has given rise to hypotheses that autism is a disorder of complex information processing (Williams, Goldstein, & Minshew, 2006). For example, Williams and colleagues (2006) found that children with high-functioning autism showed multiple impairments across cognitive domains, such as language, memory, and motor tasks, with the greatest impairments observed for complex tasks requiring integration of information. In contrast, performance on simple cognitive tasks was age-appropriate. Williams and colleagues' conceptualization of autism as a disorder of complex information processing seems applicable to the social-cognitive deficits characteristic of autism. That is, social contexts are rarely, if ever, identical; therefore, novel reasoning, a complex cognitive process, is required to guide appropriate social behavior across disparate contexts and changing settings.

Selected Neurobiological Findings

Several promising lines of neurobiological research have focused on varied brain areas and biological systems, such as overall brain size, cerebellar anomalies, and brain structures relevant to social cognition.

Brain Size. Macrocephaly (i.e., enlarged head circumference) for individuals with autism was first reported by Kanner (1943) and is found in roughly 10–30% of older children and adults with autism. In the presence of macrocephaly, however, adolescents and adults with autism show *normal* brain volume. In contrast, structural magnetic resonance imaging (MRI) has documented overall brain size 5–10% larger than normal for 2- to 4-year-olds with autism, suggesting brain overgrowth early in the developmental period followed by slowed growth later in development (Courchesne & Pierce, 2005). Brain enlargement appears greatest in the temporal and frontal lobes, with evidence for more overgrowth of white matter than gray matter. Early brain overgrowth in autism has been described as "growth without guidance," suggesting that typical patterns of synaptogenesis, neuronal growth, and neuronal differentiation guided by experience and environmental influence are disrupted for young children with ASDs. Early overgrowth of white matter may lead to abnormal connectivity within the brain, which has been documented recently for brain areas important in social cognition via diffusion tensor imaging (Barnea-Goraly et al., 2004). Compromised interconnectivity between neuronal systems may help explain the cognitive symptoms often seen in ASDs, such as heightened attention to detail, problematic conceptual reasoning, and weak central coherence (Volkmar, Lord, Klin, Schultz, & Cook, 2007).

Cerebellar Anomalies. Difficulties in the areas of repetitive motor movements and dysregulated attention have given rise to structural study of the cerebellum. Neuropathological studies have shown reduced numbers of Purkinje cells in the cerebellum, minicolumnar pathology within the cerebellum, and (less definitively) hypoplasia in parts of the cerebellum. The confounding influence of IQ and age on cerebellar size has not been accounted for in studies documenting cerebellar hypoplasia (Volkmar et al., 2007).

"Social" Brain Areas. Because social deficits are so characteristic of ASDs, research has focused on several brain areas thought to be particularly important in social cognition. Pelphrey, Adolphs, and Morris (2004) provided a thorough review of three such areas: the amygdala, the superior temporal sulcus, and the fusiform gyrus. The amygdala is implicated in emotion recognition and other "theory-of-mind" (i.e., social perspective-taking) tasks. Individuals with ASDs, versus controls, show hypoactivation of the amygdala during social inference and emotion recognition tasks. The superior temporal sulcus is implicated in social attribution tasks as well as in human speech perception. Similar to the amygdala, superior temporal sulcus regions are hypoactive during these tasks for individuals with autism. Finally, the fusiform gyrus is a fairly specialized brain area that is activated during human face processing. When compared to

age- and IQ-matched controls, individuals with ASDs have shown hypoactivation in the right fusiform gyrus during face-processing tasks (e.g., Schultz, 2005). Interestingly, the individuals with ASDs show activation in the adjacent inferior temporal gyrus, a brain area typically activated during simple object discrimination tasks. All told, findings from the field of social-cognitive neuroscience implicate varied areas of hypoactivation for individuals with ASDs during social information-processing tasks.

Vaccinations and Thimerosal

Some have argued that the increase in ASDs reflects the role of environmental factors, particularly toxins with known neurological effects, such as elemental mercury and methylmercury. This basic reasoning has implicated the potential etiological role of measles–mumps–rubella (MMR) vaccinations (Wakefield et al., 1998) in general, and of thimerosal in particular. Thimerosal has been used as a preservative in multidose MMR vaccines and is metabolized into ethylmercury. Parents have reported the onset of autistic symptomatology soon after children receive MMR vaccination; some have identified this symptomatology as a "regressive" subtype of autism (Wakefield et al., 1998). Most research does not support the etiological role of MMR vaccines or thimerosal in the causation of autism (e.g., Richler et al., 2006), and several authors of the original Wakefield and colleagues study have withdrawn their support for its findings. The co-occurrence between MMR vaccination scheduling and onset of autism symptomatology, coupled with more recent research findings, suggests a correlational rather than a causal relationship. We raise this controversy because of the likelihood that parents may inquire about the safety of vaccines.

Assessment Methods and Procedures

The American Academy of Pediatrics has recently published practice guidelines for the identification and assessment of children with ASDs (Johnson & Myers, 2007). This report outlines recommended procedures for screening, assessment, and diagnosis of ASDs; the guidelines are introduced here as an additional reference and may well represent the guidelines most familiar to referring pediatricians. In response to the call for evidence-based assessment practices within the field of psychology, Ozonoff, Goodlin-Jones, and Solomon (2005) have also recommended a core psychological assessment battery for children with suspected or confirmed ASDs. This battery includes diagnostic assessment, as well as IQ, language, and adaptive behavior assessment.

Various procedures and measures exist for documenting the core features of social and communicative dysfunction across the ASD spectrum. Historically, observation by a trained child psychiatrist or psychologist served as the "gold standard" for diagnosing ASDs, typically in the absence of formal rating scales or other assessment instruments. Over time, however, expert opinion has been supplemented by standardized diagnostic instruments, such as the Autism Diagnostic Interview—Revised (ADI-R; Rutter, LeCouteur, & Lord, 2003) and the Autism Diagnostic Observation Schedule (ADOS; Lord, Rutter, DiLavore, & Risi, 2001), which are commonly used together. The ADI-R is an extensive interview completed with a knowledgeable caregiver that assesses a range of ASD symptoms and related problems, as well as developmental history; the ADOS is a semistructured observation designed to elicit social and communicative impairments indicative of ASDs. Both the ADI-R and ADOS require specialized training for appropriate use and accurate ASD diagnosis. Given the prognostic utility of IQ and language functioning, and the treatment-planning utility of a measure of adaptive behavior, comprehensive assessment should include evaluation within each domain (Ozonoff, Goodlin-Jones, et al., 2005).

Approaches to Intervention

Due to the complex presentation of problems that overlap domains of professional expertise, such as psychology, special education, and psychiatry, involvement of a range of professionals is the norm for intervention with children with ASDs. Indeed, because of the language, social, and behavioral features of autism and other ASDs, treatment will almost invariably involve educational and clinical professionals at some point. Interventions for children with ASD are either focal (or skills-based) or comprehensive. Focal interventions are designed to target specific core ASD symptoms (e.g., increasing appropriate toy play) or associated features of ASDs (e.g., reducing self-injury). Examples of focal treatments include using differential reinforcement of alternative behavior to decrease self-injury, or prescribing a selective serotonin reuptake inhibitor (SSRI) to improve mood. In contrast to focal interventions, comprehensive interventions are designed to target a wide range of symptoms and improve the long-term outcomes of children with ASDs (Rogers & Vismara, 2008).

Psychosocial Approaches to Intervention

Approaches to intervention vary widely within the ASD literature and differ along key dimensions, such as the degree of child versus adult direction emphasized. For example, discrete-trial training is a largely adult-directed intervention, whereas relationship-focused interventions are largely child-directed. Comprehensive treatment approaches for ASDs are implemented via treatment teams, usually with high intensity (e.g., 20–40 hours per week) and over long periods of time (e.g., 2–3 years). In a systematic review, Campbell, Herzinger, and James (2008) concluded that applied behavior analysis approaches, both focal and comprehensive, have garnered the most empirical support. Regardless of intervention type, there is a consensus that high-quality ASD intervention programs are characterized by early and intensive intervention; parent training and support; a curriculum that targets core deficits; ongoing assessment of progress; transition planning; and highly trained staff (National Research Council, 2001).

Psychopharmacological Approaches to Intervention

Various psychotropic medications have been used to treat behaviors associated with autism, although none have successfully treated the core social and communicative symptoms of ASDs. In a comprehensive review, Myers and Johnson (2007) noted that 45% of children and adolescents and up to 75% of adults are treated with psychotropic medications. Stimulants (e.g., methylphenidate), SSRIs (e.g., fluoxetine), and atypical antipsychotics (e.g., risperidone), among other medications, have been used with variable success to target repetitive behaviors, aggression, symptoms of attention-deficit/ hyperactivity disorder (ADHD), anxiety, and depression. Efficacy trials for medications have improved significantly over the past two decades, with rigorous double-blind, placebo-controlled studies establishing efficacy for many medications. Even so, Myers and Johnson concluded that evidence-based consensus for pharmacological management of ASDs has yet to be reached. If medications are used, potential benefits and side effects should be explained, baseline data collected, and a quantifiable assessment approach employed to document treatment effectiveness.

Prognosis and Outcomes

Adult outcomes for individuals with autism vary widely; however, for the majority, outcomes are typically described as poor or very poor, characterized by residential living or hospital placement, limited independence, and significant social-communicative impairment (Cederlund, Hagberg, Billstedt, Gillberg, & Gillberg, 2008; Howlin, Goode, Hutton, & Rutter, 2004). Recently Cederlund and colleagues (2008) documented "poor" or "very poor" outcomes for 75% of adolescents and adults with autism, while Howlin and colleagues (2004) reported similar outcomes for 57% of adults with autism. Howlin and colleagues documented "good" to "very good" outcomes for 22% of adults with autism, characterized by independent or supported employment, at least some friendships, and living or traveling independently. Cederlund and colleagues found that only 7% of adults with autism enjoyed a "good" or "fair" outcome, such as either paid employment or significant social relationships. In contrast to these outcomes for autism, Cederlund and colleagues found that 75% of individuals with AD had achieved "fair" to "good" outcomes.

Emergence of some meaningful speech by age 5–6 and measured IQ at the time of diagnosis have been identified as fairly robust predictors of positive outcomes for individuals with autism. Howlin and colleagues (2004) found that individuals with nonverbal IQs ≥ 70 in childhood enjoyed more favorable outcomes than counterparts with IQs of 50–69. Similarly, all of the adults with "very good" outcomes in the Howlin and colleagues study had some meaningful speech by the age of 5. Although less definitive, other factors associated with poorer outcomes are being female; the presence of epilepsy; and the severity of early symptoms, particularly abnormality of language and disruptive RRB (Howlin, 2005).

Intellectual and Other Developmental Disabilities

A "developmental disability" is a severe, chronic disability that (1) is attributable to a mental or physical impairment or a combination of mental and physical impairments; (2) is present prior to 22 years of age; (3) is likely to continue indefinitely; (4) results in substantial restrictions in several life activities, such as self-care, learning, daily living skills, and economic sufficiency; and (5) reflects the person's need for a combination and sequence of lifelong interdisciplinary care, treatment, or support services (Rehabilitation, Comprehensive Services, and Developmental Disabilities Amendments, 1978). ID is one of the most common developmental disabilities and is the focus of this section of the chapter. As noted earlier, ID has replaced the term "mental retardation." This change is perhaps best exemplified by the fact that the American Association on Mental Retardation (AAMR) has recently changed its name to the American Association on Intellectual and Developmental Disabilities (AAIDD). Two classification systems used widely in the diagnosis of ID are the AAIDD guidelines and the DSM-IV-TR diagnostic criteria.

Diagnostic Standards and Epidemiology

The AAIDD has defined ID as "a disability characterized by significant limitations both in intellectual functioning and in adaptive behavior as expressed in conceptual, social, and practical adaptive skills" (Luckasson et al., 2002, p. 1). The AAIDD definition also specifies that the disability must be present prior to the age of 18. Emphasizing the eco-logical interplay among the person with ID, environments, and necessary supports, the 1992 guidelines delineated four categories (i.e., "intermittent," "limited," "extensive," and "pervasive") to describe an individual's need for intervention services within areas of delay. The 2002 guidelines continue to adhere to this general theoretical position, but define "supports" as mediators between a person's capabilities and resultant function-ing. However, the 2002 AAIDD definition allows for classification based on support intensity, IQ range, limitations in adaptive behavior, or etiology, among others. The 1992 and 2002 AAIDD guidelines were proposed in order to reduce reliance on IQ for classifying disability level, as well as to emphasize the ecological interdependency of an individual's needs, supports in the environment, and level of functioning.

Within the DSM-IV-TR, ID is defined as mental retardation; however, for consis-tency, we continue to use the term ID. As such, ID "is characterized by significantly subaverage intellectual functioning (an IQ of approximately 70 or below) with onset before age 18 years and concurrent deficits or impairments in adaptive functioning" (American Psychiatric Association, 2000, p. 39). In contrast to the 2002 AAIDD defini-tion, the DSM-IV-TR includes subcategories of ID used to describe an individual's level of impairment based on current level of intellectual functioning: "mild" (IQ of 50–55 to about 70), "moderate" (IQ of 35–40 to 50–55), "severe" (IQ of 20–25 to 35–40), and "profound" (IQ < 20–25) (American Psychiatric Association, 2000). As the AAIDD definition does, the DSM-IV-TR guidelines define ID as the combination of limitations in the domains of intellectual functioning and adaptive behavior as necessary for diag-nosis. "Adaptive functioning" is defined as the degree to which individuals cope with life demands and personal independence when compared to someone of similar age, sociocultural background and community setting (American Psychiatric Association, 2000).

Prevalence rates of ID typically hover around 1% for school-age children, although rates fluctuate depending on definitions of ID, methods used to detect individuals with ID, cutoff scores used to subgroup individuals with ID, and the size of the study popu-lation (Leonard & Wen, 2002). Average prevalence rates for severe ID (IQ < 35–50) range from 1.4 to 3.8 per 1,000; average prevalence rates for mild ID (IQ of 50–70) range from 5.4 to 10.6 per 1,000 (Leonard & Wen, 2002). Males are more frequently diagnosed with ID than females, at ratios of 1.4–1.7:1 in the severe range and 1.6–1.9:1 in the mild range (Leonard & Wen, 2002).

Etiological Considerations

For a sizable percentage of individuals diagnosed with ID (22–77%), no etiology can be determined, although etiology is more frequently identified for severe than for mild ID (Leonard & Wen, 2002). In cases where no clear etiology exists, ID is typically thought to result from multiple causal factors, such as polygenic inheritance and environmental risks. ID is associated with a large number of conditions, including genetic disorders (e.g., Down syndrome [DS], FXS), prenatal or early environmental insults (e.g., fetal alcohol syndrome [FAS]), and health-related conditions (e.g., tuberous sclerosis; Leonard & Wen, 2002). As many as 1,000 genetic disorders are associated with ID; DS and FXS are often reported as the two most frequent genetic causes (Leonard & Wen, 2002).

Phenotypic "Profiling"

By definition, individuals with ID show delayed intellectual and adaptive functioning; however, the variability within the population is remarkable. With recent technological advances in molecular genetics, research has focused on linking physical, cognitive, and behavioral phenotypes to genetic causes of ID—that is, on delineating symptom presentation with a specific genetic abnormality (Dykens & Hodapp, 2001). As such, phenotypic descriptions have been identified for many known genetic causes, such as DS, FXS, Prader–Willi syndrome, and Williams syndrome. Outside of genetic disorders, there is evidence for a phenotypic profile for children with FAS and related conditions. Phenotypes associated with three of the most common causes of ID are reviewed briefly.

Down Syndrome

DS is the most prevalent genetic cause of ID, occurring in about 1 in 730 births in the United States, or roughly 5,400 infants born annually (Silverman, 2007). DS results from trisomy of all or part of chromosome 21; approximately 95% of individuals with DS have an extra 21st chromosome and are identified as having the "trisomy 21" subtype. Roughly 3–4% of individuals with DS are classified as having the "translocation" subtype, in which a portion of chromosome 21 is attached to other chromosomes. The "mosaicism" subtype of DS refers to the presence of both normal and trisomic cells within the individual and occurs in about 1–2% of cases. Common physical characteristics associated with DS include muscle hypotonia, flat facial profile, oblique palpebral fissures, and hyperflexibility.

Individuals with DS frequently demonstrate moderate to severe intellectual delays, with several characteristic cognitive strengths and weaknesses. Cognitive-linguistic weaknesses associated with DS are relative weaknesses in auditory processing, expressive language, speech intelligibility, verbal memory, and syntactic speech (e.g., Silverman, 2007). Cognitive-linguistic strengths are often identified in the domains of receptive language, pragmatic language, visual–spatial processing, and visual memory (Fidler & Nadel, 2007). Academically, word identification has been identified as an area of relative strength in the presence of weak word attack and decoding skills, possibly associated with the visual over verbal cognitive processing advantage for individuals with DS (Fidler & Nadel, 2007).

Individuals with DS are at risk for varied health problems, such as hearing deficits, heart defects, leukemia, hypothyroidism, and gastrointestinal disorders. A well-established component of the DS phenotype is the increased risk of developing Alzheimer-type dementia (AZD). In the general population, AZD typically develops after the age of 50, with the largest prevalence rate of 5–10% in individuals over the age of 65. In contrast, 25% of individuals with DS develop AZD by the age of 35, and 50–70% of individuals with DS over the age of 60 develop it (Zigman & Lott, 2007). Although age is a risk factor for developing AZD, the role of other variables, such as IQ, has been less clearly specified.

The stereotypic representation of a child with DS is an affectionate child with an easy temperament and relative strengths in social functioning. Some findings support the notion of a behavioral adaptation advantage for DS early in development. On average, for example, children with DS exhibit reduced rates of maladaptive behavior and psychiatric disorders (18–23%), compared to other children with ID of known or "mixed" etiology (30–40%; Dykens, 2007). Nonetheless, children with DS exhibit more behavioral difficulties than either typically developing siblings or general population norms. Moreover, in contrast to children with DS, adults with DS are diagnosed with depression at rates five to six times higher than other adults with ID—a finding that may herald the onset of AZD (Dykens, 2007).

Fragile X Syndrome

FXS is the most common inherited form of ID, found in roughly 1 per 1,000 males and 1 per 2,000 females. FXS is caused by a mutated repetition of the cytosine–guanine–guanine (CGG) genetic sequence on the long arm of the X chromosome. The abnormal repetition occurs at the site of the fragile X MR-1 gene, which inhibits production of the fragile X mental retardation protein (FMRP). Reduced or absent FMRP production yields atypical brain development, with a strong relationship found between degree of FMRP deficiency and aberrant brain morphology, particularly the caudate nucleus and cerebellar vermis (e.g., Gothelf et al., 2008). Full-mutation (CGG repetitions of greater than 200) and premutation (CGG repetitions of about 50 to about 200) subtypes have been identified; the premutation subtype generally results in less severe symptoms. Characteristic physical features for boys with FXS include hyperextensible finger joints, large ears, narrow face, and macroorchidism (i.e., enlarged testicles). Although phenotypic variability exists within each group, in general females are less affected than males.

Symptoms of persistent inattention, hyperactivity, and impulsivity are common for boys with FXS (Cornish, Sudhalter, & Turk, 2004). Males with FXS often exhibit social-communicative problems similar to autism, such as perseverative and repetitive speech, pragmatic language deficits, and social anxiety. The relationship between FXS and autistic symptomatology has been established for over two decades, with autism present in up to 25% of boys with FXS; however, recent reports have documented higher rates of autism symptomatology for children with FXS. Hall, Lightbody, and Reiss (2008) found that 51.6% of boys with FXS and 20.7% of girls with FXS met ADOS criteria for autism. Interestingly, there was no relationship between ADOS scores and IQ for boys but a significant relationship for girls, indicating greater autistic symptomatology related to lower IQ (Hall et al., 2008). Cornish and colleagues (2004) have suggested that the nature of social dysfunction in FXS may be secondary to hyperarousal, inhibition deficits, anxiety, and executive dysfunction.

Self-injurious behavior, compulsive behavior, and aggression are frequent problems for children with FXS, especially boys. For example, self-injurious behavior appears more common in boys (58–79%) than in girls (17%), with hitting, biting, and scratching as frequent self-injurious behavior topographies (Hall et al., 2008; Hessl et al., 2008). Compulsive behavior is reported in 74% of boys and 55% of girls, taking the form of ordering, checking, and insisting on "completeness," such as closing doors (Hall et al., 2008). Up to 75% of boys with FXS exhibited aggressive behavior, as reported by parents over a 2-month recall period (Hessl et al., 2008). Although FXS is known as a "single-gene" disorder, research efforts have begun to examine moderating genes, such as those that influence serotonin transport (Hessl et al., 2008), to better understand individual differences within the group.

Fetal Alcohol Spectrum Disorders

Prenatal exposure to alcohol can result in a range of structural/morphological and cognitive-behavioral symptoms. Although these do not constitute a formal diagnostic category, the term "fetal alcohol spectrum disorders" (FASDs) was coined to capture the full spectrum of symptoms and severity arising from prenatal alcohol exposure. The most severely affected children exhibit FAS, which has a wide-ranging estimated prevalence rate of between 0.33 and 7.4 per 1,000 across U.S. and Western European cultures (May et al., 2006). FAS is characterized by the presence of prenatal and/or postnatal growth delay, abnormalities of the face and head (e.g., microcephaly), and central nervous system dysfunction. The characteristic facial phenotype of FAS includes small eyes, smooth philtrum (i.e., indistinct groove between upper lip and nose), and a thin upper lip (see Hoyme et al., 2005). Children with FAS are more likely to suffer from chronic otitis media, visual problems, cardiac problems, seizures, and immune system deficits (e.g., Burd, Klug, Martsolf, & Kerbeshian, 2003). In addition to physical complications, children with FAS often exhibit problems with sustained attention and overactivity; up to 73% are diagnosed with ADHD (Burd et al., 2003).

Prenatal alcohol exposure results in structural changes to the brain thought to arise as a result of decreased neuron production, abnormal migration, and premature cell death (Burd et al., 2003). Structural MRI shows particular vulnerability for reduced growth within frontal and parietal lobes, cerebellum, corpus callosum, and caudate nucleus as a result of prenatal alcohol exposure (Spadoni, McGee, Fryer, & Riley, 2007). Frontal lobe anomalies are thought to be consistent with the deficits in attention, executive functioning, and impulsive behavioral profile for individuals with FASDs (Spadoni et al., 2007). Likewise, cerebellar anomalies are hypothesized to associate with problems with balance, fine motor coordination, and attention.

Adolescents and adults with FAS are at increased risk for various educational and social problems. Streissguth and colleagues (2004) documented significant impairments in academic achievement and adaptive functioning for adolescents and adults with FASDs. Roughly 80% were raised by adults other than their mothers, and 67% were abused or subjected to domestic violence. Educational experiences were characterized by special education placement (42%), suspensions (53%), expulsions (29%), and dropping out of school (25%). Adolescents and adults experienced problems with the law (60%); shoplifting, theft, assault, burglary, and domestic violence were the most frequently reported crimes. Using a risk–resiliency approach, Streissguth and colleagues identified higher IQ, being male, and later age at diagnosis as risk factors for suffering adverse life events; being raised in a stable and nurturing home and earlier age of diagnosis were associated with lower risk for negative outcomes.

Diagnostic Assessment

Diagnostic assessment of ID involves measurement of both cognitive ability and adaptive behavior. Clinicians have an array of empirically validated IQ tests from which to choose for documenting cognitive delay (Campbell, Brown, Cavanagh, Vess, & Segall, 2008). Assessment of adaptive delays may be documented via rating scales, interview information, or observation, with multiple methods of data collection preferred (Luckasson et al., 2002). Furthermore, clinicians should collect information regarding a youth's adaptive behavior from multiple sources (e.g., parent and teacher) across multiple settings (e.g., home and school). Detailed assessment of the individual's repertoire of adaptive skill provides starting points for intervention and baseline assessment to evaluate education and treatment progress.

Assessment of Psychopathology and Diagnostic Overshadowing

Children and adolescents with ID suffer from psychopathology and behavioral problems at rates higher than those of typically developing peers (Dykens, 2000). Rates of comorbid psychopathology range widely across studies, from as low as 10% to as high as 70% (Dykens, 2000). Children and adolescents with lower IQs are usually more at risk for self-injurious behavior, motor stereotypies, or other disruptive behavior problems. Children with milder delays, on the other hand, appear to be more at risk for mood and anxiety disorders (Dykens, 2000). Historically, psychological disorders appear to have been underdiagnosed in individuals with ID, due to the phenomenon known as "diagnostic overshadowing" (i.e., the tendency to attribute symptoms of psychopathology to the presence of ID) (Jopp & Keys, 2001). Psychological assessment of individuals with ID is problematic because of their cognitive limitations and associated language delays; therefore, a focus on behavioral signs of psychopathology is typically most useful. Assessment of psychological functioning should involve a parent or caregiver interview, interview with the individual with ID, and behavior rating scales. Given the high percentage of individuals with ID who exhibit maladaptive behavior, disruptive behaviors, such as aggression to self or others, should be documented in terms of frequency, intensity, and duration. Furthermore, a functional assessment or analysis has shown to be useful for improving behavioral intervention outcomes for individuals with ID. For individuals exhibiting maladaptive behavior, identifying the function of the behavior (e.g., attention, escape) provides guidance for behavioral intervention.

Psychopharmacological Interventions

Similar to the ASD literature, no studies have found that medications have improved the core cognitive deficits defining ID; rather, psychotropic medications are used to target specific behavioral symptoms and comorbid psychological disorders encountered within this group. Also as for persons with ASDs, many types of psychotropic medications have been used to target varied symptoms for individuals with ID; these drugs include psychostimulants, antipsychotics, antidepressants, mood stabilizers, and alpha agonists. Handen and Gilchrist (2006) reviewed the efficacy of psychotropics for individuals with ID and concluded that individuals with ID generally show a poorer response and greater occurrence of side effects than samples without ID do. For example, 45–66% of children with ID respond to methylphenidate, compared to 77% of children with ADHD. The poorer response and greater chance for untoward effects call for increased monitoring, lower initial dosages, and slower increases for individuals with ID (Handen & Gilchrist, 2006).

Psychosocial and Educational Interventions

The predominant psychosocial approach to intervention with ID employs behavioral methods to increase adaptive skills and decrease maladaptive behaviors. Behavioral techniques, such as task analysis, shaping, chaining, and prompting, are frequently used in combination to teach adaptive skills in a systematic manner. Once adaptive skills are reliably performed within one setting, intervention focuses on teaching the individual to generalize the skills to other settings. Numerous single-subject research studies have documented the efficacy of behavioral teaching methods in improving self-care, social, academic, and vocational skills.

Summary and Conclusions

It is important for pediatric psychologists to appreciate the heterogeneity that exists among individuals with ASDs and ID. This heterogeneity is accompanied by varied causal factors, and diagnostic endpoints may be reached via a host of genetic, biological, and environmental influences. The heterogeneity also necessitates individualized intervention for individuals with ASDs and ID. Despite the necessary tailoring of interventions, the literature on outcomes for these individuals consistently concludes that early intervention produces the most optimal outcomes. Within the group of psychological interventions, the strongest empirical support exists for behaviorally based approaches.

The field has made considerable progress in phenotypic profiling physical, behavioral, and cognitive characteristics for the disorders reviewed in this chapter. These research efforts may be best characterized as "between-group" comparisons. There has been recent movement toward another line of research, which is focused on increased specificity to account for the variable outcomes for individuals with ASDs and ID— that is, "within-group" comparisons. The movement toward a better understanding of within-group variability has focused on both intraindividual and contextual variables. Intraindividual research has begun to document the moderating and mediating influences of gender, genes, cognitive, functioning, and comorbid psychopathology on outcomes across disorders. Studies have also turned toward examining the roles of contextual variables, such as parenting stress, adjustment, childrearing experiences, and socioeconomic status, in outcomes for various conditions. As such, ASD and ID research may benefit from explicit application of the disability–stress–coping and social-ecological frameworks that have been embraced within pediatric psychology to improve our understanding of child outcomes.

References

American Psychiatric Association. (2000). *Diagnostic and statistical manual of mental disorders* (4th ed., text rev.). Washington, DC: Author.

Barnea-Goraly, N., Kown, H., Menon, V., Eliez, S., Lotspeich, L., & Reiss, A. L. (2004). White matter structure in autism: Preliminary evidence from diffusion tensor imaging. *Biological Psychiatry, 55,* 323–326.

Burd, L., Klug, M. G., Martsolf, J. T., & Kerbeshian, J. (2003). Fetal alcohol syndrome: Neuropsychiatric phenomics. *Neurotoxicology and Teratology, 25,* 697–705.

Campbell, J. M., Brown, R. T., Cavanagh, S. E., Vess, S. F., & Segall, M. J. (2008). Evidence-based assessment of cognitive functioning in pediatric psychology. *Journal of Pediatric Psychology, 33,* 999–1014.

Campbell, J. M., Herzinger, C. V., & James, C. L. (2008). Evidence-based therapies for children with autism and pervasive developmental disorders. In R. Steele, T. Elkin, & M. Roberts, (Eds.), *Handbook of evidence based therapies for children and adolescents* (pp. 373–388). New York: Springer.

Castelli, F., Frith, C., Happé, F., & Frith, U. (2002). Autism, Asperger syndrome and brain mechanisms for the attribution of mental states to animated shapes. *Brain, 125,* 1839–1849.

Cederlund, M., Hagberg, B., Billstedt, E., Gillberg, I. C., & Gillberg, C. (2008). Asperger syndrome and autism: A comparative longitudinal follow-up study more than 5 years after original diagnosis. *Journal of Autism and Developmental Disorders, 38,* 72–85.

Centers for Disease Control and Prevention (CDC). (2007). Prevalence of autism spectrum disorders—Autism and Developmental Disabilities Monitoring Network, 14 sites, United States, 2002. *Morbidity and Mortality Weekly Report Surveillance Summaries, 56*(No. SS-1).

Cornish, K., Sudhalter, V., & Turk, J. (2004). Attention and language in fragile X. *Mental Retardation and Developmental Disabilities Research Reviews, 10,* 11–16.

Courchesne, E., & Pierce, K. (2005). Brain overgrowth in autism during a critical time in development: Implications for frontal pyramidal neuron and interneuron development and connectivity. *International Journal of Developmental Neuroscience, 23,* 153–170.

Dykens, E. M. (2000). Annotation: Psychopathology in children with intellectual disability. *Journal of Child Psychology and Psychiatry, 41,* 407–417.

Dykens, E. M. (2007). Psychiatric and behavioral disorders in persons with Down syndrome. *Mental Retardation and Developmental Disabilities Research Reviews, 13,* 272–278.

Dykens, E. M., & Hodapp, R. M. (2001). Research in mental retardation: Toward an etiologic approach. *Journal of Child Psychology and Psychiatry, 42,* 49–71.

Edelson, M. G. (2006). Are the majority of children with autism mentally retarded?: A systematic evaluation of the data. *Focus on Autism and Other Developmental Disabilities, 21,* 66–83.

Fidler, D. J., & Nadel, L. (2007). Education and children with Down syndrome: Neuroscience, development, and intervention. *Mental Retardation and Developmental Disabilities Research Reviews, 13,* 262–271.

Fombonne, E. (2005). Epidemiological studies of pervasive developmental disorders. In F. R. Volkmar, R. Paul, A. Klin, & D. Cohen (Eds.), *Handbook of autism and pervasive developmental disorders* (3rd ed., pp. 42–69). Hoboken, NJ: Wiley.

Gothelf, D., Furfaro, J. A., Hoeft, F., Eckert, M. A., Hall, S. S., O'Hara, R., et al. (2008). Neuroanatomy of fragile X syndrome is associated with aberrant behavior and the fragile X mental retardation protein (FMRP). *Annals of Neurology, 63,* 40–51.

Hall, S. S., Lightbody, A. A., & Reiss, A. L. (2008). Compulsive, self-injurious, and autistic behavior in children and adolescents with fragile X syndrome. *American Journal on Mental Retardation, 113,* 44–53.

Handen, B. L., & Gilchrist, R. (2006). Practitioner review: Psychopharmacology in children and adolescents with mental retardation. *Journal of Child Psychology and Psychiatry, 47,* 871–882.

Happé, F. (2005). The weak central coherence account of autism. In F. R. Volkmar, R. Paul, A. Klin, & D. Cohen (Eds.), *Handbook of autism and pervasive developmental disorders* (3rd ed., pp. 640–649). Hoboken, NJ: Wiley.

Happé, F., Ronald, A., & Plomin, R. (2006). Time to give up on a single explanation for autism. *Nature Neuroscience, 9,* 1218–1220.

Hessl, D., Tassone, F., Cordiero, L., Koldewyn, K., McCormick, C., Green, C., et al. (2008). Brief report: Aggression and stereotypic behavior in males with fragile X syndrome—Moderating secondary genes in a "single gene" disorder. *Journal of Autism and Developmental Disorders, 38,* 184–189.

Howlin, P. C. (2005). Outcomes in autism spectrum disorders. In F. R. Volkmar, R. Paul, A. Klin, & D. Cohen (Eds.), *Handbook of autism and pervasive developmental disorders* (3rd ed., pp. 201–220). Hoboken, NJ: Wiley.

Howlin, P., Goode, S., Hutton, J., & Rutter, M. (2004). Adult outcome for children with autism. *Journal of Child Psychology and Psychiatry, 45,* 212–229.

Hoyme, H. E., May, P. A., Kalberg, W. O., Kodituwakku, P., Gossage, P., Trujillo, P. M., et al. (2005). A practical approach to diagnosis of fetal alcohol spectrum disorders: Clarification of the 1996 Institute of Medicine criteria. *Pediatrics, 115,* 39–47.

Johnson, C. P., & Myers, S. M. (2007). Identification and evaluation of children with autism spectrum disorders. *Pediatrics, 120,* 1183–1215.

Jopp, D. A., & Keys, C. B. (2001). Diagnostic overshadowing reviewed and reconsidered. *American Journal on Mental Retardation, 106,* 416–433.

Kanner, L. (1943). Autistic disturbances of affective contact. *Nervous Child, 2,* 217–250.

Leonard, H., & Wen, X. (2002). The epidemiology of mental retardation: Challenges and opportunities in the new millennium. *Mental Retardation and Developmental Disabilities Research Reviews, 8,* 117–134.

Lord, C., Rutter, M., DiLavore, P. C., & Risi, S. (2001). *Autism Diagnostic Observation Schedule manual.* Los Angeles: Western Psychological Services.

Luckasson, R., Borthwick-Duffy, S., Buntinx, W. H. E., Coulter, D. L., Craig, E. M., Polloway, E. A., et al. (2002). *Mental retardation: Definition, classification, and systems of supports* (10th ed.). Washington, DC: American Association on Mental Retardation.

May, P. A., Fiorentino, D., Gossage, J. P., Kalberg, W. O., Hoyme, H. E., Robinson, L. K., et al. (2006). Epidemiology of FASD in a province in Italy: Prevalence and characteristics of children in a random sample of schools. *Alcoholism: Clinical and Experimental Research, 30,* 1562–1575.

Myers, S. M., & Johnson, C. P. (2007). Management of children with autism spectrum disorders. *Pediatrics, 120,* 1162–1182.

National Research Council. (2001). *Educating children with autism* (C. Lord & J. P. McGee, Eds.). Washington, DC: National Academy Press.

Ozonoff, S., Goodlin-Jones, B. L., & Solomon, M. (2005). Evidence-based assessment of autism spectrum disorders in children and adolescents. *Journal of Clinical Child and Adolescent Psychology, 34,* 523–540.

Ozonoff, S., South, M., & Provencal, S. (2005). Executive functions. In F. R. Volkmar, R. Paul,

A. Klin, & D. Cohen (Eds.), *Handbook of autism and pervasive developmental disorders* (3rd ed., pp. 606–627). Hoboken, NJ: Wiley.

Pelphrey, K., Adolphs, R., & Morris, J. P. (2004). Neuroanatomical substrates of social cognition dysfunction in autism. *Mental Retardation and Developmental Disabilities Research Reviews, 10*, 259–271.

Rehabilitation, Comprehensive Services, and Developmental Disabilities Amendments, Pub. L. 95-602, 92 Stat. 2955 (1978).

Richler, J., Luyster, R., Risi, S., Hsu, W., Dawson, G., Bernier, R., et al. (2006). Is there a 'regressive phenotype' of autism spectrum disorder associated with the measles–mumps–rubella vaccine?: A CPEA study. *Journal of Autism and Developmental Disorders, 36*, 299–316.

Rogers, S. J., & Vismara, L. A. (2008). Evidence-based comprehensive treatments for early autism. *Journal of Clinical Child Psychology, 37*, 8–38.

Rutter, M. (2005). Genetic influences and autism. In F. R. Volkmar, R. Paul, A. Klin, & D. Cohen (Eds.), *Handbook of autism and pervasive developmental disorders* (3rd ed., pp. 425–452). Hoboken, NJ: Wiley.

Rutter, M., LeCouteur, A., & Lord, C. (2003). *Autism Diagnostic Interview—Revised.* Los Angeles: Western Psychological Services.

Schultz, R. T. (2005). Developmental deficits in social perception in autism: The role of the amygdala and fusiform face area. *International Journal of Developmental Neuroscience, 23*, 125–141.

Silverman, W. (2007). Down syndrome: Cognitive profile. *Mental Retardation and Developmental Disabilities Research Reviews, 13*, 228–236.

Spadoni, A. D., McGee, C. L., Fryer, S. L., & Riley, E. P. (2007). Neuroimaging and fetal alcohol spectrum disorders. *Neuroscience and Biobehavioral Reviews, 31*, 239–245.

Streissguth, A. P., Bookstein, F. L., Barr, H. M., Sampson, P. D., O'Malley, K., & Young, J. K. (2004). Risk factors for adverse life outcomes in fetal alcohol syndrome and fetal alcohol effects. *Journal of Developmental and Behavioral Pediatrics, 25*, 228–238.

Towbin, K. E. (2005). Pervasive developmental disorder not otherwise specified. In F. R. Volkmar, R. Paul, A. Klin, & D. Cohen (Eds.), *Handbook of autism and pervasive developmental disorders* (3rd ed., pp. 165–200). Hoboken, NJ: Wiley.

Volkmar, F. R., Lord, C., Klin, A., Schultz, R., & Cook, E. H. (2007). Autism and the pervasive developmental disorders. In A. Martin & F. R. Volkmar (Eds.), *Lewis's child and adolescent psychiatry: A comprehensive textbook* (4th ed., pp. 384–400). New York: Wolters Kluwer.

Wakefield, A. J., Murch, S. H., Anthony, A., Linnell, J., Casson, D. M., Malik, M., et al. (1998). Ileal-lymphoid-nodular-hyperplasia, non-specific colitis, and pervasive developmental disorder in children. *Lancet, 351*, 634–641.

Williams, D. L., Goldstein, G., & Minshew, N. J. (2006). Neuropsychologic functioning in children with autism: Further evidence for disordered complex information-processing. *Child NeuroPsychology, 12*, 279–298.

Zigman, W. B., & Lott, I. T. (2007). Alzheimer's disease in Down syndrome: Neurobiology and risk. *Mental Retardation and Developmental Disabilities Research Reviews, 13*, 237–246.

CHAPTER 35

Behavior Problems in a Pediatric Context

SUSAN M. VᴀɴSCOYOC
EDWARD R. CHRISTOPHERSEN

Problem behaviors in children, especially externalizing behaviors, are common referral issues for psychologists (Feinfield & Baker, 2004; Sobel, Roberts, Rayfield, Barnard, & Rapoff, 2001). In fact, children with disruptive behavior disorders are the most frequently referred population for child mental health services (Kazdin, Mazurick, & Siegel, 1994). The impact of behavior problems on a child is severe and chronic, often interfering with the child's social interactions, and school performance. Furthermore, children with behavior problems often have comorbid disruptive and mood disorders (Barkley, 2006; Kazdin, 1996; McMahon & Frick, 2005). For example, in a study of 75 children ages 4–13 years, Kazdin (1996) found that a significant number of children (45–70%) diagnosed with attention-deficit/hyperactivity disorder (ADHD) or conduct disorder also met criteria for the other disorder. Thus children with behavior problems are among the most prevalent and impaired populations in the area of child mental health.

Literature reviews of emotional and behavioral adjustment for children with medical conditions show variable ranges of dysfunction from minimal to significant when such children are compared to their healthy peers (e.g., Bachanas et al., 2001; Helgeson, Snyder, Escobar, Siminerio, & Becker, 2007; Noll et al., 1997). Some studies demonstrate that children with behavior problems are referred more for psychological services while hospitalized (e.g., Carter et al., 2003) than children without these issues, and that such behaviors are a barrier to medical treatment adherence (e.g., Modi & Quittner, 2006). In addition, a relationship has been suggested between the presence of externalizing behaviors and increased medical problems, such as unintentional injury (Morrongiello & Lasenby-Lessard, 2007; Schwebel, Speltz, Jones, & Bardina, 2002) and injury severity (DiScala, Lescohier, Barthel, & Li, 1998; Mangus, Bergman, Zieger, & Coleman, 2004). Regardless of health status, problem behaviors in children represent an important area of intervention for the pediatric practitioner.

526

This chapter highlights key issues in the outpatient assessment and treatment of externalizing behavior problems in children. When possible, specific caveats or applications of findings to pediatric patients are discussed. Although many pediatric practitioners also provide services in an inpatient setting, we could find little definitive evidence of empirically valid assessment or treatment options for addressing externalizing behavioral problems in that setting. In addition, our focus on externalizing disorders does not diminish the importance of internalizing behaviors (such as anxiety and depression) as referral concerns. These disorders can also significantly affect how successfully developmental tasks and medical conditions are managed by the child and caregivers. Indeed, some pediatric patients, such as older children and adolescents with cardiac problems, are more at risk for internalizing than externalizing disorders (Karsdorp, Everaerd, Kindt, & Mulder, 2007). The reader is referred to other resources for information on how to assess and treat internalizing disorders (e.g., Compton et al., 2004; Kendall & Hedtke, 2006). Also, more specific information on managing the externalizing behaviors and other characteristics of ADHD is provided elsewhere in this volume (see Daly, Cohen, Carpenter, & Brown, Chapter 36), as well as by Barkley (2006).

Assessment

The topic of child behavior assessment is a broad and evolving one. Entire books, courses, and careers are spent in evaluating and disseminating the best practices available for measuring typical and problematic behaviors for children. The most useful assessment tools for evaluating any child behavior problem are those that will accurately and reliably measure the behaviors of concern in a manner that results in efficacious intervention. A movement is underway to investigate the availability of evidence-based instruments for assessing key areas in pediatric psychology, such as pain (Cohen et al., 2008), coping and stress (Blount et al., 2008), and cognitive functioning (Campbell, Brown, Cavanagh, Vess, & Segall, 2008). The *Journal of Clinical Child and Adolescent Psychology* devoted most of its September 2005 issue to the issue of evidence-based assessment. An article by McMahon and Frick (2005) in that issue specifically focuses on evidence-based assessment of conduct problems, concluding that assessment methods with more developmental considerations and greater clinical utility are needed.

Assessment Goals

The goals of an assessment for behavior problems are largely to determine whether a clinically significant problem exists and how to treat it. These goals are best met when the practitioner has adequate knowledge of child development and psychopathology, as well as the roles of social, cultural, and parent–child relationship variables in behavior (Barkley & Edwards, 2006; Mash & Terdal, 1988). For the assessment of a pediatric patient, a working knowledge of how the disease state, physical trauma, treatment regimen, and/or medications affect behavior is also important. For example, a child's level of behavior problems has been associated with the frequency of seizure activity (Austin et al., 2001). Children with functional abdominal pain (Huntley, Campo, Dahl, & Lewin, 2007) and atopic dermatitis (LeBovidge et al., 2007) may experience condition-related sleep disturbances, which may in turn influence affect and behavior. For a pediatric patient with behavior problems, the roles of social and cultural factors, including the child's and parent's beliefs about the impact of the child's medical condition on behavior, are important to understand as well.

Common Assessment Methods

A multimethod assessment protocol that describes both problematic and positive behavior, obtained via at least two different assessment methods (and from multiple informants), is typically necessary to provide the most accurate case conceptualization and effective treatment plan for a child with behavior problems (Morrison & Anders, 1999; Velting, Setzer, & Albano, 2004). An overview of three common assessment methods for evaluating child behavior problems—behavioral interviews, rating scales, and observations—is presented below.

Behavioral Interviews: Caregiver Interview

An interview with the caregiver is often the first step in collecting vital historical information related to the referral issue. Typically, this initial contact with the family begins the process of identifying characteristics of the child, parent, and environment that may be contributing to the child's behavior problems. For a pediatric patient, an interview with the child's teacher, school nurse, or medical care provider may also be necessary to determine whether behavior problems exist in other settings, as well as the impact of those problems on the child's medical condition, adherence, and health. An interview with teachers or other caregivers who knew the child before an illness or injury may be helpful in establishing premorbid behavioral strengths and weaknesses that may influence the treatment plan and success (cf. Christophersen & Mortweet, 2001). For example, a child who presented with significant compliance problems prior to the injury or illness is much more likely to exhibit behavior problems, and to be more difficult to treat, than a child without prior behavior problems (Irwin, Cataldo, Matheny, & Peterson, 1992).

Structured and Semistructured Interviews. Several interview format options are available to the practitioner. Structured interviews require precise questioning by the examiner with no latitude for clinical judgment, whereas semistructured formats allow some flexibility and clinical decision making based on the informant's answers to questions about symptomatology (Orvaschel, 2006). Both of these interview types emphasize criteria supported by the *Diagnostic and Statistical Manual of Mental Disorders* (DSM) criteria (e.g., DSM-IV-TR; American Psychiatric Association, 2000) or other diagnostic criteria; they are often designed for epidemiological research, with some feasibility for clinical application. Two examples of such interviews include the structured Diagnostic Interview Schedule for Children, Version IV (Shaffer, Fisher, Lucas, Dulcan, & Schwab-Stone, 2000) and the semistructured Schedule for Affective Disorders and Schizophrenia for School-Age Children (Puig-Antich & Chambers, 1978; see also Orvaschel, 2006). The time-consuming nature of such interviews, often 2 hours or more (depending on the skill of the examiner and the level of information provided by the caregivers), can make them impractical to use in the typical office or inpatient setting. Such interviews may have some clinical utility, however, as a reference source for a difficult differential diagnosis or as a guide for developing a nonstandardized interview format.

Nonstandardized Interviews. Practitioners often create their own caregiver interviews from their experience with referral issues such as behavior problems. Several authors have published suggestions for structuring these nonstandardized interviews, targeting important topics for assessing externalizing behavior problems (e.g., Barkley & Edwards, 2006; McMahon & Forehand, 2003; Merrell, 2003). At a minimum, a thorough caregiver interview should provide the practitioner with vital information about possible causes for the problematic behaviors; an estimate of when these problems started; the level of distress for the child and parent; other possible psychiatric disturbances; and ultimate target intervention areas (Barkley & Edwards, 2006). Parents may not be used to thinking about their child's behavior in the specific terms introduced by the practitioner, and thus may require extensive questioning in order to provide a description more useful than "He has a bad attitude" or "She never listens to me." Sometimes a structured observation task for the parent to complete at home is needed before an objective description of the behavioral issues requiring intervention can be reported.

It is also important to establish the potential role of environmental factors in the manifestation of behavioral problems, as well as for guidance in designing an effective intervention. In addition to family mental health history, two of the most important environmental factors to assess are current parenting techniques and parental stressors. The practitioner must have some sense of the parents' beliefs about appropriate and inappropriate behavior, of how they view discipline, and what strategies they use to manage behavior. If the child has a medical condition, a discussion about how their parenting has changed since diagnosis is vital. This may be especially relevant if the parents report changing discipline strategies because they believe that the medical condition somehow precludes the child from demonstrating appropriate behavior.

The practitioner must also assess the parents' current stressors to fully appreciate how difficult it may be to carry out the demands of a behavioral intervention. For example, parents of children with ADHD report more parenting-related stressors, such as dissatisfaction with the parenting role and greater personal distress, than parents with children without ADHD do (Barkley, Anastopoulos, Guevremont, & Fletcher, 1992; Podolski & Nigg, 2001). Many parents of children with a medical condition understandably also suffer from parenting stress and psychological distress. Descriptive and empirical research of parental adjustment to their children's illness suggest that elevated anxiety, depression, and symptoms of posttraumatic stress disorder are evident for many parents, especially mothers (Bourdeau & Mullins, 2007; Dolgin et al., 2007; Wiener, Vasquez, & Battles, 2001). Given the additional burden of managing a child's medical condition, as well as the substantial parental effort required in most behavioral interventions, it is obvious why thorough assessment and consideration of parental contributions are essential to addressing behavior problems in children.

Behavioral Interviews: Child Interview

One of the most important informants in assessing behavior problems for a child is the child. An interview with the child can provide valuable information about the child's perspective on his or her environment, behavior, and medical issues. Merrell (2003) offers five recommended areas for questioning to obtain a comprehensive view of the child's perspective: medical history, developmental history, social-emotional functioning, educational progress, and community involvement. For a pediatric patient, it is especially vital to verify what the child understands about his or her illness and treatment. In our clinical experience, oppositional behavior may be based on a misinterpretation by the child (or parent) that can be rectified with the help of the child's medical care providers. For example, a child with diabetes who is "sneaking" food may simply need a new meal plan to accommodate an increase in hunger.

The child interview also provides the practitioner a chance to observe the child and his or her behavior. Interactions with the child offer the chance to note any strengths or peculiarities in major developmental domains, such as language, cognitive, motor, and social skills (Barkley & Edwards, 2006). Behavioral observations can be made informally in the office setting, while the child is interacting with a parent or (perhaps most informatively) while the child is interacting in the waiting area. Structured parent and child interaction tasks are also helpful and are discussed later in this chapter. More extensive information about how to interview a child can be found in the literature (e.g., McConaughy & Achenbach, 1990; Merrell, 2003).

Standardized Behavior Rating Scales

Standardized behavior rating scales are an efficient way to obtain input about a child's behavior from multiple informants, including parents, teachers, and the child. When more than one informant completes a rating scale of the child's emotional and behavioral functioning, the practitioner can ascertain how consistently the child is perceived in the environment (Achenbach & McConaughy, 1996; Merrell, 2003). Such information is vital for intervention planning and success. The use of rating scales can also provide a way to repeat assessment during and after treatment to monitor progress.

Of course, responses to any rating scale are subject to the personal biases and limitations of the informant, and thus rating scales should be considered only part of a more comprehensive assessment routine (Barkley & Edwards, 2006). Additional caveats are important to mention with respect to the use of rating scales in the pediatric population. Some of the subscales, particularly those related to the expression of physical symptomatology, may skew the results of these scales (Friedman, Bryant, & Holmbeck, 2007). These instruments can lead the practitioner to erroneous conclusions regarding adjustment issues for a child with a chronic illness, the endorsement of physical symptoms in the behavioral profile, or the child's true level of social competence (Friedman et al., 2007; Mathews, Spieth, & Christophersen, 1995; Perrin, Stein, & Drotar, 1991). For example, a child or parent may endorse numerous physical symptoms or social isolation factors that are related to an illness, and thus may artificially inflate scores on subscales related to mood or social problems. With those caveats, we review four commonly used types of rating scales for the assessment of a child's behavior and emotional state.

Broadband Rating Scales. Broadband rating scales have been used extensively in research and clinical practice with children of all ages. Two psychometrically sound, comprehensive rating scale systems available for evaluating the behavioral and emotional status of a child are the Behavior Assessment System for Children, Second Edition (BASC-2; Reynolds & Kamphaus, 2004) and the Child Behavior Checklist (CBCL; Achenbach & Rescorla, 2001). Both systems have questionnaires available for parent, teacher, and self-report of both adaptive and maladaptive behaviors for children and adolescents. The BASC-2 provides an extensive, computer-generated practitioner's report, including *T* scores and percentile rankings for various individual and composite scales (Adaptive Skills, Behavioral Symptoms Index, Externalizing Problems, and Internalizing Problems); suggestions for possible DSM-IV-TR (American Psychiatric Association, 2000) diagnoses and target behaviors for treatment are also offered. The CBCL includes scales that were constructed with characteristics consistent with DSM categories, including Oppositional Defiant Problems and Attention-Deficit/Hyperactivity Problems. An updated feature of the most recent CBCL scales is the ability to interpret results using multicultural norms. The interested reader is referred to the Achenbach System for Empirically Based Assessment website for information on the current edition of the CBCL (*www.aseba.org*). More information about the BASC-2 can be found at its current publisher's website (*ags.pearsonassessments.com*).

Specific Behavior Rating Scales. The Conners Rating Scales have been used for many years to assess externalizing disorders (specifically, ADHD, oppositional defiant disorder, and conduct disorder) in school-age children. The most recent version of these scales, the Conners 3rd Edition (Conners 3; Conners, 2008a) is based on a larger, representative normative sample and has stronger connections to the DSM-IV-TR (American Psychiatric Association, 2000) than previous versions. In addition, a more comprehensive rating scale is now available from Conners. The Conners Comprehensive Behavior Rating Scales (Conners CBRS; Conners, 2008b) was developed as a way to provide a more thorough assessment of a wider range of behavioral and emotional problems in children than the externalizing disorders assessed in the Conners 3. The psychometric properties of the scale are reportedly strong and are detailed in the Conners CBRS manual (Conners, 2008b). The parent form clusters responses into scales such as Emotional Distress, Aggressive Behaviors, ADHD Symptoms, and Academic Problems. A separate set of scales related directly to the DSM-IV-TR (American Psychiatric Association, 2000) is also provided. Information about both the Conners 3 and the Conners CBRS can be found at the publisher's website (*www.mhs.com*).

The Eyberg Child Behavior Inventory (ECBI; Eyberg & Pincus, 1999; Funderburk, Eyberg, Rich, & Behar, 2003) is designed to assess parental report of conduct behavioral problems in children and adolescents ages 2–16, by measuring the number of difficult behavior problems and the frequency with which they occur. This measure also includes norms for chronically ill children, based on 345 children and adolescents representing a broad spectrum of disease types. The ECBI has been used in numerous research studies and is described in detail elsewhere (*www.pcit.org*).

Behavioral Observations

An assessment of a child's behavior problems would not be complete without some type of direct behavioral observation on the part of the practitioner. Behavioral observations are especially useful for providing "ecologically valid" data with respect to treatment planning (Merrell, 2003) and treatment effectiveness (Reid, Webster-Stratton, & Baydar, 2004). A child's behavior in the office setting may not reflect his or her disruptive behavior at home or in the classroom, but much information can be gleaned by watching the child interact with parents, professionals, and even other children in the waiting room. McMahon and Forehand (2003) provide detailed information on how to conduct structured observations in the office setting.

An observation in the setting that is most troublesome to the child can be very helpful in determining the antecedents and consequences of problem behavior. Many practitioners cannot observe a child at home or at school, however, especially with constraints on time and financial reimbursement. Practitioners with well-prepared trainees may be able to send one to observe the child in the natural setting. This arrangement can actually be beneficial, as the child does not know the observer or realize that he or she is being specifically observed, and may thus behave more naturally. It is quite common with school observations for the person doing the observations to observe the target child and one "control child," in order to determine more accurately how the child is behaving in relation to peers. In some cases, a formal functional analysis of behavior may be needed to identify the antecedents, behaviors, and consequences present in the setting. Extensive information on conducting behavioral observations can be found in Merrell (2003).

Empirically Supported Interventions

Empirically supported interventions are available for addressing behavior problems in children. A review of interventions for childhood behavior problems by Christophersen and Mortweet (2001) found that parent training, both individually and in a group format, had the most support as an effective intervention for decreasing common behavior problems. Solid empirical evidence was also found for cognitive-behavioral therapy, mainly in the form of problem-solving skills training (PSST; see below). The current state of these interventions with respect to improving behavior problems is reviewed in this section. Family-based interventions are also showing promise for addressing behavior problems and are reviewed briefly as well.

The direct application of parent training and cognitive-behavioral programs for addressing the behavior problems of children with medical issues, however, is speculative at best. Some case studies have described the effects of behavioral interventions such as parent training on the behavior problems of pediatric patients (e.g., Bagner, Fennander, & Eyberg, 2004; Carton & Schweitzer, 1996; Kanoy & Schroeder, 1985). Although behavioral and cognitive-behavioral interventions have been effective in addressing important issues for pediatric patients, such as pain management (Robins, Smith, Glutting, & Bishop, 2005) and adherence (Cipes & Miraglia, 1985; Koch, Giardina, Ryan, MacQueen, & Hilgartner, 1993; Roter et al., 1998), the role of these interventions for improving behavioral outcomes in this population remains elusive. For this reason, we focus primarily on parent training and cognitive-behavioral therapy as two mainstays in the treatment of behavior problems in children.

Parent Training

One of the primary interventions for managing disruptive behaviors in children is training parents in improved behavior management techniques and is based on the pioneering work of Patterson (1974, 1982). Parent training interventions, in both individual and group formats, have been carefully documented and have significant empirical support in the literature as an intervention for behavior problems in children of all ages (Brestan & Eyberg, 1998; Fleischman, 1981; Hood & Eyberg, 2003; Long, Forehand, Wierson, & Morgan, 1994; Patterson, 1974; Reid et al., 2004; Webster-Stratton, 1996). Long-term outcome data on the maintenance of intervention effects have been documented for individual parent training programs based in large part on the original work of Patterson and his colleagues (Long et al., 1994), as well as for Eyberg's parent–child interaction therapy (Hood & Eyberg, 2003). We now discuss group parent training in more detail.

Group Parent Training

Webster-Stratton and her colleagues have conducted numerous well-designed studies of group parent training for families with disruptive children (Reid et al., 2004; Webster-Stratton, 1990, 1996; Webster-Stratton & Hammond, 1997). One example of Webster-Stratton's group parent training program is reported by Webster-Stratton and Hammond (1997). The authors compared group child therapy alone, group parent training alone, a combination of group child and parent therapy, and a waiting-list control group for children ages 4–8 years diagnosed with conduct problems. The results showed that child therapy alone and in combination with parent training significantly improved the children's problem solving and conflict resolution skills with peers. The combined therapy also resulted in maintained improvements in functioning at a 1-year follow-up. Long-term outcome data are also available for Webster-Stratton's Incredible Years program, based on over 800 families enrolled in this program offered at Head Start locations (Reid et al., 2004). The authors' analysis indicated that changes in parenting behavior related to the group parenting intervention could be linked to decreases in conduct problems and increases in prosocial behavior for the children.

More recently, group therapy strategies have been extended to include parent groups and teacher groups to determine the benefits of group training for disruptive behavior management (Webster-Stratton, Reid, & Hammond, 2004). The group training format was effective in reducing conduct problems in children across parents, teachers, and peers, as well as decreasing negative parenting for the mothers and fathers involved in the study. Finally, adding teacher training to parent training or child therapy improved treatment outcome in terms of teacher behavior management in the classroom. Webster-Stratton is a key researcher in the area of group parent training, now extended to group teacher training, for improving the behavior of disruptive children. More can be found about her research program and applied outcomes at the Incredible Years website (*www.incredibleyears.com*).

Cognitive-Behavioral Therapy

Cognitive-behavioral therapy, often in the form of PSST, has been used as an effective strategy for managing disruptive behaviors in children. An example of a PSST program is offered by Kazdin, Bass, Siegel, and Thomas (1989). In this program, children ages 7–13 were taught how to use cognitive and behavioral techniques in a step-by-step approach to effectively manage interactions with peers, parents, teachers, and others. The skills were taught by using practice, modeling, role playing, and social and token reinforcement during the sessions. The authors showed that children in the PSST group showed significantly greater reductions in antisocial behavior and overall behavior problems and greater increases in prosocial behavior, compared to children in a client-centered relationship therapy group. These effects were evident on measures of child performance at home and school, obtained both immediately after treatment and at a 1-year-follow-up.

PSST is often compared to parent training to determine treatment effectiveness, or is used in combination with parent training strategies. For example, Kazdin, Siegel, and Bass (1992) conducted a large prospective study with random assignment to treatment groups to compare the effectiveness of PSST alone, PSST combined with a parent training program, and the parent training program alone. The results of the study showed that the children in all three groups improved with treatment in regard to overall functioning, prosocial skills, and reduced negative behaviors (e.g., aggression). The combined PSST and parent training resulted in the best outcomes. Another large prospective study by Kazdin and Wassell (2000) also provides support for PSST as an effective treatment option for children with conduct problems. Kazdin and his colleagues have conducted rigorous scientific evaluation of their model and offer the practitioner a promising intervention for managing difficult behaviors in all children.

Family Interventions

There is also a growing empirical literature on family-based interventions addressing severe conduct problems and other issues relevant to pediatric conditions. Two examples are brief strategic family therapy (see Santisteban, Suarez-Morales, Robbins, & Szapocznik, 2006, for a review) and multisystemic therapy (MST; Henggeler, Schoenwald, Borduin, Rowland, & Cunningham, 1998; Timmons-Mitchell, Bender, Kishna, & Mitchell, 2006). Initial research has begun on adapting MST for adolescents with poorly controlled Type 1 diabetes as well (Ellis, Naar-King, Frey, Rowland, & Greger, 2003; Ellis et al., 2005; Henggeler, 2003). The December 2005 issue of the *Journal of Pediatric Psychology* is dedicated to a discussion of research findings and future challenges for family-based interventions in pediatric psychology (e.g., Fiese, 2005). All children, including those with pediatric conditions, may benefit greatly from the growing research programs investigating family interventions.

Conclusions

Children with behavior problems are a mainstay in the practice of child psychology. If left untreated, disruptive behaviors in childhood can have long-lasting effects on a child's social, emotional, academic, and physical well-being. Children with medical conditions may suffer even more serious consequences of problem behaviors, especially nonadherence, if such behaviors interfere with their medical care and health outcomes. Thus addressing behavioral problems, preferably early in a child's life, is necessary to maintain that child's intended developmental trajectory—and, if the child is a pediatric patient, physical well-being. For the pediatric psychologist, treating general behavioral compliance issues first is often necessary to improve intervention efforts for more specific developmental or medically related problems.

In order to assist parents in managing a disruptive child, with or without a pediatric condition, a targeted (and preferably evidence-based) assessment of child and family functioning is necessary. Information should be collected from multiple informants, including parents, teachers, medical care providers (if appropriate), and the child. Interviews, rating scales, and behavioral observations provide methods for collecting data on global mental health functioning, as well as on issues specific to the child and his or her pediatric condition. Careful attention should also be paid to child and family functioning—in particular, the role of parenting stress both before and after the diagnosis of a medical condition—in order to design an effective and workable treatment plan.

Finally, effective treatments for managing disruptive behaviors in children are available to the practitioner. Parent training is at the foundation of most treatments successful in addressing noncompliant and disruptive behavior. Parent training interventions are becoming increasingly elaborate, including other caregivers such as teachers in an effort to comprehensively address the complexity surrounding the development and maintenance of behavior problems in children. Older children, who are typically more responsible for managing their behavior than younger children, may benefit from cognitive-behavioral treatment that teaches them problem-solving strategies. In addition, family-based interventions that address a wide variety of factors affecting family dynamics and behavioral issues, including medical adherence, show promise as an intervention alternative for the practitioner. The next step is to further our understanding of these effective interventions with respect to the outpatient and inpatient treatment of behavioral problems in pediatric patients.

References

Achenbach, T. M., & Rescorla, L. A. (2001). *Manual for ASEBA school-age forms and profiles.* Burlington: University of Vermont, Research Center for Children, Youth, and Families.

Achenbach, T. M., & McConaughy, S. H. (1996). Relations between DSM-IV and empirically based assessment. *School Psychology Review, 25,* 329–341.

American Psychiatric Association. (2000). *Diagnostic and statistical manual of mental disorders* (4th ed., text rev.). Washington, DC: Author.

Austin, J. K, Harezlak, J., Dunn, D. W., Huster, G. A., Rose, D. F., & Ambrosius, W. T. (2001). Behavior problems in children before first recognized seizures. *Pediatrics, 107,* 115–122.

Bachanas, P. J., Kullgren, K. A., Schwartz, K. S., Lanier, B., McDaniel, J. S., Simth, J., et al. (2001). Predictors of psychological adjustment in school-aged children infected with HIV. *Journal of Pediatric Psychology, 26,* 343–352.

Bagner, D. M., Fernandez, M. A., & Eyberg, S. M. (2004). Parent–child interaction therapy and chronic illness: A case study. *Journal of Clinical Psychology in Medical Settings, 11,* 1–6.

Barkley, R. A. (2006). *Attention-deficit hyperactivity disorder: A handbook for diagnosis and treatment* (3rd ed.). New York: Guilford Press.

Barkley, R. A., Anastopoulos, A. D., Guevremont, D. C., & Fletcher, K. E. (1992). Adolescents with attention deficit hyperactivity disorder: Mother–adolescent interactions, family beliefs and conflicts, and maternal psychopathology. *Journal of Abnormal Child Psychology, 20,* 263–288.

Barkley, R. A., & Edwards, G. (2006). Diagnostic interview, behavior rating scales and the medical examination. In R. A. Barkley, *Attention-deficit hyperactivity disorder: A handbook for diagnosis and treatment* (3rd ed., pp. 337–368). New York: Guilford Press.

Blount, R. L., Simons, L. E., Devine, K. A., Jaaniste, T., Cohen, L. L., Chambers, C. T., et al. (2008). Evidence-based assessment of coping and stress in pediatric psychology. *Journal of Pediatric Psychology, 33,* 1021–1045.

Bourdeau, T. L., & Mullins, L. L. (2007). An examination of parenting variables and child self-care behavior across disease groups. *Journal of Developmental and Physical Disabilities, 19,* 125–134.

Brestan, E. V., & Eyberg, S. M. (1998). Effective psychosocial treatments of conduct-disordered children and adolescents: 29 years, 82 studies, and 5,272 kids. *Journal of Clinical Child Psychology, 27,* 180–189.

Campbell, J. M., Brown, R. T., Cavanagh, S. E., Vess, S. F., & Segall, M. J. (2008). Evidence-based assessment of cognitive functioning in pediatric psychology. *Journal of Pediatric Psychology, 33,* 999–1014.

Carter, B. D., Kronenberger, W. G., Baker, J., Grimes, L. M., Crabtree, V. M., Smith, C., et al. (2003). Inpatient pediatric consultation–liaison: A case-controlled study. *Journal of Pediatric Psychology, 28,* 423–432.

Carton, J., & Schweitzer, J. B. (1996). Use of a token economy to increase compliance during hemodialysis. *Journal of Applied Behavior Analysis, 29,* 111–113.

Christophersen, E. R., & Mortweet, S. L. (2001). *Treatments that work with children: Empirically supported strategies for managing childhood problems.* Washington, DC: American Psychological Association.

Cipes, M. H., & Miraglia, M. (1985). Monitoring versus contingency contracting to increase compliance with home fluoride mouthrinsing. *Pediatric Dentistry, 7,* 198–204.

Cohen, L. L., Lemanek, K., Blount, R. L., Dahlquist, L. M., Lim, C. S., Palermo, T. M., et al. (2008). Evidence-based assessment of pediatric pain. *Journal of Pediatric Psychology, 33,* 939–955.

Compton, S. N., March, J. S., Brent, D., Albano, A. M., Weersing, R., & Curry, J. (2004). Cognitive-behavioral psychotherapy for anxiety and depressive disorders in children and adolescents: An evidence-based medicine review. *Journal of the American Academy of Child and Adolescent Psychiatry, 43,* 930–959.

Conners, C. K. (2008a). *Conners 3rd Edition.* North Tonawanda, NY: Multi-Health Systems.

Conners, C. K. (2008b). *Conners Comprehensive Behavior Rating Scales.* North Tonawanda, NY: Multi-Health Systems.

DiScala, C., Lescohier, I., Barthel, M., & Li, G. (1998). Injuries to children with attention deficit hyperactivity disorder. *Pediatrics, 102,* 1415–1421.

Dolgin, M. J., Phipps, S., Fairclough, D. L., Sahler, O. J. Z., Askins, M., Noll, R. B., et al. (2007). Trajectories of adjustment in mothers of children with newly diagnosed cancer: A natural history investigation. *Journal of Pediatric Psychology, 32,* 771–782.

Ellis, D. A., Naar-King, S., Frey, M., Templin, T., Rowland, M., & Cakan, N. (2005). Multisystemic treatment of poorly controlled type 1 diabetes: Effects on medical resource utilization. *Journal of Pediatric Psychology, 30,* 656–666.

Ellis, D. A., Naar-King, S., Frey, M. A., Rowland, M., & Greger, N. (2003). Case study: Feasibility of multisystemic therapy as a treatment for urban adolescents with poorly controlled Type 1 diabetes. *Journal of Pediatric Psychology, 28,* 287–294.

Eyberg, S. M., & Pincus, D. (1999). *Eyberg Child Behavior Inventory and Sutter–Eyberg Student Behavior Inventory: Professional manual.* Odessa, FL: Psychological Assessment Resources.

Feinfield, K., & Baker, B. L. (2004). Empirical support for a treatment program for families of young children with externalizing problems. *Journal of Consulting and Clinical Psychology, 33,* 182–195.

Fiese, B. H. (2005). Introduction to the special issue: Time for family-based intervention in pediatric psychology? *Journal of Pediatric Psychology, 30,* 629–630.

Fleischman, M. J. (1981). A replication of Patterson's "Intervention for boys with conduct problems." *Journal of Consulting and Clinical Psychology, 49,* 342–251.

Friedman, D., Bryant, F. B., & Holmbeck, G. N. (2007). Brief report: Testing the factorial invariance of the CBCL Somatic Complaints scale as a measure of internalizing symptoms for children with and without chronic illness. *Journal of Pediatric Psychology, 32,* 512–516.

Funderburk, B. W., Eyberg, S. M., Rich, B. A., & Behar, L. (2003). Further psychometric evaluation of the Eyberg and Behar rating scales for parents and teachers of preschoolers. *Early Education and Development, 14,* 67–81.

Helgeson, V. S., Snyder, P. R., Escobar, O., Siminerio, L., & Becker, D. (2007). Comparison of adolescents with and without diabetes on indices of psychosocial functioning for three years. *Journal of Pediatric Psychology, 32,* 794–806.

Henggeler, S. W. (2003). Commentary on Ellis et al.: Adapting multisystemic therapy for challenging clinical problems of children and adolescents. *Journal of Pediatric Psychology, 28,* 295–297.

Henggeler, S. W., Schoenwald, S. K., Borduin, C. M., Rowland, M. D., & Cunningham, P. B. (1998). *Multisystemic treatment of antisocial behavior in children and adolescents.* New York: Guilford Press.

Hood, K. K., & Eyberg, S. M. (2003). Outcomes of parent–child interaction therapy: Mothers' reports of maintenance three to six years after treatment. *Journal of Clinical Child and Adolescent Psychology, 32,* 419–429.

Huntley, E. D., Campo, J. V., Dahl, R. E., & Lewin, D. S. (2007). Sleep characteristics of youth with functional abdominal pain and a healthy comparison group. *Journal of Pediatric Psychology, 32,* 938–949.

Irwin, C. E., Cataldo, M. F., Matheny, A. P., & Peterson, L. (1992). Health consequences of behaviors: Injury as a model. *Pediatrics, 90,* 798–807.

Kanoy, K. W., & Schroeder, C. S. (1985). Suggestions to parents about common behavior problems in a pediatric primary care office: Five years follow-up. *Journal of Pediatric Psychology, 10,* 15–30.

Karsdorp, P. A., Everaerd, W., Kindt, M., & Mulder, B. J. (2007). Psychological and cognitive functioning in children and adolescents with congenital heart disease: A meta-analysis. *Journal of Pediatric Psychology, 32,* 527–541.

Kazdin, A. E. (1996). Problem solving and parent management in treating aggressive and antisocial behavior. In E. D. Hibbs & P. S. Jensen (Eds.), *Psychosocial treatments for child and adolescent disorders: Empirically based strategies for clinical practice* (pp. 377–408). Washington, DC: American Psychological Association.

Kazdin, A. E., Bass, D., Siegel, T., & Thomas, C. (1989). Cognitive-behavioral therapy and relationship therapy in the treatment of children referred for antisocial behavior. *Journal of Consulting and Clinical Psychology, 57,* 522–535.

Kazdin, A. E., Mazurick, J. L., & Siegel, T. C. (1994). Treatment outcomes among children with externalizing disorder who terminate prematurely versus those who complete psychotherapy. *Journal of the American Academy of Child and Adolescent Psychiatry, 33,* 549–557.

Kazdin, A. E., Siegel, T. C., & Bass, D. (1992). Cognitive problem-solving skills training and parent management training in the treatment of antisocial behavior in children. *Journal of Consulting and Clinical Psychology, 60,* 733–747.

Kazdin, A. E., & Wassell, G. (2000). Therapeutic changes in children, parents, and families resulting from treatment of children with conduct problems. *Journal of the American Academy of Child and Adolescent Psychiatry, 39,* 414–420.

Kendall, P. C., & Hedtke, K. A. (2006). *Cognitive-behavioral therapy for anxious children: Therapist manual* (3rd ed.). Philadelphia: Workbook.

Koch, D. A., Giardina, P. J., Ryan, M., MacQueen, M., & Hilgartner, M. W. (1993). Behavioral contracting to improve adherence in patients with thalassemia. *Journal of Pediatric Nursing, 8,* 106–111.

LeBovidge, J. S., Kelley, S. D., Lauretti, A., Bailey, E. P, Timmons, K. G., Timmon, A. K., et al. (2007). Integrating medical and psychological health care for children with atopic dermatitis. *Journal of Pediatric Psychology, 32,* 617–625.

Long, P., Forehand, R., Wierson, M., & Morgan, A. (1994). Does parent training with young noncompliant children have long term effects? *Behaviour Research and Therapy, 32,* 101–107.

Mangus, R. S., Bergman, D., Zieger, M., & Coleman, J. J. (2004). Burn injuries in children with attention deficit/hyperactivity disorder. *Burns, 30,* 148–150.

Mash, E. J., & Terdal, L. G. (1988). Behavioral assessment of child and family disturbance. In E. J. Mash & L. G. Terdal (Eds.), *Behavioral assessment of childhood disorders: Selected core problems* (2nd ed., pp. 3–65). New York: Guilford Press.

Mathews, J. R., Spieth, L. E., & Christophersen, E. R. (1995). Behavioral compliance in a pediatric context. In M. C. Roberts (Ed.), *Handbook of pediatric psychology* (2nd ed., pp. 617–632). New York: Guilford Press.

McConaughy, S. H., & Achenbach, T. M. (1990). *Guide for the semistructured clinical interview for children aged 6–11.* Burlington, VT: University Associates in Psychiatry.

McMahon, R. J., & Forehand, R. L. (2003). *Helping the noncompliant child: Family-based treatment for oppositional behavior* (2nd ed.). New York: Guilford Press.

McMahon, R. J., & Frick, P. J. (2005). Evidence-based assessment of conduct problems in children and adolescents. *Journal of Clinical Child and Adolescent Psychology, 34,* 477–505.

Merrell, K. W. (2003). *Behavioral, social and emotional assessment of children and adolescents* (2nd ed.). Mahwah, NJ: Erlbaum.

Modi, A. C., & Quittner, A. L. (2006). Barriers to treatment adherence for children with cystic fibrosis and asthma: What gets in the way? *Journal of Pediatric Psychology, 31,* 846–858.

Morrison, J., & Anders, T. F. (1999). *Interviewing children and adolescents: Skills and strategies for effective DSM-IV diagnosis.* New York: Guilford Press.

Morrongiello, B. A., & Lasenby-Lessard, J. (2007). Psychological determinants of risk taking by children: An integrative model and implications for interventions. *Injury Prevention, 13,* 20–25.

Noll, R. B., MacLean, W. E., Whitt, J. K., Kaleita, T. A., Stehbens, J. A., Waskerwitz, M. J., et al. (1997). Behavioral adjustment and social functioning of long-term survivors of childhood leukemia: Parent and teacher reports. *Journal of Pediatric Psychology, 22,* 827–841.

Orvaschel, H. (2006). Structured and semistructured interviews. In M. Hersen (Ed.), *Clinician's handbook of child behavioral assessment* (pp. 159–179). Burlington, MA: Elsevier.

Patterson, G. R. (1974). Interventions for boys with conduct problems: Multiple settings, treatments, and criteria. *Journal of Consulting and Clinical Psychology, 42,* 471–481.

Patterson, G. R. (1982). *Coercive family process.* Eugene, OR: Castalia.

Perrin, E. C., Stein, R. K. E., & Drotar, D. (1991). Cautions in using the Child Behavior Checklist: Observations based on research about children with chronic illness. *Journal of Pediatric Psychology, 16,* 411–421.

Podolski, C. L., & Nigg, J. T. (2001). Parent stress and coping in relation to child ADHD severity and associated child disruptive behavior problems. *Journal of Clinical Child Psychology, 30,* 503–513.

Puig-Antich, J., & Chambers, W. (1978). *Schedule for Affective Disorders and Schizophrenia for School-Age Children (KIDDIE-SADS).* New York: New York State Psychiatric Institute, Biometrics Research.

Reid, M. J., Webster-Stratton, C., & Baydar, N. (2004). Halting the development of conduct problems in Head Start children: The effects of parent training. *Journal of Clinical Child and Adolescent Psychology, 33,* 279–291.

Reynolds, C. R., & Kamphaus, R. W. (2004). *BASC-2: Behavior Assessment System for Children, Second Edition.* Circle Pines, MN: American Guidance Service.

Robins, P. M., Smith, S. M., Glutting, J. J., & Bishop, C. T. (2005). A randomized controlled trial of cognitive-behavioral family intervention for pediatric recurrent abdominal pain. *Journal of Pediatric Psychology, 30,* 397–408.

Roter, D. L., Hall, J. A., Merisca, R., Nordstrom, B., Cretin, D., & Svarstad, B. (1998). Effectiveness of interventions to improve patient compliance: A meta-analysis. *Medical Care, 36,* 1138–1161.

Santisteban, D. A., Suarez-Morales, L., Robbins, M. S., & Szapocznik, J. (2006). Brief strategic family therapy: Lessons learned in efficacy research and challenges to blending research and practice. *Family Process, 45,* 259–271.

Schwebel, D. C., Speltz, M. L., Jones, K., & Bardina, P. (2002). Unintentional injury in preschool boys with and without early onset of disruptive behavior. *Journal of Pediatric Psychology, 27,* 727–737.

Shaffer, D., Fisher, P., Lucas, C. P., Dulcan, M. K., & Schwab-Stone, M. E. (2000). NIMH Diagnostic Interview Schedule for Children Version IV (NIMH DISC-IV): Description, differences from previous versions, and reliability of some common diagnoses. *Journal of the American Academy of Child and Adolescent Psychiatry, 39,* 28–38.

Sobel, A. B., Roberts, M. C., Rayfield, A. D., Barnard, M. U., & Rapoff, M. A. (2001). Evaluating outpatient pediatric psychology services in a primary care setting. *Journal of Pediatric Psychology, 26,* 395–405.

Timmons-Mitchell, J., Bender, M. B., Kishna, M. A., & Mitchell, C. C. (2006). An independent effectiveness trial of multisystemic therapy with juvenile justice youth. *Journal of Clinical Child and Adolescent Psychology, 35,* 227–236.

Velting, O. N., Setzer, N. J., & Albano, A. M. (2004). Update on and advances in assessment and cognitive-behavioral treatment of anxiety disorders in children and adolescents. *Professional Psychology: Research and Practice, 35,* 42–54.

Webster-Stratton, C., Reid, M. J., & Hammond, M. (2004). Treating children with early-onset conduct problems: Intervention outcomes for parent, child, and teacher training. *Journal of Clinical Child and Adolescent Psychology, 33,* 105–124.

Webster-Stratton, C. H. (1990). Long-term follow-up of families with young conduct problem children: From preschool to grade school. *Journal of Clinical Child Psychology, 19,* 144–149.

Webster-Stratton, C. H. (1996). Early intervention with videotaped modeling: Programs for families of children with oppositional defiant disorder or conduct disorder. In E. D. Hibbs & P. S. Jensen (Eds.), *Psychosocial treatments for child and adolescent disorders: Empirically based strategies for clinical practice* (pp. 435–474). Washington, DC: American Psychological Association.

Webster-Stratton, C. H., & Hammond, M. (1997). Treating children with early-onset conduct problems: A comparison of child and parent training interventions. *Journal of Consulting and Clinical Psychology, 65,* 93–109.

Wiener, L. S., Vasquez, M. P., & Battles, H. B. (2001). Fathering a child living with HIV/AIDS: Psychosocial adjustment and parenting stress. *Journal of Pediatric Psychology, 26,* 353–358.

CHAPTER 36

Attention-Deficit/Hyperactivity Disorder in the Pediatric Context

BRIAN P. DALY
JEREMY S. COHEN
JOHANNA L. CARPENTER
RONALD T. BROWN

Attention-deficit/hyperactivity disorder (ADHD) is a chronic condition characterized by developmentally inappropriate levels of inattention, impulsivity, overactivity, or a combination of these symptoms; it results in functional impairments across a number of domains, including family relationships, school functioning, and peer problems (American Psychiatric Association, 2000). The most common ADHD diagnosis, ADHD combined type, is diagnosed when symptoms from all three groups (inattention, impulsivity, and hyperactivity) are present. The other two primary subtypes of the disorder are the predominantly inattentive type and the primarily hyperactive–impulsive type (American Psychiatric Association, 2000). Finally, ADHD not otherwise specified is diagnosed when symptoms of inattention and hyperactivity are present, but do not meet criteria for a formal diagnosis of ADHD (American Psychiatric Association, 2000).

Prevalence

It has recently been estimated that 2–8% of the school-age population (depending on whether community or clinical samples are used) in the United States can be diagnosed with ADHD, with boy-to-girl ratios ranging from 2:1 to 6:1 (Biederman, Lopez, Boellner, & Chandler, 2002; Froehlich et al., 2007). In any given year, the disorder affects 1.4 to 3 million school-age children (Barkley, 1997). In a review of studies, Egger, Kondo, and Angold (2006) report that the prevalence of ADHD among community samples of preschool-age children ranges from 2 to 7.9%. Barkley (1997) noted a recent increase in the documented prevalence of ADHD among females, which can probably be attributed to the more careful identification of specific subtypes of the disorder (particularly the predominantly inattentive type). Notably, some experts have suggested that ADHD is more prevalent than epidemiological data would suggest, with many children and adolescents not receiving access to care for appropriate identification and management of the disorder.

Cultural Issues

Cross-cultural research generally indicates similar rates of prevalence and heritability of ADHD (Rohde et al., 2005). It also should be noted that cultural backgrounds may influence teachers' appraisals of the severity of these children's symptoms and functional impairments (Havey, Olson, McCormick, & Cates, 2005). Some data indicate that individuals from ethnic minority groups may have poorer access to psychological and medical services and may be less frequently referred for diagnostic and treatment services. Hence these individuals may receive less optimal treatment for the disorder than do their majority counterparts (Brown, Fuemmeler, & Forti, 2003).

Course

Studies of the natural history of ADHD suggest a rather protracted course that begins prior to the age of 7 years and in many cases persists well into adolescence and adulthood (Barkley, 1997). Compelling data suggest that early symptoms of the disorder, including those that may be present at preschool, predict a more severe presentation of ADHD during childhood and possibly during adolescence and adulthood (Campbell, 1990). ADHD is frequently comorbid with other psychological disorders—not only other externalizing disorders (e.g., conduct disorder, oppositional defiant disorder), but internalizing disorders as well (e.g., anxiety, depression).

Developmental Issues

Symptoms associated with ADHD present very differently during childhood than in adolescence and adulthood. In recent years, criticisms of the current conceptualization of the disorder have suggested that it is primarily symptom-driven and fails to take into account important developmental issues throughout the lifespan (for a review, see Barkley, 1997). In essence, many of the symptoms associated with the disorder shift throughout the lifespan, with approximately 60% of children with ADHD continuing to have ADHD as adults (Spencer et al., 1998). Although some of the symptoms of the disorder may dissipate at adulthood (e.g., hyperactivity), symptoms such as distractibility and impulsivity may still persist throughout the lifespan, resulting in challenges in the work setting (e.g., problems with meeting work deadlines, organizing materials, prioritizing tasks, time management) (Nadeau, 2005). The symptoms of ADHD also may have a negative impact on peer relationships in children and adults. For example, adults with ADHD may find themselves experiencing marital discord and having other difficulties with relationships (Barkley, 1997). Finally, while children with ADHD have been found to be at greater risk for injury due to symptoms associated with impulsivity (Barkley, 1997), adolescents and adults with ADHD are more likely to have automobile accidents and receive traffic tickets than those without the disorder (Barkley, Guevremont, Anastopoulos, DuPaul, & Shelton, 1993; Barkley, Murphy, & Kwasnik, 1996). Hence ADHD represents a major public health concern in the United States (Pelham, Foster, & Robb, 2007). The American Academy of Pediatrics (2001) has recommended that treatment begin as soon as the disorder is identified; that treatment address functioning across multiple domains; and that therapeutic interventions be implemented across settings (e.g., home, school) over potentially long periods of time, given the chronic nature of the condition.

Referral Patterns in Pediatric and Psychiatric Practice Settings

Primary care providers (including pediatricians and family practice physicians) assume an increasingly important role in the diagnosis and management of ADHD in children, as they are frequently the first professionals approached by families of children presenting with symptoms of ADHD (Wolraich, 1999). However, much of the research literature examining ADHD has relied extensively on samples of children from psychiatric settings. Some investigators suggest that children with ADHD who have been investigated in pediatric settings differ systematically from those children with ADHD in psychiatric settings (Bussing, Zima, & Belin, 1998; Zarin, Suarez, Pincus, Kupersanin, & Zito, 1998); however, recent data from a case–control study indicate that children from pediatric and psychiatric settings present with similar symptomatology and comorbidities (Busch et al., 2002). This is noteworthy, because the presence of comorbid disorders and evidence of poorer functioning across multiple domains (i.e., social and academic functioning) are associated with poorer outcomes (Biederman et al., 1996). As such, regardless of setting, clinicians should evaluate for the presence of comorbid disorders, as they have important treatment implications.

Assessment

The goals of a comprehensive ADHD assessment are twofold: (1) to ascertain the child's diagnostic status, and (2) to develop a treatment plan. Information on the child's primary ADHD symptoms according to the *Diagnostic and Statistical Manual of Mental Disorders*, fourth edition, text revision (DSM-IV-TR; American Psychiatric Association, 2000); the age of onset and duration of symptoms; the degree of functional impairment across settings; and any situational variability in symptom presentation should be considered. It is also important to evaluate various indices of executive functioning, such as organizational skills, planning skills, and active working memory, as these areas are frequently impaired in children with ADHD compared to their typically developing peers (Geurts, Verte, Oosterlaan, Roeyers, & Sergeant, 2005). Moreover, it is important to assess for co-occurring mental health conditions; to understand various contexts in which the child's problem behaviors are embedded (e.g., the family environment); and to understand how the child's behavior is maintained or even reinforced in the environment. Any medical and neuropsychological conditions also must be ruled out, as overactivity and inattention can be symptoms of numerous medical conditions (e.g., hyperthyroidism) and developmental disorders (e.g., learning disability). Finally, the diagnostician should gain an understanding of the psychological strengths and weaknesses of the child, caregivers, and family system, as well as the family's ability to access services within the community (Barkley & Edwards, 2006). As a result, the comprehensive assessment of ADHD requires a multimethod, multi-informant approach that blends information derived from interviews, behavioral rating scales, parent self-report measures, psychoeducational testing, and medical examination.

General Considerations

A diagnosis of ADHD should not be assigned without evidence that the child's problem behavior is present across contexts (e.g., home and school) and across informants (e.g., caregivers and teachers). If symptoms of ADHD are limited to only one setting, certain features of that environment may be eliciting and perhaps reinforcing the child's behavior. Informant-specific reports of ADHD symptoms also must be interpreted with caution. Such reports may simply reflect a poor fit between the child's characteristics and the styles or expectations of teachers or caregivers. Nevertheless, it is unrealistic to expect that teacher and parent reports of specific symptoms will be in complete agreement (Antrop, Roeyers, Oosterlaan, & Van Oost, 2002). Barkley and Edwards (2006) have recommended that clinicians inquire about past and/or present ADHD symptoms in several settings and that they combine symptoms across settings to derive a diagnosis, even if some symptoms are not reported by both informants.

The clinical significance of reported ADHD symptoms must always be considered in the context of the child's gender and developmental level. The DSM-IV-TR criteria are limited by their relative subjectivity, lack of consideration of gender, developmental heterogeneity, and evidence with regard to functional impairment (American Academy of Pediatrics, 2000). Therefore, it is useful to inquire of parents, and especially teachers, whether the child's problem behaviors are more severe or occur with greater frequency than would be expected among the majority of the child's same-gender peers of the same mental age. As such, the examiner should employ a developmental perspective and employ clinical judgment when determining symptom severity. Finally, to qualify for a diagnosis of ADHD, there must be evidence of functional impairment (e.g., academic achievement, family functioning, peer relationships) that is sufficiently severe to impair quality of life (Sawyer et al., 2002).

Guidelines for the assessment and treatment for ADHD have underscored that co-occurring conditions also be assessed (American Academy of Pediatrics, 2000). Finally, care should be taken to gather assessment data on the child's caregivers, siblings, and familial interactions. This information, although not immediately relevant to diagnostic questions, sheds light on how the child's problem behaviors may be maintained or exacerbated by the home environment. Moreover, understanding how factors external to the child's symptoms of ADHD interact with the child's behavior has important implications for intervention planning and management. For example, parental disciplinary style may emerge as a point of intervention, or parental beliefs and attributions about mental health services may dictate whether interventions are behavioral or pharmacological in nature. It is also possible that parent characteristics, including parental psychopathology, stress, and marital discord, may affect parents' ability to engage in the necessary treatment process with their children (Bussing, Zima, Gary, & Garvan,

2003) and therefore should be addressed in order to optimize the children's treatment outcomes.

Assessment Tools

Behavior Rating Scales

Behavior rating scales offer a convenient and cost-effective assessment strategy that easily allows the collection of data across informants and settings. Rating scales may be either ADHD-specific (i.e., items concern only symptoms of ADHD) or broadband instruments that inquire about a wide range of internalizing and externalizing behavioral symptoms (American Academy of Pediatrics, 2000). Informants, most commonly caregivers and teachers, are asked to indicate the extent or frequency with which the child exhibits certain externalizing or internalizing problem behaviors.

Broadband instruments initially should be administered to both parents and teachers, in order to screen for co-occurring conditions and gain a broader picture of the child's psychological functioning. The Child Behavior Checklist (Achenbach & Rescorla, 2001) and the Behavior Assessment System for Children, Second Edition (Reynolds & Kamphaus, 2004) are two well-normed broadband instruments with adequate psychometric properties. Although broadband instruments may be helpful in the identification of co-occurring conditions, only ADHD-specific measures have reliably differentiated children with ADHD from those without it (Brown et al., 2001). Indeed, the American Academy of Pediatrics (2000) recommends that only well-normed ADHD-specific instruments be used to aid in the diagnosis of ADHD. Such measures include the ACTeRS rating scales (Ullman, Sleator, & Sprague, 1986); the Conners 3 ADHD/DSM-IV Scale (CADS; Conners, 2008), a component of the larger Conners Rating System—Revised (Conners, 2001); the Disruptive Behavior Rating Scale (Barkley & Murphy, 2006); the IOWA Conners Rating Scale (Loney & Milich, 1982); the Swanson, Nolan, Abikoff, and Pelham Rating Scale (Swanson, 1992); and the Vanderbilt Attention Deficit Hyperactivity Diagnostic Parent and Teacher Rating Scales (Wolraich, Hannah, Baumgaertel, & Feurer, 1998; Wolraich, Lambert, & Worley, 2003). One frequently employed rating scale that measures executive function is the Behavior Rating Inventory of Executive Function (Gioia, Isquith, Guy, & Kenworthy, 2000).

Interviews

It is recommended that thorough clinical, semistructured, or structured interviews be conducted with the child, one or both parents, and even the child's teacher at school (American Academy of Pediatrics, 2000). The child interview can provide the opportunity for the clinician to observe the child's language ability, nonverbal behaviors, social skills, and affect. Although the information attained should be interpreted judiciously, as children with ADHD are not especially astute in recognizing their symptoms associated with ADHD (Fischer, Barkley, Fletcher, & Smallish, 1993), the clinician should inquire about difficulties with school performance, peer relationships, family functioning, and extracurricular activities.

Parental report on the child's difficulties represents an important and valuable source of assessment data, particularly with regard to symptom presence (Faraone, Biederman, & Milberger, 1995). The parent interview also can be invaluable in establishing rapport; gaining descriptive information on developmental, academic, and family histories; reviewing the child's achievement in major developmental domains; permitting the observation of caregiver attitudes and possible psychopathology; and collecting information on marital discord (Barkley & Edwards, 2006).

Structured diagnostic interviews include the Diagnostic Interview Schedule for Children, Version IV, for use with children and adolescents 6–18 years of age and their caregivers (Shaffer, Fisher, Lucas, Dulcan, & Schwab-Stone, 2000). In addition, the Schedule for Affective Disorders and Schizophrenia for School-Age Children (Kaufman et al., 1997) is a semistructured psychiatric interview used in formulating the diagnosis of ADHD. These interviews are often quite time-consuming, and for this reason are primarily used in the research context.

Caregiver Self-Report

Parental psychological well-being has important implications for treatment engagement, adherence to treatment, and outcome, making its evaluation an essential component of the overall diagnostic assessment (Chronis, 2005). Given that parents of children with ADHD may evidence high rates of stress (Anastopoulos, 1992) and psychopathology, including ADHD (Biederman et al., 1995), screening for ADHD as well as other psychopathology among caregivers is particularly important. This may be accomplished through a clinical interview; with normed self-report scales for adults, such as the Conners Adult ADHD Rating Scales (Conners, Erhardt, & Sparrow, 2000); or with behavior rating scales based on psychiatric criteria for ADHD (American Psychiatric Association, 2000; Barkley & Murphy, 2006). General psychopathology among adults is frequently screened with the Symptom Checklist 90—Revised (Derogatis, 1995), whereas situational stress and life events are often measured with the Parenting Stress Index (Abidin, 1995).

Psychoeducational Testing

Psychoeducational testing can supplement the ADHD evaluation by assessing for alternative explanations of ADHD symptoms, including ruling an ADHD diagnosis in or out (particularly amidst informant disagreement) and identifying co-occurring conditions that should receive treatment (e.g., specific learning disabilities) (Gordon, Barkley, & Lovett, 2006). Intelligence and achievement testing is commonly undertaken to assist in differential diagnosis if testing has not been recently conducted. However, no individually administered test or configuration of tests has actually demonstrated sufficient diagnostic specificity to ADHD to be solely conclusive in the diagnostic process. Assessment goals should be clear prior to beginning testing, and the results should always be interpreted in the context of a comprehensive battery of measures (e.g., attention, processing, executive function). For a thorough review of the role of psychological testing in ADHD assessment, see Gordon and colleagues (2006).

Medical Interview

A pediatrician-conducted medical interview is a critical component of assessment for ADHD. In addition to a review of the child's developmental history (including genetic, prenatal, and birth histories, gross sensory–motor development, and current health), a central goal of the medical interview is to rule out medical symptoms and etiologies of ADHD (e.g., lead poisoning), as well as medical conditions (e.g., hyperthyroidism) that present similarly to ADHD (American Academy of Pediatrics, 2000). These include hypoxic–anoxic events, significant head trauma, cerebrovascular disease, infection of the central nervous system, seizure disorders, and some medications used to treat seizure disorders (Barkley & Edwards, 2006). The medical interview also should focus on determining whether comorbid medical conditions are present for which pharmacological interventions for ADHD are contraindicated (e.g., severe hypertension), as well as the evaluation of co-occurring conditions that occur with ADHD and require medical intervention (e.g., encopresis) (Barkley & Edwards, 2006).

Medical Examination

Medical examination should be conducted as part of an ADHD assessment, even though such examinations are frequently unremarkable (Barkley & Edwards, 2006). Physicians should carry out a thorough neurodevelopmental screening (motor development, cognitive functioning, visual-perceptual ability, auditory discrimination, and language), as well as routine growth examination and screening for hyper- or hypothyroidism.

Management

Evidence-based management strategies for children and adolescents with ADHD include pharmacological management, behavioral treatment, and combined or multimodal treatment approaches (Chronis, Jones, & Raggi, 2006). Although each of these strategies demonstrates efficacy, the overwhelming majority of children with ADHD (over 80%) continue to evidence symptoms of the disorder well throughout adolescence and even into adulthood (Barkley, 1997). Therefore, it is imperative that pediatric psychologists obtain a working knowledge of the strengths and limitations associated with each evidence-based approach to the management of ADHD.

Pharmacotherapy

Stimulant medication that targets the central nervous system represents the class of psychotropics most widely used and studied for the management of ADHD and its associated symptoms in school-age children and adolescents (Zito et al., 2003). The most frequently prescribed stimulants to pediatric populations are methylphenidate (MPH), dextroamphetamine (DEX), and amphetamines (AMP). Of these preparations, the various short- and long-acting versions of MPH are the most commonly prescribed stimulants (for a review, see Brown & LaRosa, 2002).

All of the stimulant formulations have generally similar adverse side effects and may be grouped according to their approximate duration of action: immediate-release or short-acting (effects lasting 3–4 hours); intermediate-acting (effects lasting 6–8 hours); and long-acting (effects lasting 8–12 hours) (Wolraich, 2003). The intermediate- and long-acting formulations were developed to control the rate of dose delivery in order to optimize the therapeutic effect for longer durations of time than immediate-release medication (Adesman, 2002), thereby eliminating the need for a second or third dose of medication during the day. Further benefits of once-daily dosing include enhanced adherence rates and reduced stigma associated with twice-daily dosing at school (Brown & La Rosa, 2002). Evidence indicates similar response rates for long-acting and short-acting versions of the various stimulants (Pliszka, 2007). Furthermore, controlled clinical trials comparing MPH, AMP, and DEX have failed to demonstrate significant group differences in efficacy and safety (Brown et al., 2005). The reported average effect size for immediate-release stimulants is 0.91, while the average effect size for long-acting versions is 0.95 (Biederman & Faraone, 2005).

The most frequently reported adverse side effects associated with the use of stimulant medication include insomnia, loss of appetite, and headaches (Pliszka, 2007). Reports indicate that these adverse side effects are frequently relatively mild, short-lived, and linearly associated with dose (McMaster University Evidence-Based Practice Center, 1999). The evidence is weak as to whether the use of stimulant medication causes severe adverse side effects, such as growth suppression, psychosis, mania, or sudden death (Pliszka, 2007).

Results from randomized clinical trials have consistently demonstrated that stimulants are effective in the short-term management of the cognitive and behavioral symptoms associated with ADHD (inattention, impulsivity, and overactivity) (Brown & Daly, 2009). There exists additional evidence to suggest that stimulants improve cognitive performance, impulse control, and academic efficiency, and diminish aggression, in adolescents diagnosed with ADHD (for a review, see Brown & Daly, 2009). Nonetheless, there is a lack of clear evidence that stimulants change the rather guarded long-term prognosis of ADHD (MTA Cooperative Group, 1999a; Weiss & Hechtman, 1993). In addition, stimulants have failed to demonstrate improvement in many of the functional outcomes associated with ADHD, particularly problems with social behavior and academic performance (for a review, see Brown et al., 2008).

More recently, atomoxetine (Strattera), a nonstimulant compound that is a selective noradrenergic reuptake inhibitor, has been used for the management of ADHD. It is usually taken either once or twice daily, in dosages based on body weight, and is the only medication that has received approval from the Food and Drug Administration to treat adult ADHD (Spencer, 2004). It is noteworthy that there is evidence for larger effect sizes for the stimulants than for the nonstimulants (0.63) on the core symptoms of ADHD (Wigal et al., 2005). The adverse effect profile for atomoxetine is similar to that of the stimulants and includes appetite disturbances as well as sleep disturbances.

Behavioral Treatment

Behavioral approaches, including behavioral modification, target the improvement of key domains of symptom impairment associated with ADHD; these include noncompliance with parental commands, academic/school functioning, and peer relationships (Pelham, Fabiano, & Massetti, 2005). As such, the most widely employed and accepted behavioral management strategies include parent training, classroom interventions, and peer interventions. An examination of the strength of evidence for behavioral interventions indicates that behavioral parent training and behavioral school interventions are classified as well-established, empirically supported treatments (Pelham, Wheeler, & Chronis, 1998). In contrast, the evidence for the effectiveness of peer interventions or social skills groups is less consistent than that for parent training or classroom interventions (Daly, Creed, Xanthopoulos, & Brown, 2007).

The primary goal of behavioral parent training is to assist caregivers in modifying antecedents and consequences of their child's behavior (Pelham et al., 1998). Components of the intervention include the introduction of contingency management strategies, emphasizing behavior modification, cues and consequences for elicited behaviors, reward systems, and contingencies for undesirable behavior (i.e., punishment, response cost) (Chronis, Chacko, Fabiano, Wymbs, & Pelham, 2004). Because ADHD is recognized as a chronic condition, behavioral treatments must be implemented consistently over the long term (Chronis et al., 2001). Results from interventions that have employed parent training with school-age populations indicate improvement across several domains: decreased parental ratings of problem behavior in the home and school setting, decreased parental reports of stress, parental reports of increased knowledge and competence, and fewer observed negative parent and child behaviors (Chronis et al., 2004; Weinberg, 1999; Wells et al., 2000). Behavioral parent training demonstrates greater effects in specific domains, such as compliance with parental requests, rule following, defiant/aggressive behavior, and parenting skills (Anastopoulos, Shelton, DuPaul, & Guevremont, 1993; Pisterman et al., 1992), than on specific symptoms of ADHD as delineated in the DSM-IV-TR (American Psychiatric Association, 2000; MTA Cooperative Group, 1999a, 2004).

Findings from classroom interventions employed with children with ADHD are consistent with the established criteria for an empirically supported treatment (Pelham et al., 1998). Behavioral classroom interventions target symptoms of ADHD and associated functional impairments, including complying with classroom rules, engaging in appropriate interactions with classmates, displaying disruptive behavior, and complying with teacher commands. Evidence indicates that direct contingency management strategies employed in the classroom setting are more effective than traditional outpatient treatment strategies or behavioral programs for ADHD-related behaviors (Pelham et al., 1998). Components of the classroom intervention frequently include verbal praise, effective commands, a point or token economy system, daily report cards, or time out (Chronis et al., 2006). Findings from a meta-analysis (DuPaul & Eckert, 1997) reveal that behavioral classroom interventions yield a very large effect size (1.44) on measures of treatment outcome, with a larger effect size on child behavior than on academic or clinic performance.

Psychosocial interventions that promote positive social functioning and the development of appropriate peer relationships are especially important for children with ADHD, given their documented social difficulties and rejection by peers (Hoza et al., 2005). Social skills training, typically conducted in a group format, represents the most common approach to managing social and peer problems in children with ADHD. This approach focuses on the promotion of prosocial behaviors that include cooperation, communication, participation, and validation (Kavale, Forness, & Walker, 1999). Psychosocial interventions that specifically target peer relationships focus on instruction in social skills, social problem solving, and behavioral competence. These interventions attempt to enhance social competence through encouraging close friendships while simultaneously decreasing undesirable and antisocial behaviors. Employing social skills training as a stand-alone treatment has demonstrated limited success in enhancing children's social status, as suggested by peer sociometric ratings (Landau, Milich, & Diener, 1998) or the children's overall social behavior (Antshel & Remer, 2003). However, when social skills interventions are combined with behavior management programs and parent training, there is some evidence to suggest improvements in children's behavior toward their peers (Chronis et al., 2004; Pelham et al., 2005). Although psychosocial interventions employed with children with ADHD demonstrate many positive effects, employing behavior therapy as a *single* treatment modality typically does not result in normalized behavioral function for children with ADHD compared to that of their typically developing peers (Whalen & Henker, 1991). Furthermore, treatment gains are not frequently maintained following the cessation of the intervention.

Multimodal Treatment

Combined or multimodal interventions are considered to be the gold standard for ADHD treatment. The National Institute of Mental Health's Multimodal Treatment Study of ADHD (MTA) presents comprehensive data regarding the efficacy of combined treatments for ADHD (MTA Cooperative Group, 1999a, 1999b). This investigation compared the effects of four interventions: (1) behavioral intervention alone; (2) state-of-the-art medication management; (3) a combination of medication and a behavioral intervention; and, finally, (4) a control condition of routine community care.

In regard to the specific impact of the four interventions on the core symptoms of ADHD, findings from the MTA indicate that the effect sizes are nearly equivalent (moderate to large) for combined treatment (medication management and behavior therapy) and for stimulant treatment alone (MTA Cooperative Group, 1999a). However, the evidence suggests that combined treatment approaches produce stronger effects than stimulant treatment alone for specific functional impairments associated with the disorder, such as behavioral problems, disruptive behaviors, and poor social skills (Hinshaw et al., 2000). Moreover, combined treatment offers additional benefits; these include enhanced teacher and parent acceptance, and potentially lower stimulant doses needed to achieve the same therapeutic benefits as with stimulant drug treatment alone (MTA Cooperative Group, 1999a). Finally, in the MTA, combined treatment was superior to medication alone for children with comorbid conditions (e.g., anxiety disorder) and in normalizing the behavior of children with ADHD (Conners et al., 2001; Jensen et al., 2001; Swanson et al., 2001). Overall, combined or multimodal treatments have been shown to be evidence-based as effective short-term treatments for ADHD (Pelham & Waschbusch, 1999).

Preschool ADHD Interventions

Effective treatments are needed for preschool children who exhibit symptoms of ADHD, because early behavior difficulties are associated with later behavioral problems that are fairly severe and with poor peer social standing in kindergarten (Keane & Calkins, 2004). The Preschool ADHD Treatment Study investigated the safety and efficacy of low-dose MPH (3.75 mg to a total of 22.5 mg daily) for treating preschoolers (ages 3–5.5 years) diagnosed with ADHD (Greenhill et al., 2006). Results indicate that low doses of MPH are effective, safe, and generally tolerable; however, effect sizes (0.4–0.8) were smaller than those ascertained for school-age children receiving the same stimulant medication. More importantly, the participants experienced more adverse side effects (i.e., emotionality and/or irritability) associated with MPH than the older children did (Greenhill et al., 2006; Wigal et al., 2006).

There is also evidence that behavioral interventions for preschoolers with ADHD can be effective. For example, findings from a psychosocial intervention for preschool students with ADHD, titled Project ACHIEVE, revealed a significant decrease in problem behavior (e.g., aggression) and a significant improvement in social skills (Kern et al., 2007). Taken together, these findings are important, as they suggest that the combination of low-dose stimulant drug therapy with behavioral management approaches is potentially efficacious for young preschool children with ADHD.

ADHD Treatment Guidelines

The American Academy of Pediatrics (2001) has developed evidence-based guidelines for the treatment of school-age children with ADHD by primary care pediatricians. These guidelines recognize that ADHD should be considered a chronic condition, and that treatment programs should be developed through collaboration with clinicians, the child, caregivers, and school personnel. The treatment program should be individualized and tailored to the child, with treatment goals focusing on target outcomes that include improving relationships at home and with peers, improving performance at school, and increasing independence and improving self-esteem, while decreasing disruptive behaviors. Stimulant medications in low doses and/or behavior therapy are considered appropriate and effective interventions. It is recommended that clinicians regularly follow up with children to evaluate progress on goals and examine any possible adverse side effects associated with either pharmacotherapy or psychotherapy. Children who do not demonstrate improvement in symptoms after appropriate intervention should be reevaluated to confirm the ADHD diagnosis and adherence to the treatment plan. Information should be obtained from multiple sources, including the caregivers, school personnel, and the child. The American Academy of Pediatrics has developed an ADHD resource toolkit for clinicians (*www.aap.org/pubserv/adhdtoolkit/index.htm*).

A Look Ahead

Much research needs to be conducted on ameliorating the functional impairments associated with ADHD. In addition, there is a dearth of data with regard to specific sequencing of treatments, such as which treatment should be administered first (e.g., pharmacotherapy or behavioral treatment) or whether both treatments should be administered together from the beginning. Moreover, current diagnostic nomenclature has not devoted sufficient attention to important developmental issues that are central to the disorder across the lifespan. Finally, research should continue to evaluate whether "sluggish cognitive tempo" is a valid subtype of ADHD (Hartman, Willcutt, Rhee, & Pennington, 2004). Clearly, addressing these types of research issues is necessary in order to enhance the quality of life for these children and adolescents and their families.

References

Abidin, R. R. (1995). *Parenting Stress Index* (3rd ed.). Odessa, FL: Psychological Assessment Resources.
Achenbach, T. M., & Rescorla, L. A. (2001). *Manual for the ASEBA school-age forms and pro-*

files. Burlington: University of Vermont, Research Center for Children, Youth, and Families.

Adesman, A. R. (2002). New medications for treatment of children with attention-deficit/hyperactivity disorder: Review and commentary. *Pediatric Annals, 31*, 514–523.

American Academy of Pediatrics. (2000). Clinical practice guideline: Diagnosis and evaluation of the child with attention-deficit/hyperactivity disorder. *Pediatrics, 105*, 1158–1170.

American Academy of Pediatrics. (2001). Clinical practice guideline: Treatment of the school-aged child with attention-deficit/hyperactivity disorder. *Pediatrics, 108*, 1033–1043.

American Psychiatric Association. (2000). *Diagnostic and statistical manual for mental disorders* (4th ed., text revision). Washington, DC: Author.

Anastopoulos, A. D. (1992). Parenting stress among families of children with attention deficit hyperactivity disorder. *Journal of Abnormal Child Psychology, 20*, 503–520.

Anastopoulos, A. D., Shelton, T. L., DuPaul, G. J., & Guevremont, D. D. (1993). Parent training for attention deficit hyperactivity disorder: Its impact on parent functioning. *Journal of Abnormal Child Psychology, 21*, 581–596.

Antrop, I., Roeyers, H., Oosterlaan, J., & Van Oost, P. (2002). Agreement between parent and teacher ratings of disruptive behavior disorders in children with clinically diagnosed ADHD. *Journal of Psychopathology and Behavior Assessment, 24*, 67–73.

Antshel, K. M., & Remer, R. (2003). Social skills training in children with attention deficit hyperactivity disorder: A randomized-controlled clinical trial. *Journal of Clinical Child and Adolescent Psychology, 32*, 153–165.

Barkley, R. A. (1997). *ADHD and the nature of self-control*. New York: Guilford Press.

Barkley, R. A., & Edwards, G. (2006). Diagnostic interview, behavior ratings scales, and the medical examination. In R. A. Barkley, *Attention-deficit hyperactivity disorder* (3rd ed., pp. 337–368). New York: Guilford Press.

Barkley, R. A., Guevremont, D. C., Anastopoulos, A. D., DuPaul, G. J., & Shelton, T. L. (1993). Driving-related risks and outcomes of attention deficit hyperactivity disorder in adolescents and young adults: A 3- to 5-year follow-up survey. *Pediatrics, 92*, 212–218.

Barkley, R. A., & Murphy, K. R. (2006). *Attention-deficit hyperactivity disorder: A clinical workbook* (3rd ed.). New York: Guilford Press.

Barkley, R. A., Murphy, K. R., & Kwasnik, D. (1996). Psychological functioning and adaptive impairments in young adults with ADHD. *Journal of Attention Disorders, 1*, 41–54.

Biederman, J., & Faraone, S. (2005). Attention-deficit hyperactivity disorder. *Lancet, 366*, 237–249.

Biederman, J., Faraone, S., Milberger, S., Curtis, S., Chen, L., Marrs, A., et al. (1996). Predictors of persistence and remission of ADHD into adolescence: Results from a four-year prospective follow-up study. *Journal of the American Academy of Child and Adolescent Psychiatry, 35*, 343–351.

Biederman, J., Faraone, S. V., Mick, E., Spencer, T., Wilens, T., Kiely, K., et al. (1995). High risk for attention deficit hyperactivity disorder among children of parents with childhood onset of the disorder: A pilot study. *American Journal of Psychiatry, 152*, 431–435.

Biederman, J., Lopez, F. A., Boellner, S. W., & Chandler, M. C. (2002). A randomized, double-blind, placebo-controlled, parallel-group study of SL1381 (Adderall XR) in children with attention-deficit/hyperactivity disorder. *Pediatrics, 110*, 258–266.

Brown, R. T., Amler, R. W., Freeman, W. S., Perrin, J. M., Stein, M. T., Feldman, H. M., et al. (2005). Treatment of attention-deficit/hyperactivity disorder: Overview of the evidence. *Pediatrics, 115*, 749–757.

Brown, R. T., Antonuccio, D. O., DuPaul, G. J., Fristad, M. A., King, C. A., Leslie, L., et al. (2008). *Childhood mental health disorders: Evidence base and contextual factors for psychosocial, psychopharmacological, and combined interventions*. Washington, DC: American Psychological Association.

Brown, R. T., & Daly, B. P. (2009). Neuropsychological effects of stimulant medication on children's learning and behavior. In C. R. Reynolds & E. Fletcher-Janzen (Eds.), *Handbook of clinical neuropsychology* (pp. 529–580). New York: Plenum Press.

Brown, R. T., Freeman, W. S., Perrin, J. M., Stein, M. T., Amler, R. W., Feldman, H. M., et al. (2001). Prevalence and assessment of attention-deficit/hyperactivity disorder in primary care settings. *Pediatrics, 107*, e43.

Brown, R. T., Fuemmeler, B. F., & Forti, E. M. (2003). Health disparity and access to care. In M. Roberts (Ed.), *Handbook of pediatric psychology* (3rd ed., pp. 683–695). New York: Guilford Press.

Brown, R. T., & La Rosa, A. (2002). Recent developments in the pharmacotherapy of attention-deficit/hyperactivity disorder. *Professional Psychology: Research and Practice, 33*, 591–595.

Busch, B., Biederman, J., Cohen, L., Sayer, J., Monuteaux, M., Mick, E., et al. (2002). Correlates of ADHD among children in pediatric and psychiatric clinics. *Psychiatric Services, 53*, 1103–1111.

Bussing, R., Zima, B. T., & Belin, T. R. (1998). Variations in ADHD treatment among special education students. *Journal of the American Academy of Child and Adolescent Psychiatry, 37*, 968–976.

Bussing, R., Zima, B. T., Gary, F. A., & Garvan, C. W. (2003). Barriers to detection, help-seeking, and service use for children with ADHD symptoms. *Journal of Behavioral Health Services and Research, 30*, 176–189.

Campbell, S. B. (1990). *Behavior problems in preschool children: Clinical and developmental issues.* New York: Guilford Press.

Chronis, A., Chacko, A., Fabiano, G., Wymbs, B., & Pelham, W. (2004). Enhancements to the behavioral parent training paradigm for families of children with ADHD: Review and future directions. *Clinical Child and Family Psychology Review, 7*, 1–27.

Chronis, A., Jones, H. A., & Raggi, V. L. (2006). Evidence-based psychosocial treatments for children and adolescents with attention-deficit/hyperactivity disorder. *Clinical Psychology Review, 26*, 486–502.

Chronis, A. M. (2005). Parents of children with ADHD. In A. Freeman (Ed.), *Encyclopedia of cognitive behavior therapy* (pp. 268–270). New York: Springer.

Chronis, A. M., Fabiano, G. A., Gnagy, E. M., Wymbs, B. T., Burrows-MacLean, L., & Pelham, W. E. (2001). Comprehensive, sustained behavioral and pharmacological treatment for attention-deficit/hyperactivity disorder: A case study. *Cognitive and Behavioral Practice, 8*, 346–358.

Conners, C. K. (2008). *Conners Rating Scales 3.* North Tonawanda, NY: Multi-Health Systems.

Conners, C. K., Epstein, J. N., March, J. S., Angold, A., Wells, K. C., Klaric, J., et al. (2001). Multimodal treatment of ADHD in the MTA: An alternative outcome analysis. *Journal of the American Academy of Child and Adolescent Psychiatry, 40*, 159–167.

Conners, C. K., Erhardt, D., & Sparrow, E. (2000). *Conners Adult ADHD Rating Scales (CAARS).* North Tonawanda, NY: Multi-Health Systems.

Daly, B. P., Creed, T. A., Xanthopoulos, M., & Brown, R. T. (2007). Psychosocial treatments for children with attention deficit/hyperactivity disorder. *Neuropsychology Review, 17*, 73–89.

Derogatis, L. R. (1995). *Manual for the Symptom Checklist 90—Revised (SCL-90-R).* Minneapolis, MN: National Computer Systems.

DuPaul, G. J., & Eckert, T. L. (1997). The effects of school-based interventions for attention deficit hyperactivity disorder: A meta-analysis. *School Psychology Review, 26*, 5–27.

Egger, H. L., Kondo, D., & Angold, A. (2006). The epidemiology and diagnostic issues in preschool attention-deficit/hyperactivity disorder: A review. *Infants and Young Children, 19*, 109–122.

Faraone, S. V., Biederman, J., & Milberger, S. (1995). How reliable are maternal reports of their children's psychopathology?: One-year recall of psychiatric diagnoses of ADHD children. *Journal of the American Academy of Child and Adolescent Psychiatry, 34*, 1001–1008.

Fischer, M., Barkley, R. A., Fletcher, K., & Smallish, L. (1993). The stability of dimensions of behavior in ADHD and normal children over an 8 year period. *Journal of Abnormal Child Psychology, 21*, 315–337.

Froehlich, T. E., Lanphear, B. P., Epstein, J. N., Barbaresi, W. J., Katusic, S. K., & Kahn, R. S. (2007). Prevalence and treatment of ADHD in a national sample of U.S. children. *Archives of Pediatrics and Adolescent Medicine, 161*, 857–864.

Geurts, H., Verte, S., Oosterlaan, J., Roeyers, H., & Sergeant, J. (2005). ADHD subtypes: Do they differ in their executive functioning profile? *Archives of Clinical Neuropsychology, 20*, 457–477.

Gioia, G. A., Isquith, P. K., Guy, S. C., & Kenworthy, L. (2000). *Behavior Rating Inventory of Executive Function*. Odessa, FL: Psychological Assessment Resources.

Gordon, M., Barkley, R. A., & Lovett, B. J. (2006). Tests and observational measures. In R. A. Barkley, *Attention-deficit hyperactivity disorder* (3rd ed., pp. 369–388). New York: Guilford Press.

Greenhill, L., Kollins, S., Abikoff, H., McCracken, J., Riddle, M., Swanson, J., et al. (2006). Efficacy and safety of immediate-release methylphenidate treatment for preschoolers with ADHD. *Journal of the American Academy of Child and Adolescent Psychiatry, 45*, 1284–1293.

Hartman, C., Willcutt, E., Rhee, S., & Pennington, B. (2004). The relation between sluggish cognitive tempo and DSM-IV ADHD. *Journal of Abnormal Child Psychology, 32*, 491–503.

Havey, M., Olson, J., McCormick, C., & Cates, G. L. (2005). Teacher perceptions of the incidence and management of attention deficit hyperactivity disorder. *Applied Neuropsychology, 12*, 120–127.

Hinshaw, S. P., Owens, E., Wells, K., Kraemer, H., Abikoff, H., Arnold, L., et al. (2000). Family processes and treatment outcome in the MTA: Negative/ineffective parenting practices in relation to multimodal treatment. *Journal of Abnormal Child Psychology, 28*, 555–568.

Hoza, B., Gerdes, A. C., Mrug, S., Hinshaw, S. P., Bukowski, W. M., Gold, J. A., et al. (2005). Peer-assessed outcomes in the multimodal treatment study of children with attention deficit hyperactivity disorder. *Journal of Clinical Child and Adolescent Psychology, 34*, 74–86.

Jensen, P. S., Hinshaw, S. P., Swanson, J. M., Greenhill, L. L., Conners, C. K., Arnold, L. E., et al. (2001). Findings from the NIMH Multimodal Treatment Study of ADHD (MTA): Implications and applications for primary care providers. *Journal of Developmental and Behavioral Pediatrics, 22*, 60–73.

Kaufman, J., Birmaher, B., Brent, D., Rao, U., Flynn, C., Moreci, P., et al. (1997). Schedule of Affective Disorders and Schizophrenia for School-Age Children—Present and Lifetime Version (KSADS-PL): Initial reliability and validity data. *Journal of the American Academy of Child and Adolescent Psychiatry, 36*, 980–988.

Kavale, K. A., Forness, S. R., & Walker, H. M. (1999). Interventions for ODD and CD in the schools. In H. Quay & A. Hogan (Eds.), *Handbook of disruptive behavior disorders* (pp. 441–454). New York: Plenum Press.

Keane, S. P., & Calkins, S. D. (2004). Predicting kindergarten peer social status from toddler and preschool problem behavior. *Journal of Abnormal Child Psychology, 32*, 409–423.

Kern, L., DePaul, G., Volpe, R., Sokol, N., Lutz, G., Arbolino, L., et al. (2007). Multisetting assessment-based intervention for young children at risk for attention deficit hyperactivity disorder: Initial effects on academic and behavioral functioning. *School Psychology Review, 36*, 237–255.

Landau, S., Milich, R., & Diener, M. B. (1998). Peer relations of children with attention-deficit hyperactivity disorder. *Reading and Writing Quarterly: Overcoming Learning Difficulties, 14,* 83–105.

Loney, J., & Milich, R. (1982). Hyperactivity, inattention, and aggression in clinical practice. In M. Wolraich & D. Routh (Eds.), *Advances in development and behavioral pediatrics* (Vol. 3, pp. 113–147). Greenwich, CT: JAI Press.

McMaster University Evidence-Based Practice Center. (1999). *Treatment of attention-deficit hyperactivity disorder* (Evidence Report/Technology Assessment no. 11, AHCPR Publication No. 99-E018). Rockville, MD: Agency for Healthcare Policy and Research.

MTA Cooperative Group. (1999a). A 14-month randomized clinical trial of treatment strategies for attention-deficit hyperactivity disorder (ADHD). *Archives of General Psychiatry, 56,* 1073–1086.

MTA Cooperative Group. (1999b). Moderators and mediators of treatment response for children with attention-deficit/hyperactivity disorder. *Archives of General Psychiatry, 56,* 1088–1096.

MTA Cooperative Group. (2004). National institute of mental health multimodal treatment study of ADHD: 24-Month outcomes of treatment strategies for ADHD. *Pediatrics, 113,* 754–760.

Nadeau, K. G. (2005). Career choices and workplace challenges for individuals with ADHD. *Journal of Clinical Psychology, 61,* 549–563.

Pelham, W. E., Burrows-MacLean, L., Gnagy, E. M., Fabiano, G. A., Coles, E. K., Tresco, K. E., et al. (2005). Transdermal methylphenidate, behavioral, and combined treatment for children with ADHD. *Experimental and Clinical Psychopharmacology, 13,* 111–126.

Pelham, W. E., Fabiano, G. A., & Massetti, G. M. (2005). Evidence-based assessment of attention deficit hyperactivity disorder in children and adolescents. *Journal of Clinical Child and Adolescent Psychology, 34,* 449–476.

Pelham, W. E., Foster, E. M., & Robb, J. A. (2007). The economic impact of attention deficit/hyperactivity disorder in children and adolescents. *Journal of Pediatric Psychology, 32,* 711–727.

Pelham, W. E., & Waschbusch, D. (1999). Behavior therapy with ADHD children. In H. Quay & A. Hogan (Eds.), *Handbook of disruptive behavior disorders* (pp. 255–278). New York: Plenum Press.

Pelham, W. E., Wheeler, T., & Chronis, A. (1998). Empirically supported psychosocial treatments for ADHD. *Journal of Clinical Child Psychology, 27,* 190–205.

Pisterman, S., Firestone, P., McGrath, P., Goodman, J. T., Webster, I., Mallory, R., et al. (1992). The role of parent training in treatment of preschoolers with ADHD. *American Journal of Orthopsychiatry, 62,* 397–408.

Pliszka, S. R. (2007). Pharmacologic treatment of attention-deficit/hyperactivity disorder (ADHD): Efficacy, safety and mechanisms of action. *Neuropsychology Review, 17,* 61–72.

Reynolds, C. R., & Kamphaus, R. W. (2004). *Behavior Assessment System for Children, Second Edition.* Circle Pines, MN: American Guidance Service.

Rohde, L. A., Szobot, C., Polanczyk, G., Schmitz, M., Martins, S., & Tramontina, S. (2005). Attention-deficit/hyperactivity disorder in a diverse culture: Do research and clinical findings support the notion of a cultural construct for the disorder? *Biological Psychiatry, 57,* 1436–1441.

Sawyer, M. G., Whaites, L., Rey, J. M., Hazell, P. L., Graetz, B., & Baghurst, P. (2002). Health-related quality of life of children and adolescents with mental disorders. *Journal of the American Academy of Child and Adolescent Psychiatry, 41,* 530–537.

Shaffer, D., Fisher, P., Lucas, C. P., Dulcan, M. K., & Schwab-Stone, M. E. (2000). NIMH Diagnostic Interview Schedule for Children Version IV (NIMH DSC-IV). *Journal of the American Academy of Child and Adolescent Psychiatry, 39,* 28–38.

Spencer, T. (2004). Adult attention-deficit/hyperactivity disorder. *Psychiatric Clinics of North America, 27,* 11–12.

Spencer, T., Biederman, J., Wilens, T., Prince, J., Hatch, M., Jones, J., et al. (1998). Effectiveness and tolerability of tomoxetine in adults with attention deficit hyperactivity disorder. *American Journal of Psychiatry, 155,* 693–695.

Swanson, J. M. (1992). *School-based assessments and interventions for ADD students.* Irvine, CA: K.C. Publishing.

Swanson, J. M., Kraemer, H. C., Hinshaw, S. P., Arnold, L. E., Conners, C. K., Abikoff, H. B., et al. (2001). Clinical relevance of the primary findings of the MTA: Success rates based on severity of ADHD and ODD symptoms at the end of treatment. *Journal of the American Academy of Child and Adolescent Psychiatry, 40,* 168–179.

Ullman, R. K., Sleator, E. K., & Sprague, R. I. (1986). *ACTeRS rating scales.* Champagne, IL: Metri Tech.

Weinberg, H. A. (1999). Parent training for attention-deficit hyperactivity disorder: Parental and child outcomes. *Journal of Clinical Psychology, 55,* 907–913.

Weiss, G., & Hechtman, L. T. (1993). *Hyperactive children grown up* (2nd ed.). New York: Guilford Press.

Wells, K. C., Epstein, J. N., Hinshaw, S. P., Conners, C. K., Klaric, J., Abikoff, H. B., et al. (2000). Parenting and family stress treatment outcomes in attention deficit hyperactivity disorder (ADHD): An empirical analysis in the MTA study. *Journal of Abnormal Child Psychology, 28,* 543–553.

Whalen, C. K., & Henker, B. (1991). Therapies for hyperactive children: Comparisons, combinations, and compromises. *Journal of Consulting and Clinical Psychology, 59,* 126–137.

Wigal, S. B., McGough, J. J., McCracken, J. T., Biederman, J., Spencer, T. J., Posner, K. L., et al. (2005). A laboratory school comparison of mixed amphetamine salts extended release (Adderall XR) and atomoxetine (Strattera) in school-aged children with attention deficit/hyperactivity disorder. *Journal of Attention Disorders, 9,* 275–289.

Wigal, T., Greenhill, L., Chuang, S., McGough, J., Vitiello, B., Skrobala, A., et al. (2006). Safety and tolerability of methylphenidate in preschool children with ADHD. *Journal of the American Academy of Child and Adolescent Psychiatry, 45,* 1294–1303.

Wolraich, M. L. (1999). Attention deficit hyperactivity disorder: The most studied and yet most controversial diagnosis. *Mental Retardation and Developmental Disabilities Research Reviews, 5,* 163–168.

Wolraich, M. L. (2003). The use of psychotropic medications in children: An American view. *Journal of Child Psychology and Psychiatry, 44,* 159–168.

Wolraich, M. L., Hannah, J. N., Baumgaertel, A., & Feurer, I. D. (1998). Obtaining systematic teacher reports of disruptive behavior disorders utilizing DSM IV. *Journal of Abnormal Child Psychology, 26,* 141–152.

Wolraich, M. L., Lambert, E. W., & Worley, K. A. (2003). Psychometric properties of the Vanderbilt ADHD Diagnostic Parent Rating Scale in a referred population. *Journal of Pediatric Psychology, 28,* 559–568.

Zarin, D. A., Suarez, A. P., Pincus, H. A., Kupersanin, E., & Zito, J. M. (1998). Clinical and treatment characteristics of children with attention deficit/hyperactivity disorder in psychiatric practice. *Journal of the American Academy of Child and Adolescent Psychiatry, 37,* 1262–1270.

Zito, J. M., Safer, D. J., DosReis, S., Gardner, J. F., Magder, L., Soeken, K., et al. (2003). Psychotropic practice patterns for youth: A 10-year perspective. *Archives of Pediatrics and Adolescent Medicine, 157,* 17–25.

CHAPTER 37

Child Maltreatment

STEPHEN R. GILLASPY
BARBARA L. BONNER

Child maltreatment, now universally recognized as a major psychological, medical, and social problem, was first brought to the attention of the medical profession in 1962 by Henry Kempe and his colleagues through the publication of an article titled "The Battered-Child Syndrome" (Kempe, Silverman, Steele, Droegemuller, & Silver, 1962). Since that time, the fields of medicine, law, psychology, social work, and law enforcement have expanded their knowledge of and focus on the identification, prosecution, treatment, and prevention of child maltreatment. This increased focus probably resulted in a higher number of reported and confirmed cases of abuse and neglect in the United States throughout the 1980s and into the 1990s.

Over the past 20 years, several major events have occurred that have had a positive impact on psychologists and other mental health professionals who provide services to abused children and their families. These include (1) the establishment of two important professional organizations, the Section on Child Maltreatment by Division 37 of the American Psychological Association (*www.apa.org*) and the American Professional Society on the Abuse of Children (APSAC; *www.apsac.org*); (2) an increased focus on child maltreatment and child advocacy by the National Association of Children's Hospitals and Related Institutions; (3) the expansion of the International Society for the Prevention of Child Abuse and Neglect (*www.ispcan.org*) to provide training to psychologists in countries worldwide; (4) the involvement of psychologists in multidisciplinary teams and children's advocacy centers to improve the investigation, prosecution, and case management of child abuse cases; (5) an increase in research, with several hundred articles being published annually since 1990; (6) an increased focus on the prevention of child maltreatment at the local, state, and national levels; and (7) the establishment of child death review boards to review cases of suspected abuse and neglect (in many states, all child deaths) and to make recommendations to improve the systems investigating child deaths.

Scope of the Problem

The actual incidence and prevalence of child maltreatment are difficult to document accurately, due to (1) a lack of standard definitions applied across professions and across state, federal, and tribal laws; and (2) considerable variation in the methods and standards of collecting data (Leeb, Paulozzi, Melanson, Simon, & Arias, 2008). Reporting or referral bias may also skew the rates of maltreatment in certain ethnic and socioeconomic groups. In the most recent national data (from 2006), an estimated 3.6 million reports of suspected abuse involving 6 million children were received by state child protective service (CPS) agencies, and 905,000 children were found to be maltreated. The national rate of child maltreatment in 2006 was 12.1 per 1,000 children under age 18 (U.S. Department of Health and Human Services [U.S. DHHS], 2008); the highest rate of maltreatment was 15.3 child victims per 1,000 in 1993, and the rate of substantiated cases has continued to decrease since 1993.

The officially documented percentages of physical abuse and psychological maltreatment have remained relatively consistent over the past 5–10 years, while the rate of neglect has continued to increase, and sexual abuse has continued to decline. In 2006, approximately 64% of the cases involved neglect, 16% physical abuse, 9% sexual abuse, and 7% psychological maltreatment (U.S. DHHS, 2008). An additional 15% were associated with "other types" of maltreatment, including abandonment, congenital drug addiction, and threats of harm to the child. (These percentages total more than 100% because children may be classified as the recipient of more than one type of maltreatment.) The highest rate of maltreatment was for children from birth to age 1 (24.4 per 1,000), followed by children ages 1–3 (14.2 per 1,000) and ages 4–7 (13.5 per 1,000). Boys and girls were equally vulnerable to physical abuse and neglect, but girls were sexually abused at a rate four times that of boys (1.7 vs. 0.4 per 1,000). African American children were at the highest risk for abuse, with a rate of 24.7 per 1,000 children.

Despite the fact that neglect has consistently been the most prevalent type of child maltreatment, it has received the least attention by professionals, the media, and the general public. Child sexual abuse has clearly dominated the field in research, treatment interventions, and prevention programs since the mid-1980s, even though the rates of child sexual abuse have shown the greatest decline over the past 10 years. Several possible reasons for the decline have been suggested, including an actual decline in the rates of child sexual abuse; a decline in the reporting of suspected sexual abuse; and changes in attitudes, standards, and policies for confirmation in these cases (Finkelhor & Jones, 2004).

The psychological and behavioral effects of child maltreatment have been well documented in the literature. A significant addition to these negative consequences was found in a major study, the Adverse Childhood Experiences Study, conducted in the 1990s by the Centers for Disease Control and Prevention and the Department of Preventive Medicine at Kaiser Permanente. This study indicated that trauma and family dysfunction experienced in childhood were associated with adult health status decades later (Edwards et al., 2005). It tracked over 17,000 typical, middle-class, employed participants and found a set of 10 risk factors associated with such chronic diseases as heart disease, cancer, stroke, diabetes, and mental illness. The risk factors included emotional, sexual, and physical abuse; emotional and physical neglect; mother treated violently in the home; substance abuse in the household; mental illness in the home;

parental separation or divorce; and an incarcerated household member. The study found that individuals who had higher numbers of adverse childhood experiences had higher numbers of adult physical diseases and severe psychological problems (e.g., depression and suicide attempts). This is particularly important information for psychologists to recognize in order to intervene effectively with maltreated children who live in families with high levels of dysfunction.

Types of Child Maltreatment

Psychological Maltreatment

Psychological maltreatment has been viewed as a core component of all forms of child maltreatment—that is, as "the embedded psychological context behind other forms of abuse and neglect" (Hart, Brassard, Binggeli, & Davidson, 2002, p. 79). It is generally defined as a repeated pattern or extreme instances in which a parent or caregiver expresses to a child or adolescent that he or she is worthless, unloved, unwanted, endangered, or of value only in meeting someone else's needs (APSAC, 1995; Brassard, Hart, & Hardy, 1991). Psychological maltreatment involves acts of both omission and commission by a caregiver, and has effects on a continuum from mild to very severe. Whether or not a caregiver's behavior constitutes psychological maltreatment or results in identifiable harm to a child is difficult to demonstrate empirically or legally.

The most commonly identified subtypes of psychological maltreatment include spurning, terrorizing, exploiting/corrupting, isolating, denying emotional responsiveness, and unwarranted denial of mental health care, medical care, or education (APSAC, 1995; Hart et al., 2002). These can be defined as follows:

- *Spurning.* Verbal or nonverbal behaviors that reject and degrade a child, such as belittling, shaming, ridiculing, humiliating in public, or singling out one child to criticize or punish.
- *Terrorizing.* Threatening to harm the child, the child's loved ones, or his or her possessions; or engaging in potentially harmful behaviors that put a child in an unpredictable, chaotic, or dangerous situation.
- *Exploiting/corrupting.* Encouraging the child to engage in inappropriate or antisocial behaviors through modeling, permitting, or otherwise condoning such behaviors, such as prostitution, pornography, substance use, or shoplifting.
- *Isolating.* Excessive confinement or unreasonable limits on freedom or socialization.
- *Denying emotional responsiveness.* Parental ignoring, uninvolvement, or withdrawal from the child; a lack of appropriate expressions of affection, caring, or love.
- *Unwarranted denial of mental health care, medical care, or education.* Acts that overlap with the definition of neglect.

Prevalence rates of psychological maltreatment are difficult to determine, because it can occur alone or in conjunction with other forms of abuse or neglect, and it is often unrecognized and underreported. In 2006, approximately 7% of substantiated child maltreatment cases exclusively involved psychological maltreatment (U.S. DHHS, 2008). This figure does not include psychological maltreatment that occurs with other forms of maltreatment, and as such is likely to be an underestimate of the prevalence (Hart et al., 2002). In addition, as psychological maltreatment rarely shows physical evidence and is often difficult to prove, it is likely to be the least reported and prosecuted form of child maltreatment. Little is known about the specific effects of each of the subtypes of psychological maltreatment or about the comorbid overlap of the subtypes with one another (e.g., when a child is both spurned and terrorized). It is believed, however, that the psychological unavailability of the parent or denying emotional responsiveness may be the most damaging to children.

Research examining the effects of psychological maltreatment on children and adolescents has found a wide range of negative outcomes, including poor peer relationships (Brassard et al., 1991), higher rates of peer aggression (Erickson, Egeland, & Pianta, 1989), and significant academic difficulties. When the long-term effects of psychological maltreatment are compared with those of physical and sexual abuse, researchers have found strong associations between psychological maltreatment and low self-esteem (Gross & Keller, 1992), depression, and bulimia (Rorty, Yager, & Rossotto, 1994). In cases of multiple forms of abuse, the presence and severity of psychological maltreatment may represent one of the most significant causes of problematic adjustment (Hart et al., 2002).

Neglect

Although neglect accounts for the majority of maltreatment cases referred to CPS, researchers and clinicians have paid significantly less attention to neglect than to physical and sexual abuse. The 2006 data show that 64.2% of all substantiated maltreatment cases involved child neglect, with 2.2% experiencing medical neglect (U.S. DHHS, 2008). Infants and toddlers make up the most at-risk developmental group, with a significant decline in neglect cases as children enter their teen years (U.S. DHHS, 2008). Neglect is typically an ongoing and chronic pattern of omission on the caretaker's part, rather than a single event (Bonner, Logue, Kaufman, & Niec, 2001). However, there are single instances of supervisory neglect that can have tragic effects on children. Despite the pervasiveness of neglect, identification is frequently missed because physical evidence is rare unless the neglect is severe enough to lead to medical problems, as in cases of failure to thrive or an exacerbation of a chronic illness (e.g., asthma or cystic fibrosis).

"Neglect" is defined as a caregiver's failure to provide for a child's basic needs, which can lead to potential or actual harm to the child (Garbarino & Collins, 1999). The basic needs of children include adequate shelter, food, clothing, hygiene, medical care, educational opportunity, protection, affection, and supervision. The various subtypes of neglect are described below.

- *Physical or environmental neglect.* A caregiver's failure to provide for a child's basic physical needs, such as adequate housing, safety, nutrition, hygiene, supervision, and clothing, as well as exposure to domestic violence or prenatal substance use.
- *Medical neglect.* A caregiver's failure to provide necessary medical treatment or a delay in seeking health care, including mental health care; this can include noncompliance with medical recommendations, medication regimens, or required immunizations, or refusal of medical treatment for religious reasons.
- *Educational neglect.* A caregiver's failure to comply with state statutes on chil-

dren's educational attendance, including not enrolling children in school, permitting excessive truancy, or failing to address a child's special education needs.

Research focusing exclusively on neglected children suggests that neglect has more severe, long-lasting developmental consequences than either physical or sexual abuse (Gaudin, 1999). Neglected children exhibit higher rates of behavior problems (Williamson, Borduin, & Howe, 1991), poorer peer and teacher relationships (Rohrbeck & Twentyman, 1986), and more academic problems (Kendall-Tackett & Eckenrode, 1996). Longitudinal research has documented the long-term negative effects of neglect at different developmental stages (Hildyard & Wolfe, 2002). For example, studies of neglected infants show significant neurological and brain development changes, including reduced brain wave activity (Dawson, Klinger, & Panagiotides, 1997) and enlarged ventricles due to limited brain growth (Perry, 1997).

Perry (2002) has described the severe, long-term outcome in brain functioning if children's needs for physical touch from primary adult caregivers, stable emotional attachments, and interactions with peers are unmet. He concludes that if the appropriate neuronal connections are lacking due to the child's unmet needs, the development of the brain for both cognitive abilities and caring behavior is damaged in a "lasting fashion" (p. 79).

Physical Abuse

"Physical abuse" is generally defined as a nonaccidental act of commission by a parent or caregiver involving shaking, beating, burning, excessive discipline, or some other form of physical violence that results in fractures, bruises, retinal hemorrhages, burns, lacerations, or internal injuries (National Center on Child Abuse and Neglect, 1981). Children of all ages, including adolescents, are physically abused, with children under age 5 being at highest risk for serious injury and death due to physical abuse. Boys are more likely to be the victims of physical abuse and specifically more likely to be severely abused.

The effects of physical abuse on children can vary by the level of severity, intensity, and duration of the abuse, and by a child's age, developmental stage, and perceptions about the abuse. The effects can include medical and health problems, difficulties in academic performance, cognitive/perceptual and attributional problems, aggressive and other behavior disorders, internalizing problems, posttraumatic stress disorder (PTSD), and interpersonal and relationship problems (Kolko, 2002). Several well-designed longitudinal studies have documented the long-term effects of physical abuse. For example, children with a history of being physically abused are at twice as much risk as the general population of being arrested for a violent crime (Widom, 1989), and they have significant problems in adolescence and adulthood (Silverman, Reinherz, & Giaconia, 1996). Another study with a 17-year follow-up showed that when compared with nonabused children, physically abused children had significantly more symptoms of anxiety and depression, emotional and behavioral problems, and suicidal ideation and attempts in adolescence and young adulthood than nonabused children (Brown, Cohen, Johnson, & Smailes, 1999).

Munchausen syndrome by proxy (MSP), or factitious disorder by proxy, is a specific and rare type of maltreatment in which a caregiver (usually the mother) fabricates, induces, or simulates symptoms of physical illness in a child (Parnell, 2002). This highly unusual form of maltreatment is particularly relevant to pediatric psychologists, as these infants and children frequently present in a hospital setting. This particular syndrome is associated with high rates of recidivism and mortality (Galvin, Newton, & Vandeven, 2005). The disorder is most often classified as physical abuse, because it involves a caregiver (again, usually the mother) manufacturing, inducing, or simulating symptoms in a child (e.g., feeding toxic substances to induce vomiting or nausea, inducing seizures by suffocation) and then bringing the child for medical treatment (Parnell, 2002; Stirling, 2007). However, it is not unusual for MSP to co-occur with other forms of maltreatment, such as neglect or psychological maltreatment, and to continue for months or years before it is detected. MSP is now recognized as a rare form of abuse that is best detected by observing the event surreptitiously (Ware, Orr, & Bond, 2001).

Sexual Abuse

"Child sexual abuse" is broadly defined as any sexual activity with a child in which consent cannot be or is not given (Berliner & Elliott, 2002). The legal definition includes touching and fondling; kissing of the genital areas; digital or penile penetration of the mouth, vagina, or anus; and noncontact abuse, such as voyeurism, exhibitionism, and child pornography. It further includes sexual contact by actual force or threat of force, regardless of the ages of the participants, and all sexual activity between a child and an adult, regardless of physical contact (Berliner & Elliott, 2002). The definition often takes several factors into account, including the age of the child (17–18 or younger); the relationship of the child to the perpetrator (intrafamilial vs. extrafamilial); the difference in age, developmental level, or power status between the child and the offender; and the type of abuse (i.e., physical contact with the child vs. no contact).

Children of all ages, including young infants, are sexually abused, and girls are approximately three to four times more likely to be abused than boys. Surveys of the general population find almost no socioeconomic effects in sexual abuse, but a disproportionate number of sexually abused children are reported to CPS from low-income families (Sedlak & Broadhurst, 1996), possibly reflecting a reporting bias.

A wide array of symptoms has been documented in children and adolescents who have experienced sexual abuse, ranging from minimal symptoms to significant levels of disturbance. In general, symptoms in sexually abused children have been found to be more severe than in nonabused children, but less severe than the symptoms of other child outpatient mental health populations (Kilpatrick & Saunders, 1999). The most frequently reported symptoms in sexually abused children include fearfulness of abuse stimuli and other symptoms of PTSD; inappropriate sexual behavior; nightmares and sleep disorders; depression; repressed anger and hostility; behavior problems; and somatic complaints (Berliner & Elliott, 2002). It should be noted, however, that inappropriate or aggressive sexual behavior should not be used as a definitive indicator of a history of sexual abuse, as studies have documented highly inappropriate and aggressive sexual behavior in children with no known history of sexual abuse (Bonner, Walker, & Berliner, 1999). In addition, all of these symptoms can appear in children and adolescents who have not been sexually abused.

A relatively rare problem in children, encopresis or soiling, has been documented in children who have experienced sexual abuse (Morrow, Yeager, & Otnow-Lewis, 1997). Two possible connections were suggested by Krisch (1980): (1) The penetration or stimulation in the anal area might cause sufficient emotional conflict for the child to develop incontinence; or (2) the repeated exposure to anal intercourse could weaken or damage the anal sphincter, causing incontinence. However, evaluators should be cautious about considering child sexual abuse in children with encopresis, as existing evidence does not support soiling as an indicator of sexual abuse (Mellon, Whiteside, & Friedrich, 2006). Pediatric psychologists should be alert to the possibility of sexual abuse in children with encopresis, but should keep in mind that the relationship is rare and that a thorough evaluation should be conducted.

It is not possible to list a set of symptoms that are exclusively associated with child sexual abuse. However, psychologists should consider that children may have experienced sexual abuse when they present with the following symptoms. In preschool and school-age children, causes for concern include symptoms of PTSD with no known antecedent event, high levels of anxiety or restlessness, sleep disorders, aggressive behavior, depression, or inappropriate sexual behavior or knowledge. In adolescents, the symptoms can include low self-esteem, depression, suicidal ideation or behavior, eating disorders, problems at school, substance abuse, and conflicts with authority figures (Hecht, Chaffin, Bonner, Worley, & Lawson, 2002). Generally, symptoms in adolescents are more closely related to those seen in adult survivors of childhood sexual abuse. (For a review of child sexual abuse, see Putnam, 2003.)

Assessment and Treatment

The clinical assessment and treatment aspects of child maltreatment cases should be clearly separate from the forensic aspects (i.e., reporting and investigating allegations of abuse). The clinical approach to child maltreatment should follow a developmental psychopathology model (Friedrich, 2002), taking into consideration a child's developmental functioning and abilities. The goal of the clinical assessment is to determine the child's and caregivers' overall functioning, adaptation, and level of symptomatology. As a first step, a thorough assessment of the family's strengths and problems should be conducted, including the types of problems that need to be addressed at the parental, child, family, and social systems levels (Kolko, 2002). Assessments may include interviews, paper-and-pencil measures, or structured observations with the child, siblings, and caregivers.

Several specific measures have been standardized to evaluate a child's symptoms and to assess the parents. These include general assessments of trauma symptoms, such as the Trauma Symptom Checklist for Young Children (Briere et al., 2001) and the Trauma Symptom Checklist for Children (Briere, 1996); and a measurement of sexual behavior problems, such as the Child Sexual Behavior Inventory (Friedrich, 1997). To assess psychological maltreatment, the Psychological Maltreatment Rating Scales (Brassard, Hart, & Hardy, 1993) provide an observational structure to evaluate mother–child interactions, and the Child Abuse Potential Inventory (Milner, 1990) evaluates parental risk for abuse and neglect.

Various treatment approaches for abused children and adolescents have been developed, and empirical evaluations of treatment interventions are increasing. Clinicians should rely on techniques and approaches that are appropriate for a child's cognitive and developmental level of functioning and that have documented effectiveness in reducing the child's targeted symptoms. Two recent reviews provide important information on the current status of evidence-based treatment approaches (Chadwick Center for Children and Families, 2004; Saunders, Berliner, & Hanson, 2004).

Pediatric psychologists also need to be familiar with evidence-based practices for the treatment of abused children, such as the three described below. Abuse-focused cognitive-behavioral therapy (AF-CBT) targets individual child and parent characteristics related to the abusive experience, as well as the family context in which coercion or aggression exists (Kolko & Swenson, 2002). AF-CBT combines elements of several different treatment approaches: cognitive therapy, behavioral and learning therapy, family therapy, and developmental victimology. Treatment is provided to school-age children and parents or caregivers, both in separate and in periodic joint sessions. This short-term treatment is typically conducted in 12–24 sessions over 3–6 months. AF-CBT is generally provided in an outpatient setting, but can be conducted in residential or other placement settings if the parent or caregiver has regular contact with the child. Research has demonstrated that AF-CBT is most appropriate for school-age children and their physically abusive or coercive parents (Kolko, 1996).

Parent–child interaction therapy (PCIT) is a treatment approach originally developed to treat children ages 2–7 with serious behavioral problems (Eyberg, 1988). PCIT utilizes live coaching and focuses on changing the behaviors of both the parent and the child. Parents learn to model positive behaviors and are trained to act as "agents of change" for their children's behavioral or emotional difficulties (Hembree-Kigin & McNeil, 1995; Herschell & McNeil, 2005). Since its initial development, PCIT has been adapted for use with families that have experienced child maltreatment and has been found effective for physically abusive parents with children ages 4–12 (Chaffin et al., 2004). In addition, PCIT has been used to support foster parents caring for children with behavioral problems by teaching the foster parents behavior management skills and enhancing the relationship between the foster parents and foster children. After completing PCIT, foster parents have reported decreased child behavior problems, less parental stress, and high levels of satisfaction with PCIT (McNeil, Hershell, Gurwitch, & Clemens-Mowrer, 2005). (For additional information about PCIT, see *www.pcit. org*.)

Trauma-focused cognitive-behavioral therapy (TF-CBT) is an evidence-based treatment approach that addresses the negative effects of sexual abuse and other traumatic events by combining elements drawn from cognitive therapy, behavioral therapy, and family therapy. TF-CBT includes a treatment component for nonabusive parents or caregivers and a treatment component for children. Children and parents participate in individual sessions and have several joint child–parent sessions. This short-term outpatient treatment is typically provided in 12–18 sessions of 60–90 minutes. TF-CBT is appropriate for use with sexually abused children ages 3–18 and parents or caregivers who did not participate in the abuse. Research has demonstrated that TF-CBT is useful in reducing symptoms of PTSD, depression, and behavioral problems in children who have experienced sexual abuse and other traumatic experiences (Cohen, Deblinger, Mannarino, & Steer, 2004; Cohen, Mannarino, & Deblinger, 2006; Deblinger, Stauffer, & Steer, 2001; King et al., 2000). (For additional information, see *www.nctsn.org*, and for free online training, see *tfcbt.musc.edu*.)

For some forms of neglect, research has shown promising results for interventions that include home visitation as a primary approach (Lutzker, Bigelow, Doctor, Gershater, & Greene, 1998; Olds et al., 1997). A model that is showing effectiveness in reducing neglect is SafeCare, a home-based program based on Lutzker's earlier 12-Ways approach (Lutzker, Frame, & Rice, 1982). The SafeCare parenting program is an evidence-based training program for parents who are at risk or have been reported for child maltreatment. The program consists of three modules: Home Safety, Infant and Child Health, and Parent–Child/Parent–Infant Interactions. All modules have a baseline assessment, an intervention, and follow-up assessments to monitor progress. The model is based on well-established social learning theory and is currently being implemented in several states. A 4-year SafeCare research and intervention program has been implemented by Lutzker and his colleagues (Gershater-Molko, Lutzker, & Wesch, 2003). The parents were trained in the three modules, and effectiveness was evaluated by changes in the parents' scores on a role-play situation for child health problems, the frequency and quality of parent–child interactions, and the hazards in the home. The results indicated that SafeCare resulted in statistically significant improvements in children's care, parent–child interactions, and home safety. A companion study indicated that, compared to a group of parents involved in a family preservation group, the SafeCare parents had significantly lower reports of child maltreatment over 36 months during and after the intervention (Gershater-Molko, Lutzker, & Wesch, 2002).

Reporting

Pediatric psychologists must be knowledgeable about the mandatory reporting laws in the state or federal setting (such as a tribal reservation) where they practice. All 50 states have mandatory child abuse and neglect reporting laws; however, individual states vary in the requirements of these laws. All states require certain individuals to report suspected child abuse, and psychologists are more often than not included in this mandate. State requirements vary about what must be reported: Some states require reporting when there is merely a suspicion of maltreatment; others require a higher degree of knowledge or certainty that maltreatment has occurred. Failure to report suspected child abuse can result in civil or criminal liability, typically a misdemeanor punishable by a fine. In most states, a person who reports suspected maltreatment in good faith is immune from criminal and civil liability, even if the maltreatment is not substantiated. Some states also have statutes that allow the prosecution of individuals who purposefully make false allegations of child maltreatment (Zellman & Fair, 2002). In addition, professional organizations (e.g., the American Psychological Association, state psychological associations) have ethical standards and practices that require reporting suspected child maltreatment.

In cases in which a pediatric psychologist is the first professional to suspect or identify maltreatment, it is rarely his or her role to investigate or assess the validity of the allegations. This function is the role of CPS or law enforcement professionals who are trained and responsible for conducting an investigation and determining whether a child should be removed from the home. In many hospitals, the social services department has trained personnel who conduct forensic interviews with suspected victims and who work closely with CPS and law enforcement. If a pediatric psychologist suspects child maltreatment, it is essential to obtain accurate, complete documentation of the allegations and the circumstances of the disclosure of suspicious events, as well as to document the course of action the psychologist takes (including contacts with CPS, other professionals, or other agencies). This attention to detail can be useful in reporting and in the investigation of the allegations, as well as in any subsequent legal or court involvement. To maintain the validity of children's reports, psychologists should be aware of their role in the reporting and investigative process, and must gain the initial information necessary for reporting without contaminating the children's reports for the subsequent investigation.

Current Approaches in Responding to Child Maltreatment

Child Death Review Boards

Child death review boards (CDRBs) have been established in 49 U.S. states and in several foreign countries to review suspicious, vague, or violent circumstances surrounding a child's death that may be due to abuse or neglect (Durfee, Durfee, & West, 2002). The goal of these reviews is to understand how and why children die and to prevent future fatalities. Although the goals of CDRBs are generally similar, the specific review process varies considerably from state to state. Some states have legislatively established boards with specified professionals as members and review all child deaths from ages 0 to 18 each year; other states' boards only review suspected child maltreatment deaths or suspicious deaths in children under age 1. According to the National Center for Child Death Review (*www.childdeathreview.org*), state and local review teams or boards utilize a multidisciplinary approach that typically includes representatives from mental health. Pediatric psychologists can be definite assets to a CDRB because of their knowledge of child development, medical conditions in children, mental illness, and research (Bonner & Kees, 2007).

Children's Advocacy Centers

A major development in the field of child maltreatment occurred in 1985 with the establishment of children's advocacy centers (CACs), with interdisciplinary staffs from CPS, law enforcement, medicine, mental health, and the legal system. The CACs were developed primarily in response to cases of child sexual abuse to streamline and more comprehensively address child maltreatment. A CAC is a child-centered, facility-based program in which professionals work as a team to conduct joint forensic interviews and decisions about the investigation, management, and prosecution of child abuse cases. The CAC is community-based in a single setting where a child can be interviewed, medically examined, and treated or triaged for mental health problems, thereby reducing the number of places and times a child is interviewed. There are currently over 400 CACs operating nationally, and the National Children's Alliance (*www.nca-online.org*) has been organized to set criteria for team structure and to provide ongoing training and technical support. Pediatric psychologists may serve as members of these multidisciplinary teams, particularly when a CAC is located in a hospital.

Child Protection Teams

Multidisciplinary teams have been used in hospital settings since the 1950s to review cases of suspected abuse (Ells, 2000). These child protection teams (CPTs) originated in large urban hospitals in Pittsburgh, Los Angeles, and Denver. CPTs were initiated by physicians encountering emergency room cases involving child abuse, and since that time CPTs have played an important part in the child welfare system.

Many hospitals have CPTs or similar groups that review cases of suspected abuse that are reported through the hospital. These multidisciplinary teams typically include psychologists, along with physicians, nurses, social workers, CPS staff, and representatives from law enforcement and the local prosecutor's office who meet on a regular basis to discuss and provide follow-up on abuse-related cases. Typically a CPT, rather than any one individual, makes the recommendation to report suspected maltreatment to CPS or law enforcement. Pediatric psychologists may be more knowledgeable than other team members about child development, children's emotional and behavioral functioning, and family dynamics, and can assist the team in differentiating normal from abnormal behaviors or situations.

Foster Care Clinics (Medical Homes)

The American Academy of Pediatrics (*www.aap.org*) has provided recommendations for the establishment of foster care clinics based on the medical home model to provide comprehensive health care to children and adolescents in the foster care system. As part of the medical home model, the clinics utilize providers with additional training and experience with foster care children, conduct routine developmental and behavioral assessments, and provide comprehensive outpatient health care. With regard to health care needs, children entering foster care frequently have a history of inadequate well-child visits and undiagnosed or poorly managed chronic health conditions (Brattistelli, 1996). Foster children have higher rates of chronic physical disabilities, birth defects, developmental delays, and poor school achievement than children of similar socioeconomic backgrounds (Institute for Research on Women and Families, 1998). In addition, children in foster care frequently have emotional and behavioral problems, with prevalence estimates ranging from 35 to 85% (Szilagyi, 1998). Given the medical and mental health needs of these children, foster care medical homes provide unique opportunities for pediatric psychologists to provide services to this underserved population.

Conclusions

The consequences of child maltreatment continue to impose a significant burden on the victims and their families, professionals attempting to protect children, and society in general. The recognition of maltreatment is increasing, but the actual reported rates continue to be underestimated. Although advances have been made in the diagnosis, mental health interventions, and multidisciplinary management of cases, significant problems continue in the foster care and CPS systems due to the increasing numbers of children entering the foster care system, a lack of foster families, and the number of cases each CPS worker manages.

Psychologists have a moral, ethical, and legal responsibility to recognize and report suspected abuse and neglect in children. The role of pediatric psychologists in child maltreatment is varied and multifocal: They may be involved in identifying, reporting, treating, or collaborating with other professionals in addressing cases of child maltreatment. Child maltreatment is a complex problem, made more so by problems in definition, the different roles of the professionals involved, and the involvement of the legal system. The combination of these elements creates highly complex situations for pediatric psychologists and other professionals who work to protect children.

Maltreatment may be a central or peripheral treatment focus with children who are seen in medical settings. Some injuries due to maltreatment require medical intervention (e.g., extensive or severe physical abuse, neglect, or sexual abuse may result in sexually transmitted diseases or physical injury), and a psychologist may be asked to evaluate and address the psychological sequelae of the abuse. In other cases, a medical illness (rather than injury due to maltreatment) may be the primary presenting complaint (e.g., diabetes mellitus or renal failure), but maltreatment plays a role in the course and prognosis for the child. For example, a young child with diabetes mellitus may require close monitoring to adhere to diet and insulin protocols. A parent's failure to implement the regimen can lead to acute and critical problems, such as diabetic ketoacidosis. Repeated episodes of ketoacidosis can be indicators of medical neglect, and the pediatric psychologist may work with the family to increase the parents' and child's adherence to the regimen.

There are numerous opportunities for pediatric psychologists to participate through training, treatment, and research in the protection of children and the prevention of future maltreatment. Through their various roles in outpatient and inpatient settings, psychologists may encounter child maltreatment cases through the inpatient consultation–liaison service, the hospital CPT, pediatric primary care clinics, or routine screening in medical subspecialty clinics. Although pediatric psychologists may not provide direct treatment to abused or neglected children, it is vitally important that they be familiar with evidence-based assessment and treatment approaches for children exposed to maltreatment, so that an accurate assessment and appropriate referral for services can be made.

References

American Professional Society on the Abuse of Children (APSAC). (1995). *Guidelines for the psychosocial evaluation of suspected psychological maltreatment in children and adolescents*. Chicago: Author.

Berliner, L., & Elliott, D. M. (2002). Sexual abuse of children. In J. E. B. Myers, L. Berliner, J. Briere, C. T. Hendrix, C. Jenny, & T. A. Reid (Eds.), *The APSAC handbook on child maltreatment* (2nd ed., pp. 55–78). Thousand Oaks, CA: Sage.

Bonner, B. L., & Kees, M. R. (2007). The role of mental health professionals. In R. Alexander (Ed.), *Child fatality review: An interdisciplinary guide and photographic reference* (pp. 661–671). St. Louis, MO: G.W. Medical.

Bonner, B. L., Logue, M. B., Kaufman, K. L., & Niec, L. N. (2001). Child maltreatment. In C. E. Walker & M. C. Roberts (Eds.), *Handbook of clinical child psychology* (3rd ed., pp. 989–1030). New York: Wiley.

Bonner, B. L., Walker, C. E., & Berliner, L. (1999). *Children with sexual behavior problems: Assessment and treatment* (Final report). Washington, DC: Office of Child Abuse and Neglect.

Brassard, M. R., Hart, S. N., & Hardy, D. B. (1991). Psychological and emotional abuse of children. In T. Ammerman & M. Hersen (Eds.), *Case studies in treating family violence* (pp. 255–270). Boston: Allyn & Bacon.

Brassard, M. R., Hart, S. N., & Hardy, D. B. (1993). The Psychological Maltreatment Rating Scale. *Child Abuse and Neglect, 17,* 715–729.

Brattistelli, E. S. (1996). *Making managed health care work for kids in foster care: A guide to purchasing services.* Washington, DC: Child Welfare League of America.

Briere, J. (1996). *Trauma Symptom Checklist for Children (TSCC): Professional manual.* Odessa, FL: Psychological Assessment Resources.

Briere, J., Johnson, K., Bissada, A., Damon, L., Crouch, J., Gil, E., et al. (2001). The Trauma Symptom Checklist for Young Children (TSCYC): Reliability and association with abuse exposure in a multi-site study. *Child Abuse and Neglect, 25,* 1001–1014.

Brown, J., Cohen, P., Johnson, J. G., & Smailes, E. M. (1999). Childhood abuse and neglect: Specificity of effects on adolescent and young adult depression and suicidality. *Journal of the American Academy of Child and Adolescent Psychiatry, 39*(6), 1490–1496.

Chadwick Center for Children and Families. (2004). *Closing the quality chasm in child abuse treatment; Identifying and disseminating best practices. The findings of the Kauffman Best Practices Project to Help Children Heal From Child Abuse.* San Diego, CA: Author.

Chaffin, M., Silovsky, J. F., Funderburk, B., Valle, L. A., Brestan, E. V., Balachova, T., et al. (2004). Parent–child interaction therapy with physically abusive parents: Efficacy for reducing future abuse reports. *Journal of Consulting and Clinical Psychology, 72*(3), 500–510.

Cohen, J. A., Deblinger, E., Mannarino, A. P., & Steer, R. (2004). A multisite, randomized controlled trial for children with sexual abuse-related PTSD symptoms. *Journal of the American Academy of Child and Adolescent Psychiatry, 43*(4), 393–402.

Cohen, J. A., Mannarino, A. P., & Deblinger, E. (2006). *Treating trauma and traumatic grief in children and adolescents.* New York: Guilford Press.

Dawson, G., Klinger, L., & Panagiotides, H. (1997). Infants of depressed mothers exhibit atypical frontal brain activity during the expression of negative emotions. *Developmental Psychology, 33,* 650–656.

Deblinger, E., Stauffer, L., & Steer, R. (2001). Comparative efficacies of supportive and cognitive behavioral group therapies for young children who have been sexually abused and their non-offending mothers. *Child Maltreatment, 6*(4), 332–343.

Durfee, M., Durfee, D. T., & West, M. P. (2002). Child fatality review: An international movement. *Child Abuse and Neglect, 26,* 619–636.

Edwards, V. J., Anda, R. F., Dube, S. R., Dong, M., Chapman, D. F., & Felitti, V. J. (2005). The wide-ranging health consequences of adverse childhood experiences. In K. Kendall-Tackett & S. Giacomoni (Eds.), *Victimization of children and youth: Patterns of abuse and response strategies* (Chap. 8, pp. 1–16). Kingston, NJ: Civic Research Institute.

Ells, M. (2000). Forming a multidisciplinary team to investigate child abuse. Retrieved January 9, 2008, from *www.ncjrs.org/html/ojjdp/portable_guides/forming/contents.html*

Erickson, M. F., Egeland, B., & Pianta, R. C. (1989). The effects of maltreatment on the development of young children. In D. Cicchetti & V. Carlson (Eds.), *Child maltreatment: Theory and research on the causes and consequences of child abuse and neglect* (pp. 647–684). New York: Cambridge University Press.

Eyberg, S. M. (1988). Parent–child interaction therapy: Integration of traditional and behavioral concerns. *Child and Family Behavior Therapy, 10,* 33–46.

Finkelhor, D., & Jones, L. M. (2004). *Explanations for the decline in child sexual abuse cases* (Juvenile Justice Bulletin No. NC199298). Washington, DC: Office of Juvenile Justice and Delinquency Prevention.

Friedrich, W. N. (1997). *Child Sexual Behavior Inventory: Professional manual.* Odessa, FL: Psychological Assessment Resources.

Friedrich, W. N. (2002). An integrated model of psychotherapy for abused children. In J. E. B. Myers, L. Berliner, J. Briere, C. T. Hendrix, C. Jenny, & T. A. Reid (Eds.), *The APSAC handbook on child maltreatment* (2nd ed., pp. 141–158). Thousand Oaks, CA: Sage.

Galvin, H. K., Newton, A. W., & Vandeven, A. M. (2005). Update on Munchausen syndrome by proxy. *Current Opinion in Pediatrics, 17*(2), 252–257.

Garbarino, J., & Collins, C. C. (1999). Child neglect: The family with a hole in the middle. In H. Dubowitz (Ed.), *Neglected children: Research, practice, and policy* (pp. 1–23). Thousand Oaks, CA: Sage.

Gaudin, J. M. (1999). Child neglect: Short-term and long-term consequences. In H. Dubowitz (Ed.), *Neglected children: Research, practice, and policy* (pp. 89–108). Thousand Oaks, CA: Sage.

Gershater-Molko, R. M., Lutzker, J. R., & Wesch, D. (2002). Using recidivism data to evaluate Project SafeCare: Teaching bonding, safety, and health care skills to parents. *Child Maltreatment, 7*(3), 277–285.

Gershater-Molko, R. M., Lutzker, J. R., & Wesch, D. (2003). Project SafeCare: Improving health, safety and parenting skills in families reported for, and at risk for, child maltreatment. *Journal of Family Violence, 18*(6), 377–386.

Gross, A. B., & Keller, H. R. (1992). Long-term consequences of childhood physical and psychological maltreatment. *Aggressive Behavior, 18*, 171–185.

Hart, S. N., Brassard, M. R., Binggeli, N. J., & Davidson, H. A. (2002). Psychological maltreatment. In J. E. B. Myers, L. Berliner, J. Briere, C. T. Hendrix, C. Jenny, & T. A. Reid (Eds.), *The APSAC handbook on child maltreatment* (2nd ed., pp. 79–104). Thousand Oaks, CA: Sage.

Hecht, D. B., Chaffin, M., Bonner, B. L., Worley, K. B., & Lawson, L. (2002). Treating sexually abused adolescents. In J. E. B. Myers, L. Berliner, J. Briere, C. T. Hendrix, C. Jenny, & T. A. Reid (Eds.), *The APSAC handbook on child maltreatment* (2nd ed., pp. 159–174). Thousand Oaks, CA: Sage.

Hembree-Kigin, T. L., & McNeil, C. B. (1995). *Parent–child interaction therapy*. New York: Plenum Press.

Herschell, A., & McNeil, C. B. (2005). Theoretical and empirical underpinnings of parent–child interaction therapy with child physical abuse populations. *Education and Treatment of Children, 28*, 142–162.

Hildyard, K. L., & Wolfe, D. A. (2002). Child neglect: Developmental issues and outcomes. *Child Abuse and Neglect, 26*, 679–695.

Institute for Research on Women and Families. (1998). *Code blue: Health services for children in foster care*. Sacramento: California State University.

Kempe, C. H., Silverman, F. N., Steele, B. F., Droegemuller, W., & Silver, H. K. (1962). The battered-child syndrome. *Journal of the American Medical Association, 181*(17), 17–24.

Kendall-Tackett, K. A., & Eckenrode, J. (1996). The effects of neglect on academic achievement and disciplinary problems: A developmental perspective. *Child Abuse and Neglect, 20*, 161–169.

Kilpatrick, D. G., & Saunders, B. E. (1999). *Prevalence and consequences of child victimization: Results from the National Survey of Adolescents* (Report No. 93-IJ-CX-0023). Charleston, SC: National Crime Victims Research and Treatment Center.

King, N., Tonge, B., Mullen, P., Myerson, N., Heyne, D., Rollings, S., et al. (2000). Treating sexually abused children with posttraumatic stress symptoms: A randomized clinical trial. *Journal of the American Academy of Child and Adolescent Psychiatry, 39*(11), 1347–1355.

Kolko, D. J. (1996). Clinical monitoring of treatment course in child physical abuse: Psychometric characteristics and treatment comparisons. *Child Abuse and Neglect, 20*(1), 23–43.

Kolko, D. J. (2002). Child physical abuse. In J. E. B. Myers, L. Berliner, J. Briere, C. T. Hendrix, C. Jenny, & T. A. Reid (Eds.), *The APSAC handbook on child maltreatment* (2nd ed., pp. 21–54). Thousand Oaks, CA: Sage.

Kolko, D. J., & Swenson, C. C. (2002). *Assessing and treating physically abused children and their families: A cognitive behavioral approach*. Thousand Oaks, CA: Sage.

Krisch, K. (1980). Encopresis as protection from homosexual annoyance. *Praxis der Kinderpsychologie und Kinderpsychiatrie, 37,* 260–265.

Leeb, R. T., Paulozzi, L., Melanson, C., Simon, T., & Arias, I. (2008). *Child maltreatment surveillance: Uniform definitions for public health and recommended data elements* (Version 1.0). Atlanta, GA: Centers for Disease Control and Prevention. National Center for Injury Prevention and Control.

Lutzker, J. R., Bigelow, K. M., Doctor, R. M., Gershater, R. M., & Greene, B. F. (1998). An ecobehavioral model for the prevention and treatment of child abuse and neglect. In J. R. Lutzker (Ed.), *Handbook of child abuse research and treatment* (pp. 239–266). New York: Plenum Press.

Lutzker, J. R., Frame, J. R., & Rice, J. M. (1982). Project 12 Ways: An ecobehavioral approach to the treatment and prevention of child abuse and neglect. *Education and Treatment of Children, 5,* 141–155.

McNeil, C., Herschell, A. D., Gurwitch, R. H., & Clemens-Mowrer, L. C. (2005). Training foster parents in parent–child interaction therapy. *Education and Treatment of Children, 28*(2), 182–196.

Mellon, M. W., Whiteside, S. P., & Friedrich, W. N. (2006). The relevance of fecal soiling as an indicator of child sexual abuse: A preliminary analysis. *Journal of Developmental and Behavioral Pediatrics, 27*(1), 25–32.

Milner, J. (1990). *An interpretive manual for the Child Abuse Potential Inventory.* DeKalb, IL: Psytec.

Morrow, J., Yeager, C., & Otnow-Lewis, D. (1997). Encopresis and sexual abuse in a sample of boys in residential treatment. *Child Abuse and Neglect, 21,* 11–18.

National Center on Child Abuse and Neglect. (1981). *Study findings: National study of the incidence and severity of child abuse and neglect* (Publication No. OHDS 81-30325). Washington, DC: U.S. Department of Health and Human Services.

Olds, D. L., Eckenrode, J., Henderson, C. R., Kitzman, H., Powers, J., Cole, R., et al. (1997). Long-term effects of home visitation on maternal life course and child abuse and neglect. *Journal of the American Medical Association, 278,* 637–643.

Parnell, T. F. (2002). Munchausen by proxy syndrome. In J. E. B. Myers, L. Berliner, J. Briere, C. T. Hendrix, C. Jenny, & T. A. Reid (Eds.), *The APSAC handbook on child maltreatment* (2nd ed., pp. 131–138). Thousand Oaks, CA: Sage.

Perry, B. (1997). Incubated in terror: Neurodevelopmental factors in the "cycle of violence." In J. D. Osofsky (Ed.), *Children in a violent society* (pp. 124–149). New York: Guilford Press.

Perry, B. (2002). Childhood experience and the expression of genetic potential: What childhood neglect tells us about nature and nurture. *Brain and Mind, 3,* 79–100.

Putnam, F. W. (2003). Ten-year research update review: Child sexual abuse. *Journal of the American Academy of Child and Adolescent Psychiatry, 42*(3), 264–278.

Rohrbeck, C. A., & Twentyman, C. T. (1986). Multimodal assessment of impulsiveness in abusing, neglectful, and nonmaltreating mothers and their preschool children. *Journal of Consulting and Clinical Psychology, 54,* 231–236.

Rorty, M., Yager, J., & Rossotto, E. (1994). Childhood sexual, physical, and psychological abuse in bulimia nervosa. *American Journal of Psychiatry, 151,* 1122–1126.

Saunders, B. E., Berliner, L., & Hanson, R. F. (Eds.). (2004, April 26). *Child physical and sexual abuse: Guidelines for treatment* (Revised report). Charleston, SC: National Crime Victims Research and Treatment Center.

Sedlak, A. J., & Broadhurst, D. D. (1996). *Executive summary of the Third National Incidence Study of Child Abuse and Neglect* (DHHS Publication No. ACF-105-94-1840). Washington, DC: U.S. Government Printing Office.

Silverman, A. B., Reinherz, H. Z., & Giaconia, R. M. (1996). The long-term sequelae of child and adolescent abuse: A longitudinal community study. *Child Abuse and Neglect*, *8*, 709–723.

Stirling, J. (2007). Beyond Munchausen syndrome by proxy: Identification and treatment of child abuse in a medical setting. *Pediatrics*, *119*(5), 1026–1030.

Szilagyi, M. (1998). The pediatrician and the child in foster care. *Pediatrics in Review*, *19*, 39–50.

U.S. Department of Health and Human Services (U.S. DHHS), Administration on Children, Youth and Families. (2008). *11 years of reporting: Child maltreatment 2006*. Washington, DC: US Government Printing Office.

Ware, J. C., Orr, W. C., & Bond, T. (2001). Evaluation and treatment of sleep disorders in children. In C. E. Walker & M. C. Roberts (Eds.), *Handbook of clinical child psychology* (3rd ed., pp. 317–337). New York: Wiley.

Widom, C. S. (1989). Child abuse, neglect, and adult behavior: Research design and findings on criminality, violence and child abuse. *American Journal of Orthopsychiatry*, *59*, 355–367.

Williamson, J. M., Borduin, C. M., & Howe, B. A. (1991). The ecology of adolescent maltreatment: A multilevel examination of adolescent physical abuse, sexual abuse, and neglect. *Journal of Consulting and Clinical Psychology*, *59*, 449–457.

Zellman, G. L., & Fair, C. C. (2002). Preventing and reporting abuse. In J. E. B. Myers, L. Berliner, J. Briere, C. T. Hendrix, C. Jenny, & T. A. Reid (Eds.), *The APSAC handbook on child maltreatment* (2nd ed., pp. 449–475). Thousand Oaks, CA: Sage.

PART IV

Public Health Issues

CHAPTER 38

Racial and Ethnic Health Disparities and Access to Care

BERNARD F. FUEMMELER
LINDSAY MORIARTY
RONALD T. BROWN

In the year 2000, racial and ethnic minorities (African American, Native American, Asian, Pacific Islander, and Hispanic) accounted for nearly 30% of the U.S. population. By 2050, this number is expected to increase to 50%. Of special interest is what this means for pediatric populations. According to the U.S. Census Bureau (2000), by 2030 there will be more minority children than non-Hispanic European American children 0–18 years old living in the United States (see also Flores, Olson, & Tomany-Korman, 2005). As the population continues to change both in size and in ethnicity, the public health community will need to examine how this demographic shift affects the patterns and distributions of disease within the nation.

A "health disparity" can be defined as a "population-specific difference in the presence of disease, health outcomes, or access to health care" (U.S. Department of Health and Human Services [U.S. DHHS], 2004). Inequalities or differences in the amount and quality of health care accorded to various racial and ethnic groups are often attributed to social injustice and its impact on lifestyle, behavior, and access to and control over commonly sought-after resources (Adler & Rehkopf, 2008; Newman Giger & Davidhizar, 2007). A burgeoning body of literature presents compelling evidence to support claims that racial and ethnic minorities are at greater risk for increased morbidity and mortality related to chronic illnesses (Kaplan, Everson, & Lynch, 2000). In 2000, the Healthy People 2010 initiative identified the elimination of health disparities as a primary objective; however, a lack of consensus on definition, pathways, and mechanisms remains a significant barrier to achieving such an aspiration (Adler & Rehkopf, 2008; U.S. DHHS, 2006).

Racial and ethnic health disparities are apparent as early as infancy and have the potential to affect a child's health status from that point onward. Because such disparities are so widespread and persistent throughout the lifespan, understanding the origin and etiology of adult chronic diseases often begins with understanding pediatric health

and development (Harris, Gordon-Larsen, Chantala, & Udry, 2006). There are many
diseases and adverse health outcomes that can be traced back to lifestyle behaviors
developed in early childhood and adolescence, but that do not become apparent until
adulthood. Diseases related to tobacco and other substance use/abuse, poor diet, inactivity, and sexual and reproductive health generally worsen with age (Flores et al., 2005;
Gordon-Larsen, Adair, & Popkin, 2003; Harris et al., 2006). Understanding how and
why these diseases affect minority populations more severely than the non-Hispanic
white majority is a complex but necessary step in eliminating racial and ethnic health
disparities in the United States.

This chapter first presents a social-ecological framework to guide the discussion.
Within this framework, it provides a brief overview of disparities within three common
pediatric health outcomes (asthma, oral health, and obesity/Type 2 diabetes) and a discussion of how access to care relates to such disparities in the United States. The second
part of the chapter discusses determinants of health disparities principally as they are
influenced by individual, family/community, and societal factors.

A Social-Ecological Framework for Understanding Health Disparities

To better understand health disparities, it is crucial to recognize that no one factor (social,
environmental, or biological) can be identified as a single cause of racial and ethnic health
disparities; rather, the causes are multifactorial. As proposed in Figure 38.1, disparities
in health outcomes are the results of access to care and an intricate interplay among
societal, familial/community, and individual-level factors. "Upstream factors," which
include such elements as social structures, federal/state policy, and the sociopolitical
climate, can have a large impact on health inequalities; however, they are often the most

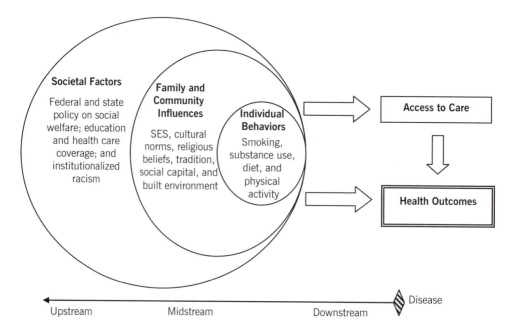

FIGURE 38.1. Understanding the determinants of racial/ethnic health disparities.

difficult to demonstrate. More proximal to health outcomes are "midstream" factors, such as family and community factors that contribute to risk of disease or poor health. Finally, "downstream" factors, which are most closely linked to the individual, include such components as behaviors and biological predispositions. The task of understanding health disparities demands the inclusion of both upstream and downstream factors.

Health Disparities within Three Common Pediatric Health Conditions

Although this is certainly not an exhaustive list, three common pediatric health outcomes (asthma, oral health, and obesity/Type 2 diabetes) show variations in prevalence and morbidity with regard to racial/ethnic groups. For example, after controlling for an extensive number of factors associated with asthma prevalence (i.e., income, education, and housing-related variables), McDaniel, Paxson, and Waldfogel (2006) found that African American children were 20% more likely than European American children to be diagnosed with asthma and to have had a recent asthmatic episode. Some experts have attributed these disparities in disease morbidity to upstream and midstream factors such as differential patterns of health care access for minority youths (Moore & Hepworth, 1994). Others have indicated that midstream and downstream factors such as family discord and stress contribute to greater difficulties in disease management (Creer & Bender, 1995).

Oral health is another condition relevant to pediatric health where disparities are present. The National Survey of Children's Health conducted in 2003–2004 found that compared to European American children, Hispanic, African American, and multiracial children had significantly greater adjusted odds of being in neither "excellent" nor "very good" oral health (Flores & Tomany-Korman, 2008). Minority children, particularly those from less affluent backgrounds, are less likely to receive appropriate preventive and restorative dental care for cavities and related dental ailments (U.S. DHHS, 1991). To eliminate such disparities, it has been recommended that greater effort be placed on remedying upstream (e.g., increasing insurance coverage), midstream (e.g., increasing access in low-income neighborhoods), and downstream (e.g., improving preventive oral health care behaviors among at-risk populations) factors (Liu, Probst, Martin, Wang, & Salinas, 2007).

With respect to obesity and Type 2 diabetes, national trends consistently show that compared to white children, children from racial and ethnic minorities have a higher point prevalence and demonstrate larger secular trends in overweight/obesity in the last 30 years (Freedman, Khan, Serdula, Ogden, & Dietz, 2006). Correspondingly, minority children bear a disproportionate burden of the rising Type 2 diabetes epidemic, with higher rates observed among minority adolescents (Dabelea, 2007). Health disparities such as these cannot be explained strictly through an examination of downstream factors such as an individual's behavior. Upstream and midstream factors linked to sociocultural, environmental, and community characteristics (e.g., crime rates, health policy, access to green space and recreational facilities, cultural norms, social capital), and their interactions with behaviors, must be considered as well.

Access to Care

Access to the health care system is more of an obstacle for some children than for others in U.S. society. Although the rates of uninsured children have been declining steadily since 1996, it is important to recognize that health insurance coverage (public and private) is not equally distributed among racial minorities and their white peers (Roberts & Rhoades, 2007). In 2006, the Hispanic youth population was identified as being more than twice as likely as non-Hispanic white youths to be uninsured (Roberts & Rhoades, 2007). The gaps in both access to care (insured vs. uninsured) and quality of care received (private vs. public health insurance) remind us that with regard to childhood and adolescent health, there is still significant room for improvement (Halfon, DuPlessis, & Inkelas, 2007). Halfon and colleagues (2007) suggest that the U.S. system of child health services is fragmented, and underperforming as a result. They urge the public health and biomedical community to work to transform the current system into one that optimizes health outcomes through disease prevention and health promotion.

Determinants of Health Disparities

As proposed in the framework, disparities in health outcomes are influenced by factors at the individual, community/family, and societal levels. We spend the remainder of the chapter examining these levels of influence and how they vary with regard to racial/ethnic groups.

Individual Behaviors

Individual behaviors and lifestyle choices initiated during childhood and adolescence are key determinants influencing later health outcomes. Some of the more common health-compromising behaviors include tobacco use, substance use, dietary practices and risk of obesity, and physical activity levels.

Tobacco Use

Tobacco use is the leading cause of preventable death in the United States and has been linked to a number of diseases, including some cancers, respiratory ailments, and cardiovascular disease (U.S. DHHS, 2000). The prevalence of cigarette smoking nationwide among high school students (grades 9–12) increased during the 1990s, peaked during 1996–1997, and since then has decreased slightly. Although smoking is more prevalent among European American youths, rates of smoking among African American youths have increased 80% relative to the decrease among their European American counterparts. Approximately 80% of tobacco users initiate use prior to the age of 18, and an estimated 6.4 million children (18 years old and younger) who are living today will die prematurely as adults because they began to smoke cigarettes during adolescence (Marshall et al., 2006). Special consideration should be given to these racial and ethnic differences, and future studies will be needed to address smoking among those who were not the traditional targets of prevention during the 1990s.

Dietary Practices and Risk of Obesity

McNutt and colleagues (1997) found that 9- to 14-year-old girls who were African American engaged in a greater frequency of dietary practices associated with weight gain (e.g., consuming foods high in fat content and calories) than a comparison group of European American children. Few differences have been found between minority ethnic/racial groups and their European American counterparts in the prevalence of obesity among infants and young children. These data have been interpreted to suggest that racial differences in dietary practices resulting in adult obesity occur during pre-adolescence and adolescence (Spear & Reinold, 1999). It is possible that differences in cultural beliefs about diet, weight, and preferential body shape influence eating behaviors, causing variation across ethnic and racial groups.

Physical Activity Levels

Multiple health benefits are associated with physical activity, such as prevention of hypertension, Type 2 diabetes, heart disease, depression, and osteoporosis (Harris, Caspersen, DeFriese, & Estes, 1989). A recent longitudinal study using direct measures of physical activity (accelerometers) found that more than 90% of the children between the ages of 9 and 11 met the current recommended level of 60 minutes or more of moderate to vigorous physical activity each day. By age 15, however, only 31% met the recommended level on weekdays, and 17% met the recommended level on weekends. The researchers estimated that physical activity declined by about 40 minutes per day each year until, by age 15, most failed to reach the daily recommended activity level (Nader, Bradley, Houts, McRitchie, & O'Brien, 2008). In general, increasing age and female gender was the largest predictor of physical activity levels. The small sample did not allow for analysis of race/ethnic differences. However, low income was a predictor of greater declines over time. Other larger studies do suggest race/ethnic differences. For instance, the U.S. Youth Risk Behavior Survey of students in grades 9–12 found that when its results were stratified by race, the prevalence of students having met current recommended levels of physical activity (participated in at least 60 minutes/day of physical activity for ≥5 of the 7 days) were higher among white (38.7%) and Hispanic (32.9%) than black (29.5%) students; higher among white female (30.2%) and Hispanic female (26.5%) than black female (21.3%) students; and higher among white male (46.9%) and Hispanic male (39.0%) than black male (38.2%) students (Eaton et al., 2006)

Family and Community Influences

In addition to the aforementioned behaviors and health-compromising lifestyle choices, community and familial factors have a significant impact on disparities in health outcomes. The identification of such influences marks an important shift in perceptions of disease etiology and places additional emphasis on the social determinants of health and disease.

Socioeconomic Status

Socioeconomic status (SES) represents a cluster of variables including education, occupation, and income; together, these serve as indicators of an individual's position within a social system (House & Williams, 2000). SES and cultural factors have in some cases been demonstrated to be salient determinants of health outcome, with health outcome being positively associated with SES (Wingood & Keltner, 1999). Low SES limits access to preventive health and adequate insurance coverage, increases exposure to less optimal environmental conditions, and makes the decision to maintain a healthy lifestyle a more difficult one due to financial constraints. Furthermore, children from less affluent families have decreased access to high-quality health care and to evidence-based diagnostic and treatment procedures (Wingood & Keltner, 1999). Although SES may account for some of the variance in health outcomes across racial and ethnic populations, studies suggest that the link between SES and health is more complicated than once believed, and that other factors (such as the social and built environment, family influences, and community-level influences) often mediate this interaction.

Family

Families are important to children's adoption of health-promoting practices and behaviors, such as a healthy diet, physical activity, and good dental hygiene (Brown, 2002). Moreover, when children are confronted with an illness, the family is a critical factor in facilitating adaptation and social support—variables that are crucial to adherence to treatment regimens, adjustment, and quality of life (Kazak, Segal-Andrews, & Johnson, 1995). Intergenerational patterns of lifestyle behaviors can have either protective or health-compromising influences on disease risk, and understanding these factors is becoming highly relevant to prevention efforts.

Community

Often referred to as "social capital," a community's resources—both relational and material—are believed to influence an array of health outcomes in both positive and negative manners. High levels of social capital, especially in lower-SES minority communities, encourage community empowerment and often provide access to political, economic, and social resources that would otherwise be overlooked and untapped. Investigating innovative strategies for improving social capital, especially for lower-SES minority communities, offers researchers the opportunity to extend the scope of community-level health interventions to include more upstream, ecological influences on racial and ethnic health disparities.

Built Environment

There is growing recognition that the built environment—the constructed physical structures and infrastructure of communities—has an impact on the patterns and distributions of diseases within any given population. It is believed that the differential distribution of recreational facilities, fast-food restaurants, affordable housing, parks, and the like in different neighborhoods can either increase or decrease an individual's (or, to a larger extent, a community's) risk for developing chronic diseases such as diabetes and asthma. The distances people travel to work or school, the convenience of purchasing healthy foods, and the safety and attractiveness of neighborhoods for walking and outdoor activities are to some extent controlled by the structural qualities of the built environment (Northridge, Sclar, & Biswas, 2003). Gorden-Larsen, Nelson, Page, and Popkin (2006) examined the relationship in adolescents among physical activity–related facilities, block-group SES, and rates of overweight and obesity. Findings revealed that higher-SES block groups had significantly greater relative odds of having one or more facilities, whereas lower-SES and high-minority block groups were less likely to have facilities. Thus the data clearly indicate that minority populations living in racially and ethnically segregated, lower-income neighborhoods have reduced access to parks, gyms, and other physical activity–related facilities; lower levels of physical activity; and increased levels of overweight compared to their white, higher-SES counterparts (Gordon-Larsen et al., 2006). Initiating a partnership between the fields of public health and city planning is essential to restoring and enhancing the health and vitality of the nation's places and people (Kochtitzhy et al., 2006).

Societal Factors

The etiology of a specific disease occurrence and its distribution within society has distal but important roots in the sociocultural practices of society. Upstream determinants of health are often viewed as the most difficult to change. They are rooted in the events, actions, and attitudes that make up the history of a nation, and continue to influence both political institutions and social thought. Such factors as historical context, racism, cultural competence, and policy provide a foundation to communities, families, and individuals, and are significant sources for the development and persistence of racial and ethnic health disparities.

Racism

Since its formation, the United States has been a race-conscious society. Oppression and discrimination throughout history have influenced federal and state laws, racial and ethnic settlement patterns, and social thought. When individuals indicate their race, they are not conceding to innate biological differences; they are taking on a label of a certain social status (Jones, 2000; Williams, Neighbors, & Jackson, 2003). In health research, racial status often has been used as a rough proxy for SES, genetics, and/or culture (Jones, LaVeist, & Lillie-Blanton, 1991). Some have hypothesized that racial and ethnic health disparities are in part the results of perceived racism and discrimination (Jones, 2000). For example, Collins and colleagues (2000) extended the explanation of why African Americans have a threefold greater rate of "very low birthweight" than European Americans by investigating the direct links between perceived racism and birthweight. They found positive associations between African American mothers' perception of exposure to racial discrimination and very low infant birthweight (Collins et al., 2000). In addition, perceived exposure to racism has been linked to increased levels of mental distress, depression, and elevated levels of blood pressure in the African American community (Williams & Williams-Morris, 2000). Racism can also affect health status indirectly by setting off a ripple-effect phenomenon, wherein a negative health status is the eventual outcome of a series of intricate interactions. An oversimplified example of this is that racism can restrict socioeconomic mobility, which can lead to differential distributions of SES and poor living conditions, which adversely affect behaviors, thereby resulting in disparities in such health outcomes as obesity and diabetes (Williams & Williams-Morris, 2000). As the proportion of minority populations continues to increase, it is likely that persistent racist ideals and institutions will levy a heavy toll on efforts to reduce health disparities in the United States.

Cultural Competence

In addition to racism, the lack of substantial levels of cultural competence demonstrated by health care workers is another social factor potentially contributing to health disparities. "Cultural competence" has been described as a set of academic, interpersonal, and clinical skills developed to help individuals increase their understanding of the differences and similarities within, among, and between groups (Williams, 2007). Culturally competent care providers establish collaborative partnerships between their patients and themselves that facilitate the successful and satisfactory delivery of medical care (Williams, 2007). The health care system of providers in the United States simply does not reflect the cultural diversity present in U.S. society. The system typically reflects white middle-class values and operates under the influences of such norms (Giachello & Arrom, 1997). Examples of this situation within health care systems include the failure to provide bilingual services in most medical centers, the lack of cultural sensitivity among some health care providers, and a shortage of minority providers. Frequently, negative stereotypes of racial and ethnic groups impede the relationships between consumers (i.e., the patients) and health care providers. Investing the necessary resources in improving the cultural competence of this country's health care system is a much-needed step in improving the access to and quality of care of racial and ethnic minorities in pediatric populations.

Summary and Future Directions for Practice, Policy, and Research

Among racial and ethnic minority populations, the following observations have been made: (1) Certain diseases and health conditions are more prevalent among racial and ethnic minority groups than among their majority counterparts; (2) individual health behavior may be associated with SES, cultural beliefs, familial influence, community structure and resources, and/or societal institutions and social thought; (3) insufficient economic, social, and political resources that severely limit insurance coverage relegate minority children and adolescents to a lower standard of care; and (4) differential patterns of health care utilization still exist.

Several federal initiatives have been launched to address the continued disparities in health among ethnic and vulnerable pediatric populations. For example, the Presidential Initiative on Race calls for a commitment to identify and address health disparities in minority and other vulnerable populations (Satcher, 2000). Total access (100%) and zero disparities are the major objectives of programs offered by many federal and state agencies. Eliminating these health disparities among minority youths will necessitate special efforts at promoting health, preventing disease, and delivering culturally appropriate care within local community settings. In addition, public programs such as Medicaid are available to increase access to and utilization of needed health services. The State Children's Health Insurance Program (SCHIP), implemented by states with federal matching funds, has increased the number of children who are eligible for health care coverage by supporting those families whose incomes are low but above Medicaid levels set by the states (Children's Defense Fund, 2000). The Women, Infants, and Children (WIC) program has been in existence for many years and provides needed resources (e.g., baby formula) for women and infants. We recommend that pediatric health care providers create and maintain linkages with Medicaid, SCHIP, and WIC through case management strategies for their pediatric patients and families.

Future research must be undertaken to examine in more detail the sources and pathways of health disparities among children. To meet the challenge of an increasingly diverse population, and to close the gaps in health among children from ethnic and racial minority groups, society and pediatric psychologists need to (1) understand culture and its relationship to health practice; (2) provide easy access to high-quality health care for all Americans; (3) collect and report data on health status indicators across race and ethnicity for comparison; (4) provide cultural competence training to all health and social service providers; and, finally, (5) develop strategies to increase the minority health care workforce. The Healthy People 2010 initiative was designed to encourage and facilitate progress toward two overarching goals: (1) to increase the quality and years of healthy life, and (2) to eliminate health disparities. Unfortunately, despite ongoing efforts, health disparities among population groups have remained relatively unchanged (U.S. DHHS, 2006). Although 2010 will not see the elimination of racial and ethnic health disparities, we will witness an increased awareness of the challenges the United States will face in reaching the aforementioned goals. It is anticipated that new research and innovative policy will offer a new understanding of what needs to, and what can be, done in years to come. The health and well-being of all U.S. residents are high-priority goals, and in time, with stronger partnerships, new insight, and renewed ambition, these goals can be realized.

References

Adler, N. E., & Rehkopf, D. H. (2008). U.S. disparities in health: Descriptions, causes, and mechanisms. *Annual Review of Public Health, 29,* 235–252.

Brown, R. T. (2002). Society of Pediatric Psychology Presidential Address: Toward a social ecology of pediatric psychology. *Journal of Pediatric Psychology, 27*(2), 191–201.

Children's Defense Fund. (2000). *The state of America's children.* Washington, DC: Author.

Collins, J. W., Jr., David, R. J., Symons, R., Handler, A., Wall, S. N., & Dwyer, L. (2000). Low-income African-American mothers' perception of exposure to racial discrimination and infant birth weight. *Epidemiology, 11*(3), 337–339.

Creer, T. L., & Bender, B. G. (1995). Pediatric asthma. In M. C. Roberts (Ed.), *Handbook of pediatric psychology* (2nd ed., pp. 219–240). New York: Guilford Press.

Dabelea, D. (2007). The predisposition to obesity and diabetes in offspring of diabetic mothers. *Diabetes Care, 30*(Suppl. 2), S169–S174.

Eaton, D., Kann, L., Kinchen, S., Ross, J., Hawkins, J., Harris, W. A., et al. (2006). *Youth risk behavior surveillance—United States, 2005.* Atlanta, GA: Centers for Disease Control and Prevention.

Flores, G., Olson, L., & Tomany-Korman, S. C. (2005). Racial and ethnic disparities in early childhood health and health care. *Pediatrics, 115*(2), e183–e193.

Flores, G., & Tomany-Korman, S. C. (2008). Racial and ethnic disparities in medical and dental health, access to care, and use of services in U.S. children. *Pediatrics, 121*(2), e286–e298.

Freedman, D. S., Khan, L. K., Serdula, M. K., Ogden, C. L., & Dietz, W. H. (2006). Racial and ethnic differences in secular trends for childhood BMI, weight, and height. *Obesity, 14*(2), 301–308.

Giachello, A. L., & Arrom, J. O. (1997). Health service access and utilization among adolescent minorities. In D. K. Wilson, J. R. Rodrigue, & W. C. Taylor (Eds.), *Health-promoting and health compromising behaviors among minority adolescents* (pp. 303–320). Washington, DC: American Psychological Association.

Gordon-Larsen, P., Adair, L. S., & Popkin, B. M. (2003). The relationship of ethnicity, socioeconomic factors, and overweight in US adolescents. *Obesity Research, 11*(1), 121–129.

Gordon-Larsen, P., Nelson, M. C., Page, P., & Popkin, B. M. (2006). Inequality in the built environment underlies key health disparities in physical activity and obesity. *Pediatrics, 117*(2), 417–424.

Halfon, N., DuPlessis, H., & Inkelas, M. (2007). Transforming the U.S. child health system. *Health Affairs, 26*(2), 315–330.

Harris, K. M., Gordon-Larsen, P., Chantala, K., & Udry, J. R. (2006). Longitudinal trends in race/ethnic disparities in leading health indicators from adolescence to young adulthood. *Archives of Pediatrics and Adolescent Medicine, 160*(1), 74–81.

Harris, S. S., Caspersen, C. J., DeFriese, G. H., & Estes, E. H., Jr. (1989). Physical activity counseling for healthy adults as a primary preventive intervention in the clinical setting: Report for the U.S. Preventive Services Task Force. *Journal of the American Medical Association, 261*(24), 3588–3598.

House, J. S., & Williams, D. R. (2000). Understanding and reducing socioeconomic and racial/ethnic disparities in health. In B. D. Smedley & S. L. Syme (Eds.), *Promoting health: Intervention strategies from social and behavioral research* (pp. 81–124). Washington, DC: National Academy Press.

Jones, C. P. (2000). Levels of racism: A theoretic framework and a gardener's tale. *American Journal of Public Health, 90*(8), 1212–1215.

Jones, C. P., LaVeist, T. A., & Lillie-Blanton, M. (1991). "Race" in the epidemiologic literature: An examination of the *American Journal of Epidemiology*, 1921–1990. *American Journal of Epidemiology, 134*(10), 1079–1084.

Kaplan, G. A., Everson, S. A., & Lynch, J. W. (2000). The contribution of social and behavioral research to an understanding of the distribution of disease: A multilevel approach. In B. D. Smedley & S. L. Syme (Eds.), *Promoting health: Intervention strategies from social and behavioral research* (pp. 37–80). Washington, DC: National Academy Press.

Kazak, A., Segal-Andrews, A. M., & Johnson, K. (1995). Pediatric psychology research and practice: A family systems approach. In M. C. Roberts (Ed.), *Handbook of pediatric psychology* (2nd ed., pp. 84–104). New York: Guilford Press.

Kochtitzhy, C., Frumkin, H., Rodriguez, R., Dannenberg, A. L., Rayman, J., Rose, K., et al. (2006). *Urban planning and public health at CDC*. Atlanta, GA: Centers for Disease Control and Prevention.

Liu, J., Probst, J. C., Martin, A. B., Wang, J. Y., & Salinas, C. F. (2007). Disparities in dental insurance coverage and dental care among U.S. children: The National Survey of Children's Health. *Pediatrics, 119*(Suppl. 1), S12–S21.

Marshall, L., Schooley, M., Ryan, H., Cox, P., Easton, A., Healton, C., et al. (2006). *Youth tobacco surveillance—United States, 2001 to 2002*. Atlanta, GA: Office on Smoking and Health, National Center for Chronic Disease Prevention and Health Promotion.

McDaniel, M., Paxson, C., & Waldfogel, J. (2006). Racial disparities in childhood asthma in the United States: Evidence from the National Health Interview Survey, 1997 to 2003. *Pediatrics, 117*(5), e868–e877.

McNutt, S. W., Hu, Y., Schreiber, G. B., Crawford, P. B., Obarzanek, E., & Mellin, L. (1997). A longitudinal study of the dietary practices of black and white girls 9 and 10 years old at enrollment: The NHBLI Growth and Health Study. *Journal of Adolescent Health, 20*, 27–37.

Moore, P., & Hepworth, J. T. (1994). Use of perinatal and infant health services by Mexican-American Medicaid enrollees. *Journal of the American Medical Association, 272*(4), 297–304.

Nader, P. R., Bradley, R. H., Houts, R. M., McRitchie, S. L., & O'Brien, M. (2008). Moderate-to-vigorous physical activity from ages 9 to 15 years. *Journal of the American Medical Association, 300*, 295–305.

Newman Giger, J., & Davidhizar, R. (2007). Eliminating health disparities: Understanding this important phenomenon. *Health Care Management Review, 26*(3), 221–233.

Northridge, M. E., Sclar, E. D., & Biswas, P. (2003). Sorting out the connections between the built environment and health: A conceptual framework for navigating pathways and planning healthy cities. *Journal of Urban Health, 80*(4), 556–568.

Roberts, M., & Rhoades, J. (2007). *Health insurance status of children in America, first half 1996–2006: Estimates for the U.S. civilian noninstitutionalized population under age 18.* Rockville, MD: Agency for Healthcare Research and Quality.

Satcher, D. (2000). Eliminating racial and ethnic disparities in health: The role of the ten leading health indicators. *Journal of the National Medical Association, 92*(7), 315–318.

Spear, B. A., & Reinold, C. (1999). Obesity and nutrition. In J. M. Raczynski & R. J. DiClemente (Eds.), *Handbook of health promotion and disease prevention* (pp. 171–190). New York: Kluwer Academic/Plenum Press.

U.S. Bureau of the Census. (2000). *Population projections of the United States by age, sex, race, and Hispanic origin: 1995–2050.* Washington, DC: Author.

U.S. Department of Health and Human Services (U.S. DHHS). (1991). *Healthy people 2000: National health promotion and disease prevention objectives* (DHHS Publication No. PHS 91-50212). Washington, DC: U.S. Government Printing Office.

U.S. Department of Health and Human Services (U.S. DHHS). (2000). *Reducing tobacco use: A report of the Surgeon General.* Washington, DC: U.S. Government Printing Office.

U.S. Department of Health and Human Services (U.S. DHHS). (2004). *Workgroup for the elimination of health disparities.* Washington, DC: U.S. Government Printing Office.

U.S. Department of Health and Human Services (U.S. DHHS). (2006). *Access to quality health services.* Washington, DC: U.S. Government Printing Office.

Williams, D. R., Neighbors, H. W., & Jackson, J. S. (2003). Racial/ethnic discrimination and health: Findings from community studies. *American Journal of Public Health, 93*(2), 200–208.

Williams, D. R., & Williams-Morris, R. (2000). Racism and mental health: The African American experience. *Ethnicity and Health, 5*(3–4), 243–268.

Williams, R. A. (2007). Cultural diversity, health care disparities, and cultural competency in American medicine. *Journal of the American Academy of Orthopaedic Surgeons, 15*(Suppl. 1), S52–S58.

Wingood, G. M., & Keltner, B. (1999). Sociocultural factors and prevention programs affecting the health of ethnic minorities. In J. M. Raczynski & R. J. DiClemente (Eds.), *Handbook of health promotion and disease prevention* (pp. 561–577). New York: Kluwer Academic/Plenum Press.

CHAPTER 39

Prevention of Unintentional Injury in Children and Adolescents

KERI J. BROWN KIRSCHMAN
SUNNYE MAYES
MICHAEL S. PERCIFUL

Unintentional injuries are the leading cause of death and disability in children and adolescents from ages 1 to 19 years, with over 8.5 million pediatric injuries reported in 2006. Each day, 27 children and adolescents die as a result of an unintentional injury, more than from all other childhood diseases combined (National Center for Injury Prevention and Control [NCIPC], 2008). Health threats due to unintentional injury have been recognized as largely preventable events (Philippakis et al., 2004). The prevailing view is that interactions of behavioral and environmental variables, rather than chance or fate, are most often responsible for childhood injury (Alexander & Roberts, 2002).

The conceptualization of pediatric injury and injury prevention is a multidisciplinary (e.g., psychology, public health, medicine, engineering) orchestration of theory and research. Although this chapter highlights several theoretical models, this review is not intended to be exhaustive. Several health behavior theories—for example, the health belief model (Becker, 1974) and the theory of reasoned action (Ajzen & Fishbein, 1980)—have been applied to the area of pediatric injury prevention. These health promotion models are reviewed by Wilson and Lawman (Chapter 40, this volume) and are discussed specifically in relation to injury by Gielen, Sleet, and DiClemente (2006). Other psychological models for conceptualizing injury prevention have been articulated and reviewed by Roberts, Brown, Boles, and Mashunkashey (2003). Although these models provide a framework for scientific investigation, Morrongiello and Schwebel (2008) have noted considerable limitations in the current state of pediatric injury research, including a dearth of studies that are theory-driven and sensitive to developmental and family process variables.

Identifying Children and Adolescents at Highest Risk of Injury

Although all children are susceptible to injury, research has been conducted to identify groups of children and adolescents who might be at the *most* risk for injury. This information is helpful in developing prevention efforts that will make the most impact in keeping children safe. The concepts and methods of psychology are clearly applicable to the prevention of injury in terms of improving the understanding of etiological causes, developmental sequences and risk factors, and situational characteristics.

Demographic Variables

Age and Development

Studies have consistently found that children's risks of sustaining specific types of injuries, as well as locations of the injury events, vary by age, developmental level, and current proficiencies. Since these variables are inextricably related, they are considered together in this section. The leading causes of injury for infants and young children are often related to inadequate supervision and/or environmental modification (Centers for Disease Control and Prevention [CDC], 2002a), coupled with the acquisition of new developmental abilities (Agran et al., 2003). Unintentional suffocation from choking or strangulation is the leading injury fatality among infants; for toddlers (i.e., children between the ages of 1 and 4), drowning is the leading cause of fatal injury (NCIPC, 2008). Both mechanisms are highly preventable with proper supervision. Motor vehicle collisions (MVCs) are the second leading cause of death for infants and toddlers, and the leading cause of death for school-age children and adolescents.

As children's cognitive abilities develop, they are increasingly able to make more appropriate safety decisions. Barton and Schwebel (2007a, 2007b) found evidence for developmental improvements in child safety behaviors with their research on pedestrian injuries. Older children were able to select safer pedestrian routes and demonstrated greater caution with street-crossing behaviors. These age effects are probably due to cognitive and motor maturation (Whitebread & Neilson, 2000). An interaction of age and behavioral effects may also be related to older children and adolescents' injury risk. Older children engage in risk-taking behaviors at a higher rate than younger children (e.g., DiLillo, Potts, & Himes, 1998), and demonstrate considerable peer influence (Christensen & Morrongiello, 1997). Many common injury risks for adolescents are associated with sensation seeking and/or impulsive, poorly considered behavioral choices (e.g., Jelalian, Alday, Spirito, Rasile, & Nobile, 2000). Thus decreasing risk-taking behaviors in older children and adolescents has been identified as a key area for intervention (Morrongiello & Lasenby-Lessard, 2007).

Gender

Male gender has consistently been identified as a risk factor for injury (e.g., Assailly, 1997). Schwebel and Gaines (2007) have noted the importance of considering engagement opportunity; boys may be more likely to engage in outdoor activities and chores, which often pose a higher risk of injury than indoor tasks. Furthermore, parenting practices may play a role in observed gender differences in injury risk behavior. Colloquial phrases such as "Boys will be boys" and "Boys don't cry" illustrate common socialization differences that have been empirically supported (e.g., Morrongiello & Dawber, 2000). Examples include encouraging boys to engage in risk-taking behaviors and providing less consolation after injuries, compared with similar situations involving girls. In addition, studies examining children's responses to injury have noted gender diversity in both injury-related cognition and behavior: Boys have been found to attribute injury more consistently to bad luck, whereas girls report a greater responsibility for behavior and are more likely to make changes to reduce injury risk in the future (Hillier & Morrongiello, 1998).

Ethnicity

Significant ethnic disparities have been noted in childhood mortality rates due to unintentional injury (Bernard, Paulozzi, & Wallace, 2007). Among all age groups, Native Americans (including American Indians and Alaska Natives) and African Americans demonstrate twice the risk of other groups. Among African American infants, suffocation was the primary mechanism of fatal unintentional injury, whereas MVCs were implicated more often in Native American populations across age groups. Native American children also demonstrate elevated rates of drowning, and African American children demonstrate elevated rates of death due to burns. Disparities across ethnic groups may be due in part to infant sleeping placements (Hauck et al., 2003); differential access to pools and states of housing disrepair (Shenassa, Stubbendick, & Brown, 2004); and higher rates of alcohol-related MVCs and lower rates of seat belt use on Native American reservations (National Highway Traffic Safety Administration [NHTSA], 2005). The reduction of health disparities is one of the two overarching goals outlined by the CDC in the *Healthy People 2010* report, which establishes health objectives for the United States through identifying preventable threats (CDC, 2000).

Socioeconomic Status

Although mortality rates for children and adolescents have declined throughout the past 30 years, children from higher-socioeconomic-status (higher-SES) families have demonstrated greater declines than their lower-SES counterparts (Bernard et al., 2007; Singh & Kogan, 2007). Between the years 1969 and 1971, children from the lowest-SES families demonstrated a 69% higher risk of sustaining unintentional injury than children from higher-SES families. This risk increased to 177% for the time period of 1998–2000. Children from low-SES backgrounds are at a greater risk of sustaining pedestrian injuries, poisonings, and burns (Groom, Kendrick, Coupland, Patel, & Hippisley-Cox, 2006; Lyons, Jones, Deacon, & Heaven, 2003). Differences in parenting practices may play a role in SES-related disparities. Previous research indicates that families from lower-SES backgrounds are more likely to allow independent outdoor play at younger ages (Soori & Bhopal, 2002). In addition, differential access to exposure opportunities, such as lack of access to safe outdoor play areas (Christie, Ward, Kimberlee, Towner, & Sleney, 2007) and resources (e.g., lower usage of bicycle helmets) (Lang, 2007), is likely to play a role in this discrepancy and may contribute to the increased prevalence of pedestrian injuries in lower-SES neighborhoods (Schwebel & Gaines, 2007). Nonetheless, it should be noted that despite the trend for higher risks in lower-SES families, families of higher SES have been found to have as many or more safety hazards in their homes as families of lower economic standing (Mayes, 2006).

Child and Parental Characteristics Associated with Injury

Child Behavior

A multinational study found that a greater number of risk-taking behaviors is associated with an increased risk of sustaining medically treated injury (Pickett et al., 2002). Furthermore, sensation-seeking behaviors have been associated with increased injury risk in adolescents (Heino, van der Molen, & Wilde, 1996). Prior experience with a given situation also plays a role in children's perceived injury risk. DiLillo and colleagues (1998) found that risk appraisal of a situation was decreased under circumstances where children had more experience with the situation. Variables such as sensation seeking and previous injury history were associated with lower risk appraisals of potentially dangerous situations. Schwebel, Speltz, Jones, and Bardina (2002) examined injury risk among boys with disruptive behavior disorders. They found that children with comorbid attention-deficit/hyperactivity disorder (ADHD) and oppositional defiant disorder evidenced twice as many injuries as individuals with ADHD alone. This study indicates that behavioral noncompliance is a separate risk variable from activity level and impulsivity, with implications for parent-centered intervention.

Child Temperament

Studies have identified temperamental characteristics with fairly consistent links to unintentional injury, such as high activity level and impulsivity (e.g., Matheny, 1987; Schwebel & Bounds, 2003). Boles, Roberts, Brown, and Mayes (2005) determined that children with higher ratings of temperamental activity were less likely to perceive themselves as vulnerable to injury under potentially hazardous circumstances. High activity levels have also been associated with decreased knowledge of safety rules (Mayes, Roberts, Boles, & Brown, 2006). Furthermore, ADHD and the poor decision making and impulsivity associated with it have been implicated in more complex risk behaviors, such as pedestrian behaviors, bicycling, and driving (Barkley, Murphy, & Kwasnik, 1996; Barton & Schwebel, 2007b; DiScala, Lescohier, Barthel, & Li, 1998). Schwebel, Brezausek, Ramey, and Ramey (2004) highlighted the interaction between child temperament and parenting behaviors. They found that environments demonstrating a "goodness of fit" between child characteristics and parenting behaviors may be protective for children who demonstrate high-risk behaviors. Barton and Schwebel (2007b) found further evidence that with increased supervision, children with lower levels of inhibitory control were able to make safer street-crossing decisions, thus lowering their risk of sustaining a pedestrian injury.

Parental Supervision

Parental supervision is certainly one of the most important injury prevention strategies for young children. Despite its consistent endorsement as an injury control mechanism, there is no "gold standard" for appropriate levels of supervision (Peterson, Ewigman, & Kivlahan, 1993), and the concept of "supervision" is ill defined in the literature (Morrongiello, 2005). One of the difficulties in decision making regarding appropriate versus inappropriate levels of supervision is that the determination is often based on the outcome (Saluja et al., 2004). Indeed, some children who are under parental supervision will sustain injury, whereas some unsupervised children will remain unharmed. In fact, Cody, Quraishi, Dastur, and Mickalide (2004) found that 88% of drownings occurred while the children were under adult supervision. Such statistics highlight the need for greater understanding of the supervision process, so that much-needed improvements can be identified and made. One area for further investigation is the influence of distraction during supervision; Boles and Roberts (2008) found that child risk behavior increased while parental attention was focused on other tasks.

Parenting beliefs and cognitions also influence supervisory behaviors. Morrongiello and Major (2002) found that parents were more likely to allow their children to take risks when the children were wearing safety equipment and when the children had more experience with a given activity (e.g., with a particular sport). Furthermore, Schwebel, Hodgens, and Sterling (2006) observed the interactions of children with behavior disorders and their parents in a "hazard room." Parental nonresponse to child risk behavior was significantly related to child injury risk. They speculated that poor supervision may be one mechanism associated with an increased risk of child injury among children with disruptive behavior disorders. These studies highlight the combined and interactive effects of parent and child characteristics in obtaining optimal levels of supervision.

Taken as a whole, the findings on supervision strategies to date indicate overwhelming evidence for reduction of child risk behaviors and injury. Furthermore, the existing literature has progressed to identify specific behaviors and characteristics that may serve to enhance or decrease the effectiveness of supervisory practices. In conclusion, these findings provide evidence that although supervision is clearly a significant mechanism of injury control for children, it is likely to be just one component in a dynamic interplay of optimal parental protective behaviors, environmental modifications, and regulatory policies.

Approaches to Preventing Pediatric Injury

"Prevention" denotes action taken in anticipation of an event, and in the case of unintentional injury, such action would result in the reduction or elimination of negative outcomes resulting from injury events (if not of the events themselves). Prevention interventions may be "primary," "secondary," or "tertiary" in nature (Caplan, 1964). Primary prevention involves strategies to keep an injury event from occurring, and fosters conditions to reduce every child's chance of injury (e.g., reduced highway speed limits). Secondary prevention applies to the prevention of injury in a high-risk situation or for high-risk individuals (e.g., window guards in high-rise apartment buildings). Tertiary prevention attempts to prevent or minimize impairment following an injury event (e.g., rapid emergency response).

These levels of prevention may be accomplished by using intervention strategies that can be conceptualized as either "passive" or "active." Passive prevention requires little or no individual effort to benefit from the prevention strategy and often involves environmental changes to build in safety (e.g., soft materials for playground surfaces). Active prevention, in contrast, requires recurrent action to obtain consistent safety benefits. Exemplars include buckling children into safety seats or actively supervising children in the bathtub. Damashek and Peterson (2002) have argued for the conceptualization of prevention on a passive–active continuum, noting that most prevention strategies are neither purely passive nor active. For example, supervising a child arguably requires more frequent and effortful action than installing child locks on cabinet doors, although both methods are classified as active strategies. Use of the entire passive–active continuum is necessary to decrease childhood injuries, as not all situations are amenable to passive approaches, and behavioral change is often required for optimal effect.

Interventions to decrease the rates of injury in infants, children, and adolescents have targeted one or more of the following areas: the environment (i.e., structural changes), legislative regulations, and human behavior. It should be recognized that these approaches overlap to some degree, and certainly interact and combine to effectively prevent injury. Representative examples for common forms of injury are described, but the following list is not exhaustive (see additional examples in Roberts, Brown, Boles, Mashunkashey, & Mayes, 2003).

Environmental and Legislative Interventions

Environmental changes are structural modifications that either remove potential hazards or separate humans from hazards to create safer conditions. Such structural changes range from abating lead paint in housing to having children wear flame-retardant sleepwear, and often are implemented as the results of legislative regulations. Of course, legislative interventions for safety are only as effective as the enforcement of these laws.

Motor Vehicle Safety

As noted earlier, MVCs are among the leading causes of childhood mortality. Proper use of child safety seats (Zaza, Sleet, Thompson, Sosin, & Bolen, 2001) and booster seats (Durbin, Elliott, & Winston, 2003) has been associated with decreased morbidity and mortality from MVC injuries. With the implementation of child restraint laws (beginning with Tennessee in 1978), use of safety seats for children has increased. By 1985, all states had passed child safety seat legislation. More recently, many states have enhanced their child passenger laws to include booster seat provisions for older children. In a large national study of children involved in MVCs, children in states with booster seat laws were 39% more likely to be appropriately restrained than children from states without comparable laws were (Winston, Kallan, Elliott, Xie, & Durbin, 2007). For adolescents, a national study of fatal MVCs between 1994 and 2004 found a reduction of 20% in mortality rates as a result of state-mandated graduated licensing programs (Chen, Baker, & Li, 2006). These programs establish nighttime driving restrictions, passenger load restrictions, and minimum requirements for supervised driving time. In addition, passive interventions, such as the implementation of daytime running lights, strengthening of side door beams in motor vehicles, and antilock braking systems, reduce injury rates for passengers of all age groups (Dewar, 2002).

In addition to MVCs, over 9,100 children were treated in hospital emergency rooms following non-traffic-related automotive incidents in a 1-year time period (CDC, 2002). Such incidents include vehicle backovers and asphyxiation by rear windows. In February 2008, the Cameron Gulbransen Kids and Cars Safety Act of 2007 was passed; as a result, all cars must now come equipped with safety features such as rear window sensors that detect obstruction and reverse direction. Furthermore, the NHTSA will establish policies to increase rear visibility standards to prevent drivers from backing over children.

Home Safety

The majority of injuries sustained by young children occur in and around the home (Phelan, Khoury, Kalkwarf, & Lanphear, 2005). The primary causes of household injury fatalities for children are fire/burns, suffocation, drowning, firearms, and poisonings, whereas falls are associated with most nonfatal residential injuries in this age group (McDonald, Girasek, & Gielen, 2006). Previous research has identified numerous vectors for household interventions. Nationwide regulations requiring 4-inch spacing between balcony rails, with the majority of codes requiring a 36-inch height regulation, have added to a stable decrease in childhood fall injuries (American Academy of Pediatrics [AAP], 2001). Window stops, which limit the opening of windows to 4 inches, may also be an effective option for fall prevention. Legislation mandating manufacturers to produce childproof containers for poisons and medications resulted in an effective reduction of childhood poisonings (Walton, 1982). Furthermore, regulations regarding the manufacture and design of cribs have helped to reduce the risk of infant strangulation and suffocation deaths in the sleeping environment (McDonald et al., 2006).

Prevention of Burn Injury

Childhood burns due to flammable sleepwear have been substantially reduced since the Flammable Fabrics Act of 1967 was signed into law (McLoughlin, Clarke, Stahl, & Crawford, 1977). Similarly, production of water heaters preset with safer temperatures (i.e., 120–125°F) have reduced household scalding injuries. Housing codes with more stringent standards for electrical wiring and smoke detectors have also initiated structural changes that have effectively reduced fire-related injury. Furthermore, Smith, Greene, and Singh (2002) revealed that 1994 legislation requiring child-resistant lighters led to a 58% annual decrease in fires, deaths, injuries, and property loss related to disposable lighters. More recently, Smith, Splaingard, Hayes, and Xiang (2006) found that smoke detectors that featured a recording of a child's mother's voice, calling the child by name and issuing specific instructions, were significantly more likely to awaken children and decrease reaction time than traditional tone alarms.

Recreational Safety

Unintentional head injuries account for about two-thirds of deaths related to bicycling (Powell, 2003). The use of helmets decreases the risk of head injury for children and adolescents by 69–74% (Thompson, Rivara, & Thompson, 1996). Although there is no federal helmet law, 21 states have laws that require riders under the age of 17 (sometimes 18) to wear a helmet while riding a bicycle (Bicycle Helmet Safety Institute, 2008). Although helmet legislation has been found to decrease the rate of pediatric head injuries (Pardi, King, Salemi, & Salvator, 2007), laws that mandate the use of helmets for other wheeled sports (e.g., skateboarding) are less common. Dannenberg, Gielen, Beilenson, Wilson, and Joffe (1993) found that rates of childhood helmet use are over two times greater in communities with helmet legislation than those relying solely on education.

Both the rate and severity of pediatric all-terrain vehicle (ATV) injuries have increased in recent years (Su, Hui, & Shaw, 2006), despite recommendations by the AAP (2000) against the use of ATVs by children under the age of 16. Pediatric ATV injuries increased 54% from 1997 to 2004 (U.S. Consumer Product Safety Commission [U.S. CPSC], 2008), with the risk of death 4–12 times greater than that of adult comparison groups. Some states have enacted mandatory helmet laws or machine-related requirements (i.e., engine size limitations for those under age 16). ATV-related death rates in these states are two times lower than in states without similar legislation (e.g., Helmkamp, 2001). Although ATV-related safety legislation is increasing, levels of compliance and enforcement remain unclear (Kirkpatrick, Puffinbarger, & Sullivan, 2007).

Playground Safety

There are 200,000 medically attended playground injuries per year (U.S. CPSC, 2003), with the majority of these injuries resulting from unintentional falls (Macarthur, Hu, Wesson, & Parkin, 2000). The prevention of playground-related injuries has largely focused on the interaction between height of fall and the playground's undersurface. Vidair, Hass, and Schlag (2007) found that structural changes to playground surfaces—including the use of shock-absorbing unitary materials (i.e., shredded tire and polyurethane binder) or loose-fill material (e.g., mulch, rubber-like materials)—are appropriate for injury reduction, as has been recommended by the CDC.

Consumer Product Safety

The U.S. CPSC was established in 1972 to improve the safety of manufactured goods marketed to the public. A number of legislative acts are enforced by this agency, with considerable evidence of their effectiveness in reducing childhood injury (e.g., the Poison Prevention Packaging Act of 1970, the Flammable Fabrics Act of 1967). However, the U.S. CPSC has relatively limited power and is restricted in its reach; not all consumer products are reviewed, although the public perceives that all marketed products have been deemed safe (Christoffel & Christoffel, 1989). One of the primary responsibilities of the U.S. CPSC is overseeing the recall of unsafe products. Over 1,000 different child products and toys have been recalled and are currently described on the U.S. CPSC website (see *www.cpsc.gov*), including over 60 million units of child products recalled in the past decade. Poorly designed children's products have been associated with suffocation, lead poisoning, entrapment, asphyxiation, burns, poisoning, falls, and lacerations. Of concern is the finding that many recalled children's products remain for sale secondhand on the Web, with a 70% resale rate to other consumers (Brown Kirschman & Smith, 2007). The Consumer Product Safety Improvement Act of 2008 was recently signed into law and will further empower the U.S. CPSC to declare mandatory recalls, as well as to enforce stricter penalties and bans for manufacturers who distribute children's products containing toxic chemicals. This legislation will also allow additional resources for U.S. CPSC product testing and establish predistribution testing standards for manufacturers.

Modification in Human Behavior

Psychological principles of behavioral change have been recognized as key components in persuading individuals to implement safety modifications or decrease risk behaviors (e.g., DiLillo, Peterson, & Farmer, 2002; Roberts, Fanurik, & Layfield, 1987). Previous behavioral injury prevention efforts have relied primarily on education. The rationale was that families would alter their behavior if provided with information that described how to prevent common injuries. Unfortunately, such interventions have not yielded empirical success (Deal, Gomby, Zippiroli, & Behrman, 2000). Rewards, incentives, and comprehensive community programs that include provision of safety gear (e.g., smoke detectors) have demonstrated greater effectiveness in behavior change.

Community Campaigns

Many community-based programs have obtained equivocal results (e.g., Terzidis et al., 2007); however, a few model programs have demonstrated improvement in safety behavior following educational campaigns. For example, the King County Booster Seat Campaign was a community-based program designed to increase the use of booster seats in children ages 4–8 (Ebel, Koepsell, Bennett, & Rivara, 2003). The program, aimed at caregivers and children, featured a focused public health message delivered via multiple media outlets and provided booster seats at reduced cost to eligible families. Observations of over 3,500 booster-eligible children 15 months after the intervention revealed a significant increase in booster seat use as a result of the campaign, doubling the preintervention use rates.

For many comprehensive community programs, the goal is to promote a culture of safety by activating schools, hospitals, service clubs, and other key community players; however, the methodological challenges of assessing multicomponent programs have been duly noted (Nilsen, 2005), and few of these programs have been evaluated empirically (Spinks, Turner, McClure, & Nixon, 2004). Furthermore, of those programs that have reported changes in knowledge of injury prevention, the extent to which increased safety knowledge translates into changes in safety behavior remains largely speculative. In a survey of the literature, Spinks and colleagues (2004) found only 9 formally evaluated community-based all-cause pediatric injury prevention programs that assessed injury outcomes using either pre–post designs ($n = 2$) or control groups ($n = 7$). The authors noted a clear need to increase efforts in establishing evidence supporting community-based injury prevention efforts. Other scholars have noted the need to identify which combination of strategies works best in what communities (Nilsen, 2005). For example, the Safe Kids/Healthy Neighborhoods program, implemented in central Harlem in New York City, involved renovating playgrounds, organizing activities for youths, educating children about injury and violence prevention, and providing safety equipment at reduced cost (Davidson et al., 1994). The program significantly decreased the number of injuries in youths in the targeted age group (5–16 years old) from the targeted injury causes (e.g., MVCs, firearms).

Physician Counseling/Anticipatory Guidance

Health care providers have multiple opportunities to provide families with injury prevention materials; these include such venues as clinics, emergency rooms, hospitals, and physicians' offices (DiGuiseppi & Roberts, 2000). Simon and colleagues (2006) found that infants of parents who received less frequent injury guidance from their pediatricians were more likely to have subsequent medically attended injuries by 16 months of age. Longitudinal studies are needed to better understand the influence of physician counseling on behavioral safety practices.

Although injury rates are rarely examined, there is support for the idea that physician counseling increases some types of parental safety behaviors, which in turn should keep their children safer. Injury messages that are tailored to the risk behaviors of a particular family (Nansel, Weaver, Jacobsen, Glasheen, & Kreuter, 2008) and are paired with additional safety and counseling instructions (Gielen et al., 2001) have been found to be most helpful in changing parental safety behaviors. A review of 22 randomized controlled trials by DiGuiseppi and Roberts (2000) found that clinical setting interventions emphasizing reinforcement of precautionary behaviors or resources to implement those behaviors demonstrated significant short-term improvement in motor vehicle restraint use; long-term effects were limited. Interventions that relied solely on education, however, revealed only modest postcounseling effects on seat belt use, helmet use, or injury outcomes. In a formal approach to integrate injury counseling into pediatric practices, the AAP initiated the Injury Prevention Project (TIPP) in 1983. TIPP includes age-appropriate injury guidelines (infancy through adolescence), safety surveys, and take-home safety sheets to be used by physicians when counseling families about injury risks (Gardner, 2007). Despite the recommendations of the AAP, fewer than 50% of families reported that they had received injury prevention counseling at their children's last well-child visit (Chen, Kresnow, Simon, & Dellinger, 2007). Counseling was reported to occur most frequently among families with infants.

Rewards and Incentive Programs

Interventions designed to reward parents and children for decreasing risky behavior have been shown to have positive effects. For instance, Roberts and Fanurik (1986) rewarded children's use of seat belts when arriving at school. Passengers who arrived at school wearing seat belts properly were awarded various prizes (e.g., stickers, coloring books, bumper stickers). A significant increase in seat belt use occurred—from 18 to 63%—in the participating schools. Roberts, Fanurik, and Wilson (1988) later implemented a community-wide intervention for 25 elementary schools with similar success. Another reward-based intervention, the Stamp-In-Safety program, was established to increase the attentiveness of preschool teachers during playground activities (Schwebel, Summerlin, Bounds, & Morrongiello, 2006). Teachers in this program rewarded children for engaging in safe play behavior. Using a quasi-experimental time series design, the investigators found that teachers demonstrated more frequent supervisory behaviors (e.g., reduced conversation among teachers) during the intervention, with continued improvement 6 months after the intervention. The use of reinforcement may be helpful in increasing safety behaviors among older children and adolescents as well. Brown Kirschman (2008) found increased helmet use in a sample of adolescent skateboarders when incentives for helmet use were provided discreetly. During the initial study session, adolescent participants were photographed individually with their skateboarding gear. These photos served as means to identify participants via observation (but not direct interaction) during the 30-day intervention period. Adolescents who were seen wearing a helmet on any given study day were notified via email, and were mailed their rewards (e.g., small-value gift certificates) to their home addresses.

Individual/Small-Group Training for Skills Building

Individual and group skills building is another behavior change method implemented to reduce the rates of injuries in children and adolescents. Behavioral interventions in small-group settings have proved to be useful in teaching children home safety skills (Peterson, 1984) and safe road-crossing skills (Barton, Schwebel, & Morrongiello, 2007). A promising application of skill-based training is the use of multimedia formats to simulate safety behaviors. Interactive computer software (i.e., Walk Smart) was used to teach children (grades K–3) fundamental street-crossing skills. Children in the program increased safety behaviors by nearly 40% in a real-life street simulation after the intervention (Glang, Noell, Ary, & Swartz, 2005). In another skills-based study, Gatheridge and colleagues (2004) examined the efficacy of two programs designed to prevent gun play among young children. The information-only Eddie Eagle Gun-Safe Program, developed by the National Rifle Association in 1988, was compared to a behavioral intervention using modeling, rehearsal, and feedback. In a naturalistic setting, 6- and 7-year-old children who received the enhanced intervention were significantly more likely to correctly demonstrate safer behavior upon finding a firearm than the information-only program recipients were.

Conclusions

The causes of unintentional injury are multifaceted, and thus interventions to decrease injury must be similarly diverse, including strategies across the passive–active continuum. In order to effectively decrease the occurrence of injury in childhood and adolescence, comprehensive approaches are needed, involving structural, behavioral, and legislative change. Pediatric psychology is a field with fundamental interest in improving the healthy development of children, and thus it has a significant role to play in formulating, implementing, and evaluating injury prevention activities (Roberts, 1986, 1994). Although some areas within the scope of unintentional injury (e.g., supervision) have received increased attention by psychologists since the third edition of this *Handbook* was published, the involvement of pediatric psychologists in injury has not been commensurate with the enormity of the problem. Pediatric psychologists are uniquely positioned to provide expertise in ameliorating this childhood injury epidemic via multifaceted and empirically supported interventions.

Acknowledgments

We thank Michael C. Roberts, Richard Boles, and Joanna Mashunkashey Shadlow for their contributions to an earlier edition of this chapter.

References

Agran, P. F., Anderson, C., Winn, D., Trent, R., Walton-Haynes, L., & Thayer, S. (2003). Rates of pediatric injuries by 3-month intervals for children 0 to 3 years of age. *Pediatrics, 111,* 683–692.

Ajzen, I., & Fishbein, M. (1980). *Understanding attitudes and predicting social behavior.* Englewood Cliffs, NJ: Prentice-Hall.

Alexander, K., & Roberts, M. C. (2002). Unintentional injuries in childhood and adolescence. In L. L. Hayman, M. M. Mahon, & J. R. Turner (Eds.), *Health and behavior in childhood and adolescence* (pp. 145–177). New York: Springer.

American Academy of Pediatrics (AAP). (2000). All-terrain vehicle injury prevention: Two-, three-, and four-wheeled unlicensed motor vehicles. *Pediatrics, 105,* 1352–1354.

American Academy of Pediatrics (AAP). (2001). Fall from heights: Windows, roofs, and balconies. *Pediatrics, 107,* 1188–1191.

Assailly, J. P. (1997). Characterization and prevention of child pedestrian accidents: An overview. *Journal of Applied Developmental Psychology, 18,* 257–262.

Barkley, R. A., Murphy, K. R., & Kwasnik, D. (1996). Motor vehicle driving competencies and risks in teens and young adults with attention deficit hyperactivity disorder. *Pediatrics, 98,* 1089–1095.

Barton, B. K., & Schwebel, D. C. (2007a). The influences of demographics and individual differences on children's selection of risky pedestrian routes. *Journal of Pediatric Psychology, 32,* 343–353.

Barton, B. K., & Schwebel, D. C. (2007b). The roles of age, gender, inhibitory control, and parental supervision in children's pedestrian safety. *Journal of Pediatric Psychology, 32,* 517–526.

Barton, B. K., Schwebel, D. C., & Morrongiello, B. A. (2007). Brief report: Increasing children's safe pedestrian behaviors through simple skills training. *Journal of Pediatric Psychology, 32,* 475–480.

Becker, M. H. (1974). The health belief model and personal health behavior. *Health Education Monographs, 2*(No. 4).

Bernard, S. J., Paulozzi, L. J., & Wallace, L. J. D. (2007). Fatal injuries among children by race and ethnicity—United States, 1999–2002. *Morbidity and Mortality Weekly Report, 56,* 1–16.

Bicycle Helmet Safety Institute. (2008). *Helmet laws for bicycle riders.* Retrieved April 7, 2008, from *www.helmets.org/mandator.htm*

Boles, R. E., & Roberts, M. C. (2008). Supervising children during parental distractions. *Journal of Pediatric Psychology, 33,* 833–841.

Boles, R. E., Roberts, M. C., Brown, K. J., & Mayes, S. (2005). Children's risk taking behaviors: The role of child-based perceptions of vulnerability and temperament. *Journal of Pediatric Psychology, 30,* 562–570.

Brown Kirschman, K. J. (2008). *An examination of two behavioral strategies to increase helmet-use among adolescent skateboarders.* Manuscript in preparation, University of Dayton.

Brown Kirschman, K. J., & Smith, G. A. (2007). Resale of children's recalled products: An examination of the world's largest yard sale. *Injury Prevention, 13,* 228–231.

Caplan, G. (1964). *The principles of preventive psychiatry.* New York: Basic Books.

Centers for Disease Control and Prevention (CDC). (2000). *Healthy People 2010*. Retrieved June 12, 2008, from *web.health.gov/healthypeople/document*

Centers for Disease Control and Prevention (CDC). (2002). Injuries and deaths among children left unattended in or around motor vehicles—United States, July 2000–June 2001. *Morbidity and Mortality Weekly Report, 51,* 570–572.

Chen, J., Kresnow, M., Simon, T. R., & Dellinger, A. (2007). Injury-prevention counseling and behavior among U.S. children: Results from the second Injury Control and Risk survey. *Pediatrics, 119,* e958–e965.

Chen, L., Baker, S. P., & Li, G. (2005). Graduated driver licensing programs and fatal crashes of 16-year-old drivers: A national evaluation. *Pediatrics, 118,* 56–62.

Christensen, S., & Morrongiello, B. A. (1997). The influence of peers on children's judgments about engaging in behaviors that threaten their safety. *Journal of Applied Developmental Psychology, 18,* 547–562.

Christie, N., Ward, H., Kimberlee, R., Towner, E., & Sleney, J. (2007). Understanding high traffic injury risks for children in low socioeconomic areas: A qualitative study of parents' views. *Injury Prevention, 13,* 394–397.

Christoffel, T., & Christoffel, K. K. (1989). The Consumer Product Safety Commission's opposition to consumer product safety: Lessons for public health advocates. *American Journal of Public Health, 79,* 336–339.

Cody, B. E., Quraishi, A. Y., Dastur, M. C., & Mickalide, A. D., (2004). *Clear danger: A national study of childhood drowning and related attitudes and behaviors.* Washington, DC: National SAFE KIDS Campaign.

Damashek, A., & Peterson, L. (2002). Unintentional injury prevention efforts for young children: Levels, methods, types, and targets. *Journal of Developmental and Behavioral Pediatrics, 23,* 443–455.

Dannenberg, A. L., Gielen, A. C., Beilenson, P. L., Wilson, M. H., & Joffe, A. (1993). Bicycle helmet laws and educational campaigns: An evaluation of strategies to increase children's helmet use. *American Journal of Public Health, 83,* 667–674.

Davidson, L. L., Durkin, M. S., Kuhn, L., O'Connor, P., Barlow, B., & Heagarty, M. C. (1994). The impact of the Safe Kids/Healthy Neighborhoods injury prevention program in Harlem, 1988 through 1991. *American Journal of Public Health, 84,* 580–586.

Deal, L. W., Gomby, D. S., Zippiroli, L., & Behrman, R. E. (2000). Unintentional injuries in childhood: Analysis and recommendations. *The Future of Children, 10,* 4–22.

Dewar, R. E. (2002). Vehicle design. In R. E. Dewar & O. L. Olson (Eds.), *Human factors in traffic safety* (pp. 303–340). Tucson, AZ: Lawyers & Judges.

DiGuiseppi, C., & Roberts, I. G. (2000). Individual-level injury prevention strategies in the clinical setting. *The Future of Children, 10,* 53–82.

DiLillo, D., Peterson, L., & Farmer, J. E. (2002). Injury and poisoning. In T. J. Boll, S. Bennett-Johnson, N. Perry, & R. H. Rozensky (Eds.), *Handbook of clinical health psychology* (pp. 555–582). Washington, DC: American Psychological Association.

DiLillo, D., Potts, R., & Himes, S. (1998). Predictors of children's risk appraisals. *Journal of Applied Developmental Psychology, 19,* 415–427.

DiScala, C., Lescohier, I., Barthel, M., & Li, G. (1998). Injuries to children with attention deficit hyperactivity disorder. *Pediatrics, 102,* 1415–1421.

Durbin, D. R., Elliott, M. R., & Winston, F. K. (2003). Belt-positioning booster seats and reduction in risk of injury among children in vehicle crashes. *Journal of the American Medical Association, 289,* 2835–2840.

Ebel, B. E., Koepsell, T. D., Bennett, E. E., & Rivara, F. P. (2003). Use of child booster seats in motor vehicles following a community campaign: A controlled trial. *Journal of the American Medical Association, 289,* 879–884.

Gardner, H. G. (2007). Office-based counseling for unintentional injury prevention. *Pediatrics*, *119*, 202–206.

Gatheridge, B. J., Miltenberger, R. G., Huneke, D. F., Satterlund, M. J., Mattern, A. R., Johnson, B. M., et al. (2004). Comparison of two programs to teach firearm injury prevention skills to 6- and 7-year-old children. *Pediatrics*, *114*, e294–e299.

Gielen, A. C., Sleet, D. A., & DiClemente, R. (2006). *Injury and violence prevention: Behavioral science theories, methods, and applications*. San Francisco: Jossey-Bass.

Gielen, A. C., Wilson, M. E., McDonald, E. M., Serwint, J. R., Andrews, J. S., Hwang, W., et al. (2001). Randomized trial of enhanced anticipatory guidance for injury prevention. *Archives of Pediatrics and Adolescent Medicine*, *155*, 42–49.

Glang, A., Noell, J., Ary, D., & Swartz, L. (2005). Using interactive multimedia to teach pedestrian safety: An exploratory study. *American Journal of Health Behavior*, *29*, 435–442.

Groom, L., Kendrick, D., Coupland, C., Patel, B., & Hippisley-Cox, J. (2006). Inequalities in hospital admission rates for unintentional poisoning in young children. *Injury Prevention*, *12*, 166–170.

Hauck, F. R., Herman, S. M., Donovan, M., Iyasu, S., Merrick Moore, C., Donoghue, E., et al. (2003). Sleep environment and the risk of sudden infant death syndrome in an urban population: The Chicago infant mortality study. *Pediatrics*, *111*, 1207–1214.

Heino, A., van der Molen, H. H., & Wilde, G. J. S. (1996). Differences in risk experience between sensation avoiders and sensation seekers. *Personality and Individual Differences*, *20*, 71–79.

Helmkamp, J. C. (2001). A comparison of state-specific all-terrain vehicle-related death rates, 1990–1999. *American Journal of Public Health*, *91*, 1792–1795.

Hillier, L. M., & Morrongiello, B. A. (1998). Age and gender differences in school-age children's appraisals of injury risk. *Journal of Pediatric Psychology*, *23*, 229–238.

Jelalian, E., Alday, S., Spirito, A., Rasile, D., & Nobile, C. (2000). Adolescent motor vehicle crashes: The relationship between behavioral factors and self-reported injury. *Journal of Adolescent Health*, *27*, 84–93.

Kirkpatrick, R., Puffinbarger, W., & Sullivan, J. A. (2007). All-terrain vehicle injuries in children. *Journal of Pediatric Orthopedics*, *27*, 725–728.

Lang, I. A. (2007). Demographic, socioeconomic, and attitudinal associations with children's cycle-helmet use in the absence of legislation. *Injury Prevention*, *13*, 355–358.

Lyons, R. A., Jones, S. J., Deacon, T., & Heaven, M. (2003). Socioeconomic variation in injury in children and older people: A population based study. *Injury Prevention*, *9*, 33–37.

Macarthur, C., Hu, X., Wesson, D. E., & Parkin, P. C. (2000). Risk factors for severe injuries associated with falls from playground equipment. *Accident Analysis and Prevention*, *32*, 377–382.

Matheny, A. P. (1987). Psychological characteristics of childhood accidents. *Journal of Social Issues*, *43*, 45–60.

Mayes, S. (2006). Protection motivation theory and knowledge of household safety hazards as predictors of parental home safety behaviors (Doctoral dissertation, University of Kansas, 2006). *Dissertation Abstracts International*, *67*, 3435–3530. (UMI No. 3222190)

Mayes, S., Roberts, M. C., Boles, R. E., & Brown, K. J. (2006). Children's knowledge of household safety rules. *Children's Health Care*, *35*, 269–280.

McDonald, E. M., Girasek, D. C., & Gielen, A. C. (2006). Home injuries. In K. DeSafey Liller (Ed.), *Injury prevention for children and adolescents* (pp. 123–162). Washington, DC: American Public Health Association.

McLoughlin, E., Clarke, N., Stahl, K., & Crawford, J. D. (1977). One pediatric burn unit's experience with sleepwear-related injuries. *Pediatrics*, *60*, 405–409.

Morrongiello, B. A. (2005). Caregiver supervision and child-injury risk: I. Issues in defining and measuring supervision; II. Findings and directions for future research. *Journal of Pediatric Psychology, 30,* 536–552.

Morrongiello, B. A., & Dawber, T. (2000). Mothers' responses to sons and daughters engaging in injury-risk behaviors on a playground: Implications for sex differences in injury rates. *Journal of Experimental Child Psychology, 76,* 89–103.

Morrongiello, B. A., & Lasenby-Lessard, J. (2007). Psychological determinants of risk taking by children: An integrative model and implications for intervention. *Injury Prevention, 13,* 20–25.

Morrongiello, B. A., & Major, K. (2002). Influence of safety gear on parental perceptions of injury risk and tolerance for children's risk taking. *Injury Prevention, 8,* 27–31.

Morrongiello, B. A., & Schwebel, D. C. (2008). Gaps in childhood injury research and prevention: What can developmental scientists contribute? *Child Development Perspectives, 2,* 78–84.

Nansel, T. R., Weaver, N. L., Jacobsen, H. A., Glasheen, C., & Kreuter, M. W. (2008). Preventing unintentional pediatric injuries: A tailored intervention for parents and providers. *Health Education Research, 23,* 656–659.

National Centers for Injury Prevention and Control. (2008). WISQARS (Web-based Injury Statistics Query and Reporting System). Retrieved July 14, 2008, from *www.cdc.gov/ncipc/wisqars*

National Highway Traffic Safety Administration (NHTSA). (2005). *Safety belt use estimate for Native American tribal reservations* (DOT Publication No. HS 809 921). Washington, DC: Author.

Nilsen, P. (2005). Evaluation of community-based injury prevention programmes: Methodological issues and challenges. *International Journal of Injury Control and Safety Promotion, 12,* 143–156.

Pardi, L. A., King, B. P., Salemi, G., & Salvator, A. E. (2007). The effect of bicycle helmet legislation on pediatric injury. *Journal of Trauma Nursing, 14,* 84–87.

Peterson, L. (1984). The "Safe-at-Home" game: Training comprehensive prevention skills in latchkey children. *Behavior Modification, 8,* 474–494.

Peterson, L., Ewigman, B., & Kivlahan, C. (1993). Judgments regarding appropriate child supervision to prevent injury: The role of environmental risk and child age. *Child Development, 64,* 934–950.

Phelan, K. J., Khoury, J., Kalkwarf, H., & Lanphear, B. (2005). Residential injuries in U.S. children and adolescents. *Public Health Reports, 120,* 63–70.

Philippakis, A., Hemenway, D., Alexe, D. M., Dessypris, N., Spyridopoulos, T., & Petridou, E. (2004). A quantification of preventable unintentional childhood injury mortality in the United States. *Injury Prevention, 10,* 79–82.

Pickett, W., Schmid, H., Boyce, W. F., Simpson, K., Scheidt, P. C., Mazur, J., et al. (2002). Multiple risk behavior and injury: An international analysis of young people. *Archives of Pediatrics and Adolescent Medicine, 156,* 786–793.

Powell, E. C. (2003). Non-motorized vehicles and walkers: Going for broke. *Clinical Pediatric Emergency Medicine, 4,* 103–111.

Roberts, M. C. (1986). Health promotion and problem prevention in pediatric psychology: An overview. *Journal of Pediatric Psychology, 11,* 147–161.

Roberts, M. C. (1994). Prevention/promotion in America: Still spitting on the sidewalk. *Journal of Pediatric Psychology, 19,* 267–281.

Roberts, M. C., Brown, K. J., Boles, R. E., & Mashunkashey, J. O. (2003). Prevention of injuries: Concepts and interventions for pediatric psychology in the schools. In R. Brown (Ed.), *Handbook of pediatric psychology in school settings* (pp. 65–80). Mahwah, NJ: Erlbaum.

Roberts, M. C., Brown, K. J., Boles, R. E., Mashunkashey, J. O., & Mayes, S. (2003). Prevention of disease and injury in pediatric psychology. In M. C. Roberts (Ed.), *Handbook of pediatric psychology* (3rd ed., pp. 84–98). New York: Guilford Press.

Roberts, M. C., & Fanurik, D. (1986). Rewarding elementary schoolchildren for their use of safety belts. *Health Psychology, 5,* 185–196.

Roberts, M. C., Fanurik, D., & Layfield, D. (1987). Behavioral approaches to prevention of childhood injuries. *Journal of Social Issues, 43,* 105–118.

Roberts, M. C., Fanurik, D., & Wilson, D. R. (1988). A community program to reward children's use of seat belts. *American Journal of Community Psychology, 16,* 395–407.

Saluja, G., Brenner, R., Morrongiello, B. A., Haynie, D., Rivera, M., & Cheng, T. L. (2004). The role of supervision in child injury risk: Definition, conceptual and measurement issues. *Injury Control and Safety Promotion, 11,* 17–22.

Schwebel, D. C., & Bounds, M. L. (2003). The role of parents and temperament on children's estimation of physical ability: Links to unintentional injury prevention. *Journal of Pediatric Psychology, 28,* 505–516.

Schwebel, D. C., Brezausek, C. M., Ramey, S. L., & Ramey, C. T. (2004). Interactions between child behavior patterns and parenting: Implications for children's unintentional injury risk. *Journal of Pediatric Psychology, 29,* 93–104.

Schwebel, D. C., & Gaines, J. (2007). Pediatric unintentional injury: Behavioral risk factors and implications for prevention. *Journal of Developmental and Behavioral Pediatrics, 28,* 245–254.

Schwebel, D. C., Hodgens, J. B., & Sterling, S. (2006). How mothers parent their children with behavior disorders: Implications for unintentional injury risk. *Journal of Safety Research, 37,* 167–173.

Schwebel, D. C., Speltz, M. L., Jones, K., & Bardina, P. (2002). Unintentional injury in preschool boys with and without early onset of disruptive behavior. *Journal of Pediatric Psychology, 27,* 727–737.

Schwebel, D. C., Summerlin, A. L., Bounds, M. L., & Morrongiello, B. A. (2006). The Stamp-in Safety program: A behavioral intervention to reduce behaviors that can lead to unintentional playground injury in a preschool setting. *Journal of Pediatric Psychology, 31,* 152–162.

Shenassa, E. D., Stubbendick, A., & Brown, M. J. (2004). Social disparities in housing and related pediatric injury: A multilevel study. *American Journal of Public Health, 94,* 633–639.

Simon, T. D., Phibbs, S., Dickinson, L. M., Kempe, A., Steiner, J. F., Davidson, A. J., et al. (2006). Less anticipatory guidance is associated with more subsequent injury visits among infants. *Ambulatory Pediatrics, 6,* 318–325.

Singh, G. K., & Kogan, M. D. (2007). Widening socioeconomic disparities in U.S. childhood mortality, 1969–2000. *American Journal of Public Health, 97,* 1658–1665.

Smith, G. A., Splaingard, M., Hayes, J. R., & Xiang, H. (2006). Comparison of a personalized parent voice smoke alarm with a conventional residential tone smoke alarm for awakening children. *Pediatrics, 118,* 1623–1632.

Smith, L. E., Greene, M. A., & Singh, H. A. (2002). Study of the effectiveness of the U.S. safety standard for child resistant cigarette lighter. *Injury Prevention, 8,* 192–196.

Soori, H., & Bhopal, R. S. (2002). Parental permission for children's independent outdoor activities: Implications for injury prevention. *European Journal of Public Health, 12,* 104–109.

Spinks, A., Turner, C., McClure, R., & Nixon, J. (2004). Community based prevention programs targeting all injuries for children. *Injury Prevention, 10,* 180–185.

Su, W., Hui, T., & Shaw, K. (2006). All-terrain vehicle injury patterns: Are current regulations effective? *Journal of Pediatric Surgery, 41,* 931–934.

Terzidis, A., Koutroumpa, A., Skalkidis, I., Matzavakis, I., Malliori, M., Frangakis, C. E., et al. (2007). Water safety: Age-specific changes in knowledge and attitudes following a school-based intervention. *Injury Prevention, 13,* 120–124.

Thompson, D. C., Rivara, F. P., & Thompson, R. S. (1996). Effectiveness of bicycle helmets in preventing head injuries. A case-control study. *Journal of the American Medical Association, 276,* 1968–1973.

U.S. Consumer Product Safety Commission (U.S. CPSC). (2003). *Handbook for public playground safety.* Washington, DC: Author.

U.S. Consumer Product Safety Commission (U.S. CPSC). (2008). *2006 annual report of ATV deaths and injuries.* Washington, DC: Author.

Vidair, C., Hass, R., & Schlag, R. (2007). Testing impact attenuation of California playground surfaces made of recycled tires. *International Journal of Injury Control and Safety Promotion, 14,* 225–230.

Walton, W. W. (1982). An evaluation of the Poison Prevention Packaging Act. *Pediatrics, 69,* 363–370.

Whitebread, D., & Neilson, K. (2000). The contribution of visual search strategies to the development of pedestrian skill by 4–11-year-old children. *British Journal of Educational Psychology, 70,* 539–557.

Winston, F. K., Kallan, M. J., Elliott, M. R., Xie, D., & Durbin, D. R. (2007). Effect of booster seat laws on appropriate restraint use by children 4 to 7 years old involved in crashes. *Archives of Pediatrics and Adolescent Medicine, 161,* 270–275.

Zaza, S., Sleet, D. A., Thompson, R. S., Sosin, D. M., & Bolen, J. C. (2001). Reviews of evidence regarding interventions to increase use of child safety seats. *American Journal of Preventive Medicine, 21,* 31–47.

CHAPTER 40

Health Promotion in Children and Adolescents

An Integration of the Biopsychosocial Model and Ecological Approaches to Behavior Change

DAWN K. WILSON
HANNAH G. LAWMAN

Clinicians and health care providers are interested in understanding the health-related problems that children and adolescents face, particularly as they relate to the prevention of chronic disease. Given the increasing prevalence of chronic diseases (e.g., Type 2 diabetes, cardiovascular disease, obesity) and other health-related problems among youths (Ogden et al., 2006; Weiss et al., 2004), there is an urgent need for effective intervention strategies to promote long-term healthy lifestyles that will ultimately result in disease prevention. Although some progress has been made in developing such effective interventions, sound theoretical approaches have not been well integrated in advancing the field. This chapter highlights the importance of developing theory-based interventions both for promoting healthy lifestyle behaviors (e.g., healthy diet, physical activity) and for preventing health-compromising behaviors (e.g., substance abuse, risky sexual behaviors) that are particularly relevant to children and adolescents. Our review of promising conceptual approaches for promoting healthy lifestyles in children and adolescents integrates the biopsychosocial model with ecological approaches to behavior change (Bronfrenbrenner, 1979; Schwartz, 1982). This integration is consistent with the perspective that health behaviors are multifaceted and dynamic, and are developed in a social context through personal, interpersonal, and environmental interactions.

The Need to Target Health-Promoting and Health-Compromising Behaviors

As other chapters of this book have made clear, several health-related behaviors of U.S. children and adolescents are matters of serious concern today. For example, a major challenge in the United States at present is the increasing rate of obesity among children and adolescents (Ogden et al., 2006; U.S. Department of Health and Human Services [U.S. DHHS], 1999). An estimated 17% of children and adolescents have been identi-fied as overweight or obese (Ogden et al., 2006), and the increasing rate of childhood obesity has also been associated with precursors for cardiovascular disease, Type 2 diabetes, metabolic syndrome, orthopedic complications, and certain cancers (Must & Strauss, 1999; Weiss et al., 2004). National studies indicate that the increasing obesity rate may in part be attributable to the fact that youths are engaging in more sedentary lifestyle behaviors and eating unhealthy diets (Wilson, in press). The prevalence rates of other health-compromising behaviors (e.g., substance abuse, risky sexual behaviors) among youths also continue to be challenging public health problems in the United States. Specifically, recent national studies show that 25% of high school students have reported engaging in episodic heavy drinking and that 23% of high school students report having smoked cigarettes (Centers for Disease Control and Prevention [CDC], 2006). With respect to risky sexual behaviors, national statistics indicate that over 37% of sexually active high school students have reported not using condoms during sexual encounters (CDC, 2006).

Previous research indicates that increasing health-promoting behaviors (e.g., healthy diet, physical activity) and decreasing health-compromising behaviors (e.g., smoking, drug use, risky sexual behavior) are both important in preventing the development of chronic disease in early adulthood. As an example of a health-promoting behavior, reg-ular physical activity has been positively associated with various health benefits, includ-ing decreased risk for cardiovascular disease, colon cancer, Type 2 diabetes, high blood pressure, high blood lipids, and obesity (CDC, 1996; U.S. DHHS, 2000). Healthy diets that are low in fat and calories have also been shown to reduce the risk of cardiovascular disease, obesity, diabetes, and cancer (Kaplan, Wilson, Hartwell, Merino, & Wallace, 1985; Stone, Baranowski, Sallis, & Cutler, 1995). In regard to health-compromising behaviors, interventions to decrease risky sexual behavior among adolescents have been successful at increasing contraceptive use as well as delaying the initiation of intercourse (Bennett & Assefi, 2005). As another example, drug prevention research has shown that adolescents reported less illicit drug use 6½ years after a comprehensive multilevel inter-vention (Botvin et al., 2000). Given the need to continue developing and demonstrating the effectiveness of both types of health promotion interventions for youths, investiga-tors must thoroughly understand the mechanisms that underlie health behavior change. A key aim of this chapter, therefore, is to review and highlight promising theoretical approaches that have been used by leaders in the field and that show promise for future research.

An Integrated Model of Health Promotion

Figure 40.1 presents an integrated model for understanding factors that affect health-promoting and health-compromising behaviors in children and adolescents. This inte-grated model is derived from biopsychosocial and ecologically based models, and con-siders the interactions between individuals and their environments (Brofenbrenner, 1979; Schwartz, 1982; see also DuPaul, Power, & Shapiro, Chapter 46, Kazak, Rourke, & Navsaria, Chapter 44, Reiter-Purtill, Waller, & Noll, Chapter 45, Seid, Opipari-Arrigan, & Sobo, Chapter 47, and Steele & Aylward, Chapter 43, this volume). Figure

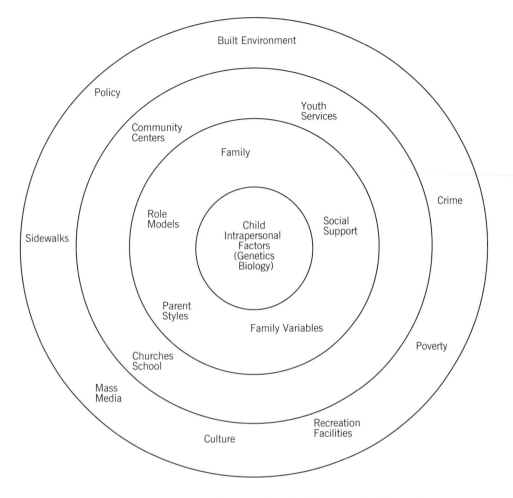

FIGURE 40.1. An ecological approach to health promotion in youths.

40.1 illustrates that health behaviors are affected by genetic/biological, intrapersonal, social, cultural, and physical environmental variables. The ecological approach as outlined by Bronfenbrenner (1979) assumes that health and health behaviors are shaped by the integration and interaction of environmental subsystems at various levels: "intrapersonal" factors (characteristics of the individual), "microsystemic" factors (families and institutions), "mesosystemic" factors (interactions between families and institutions), "exosystemic" factors (communities, policies), and "macrosystemic" effects (all systems [micro-, meso-, exo-] in relation to a culture or subculture). This approach suggests that multiple subsystems must be considered in order to reach a better understanding of what factors influence health behaviors in youths. However, investigators employing this ecological perspective have given less attention to understanding factors at the genetic and biological levels, and their interactions with factors at other levels. Thus we believe it is important to integrate the biopsychosocial model into this perspective, to give greater attention to genetic and biological factors that may influence the initiation and maintenance of specific health-promoting and health-compromising behaviors.

The biopsychosocial model integrates biological factors within the context of under-standing psychological and social factors related to health behaviors (Schwartz, 1982; Taylor, 2006). This model proposes that biological, psychological, and social factors interact in influencing youths' overall health behaviors through a dynamic reciprocal process. In particular, this model incorporates a strong focus on understanding the mechanisms by which genetics influence behaviors; it suggests that genetic influences are complex and involve the effects of multiple genes (see, e.g., Howarth, Diano, & Tschop, 2004). Previous research has shown that genetic factors play a role in regulating dietary intake (Faith & Keller, 2004) energy expenditure (Howarth et al., 2004), and physical activity (Rankinen et al., 2006). In addition, genetics have also been shown to be impor-tant in understanding the origins of alcoholism and problem drinking. For example, research based on twin studies has demonstrated a greater frequency of alcoholism in sons of alcoholic fathers than in sons of nonalcoholic fathers (Hutchison, McGeary, Smolen, Bryan, & Swift, 2002).

Given the interaction of the broad range of variables that we have outlined from our conceptual perspective, it is important to provide a review of related theories that have continued to be prominent in the field of health promotion within this context. The theoretical perspectives include models that have examined the relevance of intrap-ersonal and psychosocial factors relevant to health behavior change (see the inner circles of Figure 40.1). Below, we provide a review of these key theories and highlight how researchers have integrated these theories within the context of understanding and pro-moting complex health behavior changes in children and adolescents. Specific studies are reviewed that highlight the relevance of each theory, although the studies we have selected are not meant to provide a comprehensive perspective of the field.

Applications of Intrapersonal Theories of Behavior Change for Health Promotion

During the past decade, various psychosocial approaches have been implemented as strategies for changing health behaviors in youth. We begin this section by examining specific aspects of social-cognitive theory (SCT), such as self-efficacy theory, behavioral control theory, and outcome expectancy models (Bandura, 1986; Karoly & Kanfer, 1982). Other relevant theoretical approaches include self-determination theory (Ryan & Deci, 2000) and other motivational approaches (Resnicow et al., 2001; Wilson et al., 2002, 2005), the transtheoretical model (TTM; Prochaska & DiClemente, 1984), and the theory of planned behavior (TPB; Ajzen & Fishbein, 1980). We provide a brief review of each theory and highlight the need to expand on these theoretical models in the context of our integrated model (Figure 40.1).

Interventions Based on SCT

One of the most frequently utilized models for explaining health promotion behavior change has been Bandura's (1986) SCT. Bandura's SCT assumes that individual cogni-tive factors, environmental events, and behavior are interacting and reciprocal determi-nants of each other. The cognitive factors influencing behavioral control are said to be expectancies about outcomes and confidence in one's personal ability ("self-efficacy") to make the desired behavior change. According to Bandura, individuals who adopt challenging goals and are confident (have high self-efficacy) attain their goals more effectively than individuals who have little confidence in their ability to perform the desired behaviors.

SCT-based interventions have typically included common behavior modification components, including self-monitoring, goal setting, and behavioral skills training. For example, in a randomized trial, an intervention called Draw the Line/Respect the Line used an SCT curriculum and social inoculation approach to reduce risky sexual behavior among middle school adolescents (Coyle, Kirby, Marin, Gomez, & Gregorich, 2004). The social inoculation intervention included discussion of social pressures, developing personal sexual limits, and practicing skills needed to maintain those limits when they were challenged. The intervention helped students develop refusal skills, understand consequences of risky sexual behavior, and develop other related behavioral skills (e.g., condom use) to reduce risky sexual activities. The results showed delayed sexual initiation and significant psychosocial effects for boys receiving the intervention. Boys in the school receiving the intervention (vs. comparison schools) perceived fewer social norms supporting sexual intercourse, had more positive attitudes toward not having sex, endorsed stronger sexual limits, and were less likely to be in situations that could lead to sexual behavior. There were no significant effects of this intervention on sexual practices in girls.

This study demonstrates the usefulness of integrating SCT concepts into large-scale randomized trials for modifying long-term lifestyle habits and is consistent with other trials that have demonstrated effects on improving dietary intake and physical activity in youths (Gortmaker et al., 1999; Kelder, Perry, & Klepp, 1993). Future research is needed, however, to further our understanding of the mechanisms and mediators that are specifically linked to understanding SCT intervention components in the context of large multilevel interventions. In addition, more research is needed to explore whether biological or genetic factors may explain some of the sex differences that have been demonstrated in large-scale trials that have used SCT approaches.

Interventions Based on Motivational Theories

There have been several approaches to integrating motivational theories into health promotion interventions for youths. These theories are extensions of SCT and include cognitive dissonance theory, self-determination theory, and intrinsic motivational theory (Ryan & Deci, 2000, Wilson et al., 2005, 2008). One motivational approach to intervention involves increasing motivation by creating cognitive dissonance (inconsistency between attitudinal beliefs and behavior) and by increasing intrinsic (self-initiated) motivation (Eitel & Friend, 1999; Ryan & Deci, 2000; Wilson et al., 2002). This approach is based on a large body of research that integrates concepts from role play and commitment (Lewin, 1958), self-perception theory (Bem, 1972), and cognitive dissonance theory (Aronson, Fried, & Stone, 1991). The underlying premise of this approach is that how individuals present themselves to others has a powerful influence on how they perceive themselves and subsequently behave (Rhodewalt, 1998). Thus individuals who freely choose to commit themselves publicly to a particular identity ("I don't smoke") and a course of action (e.g., saying no to an offer for a cigarette) should be more likely to do so than individuals who only hold such beliefs privately. Findings from experimental research have demonstrated that public self-presentation has a strong influence on private self-appraisal, which in turn influences behavior (Bem, 1972). This methodology, known as "strategic self-presentation" (Wilson et al., 2002), has specifically been tested in our previous studies and has demonstrated significant increases in physical activity and healthy dietary intake in underserved adolescents (Wilson et al., 2002, 2005).

Self-determination theory is another motivational theory, which primarily focuses on behaviors that are motivated by intrinsic factors and argues that those behaviors are more likely to be sustained than behaviors that are extrinsically motivated (Ryan & Deci, 2000). That is, behavior changes motivated by intrinsic factors (such as novel, enjoyable, self-driven, and satisfying experiences) are more likely to be sustained than changes produced by extrinsic factors (such as external reward or coercion) (Ryan & Deci, 2000). Because adolescence is a time of increasing autonomy, this approach is developmentally appropriate for teens, in that it acknowledges the need for independence and self-initiated behavior change. In one study, Ferrer-Caja and Weiss (2000) examined the relationships among cognitions, intrinsic motivation, and effort/persistence in the physical education context in high school students. Teacher ratings of physical activity performance demonstrated that perceived competence and goal orientations directly predicted intrinsic motivation, and that intrinsic motivation directly predicted effort and persistence.

In summary, motivational approaches are becoming increasingly popular in health promotion interventions targeted at youths. In particular, investigators are integrating motivational strategies into multicomponent intervention trials for health behavior change. Further research is needed, however, to demonstrate what conceptual elements of motivational approaches are most effective in changing behavior and how these intrapersonal factors may interact with genetic, social, and environmental factors.

Interventions Based on the TTM

The TTM (Prochaska & Diclemente, 1984) is based on stages of readiness for behavioral change, including precontemplation, contemplation, preparation, action, and maintenance. This model proposes that tailoring an intervention to an individual's stage of readiness may be the most effective approach to promoting behavior change. The TTM has been applied to a variety of behavioral interventions for promoting long-term change in health behaviors. In a recent study, an alcohol prevention program known as Start Taking Alcohol Risks Seriously (STARS) for families was tested in a randomized controlled trial involving sixth-grade students from two urban middle schools (Werch et al., 2003). The 2-year intervention utilized family-based lessons that assessed risk factors to be targeted for reduction and protective factors (e.g., perceived susceptibility, self-efficacy, behavioral capability) to be targeted for enhancement. Together, parents and children received a program tailored to their risk/protective factors and stages of change; and they then signed contracts in which children committed themselves to avoiding alcohol and parents committed themselves to reminding children of their pledge. Results from a 1-year follow-up showed that students in the intervention had less intention to drink in the future, greater motivation to avoid drinking, and less total alcohol risk than control students. This study demonstrates that a TTM-based intervention can be effective at decreasing alcohol intake in youths, when used with a tailored motivational approach that incorporates parent support.

Relatively few studies have used TTM to promote health behaviors in children and adolescents. Some investigators have criticized the TTM by suggesting that individualized stage-based interventions are sometimes difficult to operationalize and may not be any more effective than control conditions (Miilunpalo, Nupponen, Laitakari, & Paronen, 2000). However, further research is needed to determine more clearly whether TTM approaches are useful across children and adolescents of varying ages. At younger ages, youths may not have the cognitive capacity to comprehend tailored feedback and may need the assistance and encouragement of parents in altering their health behaviors.

Interventions Based on the TPB

Ajzen and Fishbein's (1980) TPB has been applied in a number of studies evaluating health promotion interventions, albeit primarily in adult populations. The TPB focuses on identifying personal intentions as immediate determinants of behavior. Intentions are directly influenced by attitudes and subjective norms (social influence about what persons think significant others want them to do, and the motivation to conform). Attitudes and beliefs about a target behavior and consequences of performing the behavior are evaluated as either positive or negative in the context of social norms. Meta-analytic reviews of studies using the TPB have provided empirical support for the predictive capacity of a number of health behaviors (Armitage & Conner, 2001; Hardeman et al., 2002). A recent study among high school students demonstrated that a Web-based intervention incorporating TPB constructs resulted in an increase in knowledge of the importance of organ donation (Vinokur, Merion, Couper, Jones, & Dong, 2006). Although recent studies have provided support for the mediational role of intentions in enhancing health behavior change in adults (Chatzisarantis & Hagger, 2005), few studies have addressed the relevance of this approach in pediatric populations.

Critique of Intrapersonal Theories of Health Promotion

Some investigators have suggested that intrapersonal approaches to behavior change may be limited in producing long-term change in health behaviors (Wilson, 2008). In addition, only a few studies have demonstrated theoretical mediators of health behavior change in children and adolescents (Baranowski, Anderson, & Carmack, 1998). Several investigators (Sallis, Bauman, & Pratt, 1998; Wilson, 2008) have argued that investigations and applications of intrapersonal-level theoretical factors are not sufficient to alter complex health behavior patterns. Macro-level conceptual perspectives are also required, as shown in Figure 40.1; that is, the field must be expanded to include biological, social, and physical environmental factors. Thus we argue for an approach that takes into consideration a broader environmental context than many past studies have included.

Ecological and Biopsychosocial Approaches to Health Promotion

Researchers are extending the field of health promotion to include ecological perspectives (Sallis et al., 1998). To date, much of our knowledge of environmental influences on health behaviors comes from cross-sectional studies that have examined the relationship between health behaviors and actual or perceived environmental characteristics. For example, some investigators have specifically examined the relationship among neighborhood safety, availability of play space, and outdoor physical activity in adolescents (Gomez, Johnson, Selva, & Sallis, 2004). In this study, outdoor physical activity was evaluated in relation to density of violent crimes and access to play space within ½ mile of each adolescent's home. For girls, density of violent crimes within ½ mile of their homes was negatively associated with outdoor physical activity and explained 9.4% of the variance in girls' behaviors. For boys, distance to the nearest play space was inversely associated with outdoor physical activity and explained 8.8% of the variance in boys' behavior. Thus, whereas access to play space was important for predicting physical activity behaviors in boys, crime was more strongly associated with physical activity behaviors in girls.

In a study by Kelly, Comello, and Slater (2006), an in-school social marketing campaign was integrated with a community-based media intervention to decrease marijuana and alcohol use among young adolescents. Eight schools were randomly assigned to the school intervention plus community intervention, and eight schools served as the control schools. Youths in the combined intervention communities showed less use of marijuana and alcohol at posttest than youths in the control communities did. This study demonstrates the effectiveness of combining two levels of environmental factors (school and community variables) into interventions targeting reductions in health-compromising behaviors among youths.

Incorporating multiple levels of environmental variables in understanding adolescent health behavior change is important; however, further research is needed to determine how variables may interact across levels of the model presented in Figure 40.1. Below, we summarize multiple levels of our integrated model, to further our understanding of how to change health behaviors effectively in children and adolescents. We provide examples of studies that have successfully utilized microsystemic factors (families and institutions), mesosystemic factors (interactions between family and institutions), exosystemic factors (communities, policies), and macrosystemic effects (all systems [micro-, meso-, exo-] in relation to a culture or subculture).

Family-Based Approaches (Microsystemic Factors)

Several studies have examined the relationship between parental factors (social support, self-efficacy) and children's health behaviors. In a qualitative study, low-income African American adolescents reported that their parents and grandparents provided positive social support (encouragement) for eating fruits and vegetables, although they did not always provide such foods in the home (Molaison, Connell, Stuff, Yadrick, & Bogle, 2005). Adkins, Sherwood, Story, and Davis (2004) also found that parental social support (tangible) was associated with greater engagement in physical activity in African American girls ages 8–10. Interestingly, parental self-efficacy for supporting daughters to be physically active was also significantly related to higher levels of activity in daughters. A longitudinal study following children from fifth through ninth grade also showed that mothers' self-efficacy for physical activity and mothers' perceived barriers to exercise were important predictors of physical activity in girls (DiLorenzo, Stucky-Ropp, Vander Wal, & Gotham, 1998).

In an example of a study targeting health-compromising behaviors, the Chicago HIV Prevention and Adolescent Mental Health Project (CHAMP) was a family-based intervention for reducing youths' HIV exposure (McKay et al., 2004). The program delivered curriculum created to support positive family processes, such as family communication, social support, parental supervision and monitoring, and problem-solving skills. Families receiving the CHAMP intervention showed significantly better family decision making, parental monitoring, family communication regarding sensitive issues, and communication effort than comparison program families did.

In a study discussed previously, the STARS alcohol prevention program for families was tested in a randomized controlled trial with sixth-graders from two urban middle schools (Werch et al., 2003). This 2-year intervention utilized family-based lessons, as described earlier. The 1-year follow-up results were encouraging.

In summary, the studies on family-based interventions have typically addressed multiple levels of the home, family, and school environments in influencing youths' health behaviors. These studies demonstrate that involving families in programs that target health-promoting and health-compromising behaviors is an effective strategy.

Peer-Based Interventions (Microsystemic Factors)

The influence of peers on youths' behavior choices is often utilized in drug prevention programs. A review on the effectiveness of drug prevention programs indicated that peer leaders should be used to strengthen the short-term effects of such programs (Cuijpers, 2002). Furthermore, education about peer norms has been shown to decrease alcohol misuse. In the school-based Alcohol Misuse Prevention Study (AMPS; Wynn, Schulenberg, Maggs, & Zucker, 2000), middle and high school students received normative education (i.e., how common alcohol use is among peers) and peer resistance skills training. Results showed that education about peer norms concerning alcohol use mediated the effectiveness of the AMPS program. That is, such education was a specific mechanism responsible for positive behavior change in the AMPS program. This finding demonstrates the influence of perceptions of peer behavior.

This study demonstrates in particular the importance of integrating peers and school systems into health behavior change strategies. Further research is need that specifically addresses social norms and peers, given the importance of these influences as children make the transition to adolescence.

School-Based Approaches (Mesosystemic Factors)

The school environment has significant proximal influences on adolescent health behaviors, because the educational system is the main formal community institution that is responsible for the socialization of adolescents. One of the most successful drug prevention programs is Project ALERT, a school-based prevention program integrating cognitive, social, and behavioral skills theories into middle school curriculum for seventh- and eighth-graders (Ellickson, McCaffrey, Ghosh-Dastidar, & Longshore, 2003). The intervention sought to change students' beliefs about drug norms and the social, emotional, and physical consequences of using drugs; to help them resist pro-drug social pressures; and to increase their self-efficacy for resisting drugs. Eighteen months after baseline, students receiving the Project ALERT prevention intervention had lower rates of cigarette smoking initiation, marijuana initiation, and alcohol misuse than students in comparison schools.

In general, school-based intervention studies have demonstrated only modest changes in students' health-promoting behaviors. For example, the Planet Health project (Gortmaker et al., 1999) evaluated a school-based intervention in sixth- and seventh-graders over 2 years. The intervention was a physical education curriculum-based program to decrease consumption of high-fat foods and television watching, and to increase fruit and vegetable intake and moderate to vigorous physical activity. Although the intervention did reduce the overall prevalence of obesity in girls, there were no significant changes in physical activity due to the intervention, and only changes in television viewing predicted changes in obesity prevalence in this study.

Taken together, school-based approaches have demonstrated some success at influencing long-term change of both health-promoting and health-compromising behaviors in youths. However, more research is needed that evaluates the impact of integrating intervention approaches across school, home, and community environments. In addition, while a number of studies have demonstrated sex differences in outcomes, little attention has been given to understanding genetic or biological influences that may be important. Further efforts are needed to evaluate the interactions between these systems in understanding health behavior change in youths.

Community-Based Approaches (Exosystemic Factors)

Researchers have shown that community interventions through churches, supermarkets, and restaurants can influence children's and adolescents' health behaviors. A recent study by Resnicow, Taylor, Baskin, and McCarty (2005) randomly assigned 10 churches to either a high-intensity group or a moderate-intensity group targeting African American adolescent girls. The high-intensity group participated in a weekly behavioral session that included a behavioral activity, engaging in physical activity, preparing healthy snacks, and attending a retreat on group cohesion. Participants in the high-intensity group also received promotional messages via a two-way pager and telephone calls based on motivational interviewing. Participants in the moderate-intensity group received information on barriers and benefits to physical activity, fad diets, and trying new foods. No significant differences were found between the groups; however, participants in the high-intensity group who attended more than 75% of sessions had significant reductions in body mass index, compared to participants who attended fewer than 75% of sessions.

In a study evaluating health-compromising behaviors, Villarruel, Jemmott, and Jemmott (2006) conducted a randomized controlled trial of a community-based HIV prevention intervention with Latino/Latina adolescents. Six modules were delivered by adult facilitators in community-based organizations that promoted increasing positive attitudes about HIV/AIDS prevention, as well as safer sex, condom use skills, and negotiation/refusal skills (Villarruel, Jemmott, & Jemmott, 2005). Results showed that adolescents in the intervention were less likely to report having sexual intercourse, having multiple partners, or engaging in unprotected intercourse, and were more likely to report using condoms consistently, compared to adolescents in a health promotion comparison program. This study demonstrates that community-level interventions can be an effective modality for decreasing risky sexual behavior in youths.

In general, few investigators have conducted community-based interventions in children and adolescents, and more research is needed to expand this focus in this area of health promotion among youths. Limited resources make it difficult to conduct a large-scale trial of this nature, but long-term behavior change will require these broader-level approaches in order to decrease barriers to health promotion efforts.

Mass Media Approaches (Exosystemic Factors)

Messages communicated through the mass media may be particularly salient in adolescence, as decisions about adult values and lifestyles are being made and responsibility is being assumed. Kelly and colleagues (2006) tested an integrated drug prevention program in middle school students. Sixteen middle schools participated in a school-based communication campaign based on social marketing principles, combined with a community-based media effort to reduce marijuana, alcohol, and tobacco use. The message strategy of the intervention focused on greater independence and autonomy for adolescents. The "Be Under Your Own Influence" campaign utilized a variety of promotional products (e.g., book covers, tray liners, T-shirts, water bottles, and posters) and placements to accomplish individual and schoolwide behavior change. The community participated in prevention efforts by helping to identify prevention strategies appropriate to that community. In addition, community media promoted the campaign via press releases, posters, and radio public service announcements. Intervention communities had fewer users of marijuana, alcohol, and cigarettes at posttest, and growth trajectory results were significantly reduced for marijuana and marginally for alcohol.

In the area of youth pregnancy and sexually transmitted disease (STD) prevention, Roberto, Zimmerman, Carlyle, and Abner (2007) tested a computer- and Internet-based approach in rural high school adolescents. Two schools were randomly assigned to receive either an intervention or a comparison program. The intervention included interactive computer lessons on sensation seeking, truths and myths about pregnancy and STDs, impulsive decision making, risky behavior, and refusal skills, as well as a radio contest activity. Results showed that the majority of adolescents (89%) completed at least one of the computer lessons. Students receiving the computer-based intervention were less likely to initiate sexual activity, and had greater self-efficacy for condom negotiation, more favorable attitudes toward waiting to have sex, and greater situational self-efficacy, than students in the comparison program.

These results show that mass media influences can be utilized in interventions seeking to promote positive health behaviors and to decrease health-compromising behaviors. Furthermore, mass media can have positive effects on behavior not only through media-intensive interventions like the "Be Under Your Own Influence" campaign (Kelly et al., 2006), but also in more cost-effective and feasible interventions like that conducted by Roberto and colleagues (2007).

Public Policy Approaches (Macrosystemic Effects)

The field of health promotion has long endorsed the value of policy interventions. Such interventions can play a large role in health promotion efforts, as the enactment of legislation ensuring food safety and requiring seat belts to be worn has shown. However, the study of how policies affect adolescent health behaviors is relatively new, and much more work is needed to conceptualize the relevant policy variables for individuals' behaviors among this population group.

Policy concerning public schools' sex education curricula has been a topic of heated debate. Federal funding for abstinence-only programs reached its highest level in 2001 (Gold & Nash, 2001). In addition, results from a review of school superintendents showed that one-third of school districts in the country prohibited education about contraceptives unless it was to emphasize their limitations (Landry, Kaeser, & Richards,

1999). This orientation has obvious influences on the kinds of information that youths receive, which may result in differential changes in behavior. Specifically, a review was published comparing randomized controlled trials of abstinence-only programs to those including contraceptive information (Bennett & Assefi, 2005). The authors concluded that neither type of program is very effective in delaying initiation of sexual activity, but that the majority of abstinence-plus programs result in an increase of contraceptive use among youths. These studies show how public policy restricting contraceptive education can have an effect on youths' health behaviors.

Summary and Conclusions

The studies reviewed in this chapter illustrate how the field has expanded from using intrapersonal models of health promotion to incorporating social, environmental, and policy-based interventions. Furthermore, we have highlighted throughout this chapter the importance of considering genetic and biological factors in developing health promotion interventions for youths. Given that the transition into adolescence is developmentally a time of biological and social transition, all these factors will need to be incorporated into multilevel models that integrate the biopsychosocial model and ecological approaches to health behavior change. This chapter promotes the use of multiple-level approaches that also examine mediators of behavior change. This approach will help health care providers and scientists to determine why interventions are effective and under what circumstances effects can be maximized. Future research should continue to focus on integrated theoretical approaches in developing interventions that include genetic/biological, intrapersonal, social, cultural, and physical environmental variables in changing long-term health behaviors in children and adolescents.

Acknowledgment

Preparation of this chapter was partially supported by a grant (No. R01 HD 045693) funded by the National Institutes of Child Health and Human Development to Dawn K. Wilson.

References

Adkins, S., Sherwood, N., Story, M., & Davis, M. (2004). Physical activity among African-American girls: The role of parents and the home environment. *Obesity Research, 12,* 38S–45S.

Ajzen, I., & Fishbein, M. (1980). *Understanding attitudes and predicting social behavior.* Englewood Cliffs, NJ: Prentice-Hall.

Armitage, C. J., & Conner, M. (2001). Efficacy of the theory of planned behaviour: A meta-analytic review. *British Journal of Social Psychology, 40,* 471–499.

Aronson, E., Fried, C. B., & Stone, J. (1991). Overcoming denial and increasing the intention to use condoms through the induction of hypocrisy. *American Journal of Public Health, 81,* 1636–1638.

Bandura, A. (1986). *Social foundations of thought and action.* Englewood Cliffs, NJ: Prentice-Hall.

Baranowski, T., Anderson, C., & Carmack, C. (1998). Mediating variable framework in physical activity interventions: How are we doing? How might we do better? *American Journal of Preventive Medicine, 15,* 266–297.

Bem, D. J. (1972). Self-perception theory. In L. Berkowitz (Ed.), *Advances in experimental social psychology* (Vol. 6, pp. 1–62). New York: Academic Press.

Bennett, S. E., & Assefi, N. P. (2005). School-based teenage pregnancy prevention programs: A systematic review of randomized controlled trials. *Journal of Adolescent Health, 36,* 72–81.

Botvin, G. J., Griffin, K. W., Diaz, T., Scheier, L. M., Williams, C., & Epstein, J. A. (2000). Preventing illicit drug use in adolescents: Long-term follow-up data from a randomized control trial of a school population. *Addictive Behaviors, 25*(5), 769–774.

Bronfenbrenner, U. (1979). *The ecology of human development: Experiments by nature and design.* Cambridge, MA: Harvard University Press.

Centers for Disease Control and Prevention (CDC). (1996). *Physical activity and health: A report of the Surgeon General.* Atlanta, GA: Author.

Centers for Disease Control and Prevention (CDC). (2006). Youth risk behavior surveillance: United States, 2005. *Morbidity and Mortality Weekly Report, 55*(SS-5).

Chatzisarantis, N. L. D., & Hagger, M. S. (2005). Effects of a brief intervention based on the theory of planned behaviour on leisure-time physical activity participation. *Journal of Sport and Exercise Psychology, 27,* 470–487.

Coyle, K. K., Kirby, D. B., Marin, B. B., Gomez, C. A., & Gregorich, S. E. (2004). Draw the Line/Respect the Line: A randomized trial of a middle school intervention to reduce sexual risk behaviors. *American Journal of Public Health, 94,* 843–851.

Cuijpers, P. (2002). Effective ingredients of school-based drug prevention programs: A systematic review. *Addictive Behaviors, 27,* 1009–1023.

DiLorenzo, T. M., Stucky-Ropp, R. C., Vander Wal, J. S., & Gotham, H. J. (1998). Determinants of exercise among children: II. A longitudinal analysis. *Preventive Medicine, 27,* 470–477.

Eitel, P., & Friend, R. (1999). Reducing denial of STD and HIV risk in college students: A comparison of a cognitive and motivational approach. *Annals of Behavioral Medicine, 21,* 12–19.

Ellickson, P. L., McCaffrey, D. F., Ghosh-Dastidar, B., & Longshore, D. L. (2003). New inroads in preventing adolescent drug use: Results from a large-scale trial of Project ALERT in middle schools. *American Journal of Public Health, 93,* 1830–1836.

Faith, M. S., & Keller, K. L. (2004). Genetic architecture of ingestive behavior in humans. *Nutrition, 20*(1), 127–133.

Ferrer-Caja, E., & Weiss, M. R. (2000). Predictors of intrinsic motivation among adolescent students in physical education. *Research Quarterly for Exercise and Sport, 71,* 267–279.

Gold, R. B., & Nash, B. (2001). State-level policies on sexuality, STD education. *Issues in Brief, 5,* 1–4.

Gomez, J. E., Johnson, B. A., Selva, M. S., & Sallis, J. F. (2004). Violent crime and outdoor physical activity among inner-city youth. *Preventive Medicine, 39,* 876–881.

Gortmaker, S. L., Peterson, K., Wiecha, J., Sobol, A. M., Dixit, S., Fox., M. K., et al. (1999). Reducing obesity via a school-based interdisciplinary intervention among youth. *Archives of Pediatrics and Adolescent Medicine, 153,* 409–418.

Hardeman, W., Johnston, M., Johnston, D. W., Bonetti, D., Wareham, N. J., & Kinmonth, A. L. (2002). Application of the theory of planned behaviour in behaviour change interventions: A systematic review. *Psychology and Health, 17,* 123–158.

Howarth, T., Diano, S., & Tschop, M. (2004). Brain circuits regulating energy homeostasis. *The Neuroscientist, 10*(3), 235–246.

Hutchison, K. E., McGeary, J., Smolen, A., Bryan, A., & Swift, R. M. (2002). The DRD4

VNTR polymorphism moderates craving after alcohol consumption. *Health Psychology*, *21*, 139–146.

Kaplan, R. M., Wilson, D. K., Hartwell, S. L., Merino, K. L., & Wallace, J. P. (1985). Prospective evaluation of HDL cholesterol changes after diet and physical conditioning programs for patients with type II diabetes mellitus. *Diabetes Care*, *8*(4), 343–348.

Karoly, P., & Kanfer, F. H. (Eds.). (1982). *Self management and behavior change: From theory to practice*. New York: Pergamon Press.

Kelder, S. H., Perry, C. L., & Klepp, K. I. (1993). Community wide youth exercise promotion: Long-term outcomes of the Minnesota Heart Health Program and the Class of 1989 Study. *Journal of School Health*, *63*, 218–223.

Kelly, K. J., Comello, M. L. G., & Slater, M. D. (2006). Development of an aspirational campaign to prevent youth substance use: "Be Under Your Own Influence." *Social Marketing Quarterly*, *12*(2), 14–27.

Landry, D. J., Kaeser, L., & Richards C. L. (1999). Abstinence promotion and the provision of information about contraception in public school district sexuality education policies. *Family Planning and Perspectives*, *31*, 280–286.

Lewin, K. (1958). Group decision and social change. In E. E. Maccoby, T. M. Newcomb, & E. L. Hartley (Eds.), *Readings in social psychology* (pp. 197–212). New York: Holt.

McKay, M. M., Chasse, T. K., Paikoff, R., McKinney, L. D., Baptiste, D., Coleman, D., et al. (2004). Family-level impact of the CHAMP family program: A community collaborative effort to support urban families and reduce youth HIV risk exposure. *Family Process*, *43*, 79–93.

Miilunpalo, S., Nupponen, R., Laitakari, J., & Paronen, O. (2000). Stages of change in two modes of health-enhancing physical activity: Methodological aspects and promotional implications. *Health Education Research*, *15*, 435–448.

Molaison, E., Connell, C., Stuff, J., Yadrick, K., & Bogle, M. (2005). Influences on fruit and vegetable consumption by low-income black American adolescents. *Journal of Nutrition Education and Behavior*, *37*, 246–251.

Must, A., & Strauss, R. S. (1999). Risk and consequences of childhood and adolescent obesity. *International Journal of Obesity*, *23*(Suppl. 2), S2–S11.

Ogden, C. L., Carroll, M. D., Curtin, L. R., McDowell, M. A., Tabak, C. J., & Flegal, K. M. (2006). Prevalence of overweight and obesity in the United States, 1999–2004. *Journal of the American Medical Association*, *295*, 1549–1555.

Prochaska, J. O., & DiClemente, C. C. (1984). *The transtheoretical approach: Crossing traditional boundaries of change*. Homewood, IL: Dow Jones-Irwin.

Rankinen, T., Bray, M. S., Hagberg, J. M., Perusse, L., Roth, S. M., Wolfarth, B., et al. (2006). The human gene map for performance and health-related fitness phenotypes: The 2005 update. *Medicine, Science, and Sports Exercise*, *38*(11), 1863–1888.

Resnicow, K., Jackson, A., Wang, T., De, K. A., McCarty, F., Dudley, W., et al. (2001). A motivational interviewing intervention to increase fruit and vegetable intake through black churches: Results of the Eat for Life Trial. *American Journal of Public Health*, *9*, 1686–1693.

Resnicow, K., Taylor, R., Baskin, M., & McCarty, F. (2005). Results of Go Girls: A weight control program for overweight African-American adolescent females. *Obesity Research*, *13*, 1739–1748.

Rhodewalt, F. (1998). Self-presentation and the phenomenal self: The "carryover effect" revisited. In J. Cooper & J. M. Darley (Eds.), *Attributional processes, person perception, and social interaction: The legacy of Edward E. Jones* (pp. 373–421). Washington, DC: American Psychological Association.

Roberto, A. J., Zimmerman, R. S., Carlyle, K. E., & Abner, E. L. (2007). A computer-based approach to preventing pregnancy, STD, and HIV in rural adolescents. *Journal of Health Communication, 12*, 53–76.

Ryan, D. M., & Deci, E. L. (2000). Self-determination theory and the facilitation of intrinsic motivation, social development, and well-being. *American Psychologist, 55*, 68–78.

Sallis, J. F., Bauman, A., & Pratt, M. (1998). Environmental policy interventions to promote physical activity. *American Journal of Preventive Medicine, 15*, 379–397.

Schwartz, G. E. (1982). Testing the biopsychosocial model: The ultimate challenge facing behavioral medicine? *Journal of Consulting and Clinical Psychology, 50*, 1040–1053.

Stone, E., Baranowski, T., Sallis, J., & Cutler, J. (1995). Review of behavioral research for cardiopulmonary health: Emphasis on youth, gender, and ethnicity. *Journal of Health Education, 26*(Suppl.), 9–17.

Taylor, S. E. (2006). *Health psychology* (6th ed.). New York: McGraw-Hill.

U.S. Department of Health and Human Services (U.S. DHHS). (1999). *Child health USA*. Washington, DC: Author.

U.S. Department of Health and Human Services (U.S. DHHS). (2000). *Healthy people 2010*. Washington, DC: U.S. Government Printing Office.

Villarruel, A. M., Jemmott, J. B., & Jemmott, L. S. (2005). Designing a culturally based intervention to reduce HIV sexual risk for Latino adolescents. *Journal of the Association of Nurses in AIDS Care, 16*(2), 23–31.

Villarruel, A. M., Jemmott, J. B., & Jemmott, L. S. (2006). A randomized controlled trial for testing an HIV prevention intervention for Latino youth. *Archives of Pediatrics and Adolescent Medicine, 160*(8), 772–777.

Vinokur, A. D., Merion, R. M., Couper, M. P., Jones, E. G., & Dong, Y. H. (2006). Educational Web-based intervention for high school students to increase knowledge and promote positive attitudes toward organ donation. *Health Education and Behaviour, 33*, 773–786.

Weiss, R., Dziura, J., Burgert, T. S., Tamborlane, W. V., Taksali, S. E., Yeckel, C. W., et al. (2004). Obesity and the metabolic syndrome in children and adolescents. *New England Journal of Medicine, 350*, 2362–2374.

Werch, C. E., Owen, D. M., Carlson, J. M., DiClemente, C. C., Edgemon, P., & Moore, M. (2003). One-year follow-up results of the STARS for families alcohol prevention program. *Health Education Research, 18*(1), 74–87.

Wilson, D. K. (2008). Theoretical advances in diet and physical activity interventions. *Health Psychology, 27*, S1–S2.

Wilson, D. K. (in press). New perspectives on health disparities and obesity in youth. *Journal of Pediatric Psychology*.

Wilson, D. K., Evans, A. E., Williams, J., Mixon, G., Minette, C., Sirad, J., et al. (2005). A preliminary test of a student-centered intervention on increasing physical activity in underserved adolescents. *Annals of Behavioral Medicine, 30*, 119–124.

Wilson, D. K., Kitzman-Ulrich, H., Williams, J. E., Saunders, R., Griffin, S., Pate, R. R., et al. (2008). An overview of "The Active by Choice Today" (ACT) trial for increasing physical activity. *Contemporary Clinical Trials, 29*, 21–31.

Wilson, D. K., Teasley, N., Friend, R., Green, S., Reeves, L., & Sica, D. A. (2002). Motivational versus social cognitive interventions for promoting fruit and vegetable intake and physical activity in African American adolescents. *Annals of Behavioral Medicine, 24*, 310–319.

Wynn, S. R., Schulenberg, J., Maggs, J. L., & Zucker, R. A. (2000). Preventing alcohol misuse: The impact of refusal skills and norms. *Psychology of Addictive Behaviors, 14*(1), 36–47.

CHAPTER 41

Enhancing Adoption of Preventive Behaviors
Vaccination as an Example

MARY B. SHORT
SUSAN L. ROSENTHAL
LYNNE STURM
GREGORY D. ZIMET

Pediatric psychologists typically focus on treating behavioral problems with health-related outcomes (e.g., encopresis), enhancing adherence to medical regimens, and helping individuals cope with health conditions. However, opportunities also exist for pediatric psychologists to develop evidence-based strategies at the societal, institutional, and individual levels to enhance adoption of preventive behaviors (Tercyak, 2008). Immunization is one of the preventive strategies on which pediatric psychology can have a major impact. From a public health standpoint, immunization has been among the most successful strategies, leading to decreases in the morbidity and mortality of many diseases. For example, vaccines have eradicated smallpox and led to the virtual elimination of polio (Centers for Disease Control and Prevention [CDC], 1999). This chapter reviews vaccination practices in the United States, social-environmental factors influencing beliefs about vaccination, and ways in which psychologists and others can intervene to increase vaccination.

Vaccination Practices in the United States

Vaccines have become a standard part of well-child care. In 2007, there were 14 vaccines given to U.S. children and adolescents, resulting in a total of 30–40 doses of vaccine between birth and 18 years. Several of these vaccines have been added over the last few years, including the meningococcal conjugate vaccine, a pertussis vaccine booster for adolescents, and the human papillomavirus (HPV) vaccine for adolescent girls (CDC, 2008). Overall, most parents support vaccination of their children and believe that vaccines are an important part of protecting their children (Constantine & Jerman, 2007; Gellin, Maibach, Marcuse, & the National Network for Immunization Information Steering Committee, 2000). Although most parents have their children vaccinated on the recommended schedule, approximately 36.9% of children ages 19–35 months are undervaccinated, and 0.3% of these children do not receive any vaccines. Unvaccinated and undervaccinated children are more likely to contract vaccine-preventable infections and to create public health problems by spreading these infections to others (Smith, Chu, & Barker, 2004).

Undervaccination is associated with belonging to a racial/ethnic minority, having a parent with low educational status, living in poverty or near-poverty, and having parents who are single (widowed, divorced, separated, unmarried) (Darling, Barker, Shefer, & Chu, 2005; Gore et al., 1999; Herrera, Zhao, & Klevens, 2001; Klevens & Luman, 2001; Luman, McCauley, Shefer, & Chu, 2003; Rosenthal et al., 2004; Smith et al., 2004). In one study examining vaccine coverage of U.S. children ages 19–35 months, data showed a 10–13% difference between those children living in poverty and those living above poverty (Klevens & Luman, 2001). It is unclear why these demographic variables are associated with low immunization rates; however, these parents may encounter practical barriers to getting their children vaccinated (e.g., they cannot afford the vaccine, do not get routine health care, or have less knowledge about the appropriate vaccines to get their children).

Unvaccinated children come from families with very different demographics from those of undervaccinated children, and many unvaccinated children have parents who are opposed to vaccination. A large, population-based national survey found that compared to undervaccinated children, unvaccinated children were more likely to be non-Hispanic white, to have an older mother (over age 29), to have a college-educated mother, to live in a household with a higher income ($75,000), and to live in a household with more than three children (Smith et al., 2004). In the United States, the antivaccine movement is fairly powerful, and implementing interventions to enhance immunization among these individuals has proven difficult. In addition, these parents are significantly more likely to report that doctors have little or no influence on their decision to vaccinate their children (Smith et al., 2004).

Beyond the practical issues associated with getting children vaccinated, general health beliefs, as well as specific beliefs about the safety and efficacy of vaccines, have emerged as important determinants of parental decision making. An understanding of the factors that affect parental acceptance and rejection of available immunizations for children will be critical to the development of interventions to increase acceptance and uptake (physically getting the vaccines into the children's arms) of childhood/adolescent vaccines (Sturm, Mays, & Zimet, 2005). Beliefs may be related to vaccines in general (e.g., the antivaccination movement, as noted above) or to specific vaccines. For example, parents with positive attitudes about vaccines in general may delay acceptance of a new vaccine because they do not believe there are sufficient data about safety. Parents also may reject a vaccine if they believe that their children are not at risk for the infection targeted by the vaccine, and/or if they view the infection/disease as not serious

(Bedford & Lansley, 2007; Mills, Jadad, Ross, & Wilson, 2005). Beliefs that vaccine combinations lead to "overload" of the immune system may lead to delays in immunization as well (Hilton, Petticrew, & Hunt, 2006).

Social-Environmental Factors Influencing Beliefs

Psychological research has helped in understanding the vaccine decision-making process for parents. When making this decision, parents have to balance protecting their children from possible diseases in the future with the perceived negative effects associated with having their children get the vaccine. Based on the information parents have, they form opinions and develop perceptions about whether or not a vaccine is in the best interest of their children. Most parents receive information and develop vaccine perceptions from different social-environmental sources, including the mass media, their peer groups, and their health care providers (HCPs). The accuracy of vaccine information from these sources can be quite variable, as exemplified by the frequent but inaccurate media messages suggesting that childhood immunization causes autism.

Health Beliefs

The health belief model (HBM) proposes that certain beliefs may influence acceptance or nonacceptance of vaccines, including perceived severity of and susceptibility to the disease, as well as perceived benefits of and obstacles to vaccination. The theory of reasoned action extends this model by including the beliefs of normative others (Fishbein, 1980). Overall, these health behavior theories are the most widely represented in the research on parental acceptance of child and adolescent immunization. Various studies have found that the components of the HBM predict vaccine uptake (Daley, Crane, et al., 2006a; Daley, Liddon, et al., 2006; Flynn & Ogden, 2004; Kempe et al., 2007; Rosenthal, Kottenhahn, Biro, & Succop, 1995; Short, Rupp, Stanberry, & Rosenthal, 2005). Severity of the disease and efficacy of the vaccine (a benefit) have been shown to be two of the most influential factors in vaccine decision making (Brabin, Roberts, Farzaneh, & Kitchener, 2006; Rosenthal et al., 1995; Webb, Zimet, Mays, & Fortenberry, 1999; Zimet et al., 2005). These two factors have been clearly seen with the new vaccine for HPV, in that most parents are interested in the vaccine because it protects against a serious illness (i.e., cervical cancer) and is highly effective.

Perceived social norms (i.e., health behaviors that the parents' social group considers appropriate) have been shown to be important factors in parental decision making regarding vaccines (Daley, Crane, et al., 2006b). Furthermore, acceptance within the peer group may be extremely important for the acceptability of vaccines targeting sexually transmitted infections (STIs), since some people may view getting an STI vaccine as stigmatizing (Barrington, Moreno, & Kerrigan, 2007; Ogilvie et al., 2007). To date, the research suggests that most parents' decisions about STI vaccines are independent of their views of the stigma associated with STIs.

A more complicated relationship is that between STI vaccine acceptance and concern about sexual disinhibition (i.e., the belief that those who are vaccinated will engage in riskier sexual behavior). For most parents, the decision to have their children vaccinated for STIs is based on views of disease severity and vaccine efficacy, but those parents who believe that such vaccination will have a disinhibiting effect are less likely to vaccinate their children (Brabin et al., 2006; Constantine & Jerman, 2007).

Perceptions that a vaccine might not be safe are a consistent barrier to uptake (Brabin et al., 2006). The decision to accept any side effects associated with vaccination is difficult, since the vaccine is given to normal, healthy children, and some parents express concerns about the anticipated regret and guilt they might feel if their children were harmed or had an adverse reaction (Flynn & Ogden, 2004; Wallace, Leask, & Trevena, 2005; Wroe, Turner, & Salkovskis, 2004). As the prevalence of the disease drops and individuals become less aware of the severity of the illness, vaccine uptake often decreases.

Media Coverage

Other sources of information for parents as they form their beliefs are the mass media. The less knowledgeable parents are about the vaccine or the vaccine-preventable disease, the less likely they are to have their children vaccinated (Daley, Crane, et al., 2006b; Freeman & Freed, 1999; Gust et al., 2005). Although HCPs can be very influential sources of information for parents, it is important to recognize that the mass media, including the Internet, are major sources of information related to vaccines and vaccine-preventable diseases. One study found that the media were the most frequently mentioned sources of information regarding the varicella vaccine (Freeman & Freed, 1999). With regard to vaccine-preventable diseases, the media can be informative in different ways, including reporting increases in disease outbreaks or negative outcomes related to getting the disease. This in turn can lead to parents viewing their children as being at greater risk and to their viewing the disease as more severe—two factors known to be associated with vaccine uptake (Brabin et al., 2006; Daley, Crane, et al., 2006b). A review of the content of media messages about vaccine-preventable diseases suggests that they may overuse panic language, disease personification, and stories of personal tragedies (Leask & Chapman, 2002). A promising research direction explores how parents negotiate and respond to competing media messages about vaccine safety (Leask, Chapman, Hawe, & Burgess, 2006).

It may be difficult for parents to sort out misinformation from accurate information. For instance, a study of Internet search engine results for the terms "immunization" and "vaccination" found that the first 10 sites identified by Google were all antivaccine in orientation (Davies, Chapman, & Leask, 2002). Overall, 43% of Internet sites identified had an antivaccine slant and contained significant misinformation. Some parents may have become aware of this issue, as indicated by the number of visitors to the National Network for Immunization Information webpage who click on the "Vaccine misinformation" section (Myers & Pineda, 2007). In New Zealand, there has been an overall positive trend toward reduction of strong antiimmunization messages in the media (Goodyear-Smith, Petousis-Harris, Vanlaar, Turner, & Ram, 2007). These changes are thought to result from preventive strategies employed by a university-based communication team that proactively involves itself with media coverage. There is some support for the concern that the media may have a negative effect on vaccine uptake (Gangarosa et al., 1998). For example, a study in Wales found that measles–mumps–rubella (MMR) vaccine uptake was lower in areas where negative information about the vaccine was printed in a local newspaper (Mason & Donnelly, 2000).

Influence of Others

In addition to the mass media, the beliefs and recommendations of influential others, such as a family's HCP, may be critical to whether or not parents get their children vaccinated. Studies of parents' acceptance of vaccines repeatedly document the importance of HCPs' attitudes and recommendations for parents' beliefs and acceptance of vaccines (Daley, Liddon, et al., 2006; Freeman & Freed, 1999; Gellin et al., 2000; Rosenthal et al., 1995; Smith, Kennedy, Wooten, Gust, & Pickering, 2006). It is important, however, that physicians listen to parents' concerns about vaccines, as research has demonstrated that parents are more likely to accept a vaccine when they trust that their HCPs have taken their vaccine concerns seriously (Leask et al., 2006; Marlow, Waller, & Wardle, 2007).

The children of parents who look to their HCPs for recommendations have a vaccination coverage rate significantly higher than children of parents whose decision is not influenced by their HCPs (Smith et al., 2006), and HCPs may have little influence on parents who are vaccine refusers. For example, one study found that among those parents who intended to get the varicella vaccine, 60% reported that a doctor's recommendation was influential in their decision, whereas only 17% of the refusers cited HCPs' recommendation as important. (Freeman & Freed, 1999) For these parents, most HCPs give additional information and discuss vaccination again at a later visit, and 20% ask parents to seek care from another physician (Freed, Clark, Hibbs, & Santoli, 2004). Provider–parent communication is most effective when an HCP takes into account the level of parents' knowledge, and then engages parents in a decision-making partnership (Ball, Evans, & Bostrom, 1998). However, this approach can be challenging for a pediatrician in a clinic with limited time to see patients.

Interventions to Increase Vaccination

A number of strategies have been used to change parental and personal attitudes and to reduce institutional and practical barriers to uptake of childhood and adolescent vaccines. Psychologists have the potential to play a role in this important public health strategy by conducting the relevant research, as well as by developing and evaluating interventions designed to increase vaccine uptake.

HCP Interventions

Some of the existing vaccines and those under development will protect against diseases with which HCPs may have little experience. For example, pediatricians often have limited experience and knowledge of HPV and the vaccine, because most pediatric patients do not present with HPV-related diseases (Kahn et al., 2007). Yet improving parents' knowledge about vaccines has been linked to increases in vaccination rates (Tung & Middleman, 2005). Thus pediatricians must be prepared to educate parents even if the HCPs know little about disease. Furthermore, for vaccines for STIs, pediatricians may need to discuss sexuality and address any parental concerns about sexual disinhibition after vaccination—concerns that may be shared by some pediatricians (Brabin et al., 2006; Constantine & Jerman, 2007; Kahn et al., 2007; Webb et al., 1999). HCPs rely heavily on the information and recommendations of the Advisory Committee on Immunization Practices and other professional organizations, such as the American Academy of Pediatrics and the Society for Adolescent Medicine (Kahn et al., 2007; Kempe et al., 2007; Mays & Zimet, 2004; Riedesel et al., 2004).

Developing and implementing effective educational programs to increase HCPs' knowledge will be important for optimizing parental acceptance of HPV vaccine. Education-based tutorials to improve providers' knowledge of and comfort with addressing parents' concerns about childhood immunizations are examples of this promising approach (Levi, 2006). One study evaluating a peer education intervention found that HCPs' scores on a knowledge questionnaire and their immunization behaviors (i.e., screening, talking with patients) increased significantly from pre- to postintervention (Boom, Nelson, Laugman, Kohrt, & Kozinetz, 2007). Pediatric psychologists can take a lead both in developing these interventions and in testing their effectiveness. For example, pediatric psychologists could use their skills to develop programs to enhance the skills of HCPs in discussing vaccine-related issues with parents and children/adolescents, particularly vaccine safety and risk of infection. In addition, pediatric psychologists can help HCPs understand the flaws in the reasoning regarding the risk of sexual disinhibition following HPV vaccination, so that they can discuss this with parents in a sensitive manner (Tissot, Zimet, Rosenthal, Bernstein, Wetzel, & Kahn, 2007).

Even with new information, pediatricians may not always adopt new vaccines. For example, one study examined the changes in provider practices after a combination vaccine (diphtheria, tetanus toxoids, acellular pertussis adsorbed, hepatitis B, and inactivated poliovirus) was introduced. Even though this combination vaccine would reduce the number of injections and office visits for a child, 40% of pediatricians would not order it for their practice because of a variety of practical reasons, such as the unavailability of the vaccine through their state program, the need to use different vaccines for their public and private patients, and questions regarding the compatibility of this vaccine with other vaccines (Freed, Cowen, Clark, Santoli, & Bradley, 2006).

Structural Interventions

The most effective structural strategies for enhancing uptake appear to be multicomponent interventions that combine strategies to enhance access by reducing concrete barriers with strategies to prevent missed opportunities (Niederhauser, Walters, & Ganeko, 2007; Zimmerman et al., 2006). For example, one study was successful at increasing influenza vaccinations in children and adolescents through use of posters; a Web-based registry; advance planning with suppliers to order vaccines; reminders to patients; reminders to HCPs to address vaccine issues; walk-in or weekend vaccine clinics; and same-day vaccinations (Britto, Schoettker, Pandzik, Weiland, & Mandel, 2006). Therefore, HCPs and health care clinics may need to implement as many specialized interventions as possible, while still staying within the clinics' time and workload limits.

Perhaps the single intervention with the most impact at the institutional level has been school entry requirements. All states have some school-entry laws, although the specific requirements vary from state to state. Laws may mandate certain vaccines for child care attendance, as well as for entry into elementary school, middle school, or college. Since the enactment and enforcement of state laws, over 95% of school-age children are being appropriately vaccinated, and there have been subsequent reductions in vaccine-preventable disease rates (Averhoff et al., 2004; Wilson, Fishbein, Ellis, & Edlavitch, 2005). In all states, parents can "opt out" of having their children vaccinated, but the ease with which they can do this varies from state to state. When opt-out policies are relaxed, however, vaccine coverage decreases markedly (Thompson et al., 2007).

Other structural interventions have been found to be helpful as well. Immunization registries provide a computerized record of the vaccination status of all children in the region or state. These registries have proven to be effective in identifying unvaccinated children and increasing vaccine uptake (Enger & Stokley, 2007; Hinman, Urquhart, Strikas, & the National Vaccine Advisory Committee, 2007). Various reminder strategies have been used, including calendars, automated phone messages, personal phone calls, letters/cards, and posters in clinics (Zimmerman et al., 2006). These strategies have been shown to be at least somewhat effective; however, reminders are probably not sufficient by themselves (Hicks, Tarr, & Hicks, 2007; Niederhauser et al., 2007; Szilagyi et al., 2000, 2006).

Another component to enhancing vaccination rates is to utilize alternative settings for delivery, which allow for easier access. One strategy is to use traditional medical settings, but to take advantage of sick visits or sports physicals (Szilagyi et al., 1994). Providing vaccines in easily and frequently accessed locations, such as grocery stores or pharmacies, has been shown to be effective in increasing vaccinations (Niederhauser et al., 2007). Other effective settings for providing vaccines are schools (on dedicated vaccine days) or school-based clinics. School-based influenza immunization has been shown to be an effective approach for reducing the morbidity and costs associated with influenza infection (King et al., 2006). The success of school-based immunization may depend on the active involvement of school personnel. For example, when teachers were involved, more children returned signed consent forms and were more likely to be fully vaccinated (three doses) against hepatitis B (Tung & Middleman, 2005). Overall, vaccinating in school-based clinics may be easier, since the infrastructure for delivering vaccine already exists; studies have also demonstrated that vaccination in this setting increases the rate of vaccine uptake and decreases the outbreak of vaccine-preventable diseases (Allison et al., 2007; King et al., 2005, 2006).

Pediatric psychologists can play several roles in the development and evaluation of structural interventions. Their knowledge of those factors that increase the likelihood of implementing a new behavior or that serve as a barrier to a behavior may be useful in choosing effective types of reminders or the best alternative locations for vaccination. Conducting research to identify the specific elements that make intervention strategies successful is also a valuable role for pediatric psychologists.

Parental Interventions

Pediatric psychologists, with their expertise in health communication and the social psychological determinants of health behavior, can also develop effective interventions to improve parents' attitudes toward vaccination (Gerend & Shepherd, 2007; Sturm et al., 2005). Jacobson, Targonski, and Poland (2007) outlined cognitive flaws in anti-vaccine reasoning. They recommended that in the introduction of new vaccines, educational materials and provider–parent communication should anticipate these errors and directly address cognitive distortions that are likely to arise. Psychologists can lead the way in research on communication interventions to help HCPs identify parental discomfort about safety issues with vaccines and then address worry-based cognitive reasoning errors during clinic encounters. Furthermore, because they can draw on the established research literature on systematic biases in risk appraisal, pediatric psychologists are well positioned to develop interventions to influence parents' understanding of risks and probabilities related to vaccines and vaccine-preventable diseases. For example, Wallace and colleagues (2006) reported that an interactive, Web-based decision support tool, which included graphic displays to anchor risk probabilities, significantly improved parental attitudes toward MMR vaccination.

Conclusions

Pediatric psychologists have a responsibility to help prevent illness and disease, as well as to help children and their families cope with medical illnesses and conditions. Vaccination is an excellent example of a biomedical prevention for which the involvement of psychologists in research and implementation programs is valuable. Their knowledge about the development of attitudes and beliefs, the importance of working within a cultural context, and the elements necessary for development of effective behavioral interventions make pediatric psychologists potentially very helpful in efforts to ensure maximum protection for all children against vaccine-preventable diseases.

References

Allison, M. A., Crane, L. A., Beaty, B. L., Davidson, A. J., Melinkovich, P., & Kempe, A. (2007). School-based health centers: Improving access and quality of care for low-income adolescents. *Pediatrics*, 120(4), e887–e894.

Averhoff, F., Linton, L., Peddecord, K. M., Edwards, C., Wang, W., & Fishbein, D. (2004). A middle school immunization law rapidly and substantially increases immunization coverage among adolescents. *American Journal of Public Health*, 95(6), 978–984.

Ball, L. K., Evans, G., & Bostrom, A. (1998). Risky business: Challenges in vaccine risk communication. *Pediatrics*, 101(3), 453–458.

Barrington, C., Moreno, L., & Kerrigan, D. (2007). Local understanding of an HIV vaccine and its relationship with HIV-related stigma in the Dominican Republic. *AIDS Care*, 19(7), 871–877.

Bedford, H., & Lansley, M. (2007). More vaccines for children?: Parents' views. *Vaccine*, 25(45), 7818–7823.

Boom, J. A., Nelson, C. S., Laugman, L. E., Kohrt, A. E., & Kozinetz, C. A. (2007). Improvement in provider immunization knowledge and behaviors following a peer education intervention. *Clinical Pediatrics*, 46(8), 706–717.

Brabin, L., Roberts, S. A., Farzaneh, F., & Kitchener, H. C. (2006). Future acceptance of adolescent human papillomavirus vaccination: A survey of parental attitudes. *Vaccine*, 24(16), 3087–3094.

Britto, M. T., Schoettker, P. J., Pandzik, G. M., Weiland, J., & Mandel, K. E. (2007). Improving influenza immunisation for high-risk children and adolescents. *Quality and Safety in Health Care*, 16(5), 363–368.

Centers for Disease Control and Prevention (CDC). (1999) Achievements in public health, 1900–1998. *Morbidity and Mortality Weekly Report*, 48, 243–248.

Centers for Disease Control and Prevention (CDC). (2008). Recommended immunization schedule for persons aged 7–18 years—United States. *Morbidity and Mortality Weekly Report, 48,* 243–248.

Constantine, N. A., & Jerman, P. (2007). Acceptance of human papillomavirus vaccination among Californian parents of daughters: A representative statewide analysis. *Journal of Adolescent Health, 40*(2), 108–115.

Daley, M. F., Crane, L. A., Chandramouli, V., Beaty, B. L., Barrow, J., Alfred, N., et al. (2006a). Influenza among healthy young children: Changes in parental attitudes and predictors of immunization during the 2003 to 2004 influenza season. *Pediatrics, 117*(2), e268–e277.

Daley, M. F., Crane, L. A., Chandramouli, V., Beaty, B. L., Barrow, J., Alfred, N., et al. (2006b). Misperceptions about influenza vaccination among parents of healthy young children. *Clinical Pediatrics, 46*(5), 408–417.

Daley, M. F., Liddon, N., Crane, L. A., Beaty, B. L., Barrow, J., Babbel, C., et al. (2006). A national survey of pediatrician knowledge and attitudes regarding human papillomavirus vaccination. *Pediatrics, 118*(6), 2280–2289.

Darling, N. J., Barker, L. E., Shefer, A. M., & Chu, S. Y. (2005). Immunization coverage among Hispanic ancestry: 2003 National Immunization Survey. *American Journal of Preventive Medicine, 29*(5), 421–427.

Davies, P., Chapman, S., & Leask, J. (2002). Antivaccination activists on the World Wide Web. *Archives of Disease in Childhood, 87*(1), 22–25.

Enger, K. S., & Stokley, S. (2007). Meningococcal conjugate vaccine uptake, measured by Michigan's immunization registry. *Journal of Adolescent Health, 40*(5), 398–400.

Fishbein, M. (1980). A theory of reasoned action: Some applications and implications. In *Nebraska Symposium on Motivation* (Vol. 27, pp. 65–116). Lincoln: University of Nebraska Press.

Flynn, M., & Ogden, J. (2004). Predicting uptake of MMR vaccination: A prospective questionnaire study. *British Journal of General Practice, 54*(504), 526–530.

Freed, G. L., Clark, S. J., Hibbs, B. F., & Santoli, J. M. (2004). Parental vaccine safety concerns: The experiences of pediatricians and family physicians. *American Journal of Preventive Medicine, 26*(10), 11–14.

Freed, G. L., Cowen, A. E., Clark, S. J., Santoli, J., & Bradley, J. (2006). Use of a new combined vaccine in pediatric practices. *Pediatrics, 118*(2), e251–e257.

Freeman, V. A., & Freed, G. L. (1999). Parental knowledge, attitudes, and demand regarding a vaccine to prevent varicella. *American Journal of Preventive Medicine, 17*(2), 153–155.

Gangarosa, E. J., Galazka, A. M., Wolfe, C. R., Phillips, L. M., Gangarosa, R. E., Miller, E., et al. (1998). Impact of anti-vaccine movements on pertussis control: The untold story. *Lancet, 351,* 356–351.

Gellin, B. G., Maibach, E. W., Marcuse, E. K., & the National Network for Immunization Information Steering Committee. (2000). Do parents understand immunizations?: A national telephone survey. *Pediatrics, 106*(5), 1097–1102.

Gerend, M. A., & Shepherd, J. E. (2007). Using message framing to promote acceptance of the human papillomavirus vaccine. *Health Psychology, 26*(6), 745–752.

Goodyear-Smith, F., Petousis-Harris, H., Vanlaar, C., Turner, N., & Ram, S. (2007). Immunization in the print media: Perspectives presented by the press. *Journal of Health Communication, 12*(8), 759–770.

Gore, P., Madhavan, S., Curry, D., McClung, G., Castiglia, M., Rosenbluth, S. A., et al. (1999). Predictors of childhood immunization completion in a rural population. *Social Science and Medicine, 48*(8), 1011–1027.

Gust, D. A., Kennedy, A., Shui, I., Smith, P. J., Nowak, G., & Pickering, L. K. (2005). Parental attitudes toward immunizations and healthcare providers: The role of information. *American Journal of Preventive Medicine, 29*(2), 105–112.

Herrera, G. A., Zhao, S., & Klevens, M. (2001). Variation in vaccination coverage among children of Hispanic ancestry. *American Journal of Preventive Medicine, 20*(4S), 69–74.

Hicks, P., Tarr, G. A. M., & Hicks, X. P. (2007). Reminder cards and immunization rates among Latinos and the rural poor in northeast Colorado. *Journal of the American Board of Family Medicine, 20*(6), 581–586.

Hilton, S., Petticrew, M., & Hunt, K. (2006). "Combined vaccines are like a sudden onslaught to the body's immune system": Parental concerns about vaccine "overload" and "immune-vulnerability." *Vaccine, 24*(20), 4321–4327.

Hinman, A. R., Urquhart, G. A., Strikas, R. A., & the National Vaccine Advisory Committee. (2007). Immunization information systems: National Vaccine Advisory Committee Progress Report. *Journal of Public Health Management and Practice, 13*(6), 553–558.

Jacobson, R. M., Targonski, P. V., & Poland, G. A. (2007). A taxonomy of reasoning flaws in the anti-vaccine movement. *Vaccine, 25*(16), 3146–3152.

Kahn, J. A., Rosenthal, S. L., Tissot, A. M., Bernstein, D. I., Wetzel, C., & Zimet, G. D. (2007). Factors influencing pediatricians' intention to recommend human papillomavirus vaccines. *Ambulatory Pediatrics, 7*(5), 367–373.

Kempe, A., Daley, M. F., Parashar, U. D., Crace, L. A., Beaty, B. L., Stokley, S., et al. (2007). Will pediatricians adopt the new rotavirus vaccine? *Pediatrics, 119*(1), 1–10.

King, J. C., Cummings, G. E., Stoddard, J., Readmond, B. X., Madger, L. S., Strong, M., et al. (2005). A pilot study of the effectiveness of a school-based influenza vaccination program. *Pediatrics, 116*(6), e868–e873.

King, J. C., Stoddard, J. J., Gaglani, M. J., Moore, K. A., Magder, L., McClure, E., et al. (2006). Effectiveness of school-based influenza vaccination. *New England Journal of Medicine, 355*, 2523–2532.

Klevens, R. M., & Luman, E. T. (2001). U.S. children living in and near poverty: Risk of vaccine-preventable diseases. *American Journal of Preventive Medicine, 20*(4S), 41–46.

Leask, J., & Chapman, S. (2002). 'The cold hard facts': Immunization and vaccine preventable diseases in Australia's newsprint media 1993–1998. *Social Science and Medicine, 54*(3), 445–457.

Leask, J., Chapman, S., Hawe, P., & Burgess, M. (2006). What maintains parental support for vaccination when challenged by anti-vaccination messages?: A qualitative study. *Vaccine, 24*(49–50), 7238–7245.

Levi, B. H. (2006). Addressing parents' concerns about childhood immunizations: A tutorial for primary care providers. *Pediatrics, 120*(1), 18–26.

Luman, E. T., McCauley, M. M., Shefer, A., & Chu, S. Y. (2003). Maternal characteristics associated with vaccination of young children. *Pediatrics, 111*(5), 1215–1218.

Marlow, L. A. V., Waller, J., & Wardle, J. (2007). Trust and experience as predictors of HPV vaccine acceptance. *Human Vaccines, 3*(5),171–175.

Mason, B. W., & Donnelly, P. D. (2000). Impact of a local newspaper campaign on the uptake of the measles mumps and rubella vaccine. *Journal of Epidemiology and Community Health, 54*(6), 473–474.

Mays, R. M., & Zimet, G. D. (2004). Recommending STI vaccination to parents of adolescents: The attitudes of nurse practitioners. *Sexually Transmitted Diseases, 31*(7), 428–432.

Mills, E., Jadad, A. R., Ross, C., & Wilson, K. (2005). Systematic review of qualitative studies exploring parental beliefs and attitudes toward childhood vaccination identifies common barriers to vaccination. *Journal of Clinical Epidemiology, 58*(11), 1081–1088.

Myers, M. G., & Pineda, D. I. (2007, May). *Widely publicized misinformation about vaccine safety causes searches for information.* Abstract presented at the annual meeting of the Pediatric Academic Societies, Toronto.

Niederhauser, V., Walters, M., & Ganeko, R. (2007). Simple solutions to complex issues: Minimizing disparities in childhood immunization rates by providing walk-in shot clinic access. *Family Community Health, 30*(25), S80–S91.

Ogilvie, G. S., Remple, V. P., Marra, F., McNeil, S. A., Naus, M., Pielak, K. L., et al. (2007). Parental intention to have daughters receive the human papillomavirus vaccine. *Canadian Medical Association Journal, 177*(12), 1506–1512.

Riedesel, J. M., Rosenthal, S. L., Zimet, G. D., Bernstein, D. I., Huang, B., Lan, D., et al. (2005). Attitudes about human papillomavirus vaccine among family physicians. *Journal of Pediatric and Adolescent Gynecology, 18*(6), 391–398.

Rosenthal, J., Rodewald, L., McCauley, M., Berman, S., Irigoyen, M., Sawyer, M., et al. (2004). Immunization coverage levels among 19- to 35-month-old children in 4 diverse, medically underserved areas of the United States. *Pediatrics, 113*(4), e296–e302.

Rosenthal, S. L., Kottenhahn, R. K., Biro, F. M., & Succop, P. A. (1995). Hepatitis B vaccine acceptance among adolescents and their parents. *Journal of Adolescent Health, 17*(4), 248–254.

Short, M. B., Rupp, R., Stanberry, S. L., & Rosenthal, S. L. (2005). Parental acceptance of adolescent vaccines within school based health centres. *Herpes, 12*(1), 23–27.

Smith, P. J., Chu, S. Y., & Barker, L. E. (2004). Children who have received no vaccines: Who are they and where do they live? *Pediatrics, 114*(1), 187–195.

Smith, P. J., Kennedy, A. M., Wooten, K., Gust, D. A., & Pickering, L. K. (2006). Association between health care providers' influence on parents who have concerns about vaccine safety and vaccination coverage. *Pediatrics, 118*(5), e1287–e1292.

Sturm, L. A., Mays, R. M., & Zimet, G. D. (2005). Parental beliefs and decision making about child and adolescent immunization: From polio to sexually transmitted infection. *Journal of Developmental and Behavioral Pediatrics, 26*, 441–451.

Szilagyi, P. G., Bordley, C., Vann, J. C., Chelminski, A., Kraus, R. M., Margolis, P. A., et al. (2000). Effect of patient reminder/recall interventions on immunization rates: A review. *Journal of the American Medical Association, 284*(14), 1820–1827.

Szilagyi, P. G., Rodewald, L. E., Humiston, S. G., Hager, J., Roghmann, K. J., Doane, C., et al. (1994). Immunization practices of pediatricians and family physicians in the United States. *Pediatrics, 94*(4), 517–523.

Szilagyi, P. G., Schaffer, S., Barth, R., Shone, L. P., Humistron, S. G., Ambrose, S., et al. (2006). Effect of telephone reminder/recall on adolescent immunization and preventive visits. *Archives of Pediatric and Adolescent Medicine, 160*(2), 157–163.

Tercyak, K. P. (2008). Editorial: Prevention in child health psychology and the *Journal of Pediatric Psychology. Journal of Pediatric Psychology, 33*(1), 31–34.

Thompson, J. W., Tyson, S., Card-Higginson, P., Jacobs, R. F., Wheeler, J. G., Simpson, P., et al. (2007). Impact of addition of philosophical exemptions on childhood immunization rates. *American Journal of Preventive Medicine, 32*(3), 194–201.

Tissot, A. M., Zimet, G. D., Rosenthal, S. L., Bernstein, D. I., Wetzel, C., & Kahn, J. A. (2007). Effective strategies for HPV vaccine delivery: The views of pediatricians. *Journal of Adolescent Health, 41*(2), 119–125.

Tung, C. S., & Middleman, A. B. (2005). An evaluation of school-level factors used in a successful school-based hepatitis B immunization initiative. *Journal of Adolescent Health, 37*(1), 61–68.

Wallace, C., Leask, J., & Trevena, L. J. (2006). Effects of a Web based decision aid on parental attitudes to MMR vaccination: A before and after study. *British Medical Journal, 332*, 146–149.

Webb, P. M., Zimet, G. D., Mays, R., & Fortenberry, J. D. (1999). HIV immunization: Acceptability and anticipated effects on sexual behavior among adolescents. *Journal of Adolescent Health, 25*(5), 320–322.

Wilson, T. R., Fishbein, D. B., Ellis, P. A., & Edlavitch, S. A. (2005). The impact of a school entry law on adolescent immunization rates. *Journal of Adolescent Health, 37*(6), 511–516.

Wroe, A. L., Turner, N., & Salkovskis, P. M. (2004). Understanding and predicting parental decisions about early childhood immunizations. *Health Psychology, 23*(1), 33–41.

Zimet, G. D., Mays, R. M., Sturm, L. A., Ravert, A. A., Perkins, S. M., & Juliar, B. E. (2005). Parental attitudes about sexually transmitted infection vaccination for their adolescent. *Archives of Pediatrics and Adolescent Medicine, 159*(2), 132–137.

Zimmerman, R. K., Hoberman, A., Nowalk, M. P., Lin, C. J., Greenberg, D. P., Weinberg, S. T., et al. (2006). Improving influenza vaccination rates of high-risk inner-city children over 2 intervention years. *Annals of Family Medicine, 4*(6), 534–540.

CHAPTER 42

Pediatric Psychology and Primary Care

TERRY STANCIN
ELLEN C. PERRIN
LISA RAMIREZ

Most children seen for pediatric care are not in hospitals and do not have serious chronic illnesses or debilitating medical issues, which historically have constituted the primary focus of pediatric psychology. Most health care services for children take place in outpatient pediatric and primary care settings. "Primary care" refers to a broad spectrum of health care services, both preventive and curative, delivered in outpatient (ambulatory) medical settings. The primary care clinician and office serve, among other things, as the "medical home" for a child—ideally providing continuity and integration of health care services over time, with activities that focus on prevention of illness, promotion of health and wellness, and amelioration of consequences of chronic health conditions. Primary care can be contrasted with acute and urgent care health services that are directed toward sick or injured children. In the United States, pediatric primary care providers (PPCPs) are usually pediatricians and family medicine physicians, with some care also delivered by nurse practitioners, nurse clinicians, or physician assistants. Ideally, PPCPs serve as health care coordinators of all care that young patients receive.

Primary care settings that include onsite mental health services are referred to as "integrated" or "collaborative care" settings (Stancin, 2005). Although pediatric psychologists would appear to be ideally suited to partner with PPCPs and lead the development of mental health services in primary care settings, the reality is that pediatric psychology has had a fairly limited presence in these settings, perhaps because of its historical focus on inpatient collaboration in the care of children with chronic medical conditions. This chapter describes past and present behavioral health activities in pediatric primary care settings, and outlines opportunities for pediatric psychology to have an impact on the mental health care of children and adolescents.

Historical Context

The idea for providing psychological services in primary care settings was presented more than 40 years ago by Don Freedheim and colleagues (Smith, Rome, & Freedheim, 1967), who described a pediatric practice with "colocated" mental health activities (i.e., behavioral and primary care services provided in the same place). Other psychologists have advocated primary care mental health services for many years (e.g., see Christophersen, 1982; Drotar, 1993; Roberts & Wright, 1982; Routh, Schroeder, & Koocher 1983; Stancin, 1999). However, it was Carolyn Schroeder who raised the greatest awareness of the potential scope and impact of a primary care psychology practice (Schroeder, 1979, 1999, 2004).

Schroeder established a visionary pediatric psychology practice in the 1970s in Chapel Hill, North Carolina. The practice included clinical, teaching, research, community advocacy, and public health components that continue to serve as models for such components today. Among her innovations were telephone "call-in hours" for parents, evening parent education groups, brief "come-in" sessions for parents to discuss individual concerns, and a developmental screening program. Later, services were expanded into an integrated, collaborative private practice that added prevention programs (e.g., a parent resource library and a series of parent handouts on such common behavioral concerns as toilet training) and direct clinical services for a variety of problems (e.g., negative behaviors, anxiety, attention-deficit/hyperactivity disorder [ADHD], adjustment issues). Interventions emphasized the use of brief, problem-focused treatments; protocols for more commonly seen problems (e.g., enuresis, sleep problems, negative behaviors); and parent–child groups—all of which proved to be cost-effective and efficient modalities. A pediatric psychologist in this practice had multiple roles besides therapist, including educator (of physicians, parents, and teachers); consultant; advocate (in court, schools, and community); case manager (coordinating services among various medical, school, and community providers); and outcomes researcher.

There has been ongoing interest in pediatric psychology in primary care applications. Dennis Drotar (1995) featured descriptions of collaborative outpatient pediatric practices in Consulting with Pediatricians (e.g., Hurley, 1995). A special issue of the Journal of Pediatric Psychology was devoted to pediatric mental health services in primary care settings (see Stancin, 1999). Maureen Black (2002) advocated for pediatric psychologists to develop and evaluate health promotion programs for use in primary care in her Society of Pediatric Psychology presidential address. A section on primary care was included in a chapter on professional roles and practice patterns in the third edition of this handbook (Drotar, Spirito, & Stancin, 2003). Spirito and colleagues (2003) and others (e.g., Perrin 1999a, 1999b; Stancin, 2005; Wildman & Stancin, 2004) have recommended expansions of pediatric primary care services by pediatric psychologists.

Pediatricians themselves have become concerned about the huge level of unmet need in the area of child mental health services. They recognize the need for prevention, early detection, and prompt and effective intervention, and have begun to explore and address this need through a number of initiatives (e.g., American Academy of Pediatrics [AAP], 2000, 2001, 2006; Johnson, Myers, & AAP Council on Children with Disabilities, 2007). Although some of these programs have included a handful of pediatric psychologists, many more opportunities for collaboration exist and await participation by psychologists in greater numbers.

Why Should Pediatric Psychologists Consider Work in Primary Care Settings?

Shorter hospitalizations for children have limited the opportunities to provide inpatient consultation and intervention services, previously a mainstay for pediatric psychologists. However, there is a great need for additional child mental health services in primary care settings. PPCPs are the health care professionals most likely to come in contact with youths with behavioral and emotional problems, and they are seeking broader assistance in addressing children's psychosocial concerns in the primary care setting. Pediatricians neither are trained nor have time to address all the behavioral problems that arise in their practices, and many lament the scarcity of well-qualified child mental health care providers or community services. Without much support being offered by psychologists, pediatricians are left managing many difficult psychological concerns alone, or look to other mental health professionals such as child psychiatrists and social workers for help. Furthermore, referral to community mental health care providers may be difficult for parents to accept; some data suggest that 40% of children identified never receive behavioral services in any setting (Rushton, Bruckman, & Kelleher, 2002).

Mental health services that are provided in primary care settings appear to be more acceptable to families. Parents and children have long-term relationships with their PPCPs and are more comfortable in that setting. Worrisome aspects of children's development and behavior may manifest themselves in vague concerns or by way of physical symptoms. Therefore, an integrated approach that includes attention to the physical, developmental, and emotional aspects of each child and family system is optimal. Thus primary care settings promote a nonstigmatizing service delivery with easy access.

Providing mental health services in primary care settings can have direct advantages for psychologists as well. There are opportunities to develop and implement prevention and early intervention programs, as well as services to promote mental health and to screen for early signs of psychosocial problems. Primary care treatment of mental health problems results in better adherence and provides good training and research laboratories for psychologists (Schroeder, 2004). Finally, such treatment offers endless opportunities for multidisciplinary collaboration with medical care providers in clinical and research efforts.

How Do Integrated Mental Health Primary Care Services Differ from Traditional Care?

Mental health services provided in primary care differ from traditional care in many important ways. In traditional primary care settings, care is delivered by physicians and nurse practitioners, and mental health care is all delivered by referral to outside mental health providers. Offices, records, schedules, and treatments are entirely separate. If there is any behavioral health emphasis in a traditional primary care office, it is on screening and referral, with limited pharmacological management for selected conditions (e.g., ADHD).

In a primary care center with integrated mental health services, there are medical and mental health professionals collaborating as a team on patient care, all of whom are office staff. Office space and records are shared, and schedules overlap. Mental health services include direct patient care as well as prevention and screening. Psychopharmacological care is monitored and managed collaboratively. Key factors that define how services are delivered are the extent to which they are colocated and integrated into practice procedures (Stancin, 2005).

Primary care mental health services tend to be delivered differently from interventions in traditional outpatient mental health settings, which typically consist of relatively small client loads, 50-minute sessions over many sessions, fairly extensive documentation, and case closure at termination. Psychologists in an integrated primary care setting tend to have larger client loads offset by flexible time limits; brief, short-term treatments; less extensive documentation; and open-ended case plans (i.e., children are followed as needed).

Several studies have described the most common behavioral problems addressed in primary care settings. In contrast to more traditional outpatient mental health settings, where providers often treat multiple, severe problems with complex psychosocial factors, primary care interventions tend to focus more on targeted, specific problems that are of mild to moderate severity and involve less complex psychosocial factors. One reason for this difference is age. Although children of all ages are seen in primary care settings, the majority are infants and very young children; healthy children over age 2 years usually see their PPCPs only once per year unless they have an acute illness or their parents have a particular concern. This predominantly infant and toddler population offers important opportunities for prevention and early intervention, such as developmental monitoring, screening for delays, promotion of healthy parent–child interactions, and detection of parental mental health problems (Roberts & Brown, 2004; Stancin, 2005).

Studies describing the nature of problems of children seen for primary care behavioral services have shown that the most frequently referred problems are negative behaviors, such as tantrums, oppositional behavior, defiance, noncompliance, and aggression. For example, Finney, Riley, and Cataldo (1991) reported that 56% of children were referred to their primary care psychology clinic for aggression and sleep/mealtime struggles, and that toileting (e.g., enuresis) and somatic (e.g., recurrent abdominal pain) problems were also common reasons for referral. Similarly, Sobel, Roberts, Rayfield, Barnard, and Rapoff (2001) reported that most children seen for psychological services at two primary care settings were diagnosed with oppositional defiant disorder (ODD) (22%), ADHD (22%), and adjustment disorder (14.4%).

Roles and communication patterns in primary care practices also differ from those in a more traditional mental health setting, which emphasizes a single therapist role with little or no direct communication with a PPCP. As noted above, primary care–based psychologists often adopt multiple roles, including consultant, educator, liaison to community settings, and therapist. The primary care psychologist is visible and accessible to the PPCP because the two encounter one another on a regular basis. There are ample opportunities for prompt, frequent feedback and discussion.

Opportunities for Pediatric Psychologists in Primary Care Settings

Pediatric psychologists in primary care settings may be involved at every level of care— for example, developing and carrying out screening programs; organizing and running educational and therapeutic groups for parents and for children; providing individual psychotherapy to parents and to children; and facilitating effective referrals to community-based mental health and developmental resources. They may also be extremely valuable in helping the practice to coordinate the medical, mental health, and family/ community care of children with chronic health conditions and their families—an area of increasing focus within pediatric primary care (McMenamy & Perrin, 2002). Moreover, behavioral research in primary care would be greatly advanced by more pediatric psychology involvement (Wildman & Stancin, 2004).

Screening: Identifying and Monitoring Children with Developmental and Behavioral Problems

It has been shown that using a standardized developmental screening test in children 24 months and younger enhances the detection of developmental delays and increases referrals to mental health providers by over 200% (Hix-Small, Marks, Squires, & Nickel, 2007). However, recent evaluations of pediatrician developmental screening practices revealed that up to 71% of PPCPs reported not routinely using a formal screening instrument (Gardner, Kelleher, Pajer, & Campo, 2003; Sand et al., 2005). In addition, most pediatricians report finding broad screening valuable but are burdened by systemic factors, including limited access to mental health specialists (Brown, Riley, & Wissow, 2007). Indeed, limited access to effective sources for referral has probably impeded some pediatricians from embarking on a systematic screening program (Perrin, 1998).

There is considerable pressure on pediatricians to screen for a variety of developmental and behavioral conditions, and they are actively seeking advice about tools and procedures. For example, the AAP (2006) has published guidelines on developmental screening, recommending administration of a standardized screening measure at the 9-, 18-, and 24- or 30-month visits for every child. Although there are many standardized screening methods, few have been subjected to rigorous empirical study, and many have limited norms or evidence of validity for use in primary care. In addition, some are limited by practical considerations of cost, administration requirements, and/or scoring. Training of pediatricians has traditionally lacked attention to the typical and unusual processes of development of language, motor, cognitive, self-regulation, and emotional skills, let alone instruction on psychometric methods. Even as the pediatric subspecialty of developmental–behavioral pediatrics has improved pediatric training considerably, the vast breadth of this field, its unending clinical needs, and the short time allocated to it in pediatric training programs results in many PPCPs' remaining unsure about how to evaluate and select an appropriate screening test for a particular age and problem, and also about appropriate follow-up if a possible problem is identified. Pediatric practitioners need guidance on selecting among the array of available instruments, which differ in important ways, including their purposes (e.g., general developmental screening vs. autism screening) as well as methods (e.g., parent report of concerns vs. report of skills vs. practitioner administered).

With training in psychometrics as well as medical collaboration, pediatric psychologists are uniquely qualified to guide pediatricians in selecting valid and feasible methods for developmental and behavioral screening in their practice (Stancin & Palermo, 1997). Recently, Drotar, Stancin, Dworkin, Sices, and Wood (2008) conducted a scientific review of developmental screening instruments for children less than 3 years of age. They developed guides to address the need to provide a scientifically valid yet user-friendly synthesis of the research on developmental screening instruments, in order to inform practitioners' selection and application of screening instruments in a range of practice settings.

One of the barriers to the institution of routine screening in pediatric office settings, despite their acknowledged appropriateness for routine developmental surveillance, has been the process necessary to follow up on any suspicious or abnormal findings so identified. Common errors made by PPCPs faced with positive screening test results include (1) disbelieving the results, and thus not initiating further evaluation or referral; or (2) acting as if (while knowing better) the screening test results were tantamount to a diagnosis. These errors may lead to a series of unfortunate outcomes, including late and/or inappropriate referrals and unnecessary worry for parents. Another deficit in many PPCPs' training is the ability to provide "bad news" to parents in a manner that is supportive and empowers parents to advocate appropriately for their children. Moreover, identification of psychosocial issues may have implications about additional clinician responsibilities and costs, and reimbursement restrictions once problems are identified (Perrin & Stancin, 2002; Weitzman & Leventhal, 2006).

Screening instruments and procedures that are feasible in a pediatric primary care setting might differ from what a pediatric psychologist might recommend initially. It is critical for psychologists working with PPCPs to consider the impact of even very brief procedures on primary care visits that are often scheduled for 15–20 minutes, during which time an entire review of medical, behavioral, developmental and physical examination findings is supposed to occur (Perrin & Stancin, 2002; Riekert, Stancin, Palermo, & Drotar, 1999; Stancin & Palermo, 1997). Innovative methods, such as computer-based behavioral screening in primary care, have demonstrated success at alleviating some of the burden associated with broad psychosocial screening (Chisolm, Gardner, Julian, & Kelleher, 2008).

Identifying Resources Available for Evaluation and Treatment

Typically, when a developmental or behavioral concern is suspected or identified in the process of formal or informal screening by the pediatric office, the traditional PPCP has a number of options: (1) initiating some counseling if the PPCP or another pediatrician in the office is trained and competent (e.g., guidance regarding methods to support language development or disciplinary structures); (2) requesting consultation with a mental health colleague; and/or (3) referring the child and family to a child development or mental health colleague in the community. Some pediatric practices have worked out arrangements with community-based colleagues that make such consultation and referral options easier. For very young children (<3 years), the early intervention services of most states provide some accessible resources, though they are usually inadequate for the wide range of problems that may be encountered.

Few pediatric offices have initiated a model of integrated or collaborative care in which a pediatric psychologist may direct screening programs, provide individual and/or family therapy, and serve as a resource to families regarding additional services for their children. Onsite mental health services can facilitate access, provide greater continuity of care, confer trust by the PPCP, increase communication between medical and mental health clinicians, and ease the stigma associated with mental health services.

Furthermore, up to 66% of families referred for onsite counseling followed through with mental health referrals, compared to 2.6% of families referred for offsite counseling (Lieberman, Adalist-Estrin, Erinle, & Sloan, 2006). If psychopharmacological agents are indicated for a child, an office-based psychologist may have an additional role to ensure coordination of the pharmacological and psychological interventions.

Colocating mental health services within primary care offices can provide other opportunities as well. Recent examples include a program for routing children with identified psychosocial problems through nurse practitioners to a team social worker or psychologist for further evaluation (Campo et al., 2005), and another program giving primary care physicians direct telephone access to child psychiatrists for consultation (Connor et al., 2006). Williams, Shore, and Foy (2006) have described three additional models: (1) stationing community mental health employees within practices and generating revenue based on billing for services; (2) employing mental health professionals in pediatric private practices; and (3) having independent mental health practices coexist with independent pediatric practices. Outcome data for all models have demonstrated increased levels of access to mental health providers, increased referral follow-through for mental health services, and increased communication between mental health and medical providers. Despite demonstrated success, drawbacks to colocated services included increased work for office staff, increased demand for space, and long-term salary sustainability questions (Williams et al., 2006).

Delivering Psychological Services in Nontraditional Ways

Schroeder (2004) has noted that psychological services provided in primary care settings are often similar to more traditional interventions, but they are delivered in nontraditional ways. Such services as diagnostic assessments and testing, brief counseling, and parent groups are important in primary care, but may be scheduled with more flexibility. Psychologists in primary care settings often assist PPCPs in preparing families for referral to other specialists or community resources, and often also serve as primary liaisons to schools. They may also serve as anchors in the primary care setting for families of children with chronic health conditions—a population that has traditionally been a focus for pediatric psychologists' training and practice. Psychologists have empirically supported interventions available for the treatment of common childhood problems (disruptive behavior disorders, mood disorders, etc.), and primary care settings are proving to be appropriate environments for adapting some of these programs. For example, one study found that a telephone-based manualized intervention for disruptive behavior problems was more effective than standard screening, referral, and follow-up care in a primary care setting (Borowsky, Mozayeny, Stuenkel, & Ireland, 2004). Recently, Lavigne and colleagues (2008) compared three interventions for ODD in primary care. Twenty-four pediatric practices were randomly assigned to receive (1) nurse-led or (2) psychologist-led group manualized parent training treatment, or (3) a minimum intervention consisting of just the companion treatment book. Results indicated sustained improvements in all three conditions, with better results for parents who attended more of the intervention sessions. The authors also noted improvements with minimal interventions in this relatively more educated parent population, suggesting that intensive interventions may not be the first-line treatment of choice for all children identified with ODD in primary care.

Other recent studies are demonstrating how interventions can be tailored to the primary setting. For example, several studies have identified both patient and clinician characteristics that affect the likelihood of problem identification and/or referrals (e.g., Sices, Feudtner, McLaughlin, Drotar, & Williams, 2004). Interesting trends that have emerged include lower rates of screening by female clinicians or family practitioners (Gardner et al., 2003); of African American youths (Gardner et al., 2003); or when treating problems was associated with greater burden (Brown et al., 2007). Studies have also shown that physicians with less training in psychosocial issues were more likely to report barriers to identifying childhood psychosocial problems (Horwitz et al., 2007).

It is well known that children with chronic physical health conditions experience secondary psychological and social morbidity. Many studies have found approximately double the prevalence of school, interpersonal, and emotional difficulties among these children, compared to children without a chronic condition. The notion that a PPCP can provide a "medical home" for children with complex health conditions is appealing, but seldom sufficient for the breadth of needs these families experience. Innovative ideas for coping with concerns can be beneficial but costly. One practice in rural Nebraska provides parents with a call-in service to address concerns about their children; although parents reported high levels of satisfaction with the service and advice received, calls averaged about 21 minutes apiece (Polaha, Volkmer, & Valleley, 2007), and the service was not reimbursed.

Pediatricians' Responses to Needs for Care of Children with Mental Health Concerns

Recently, a surge of interest by pediatricians on the identification and care of children with mental health problems has resulted from the recognition that:

- Precursors of mental health disorders in adulthood can often be identified in early childhood (e.g., Anda et al., 2007).
- At least 10% of children and adolescents have functional impairment due to a diagnosed mental health and/or substance abuse disorder (U.S. Department of Health and Human Services, 1999), and up to 25% have clinically significant problems that may not (yet) rise to the level of a diagnosable psychiatric disorder (Briggs-Gowan et al., 2003).
- There is a shortage of qualified mental health clinicians, especially for children younger than 5, and for families in middle- and low-income groups and/or of minority background.
- Primary care settings provide the most accessible and least stigmatizing resources for many families who have concerns about their children's developmental and/or behavior.

The importance of pediatricians' understanding and assuming the care of children with ADHD has been highlighted by the AAP guidelines for the diagnosis (AAP, 2000) and treatment (AAP, 2001) of ADHD. Pediatric psychologists were involved in developing and disseminating these guidelines, which have radically changed the care of children and adolescents with this condition in pediatric settings. These guidelines highlight the importance of, and provide strategies for, obtaining observations from teachers and child care providers about a child's behavior, both at the time of diagnosis and for ongoing monitoring. They also emphasize the importance of assessing and treating any coexisting mental health conditions.

General surveys demonstrate that while PPCPs are increasingly comfortable with diagnosing and treating children with ADHD, there is much more variability in responses about diagnosing and treating anxiety, depression and other behavioral problems (Williams, Klinepeter, Palmes, Pulley, & Foy, 2004). The Resource for Advancing Children's Health Institute has taken on as one of its missions the challenge of teaching and encouraging pediatricians to identify, treat, and monitor children's mental health disorders with only occasional consultation with child and adolescent psychiatrists. Its first effort, "Guidelines for Adolescent Depression in Primary Care," provided recommendations for identification and treatment of depression among adolescents in the primary care context (Cheung et al., 2007). Subsequent efforts include the Warning Signs Project, which promotes recognition by families, schools, and communities of symptoms of mental health disorders, and the Pediatric Psychopharmacology Mini-Fellowship Program, which helps interested PPCPs to refine and improve psychopharmacological management of adolescents with mental illness.

In response to growing concerns about mental health, the AAP has created a Task Force on Mental Health to organize a comprehensive assessment of pediatricians' responsibilities and mechanisms for identifying, monitoring, and treating children with mental health concerns. The final Task Force report is likely to provide guidance to pediatricians about screening methods; to furnish a "toolkit" to enhance care; and to suggest the development of integrated, collaborative care practices to improve recognition and management of mental health disorders among their patients.

The AAP and other organizations and individuals have also recently focused on the development of recommendations and advice regarding universal and systematic screening in the context of pediatric practices; however, but most of the focus has been on screening for developmental progress rather than for emerging mental health concerns (AAP, 2006; Drotar et al., 2008; Johnson et al., 2007). An exception has been a policy mandated by Massachusetts Medicaid as a result of a court challenge. This policy, which began January 1, 2008, requires every pediatrician in the state to administer a behavioral health screening instrument to every child who is covered by the Medicaid program, at every well-child visit from birth to age 21. A tangential outcome of the initiation of this program has been the recognition of serious shortcomings in validity and feasibility characteristics of all current mental health screening instruments for children less than 6 years of age.

Training physicians on specific strategies to treat psychosocial issues during primary care visits is one option available to address the underdetection and treatment of childhood mental health problems. Pediatric psychologists have long been involved in the training of pediatricians in primary care (Coury, Berger, Stancin, & Tanner, 1999; Drotar, 1995), but economic constraints have decreased the amount of time many academic psychologists are able to devote to the time intensive nature of this activity. One recent effort to educate PPCPs to better address psychosocial concerns in primary care includes incorporating motivational interviewing techniques in practice (Suarez & Mullens, 2008).

Other innovative models of care that include psychologists working alongside pediatricians are the Guiding Appropriate Pediatric Services project, which focused on the care of children with chronic health conditions (a population about which pediatric psychologists are generally expert) (McMenamy & Perrin, 2004), and the ongoing Advanced Parenting Education in Pediatrics project, which focuses on providing parenting advice and support within the pediatric primary care setting to parents of very young children with early evidence of disruptive behavior. The Positive Parenting Program (Sanders, 1999) and the Community Parent Education Program (Cunningham, Bremner, Secord, & Chedoke-McMaster Hospitals, 1997) also provide strategies for pediatric practices to provide brief mental health interventions in their offices for children with disruptive behaviors, primarily through manualized treatment protocols for working with their parents. The Well-child Care Visit, Evaluation, Community Resources, Advocacy, Referral, Education (WE-CARE) program (Garg et al., 2007) was developed to be a comprehensive intervention available for low-income children seeking treatment in an urban hospital and included formal screening materials, community resource booklets, and dedicated time with a physician dedicated to discussing psychosocial concerns. Outcome data for WE-CARE demonstrated that this broad intervention was successful in encouraging communication centered around diverse psychosocial issues affecting the pediatric patients; it also increased the number of referrals given by PPCPs, as well as the amount of caregiver follow-through with referrals (Garg et al., 2007). A program in North Carolina developed a generalizable model for providing developmental and behavioral screening in primary care practices that included recommendations for office resources for the office, providing anticipatory guidance, providing posters in the waiting rooms, and training materials for office staff (Earls & Hay, 2006).

Cultural Competency in Providing Mental Health Services

Patient demographics in primary care settings vary widely by geographical region and even within the same region. Pediatric psychologists have an opportunity to contribute to understanding of how different cultures may express psychosocial symptoms or react to psychosocial problems in their children and present them in primary care. For instance, when Mexican children in a California clinic were screened for problems, almost 40% of caregivers reported concerns about aggression and attention, but no anxiety or depression symptoms were identified, despite the tendency for internalizing symptoms to be pronounced in Hispanic populations (Tarshis, Jutte, & Huffman, 2006). MetroHealth Medical Center in Cleveland, Ohio has integrated psychological services into its Hispanic clinic by offering onsite bilingual psychological services and consultation for bilingual and Spanish-speaking families and clinicians (El-Ghoroury & Bonny, 2007).

Training Pediatric Psychologists to Work in Primary Care

The model of integrating mental and medical mental health care in primary care settings requires a different emphasis than is found in most pediatric psychology training programs (Spirito et al., 2003). McDaniel, Belar, Schroeder, Hargrove, and Lerman Freeman (2002) have proposed a training curriculum in primary care psychology to supplement standard core graduate psychology training. This curriculum includes 12 areas of core knowledge and skills, as well as specific training objectives pertaining to health and illness. In addition to a broad clinical child and pediatric psychology background, the successful psychologist in a primary care setting needs a solid knowledge of normal child development and behavioral concerns; facility with behavioral and developmental screening and assessment techniques; and competence to deliver brief, solution-focused individual and family systems treatments. Psychoeducational assessment and intervention skills related to topics of parenting behavior and discipline are essential. Moreover, primary care psychologists must be knowledgeable about general pediatric medical issues, including anatomy, disease processes, and preventive medicine (Blount, 1998). Knowledge about the evaluation and treatment of psychosocial aspects of child and adolescent chronic and acute medical conditions is likewise essential. The primary care psychologist also needs to be comfortable about discussing a patient's need for psychopharmacology, although not as a replacement for a psychiatrist (Blount, 1998). The importance of this issue is highlighted by Sobel and colleagues (2001), who reported that 44% of the children receiving psychological services in their primary care setting were taking medication related to their psychological diagnoses.

Challenges to Collaborative Care

If establishing collaborative care practices were simple, then there might be more of them. As was generally noted when psychology first entered the pediatric arena, there may be differences in theoretical and cultural assumptions about health and wellness, as well as in practice parameters. Collaboration across disciplines and training models is complex and difficult at best (McDaniel, Campbell, & Seaburn, 1995), and requires motivation and patience to be successful. Such apparently simple issues as assumptions about scheduling and time management, and the use of questionnaires and collateral sources of information, can become major stumbling blocks in collaborative practice.

One major issue is confidentiality. Mental health care providers tend to be so protective of patient disclosures during sessions that they refuse to share any information with another care provider unless it is specifically released by a patient or guardian. This can be very frustrating to a PPCP who also respects confidentiality but seeks access to information that a psychologist has in order to respond better to a patient's medical needs. Integrated practices assume that there will be open communication between mental health and medical professionals. Patients and families should be informed about communication so that they can provide informed consent to treatment. Confidentiality concerns may extend to access to medical records. Providing mental health services in primary care raises challenging issues related to the protection of the privacy of mental health records and protected information, as dictated by mandates of the federal Health Insurance Portability and Accountability Act of 1996 (HIPAA). An integrated practice should permit open access to medical and psychological records by the providers, so charting style will need to take this into consideration. In addition, with more practices utilizing electronic medical records, there are increased potential risks of unintentional access to protected private information by personnel and third-party payers.

There are considerable economic challenges to integrating care in primary care settings. There are personnel costs to consider if staff is added; there may be additional integrated training expenses for all providers, including office staff along with physicians, nurses, and mental health professionals. Well-integrated primary behavioral health care services should focus on controlling medical costs while optimizing health care outcomes (Strosahl, 1998). Reduced medical costs, higher rates of patient satisfaction, lower provider turnover, and increased productivity have been attributed to integrated care models in adults, although data demonstrating medical cost savings in pediatric populations have been less available (Blount, 1998). Research evaluating patient and provider satisfaction and effectiveness of mental health services in primary care has been supportive of interventions (e.g., Finney et al., 1991; Sobel et al., 2001; Tynan, Schuman, & Lampert, 1999). However, these studies have been primarily descriptive in nature, and few randomized controlled trials that would empirically evaluate the efficacy of primary care interventions compared with other service systems have been reported.

Despite recognition of the importance of delivering mental health care in pediatric outpatient settings, providers have faced difficult challenges when trying to obtain reimbursement for services. Psychologists need to demonstrate the necessity for and effectiveness of primary care interventions if they hope to convince insurance payers to reimburse services (Drotar & Lemanek, 2001). Coding and billing are complex issues in any mental health setting, but are particularly troublesome in primary care. Insurance reimbursement is driven by codes for diagnoses and procedures (see Tynan, Stehl, & Pendley, Chapter 5, this volume), and mental health services in primary care settings do not always fit neatly into recognizable codes. Many insurance companies and other third-party payers are unfamiliar with the range of mental health services in primary care practices and may be reluctant to agree to payment. For example, brief intervention services may be recommended for behavioral problems at early stages (e.g., parent training in behavior management for a preschool child with oppositional behavior). In this case, reimbursement may be denied because services are provided for mental health conditions that do not meet diagnostic criteria for a mental disorder. *The Diagnostic and Statistical Manual for Primary Care* (DSM-PC), *Child and Adolescent Version* (Wolraich, Felice, & Drotar, 1996), is a coding system developed as a way to describe the child mental health problems most often treated in primary care settings. This system not only allows child symptoms to be coded even if they are subthreshold for a *disorder* (e.g., anxiety), but also incorporates the child's environmental stresses (e.g., divorce). One of the intentions for developing the DSM-PC was the expectation that with increased number of diagnostic classifications for children, it would be easier to identify children, thus leading to more requests for reimbursement. Unfortunately, the DSM-PC does not appear to have been adopted by most pediatric practices, in part because most insurers have been unwilling to reimburse for these conditions (Drotar, 1999; Drotar, Sturner, & Nobile, 2004).

A major roadblock to fiscal viability of integrated care is the system of mental health "carve-outs" favored over the past decade by most insurance payers. Access to "approved panels" of mental health clinicians has been restricted, and considerable effort has often been required to join these panels. Thus a pediatrician's office may provide access to patients with insurance coverage from many payers, but a psychologist practicing in the same office may be paid to see patients with only certain coverage policies. The added administrative inefficiency of this system has impaired the ability of PPCPs to embrace the notion of collaborative care with enthusiasm.

Concluding Comments

Among behavioral health professionals, pediatric psychologists bring a unique perspective to primary care, including a background in systematic research and advanced clinical training in the health care of children (McDaniel et al., 2002). Quality of care, access to services, availability of empirically supported interventions, and economic factors (to name a few) are important issues in primary care as well as in other treatment settings. For integrated practices to survive, pediatric psychologists will need to expand advocacy efforts to enhance reimbursement of mental health services on state and national levels.

Pediatric organizations have responded loudly to the need to address mental health in primary care with national initiatives, and medical care providers have done so by learning skills or using tools that traditionally "belong" to psychology. However, a comparable response by psychologists has been missing. Psychologists need to advocate and collaborate more directly with medical colleagues to develop and test models that incorporate broad mental health considerations within the primary care setting. They also need to take advantage of the rich opportunities available for innovation with prevention, intervention, and public health initiatives.

References

American Academy of Pediatrics (AAP). (2000). Clinical practice guideline: Diagnosis and evaluation of the child with attention-deficit/hyperactivity disorder. *Pediatrics, 105,* 1158–1170.

American Academy of Pediatrics (AAP). (2001). Clinical practice guideline: Treatment of the school-aged child with attention-deficit/hyperactivity disorder. *Pediatrics, 108,* 1033–1044.

American Academy of Pediatrics (AAP). (2006). Identifying infants and young children with developmental disorders in the medical home: An algorithm for developmental surveillance and screening. *Pediatrics, 118,* 405–420.

Anda, R. F., Brown, D. W., Felitti, V. J., Bremner, J. D., Dube, S. R., & Giles, W. H. (2007). Adverse childhood experiences and prescribed psychotropic medications in adults. *American Journal of Preventive Medicine, 32,* 389–394.

Black, M. M. (2002). Society of pediatric psychology presidential address: Opportunities for health promotion in primary care. *Journal of Pediatric Psychology, 27,* 637–646.

Blount, A. (1998). Introduction to integrated primary care. In A. Blount (Ed.), *Integrated primary care: The future of medical and mental health collaboration* (pp. 1–43). New York: Norton.

Borowsky, I. W., Mozayeny, S., Stuenkel, K., & Ireland, M. (2004). Effects of a primary care-based intervention on violent behavior and injury in children. *Pediatrics, 114,* e392–e399.

Briggs-Gowan, M. J., Owens, P. L., Schwab-Stone, M. E., Leventhal, J. M., Leaf, P. J., & Horwitz, S. M. (2003). Persistence of psychiatric disorders in pediatric settings. *Journal of the American Academy of Child and Adolescent Psychiatry, 42,* 1360–1369.

Brown, J. D., Riley, A. W., & Wissow, L. S. (2007). Identification of youth psychosocial problems during pediatric primary care visits. *Administration and Policy in Mental Health and Mental Health Services Research, 34,* 269–281.

Campo, J. V., Shafer, S., Strohm, J., Lucas, A., Cassesse, C. G., Shaeffer, D., et al. (2005). Pediatric behavioral health in primary care: A collaborative approach. *Journal of the American Psychiatric Nurses Association, 11,* 276–282.

Cheung, A. H., Zuckerbrot, R. A., Jensen, P. S., Ghalib, K., Laraque, D., Stein, R. E. K., et al. (2007). Guidelines for adolescent depression in primary care (GLAD-PC): II. Treatment and ongoing management. *Pediatrics, 120*, e1313–e1326.

Chisolm, D. J., Gardner, W., Julian, T., & Kelleher, K. (2008). Adolescent satisfaction with computer-assisted behavioural risk screening in primary care. *Child and Adolescent Mental Health, 13*(4), 163–168.

Christophersen, E. R. (1982). Incorporating behavioral pediatrics into primary care. *Pediatric Clinics of North America, 29*, 261–296.

Connor, D. F., McLaughlin, T. J., Jeffers-Terry, M., O'Brien, W. H., Stille, C. J., Young, L. M., et al. (2006). Targeted child psychiatric services: A new model of pediatric primary clinical–child psychiatry collaborative care. *Clinical Pediatrics, 45*, 423–434.

Coury, D., Berger, S., Stancin, T., & Tanner, L. (1999). Curricular guidelines for residency training in developmental and behavioral pediatrics. *Journal of Developmental and Behavioral Pediatrics, 20*, S1–S38.

Cunningham, C. E., Bremner, R., Secord, M., & Chedoke-McMaster Hospitals. (1997). *COPE: The Community Parent Education program. A school-based family systems oriented workshop for parents of children with disruptive behavior disorders: Leader's manual.* Hamilton, ON, Canada: Chedoke-McMaster Hospitals.

Drotar, D. (1993). Influences on collaborative activities among psychologists and physicians: Implications for practice, research, and training. *Journal of Pediatric Psychology, 18*, 159–172.

Drotar, D. (Ed.). (1995). *Consulting with pediatricians: Psychological perspectives for research and practice.* New York: Plenum Press.

Drotar, D. (1999). *The Diagnostic and Statistical Manual for Primary Care (DSM-PC), Child and Adolescent Version*: What pediatric psychologists need to know. *Journal of Pediatric Psychology, 24*, 369–380.

Drotar, D., & Lemanek, K. (2001). Steps toward a clinically relevant science of interventions in pediatric settings. *Journal of Pediatric Psychology, 26*, 385–394.

Drotar, D., Spirito, A., & Stancin, T. (2003). Professional roles and practice patterns. In M. C. Roberts (Ed.), *Handbook of pediatric psychology* (3rd ed., pp. 50–66). New York: Guilford Press.

Drotar, D., Stancin, T., Dworkin, P. H., Sices, L., & Wood, L. (2008). Selecting developmental surveillance and screening tools. *Pediatrics in Review, 29*, e52–e58.

Drotar, D., Sturner, R., & Nobile, C. (2004). Diagnosing and managing behavioral and developmental problems in primary care: Current applications of the DSM-PC. In B. W. Wildman & T. Stancin (Eds.), *New directions for research and treatment of pediatric psychosocial problems in primary care* (pp. 199–224). Westport, CT: Greenwood Press.

Earls, M. F., & Hay, S. S. (2006). Setting the stage for success: Implementation of developmental and behavioral screening and surveillance in primary care practice—the North Carolina Assuring Better Child Health and Development (ABCD) Project. *Pediatrics, 118*, e183–e188.

El-Ghoroury, N. H., & Bonny, A. (2006, October). *Integrating psychological services for Hispanic youth in primary care: The Cleveland Hispanic Child and Adolescent Clinic at MetroHealth Medical Center.* Paper presented at the meeting of the National Latino Psychological Association, Milwaukee, WI.

Finney, J. W., Riley, A. W., & Cataldo, M. F. (1991). Psychology in primary care: Effects of brief targeted therapy on children's medical care utilization. *Journal of Pediatric Psychology, 16*, 447–461.

Gardner, W., Kelleher, K. A., Pajer, K. A., & Campo, J. V. (2003). Primary care clinicians' use of standardized tools to assess child psychosocial problems. *Ambulatory Pediatrics, 3*, 191–195.

Garg, A., Butz, A. M., Dworkin, P. H., Lewis, R. A., Thompson, R. E., & Serwint, J. R. (2007). Improving the management of family psychosocial problems at low-income children's well child care visits: The WE CARE project. *Pediatrics, 120,* 547–558.

Hix-Small, H., Marks, K., Squires, J., & Nickel, R. (2007). Impact of implementing developmental screening at 12 and 24 months in a pediatric practice. *Pediatrics, 120,* 381–389.

Horwitz, S. M., Kelleher, K. J., Stein, R. E., Storfer-Isser, A., Youngstrom, E. A., Park, E. R., et al. (2007). Barriers to the identification and management of psychosocial issues in children and maternal depression. *Pediatrics, 119,* e208–e218.

Hurley, L. K. (1995). Developing a collaborative pediatric psychology practice in a pediatric primary care setting. In D. Drotar (Ed.), *Consulting with pediatricians: Psychological perspectives* (pp. 159–184). New York: Plenum Press.

Johnson, C. P., Myers, S. M., & American Academy of Pediatrics (AAP) Council on Children with Disabilities. (2007). Identification and evaluation of children with autism spectrum disorders. *Pediatrics, 120,* 1183–1215.

Lavigne, J. V., Lebailly, S. A., Gouze, K. R., Cicchetti, C., Jessup, B. W., Arend, R., et al. (2008). Treating oppositional defiant disorder in primary care: A comparison of three models. *Journal of Pediatric Psychology, 33,* 449–461.

Lieberman, A., Adalist-Estrin, A., Erinle, O., & Sloan, N. (2006). On-site mental health care: A route to improving access to mental health services in an inner-city, adolescent medicine clinic. *Child: Care, Health, and Development, 32,* 407–413.

McDaniel, S. H., Belar, C. D., Schroeder, C., Hargrove, D. S., & Lerman Freeman, E. (2002). A training curriculum for professional psychologists in primary care. *Professional Psychology: Research and Practice, 33,* 65–72.

McDaniel, S. H., Campbell, T. L., & Seaburn, D. B. (1995). Principles for collaboration between health and mental health providers in primary care. *Family Systems Medicine, 13,* 283–298.

McMenamy, J. M., & Perrin, E. C. (2002). Integrating psychology into pediatrics: The past, the present, and the potential. *Families, Systems, and Health, 20,* 153–160.

McMenamy, J. M., & Perrin, E. C. (2004). Filling the GAPS: Evaluation of a primary care intervention for children with chronic health conditions. *Ambulatory Pediatrics, 4,* 249–256.

Perrin, E. C. (1998). Ethical questions about screening. Commentary. *Journal of Developmental and Behavioral Pediatrics, 19,* 350–352.

Perrin, E. C. (1999a). Collaboration in pediatric primary care: A pediatrician's view. *Journal of Pediatric Psychology, 24,* 453–458.

Perrin, E. C. (1999b). The promise of collaborative care. *Journal of Developmental and Behavioral Pediatrics, 20,* 57–62.

Perrin, E. C., & Stancin, T. (2002). A continuing dilemma: Whether and how to screen for concerns about children's behavior. *Pediatrics in Review, 23,* 264–282.

Polaha, J., Volkmer, A., & Valleley, R. J. (2007). A call in service to address parent concerns about child behavior in rural primary care. *Families, Systems, and Health, 25,* 333–343.

Riekert, K. A., Stancin, T., Palermo, T. M., & Drotar, D. (1999). A psychological behavioral screening service: Use, feasibility, and impact in a primary care setting. *Journal of Pediatric Psychology, 24,* 405–414.

Roberts, M., & Wright, L. (1982). The role of the pediatric psychologist as consultant to pediatricians. In J. Tuma (Ed.), *Handbook for the practice of pediatric psychology* (pp. 251–289). New York: Wiley-Interscience.

Roberts, M. C., & Brown, K. J. (2004). Primary care, prevention and pediatric psychology: Challenges and opportunities. In B. W. Wildman & T. Stancin (Eds.), *New directions for research and treatment of pediatric psychosocial problems in primary care* (pp. 35–59). Westport, CT: Greenwood Press.

Routh, D. K., Schroeder, C. S., & Koocher, G. P. (1983). Psychology and primary health care for children. *American Psychologist, 38,* 95–98.

Rushton, J., Bruckman, D., & Kelleher, K. (2002). Primary care referral of children with psychosocial problems. *Archives of Pediatrics and Adolescent Medicine, 156,* 592–598.

Sand, N., Silverstein, M., Glascoe, F. P., Gupta, V., Tonniges, T. P., & O'Connor, K. G. (2005). Pediatricians' reported practices regarding developmental screening: Do guidelines work? Do they help? *Pediatrics, 116,* 174–179.

Sanders, M. R. (1999). The Triple P Positive Parenting Program: Towards an empirically validated multilevel parenting and family support strategy for the prevention of behavior and emotional problems in children. *Clinical Child and Family Psychology, 2,* 71–90.

Schroeder, C. S. (1979). Psychologists in a private pediatric practice. *Journal of Pediatric Psychology, 4,* 5–18.

Schroeder, C. S. (1999). Commentary: A view from the past and a look to the future. *Journal of Pediatric Psychology, 24*(5), 447–452.

Schroeder, C. S. (2004). Reaching beyond the guild. In B. W. Wildman & T. Stancin (Eds.), *New directions for research and treatment of pediatric psychosocial problems in primary care* (pp. 1–32). Westport, CT: Greenwood Press.

Sices, L., Feudtner, C., McLaughlin, J., Drotar, D., & Williams, M. (2004). How do primary care physicians manage children with possible developmental delays?: A national survey with an experimental design. *Pediatrics, 113,* 274–282.

Smith, E. E., Rome, L. P., & Freedheim, D. K. (1967). The clinical psychologist in the pediatric office. *Journal of Pediatric Psychology, 71,* 48–51.

Sobel, A. B., Roberts, M. C., Rayfield, A. D., Barnard, M. U., & Rapoff, M. D. (2001). Evaluating outpatient pediatric psychology services in a primary care setting. *Journal of Pediatric Psychology, 26,* 395–405.

Spirito, A., Brown, R. T., D'Angelo, E., Delamater, A., Rodrique, J., & Siegel, L. (2003). Society of Pediatric Psychology Task Force Report: Recommendations for the training of pediatric psychologists. *Journal of Pediatric Psychology, 28,* 85–98.

Stancin, T. (1999). Special issue on pediatric mental health services in primary care settings [Introduction]. *Journal of Pediatric Psychology, 24,* 367–368.

Stancin, T. (2005). Mental health services for children in pediatric primary care settings. In R. G. Steele, Jr. & M. C. Roberts (Eds.), *Handbook of mental health services for children, adolescents, and families* (pp. 85–101). New York: Kluwer Academic/Plenum.

Stancin, T., & Palermo, T. M. (1997). A review of behavioral screening practices in pediatric settings: Do they pass the test? *Journal of Developmental and Behavioral Pediatrics, 18,* 183–194.

Strosahl, K. (1998). Integrating behavioral health and primary care services: The primary mental health care model. In A. Blount (Ed.), *Integrated primary care: The future of medical and mental health collaboration* (pp. 139–166). New York: Norton.

Suarez, M., & Mullins, S. (2008). Motivational interviewing and pediatric health behavior interventions. *Journal of Developmental and Behavioral Pediatrics, 29,* 417–428.

Tarshis, T. P., Jutte, D. P., & Huffman, L. C. (2006). Provider recognition of psychosocial problems in low-income Latino children. *Journal of Health Care for the Poor and Underserved, 17,* 342–357.

Tynan, W. D., Schuman, W., & Lampert, N. (1999). Concurrent parent and child therapy groups for externalizing disorders: From the laboratory to the world of managed care. *Cognitive and Behavioral Practice, 6,* 3–9.

U.S. Department of Health and Human Services. (1999). *Mental health: A Report of the Surgeon General.* Washington, DC: U.S. Government Printing Office.

Weitzman, C. C., & Leventhal, J. M. (2006). Screening for behavioral health problems in primary care. *Current Opinion in Pediatrics, 18,* 641–648.

Wildman, B. W., & Stancin, T. (Eds.). (2004). *New directions for research and treatment of pediatric psychosocial problems in primary care*. Westport, CT: Greenwood Press.

Williams, J., Klinepeter, K., Palmes, G., Pulley, A., & Foy, J. M. (2004). Diagnosis and treatment of behavioral health disorders in pediatric practice. *Pediatrics, 114*, 601–606.

Williams, J., Shore, S. E., & Foy, J. M. (2006). Co-location of mental health professionals in primary care settings: Three North Carolina models. *Clinical Pediatrics, 45*, 537–543.

Wolraich, M. L., Felice, M. E., & Drotar, D. (Eds.). (1996). *The classification of child and adolescent mental diagnoses in primary care: Diagnostic and Statistical Manual for Primary Care (DSM-PC), Child and Adolescent Version*. Elk Grove, IL: American Academy of Pediatrics.

PART V

Systems

CHAPTER 43

An Overview of Systems
in Pediatric Psychology Research and Practice

RIC G. STEELE
BRANDON S. AYLWARD

Despite a long-standing conceptual systems orientation in the field (see Roberts & McNeal, 1995), the practice of pediatric psychology has remained relatively individually oriented throughout much of the 20th century (Kaufman, Holden, & Walker, 1989). Recognizing this discrepancy, a number of authors have called for the field to renew its emphasis on systems-level research and practice. For example, Brown and Roberts (2000) identified "addressing changes in larger societal and socioeconomic conditions that affect child development, education, medical care, and psychological services" (p. 8) as one of the top issues facing the field. Similarly, in his Society of Pediatric Psychology presidential address, Brown (2002) noted the need for more systemic approaches in the study of the reciprocal influences between children with chronic illnesses and health care providers, peers, and schools. Such calls have been regularly noted in the recent pediatric literature (e.g., Freier & Aylward, 2007; Kazak, Rourke, & Crump, 2003) and underscore the importance of incorporating broader contextual perspectives as a means of more effectively addressing the physical and psychological needs of children and youths.

Broadly characterized, a systems-oriented perspective in psychology assumes a reciprocal influence between an individual's behavior and the behavior of other individuals within the system (Hobbs, 1966). This framework has been applied to understanding the functioning of the child in the family and other systems, such as the school and health care network (Power & Bartholomew, 1987; Power, DuPaul, Shapiro, & Kazak, 2003). Among the conceptual models that illustrate a systems-oriented approach to child development, Bronfenbrenner's (1979) social-ecological model of development is perhaps the most recognizable. In brief, the theory posits that human development is the product of psychological, familial, social, cultural, political, and biological factors, none of which can be considered in isolation. Graphically, the model is often represented as a set of concentric rings, each representing more distal influences on the child (see Figure 43.1). As described in more detail below, relatively distal forces (e.g., culture, political movements) are hypothesized to exert their influence on child development by affecting the contexts within which proximal influences operate (e.g., relationships with parents).

Originally proposed to explain human developmental processes, Bronfenbrenner's social-ecological theory has been adopted within applied psychology as a way of understanding clinical issues, processes, and outcomes (see Fiese, Spagnola, & Everhart, 2008; Kazak et al., 2003). With this in mind, an overview of Bronfenbrenner's four systems, with particular attention to how they have informed the pediatric psychology literature, is appropriate.

Microsystems

At the most proximal level, "microsystems" contain the child and those individuals with direct influence on the child. Bronfenbrenner (1994) noted that microsystems include the patterns of "activities, roles, and interpersonal relations experienced by the developing person in a given face-to-face setting" (p. 1645). In the developmental literature, these include the child's reciprocal relationships with parents and caregivers, siblings, teachers, peers, health care and mental health care providers, and others with direct influence on the youth's development. Consistent with Bronfenbrenner's later addition of "bio-" to his ecological systems theory (see Ceci, 2006), Kazak, Segal-Andrews, and Johnson

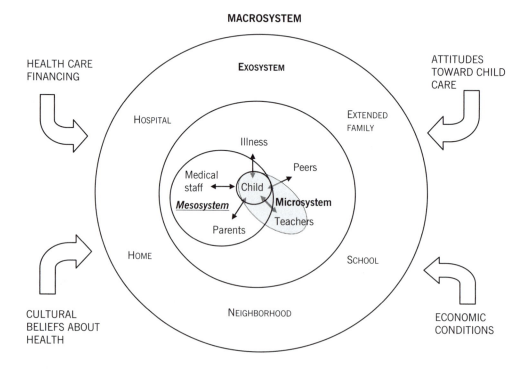

FIGURE 43.1. Bronfenbrenner's social-ecological systems theory.

(1995) noted that in the pediatric health setting, the interactions between the child and the illness and between the child and the treatment team also constitute microsystems that can have direct effects on the child, and can interact with other microsystems to affect the context of development.

A child's or adolescent's reciprocal interactions with parents and siblings (e.g., Kazak, Rourke, & Navsaria, Chapter 44, this volume) or peers (Reiter-Purtill, Waller, & Noll, Chapter 45, this volume) constitute the most proximal influences on the youth's well-being in the context of medical illness. As such, much of the research that has been conducted within populations of concern to pediatric psychology falls within the microsystem. Following Kazak and colleagues' (1995) reconceptualization of Bronfenbrenner's (1979) model, characteristics of the illness itself and the child's understanding of and attitude toward the illness also fall within the microsystem.

Mesosystems

One step removed from these direct relationships are the interactions between two or more microsystems that have an effect on a child's care, adjustment, or outcome. As identified by Bronfenbrenner (1993), these "mesosystems" comprise the relationships that exist among individuals from two or more settings in which the child functions. More plainly, Bronfenbrenner and Morris (1998) noted that a mesosystem is "a system of two or more microsystems" (p. 1016)—for example, the system comprising the child–parent microsystem and the child–teacher microsystem. With the addition of relevant microsystems, the mesosystem becomes increasingly complex (e.g., a mesosystem including parents, teachers, and peers), but provides a sense of the context within which the child develops.

In the clinical arena, much of what constitutes a "system of care" (SOC) can be characterized as existing within the mesosystem. Stroul and Friedman (1986) defined an SOC as "a comprehensive spectrum of mental health and other necessary services which are organized into a coordinated network to meet the multiple and changing needs of children and adolescents" (p. xxii). Similarly, Winters, Pumariga, the Work Group on Community Child and Adolescent Psychology, and the Work Group on Quality Issues (2007) have underscored the importance of services for children that are coordinated and integrated to promote optimal care. Consistent with this view, we argue that an SOC approach to care in pediatric psychology is both *interdisciplinary* and *intersystemic* (in which the child is the beneficiary of multiple disciplines working together across system boundaries), rather than simply *multidisciplinary* (in which multiple disciplines independently work with a child). For example, a child's reintegration into a school system following an extended illness necessitates well-functioning mesosystems (perhaps including families, school personnel, medical staff, and peers) to increase the child's likelihood of success (see DuPaul, Shapiro, & Power, Chapter 46, this volume).

Exosystems

The complex interactions between the microsystems that constitute mesosystems do not occur within a vacuum. Indeed, a number of factors ostensibly unrelated to a child or family can have significant effects on the child's development and outcome. Bronfenbrenner (1993) conceptualized the "exosystem" as "the linkages and processes taking place between two or more settings, at least one of which does not contain the developing person, but in which events occur that indirectly influence processes within the immediate setting in which the developing person lives" (p. 24). As such, even though the exosystem may not include the child, it nevertheless affects the microsystems that do include the child. For example, work environments, extended family supports, the mass media, community services, and neighbors can all affect components of the microsystems that include the developing child, and can also affect the nature and extent of the various microsystems' interactions with one another. Within pediatric settings, structured or unstructured parent support groups, hospital programs that help reintegrate children into schools, extended family supports, and parental workplace policies and programs may all indirectly affect the child by enhancing the resources of the direct caregivers.

Macrosystems

Most distal from the child is the "macrosystem," which encompasses cultural and subcultural values, norms, and expectations relating to child care and development. As noted by Bronfenbrenner (1993) the macrosystem encompasses "the overarching pattern of micro-, meso-, and exosystemic characteristics of a given culture" (p. 25), which influences the opportunities, expectations, and social interaction patterns that directly influence child development. For example, the cultural values that have prompted universal health insurance for children in some countries, or those that prompted the passage of the Family and Medical Leave Act (FMLA) in the United States, represent positive macrosystemic influences on child development. FMLA legislation, for example, may facilitate decreased levels of job stress in the family of a child with a serious medical illness, which may translate into better parental functioning, better family communication with health care providers, and ultimately better child health outcomes.

Both Brown (2002) and Kazak and colleagues (2003) have noted that despite its influence on child development, the macrosystem is frequently overlooked in the pediatric literature. We assume that the paucity of research on the macrosystem is related to the difficulty of adequately characterizing and measuring values at the community level. Nevertheless, some work that approximates research at this level has been reported. For example, the effects of discriminatory beliefs and attitudes about children with HIV may represent negative macrosystemic influences on the children's development (e.g., Jessee, Nagy, & Gresham, 2001; Stinnett, Cruce, & Choate, 2004).

Social-Ecological Theory in Practice Settings

If one considers the tertiary care hospital setting as a stand-alone microcosm, one can easily see the various ecological systems at work. The child comes to the hospital with already developing microsystems with parents, teachers, peers, a referring pediatrician, and the illness itself. To these existing microsystems are added new microsystems with physicians, nurses, physical therapists, child life specialists, pediatric psychologists, and social workers. The reciprocal relationships that exist among these various health care providers and between the providers and the family constitute mesosystemic relationships that can dramatically affect a child's health status (e.g., via adherence), academic performance (e.g., via school attendance and service), and social functioning (e.g., via social support networks; see Seid, Opipari-Arrigan, & Sobo, Chapter 47, this volume, for a more detailed analysis of the family within the health care system). Much of what constitutes interdisciplinary or "child-centered" care is accurately described within a social-ecological framework. The degree to which an institution values and fosters such interdisciplinary and intersystemic care (i.e., the macrosystem) directly affects the institutional structures and opportunities that enhance collaboration within and among multidisciplinary treatment teams (i.e., the exosystems). As briefly discussed below, successful navigation of these interrelated systems can be benefited by systems-related training and by ecologically informed research.

Implications for Training and Research in Pediatric Psychology

In his seminal article outlining the parameters of the discipline, Wright (1967) underscored the importance of collaboration within multiple settings to develop and utilize interventions that best fit within the settings. This is no less true today. The collaborations and synergies between and within systems and settings can optimize programs of intervention and prevention, as well as the overall development of the child within each system (e.g., parent–child relationship, school performance; Patrikakou, Weissberg, & Rubenstein, 1999). Consistent with this view, Power, Shapiro, and DuPaul (2003) reaffirmed the value of training psychologists to link health, educational, and family systems, and also highlighted several predoctoral programs that have been established to train students to provide comprehensive care to children. Generally, these programs aim to prepare students to work in multiple contexts and to be effective in linking systems of care for children and families through an integrated set of interdisciplinary courses and practicum placements, which expose trainees to interaction and collaboration with multidisciplinary teams and to a number of different service models (e.g., inpatient, outpatient, consultation–liaison services; see also Drotar, 1998; Power, Shapiro, et al., 2003; Roberts & Steele, 2003).

On the research side, a number of authors (e.g., Kazak et al., Chapter 44, and Seid et al., Chapter 47, this volume) have called for further research examining the reciprocal relationships among various systems in pediatric populations, to more clearly identify the factors that may influence adjustment and adaptation of children with chronic illnesses. Similarly, Brown (2002) has outlined several important areas of research for the future. For example, although there has been research examining the profound influence of the family on child adjustment, the means by which other contextual factors (e.g., relationships with health care providers and schools) mediate or moderate this relationship have been largely unexamined. In addition, such areas as school reentry of children with chronic illness, as well as issues related to the influence of health care providers on treatment outcome (e.g., provider attitude, parent–provider communication), have received little attention in the pediatric psychology literature.

Systems-based research, such as that called for above, will almost certainly involve the collection of data from a number of sources and by a number of different means (methods). As discussed by Holmbeck, Li, Schurman, Friedman, and Coakley (2002), there are a number of ways of handling multisource data, each with its advantages and disadvantages. For example, although keeping data from within or across systems disaggregated allows for easy examination of each source, it also increases the number of discrete analyses that are necessary to address the research questions. Alternatively, Holmbeck and colleagues (2002) note that the use of source/method aggregation via latent variable modeling allows for a greater understanding of "shared perspective" (p. 10) across reporters. This will require the use of advanced statistical approaches, such as structural equation modeling (SEM) techniques, to examine the multiple interacting relationships in complex social-ecological systems models in their entirety rather than in a piecemeal fashion (see Nelson, Aylward, & Steele, 2008).

Summary

Recent commentaries and editorial vale dicta in the *Journal of Pediatric Psychology* (e.g., Brown, 2007; Freier & Aylward, 2007; Kazak, Simms, & Rourke, 2002) have noted that the field of pediatric psychology is expanding in terms of the illnesses that have been researched, as well as in terms of the participant focus of the research (individual → families). Nevertheless, investigations incorporating the broader context of the child and family are still relatively rare. Although Bronfenbrenner's microsystems have been investigated in a number of populations, research into the mesosystems, exosystems, and macrosystems that influence the microsystems has only just begun to emerge. In order to develop and provide the most effective and sustainable interventions for children with chronic illness, research into these broader systems must be given greater attention (Freier & Aylward, 2007).

References

Bronfenbrenner, U. (1979). *The ecology of human development.* Cambridge, MA: Harvard University Press.

Bronfenbrenner, U. (1993). The ecology of cognitive development: Research models and fugitive findings. In R. H. Wozniak & K. Fischer (Eds.), *Scientific environments* (pp. 3–44). Hillsdale, NJ: Erlbaum.

Bronfenbrenner, U. (1994). Ecological models of human development. In T. Husen & T. N. Postlethaite (Eds.), *International encyclopedia of education* (2nd ed., Vol. 3, pp. 1643–1647). Oxford, UK: Pergamon Press/Elsevier Science.

Bronfenbrenner, U., & Morris, P. A. (1998). The ecology of developmental processes. In W. Damon (Series Ed.) & L. M. Lerner (Vol. Ed.), *Handbook of child psychology: Vol. 1. Theoretical models of human development* (5th ed., pp. 993–1028). New York: Cambridge University Press.

Brown, K. J., & Roberts, M. C. (2000). Future issues in pediatric psychology: Delphic survey. *Journal of Clinical Psychology in Medical Settings, 7,* 5–15.

Brown, R. T. (2002). Society of Pediatric Psychology presidential address: Toward a social ecology of pediatric psychology. *Journal of Pediatric Psychology, 27,* 191–201.

Brown, R. T. (2007). *Journal of Pediatric Psychology (JPP),* 2003–2007: Editor's vale dictum. *Journal of Pediatric Psychology, 32,* 1165–1178.

Ceci, S. J. (2006). Urie Bronfenbrenner (1917–2005). *American Psychologist, 61,* 173–174.

Drotar, D. (1998). Training students for careers in medical settings: A graduate program in pediatric psychology. *Professional Psychology: Research and Practice, 29,* 402–404.

Fiese, B. H., Spagnola, M., & Everhart, R. S. (2008). Family context in developmental–behavioral pediatrics. In M. L. Wolraich, D. D. Drotar, P. H. Dworkin, & E. C. Perrin (Eds.), *Developmental and behavioral pediatrics: Evidence and practice* (pp. 79–108). Philadelphia: Mosby.

Freier, M. C., & Aylward, G. P. (2007). Commentary: Broadening the scope of practice and research in pediatric psychology. *Journal of Pediatric Psychology, 32,* 875–876.

Hobbs, N. (1966). Helping disturbed children: Psychological and ecological strategies. *American Psychologist, 21,* 1105–1115.

Holmbeck, G. N., Li, S. T., Schurman, J. V., Friedman, D., & Coakley, R. M. (2002). Collecting and managing multisource and multimethod data in studies of pediatric populations. *Journal of Pediatric Psychology, 27,* 5–18.

Jessee, P. O., Nagy, M., & Gresham, C. (2001). Public opinion concerning group involvement for children with AIDS. *Early Child Development and Care, 166,* 29–38.

Kazak, A. E., Rourke, M. T., & Crump, T. A. (2003). Families and other systems in pediatric psychology. In M. C. Roberts (Ed.), *Handbook of pediatric psychology* (3rd ed., pp. 159–175). New York: Guilford Press.

Kazak, A. E., Segal-Andrews, A. M., & Johnson, K. (1995). Pediatric psychology research and practice: A family/systems approach. In M. C. Roberts (Ed.), *Handbook of pediatric psychology* (2nd ed., pp. 84–104). New York: Guilford Press.

Kazak, A. E., Simms, S., & Rourke, M. T. (2002). Family systems practice in pediatric psychology. *Journal of Pediatric Psychology, 27,* 133–143.

Kaufman, K. L., Holden, E. W., & Walker, C. E. (1989). Future directions in pediatric and clinical child psychology. *Professional Psychology: Research and Practice, 20,* 148–152.

Nelson, T. D., Aylward, B. S., & Steele, R. G. (2008). Structural equation modeling in pediatric psychology: Overview and review of applications. *Journal of Pediatric Psychology, 33,* 679–687.

Patrikakou, E. N., Weissberg, R. P., & Rubenstein, M. I. (1999). School–family partnerships. In A. J. Reynolds, R. P. Weissberg, & H. J. Walberg (Eds.), *Promoting positive outcomes in children and youth* (pp. 95–127). Washington, DC: Child Welfare League of America.

Power, T. J., & Bartholomew, K. L. (1987). Family–school relationship patterns: An ecological assessment. *School Psychology Review, 14,* 222–229.

Power, T. J., DuPaul, G. J., Shapiro, E. S., & Kazak, A. E. (2003). *Promoting children's health: Integrating school, family, and community.* New York: Guilford Press.

Power, T. J., Shapiro, E. S., & DuPaul, G. J. (2003). Preparing psychologists to link systems of care in managing and preventing children health problems. *Journal of Pediatric Psychology, 28,* 147–155.

Roberts, M. C., & McNeal, R. E. (1995). Historical and conceptual foundations of pediatric psychology. In M. C. Roberts (Ed.), *Handbook of pediatric psychology* (2nd ed., pp. 3–18). New York: Guilford Press.

Roberts, M. C., & Steele, R. G. (2003). Predoctoral training in pediatric psychology at the University of Kansas Clinical Child Psychology Program. *Journal of Pediatric Psychology, 28,* 99–103.

Stinnett, T. A., Cruce, M. K., & Choate, K. T. (2004). Influences on teacher education student attitudes toward youth who are HIV. *Psychology in the Schools, 41,* 211–219.

Stroul, B. A., & Friedman, R. M. (1986). *A system of care for children and youth with severe emotional disturbances* (rev. ed.). Washington, DC: Georgetown University Child Development Center, CASSP Technical Assistance Center.

Winters, N. C., Pumariga, A., the Work Group on Community Child and Adolescent Psychiatry, & the Work Group on Quality Issues. (2007). Practice parameter on child and adolescent mental health care in community systems of care. *Journal of the American Academy of Child and Adolescent Psychiatry, 46,* 284–299.

Wright, L. (1967). The pediatric psychologist: A role model. *American Psychologist, 22,* 323–325.

CHAPTER 44

Families and Other Systems in Pediatric Psychology

ANNE E. KAZAK
MARY T. ROURKE
NEHA NAVSARIA

A child's health-related concerns inherently and unquestionably affect not only the child, but also parents, siblings, extended family, classmates, school personnel, and the health care team. Likewise, these groups, or subsystems reciprocally interact with one another, and all of them both influence and are influenced by the child. Children with chronic illness and their families must balance the complicated tasks of growing up with the symptoms of their disease and implications of their treatment. The course of a child's life and a family's development may be both subtly and profoundly shaped by a shortened lifespan, a lifetime of unpredictable medical issues, cognitive impairments, and/or the financial impact of long-term illness.

There is much to be learned from a broader inclusion of families and other systems in our conceptualization of children and health. Historically, families of ill children tended to be viewed as disrupted or even pathological. This idea remains remarkably entrenched, although the empirical literature supporting the competence of families and clarifying the substantial but understandable distress associated with child health problems is growing. As the broad range of responses—along the continuum from normative/adaptive to maladaptive—has begun to be elaborated, models that foster understanding the distribution of responses along this continuum are essential. Similarly, research on extrafamilial systems (e.g., schools, the health care system) is also expanding. When families, as well as other relevant developmental contexts, are viewed as essential and inseparable from young patients in understanding illness and adaptation, the systemic complexity of pediatric psychology becomes evident.

In this chapter, we use a social-ecological model to organize family and contextual factors related to child health. After discussing relevant family subsystems and major systems external to the family, we address current knowledge regarding family assessment and intervention. In doing so, we recognize the importance of conceptual frameworks (e.g., Fiese & Sameroff, 1989; Wallander, Thompson, & Alriksson-Schmidt, 2005; Wood, 1995), as well as recent advances in family research methodology, including multilevel modeling approaches, survival analysis, process research, and narrative and qualitative approaches (see the *Journal of Family Psychology* special issue "Methodology in Family Science" [Snyder & Kazak, 2005]).

A Social-Ecological Framework Applied to Pediatric Psychology

Social ecology is a useful model for conceptualizing the complex ways in which systems relevant to the lives of pediatric patients and their families interact to shape development and adaptation (Kazak, 1989). Based on the work of developmental psychologist Urie Bronfenbrenner (1979), social ecology maps systems at varying levels of distance from a child, and provides a framework for understanding relationships among these systems. At the most basic level are the immediate settings in which a child directly participates (or "microsystems"), such as the family, school, and health care system, as well as subsystems of these settings, including the parent–child relationship or siblings.

At the next level of influence, multiple microsystems interact to affect a child's development and adaptation. For chronically ill children, these "mesosystem" influences include family–health care team interactions and family–school interactions—allowing psychologists to explore, for example, how interactions among families, health care teams, and school personnel affect children with chronic illness and their families. At a more distal level, systems in which a child does not directly participate, but that indirectly affect the child (i.e., "exosystems"), include parental social networks and parental employment. For children with chronic illness, relevant exosystems may include the health care environment, or morale among the inpatient medical team (or other families on the unit).

At the outermost level of social ecology is the "macrosystem," which refers to the impact of subculture, culture, and general belief patterns throughout the ecology. Although broader systems issues are frequently not considered within the realm of psychological theory or intervention, neglect of these issues can result in a dangerously myopic view of families. Culture and ethnicity have a significant role in shaping the values and beliefs that are embedded within a family unit. Within the medical context, a family's belief system is cultivated and maintained through its members' interactions with health care systems and its problem-solving efforts (McCubbin, Thompson, Thompson, McCubbin, & Kaston, 1993). An assessment of cultural domains can elucidate the processes that form paradigms of family functioning. An evaluation of cultural domains should include an understanding of the meaning, source, and language of illness for a family; exploration of religious and spiritual beliefs; and, on a broader level, assessment of the impacts of socioeconomic status (SES), discrimination, immigration, and political history (Maloney, Clay, & Robinson, 2005).

On a broader systemic level, local, state, and federal laws and policies, including mental health insurance coverage for children with medical illness, have direct implications for the types of care and services available to children and families. Over the past two decades, we have witnessed the impact of dramatic changes in health care on families, as well as the passage of legislation (e.g., the Family and Medical Leave Act) that provides options for balancing family and work demands. Understanding ways in which broader systems constrain or support family adaptation during the course of an illness is critical to designing more effective interventions.

We use the social-ecological model as a map for presenting relevant research to examine the developmental context of the child with chronic illness, and to review the development and evaluation of interventions. We focus on the family as the child's primary microsystem and, whenever possible, include studies that frame research questions and methodologies in ways acknowledging the complex interplay of ecological variables. Because our approach also emphasizes family strength or competence, we include studies that focus on the presumably adaptive processes families demonstrate when confronted with illness.

The Developmental Context of the Child with Chronic Illness

The Child

The child is at the center of a series of concentric and interactive circles, each representing a system in the child's ecology (e.g., family, health care environment, illness). This ecological context is highly interactional. For example, parents must provide consent to initiate treatment for a child; even for an adolescent, family members assume responsibility for managing medical care and for setting the tone of interactions between the medical team and the adolescent. Despite the family's broad and powerful impact throughout the course of treatment, however, most of what is known about child adjustment to illness focuses on the individual child.

The substantial literature on child adjustment demonstrates that children with chronic illness are at some elevated risk for psychological difficulties (Cadman, Boyle, Szatmari, & Offord, 1987). However, there is a discernible need for methodologically rigorous research that identifies the contextual variables placing a chronically ill child and family at risk for ongoing difficulties across all phases of illness and treatment. In addition, consistent with medicine's organization by organ systems and diseases, much of the existing literature focuses on specific illnesses. An ecological perspective, considering the concurrent interaction of many systems, provides an opportunity to identify common parameters of illness, treatment, and family responses across conditions.

A key social-ecological concept involves understanding how reciprocal interactions provide a context for development. Children with illnesses continue to grow and develop as they adjust to and cope with their health-related concerns, but this developmental progress may be affected by the interplay of the illness/treatment with more normative developmental influences. For example, early in the illness trajectory or after a significant exacerbation, as family members cope and adjust to the realities of their child's health concerns, they may (perhaps appropriately) treat the child differently. A child who is not feeling well may be excused temporarily from some developmentally appropriate expectations, and may seek comfort and emotional support in a way similar to a younger child. As treatment progresses, the child is expected to participate in a developmentally appropriate manner. As at diagnosis, the child and family reorganize around the illness, perhaps shifting roles, with a common goal of achieving successful treatment while supporting general development. Occasionally, however, this reorganization becomes rigid and static: A child is unable to move on to more developmentally appropriate behaviors, and parents are unable to support more independent behavior in their child.

Similarly, normative developmental changes require families to renegotiate illness-specific issues frequently. For example, as adolescence unfolds, the parents and child need to be flexible and gradually shift roles in order to accommodate, or even encourage, the child's increasing independence. This extended period of shared, but shifting, responsibility for illness management can set the stage for significant parent–child conflict over adherence. As prognoses improve for many serious childhood illnesses, long-term survivorship is an important developmental phase for patients and families; it presents such new challenges as facing long-term medical effects of intense treatments, complicated but potentially disruptive medical regimens that are necessary for health maintenance, and real or perceived functional impairment.

The Illness and Treatment

The illness and its treatment form a critical microsystem in the lives of children and families. Diseases and treatments differ vastly and can assume different roles within the family context. Likewise, the impact of the very same disease/treatment can vary, depending on the child or family managing it. As discussed above, an illness also interacts with development, causing the nature of the illness and its impact to shift over time.

Illnesses vary in important ways. Some conditions are highly visible (e.g., cerebral palsy, amputation), while others, though significant, are not apparent to others. Illnesses also vary in severity, although it can be difficult to characterize severity. In general illness, severity is not associated with adjustment, although it may affect the demands placed on the child and family for treatment (Rodrigues & Patterson, 2007). There are also potential indirect effects; for example, disease severity may influence parental behavior, but may not be directly associated with health care utilization (Logan, Radcliffe, & Smith-Whitley, 2002). An exception is a case in which the child's illness affects the central nervous system (Wade et al., 2006).

Subjective factors (e.g., what the patient and family believe about the illness and its treatment) are generally more powerful predictors of outcome than are typical "objective" measures of illness severity (e.g., physician ratings). In a sample with congenital heart disease, mothers' perceptions, but not physician ratings, of illness severity were correlated with psychological distress (Van Horn, DeMaso, Gonzalez-Heydrich, & Erickson, 2001). Similarly, sibling adjustment was not associated with severity of the illness, although more negative adjustment was evident with conditions in which daily functioning was more heavily affected (Sharpe & Rossiter, 2002).

The lack of association between distress and more objective measures of illness severity emphasizes the importance of focusing on the subjective illness experience of children and their caregivers. Even in diseases with more positive prognoses, family members must confront the losses associated with the illness and treatments. That is, a child's illness experience is a product of the complex interaction of micro-, meso-, exo-, and macrosystem influences, rather than a clear reflection of "medical facts" that may more objectively indicate severity.

Siblings

Although siblings have received relatively little attention in the literature, pediatric illnesses and their treatments have many effects on siblings, and siblings in turn affect the ill child and family in multiple ways. On an individual level, distress in siblings has been demonstrated (Sharpe & Rossiter, 2002); age, birth order, gender, and disease characteristics have all been linked to sibling adaptation. Family factors also affect sibling adaptation. For example, Williams and colleagues (1999) found that family cohesion mediated the relationship between maternal and sibling mood. Having a sibling with chronic illness may also be associated with positive outcomes, including potential benefits for those who donate bone marrow (Packman, 1999). High levels of social support appear to play a protective role as well, supporting the development of interventions for siblings (Barerra, Chung, & Fleming, 2004).

Parents

Parents are central to effective family functioning and are the usual informants about the child's health, history, and functioning. When parents have been the focus of pediatric investigations, the main aim has been to describe parental adaptation to the child's illness and related demands. In general, distress around the time of diagnosis of illnesses such as cancer has been well documented, with meta-analyses supporting the natural course of adaptation and adjustment over time (Pai et al., 2007). Less well understood are the myriad of ways that parental moods, attitudes, functioning, and behavior promote or confound health outcomes in children. For example, parental mood and management of family activities related to bedtime were associated with the likelihood that children with asthma would awaken during the night (Fiese, Winter, Sliwinski, & Anbar, 2007). In samples of children with spina bifida and with cancer, parental distress has been found to be related to distress in the ill child (Friedman, Holmbeck, Jandasek, Zukerman, & Abad, 2004; Robinson, Gerardt, Vannatta, & Noll, 2007).

An understanding of parenting in pediatric psychology remains biased by reliance on maternal report. Although this bias reflects the general focus on mothers and children in pediatric health care services, its persistence is remarkable; it limits professionals' understanding of how families function, and maintains a view of fathers as peripheral to the well-being of children. Studies documenting paternal distress in HIV/ AIDS (Wiener, Vasquez, & Battles, 2001) and injuries (Schwebel & Brezausek, 2004) are welcome developments. Including fathers is important; however, assuring that study design and methods support the analysis and interpretation of father "effects" on outcomes is also critical (Phares, Lopez, Fields, Kamboukos, & Duhig, 2005).

Marital Relationships

One of the most frequently heard comments about the impact of serious childhood illness on families is the suggestion that marital separation and divorce are inevitable, despite compelling evidence over the past two decades that overall levels of marital satisfaction are not different between families with and without chronically ill children (Berge, Patterson, & Rueter, 2006; Sabbeth & Leventhal, 1984). More recent research has moved beyond simple group comparisons to explore systemic factors related to marital satisfaction in parents of children with chronic illness or disability. Some research has documented different processes of communication among parents of such children. For example, although parents of children with asthma did not differ in marital satisfaction from parents of never-ill children, they expressed less disagreement, more frequently detoured potentially conflictual conversations, and more often drew the children into parental disputes (Northey, Griffin, & Krainz, 1998).

Role strain—or parents' experience of illness-related demands, including frustration about the division of labor, role conflict, and affective exchanges (Quittner et al., 1998)—can contribute to marital strain. Parents of children with cystic fibrosis report more role strain than parents of well children do (Quittner et al., 1998). Similarly, parents of children with spina bifida (Friedman et al., 2004) and developmental disabilities (Stoneman & Gavidia-Payne, 2006) report more daily stressors, and this distress is related to marital dissatisfaction. As research on marital satisfaction has begun to include reports from both fathers and mothers, it has become clear that specific stressors vary according to parental role (Holmbeck et al., 1997), and that the ways in which illness-related stressors may relate to marital satisfaction may differ for fathers and mothers (Berge et al., 2006).

Research on marital satisfaction in families documents the relational interdependence of family members. In a study of parents of children with cancer, marital adjustment was predicted not only by each parent's own affective functioning, but also by the spouse's marital satisfaction (Dahlquist, Czyzewski, & Jones, 1996). Similarly, in a study of parents of children with disabilities, mothers' reports of marital adjustment were higher when fathers reported a higher use of problem-focused coping (Stoneman & Gavidia-Payne, 2006). The impact of marital satisfaction on the ill child has also been explored. Friedman and colleagues (2004) found that marital adjustment, along with parental psychopathology and parenting stress, predicted child adjustment. There is even some evidence that the marital relationship may affect disease control. In adolescents with diabetes, higher levels of mother-reported spousal support were related to less conflict and better treatment adherence (Lewandowski & Drotar, 2007).

Families

It is important to think broadly about family composition and function, and to develop inclusive definitions of "families." There are many different types of families; single-parent families, remarried families, gay/lesbian families, adoptive families, and foster care families are among the most commonly encountered. There are literatures on each that provide cogent summaries based on empirical studies and clinical experience. In most cases, however, illness-specific issues confronting more diverse families have not been addressed. For example, the family members who mobilize in a crisis; the family members who help ensure that the family functions as routinely as possible; or the family as defined by ethnic, religious, or other cultural parameters may vary.

Research on families and childhood illness examines some of the consistent predictors of well-being. These include, for example, family flexibility; integration into a supportive social network; being able to balance the demands of the illness with other family needs and responsibilities; clear family boundaries; effective communication; positive attributions; active coping; and the encouragement of development of individuals within the family. Across a series of studies, families of children with cancer were more like other, nonaffected families than different, with only a subset of families demonstrating psychosocial difficulties at a clinical level (Kazak, 2001). This is not meant to imply that families do not "need" or benefit from assistance. Rather, it underscores family competence and the many possibilities for including family members as partners in the development and delivery of interventions in child health.

Understanding family-level variables can clarify the complex process of adaptation to a child's illness. For example, lower levels of family function were observed in families of school-age children with cystic fibrosis than in families of well children (Janicke, Mitchell, & Stark, 2005). Lower levels of cohesion were observed in families of children with spina bifida than in a matched sample, although there were no group differences in family conflict (Holmbeck, Coakley, Hommeyer, Shapera, & Westhoven, 2002). While illness may disrupt family cohesion, families are resilient and adapt to illness-related issues, which may avert higher levels of family conflict. Interestingly, in this study, families of lower SES evidenced less cohesion, more conflict, and more stressful life events than higher-SES families, suggesting how an exosystemic factor (i.e., SES) may shape a family's illness experience. This same line of research highlights how normative developmental events may be experienced differently by families managing chronic illness. Early puberty was associated with higher levels of family conflict and lower levels of family cohesion for well children, but not for those with spina bifida (Coakley, Holmbeck, Friedman, Greenley, & Thill, 2002). These kinds of developmental differences, their meanings for individuals and for families, and similarities and differences across illnesses need to be explored further.

Some research suggests the potential for individual or family dysfunction to influence disease course and even outcome. For example, patterns of family interaction have been linked to disease activity in families of children with diabetes (Martin, Miller-Johnson, Kitzmann, & Emery, 1998). In families of children with asthma, family emotional climate has been shown to influence child depressive symptoms, which in turn were associated with triggering asthma attacks and with overall disease severity (Wood et al., 2007). Family environment may also affect a child's experience of illness. For example, in a sample of children with recurrent pain syndromes, the experience of pain led to more functional disability for children in more disruptive families (Logan & Scharff, 2005).

Families may also play an indirect role in illness management. Family functioning, for example, has been shown to predict treatment adherence in children and adolescents with diabetes, which in turn predicted metabolic control (Lewin et al., 2006). Parenting style and parent–child relatedness have been suggested as relevant variables in illness management. Authoritative parenting, characterized by warmth, support, and control, was associated with better adherence in preschool and school-age children with diabetes (Davis et al., 2001). Parent–child conflict has been associated with adherence difficulties in adolescents with diabetes (Jacobson et al., 1994), whereas close parental supervision of diabetes care in adolescents, coupled with higher levels of parental support, predicted better treatment adherence (Ellis et al., 2007). Parenting variables have also been implicated in the development of coping skills in children with spina bifida. Specifically, parental responsiveness predicted 8- and 9-year-old children's use of problem-focused coping, both concurrently and 2 years later (McKernon et al., 2001). In asthma, there is also evidence that attachment styles between mothers and children mediate the relationship between a child's functional health status and depressive symptoms (Bleil, Ramesh, Miller, & Wood, 2000).

Using the example of childhood asthma, Fiese and Wamboldt (2000) describe family rituals—patterns of family behavior ranging from highly structured religious activities to daily household routines—as potential mediating factors in treatment adherence. Rituals may help families maintain disease-related treatment regimens by reducing anxiety, increasing predictability, or helping families adapt and apply effective problem solving to new demands.

Schools

For children, schools are essential ecologies that interact with other systems (e.g., families, hospitals, communities). However, though schools represent important contexts, consistent integration of interventions across the child, family, and school remains the exception rather than the rule. Furthermore, there is little research examining this process as it relates to children with chronic illness.

At the broadest level, active collaborations among families, schools, and health care systems necessitate thoughtful consideration of the resources and challenges associated with meeting the health care needs of children within each system. Identifying and developing such approaches are particularly important, given changes in health care delivery and the increasing responsibility placed on communities for caring for children with health care needs (Power, DuPaul, Shapiro, & Kazak, 2003).

Peers

The peer system is critical in the process of socialization, and thorough reviews document what is known about the risks and potential benefits that the peer subsystem can represent in the lives of children with chronic illness (see Reiter-Purtill, Waller, & Noll, Chapter 45, this volume). Despite this potentially rich resource, peers are generally invisible in health care settings, and there are few studies of how children with chronic illness operate within the peer subsystem. Two existing studies, both in the area of diabetes, suggest that peer issues can relate in important ways to disease management (Hains et al., 2007) and to family conflict centering around disease management (Greco, Pendley, McDonell, & Reeves, 2001). Clearly, this underexplored system may offer tremendous opportunity in understanding variables that may affect disease management and adjustment, as well as providing an arena for creative interventions.

The Health Care System

Given the prominence of the health care system in pediatric psychology, it is surprising how little has been written describing models of hospital–family collaboration. Family-centered care is perhaps the most widely described model (e.g., Johnson, 2000), with its clearly articulated principles affirming the importance and role of families in pediatric health care. This model is also widely accepted, with many of its recommendations implemented in children's hospitals nationwide.

Another movement advocating for consideration of families and healthcare teams in patient care is the Collaborative Family Healthcare Association (CFHA; *www.cfhcc. org*), a movement that advocates for collaboration between families and health care teams in patient care. Specifically, the CHFA's statement of its approach highlights the need for "seamless collaboration between psychosocial, biomedical, nursing, and other healthcare providers, and views patient, family, community, and provider systems as equal participants in the healthcare process" (*www.cfhcc.org/pages/CFHA-Approach*). In addition, the CFHA emphasizes the potential for this care model to have an impact on fiscal resources. That is, a coordinated, collaborative approach, viewing clinical medicine within a biopsychosocial framework, may result in cost savings by reducing duplicative care, by ending the practice of treating "medical" issues in isolation from "psychosocial" ones, and by building on the adaptive competencies of patients and families.

Most literature on parent–physician interaction has focused on this conflicts in this relationship, and typically proposes approaches to prevent escalation. There are data showing, for example, that pediatricians view verbal, cooperative, and compliant mothers more positively than those who demonstrate fewer of these attributes (Tellerman & Medio, 1988). This is often viewed as a training issue, in that pediatricians may not have the skills to deal with families they find difficult and may not utilize approaches that can facilitate these relationships (Sunde, Mabe, & Josephson, 1993). Cohen and Wamboldt (2000) analyzed speech samples of parents of children with asthma and their asthma specialists talking about their perceptions of one another and their relationships. They found relationship difficulties in 15–40% of these interactions.

Waters (2001) describes the lack of attention to the relationship aspects of the doctor–patient–family interaction as "medicine's dirty secret." Noting that this lack of attention is widely known (but not discussed), Waters notes that collaborative models of health care are "revolutionary" in offering a solution. For example, health care providers can improve family–health care system relations by identifying tasks that are common to families and to staff. These include self-soothing in the face of stress, developing trust (in the relationships that must be formed to ensure optimal health care), and managing the inevitable conflicts that arise in modern health care (Kazak, Simms, & Rourke, 2002). Focusing on facilitating family and team resolution of these tasks, a consultant can develop a specific clinical protocol to help the health care team address situations in which relationships between families and health care providers become strained.

Family/Systems Assessments and Interventions in Pediatric Psychology

Translation of research on families in pediatric psychology into evidence-based interventions is underway, with some modest yet significant advances in the past decade. The first step in effective intervention is accurate assessment. In a recent review of evidence-based family assessment in pediatric psychology, 19 of 29 published measures met criteria as "well established," highlighting the availability of reliable and valid measures for family constructs relevant to pediatric health (Alderfer et al., 2008). Other measures specific to the families of children with pediatric health concerns are emerging.

Most interventions for children with pediatric illness either have focused on the individual child or have included members of the family system without an explicit family framework that integrates these other family members in the treatment. In order to promote family intervention research in child health, conceptual and methodological challenges must be addressed, such as measuring change in multiple family members and conceptualizing change in related individuals. Although family interventions are often discussed as if they were one type of intervention, it is important to distinguish among the various types, including therapy, psychoeducation, information and support, and direct service (Campbell & Patterson, 1995), each with potentially differing goals, approaches, and outcomes.

Behavioral treatment for children with cystic fibrosis and their families has been effective in increasing adherence to a high-energy, high-fat diet to treat pancreatic insufficiency (Powers et al., 2005; Stark, 2001). The treatment protocols provide interventions for parents and patients separately, in each case emphasizing nutritional information, calorie goals, and developmentally appropriate behavioral approaches for encouraging intake of targeted foods. Comparatively, family-based behavioral treatment for childhood obesity that focuses on eating and exercise behaviors in both parents and children has been shown to be effective in achieving long-term child weight reduction (i.e., 2 years) and diminished child behavior problems. Furthermore, when this treatment is expanded to incorporate problem-solving training, improvements in parents' distress have been observed over time (Epstein, Paluch, Gordy, Saelens, & Ernst, 2000). A family psychoeducational approach integrating biological (e.g., knowledge about sickle cell disease), psychological (e.g., psychological symptoms, cognitive functioning), and sociocultural (e.g., racial identity, family resources) issues related to disease management has been pilot-tested with families of children with sickle cell disease (Kaslow et al., 2000). Relative to standard treatment, this intervention has been associated with increased knowledge about sickle cell disease for both children and parents; for the child participants, enhanced disease knowledge was maintained over time (6 months). Although findings about the efficacy of this treatment in addressing psychological adjustment and family functioning are equivocal, there is evidence that an intervention of this kind might be beneficial for children and families with sickle cell disease.

One of the earliest family interventions in pediatric psychology used a multifamily model and included parental simulation of diabetes (Satin, La Greca, Zigo, & Skyler, 1989). Subsequent interventions that promote adherence in children with diabetes are among the most advanced in their incorporation of families. Wysocki and colleagues (2000) compared behavioral family systems therapy (BFST) to a standard treatment and to an educational support condition for adolescents with diabetes. BFST targets family conflict by emphasizing problem solving and negotiation, communication skills, cognitive restructuring of beliefs that may maintain conflicts, and intervention in family patterns that are contradictory to adaptive functioning. BFST was associated with improvements in family relationships and reduced conflict, but was not strongly associated with diabetes control and adherence. A recent revision added a more specific behavior management component and included parent simulation. Compared to standard care and an educational support group, the revised BFST was related to decreased family conflict and improved adherence; both the new BFST and the educational support group were related to improved metabolic control (Wysocki et al., 2006). The data reflect the complications inherent in taking a broader perspective on adherence. That is, improvements in conflict are important and may relate indirectly to adherence (although they may not show direct and clear relationships), and interventions may need to include simultaneous attention to more generic family functioning factors and to more specific disease-related "problems."

Anderson and her team have developed brief, systemically oriented interventions that include family psychoeducation aimed at preventing the increase in conflict over diabetes care that is typically seen in the early adolescent years (Anderson, Svoren, & Laffel, 2007). Success with these approaches has led to recent investigations to test whether long-term changes can be maintained, and to further evaluate individual and group administration of interventions.

Interventions for families can be based on integrative models. For example, given evidence for posttraumatic stress symptoms in mothers and fathers of childhood cancer survivors, an intervention that integrated cognitive-behavioral and multiple-family therapy was developed and tested in a randomized clinical trial of 150 families. Families randomized to the Surviving Cancer Competently Intervention Program showed significant improvements in posttraumatic stress symptoms over those in a waiting-list control condition (Kazak et al., 2004).

Family and systems interventions can also be integrated into other areas of pediatric psychology practice. In the area of procedural pain, for example, parents can be active and effective interventionists with their children (Kazak, Penati, Brophy, & Himelstein, 1998). It is possible to conceptualize change at the level of the health care team and to anticipate systemic forces that can help or hinder the introduction of interventions (Kazak, Blackall, Himelstein, Brophy, & Daller, 1995). In addition, emotionally focused therapy has strong empirical support for addressing family adjustment to chronic illness. This marital intervention, which targets a couple's negative patterns of interaction and attachment bond, has been shown to reduce marital distress; improvements have been reported to be stable over a 2-year period (Cloutier, Manion, Walker, & Johnson, 2002; Walker, Johnson, Manion & Cloutier, 1996). The emotionally focused model offers an opportunity to examine not only how the marital relationship is affected by the illness, but how the disease course and the child's functioning is influenced by the marital relationship. Multisystemic therapy, an effective intervention across an array of childhood and adolescent problems, has also shown to be effective in families of youths with diabetes (Ellis et al., 2005).

The examples of family intervention research provided above exhibit some commonalities, despite differences in patient groups and theoretical orientations. That is, these findings represent work that has evolved from more basic research in pediatric psychology. These researchers are all also applying family interventions to problems that are central to pediatric health care and that are concerns shared by families and healthcare teams (e.g., adherence, knowledge about disease and treatment, long-term sequelae of treatment). They are responding to the challenges of conducting research in "real-world" settings, including difficulties with small sample sizes and recruitment and attrition concerns. Furthermore, there are no published family-based interventions specific to many chronic conditions (e.g., spina bifida), and it is not clear to what degree existing interventions might apply across illness categories. These are important challenges, and ones that we hope will continue to be refined and evaluated empirically.

Some elements that are missing from current pediatric family research are the rich clinical perspectives from family therapy models. These include structural family therapy, which was among the earliest models applied to pediatric samples (Minuchin et al., 1975), and others that are highly applicable, such as medical family therapy (McDaniel, Hepworth, & Doherty, 1992). Although this situation is unlikely to change in the near future, with the current and important focus on evidence-based practice, these family therapy frameworks provide important perspectives for treating ill children and their families. The medical family therapist, for example, will supplement behavioral strategies with an awareness of such family/systems issues as perceived closeness in the family, interactional patterns, and generational boundaries. Similarly, therapy goals are likely to include a consideration of individual and family developmental tasks that are affected by and/or that change in the presence of illness. Opportunities exist for the development of family therapy–based interventions that could be manualized and tested in pediatric practice Furthermore, it will be important for researchers to address some challenges that have impeded the development of this field, such as utilizing the descriptive and explicative research on family variables to identify malleable risk and protective factors associated with disease management, and to develop family assessment strategies that provide focused information to gauge the type and target of intervention.

Summary

Perhaps the most important "take-home" message with respect to families and other systems in pediatric psychology is that we strongly encourage pediatric psychologists to incorporate broader perspectives in their work. Clinically, children facing health challenges live in systems, the most prominent of which are families, schools, and hospital systems. More systemic conceptualizations of adaptation within pediatric psychology and interventions that are concordant with these systemic conceptualizations have the potential to change not only the specific individuals, but also the broader contexts in which children grow and develop.

One of the most obvious steps is to ask research questions that incorporate the perspective of other important individuals in the child's life, and to view these questions from an interactional perspective. For example, how does the behavior among and between parents and staff affect the child's coping ability in the procedural context? What impact do family patterns and the family's relationships with schools and community support systems have on an adolescent's diabetes management? Should psychologists be changing only the behavior of a disruptive pediatric inpatient, or should they also be asking that parents and staff shift their perceptions and behaviors to understand the family and systemic factors contributing to the behavior? These are questions that are easier asked than answered. Indeed, the relatively small body of research in this area speaks to the difficulty of conducting these studies.

However, a few general recommendations can be made. First, assuring that multi-disciplinary family and systems perspectives are integrated into curricula (in terms of both didactics and supervised clinical experience) will expose more pediatric psychologists to these approaches. Second, pediatric psychologists can and should assume an optimistic and energetic approach to including other members of the family in their studies. At a minimum, psychologists should no longer tolerate generalizations made from mother-only data to represent the perspective of parents more broadly, but rather should consider how exclusion of fathers and other family members limits the knowledge contributed. Third, children do not receive health care in isolation from the broader contexts in which they live. Pediatric psychologists must identify ways to better account not just for family processes, but for the broader impact of peers, schools, culture/ethnicity, health care systems, and factors that affect access to care. Addressing these issues will ultimately improve the ability of psychologists to provide clinical care to individual families, to consult with medical teams about family-focused treatment approaches, and to advocate more effectively for the inclusion of the needs of children and families in local and national health care policy.

References

Alderfer, M. A., Fiese, B., Gold, J., Cutuli, J. J., Holmbeck, G., Goldbeck, L., et al. (2008). Evidence-based assessment in pediatric psychology: Family measures. *Journal of Pediatric Psychology, 33*, 1046–1061.

Anderson, B., Svoren, B., & Laffel, L. (2007). Initiatives to promote effective self-care skills in young patients with diabetes. *Disease Management and Health Outcomes, 15,* 101–108.

Barerra, M., Chung, J., & Fleming, C. F. (2004). A group intervention for siblings of pediatric cancer patients. *Journal of Psychosocial Oncology, 22,* 21–39.

Berge, J. M., Patterson, J. M., & Rueter, M. (2006). Marital satisfaction and mental health of couples with children with chronic health conditions. *Families, Systems, and Health, 24,* 267–285.

Bleil, M., Ramesh, S., Miller, B., & Wood, B. (2000). The influence of parent–child relatedness on depressive symptoms in children with asthma: Tests of moderator and mediator models. *Journal of Pediatric Psychology, 25,* 481–491.

Bronfenbrenner, U. (1979). *The ecology of human development.* Cambridge, MA: Harvard University Press.

Cadman, D., Boyle, M., Szatmari, P., & Offord, D. (1987). Chronic illness, disability, and mental and social well-being: Findings of the Ontario Child Health Study. *Pediatrics, 79,* 805–813.

Campbell, T., & Patterson, J. (1995). The effectiveness of family interventions in the treatment of physical illness. *Journal of Marital and Family Therapy, 21,* 545–583.

Coakley, R., Holmbeck, G., Friedman, D., Greenley, R., & Thill, A. (2002). A longitudinal study of pubertal timing, parent–child conflict, and cohesion in families of young adolescents with spina bifida. *Journal of Pediatric Psychology, 27,* 461–473.

Cloutier, P. F., Manion, I. G., Walker, J. G., & Johnson, S. M. (2002). Emotionally focused interventions for couples with chronically ill children: A 2-year follow-up. *Journal of Marital and Family Therapy, 28,* 391–398.

Cohen, S., & Wamboldt, F. (2000). The parent–physician relationship in pediatric asthma care. *Journal of Pediatric Psychology, 25,* 69–77.

Dahlquist, L. M., Czyzewski, D. I., & Jones, C. L. (1996). Parents of children with cancer: A longitudinal study of emotional distress, coping style, and marital adjustment two and twenty months after diagnosis. *Journal of Pediatric Psychology, 21,* 541–554.

Davis, C., Delamater, A., Shaw, K., La Greca, A., Eidson, M., Perez-Rodriques, J., et al. (2001). Brief report: Parenting styles, regimen adherence and glycemic control in 4–10 year old children with diabetes. *Journal of Pediatric Psychology, 26,* 123–129.

Ellis, D., Frey, M., Naar-King, S., Templin, T., Cunningham, P., & Cakan, N. (2005). The effects of multisystemic therapy on diabetes stress in adolescents with chronically poorly controlled Type 1 diabetes: Findings from a randomized controlled trial. *Pediatrics, 116,* e826–e832.

Ellis, D., Podolski, C., Frey, M., Near-King, S., Wang, B., & Moltz, K. (2007). The role of parental monitoring in adolescent health outcomes: Impact on regimen adherence in youth with type 1 diabetes. *Journal of Pediatric Psychology, 32,* 907–917.

Epstein, L., Paluch, R., Gordy, C., Saelens, B., & Ernst, M. (2000). Problem solving in the treatment of childhood obesity. *Journal of Consulting and Clinical Psychology, 68,* 717–721.

Fiese, B., & Sameroff, A. (1989). Family context in pediatric psychology: A transactional perspective. *Journal of Pediatric Psychology, 14,* 293–314.

Fiese, B., & Wamboldt, F. (2000). Family routines, rituals and asthma management: A proposal for family-based strategies to increase treatment adherence. *Families, Systems, and Health, 18,* 405–418.

Fiese, B., Winter, M., Sliwinski, M., & Anbar, R. (2007). Nighttime waking in children with asthma: An exploratory study of daily fluctuations in family climate. *Journal of Family Psychology, 21,* 95–103.

Friedman, D., Holmbeck, G. N., Jandasek, B., Zukerman, J., & Abad, M. (2004). Parent functioning in families of preadolescents with spina bifida: Longitudinal implications for child adjustment. *Journal of Family Psychology, 18,* 609–619.

Greco, P., Pendley, J. S., McDonell, J., & Reeves, G. (2001). A peer group intervention for adolescents with Type I diabetes and their best friends. *Journal of Pediatric Psychology, 26,* 485–490.

Hains, A. A., Berlin, K. S., Davies, W. H., Smothers, M. K., Sato, A. F., & Alemzadeh, R. (2007). Attributions of adolescents with Type I diabetes related to performing diabetes care around friends and peers: The moderating role of friend support. *Journal of Pediatric Psychology, 32,* 561–570.

Holmbeck, G., Coakley, R., Hommeyer, J., Shapera, W., & Westhoven, V. (2002). Observed and perceived dyadic and systemic functioning in families of preadolescents with spina bifida. *Journal of Pediatric Psychology, 27,* 177–189.

Holmbeck, G., Gorey-Ferguson, L., Hudson, T., Seefeldt, T., Shapera, W., Turner, T., et al. (1997). Maternal, paternal and marital functioning in families of preadolescents with spina bifida. *Journal of Pediatric Psychology, 22,* 167–181.

Jacobson, A., Hauser, S., Lavori, P., Willett, J., Cole, C. F., Wolfsdorf, J. I., et al. (1994). Family environment and glycemic control: A four year prospective study of children and adolescents with insulin-dependent diabetes mellitus. *Psychosomatic Medicine, 56,* 401–409.

Janicke, D. M., Mitchell, M. J., & Stark, L. J. (2005). Family functioning in school-aged children with cystic fibrosis: An observational assessment of family interaction in the mealtime environment. *Journal of Pediatric Psychology, 30,* 179–186.

Johnson, B. (2000). Family-centered care: Four decades of progress. *Families, Systems, and Health, 18,* 137–156.

Kaslow, N., Collins, M., Rashid, F., Baskin, M., Griffith, J., Hollins, L., et al. (2000). The efficacy of a pilot family psychoeducational intervention for pediatric sickle cell disease. *Families, Systems, and Health, 18,* 381–404.

Kazak, A. (1989). Families of chronically ill children: A systems and social ecological model of adaptation and challenge. *Journal of Consulting and Clinical Psychology, 57,* 25–30.

Kazak, A. (2001). Comprehensive care for children with cancer and their families: A social ecological framework guiding research, practice and policy. *Children's Services: Social Policy, Research and Practice, 4,* 217–233.

Kazak, A., Alderfer, M., Streisand, R., Simms, S., Rourke, M. T., Barakat, L. M., et al. (2004). Treatment of posttraumatic stress symptoms in adolescent survivors of childhood cancer and their families: A randomized clinical trial. *Journal of Family Psychology, 18,* 493–504.

Kazak, A., Blackall, G., Himelstein, B., Brophy, P., & Daller, R. (1995). Producing systemic change in pediatric practice: An intervention protocol for reducing distress during painful procedures. *Family Systems Medicine, 13,* 173–185.

Kazak, A., Penati, B., Brophy, P., & Himelstein, B. (1998). Pharmacologic and psychologic interventions for procedural pain. *Pediatrics, 102,* 59–66.

Kazak, A., Simms, S., & Rourke, M. (2002). Family systems practice in pediatric psychology. *Journal of Pediatric Psychology, 27,* 133–143.

Lewandowski, A., & Drotar, D. (2007). The relationship between parent-reported social support and adherence to medical treatment in families of adolescents with Type I diabetes. *Journal of Pediatric Psychology, 32,* 427–436.

Lewin, A., Heidgerken, A., Geffken, G., Williams, L., Storch, E. A., Gelfand, K. M., et al. (2006). The relation between family factors and metabolic control: The role of diabetes adherence. *Journal of Pediatric Psychology, 31,* 174–183.

Logan, D., Radcliffe, J., & Smith-Whitley, K. (2002). Parent factors and adolescent sickle cell disease: Associations with patterns of health service use. *Journal of Pediatric Psychology, 27,* 475–484.

Logan, D. E., & Scharff, L. (2005). Relationships between family and parenting characteristics and functional abilities in children with recurrent pain syndromes: An investigation of moderating effects on the pathway from pain to disability. *Journal of Pediatric Psychology, 30*, 698–707.

Maloney, R. M., Clay, D. L., & Robinson, J. (2005). Sociocultural issues in pediatric transplantation: A conceptual model. *Journal of Pediatric Psychology, 30*, 235–246.

Martin, M., Miller-Johnson, S., Kitzmann, K., & Emery, R. (1998). Parent–child relationships and insulin-dependent diabetes mellitus: Observational ratings of clinically relevant dimensions. *Journal of Family Psychology, 12*, 102–111.

McCubbin, H. I., Thompson, E. A., Thompson, A. I., McCubbin, M. A., & Kaston, A. J. (1993). Culture, ethnicity, and the family: Critical factors in childhood chronic illnesses and disabilities. *Pediatrics, 91*, 1063–1070.

McDaniel, S., Hepworth, J., & Doherty, W. (1992). *Medical family therapy.* New York: Basic Books.

McKernon, W., Holmbeck, G., Colder, C., Hommeyer, J., Shapera, J., & Westhoven, V. (2001). Longitudinal study of observed and perceived family influences on problem-focused coping behaviors of preadolescents with spina bifida. *Journal of Pediatric Psychology, 26*, 41–54.

Minuchin, S., Baker, L., Rosman, B., Liebman, R., Millman, L., & Todd, T. (1975). A conceptual model of psychosomatic illness in children: Family organization and family therapy. *Archives of General Psychiatry, 32*, 1031–1038.

Northey, S., Griffin, W., & Krainz, S. (1998). A partial test of the psychosomatic family model: Marital interaction patterns in asthma and nonasthma families. *Journal of Family Psychology, 12*, 220–223.

Packman, W. L. (1999). Psychosocial impact of pediatric BMT on siblings. *Bone Marrow Transplantation, 24*, 701–706.

Pai, A., Greenley, R., Lewandowski, A., Drotar, D., Youngstrom, E., & Peterson, C. (2007). A meta-analytic review of the influence of pediatric cancer on parent and family functioning. *Journal of Family Psychology, 21*, 407–415.

Phares, V., Lopez, E., Fields, S., Kamboukos, D., & Duhig, A. (2005). Are fathers involved in pediatric psychology research and treatment? *Journal of Pediatric Psychology, 30*, 631–643.

Power, T., DuPaul, G., Shapiro, E., & Kazak, A. (2003). *Promoting children's health: Integrating school, family, and community.* New York: Guilford Press.

Powers, S. W., Jones, J. S., Ferguson, K. S., Piazza-Waggoner, C., Daines, C., & Acton, J. D. (2005). Randomized clinical trial of behavioral and nutritional treatment to improve energy intake and growth in toddlers and preschoolers with cystic fibrosis. *Pediatrics, 116*(6), 1442–1450.

Quittner, A., Espelage, D., Opipari, L., Carter, B., Eid, N., & Eigen, H. (1998). Role strain in couples with and without a child with a chronic illness: Associations with marital satisfaction, intimacy, and daily mood. *Health Psychology, 17*, 112–124.

Robinson, K. E., Gerdardt, C. A., Vannatta, K., & Noll, R. B. (2007). Parent and family factors associated with child adjustment to pediatric cancer. *Journal of Pediatric Psychology, 32*(4), 400–410.

Rodrigues, N., & Patterson, J. M. (2007). Impact of severity of a child's chronic condition on the functioning of two-parent families. *Journal of Pediatric Psychology, 32*(4), 417–426.

Sabbeth, B., & Leventhal, J. (1984). Marital adjustment to chronic childhood illness. *Pediatrics, 73*, 762–768.

Satin, W., La Greca, A., Zigo, M., & Skyler, J. (1989). Diabetes in adolescence: Effects of multifamily group intervention and parent simulation of diabetes. *Journal of Pediatric Psychology, 14*, 259–569.

Schwebel, D., & Brezausek, C. (2004). The role of fathers in toddlers' unintentional injuries. *Journal of Pediatric Psychology, 29*, 19–28.

Sharpe, D., & Rossiter, L. (2002). Siblings of children with a chronic illness: A meta-analysis. *Journal of Pediatric Psychology, 27,* 699–710.

Snyder, D., & Kazak, A. (2005). Methodology in family science: Introduction to the special issue. *Journal of Family Psychology, 19,* 3–5.

Stark, L. (2001). Adherence to diet in chronic conditions. In D. Drotar (Ed.), *Promoting adherence to medical treatment and chronic childhood illness* (pp. 409–427). Mahwah, NJ: Erlbaum.

Stoneman, Z., & Gavidia-Payne, S. (2006). Marital adjustment in families of young children with disabilities: Associations with daily hassles and problem-focused coping. *American Journal of Mental Retardation, 111*(1), 1–14.

Sunde, E., Mabe, P., & Josephson, A. (1993). Difficult parents: From adversaries to partners. *Clinical Pediatrics, 32,* 213–219.

Tellerman, K., & Medio, F. (1988). Pediatrician opinions of mothers. *Pediatrics, 81,* 186–189.

Van Horn, M., DeMaso, D., Gonzalez-Heydrich, J., & Erickson, J. (2001). Illness-related concerns of mothers of children with congenital heart disease. *Journal of the American Academy of Child and Adolescent Psychiatry, 40,* 847–854.

Wade, S., Taylor, H., Yeates, K., Drotar, D., Stancin, T., Minich, N. M., et al. (2006). Long-term parental and family adaptation following pediatric brain injury. *Journal of Pediatric Psychology, 31,* 1072–1083.

Walker, J., Johnson, S., Manion, I., & Cloutier, P. (1996). Emotionally focused marital intervention for couples with chronically ill children. *Journal of Consulting and Clinical Psychology, 64,* 1029–1036.

Wallander, J., Thompson, R. J., Jr., & Alriksson-Schmidt, A. (2003). Psychosocial adjustment of children with chronic physical conditions. In M. C. Roberts (Ed.), *Handbook of pediatric Psychology* (3rd ed., pp. 141–158). New York: Guilford Press.

Waters, D. (2001). Commentary: The revolutionary subtext of collaborative care. *Families, Systems, and Health, 19,* 59–63.

Wiener, L., Vasquez, M. J., & Battles, H. (2001). Brief report: Fathering a child living with HIV/AIDS: Psychosocial adjustment and parenting stress. *Journal of Pediatric Psychology, 26,* 353–358.

Williams, P., Williams, A., Hanson, S., Gruff, C., Ridder, L., Curry, H., et al. (1999). Maternal mood, family functioning, and perceptions of social support, self-esteem, and mood among siblings of chronically ill children. *Children's Health Care, 28,* 297–310.

Wood, B. (1995). A developmental biopsychosocial approach to the treatment of chronic illness in children and adolescents. In R. H. Mikesell, D. D. Lusterman, & S. H. McDaniel (Eds.), *Integrating family therapy* (pp. 437–455). Washington, DC: American Psychological Association.

Wood, B., Lim, J., Miller, B., Cheah, P., Simmens, S., Stern, T., et al. (2007). Family emotional climate, depression, emotional triggering of asthma, and disease severity in pediatric asthma: Examination of pathways and effect. *Journal of Pediatric Psychology, 32,* 542–551.

Wysocki, T., Harris, M., Buckloh, L., Mertlich, D., Lochrie, A., Taylor, A., et al. (2006). Effects of behavioral family systems therapy for diabetes on adolescents' family relationships, treatment adherence, and metabolic control. *Journal of Pediatric Psychology, 31,* 928–938.

Wysocki, T., Harris, M., Greco, P., Bubb, J., Danda, C. E., Harvey, L. M., et al. (2000). Randomized controlled trial of behavioral therapy for families of adolescents with insulin-dependent diabetes mellitus. *Journal of Pediatric Psychology, 25,* 23–33.

CHAPTER 45

Empirical and Theoretical Perspectives on the Peer Relationships of Children with Chronic Conditions

JENNIFER REITER-PURTILL
JENNIFER M. WALLER
ROBERT B. NOLL

Considerable research has highlighted the importance of peer relationships to healthy psychological development for all children, regardless of health status. Work focusing on children's social reputation (What are the children like?) and social acceptance (Are the children liked?) has demonstrated the stability and predictive validity of peer relationships when these are assessed by peer nominations (e.g., Zeller, Vannatta, Schafer, & Noll, 2003). Poor peer adjustment is a risk factor for later academic difficulties, externalizing symptoms, delinquency, negative self-perceptions, depressive symptoms, leaving school early, and a less active social life (Bagwell, Newcomb, & Bukowski, 1998; French & Conrad, 2001; Laird, Pettit, Dodge, & Bates, 2005). In contrast, friendships in childhood have been demonstrated to be concurrently and longitudinally associated with less loneliness, less depression, and more positive self-concept (Bagwell et al., 1998; Nangle, Erdley, Newman, Mason, & Carpenter, 2003; Parker & Asher, 1993), and may offer protection against the effects of victimization (Hodges, Boivin, Vitaro, & Bukowski, 1999).

Although the importance of peer relationships for typically developing children (i.e., youths ages 0–18 years) has been well documented, this chapter focuses on peer relationships for children with chronic health conditions. We make the assumption that social relationships for children with chronic health conditions are important, and that measurement strategies used to assess typically developing peers have similar psychometric qualities when used with children experiencing chronic illness. Consistent evidence has demonstrated a significant increase in childhood chronic health conditions in the United States (Perrin, Bloom, & Gortmaker, 2007)—presumably a result of improvements in pediatric and neonatal care, as well as of changes in diet, decreases in physical activity, and increased mass media exposure. A recent review of approaches utilized to determine the prevalence of pediatric chronic health conditions suggests the following criteria: Professional standards exist to diagnose the disease; the duration of the disease is greater than 3 months; and children with the disease typically have some functional limitations (van der Lee, Mokkink, Grootenhuis, Heymans, & Offringa, 2007).

The purposes of this chapter are to review some of the most recent empirical studies on the social functioning of children with chronic conditions (see Table 45.1) and to discuss theoretical and methodological issues pertinent to this literature. Children with chronic conditions commonly experience school absences, changes in appearance, restrictions on activities, physical complaints, and/or cognitive impairments; all have the potential to interfere with social functioning. Our review has included studies that have addressed many aspects of children's social functioning and peer relationships, including social competence, social behavior, social acceptance, social quality of life, and social self-concept. Empirical studies prior to 2003 are not included in this review; please see our earlier work (Reiter-Purtill & Noll, 2003).

Why Might Chronic Illness Adversely Affect Peer Relationships?

La Greca (1990) has suggested that chronic illness and its treatment may produce a number of challenges to children as a consequence of physical restrictions on activities or changes in physical appearance. Cognitive impairment as a result of illness or treatment may also result in increased susceptibility to experiencing difficulties in peer relationships (Nassau & Drotar, 1997; Schuman & La Greca, 1999). In the following sections, we have reviewed empirical studies addressing both social functioning and these repercussions of chronic illness. In addition, we have included a section on the social functioning of children experiencing chronic conditions without a known biological mechanism.

Physical Restrictions

Chronic illness in childhood is often associated with restrictions on physical activities. Multiple studies, both in our earlier review (Reiter-Purtill & Noll, 2003) and more recently (Feldmann, Weglage, Roth, Foell, & Frosch, 2005; Gerhardt, Vannatta, Valerius, Correll, & Noll, 2007), have indicated fewer social and physical activities for youths with a chronic illness than for children without a chronic condition. This is not surprising, as many affected children experience pain, fatigue, or disability. Fewer activities may mean less contact with peers, and thus fewer opportunities to develop important social skills. Little research has directly and longitudinally examined the impact of limited activities on social functioning for children with chronic illness. However, several cross-sectional studies have indicated minimal social problems for children with a chronic illness even when they experience limitations to their activities (Feldman et al., 2005; Huygen, Kuis, & Sinnema, 2000). For instance, Huygen and colleagues (2000) reported that youths with juvenile chronic arthritis have lower self-perceptions of athletic competence and report fewer physical and social activities than comparison peers without a chronic illness. However, these children did not differ in parent- or self-reported social functioning. These authors suggest that the primary difference between groups is that

TABLE 45.1. Peer Relationships and Children with Chronic Illness

Reference	Sample (age)	Comparison	Measure of social functioning	Findings
Barton & North (2004)	NF1 with and without ADHD (*n* = 79), R = 8–16	Yes (unaffected siblings, *n* = 46)	*Parent:* CBCL, SSRS *Teacher:* TRF, SSRS *Child:* SSRS	Parents reported greater social problems for children with NF1 than for siblings; parents and teachers reported poorer social skills for children with NF1 than for norm group, but children rated themselves higher; in the group with NF1, social skills/outcomes were poorer in children with comorbid ADHD than in those with only NF1 or NF1 and learning disability.
Gerhardt, Vannatta, Valerius, Correll, & Noll (2007)	Cancer survivors (*n* = 56), *M* age = 18.7 years	Yes (nonchronically ill, *n* = 60)	*Parent:* CBCL-SCS *Child:* Status Questionnaire (Social Competence and Family Relationships), SPPA	No significant group differences for self-reports of social self-concept, social competence, friendships, romantic relationships, activities, or popularity; mothers reported fewer activities for survivors; time since diagnosis and treatment intensity were associated with greater activities (father report); more severe late effects were associated with fewer activities (mother report) and not having a confidant (self-report).
Greco, Freeman, & Dufton (2006)	Frequent abdominal pain (*n* = 60), *M* age = 12.2 years	Yes (pain-free, *n* = 60)	*Teacher:* SSRS *Peer:* Children's Social Experiences Questionnaire	Relative to comparison group, children with abdominal pain experienced more relational victimization; for overt victimization, a significant group × gender interaction showed boys with abdominal pain experiencing the greatest levels; greater pain was associated with more victimization and with lower teacher-rated social skills and academic competence.
Hayden-Wade et al. (2005)	Overweight (*n* = 70), R = 10–14	Yes (nonoverweight, *n* = 86)	*Child:* Perception of Teasing Scale, ATI, LSDQ, SPPC, MLTA	Relative to comparison group, significantly more overweight children reported experiencing appearance-related teasing and a greater frequency of teasing; they also felt that teasing was more "upsetting." In overweight children, greater weight-related teasing was associated with lower self-perceived social ability, loneliness, and preference for sedentary and isolative activities.
Hoie et al. (2006)	Epilepsy, without severe cognitive deficits (*n* = 117), R = 6–13	Yes (nonchronically ill, *n* = 117)	*Parent:* CBCL *Teacher:* TRF *Child:* YSR (if age > 11 years)	Mothers and teachers reported greater social problems and withdrawn behavior in children with epilepsy than in comparison children; mothers reported more delinquent and aggressive behavior in both girls and boys with epilepsy, while teachers reported this in boys only. Girls with epilepsy reported more social problems and withdrawn behavior than comparison girls; no group differences in self-reports for boys.
Holmbeck et al. (2003)	SB (*n* = 68), R = 8–9	Yes (nonchronically	*Parent:* SPPC, CBCL	Parents reported that children with SB had lower social competence and activity involvement than comparisons; both parents and teachers viewed children with

674

Citation	Group	Comparison group	Measures	Findings
		ill, *n* = 68	*Teacher:* SPPC, TRF *Child:* SPPC	SB as having more somatic complaints, social problems, and attention problems; all raters perceived children with SB as lower in athletic competence and physical appearance.
Hunt, Burden, Hepper, Stevenson, & Johnston (2006)	CLP (*n* = 160), R = 8–21	Yes (no CLP, *n* = 113)	*Child:* Interview, YSR/YASR	Adolescents with CLP (ages 11–18 years) reported more behavior problems than comparisons; individuals with CLP were significantly more likely to have been teased or bullied by peers than comparison group; in both groups, behavior problems were predicted by greater age, female gender, and history of teasing.
Hunt et al. (2007)	Cleft lip and/or palate (*n* = 129), R = 8–18	Yes (no CLP, *n* = 96)	*Parent:* CBCL, semistructured interview	Relative to comparison group, children with CLP had more behavior problems and were more likely to experience teasing. History of teasing, presence of visible scars, and family history of CLP were predictive of greater behavior problems.
Kashikar-Zuck et al. (2007)	JPFS (*n* = 55), R = 12–18	Yes (nonchronically ill, *n* = 55)	*Teacher:* RCP *Peer:* RCP, Three Best Friends, Like Rating Scale *Child:* RCP	Relative to comparison group, adolescents with JPFS were more sensitive–isolated, according to all raters; peer and self-reports indicated less leadership, and teachers reported less aggressive–disruptive behavior; youths with JPFS were less well liked by peers, chosen as best friends less often, and had fewer reciprocated friendships; peers perceived them as being sick a lot, less attractive, and less athletically competent.
Noll, Reiter-Purtill, Moore, et al. (2007)	NF1 (*n* = 58), R = 7–15	Yes (nonchronically ill, *n* = 51)	*Peer:* RCP, Three Best Friends, Like Rating Scale *Teacher:* RCP *Parent:* CBCL *Child:* LSDQ, SPPC	Children with NF1 were viewed by teachers as more prosocial than comparison children, but had fewer friendships, were less well liked by peers, and were viewed by teachers and peers as exhibiting less leadership and more sensitive–isolated behavior. Greater neurological severity was associated with fewer friendships, lower likeability, and peer reports of less leadership and more sensitive–isolated behavior. Parents viewed children with NF1 as less socially competent than comparison group; mothers rated them as more withdrawn and aggressive; no group differences in social self-concept or self-reported loneliness.
Noll, Reiter-Purtill, Vannatta, Gerhardt, & Short (2007)	SCD (*n* = 42), R = 8–15	Yes (nonchronically ill, *n* = 42)	*Peer:* RCP, Three Best Friends, Like Rating Scale *Child:* LSDQ	Relative to comparisons, peers described children with SCD as having fewer friends, being less athletic, being ill more often, and missing more school; no group differences for self-reported loneliness.
Reiter-Purtill, Vannatta, Gerhardt, Correll, & Noll (2003)	Completed treatment for cancer (*n* = 69), R = 9–17	Yes (nonchronically ill, *n* = 77)	*Teacher:* RCP *Peer:* RCP, Three Best Friends, Like Rating Scale *Child:* RCP	Two-year follow-up; relative to comparison group, survivors described themselves as more prosocial; they were perceived by teachers as less aggressive and by peers as more sick, more tired, and missing more school; children who received more intense treatment were perceived by peers as more prosocial and less aggressive, but also had fewer best-friend nominations 2 years after treatment ended.

TABLE 45.1. (cont.)

Reference	Sample (age)	Comparison	Measure of social functioning	Findings
Rose & Holmbeck (2007)	SB (n = 68), R = 8–9	Yes (nonchronically ill, n = 68)	*Parent:* SPPC Social Scale, SSRS, BRIEF *Teacher:* SPPC Social Scale, SSRS, BRIEF	Parent-reported social skills and both parent and teacher-reported social competence were lower for children with SB than for comparison children; attention and executive functioning were significantly more impaired in children with SB, according to parents, teachers, and objective assessments. Impairments in attention and executive functioning predicted difficulties in social skills and social competence.
Sandberg, Bukowski, Fung, & Noll (2004)	Short stature or tall stature (n = 126), grades 6–12	Yes (average height, n = 123)	*Peer:* Best Friend Nominations, Like Rating Scale, RCP *Child:* RCP	No significant associations between height and peer- or self-reported peer relations; peers perceived children of short stature as looking younger than their age; this effect was stronger in younger children; significant associations between "looking young" and social behaviors accounted for little more than 1% of variance.
Slifer et al. (2004)	Oral cleft (n = 34), R = 8–15	Yes (no oral cleft, n = 34)	*Parent:* CBCL *Child:* SPPC/A, semistructured social interaction	Relative to comparison group, children with oral clefts were rated by parents as being significantly less socially competent; no group differences in self-perceived social acceptance. During interaction with a peer confederate, children with oral clefts were less likely to participate in an activity or respond to direct questions than comparison children.
Slifer et al. (2006)	Oral cleft (n = 24), R = 7–16.5	Yes (no oral cleft, n = 25)	*Child:* SPPC/A (Social Acceptance subscale), semistructured social interaction	In a semistructured interaction with a peer confederate, children with oral clefts demonstrated more prosocial nonverbal behaviors than comparison children; no group differences in self-reports of perceived social acceptance; in the group with oral cleft, low self-perceived social acceptance was related to greater eye contact avoidance.
Storch et al. (2004)	Type 1 diabetes (n = 32), R = 8–18	Yes (nonchronically ill, n = 32)	*Child:* SEQ, CDI, Social Anxiety Scale for Children— Revised, Asher Loneliness Scale	Children with diabetes reported experiencing more relational victimization and less prosocial peer support than comparison children; no group differences in overt victimization; children with diabetes who experienced higher rates of relational victimization were more likely to report symptoms of depression, social anxiety, and loneliness.
Storch et al. (2007)	Overweight (n = 90) and overweight-risk (n = 2), R = 8–18	No	*Parent:* CBCL *Child:* SPVS, CDI, Asher Loneliness Scale, MASC, SPA, PACE+	Higher rates of child-reported peer victimization were associated with lower physical activity and greater depressive symptoms, social anxiety, and loneliness, as well as greater parent reported internalizing and externalizing problems; body mass index was not related to peer victimization or psychosocial outcomes; physical activity was negatively associated with loneliness; loneliness and depression mediated the relationship between peer victimization and physical activity.
Strauss & Pollack (2003)	Overweight (n = 1,852), R = 13–18	Yes (normal-weight, n = 15,705)	*Peer:* Friendship nominations	Overweight adolescents were nominated as friends less often than normal-weight peers and had fewer reciprocated friends; youths who nominated overweight adolescents as friends received fewer nominations than friends of normal-weight peers.

Study	Group	Comparison	Measures	Findings
Strine, Okoro, McGuire, & Balluz (2006)	Frequent or severe headaches (n = 621), R = 4–17	Yes (children without frequent or severe headaches, n = 8,643)	*Parent:* National Health Interview Survey, extended version of the SDQ	Relative to comparison group, children with headaches were significantly more likely to have parent-reported peer difficulties, emotional symptoms, conduct problems, and hyperactivity–inattention than children without headaches; children with headaches were significantly more likely to be distressed by these problems and more likely to have these problems interfere with their daily lives, including friendships.
Trzepacz, Vannatta, Davies, Stehbens, & Noll (2003)	Hemophilia (n = 40), R = 8–15	Yes (nonchronically ill, n = 40)	*Parent:* CBCL-SCS; *Peer:* RCP, Three Best Friends, Like Rating Scale; *Child:* LSDQ, SPPC	No significant group differences for peer report measures of social reputation or social acceptance; no significant group differences in parent reports of social competence, self-reported loneliness, or self-perceived social acceptance; children with moderate to severe hemophilia were perceived by peers as significantly less aggressive and disruptive than children with mild disease.
Vannatta, Gerhardt, Wells, & Noll (2007)	Cancer survivors (n = 82), R = 9–17	No	*Teacher:* RCP; *Peer:* RCP, Three Best Friends, Like Rating Scale; *Child:* RCP	Greater intensity of CNS-directed treatment was associated with lower peer acceptance, fewer best-friend nominations, lower peer ratings of leadership behavior, and more peer-reported sensitive–isolated behavior; these associations were stronger for males and children <10 years of age at diagnosis; for children diagnosed at age 10 or younger, higher-intensity CNS-directed treatment was associated with teacher reports of greater aggressive–disruptive behavior.
Vannatta et al. (2008)	Migraine (n = 69), R = 8–14	Yes (nonchronically ill, n = 69)	*Teacher:* RCP; *Peer:* RCP, Three Best Friends, Like Rating Scale; *Child:* RCP	Elementary school children with migraines were nominated less often as best friends and had fewer reciprocated friendships than comparison peers; middle school children were perceived by peers as displaying greater leadership behaviors than comparison children; peers perceived children with migraine as missing more school and as sick more often; children with migraine self-reported higher leadership behavior; teachers perceived children with migraine as less aggressive and disruptive; migraine frequency and severity were not significantly associated with any outcome.
Zeller, Reiter-Purtill, & Ramey (2008)	Obese (n = 90), R = 8–16	Yes (nonoverweight, n = 76)	*Teacher:* RCP; *Peer:* Three Best Friends, Like Rating Scale, RCP; *Child:* RCP	Relative to comparisons, obese children received fewer best-friend nominations, were less well liked, and were described by peer, teacher, and self-report as more sensitive–isolated; according to peers, obese children displayed less leadership and more aggressive behavior, were less attractive and athletic, and were more sick, tired, and absent from school. Peer-rated attractiveness and athleticism mediated the association between obesity status and peer acceptance.

Note. ATI, Appearance Teasing Inventory; BRIEF, Behavior Rating Inventory of Executive Function; CBCL, Child Behavior Checklist; CBCL-SCS, Child Behavior Checklist—Social Competence scale; CDI, Children's Depression Inventory; CLP, cleft lip and/or palate; JPFS, juvenile primary fibromyalgia syndrome; LSDQ, Loneliness and Social Dissatisfaction Questionnaire; MASC, Multidimensional Anxiety Scale for Children; MLTA, Minnesota Leisure Time Activity Questionnaire; NF1, neurofibromatosis Type 1; PACE+, Adolescent Physical Activity Measure; R, age range (in years); RCP, Revised Class Play; SB, spina bifida; SCD, sickle cell disease; SDQ, Strengths and Difficulties Questionnaire; SEQ, Social Experience Questionnaire; SPA, Social Physique Anxiety Scale; SPPA, Self-Perception Profile for Adolescents; SPPC, Self-Perception Profile for Children; SPVS, Schwartz Peer Victimization Scale; SSRS, Social Skills Rating System; TRF, Teacher Report Form; YASR, Young Adult Self-Report; YSR, Youth Self-Report.

677

youths with arthritis have fewer opportunities to participate in activities due to physical limitations, but that this does not seem to negatively affect their social functioning.

Some studies have indicated that peers perceive children with a chronic illness as more sick, as more tired, and as missing more school than comparison peers without a chronic illness (Noll, Reiter-Purtill, Vannatta, Gerhardt, & Short, 2007; Reiter-Purtill, Vannatta, Gerhardt, Correll, & Noll, 2003). Despite this recognition by peers of the physical limitations of affected children, these studies demonstrated that children with chronic conditions had few functional social difficulties relative to comparison peers.

These results seem consistent with findings regarding disease severity. Objective measures of disease severity have been primarily associated with school absences and fewer activities, but have not been consistently associated with functional problems with peers (Reiter-Purtill & Noll, 2003). However, there are two exceptions. First, when the measure of disease severity focuses on a child's central nervous system (CNS), significant associations are reported between CNS disease/treatment intensity and social functioning (Noll, Reiter-Purtill, Moore, et al., 2007; Vannatta, Gerhardt, Wells, & Noll, 2007). Second, significant associations are found when assessments of disease severity and social functioning are made by the same reporter, usually a parent.

It is noteworthy that the physical limitations and fatigue that accompany some illnesses may serve a protective function, making some children less likely to be contentious with peers (Gartstein, Noll, & Vannatta, 2000). This may result in the disruption of developmental pathways to future externalizing behaviors or conduct problems. Several studies have shown that greater disease severity or more intense treatment are associated with peer perceptions of less aggressive behavior (Feldmann et al., 2005; Reiter-Purtill et al., 2003; Trzepacz, Vannatta, Davies, Stehbens, & Noll, 2003).

Physical Appearance

Physical attractiveness has consistently been shown to be a strong predictor of friendships and peer acceptance (Vannatta, Gartstein, Zeller & Noll, in press). Thus those chronic conditions and their treatments that adversely affect a child's appearance may negatively affect a child's peer relationships. For instance, appearance changes can create body image concerns for a child with a chronic condition. Indeed, even among children without a chronic illness, dissatisfaction with appearance may result in some children limiting their peer interactions (Cobb, Cohen, Houston, & Rubin, 1998). Changes in appearance may also affect how peers perceive children with chronic conditions, eliciting negative reactions from the peer group, including teasing and peer rejection. In several studies, Hunt, Burden, Hepper, Stevenson, and Johnston (2006, 2007) reported that more children with cleft lip and/or palate than comparison peers had experienced teasing or bullying (according to both parent and self-reports), and that this teasing was typically associated with their facial appearance or speech. Notably, these researchers found that the experience of teasing was significantly associated with poorer psychological outcomes, rather than the presence of the condition alone.

Another highly visible condition, obesity, has been steadily increasing in prevalence in the United States (Freedman, Khan, Serdula, Ogden, & Dietz, 2006). Obese children have been demonstrated to have fewer friends, to be less well liked, and to be perceived by peers as sensitive and isolated (Strauss & Pollack, 2003; Zeller, Reiter-Purtill, & Ramey, 2008). Obese youths report numerous social difficulties, such as stigmatization, teasing, and victimization (Hayden-Wade et al., 2005; Puhl & Latner, 2007; Thompson et al., 2007). Hayden-Wade and colleagues (2005) found that relative to nonoverweight peers, a greater percentage of overweight children experienced teasing related to their appearance; this teasing also came most often from the general peer group, whereas nonoverweight children reported "a specific peer" as the most common teasing source. These authors suggest that this difference may indicate that teasing associated with weight status is "normative" and "acceptable" (p. 1387). Indeed, weight bias has been identified in very young children and seems to worsen with age, with multiple studies suggesting that peers consistently choose negative qualities related to appearance (e.g., "ugly") and behavior (e.g., "lazy," "stupid") to describe obese children (for a review, see Puhl & Latner, 2007).

In contrast to the aforementioned studies, some research has found that some children who are visibly different have few social difficulties. In a study examining the peer relationships of children with idiopathic short stature (Sandberg, Bukowski, Fung, & Noll, 2004), minimal effects of height on peer report measures of social behaviors, friendship, or acceptance were detected.

Cognitive Impairment

The literature examining the social functioning of children with chronic conditions that negatively affect CNS functioning is consistent: Children with these conditions are at considerable risk for social difficulties (Nassau & Drotar, 1997; Reiter-Purtill & Noll, 2003). Nassau and Drotar (1997) suggested several reasons accounting for this risk, including visible appearance changes and restrictions on activities, or cognitive impairments (e.g., memory, attention) that affect social understanding or social skills.

Some CNS conditions can be stigmatizing to children because of their high visibility. Freilinger and colleagues (2006) found a significant association between more symptomatic epilepsy and higher Social Competence scores, according to parent report on the Child Behavior Checklist (CBCL). Similarly, Curtin and Siegel (2003) reported that more visible epilepsy in adolescents was associated with greater self-perceived loneliness.

Chronic conditions that affect CNS functioning often affect children's attentional skills. In the general developmental literature, attentional skills have been suggested to be central to children's overall adjustment, and to their social functioning in particular, because of their importance to self-regulation (Rothbart, Ahadi, & Hershey, 1994). Children with attention-deficit/hyperactivity disorder (ADHD) have been reported to experience numerous social difficulties, including peer rejection and fewer friendships (see Hoza, 2007). Several studies of children with epilepsy (Freilinger et al., 2006; Hoie et al., 2006) or with congenital heart disease (Miatton, De Wolf, Francois, Thiery, & Vingerhoets, 2007) have indicated a number of difficulties, but particularly in the domains of social problems and attention. Unfortunately, few studies have directly examined the impact of attentional deficits on social functioning for children with chronic conditions. One exception is Rose and Holmbeck's (2007) recent longitudinal study of adolescents with spina bifida (SB), who had more social difficulties and problems with attention and executive functioning than comparison adolescents without a chronic illness did. These researchers found that the association between SB and social difficulties was mediated or explained by these neurocognitive problems.

Children with neurofibromatosis Type 1 (NF1), a genetic disorder associated with numerous CNS complications (Hyman, Shores, & North, 2005), also seem to be at risk for social difficulties. Data from peers suggest significant social problems related to social isolation and lack of friendships (Noll, Reiter-Purtill, Moore, et al., 2007); data from parents and teachers are consistent with reports from peers (Barton & North, 2004). Interestingly, data from both of the research groups cited above show a consistent pattern of associations linking greater neurological involvement (i.e., attention problems, learning disabilities) with social dysfunction.

Illnesses without a Known Biological Mechanism

In addition to research on children with chronic illnesses that have a clearly identified biological cause, some work has focused on peer relationships of children with diseases that have less clearly defined origins. In general, many of these studies have found that children affected by these conditions experience numerous peer difficulties. For instance, adolescents with juvenile primary fibromyalgia syndrome (JPFS)—a pain condition that lacks a specific biological marker and is often associated with psychological distress—were found to exhibit less leadership behavior, were more sensitive and isolated, had fewer best-friend nominations and reciprocated friendships, and were less well liked than comparison peers without a chronic illness, according to peer report (Kashikar-Zuck et al., 2007). Similarly, Greco, Freeman, and Dufton (2006) reported social difficulties for a group of children experiencing frequent abdominal pain without a specific medical diagnosis. Relative to comparison peers, these children experienced greater levels of victimization, and boys with abdominal pain had the greatest levels of overt victimization. Among affected children, greater self-reported abdominal pain symptoms were significantly associated with lower teacher-rated social skills and academic competence. These authors suggested that children may develop physical symptoms in response to victimization, or that children with abdominal pain may exhibit behaviors that lead peers to perceive them as "sickly" or "weak," potentially resulting in greater peer harassment (Greco et al., 2006, p. 326; see also Nishina, Juvonen, & Witkow, 2005).

Strine, Okoro, McGuire, and Balluz (2006) studied a group of children who experienced frequent or severe headaches (e.g., migraine), according to their parents. These children were reported by parents to be more likely to have peer difficulties, as well as emotional symptoms, conduct problems, and hyperactivity–inattention, than children without headaches. In contrast to this work is a study of children with migraine headaches who had been referred to a multidisciplinary headache clinic in a pediatric hospital (Vannatta et al., 2008). These researchers found that although elementary school children with migraines had fewer best friends than comparison peers, middle school children with migraines were viewed by peers as displaying more leadership behaviors.

Theoretical Models

A number of theoretical models have been proposed to explain the effects of chronic illness on children's adjustment, including their social functioning. In one group of models, chronic illness is considered a stressor or trauma. Wallander and Varni's (1998) disability–stress–coping model suggests that ongoing strain is created by chronic illness. How well a child fares depends on the presence of risk (e.g., disease severity) and resistance (e.g., cognitive abilities, family environment) factors. Similarly, in Thompson's (Wallander & Thompson, 1995) transactional stress and coping model, adjustment or dysfunction is a consequence of the transactions of illness factors (e.g., disease severity), demographic factors (e.g., age, gender), and adaptational processes (e.g., child coping, maternal adjustment). These models posit a main effect of the challenge of illness on a child's functioning. In addition, these models suggest the presence of an interaction: The adverse impact may be slight if the disease is mild and the child has resources; the impact may be greater with more disease burden and fewer resources.

Other models have suggested that psychosocial dysfunction in children resulting from such adversities as chronic illness is relatively rare (Masten, 2001). Recently, Noll and Kupst (2007) have proposed the Human EvolutionAry Response to Trauma/Stress (HEART), a model using evolutionary theory to account for children's lack of dysfunction after exposure to chronic illness or other randomly occurring traumatic life events. Within an evolutionary framework, human behavior is shaped by natural selection. When early humans were faced with a dangerous environment, their behaviors were subject to natural selection to maximize adaptation, and thereby to ensure the survival of the species. Noll and Kupst contend that the "symptoms" of posttraumatic stress may be expected to maximize fit. Exposure to trauma should cause a series of reactions that include increased alertness, vigilance, and remaining closer to trusted significant others. In contrast, social isolation and social withdrawal are not responses that should maximize adaptation. Similar to Masten (2001), Noll and Kupst have suggested that the pathway between exposure to a random traumatic medical event(s) and dysfunction (e.g., social difficulties) does *not* occur unless the trauma involves a child's CNS (e.g., brain tumors, closed head injury) or if the trauma for the child is directly related to his or her family (e.g., death of parent[s], abuse, or neglect).

How Is Peer Functioning Assessed?

Various methods and sources are available to assess the social functioning of children and adolescents. Arguably, peers are the best judges of a child's social functioning, as they have the most daily interactions with the child. Peer report often consists of multiple raters (e.g., a child's classmates), thereby providing a more stable measure of social functioning than single-rater sources. In addition, data from peers can be obtained without focusing on the child with a chronic condition.

Unfortunately, few studies in the pediatric literature have obtained social functioning data from peers. In fact, parent (typically mother) report remains one of the most common sources of information for multiple domains of children's medical and psychosocial outcomes. Our review of the literature indicates that many pediatric researchers have used the CBCL (Achenbach & Rescorla, 2001) to assess children's adjustment, including social functioning, rather than data from peers. Our research group has considerable data from peer report measures of social functioning as well as data from mothers and fathers using the CBCL, both for children with a chronic condition (e.g., cancer, sickle cell disease [SCD], juvenile rheumatoid arthritis, NF1, or migraines) and children without a chronic illness (for information regarding participants, measures, and procedures, see Noll et al., 1996, 1999, 2000; Noll, Reiter-Purtill, Moore, et al., 2007; Vannatta et al., 2008). Unfortunately, simple bivariate correlations between parent reports on the Social Problems subscale of the CBCL and peer nomination data are modest (see also Schneider & Byrne, 1989). (See Table 45.2.)

Compared with parents, teachers may have greater opportunities to observe the social functioning of children. Still, they primarily interact with children in classroom settings where peer interactions are limited, and they may be biased by other knowledge about the children (e.g., academic success) (Newcomb, Bukowski, & Pattee, 1993; Parker & Asher, 1987). In fact, Gest (2006) found only moderate teacher–peer agreement regarding school-age children's reciprocated friendships and social group affiliations.

Finally, self-report measures are especially important for understanding a child's perspectives on experiences of social acceptance, friendship, loneliness, victimization, or teasing. However, self-report may also be difficult to interpret for some populations. For instance, Owens, Goldfine, Evangelista, Hoza, and Kaiser (2007) have recently discussed the positive illusory bias present in the self-reports of children with ADHD regarding perceptions of functioning, including social competence. Specifically, children with ADHD often give overly positive self-perceptions of their own competence, relative to perceptions from other sources. Despite the limitations of self-report, the perspective of the child is especially important if interventions are to be successfully initiated. For example, if brain tumor survivors are perceived by peers as withdrawn and are rejected by those peers, but they are not identifying peer relationships as a problem, it is very challenging to gain their involvement in interventions.

In summary, the majority of empirical studies reviewed (Table 45.1) suggest that children with chronic conditions have social difficulties, according to parent report. In contrast, peer report suggests that children with chronic conditions do not have peer difficulties unless they have a condition that impairs their CNS functioning, affects their appearance, or is more somatic in nature.

TABLE 45.2. Correlations among Parent-Reported Scores on the Social Subscale of the CBCL and Peer Report Measures of Friendship and Social Acceptance for Children with a Chronic Illness and Comparison Peers without a Chronic Illness

| Peer report measures | CBCL-Social Mother Report | | | CBCL-Social Father Report | | |
	Chronic illness $n = 305–309$ r^a	Comparison $n = 309–312$ r^a	z^b	Chronic illness $n = 193–195$ r^a	Comparison $n = 195–198$ r^a	z^b
Best-friend nominations	0.23***	0.13*	1.28	−0.06	0.11	−1.68*
Reciprocated friendships	0.16**	0.09	0.88	−0.08	0.12	−1.96*
Like ratings	0.21***	0.19**	0.26	−0.06	0.14*	−1.97*

Note. CBCL, Child Behavior Checklist. [a]Pearson's r reported; [b]Z test comparing correlations between groups, two-tailed tests; *$p < .05$; **$p < .01$; ***$p < .001$.

Pathways between Chronic Illness and Social Functioning

What Do We Know?

The seminal work of La Greca (1990) identified a number of potential pathways linking chronic illness to peer dysfunction. Specifically, she suggested that restrictions on activities, missing a lot of school, pain, chronic fatigue, cosmetic changes, or CNS dysfunction could be linked to problematic peer relationships. Several of these pathways do not receive strong empirical support from our review of the literature. Considerable evidence now exists suggesting that children who experience restrictions on activities, school absences, pain, or chronic fatigue as a result of a disease with identified biological causes do not appear to have problematic social functioning from the perspective of peers. In contrast, investigations focusing on the social functioning of children with CNS involvement consistently report dysfunction with friendship, social acceptance, and social isolation from the perspectives of peers, teachers, and parents. In addition, some work indicates that children with a chronic health condition that adversely affects their appearance have more problematic peer relationships, but the evidence is less robust. Finally, recent work has begun to examine the social functioning of children with more somatic types of problems; these children seem to be at risk for difficulties.

What Do We Need to Know?

Despite significant advances over the past 20 years in clarifying disease-related variables associated with peer dysfunction, much work is still needed. First, identification of specific pathways (mediators) linking chronic illness to peer dysfunction is essential. Empirical work needs to hone in on these specific pathways so that interventions can be targeted toward the correct pathway (Yeates et al., 2007). Although the evidence is compelling that CNS involvement is linked to problematic peer relationships, the field needs to clarify precisely why this occurs. Do children with chronic illness that includes CNS involvement have poor social problem-solving skills? If yes, what aspect of social problem solving (e.g., conflict resolution, cooperation) is affected? Alternatively, is CNS involvement associated with social dysfunction only when attention and/ or executive functioning is disrupted? Or perhaps children with CNS involvement are more depressed, leading to social problems?

Second, for the vast majority of chronic illnesses in children, little work has been done obtaining information from peers. Where data have been reported, work is typically done with small samples ($N < 100$) and from only one site. Longitudinal studies remain rare. Even more problematic are the lack of data from peers for many chronic conditions of childhood. With few exceptions (e.g., Verduin & Kendall, 2008), little work has examined peer nomination data for children with many psychiatric disorders. Although children with these problems are often described by teachers, parents, or clinicians as socially dysfunctional, the lack of data from peers is egregious. It seems feasible that children who present with depression but have friends at school may respond differently to treatment than those with no friends may.

Third, data on social competence from parents do not correspond strongly to data on social competence from peers. Insofar as peer nomination data or direct observations of peer interactions are considered the "gold standard" for information about peer functioning, we strongly suggest caution in using data from other sources. When a measure with the strong psychometrics of the CBCL shows meager correspondence between parent-reported social functioning and peer reports, we are very concerned about cursory questions from health-related quality-of-life measures. If it is not feasible to obtain peer reports of social functioning, then multisource and multimethod data collection strategies should be employed, especially with input from teachers (Holmbeck, Li, Schurman, Friedman, & Coakley, 2002).

Fourth, contextual variables may play a pivotal role during assessments of subjective functioning (Noll & Fairclough, 2004). For instance, using disease-specific measures that ask questions about disease status and functional impairments, or obtaining data in clinic settings, may create a focusing illusion or misallocation of attention (Schkade & Kahneman, 1998) on health and disease when assessments of psychosocial adjustment are conducted. Thus responses to questions about day-to-day well-being may be altered when cognition has been primed or focused on disability (Smith, Schwarz, Roberts, & Ubel, 2006). We endorse the use of functional measures and data collection in neutral sites (e.g., classrooms), to minimize contextual cues that could artificially inflate reports of dysfunction.

Although the field has gained a better understanding of the functional impact of chronic illness on children's peer relationships, more work is clearly needed. When children with a chronic illness report social problems, alternative risk factors should be carefully investigated unless the disease involves a child's CNS. Interventions successfully utilized for typically developing children with no chronic health condition (Mayer, Van Acker, Lochman, & Gresham, 2009) should be implemented for children with CNS involvement in a preventive manner.

References

Achenbach, T. M., & Rescorla, L. A. (2001). *Manual for ASEBA school-age forms and profiles*. Burlington: University of Vermont, Research Center for Children, Youth, and Families.

Bagwell, C. L., Newcomb, A. F., & Bukowski, W. M. (1998). Preadolescent friendship and peer rejection as predictors of adult adjustment. *Child Development, 69,* 140–153.

Barton, B., & North, K. (2004). Social skills of children with neurofibromatosis Type 1. *Developmental Medicine and Child Neurology, 46,* 553–563.

Cobb, J. C., Cohen, R., Houston, D. A., & Rubin, E. C. (1998). Children's self-concepts and peer relationships: Relating appearance self-discrepancies and peer perceptions of social behaviors. *Child Study Journal, 28,* 291–308.

Curtin, L. S., & Siegel, A. W. (2003). Social functioning in adolescents with epilepsy. *Children's Health Care, 32,* 103–114.

Feldmann, R., Weglage, J., Roth, J., Foell, D., & Frosch, M. (2005). Systemic juvenile rheumatoid arthritis: Cognitive function and social adjustment. *Annals of Neurology, 58,* 605–609.

Freedman, D. S., Khan, L. K., Serdula, M. K., Ogden, C. L., & Dietz, W. H. (2006). Racial and ethnic differences in secular trends for childhood BMI, weight, and height. *Obesity, 14,* 301–308.

Freilinger, M., Reisel, B., Reiter, E., Zelenko, M., Hauser, E., & Seidl, R. (2006). Behavioral and emotional problems in children with epilepsy. *Journal of Child Neurology, 21,* 939–945.

French, D. C., & Conrad, J. (2001). School dropout as predicted by peer rejection and antisocial behavior. *Journal of Research on Adolescence, 11,* 225–245.

Gartstein, M. A., Noll, R. B., & Vannatta, K. (2000). Childhood aggression and chronic illness: Possible protective mechanisms. *Journal of Applied Developmental Psychology, 21,* 315–333.

Gerhardt, C .A., Vannatta, K., Valerius, K. S., Correll, J., & Noll, R. B. (2007). Social and romantic outcomes in emerging adulthood among survivors of childhood cancer. *Journal of Adolescent Health, 40,* 462.e9–462.e15.

Gest, S. D. (2006). Teacher reports of children's friendships and social groups: Agreement with peer reports and implications for studying peer similarity. *Social Development, 15,* 248–259.

Greco, L. A., Freeman, K. E., & Dufton, L. (2006). Overt and relational victimization among children with frequent abdominal pain: Links to social skills, academic functioning, and health service use. *Journal of Pediatric Psychology, 32,* 319–329.

Hayden-Wade, H. A., Stein, R. I., Ghaderi, A., Saelens, B. E., Zabinski, M. F., & Wilfley, D. E. (2005). Prevalence, characteristics, and correlates of teasing experiences among overweight children vs. non-overweight peers. *Obesity Research, 13,* 1381–1392.

Hodges, E. V., Boivin, M., Vitaro, F., & Bukowski, W. M. (1999). The power of friendship: Protection against an escalating cycle of peer victimization. *Developmental Psychology, 35,* 94–101.

Hoie, B., Sommerfelt, K., Waaler, P. E., Alsaker, F. D., Skeidsvoll, H., & Mykletun, A. (2006). Psychosocial problems and seizure-related factors in children with epilepsy. *Developmental Medicine and Child Neurology, 48,* 213–219.

Holmbeck, G. N., Li, S. T., Schurman, J. V., Friedman, D., & Coakley, R. M. (2002). Collecting and managing multisource and multimethod data in studies of pediatric populations. *Journal of Pediatric Psychology, 27,* 5–18.

Holmbeck, G. N., Westhoven, V. C., Phillips, W. S., Bowers, R., Gruse, C., Nikolopoulos, T., et al. (2003). A multimethod, multi-informant, and multidimensional perspective on psychosocial adjustment in preadolescents with spina bifida. *Journal of Consulting and Clinical Psychology, 71*(4), 782–796.

Hoza, B. (2007). Peer functioning in children with ADHD. *Journal of Pediatric Psychology, 32,* 655–663.

Hunt, O., Burden, D., Hepper, P., Stevenson, M., & Johnston, C. (2006). Self-reports of psychosocial functioning among children and young adults with cleft lip and palate. *Cleft Palate–Craniofacial Journal, 43,* 598–605.

Hunt, O., Burden, D., Hepper, P., Stevenson, M., & Johnston, C. (2007). Parent reports of the psychosocial functioning of children with cleft lip and/or palate. *Cleft Palate–Craniofacial Journal, 44,* 304–311.

Huygen, A. C. J., Kuis, W., & Sinnema, G. (2000). Psychological, behavioral, and social adjustment in children and adolescents with juvenile chronic arthritis. *Annals of the Rheumatic Diseases, 59,* 276–282.

Hyman, S. L., Shores, A., & North, K. (2005). The nature and frequency of cognitive deficits in children with neurofibromatosis Type 1. *Neurology, 65,* 1037–1044.

Kashikar-Zuck, S., Lynch, A. M., Graham, B., Swain, N. F., Mullen, S. M., & Noll, R. B. (2007). Social functioning and peer relationships of adolescents with juvenile fibromyalgia syndrome. *Arthritis and Rheumatism, 57,* 474–480.

La Greca, A. M. (1990). Social consequences of pediatric conditions: Fertile area for future investigation and intervention? *Journal of Pediatric Psychology, 15,* 285–307.

Laird, R. D., Pettit, G. S., Dodge, K. A., & Bates, J. E. (2005). Peer relationship antecedents of delinquent behavior in late adolescence: Is there evidence of demographic group differences in developmental processes? *Development and Psychopathology, 17,* 127–144.

Masten, A. S. (2001). Ordinary magic: Resilience processes in development. *American Psychologist, 56,* 227–238.

Mayer, M., Van Acker R., Lochman, J., & Gresham, F. M. (2009). *Cognitive-behavioral interventions for emotional and behavioral disorders.* New York: Guilford Press.

Miatton, M., De Wolf, D., Francois, K., Thiery, E., & Vingerhoets, G. (2007). Behavior and self-perception in children with a surgically corrected congenital heart disease. *Journal of Developmental and Behavioral Pediatrics, 28,* 294–301.

Nangle, D. W., Erdley, C. A., Newman, J. E., Mason, C. A., & Carpenter, E. M. (2003). Popularity, friendship quantity and friendship quality: Interactive influences on children's loneliness and depression. *Journal of Clinical Child and Adolescent Psychology, 32,* 546–555.

Nassau, J. H., & Drotar, D. (1997). Social competence among children with central nervous system–related chronic health conditions: A review. *Journal of Pediatric Psychology, 22,* 771–793.

Newcomb, A. F., Bukowski, W. M., & Pattee, L. (1993). Children's peer relations: A meta-analytic review of popular, rejected, neglected, controversial, and average sociometric status. *Psychological Bulletin, 113,* 99–128.

Nishina, A., Juvonen, J., & Witkow, M. R. (2005). Sticks and stones may break my bones, but names will make me feel sick: The psychosocial, somatic, and scholastic consequences of peer harassment. *Journal of Clinical Child and Adolescent Psychology, 34,* 37–48.

Noll, R. B., & Fairclough, D. (2004). Health related quality of life: Developmental and psychometric issues. *Journal of Pediatrics, 145,* 8–9.

Noll, R. B., Gartstein, M. A., Vannatta, K., Correll, J., Bukowski, W. M., & Davies, W. H. (1999). Social, emotional, and behavioral functioning of children with cancer. *Pediatrics, 103,* 71–78.

Noll, R. B., Kozlowski, M. A., Gerhardt, C. A., Vannatta, K., Taylor, J., & Passo, M. H. (2000). Social, emotional, and behavioral functioning of children with juvenile rheumatoid arthritis. *Arthritis and Rheumatism, 43,* 1387–1396.

Noll, R. B., & Kupst, M. J. (2007). Commentary: The psychological impact of pediatric cancer hardiness: The exception or the rule? *Journal of Pediatric Psychology, 32,* 1089–1098.

Noll, R. B., Reiter-Purtill, J., Moore, B. D., Schorry, E. K., Lovell, A. M., Vannatta, K., et al. (2007). Social, emotional, and behavioral functioning of children with NF1. *American Journal of Medical Genetics, 143A,* 2261–2273.

Noll, R. B., Reiter-Purtill, J., Vannatta, K., Gerhardt, C. A., & Short, A. (2007). Peer relationships and emotional well-being of children with sickle cell disease: A controlled replication. *Child Neuropsychology, 13,* 173–187.

Noll, R. B., Vannatta, K., Koontz, K., Kaylinyak, K., Bukowski, W. M., & Davies, W. H. (1996). Peer relationships and emotional well-being of youngsters with sickle cell disease. *Child Development, 67,* 423–436.

Owens, J. S., Goldfine, M. E., Evangelista, N. M., Hoza, B., & Kaiser, N. M. (2007). A critical review of self-perceptions and the positive illusory bias in children with ADHD. *Clinical Child and Family Psychology Review, 10,* 335–351.

Parker, J. G., & Asher, S. R. (1987). Peer relations and later personal adjustment: Are low-accepted children at risk? *Psychological Bulletin, 102,* 357–389.

Parker, J. G., & Asher, S. R. (1993). Friendship and friendship quality in middle childhood: Links with peer group acceptance and feelings of loneliness and social dissatisfaction. *Developmental Psychology, 29,* 611–621.

Perrin, J. M., Bloom, S. R., & Gortmaker, S. L. (2007). The increase of childhood chronic conditions in the United States. *Journal of the American Medical Association, 297,* 2755–2759.

Puhl, R. M., & Latner, J. D. (2007). Stigma, obesity, and the health of the nation's children. *Psychological Bulletin, 133,* 557–580.

Reiter-Purtill, J., & Noll, R. B. (2003). Peer relationships of children with chronic illness. In M. C. Roberts (Ed.), *Handbook of pediatric psychology* (3rd ed., pp. 176–197). New York: Guilford Press.

Reiter-Purtill, J., Vannatta, K., Gerhardt, C. A., Correll, J., & Noll, R. B. (2003). A controlled longitudinal study of the social functioning of children who completed treatment of cancer. *Journal of Pediatric Hematology/Oncology, 25*, 467–473.

Rose, B. M., & Holmbeck, G. N. (2007). Attention and executive functions in adolescents with spina bifida. *Journal of Pediatric Psychology, 32*, 983–994.

Rothbart, M. K., Ahadi, S. A., & Hershey, K. L. (1994). Temperament and social behavior in childhood. *Merrill–Palmer Quarterly, 40*, 21–39.

Sandberg, E. E., Bukowski, W. M., Fung, C. M., & Noll, R. B. (2004). Height and social adjustment: Are extremes a cause for concern and action? *Pediatrics, 114*, 744–750.

Schkade, D. A., & Kahneman, D. (1998). Does living in California make people happy?: A focusing illusion in judgments of life satisfaction. *Psychological Science, 9*, 340–346.

Schneider, B. H., & Byrne, B. M. (1989). Parents rating children's social behavior: How focused the lens? *Journal of Clinical Child Psychology, 18*, 237–241.

Schuman, W. B., & La Greca, A. M. (1999). Social correlates of chronic illness. In R. T. Brown (Ed.), *Cognitive aspects of chronic illness in children* (pp. 289–311). New York: Guilford Press.

Slifer, K. J., Amari, A., Diver, T., Hilley, L., Beck, M., Kane, A., et al. (2004). Social interaction patterns of children and adolescents with and without oral clefts during a videotaped analogue social encounter. *Cleft Palate–Craniofacial Journal, 41*, 175–184.

Slifer, K. J., Pulbrook, V., Amari, A., Vona-Messersmith, N., Cohn, J. F., Ambadar, Z., et al. (2006). Social acceptance and facial behavior in children with oral clefts. *Cleft Palate–Craniofacial Journal, 43*, 226–236.

Smith, D. M., Schwarz, N., Roberts, T. R., & Ubel, P. A. (2006). Why are you calling me?: How study introductions change response patterns. *Quality of Life Research, 15*, 621–630.

Storch, E. A., Lewin, A., Silverstein, J. H., Heidgerken, A. D., Strawser, M. S., Baumeister, A., et al. (2004). Peer victimization and psychosocial adjustment in children with Type 1 diabetes. *Clinical Pediatrics, 43*, 467–471.

Storch, E. A., Milsom, V. A., DeBranganza, N., Lewin, A. B., Geffken, G. R., & Silverstein, J. H. (2007). Peer victimization, psychosocial adjustment, and physical activity in overweight and at-risk-for-overweight youth. *Journal of Pediatric Psychology, 32*, 80–89.

Strauss, R. S., & Pollack, H. A. (2003). Social marginalization of overweight children. *Archives of Pediatrics and Adolescent Medicine, 157*, 746–752.

Strine, T. W., Okoro, C. A., McGuire, L. C., & Balluz, L. S. (2006). The associations among childhood headaches, emotional and behavioral difficulties, and health care use. *Pediatrics, 117*, 1728–1735.

Thompson, J. K., Shroff, H., Herbozo, S., Cafri, G., Rodriguez, J., & Rodriguez, M. (2007). Relations among multiple peer influences, body dissatisfaction, eating disturbance, and self-esteem: A comparison of average weight, at risk of overweight, and overweight adolescent girls. *Journal of Pediatric Psychology, 32*, 24–29.

Trzepacz, A. M., Vannatta, K., Davies, W. H., Stehbens, J. A., & Noll, R. B. (2003). Social, emotional, and behavioral functioning of children with hemophilia. *Journal of Developmental and Behavioral Pediatrics, 24*, 225–232.

van der Lee, J. H., Mokkink, L. B., Grootenhuis, M. A., Heymans, H. S., & Offringa, M. (2007). Definitions and measurement of chronic health conditions in childhood: A systematic review. *Journal of the American Medical Association, 297*, 2741–2751.

Vannatta, K., Gartstein, M. A., Zeller, M., & Noll, R. B. (in press). Peer acceptance during childhood and adolescence: How important are appearance, athleticism, and academic competence? *International Journal of Behavioral Development.*

Vannatta, K., Gerhardt, C. A., Wells, R. J., & Noll, R. B. (2007). Intensity of CNS treatment for pediatric cancer: Prediction of social outcomes in survivors. *Pediatric Blood and Cancer, 49*, 716–722.

Vannatta, K., Getzoff, E. A, Powers, S. W., Noll, R. B., Gerhardt, C. A., & Hershey, A. D. (2008). Friendships and social interactions of school-aged children with migraine. *Cephalalgia, 28*, 734–743.

Verduin, T. L., & Kendall, P. C. (2008). Peer perceptions and liking of children with anxiety disorders. *Journal of Abnormal Child Psychology, 36*, 459–469.

Wallander, J. L., & Thompson, R. J. (1995). Psychosocial adjustment of children with chronic physical conditions. In M. C. Roberts (Ed.), *Handbook of pediatric psychology* (2nd ed., pp. 124–141). New York: Guilford Press.

Wallander, J. L., & Varni, J. W. (1998). Effects of pediatric chronic physical disorders on child and family adjustment. *Journal of Child Psychology and Psychiatry, 39*, 29–46.

Yeates, K. O., Bigler, E. D., Dennis, M., Gerhardt, C. A., Rubin, K. H., Stancin, T., et al. (2007). Social outcomes in childhood brain disorder: A heuristic integration of social neuroscience and developmental psychology. *Psychological Bulletin, 133*, 535–556.

Zeller, M., Reiter-Purtill, J., & Ramey, C. (2008). Negative peer perceptions of obese children in the classroom environment. *Obesity, 16*, 755–762.

Zeller, M., Vannatta, K., Schafer, J., & Noll, R. B. (2003) Behavioral reputation: A cross-age perspective. *Developmental Psychology, 39*, 129–139.

CHAPTER 46

Schools and Integration/Reintegration into Schools

GEORGE J. DuPAUL
THOMAS J. POWER
EDWARD S. SHAPIRO

Other than their homes, children and adolescents spend more time in school settings than any other environment. In fact, the average student will spend at least 14,000 hours in school (assuming a 6-hour school day) from kindergarten through 12th grade. Schools are not only the major venue for acquisition and growth of academic skills; they also are primary settings for the development of appropriate social, emotional, and behavioral functioning. It is critical for pediatric psychologists to understand the educational system and the potential impact of physical health issues on students' school functioning, as well as the role schools can play in fostering healthy outcomes for all children.

A multisystemic perspective is needed to address children's functioning in a comprehensive manner. Ideally, personnel from the health care and educational systems will collaborate with families to develop and implement preventive and palliative strategies that promote healthy development (Power, DuPaul, Shapiro, & Kazak, 2003). Given their knowledge of child development as well as critical psychological and health issues, pediatric psychologists are in an excellent position to promote communication and cooperation across systems. Knowledge of schools as a system, as well as how children's health status will affect school functioning, will be important in the development of cross-system partnerships.

The purpose of this chapter is to provide an overview of the K–12 educational system with an emphasis on issues relevant to pediatric psychology. First, a brief description of systemic reform efforts in the context of a public health model is provided. Next, the impact of pediatric illness on academic, behavioral, and social functioning in school settings is delineated. Interventions designed to improve school functioning are described, including monitoring medication, promoting treatment adherence, and facilitating integration/reintegration into the school environment. Finally, school-based prevention and health promotion strategies are detailed, including ones related to nutrition education, physical fitness development, violence prevention, promotion of social-emotional development, and prevention of sexually transmitted diseases.

Overview of Schools from a Multisystemic Perspective

As of 2003, approximately 55 million children and adolescents attend schools in the United States, with over 88% of students attending public schools (Federal Interagency Forum on Child and Family Statistics, 2007). The school population is projected to continue growing through at least 2014 (Federal Interagency Forum, 2007). Furthermore, the student population has become increasingly diverse over the past several decades. For example, there has been tremendous growth in the percentage of students from nonwhite ethnic backgrounds. Nonwhite students made up about 22% of the school population in 1972, and that figure has nearly doubled to just over 42% of the population as of 2005 (Federal Interagency Forum, 2007, Table 5-1). By 2050, nonwhite students will be in the majority (Passel & Cohn, 2008). The percentage of the school population consisting of students with disabilities has also steadily grown over the past few decades, due to increased identification and greater emphasis on including such students in general education settings. Of particular note is the increase in students identified with "other health impairments" (e.g., asthma, diabetes), rising from 0.1% of the general student population in 1992 to 0.6% in 2002 (U.S. Department of Education, 2005).

Educational Reform Efforts

Over the past decade, a strong focus on improving the academic achievement of students has been evident in schools across the United States. In particular, an emphasis on increasing the reading performance of young children has been one of the most pervasive national educational reform efforts. Research has consistently demonstrated that students who do not develop adequate skills in reading by the end of first grade have a high probability of school struggles throughout their careers (e.g., Juel, 1988). Serious concern about developing the literacy of young children resulted in the No Child Left Behind (NCLB) Act of 2001. As a result, schools have begun to focus on the prevention of future problems in reading by bolstering instruction within the core academic program, together with providing needed remediation and intervention at the earliest point possible to those identified as potentially at risk for failure. Although the outcomes of the NCLB Act and prevention efforts have yet to be fully determined, it is clear that schools have shifted extensive energies toward data-driven decisions related to instruction. The increase in accountability for schools to improve student outcomes was a direct outgrowth of the NCLB Act (Ravitch, 1999).

Another major reform effort linked to the perspectives of the NCLB Act was evident in the passage of the 2004 Individuals with Disabilities Education Improvement Act. This law, which governs the decision-making process for identifying students in need of special education, contains a particular provision related to the identification of learning disabilities that has the potential to fully change the conceptualization of these disabilities.

Historically, a "learning disability" has been defined as unexpected underachievement in a student. Students are considered to have a learning disability when there is evidence that their capacity for achievement is much greater than what they are actually displaying. The assumption is that unexpected underachievement is due to a difficulty with the neuropsychological processing of information, and that such children need specific accommodations to the learning process that exceed what can be provided within the general education system alone. Based on these assumptions, the model for identifying a learning disability was to identify a discrepancy between a child's level of intellectual functioning and his or her current achievement (Fletcher et al., 1998). Unfortunately, research has shown that although the discrepancy model may have had logical and conceptual soundness, it has not held up to empirical scrutiny (Fletcher et al., 1998).

As a function of the dissatisfaction with the discrepancy model of identification, a method known as "response to intervention" (RTI) has been developed. Proponents of RTI believe that the basis for a learning disability is the failure to respond adequately to effective, research-based interventions delivered within the context of the general education environment (Gersten & Dimino, 2006). The essential concept is that if good instruction results in adequate gains for most children, those who do not respond to this type of instruction, as well as instruction that is intensified and individualized to address specific needs, are viewed as "not responding to instruction" and therefore as potentially eligible for services under the learning disability classification.

All of these reform efforts in the schools reflect a clear recognition that academic success is linked to favorable developmental and health outcomes. The development of strong academic skills is known to diminish the presence of many emotional and behavioral difficulties of students (e.g., Lane, Barton-Arwood, Nelson, & Wehby, 2008; Lane, Wehby, Little, & Cooley, 2005), as well as to serve as a protective factor for many adolescent mental health concerns (Brindis, 2005). The connection among academic health, prevention, and overall wellness is clearly an area of substantial overlap between pediatric psychology and school psychology.

The Public Health Model and Positive Behavior Support

The public health model is highly consonant with the mission of schools. Consistent with the public health framework, educational professionals have a responsibility to address the developmental needs of all students, including children with problems, those at risk, and those who are performing competently in all domains. Within the educational system, there is widespread recognition that health conditions, including mental health problems, can serve as obstacles to the development of academic competence. As such, strategies to promote health, and to address disorders and risk when they arise, are often required to promote the academic competence of all individuals (Hoagwood & Johnson, 2003).

The "positive behavior support" (PBS) framework, which has been applied in thousands of schools throughout the nation, is closely aligned with the public health model. The PBS model provides prevention along a continuum with three tiers: primary or universal prevention for all students; secondary or selective/indicated prevention for individuals at risk for behavioral and academic difficulties; and tertiary prevention for students who have clearly identified problems (Sugai & Horner, 2006). Although this framework has been developed primarily to address behavioral and instructional issues in schools, the PBS model can be applied to address issues at the intersection of children's health and academic competence. For example, primary prevention addresses the needs of all students; secondary prevention is targeted for children with health problems that are likely to affect academic competence; and tertiary prevention is focused on individuals with health conditions that have an effect on academic performance (e.g., asthma resulting in frequent school absence and poor school performance).

An essential component of the public health model is the identification of factors that contribute to risk, as well as factors that protect against risk (Strein, Hoagwood, & Cohn, 2003). The need to identify mutable variables that can be changed at the child, family, and classroom levels is critical to prevention efforts. Examples of mutable variables include knowledge of health issues and their treatment on the part of family members and educators; acceptability of interventions to children, parents, and educators; availability of bilingual educators and care providers; and qualities of the social network available to families (Eiraldi, Mazzuca, Clarke, & Power, 2006).

Impact of Pediatric Illness on School Functioning

Chronic illness can be associated with significant activity limitations. Given that approximately 8% of the child population is reported by parents to experience some activity limitation due to a chronic health condition (Federal Interagency Forum, 2007), it is not surprising that chronic illness may have a significant impact on academic, social, and behavioral functioning. In fact, children with chronic illnesses are about twice as likely to experience adjustment difficulties as healthy controls (Sexson & Madan-Swain, 1995).

Academic Functioning

The educational achievement of children with a chronic illness may be compromised by direct effects of the condition (e.g., impact of symptoms or treatment on central nervous system functioning) and/or the secondary consequences of the illness (e.g., fatigue, stress, or frequent absences from school) (Shapiro & Manz, 2004). In addition, an increased risk of grade retention (Byrd & Weitzman, 1994) and of identification for special education services (U.S. Department of Education, 2005) may be associated with chronic illness. The potential impact on educational achievement is characterized by substantial between-disease and within-disease variability. Specifically, deficits in academic functioning are particularly apparent for children with chronic illnesses that affect the central nervous system, receive treatment that affects cognitive functioning, or have a physical disability in addition to the chronic illness (Shapiro & Manz, 2004).

Despite the risks for academic impairment, it is important to note that the impact of a chronic illness on educational functioning is variable across children, with most students functioning in the average range. For example, McNelis, Johnson, Huberty, and Austin (2005) found variable levels of academic achievement in a large sample of children with seizure disorders; milder severity of seizures was associated with greater achievement. Given the heterogeneity of academic outcomes in children with chronic illness, it will be important for educational and health care professionals to identify those children who are at greatest risk for educational impairment as a function of their illness.

Behavioral Functioning

Children with chronic illness may be at risk for behavioral difficulties, although this risk appears minimal for most illnesses. In general, symptoms of internalizing disorders (e.g., anxiety and depression) are more likely than are problems related to externalizing disorders (e.g., attention-deficit/hyperactivity disorder [ADHD] and conduct disorder) (Lavigne & Faier-Routman, 1992). Although the research in this area is somewhat dated, it appears that children with chronic illness are more likely to experience separation fears and school avoidance than their healthy peers (Henning & Fritz, 1983). Several factors are linked to behavioral difficulties among children with chronic illness, including disease impact on brain functioning, increased maternal stress, low family cohesion and support, and children's perceived level of stress (Shapiro & Manz, 2004).

Social Functioning

It is possible that chronic illness may interfere with children's opportunities for typical social development by limiting independence from parents, exposure to healthy peers, participation in peer activities (e.g., athletics), and/or development of self-efficacy in peer interactions (Schuman & La Greca, 1999; Shapiro & Manz, 2004). Although there is a growing research literature on the social development of children with chronic illness, it remains unclear whether specific diseases carry more social risk or whether the general status of having a chronic illness confers risk (Meijer, Sinnema, Bijstra, Mellenbergh, & Wolters, 2000). The risk for social functioning deficits appears greatest for males, children with more severe and disabling symptoms of chronic illness, and those who are submissive and/or restricted in their social activities (Cadman, Boyle, Szatmari, & Offord, 1987; Meijer et al., 2000).

Interventions to Improve School Functioning

Given the potential impact of chronic illness on important areas of functioning, school-based interventions are often utilized, including medication, behavioral treatments, and cognitive-behavioral strategies. Three examples of important treatment directions are discussed here: monitoring medication effects, promoting treatment adherence, and facilitating school integration/reintegration following hospitalization.

Monitoring Medication Effects

The behavioral, academic, social, and cognitive effects of medication can be evaluated through a variety of methods, including behavior rating scales, direct observations of classroom behavior, review of school archival data (e.g., completion and accuracy rates on academic assignments), direct measures of academic performance (e.g., curriculum-based measurement), and cognitive tests when necessary (Brown, Carpenter, & Simerly,

2005; Phelps, Brown, & Power, 2001; Power et al., 2003). Multiple models for school-based medication evaluation have been proposed (e.g., Gadow, 1993; Power et al., 2003; Volpe, Heick, & Gureasko-Moore, 2005).

All of the proposed school-based medication-monitoring protocols share several important features: (1) Timelines, procedures, and measures are specified prior to the evaluation; (2) brief, psychometrically sound measures are used to assess targeted areas of functioning; (3) medication and/or dosage decisions are guided by obtained data; (4) potential adverse side effects are assessed prior to and following receipt of medication; (5) data on school functioning are gathered for both nonmedication and medication conditions; and (6) data are communicated in a clear, concise fashion to physicians and parents (Power et al., 2003).

Promoting Adherence

Interventions for many health conditions involve components that are applied in school. For example, children with asthma and ADHD are commonly prescribed medications to be taken while they are at school. Furthermore, medical interventions applied at home often have an effect on how children function in school. Because adherence to medical treatments can be highly variable across and within families, and because treatment adherence is generally considered to be critical to effective care, interventions to improve adherence are important for promoting academic and social competence (for details regarding such interventions, see La Greca & Mackey, Chapter 9, this volume).

Facilitating School Integration/Reintegration

Children with chronic health conditions often have difficulty being integrated into school early in their education, as well as during transitions into middle school, high school, and young adulthood. School reintegration is also typically a challenge for students after periods of acute problems resulting in temporary removal from school. Systematic efforts to support school integration/reintegration have been developed for children with a wide range of chronic health problems, but most of the work has been conducted on behalf of children coping with cancer and brain injury.

Intervention programs designed to support school integration/reintegration include those focused on skill building (e.g., social skills, cognitive retraining), teacher education, and peer education (for a review, see Prevatt, Heffer, & Lowe, 2000). Generally, the empirical support for these approaches is limited, and concerns have been raised about the effectiveness of these approaches in improving child outcomes in actual school settings (Power et al., 2003). Comprehensive, multicomponent programs have shown the greatest promise with regard to improving child outcomes (Madan-Swain, Katz, & LaGory, 2004). These programs typically include the following components: (1) family support to maintain strong parent–child relationships and prepare the family for school entry or reentry; (2) education of school staff regarding the child's illness and effective school-based approaches to intervention; (3) peer education and support programs; and (4) sustained follow-up to monitor progress and adjust the educational plan as needed.

Elsewhere, we (Power et al., 2003) have emphasized a staged model that includes interventions to prepare systems for integration/reintegration and to guide participants through an extended (re)integration process. The four steps in this process are described

TABLE 46.1. Steps to School Integration/Reintegration, Using a Multisystemic Model

Steps to school (re)integration	Purpose of each step
Step 1: Strengthen the family	• Strengthen the parent–child relationship. • Sustain the parent partnership. • Strengthen sibling relationships. • Support the family in collaborating with the health care system.
Step 2: Prepare the family to work with the school	• Assist the family in coping with anxiety about working with the school. • Educate the family about school ecology and educational rights. • Provide families with a framework to guide school collaboration.
Step 3: Prepare the school to partner with the family and health care system	• Educate school professionals about the child's needs and effective strategies for meeting these needs. • Assist school professionals to understand the perspective of the family. • Provide school professionals with a framework to guide family collaboration.
Step 4: Engage the family, school, and health care system in a collaborative process	• Strengthen the family–school relationship. • Support the development of a school–health care system relationship. • Guide participants through the steps of conjoint behavioral consultation.

Note. For a further description of these steps, see Power, DuPaul, Shapiro, and Kazak (2003).

in Table 46.1. Step 1 focuses on efforts to strengthen the family; Step 2 involves preparing the family to partner with the school; Step 3 emphasizes preparing school professionals to partner with the family and health care system; and Step 4 focuses on engaging the family, school, and health care system in a conjoint process of planning and implementation, which is based on the principles of conjoint behavioral consultation (Sheridan & Kratochwill, 2008). Although intervention programs typically focus on intervention design and strategy implementation (Step 4), efforts to prepare systems for multisystemic collaboration (Steps 1–3) are essential for successful school adaptation. Step 4 is viewed as an ongoing, recursive process involving intervention design, implementation, progress monitoring, intervention modification, and continuing monitoring and fine-tuning of the intervention. The purposes of Step 4 are to identify and build upon child strengths and system resources, to address anticipated challenges, and to solve problems when they arise.

School-Based Prevention and Health Promotion

Nutrition Education and Physical Fitness Development

Perhaps the major public health concern today involving children and adolescents in the United States is the issue of pediatric overweight. Data from the National Health and Nutrition Examination Survey show that 17.1% of children and adolescents are overweight (Ogden et al., 2006). The problem extends to preschool-age children as well, with estimates that over 10% of preschoolers have a body mass index above the 95th percentile. Pediatric overweight is associated with both immediate and long-term health problems, including hypertension, asthma, musculoskeletal problems, sleep disorders,

Type 2 diabetes, depression, and social stigmatization (Cruz et al., 2005; Kiess et al., 2001). Problems involving both physical and psychological difficulties persist into adolescence and can establish significant risk for adult obesity and other chronic diseases (Engeland, Bjorge, Tverdal, & Sogaard, 2004).

Schools have attempted to design and implement programs to halt the alarming trend toward obesity by directly curbing the food items available for students. In addition, efforts to alter the knowledge and eating lifestyles of students have been common. For example, Blom-Hoffman, Kelleher, Power, and Leff (2004) examined the implementation of the Five a Day for Better Health program, a national campaign sponsored by the U.S. Department of Education to encourage children to eat five servings of fruits and vegetables daily. The study reported on the inclusion of paraprofessionals to assist in the implementation of the intervention during lunch. Outcomes showed significant change in knowledge, but more variable change in behavior.

A consistent theme across studies addressing children's nutrition and eating habits is that while change in knowledge appears to be very possible, altering behavior is much more difficult. Although impact on knowledge may be a precursor to behavior change, without improvement in behavior the risk factors for child overweight will remain very high and be of substantial concern for the future health of our children (for additional consideration of these issues, see Jelalian & Hart, Chapter 30, and Wilson & Lawman, Chapter 40, this volume).

Perhaps equally important to weight control and nutrition are efforts to improve overall physical wellness among students. The Centers for Disease Control and Prevention (CDC, 2004) reported that since 2000, there has been an increase from 4 to 12% in elementary schools with regularly scheduled recess periods. At the same time, the School Health Policies and Programs Study (Federal Interagency Forum, 2007) reported that 22% of schools did not require students to take any physical education.

Some studies have focused specifically on adolescent physical health. For example, research has shown that participation in sports has been associated with decreased use of cigarettes and "other drugs" (e.g., Melnick, Miller, Sabo, Farrell, & Barnes, 2001). Physical fitness has been identified as a potential protective factor for adolescent health difficulties (Kirkcaldy, Shephard, & Siefen, 2002). Werch, Moore, DiClemente, Bledsoe, and Jobli (2005) describe the implementation of Project SPORT, which consisted of an in-person health behavior screen; a one-on-one consultation; a take-home fitness prescription targeting adolescent health-promoting behaviors and alcohol use risk and protective factors; and a flyer reinforcing key content provided during the consultation, mailed to the home. Project SPORT participants demonstrated significant positive effects at 3 months after the intervention for alcohol consumption, alcohol initiation behaviors, alcohol use risk and protective factors, drug use behaviors, and exercise habits, and at 12 months for alcohol use risk and protective factors, cigarette use, and cigarette use initiation. The results of this study support the use of brief, short-term interventions that may have a sustained impact on the health-related behaviors of adolescents.

Social and Emotional Development/Violence Prevention

Youth violence is recognized as a major public health problem in the United States and around the world (Williams, Rivera, Neighbours, & Reznik, 2007). In a nationwide survey of high school students (CDC, 2004), 33% reported being in a physical fight one or more times in the 12 months preceding the survey, and 17% reported carrying a weapon (e.g., gun, knife, or club) on one or more of the 30 days preceding the survey. An estimated 30% of 6th- to 10th-graders in the United States have been involved in bullying as a bully, a target of bullying, or both (Nansel, Overpeck, Haynie, Ruan, & Scheidt, 2001).

Efforts to reduce school violence have focused on such measures as increased security or more aggressive prosecution of violent school offenders (e.g., expulsion and zero tolerance policies). However, there has been a significant shift from an approach emphasizing intervention after violent acts have occurred to one that stresses the importance of prevention. Among the efforts in schools that are preventive in nature and focus on reducing the future of violent school behavior has been the implementation of bullying prevention. "Bullying" is defined as "repeated acts of aggression, intimidation, or coercion against a victim who is weaker than the perpetrator in terms of physical size, psychological/social power, or other factors that result in a notable power differential" (Merrell, Gueldner, Ross, & Isava, 2008, p. 26). Beyond physical acts of aggression, bullying may also occur through relational aggression (i.e., social exclusion or injuring the reputations of others), as well as verbal intimidation (Merrell et al., 2008). In addition, with the increased use of technological communication, "cyberbullying" has become more evident (Mason, 2008). Substantial research has shown that bullying can have immediate as well as long-term physical and psychological consequences for bullies and their victims (e.g., Carney & Merrell, 2001).

Bullying prevention efforts typically involve schoolwide implementation, as well as increased adult monitoring in areas (e.g., playground) where bullying is likely to happen. Most prevention programs work at educating students about myths related to confronting bullies and efforts to improve classroom climate through use of behavior management strategies, such as modeling and reinforcing prosocial role models (Felix, Furlong, Sharkey, & Osher, 2008). In their meta-analysis of bullying intervention research, Merrell and colleagues (2008) reported that for approximately 33% of the targeted variables, meaningful and clinically important positive effects for the programs were found. However, for the majority of outcomes, no effects (either positive or negative) were evident.

Concern in schools about cyberbullying has risen significantly in recent years. The effects on victims of cyberbullying are identical to those of in-person bullying and include psychological (e.g., depression, suicide) as well as physical (e.g., eating disorders, chronic illness) sequelae (Finkelhor, Mitchell, & Wolak, 2000). At present, no specific intervention program for cyberbullying has been identified. Thus recommended practices for reducing cyberbullying are no different than for in-person bullying.

Another, more subtle form of school violence is relational aggression. In contrast to physical aggression, relational aggression involves behaviors that damage the relationships between individuals. Included are direct and indirect acts such as threats to end friendship, retaliation such as purposeful ignoring of an individual, or spreading false rumors (Crick & Grotpeter, 1995). This form of aggression is often found among girls, and its impact on peers can be as devastating as those of physical aggression (e.g., Crick, Ostrov, & Werner, 2006). Intervention efforts to target relational aggression are typically focused on primary prevention programs aimed at altering the general school climate to be more inclusionary (Harrist & Bradley, 2003), using modeling and role-play techniques to teach appropriate responses to attempts at relational aggression (Leff, Power, Manz, Costigan, & Nabors, 2001), or systematically teaching prosocial skills (Van Schoiack-Edstrom, Frey, & Beland, 2002). Although some of these studies have obtained positive results, the research is still very preliminary, and more research in this area is clearly needed.

Finally, a substantial and well-developed school-based strategy for reducing school violence has been the schoolwide PBS model developed by Sugai, Sprague, Horner, and Walker (2001). Founded on the previously described PBS model of primary, secondary, and tertiary prevention, the basis of the intervention is to implement schoolwide practices that support and encourage positive school interaction, and then to use targeted and selected intervention strategies for nonresponders to the schoolwide effort. The outcomes of schoolwide PBS have been well established through multiple replications, and this model is viewed as a high-quality, evidence-based practice to reduce school violence (Sugai & Horner, 2006).

Promoting Sexual Health

An important target of prevention efforts for adolescents is the promotion of healthy sexual behavior. Universal prevention programs designed to promote sexual health have been implemented in school districts throughout the nation. Low-income children of ethnic minority status have commonly been targeted for systematic, selective prevention programs, given their increased risk for contracting sexually transmitted diseases (STDs) (Wilson, Rodrique, & Taylor, 1997). Providing these programs in public school settings raises complicated ethical issues in many communities; specifically, a community may be divided with regard to using an abstinence versus safer-sex approach in its schools. An abstinence approach emphasizes abstinence as the way to promote sexual health and to prevent pregnancy and STDs. A safer-sex approach acknowledges that abstinence is the safer approach, but affirms that using condoms can be effective in reducing the risk of pregnancy and STDs if students do engage in sex (Jemmott, Jemmott, & Fong, 1992).

Programs to promote healthy sexual behavior have been based on both the abstinence and safer-sex approaches. One program that serves as a model is Be Proud! Be Responsible, a universal approach that has been designed specifically for African American youths residing in inner-city settings (for a description, see Jemmott et al., 1992). Adolescents at the middle school and high school levels have been targeted for this program. Program facilitators are typically adults or peers from the neighborhood. Although the program can be provided in school settings, it is typically conducted in after-school and Saturday programs. The program emphasizes to youths the themes of taking pride in oneself and the community, and acting in a responsible way that will be beneficial to self and others. Program facilitators encourage youths to identify their goals in life and consider how unhealthy patterns of behavior may preclude them from achieving their goals. The program uses educational and cognitive-behavioral strategies to change both attitudes and behavior. Randomized clinical trials have demonstrated the effectiveness of both the abstinence and safer-sex approaches to prevention, although the data suggest that the safer-sex approach may be more effective with youths who are sexually experienced (Jemmott, Jemmott, & Fong, 1998).

Conclusions

Given the potential impact of chronic illness and unhealthy behavior on academic, behavioral, and social functioning, schools are a critical setting for health-related prevention and intervention efforts. Substantial progress has been made in the identification of school-related deficits associated with chronic illness; however, disease-specific risk factors and predictors of outcome must be more clearly identified, in order to aid prevention and intervention efforts. Systemic efforts at school reform also must be considered in addressing the needs of students with or at risk for health difficulties. In particular, the adoption of a public health perspective in the context of the RTI model may be a particularly effective strategy for identifying and working with students whose health difficulties significantly affect school functioning. Pediatric and school psychologists can engage in both intervention (e.g., medication monitoring) and health promotion (e.g., violence prevention) activities at the individual, classroom, or schoolwide level. Empirical studies documenting effective strategies that not only change understanding and knowledge, but also have an impact on key health-related behaviors, will be critical in promoting successful outcomes for all students who experience or are at risk for health difficulties.

References

Blom-Hoffman, J., Kelleher, C., Power, T. J., & Leff, S. S. (2004). Promoting healthy food consumption among young children: Evaluation of a multi-component, nutrition education program. *Journal of School Psychology, 42*, 45–60.

Brindis, C. D. (2005). Moving upstream: The role of schools in improving population health. *Journal of Adolescent Health, 37*, 263–265.

Brown, R. T., Carpenter, L. A., & Simerly, E. (2005). *Mental health medications for children: A primer.* New York: Guilford Press.

Byrd, R. S., & Weitzman, M. L. (1994). Predictors of early grade retention among children in the United States. *Pediatrics, 93*, 481–487.

Cadman, D., Boyle, M., Szatmari, P., & Offord, D. R. (1987). Chronic illness, disability, and mental and social well-being: Findings of the Ontario Child Health Study. *Pediatrics, 79*, 805–813.

Carney, A. G., & Merrell, K. W. (2001). Bullying in schools: Perspectives on understanding and preventing an international problem. *School Psychology International, 22*, 364–382.

Centers for Disease Control and Prevention (CDC). (2004). *Youth risk behavior surveillance— United States, 2003.* Atlanta, GA: Author.

Crick, N. R., & Grotpeter, J. K. (1995). Relational aggression, gender, and social psychological adjustment. *Child Development, 66*, 710–722.

Crick, N. R., Ostrov, J. M., & Werner, N. E. (2006). A longitudinal study of relational aggression, physical aggression, and children's social-psychological adjustment. *Journal of Abnormal Child Psychology, 34*, 131–142.

Cruz, M. L., Shaibi, G. Q., Weigensberg, M. J., Spruijt-Metz, D., Ball, G. D., & Goran, M. I. (2005). Pediatric obesity and insulin resistance: Chronic disease risk and implications for treatment and prevention beyond body weight modification. *Annual Review of Nutrition, 25*, 435–468.

Eiraldi, R. B., Mazzuca, L. B., Clarke, A. T., & Power, T. J. (2006). Service utilization among ethnic minority children with ADHD: A model of help-seeking behavior. *Administration and Policy in Mental Health and Mental Health Services Research, 33*, 607–622.

Engeland, A., Bjorge, T., Tverdal, A., & Sogaard, A. J. (2004). Obesity in adolescence and adulthood and the risk of adult mortality. *Epidemiology, 5*, 79–85.

Federal Interagency Forum on Child and Family Statistics. (2007). *America's children: Key national indicators of well-being 2007.* Washington, DC: Author.

Felix, E., Furlong, M., Sharkey, J., & Osher, D. (2007). Implications for evaluating multicomponent, complex prevention initiatives: Taking guidance from the Safe Schools/Healthy Students Initiative. *Journal of School Violence, 6(2)*, 3–20.

Finkelhor, D., Mitchell, K. J., & Wolak, J. (2000, June). *Online victimization: A report on the nation's youth.* Retrieved March 5, 2009, from *www.new.vawaet.org/category/Documents.php?doid=523&categoryid=93*

Fletcher, J. M., Francis, D. J., Shaywitz, S. E., Lyon, G. R., Foorman, B. R., Stuebing, K. K., et al. (1998). Intelligence testing and the discrepancy model for children with learning disabilities. *Learning Disabilities Research and Practice, 13*, 186–203.

Gadow, K. D. (1993). A school-based medication evaluation program. In J. L. Matson (Ed.), *Handbook of hyperactivity in children* (pp. 186–219). Needham Heights, MA: Allyn & Bacon.

Gersten, R., & Dimino, J. A. (2006). RTI (response to intervention): Rethinking special education for students with reading difficulties (yet again). *Reading Research Quarterly, 41*, 99–108.

Harrist, A. W., & Bradley, K. D. (2003). "You can't say you can't play": Intervening in the process of social exclusion in the kindergarten classroom. *Early Childhood Research Quarterly, 18*, 185–205.

Henning, J., & Fritz, G. K. (1983). School reentry in childhood cancer. *Psychosomatics, 24*, 261–269.

Hoagwood, K., & Johnson, J. (2003). School psychology: A public health framework. I. From evidence-based practices to evidence-based policies. *Journal of School Psychology, 41*, 3–21.

Jemmott, J. B., Jemmott, L. S., & Fong, G. T. (1992). Reduction in HIV risk-associated sexual behaviors among black male adolescents: Effects of an AIDS prevention intervention. *American Journal of Public Health, 82*, 372–377.

Jemmott, J. B., Jemmott, L. S., & Fong, G. T. (1998). Abstinence and safer sex: HIV riskreduction interventions for African American adolescents. *Journal of the American Medical Association, 279*, 1529–1536.

Juel, C. (1988). Learning to read and write: A longitudinal study of 54 children from first through fourth grades. *Journal of Educational Psychology, 80*, 437–447.

Kiess, W., Galler, A., Reich, A., Muller, G., Kapellen, T., Deutscher, J., et al. (2001). Clinical aspects of obesity in childhood and adolescence. *Obesity Review, 2*, 29–36.

Kirkcaldy, B. D., Shephard, R. J., & Siefen, R. G. (2002). The relationship between physical activity and self-image and problem behavior among adolescents. *Social Psychiatry and Psychiatric Epidemiology, 37*, 544–550.

Lane, K. L., Barton-Arwood, S. M., Nelson, J. R., & Wehby, J. (2008). Academic performance of students with emotional and behavioral disorders served in a self-contained setting. *Journal of Behavioral Education, 17*, 43–62.

Lane, K. L., Wehby, J. H., Little, M. A., & Cooley, C. (2005). Academic, social, and behavioral profiles of students with emotional and behavioral disorders educated in self-contained classrooms and self-contained schools: Part I. Are they more alike than different? *Behavioral Disorders, 30*, 349–361.

Lavigne, J. V., & Faier-Routman, J. (1992). Psychosocial adjustment to pediatric physical disorders: A meta-analytic review. *Journal of Pediatric Psychology, 17*, 133–157.

Leff, S. S., Power, T. J., Manz, P. H., Costigan, T. E., & Nabors, L. A. (2001). School-based aggression prevention programs for young children: Current status and implications for violence prevention. *School Psychology Review, 30,* 343–360.

Madan-Swain, A., Katz, E. R., & LaGory, J. (2004). School and social reintegration after a serious illness or injury. In R. T. Brown (Ed.), *Handbook of pediatric psychology in school settings* (pp. 637–655). Mahwah, NJ: Erlbaum.

Mason, K. L. (2008). Cyberbullying: A preliminary assessment for school personnel. *Psychology in the Schools, 45*(4), 323–348.

McNelis, A. M., Johnson, C. S., Huberty, T. J., & Austin, J. K. (2005). Factors associated with academic achievement in children with recent-onset seizures. *Seizure, 14,* 331–339.

Meijer, S. A., Sinnema, G., Bijstra, J. O., Mellenbergh, G. J., & Wolters, W. H. G. (2000). Social functioning in children with a chronic illness. *Journal of Child Psychology and Psychiatry, 41,* 309–317.

Melnick, M. J., Miller, K. E., Sabo, D. F., Farrell, M. P., & Barnes, G. M. (2001). Tobacco use among high school athletes and non-athletes: Results of the 1997 Youth Risk Behavior Survey. *Adolescence, 36,* 727–747.

Merrell, K. W., Gueldner, B. A., Ross, S. W., & Isava, D. M. (2008). How effective are school bullying programs?: A meta-analysis of intervention research. *School Psychology Review, 23,* 26–42.

Nansel, T. R., Overpeck, M. D., Haynie, D. L., Ruan, W. J., & Scheidt, P. C. (2003). Relationships between bullying and violence among US youth. *Archives of Pediatrics and Adolescent Medicine, 157,* 348–353.

Ogden, C. L., Carroll, M. D., Curtin, L. R., McDowell, M. A., Tabak, C. J., & Flegal, K. M. (2006). Prevalence of overweight and obesity in the United States, 1999–2004. *Journal of the American Medical Association, 295,* 1549–1555.

Passel, J. S., & Cohn, D. (2008). *U.S. population projections: 2005–2050.* Washington, DC: Pew Research Center.

Phelps, L., Brown, R. T., & Power, T. (2001). *Pediatric psychopharmacology: Combining medical and psychological interventions.* Washington, DC: American Psychological Association.

Power, T. J., DuPaul, G. J., Shapiro, E. S., & Kazak, A. E. (2003). *Promoting children's health: Integrating school, family, and community.* New York: Guilford Press.

Prevatt, F. F., Heffer, R. W., & Lowe, P. A. (2000). A review of school integration programs for children with cancer. *Journal of School Psychology, 38,* 447–467.

Ravitch, D. (1999). Student performance: The national agenda in education. In M. Kanstorooom & C. E. Finn (Eds.), *New directions: Federal education policy in the twenty-first century.* Washington, DC: Thomas B. Fordham/Manhattan Policy Institute.

Schuman, W. B., & La Greca, A. M. (1999). Social correlates of chronic illness. In R. T. Brown (Ed.), *Cognitive aspects of chronic illness in children* (pp. 289–311). New York: Guilford Press.

Sexson, S. B., & Madan-Swain, A. (1995). The chronically ill child in the school. *School Psychology Quarterly, 10,* 359–368.

Shapiro, E. S., & Manz, P. H. (2004). Collaborating with schools in the provision of pediatric psychological services. In R. T. Brown (Ed.), *Handbook of pediatric psychology in school settings* (pp. 49–64). Mahwah, NJ: Erlbaum.

Sheridan, S. M., & Kratochwill, T. R. (2008). *Conjoint behavioral consultation: Promoting family–school connections and interventions* (2nd ed.). New York: Springer.

Strein, W., Hoagwood, K., & Cohn, A. (2003). School psychology: A public health perspective. I. Prevention, populations, and systems change. *Journal of School Psychology, 41,* 3–28.

Sugai, G., & Horner, R. R. (2006). A promising approach for expanding and sustaining school-wide positive behavior support. *School Psychology Review, 35,* 245–259.

Sugai, G., Sprague, J. R., Horner, R., & Walker, H. M. (2001). Preventing school violence: The use of office discipline referrals to assess and monitor school-wide discipline interventions. In H. M. Walker & M. H. Epstein (Eds.), *Making schools safer and violence free: Critical issues, solutions, and recommended practices* (pp. 50–57). Austin, TX: PRO-ED.

U.S. Department of Education, Office of Special Education and Rehabilitative Services, Office of Special Education Programs. (2005). *26th annual (2004) report to Congress on the implementation of the Individuals with Disabilities Education Act.* Washington, DC: Author.

Van Schoiack-Edstrom, L., Frey, K. S., & Beland, K. (2002). Changing adolescents' attitudes about relational and physical aggression: An early evaluation of a school-based intervention. *School Psychology Review, 31,* 201–216.

Volpe, R. J., Heick, P. F., & Gureasko-Moore, D. (2005). An agile behavioral model for monitoring the effects of stimulant medication in school settings. *Psychology in the Schools, 42,* 509–523.

Werch, C., Moore, M. J., DiClemente, C. C., Bledsoe, R., & Jobli, E. (2005). A multihealth behavior intervention integrating physical activity and substance use prevention for adolescents. *Prevention Science, 6,* 213–226.

Williams, K., Rivera, L., Neighbours, R., & Reznik, V. (2007). Youth violence prevention comes of age: Research, training and future directions. *Annual Review of Public Health, 28,* 195–211.

Wilson, D. K., Rodrique, J. R., & Taylor, W. C. (Eds.). (1997). *Health-promoting and health-compromising behaviors among minority adolescents.* Washington, DC: American Psychological Association.

CHAPTER 47

Families' Interactions with the Health Care System

Implications for Pediatric Psychology

MICHAEL SEID
LISA OPIPARI-ARRIGAN
ELISA J. SOBO

In recognition of the interplay between a child's physical and psychological health and development, pediatric psychologists pursue research and practice addressing the complex relationship between children's cognitive, social, and emotional functioning and their physical well-being. In much of that research and practice, they focus directly on children and their families. A vast segment examines the relationship between chronic conditions and psychosocial well-being. For example, a search of PubMed, the National Library of Medicine's online bibliographic database, on such factors as social support, maternal depression, and family functioning in relation to adherence or outcomes of pediatric chronic conditions reveals almost 3,500 published articles in the last 10 years. Relatively little attention has been paid, however, to the effects of the health care system itself on children's well-being and health outcomes.

This chapter explores the ramifications that the health care system itself has for child and family well-being. More specifically, we discuss how experiences of interacting with the health care system can directly affect the psychosocial functioning of children with chronic health conditions and their families, adherence to recommended care plans, and health-related quality of life (HRQOL). That is, just as scholars have demonstrated that social support (La Greca & Bearman, 2002; La Greca, Bearman, & Moore, 2002), parental distress (Drotar, 1997), family functioning (Lewin et al., 2006), and quality of coping (Fredericks, Lopez, Magee, Shieck, & Opipari-Arrigan, 2007; Sales, Fivush, & Teague, 2008) can affect adherence and outcomes for children with chronic health conditions, here we argue that so can interactions between families and the health care system. Furthermore, each interaction can affect not only the ways that families navigate self-management at home, but the ways that families approach their next interaction with the system. Because families of children with chronic health conditions interact with the health care system repeatedly, they are especially vulnerable to the accretion of poor interactions. Thus these interactions over time can become a trajectory, with prior experiences influencing the next.

To explore our central thesis, we first present a framework for describing the ways that children with chronic health conditions and their families interact with the health care system. This framework highlights the role that barriers to care can play at each stage of a family's interaction with the health care system—accessing and navigating the system, experiencing the clinical encounter, and implementing (or trying to implement) the care plan. We also review what is known about interventions to improve patients' and parents' health care experiences. We describe research needs, highlighting concerns raised in patient/family–provider interactions and discussing the efficacy and effectiveness of interventions at the patient/family and at the system/provider levels. We conclude with a comment on future directions and implications for the roles pediatric psychologists can play in studying and improving the health care delivery system.

Although our conceptual framework and its implications are applicable across pediatric chronic conditions, many of our examples are drawn from pediatric asthma. Asthma is widely studied because of its prevalence; the existence of well-accepted guidelines for diagnosis, treatment, and management; and the potential that high-quality care has to reduce inpatient costs.

Interacting with the Health Care System

If children and their families are to utilize a health care system to improve the children's health, (1) a health care system must be available for them to access; (2) children, with the assistance of their parents, must access this system and (3) use needed services; (4) these services must be both technically and interpersonally of high quality; and (5) children and their families must implement the recommended health care interventions. If these steps proceed smoothly, the likelihood of improved health is maximized (Donabedian, 1966, 1988; Seid, Varni, & Kurtin, 2000).

However, all families and children face at least some barriers to health care (Aday, 1993). Although these barriers vary in their nature and seriousness, any of them can disrupt this pathway and serve to reduce the likelihood of improved health. Seid and colleagues (Seid, Sobo, Zivkovic, Nelson, & Davodi-Far, 2003; Seid et al., 2000) have proposed that barriers are multifaceted and can affect all four stages of interaction with the health care system: access, navigation, the clinical encounter, and implementation of the care plan. In this scheme, barriers to care are related to, but distinct from, vulnerability factors (e.g., race/ethnicity, socioeconomic status, limited English proficiency). Although vulnerability factors have indeed been shown to be related to access, quality of care, and outcomes, a key point is that vulnerability factors are seen as "marker" variables of other sociobehavioral processes—the barriers to care. Thus barriers are hypothesized to moderate a child's and family's journey through the health care system. As such, refocusing away from vulnerability factors (or markers) and on barriers to care entails a shift in attention to *process* variables, which theoretically link patient experience to quality of care. That is, instead of merely knowing *which* groups are experiencing *what* disparities, we can begin to determine *why* and *how* these disparities happen by focusing on processes (barriers).

This framework has several implications for understanding and improving families' and children's interactions with the health care system. First, the framework emphasizes the importance of a child's and parent's subjective experience of the health care system. Second, given that several different types of barriers may exist at several stages of the journey through the health system, this framework highlights the multidimensional context in which barriers occur. Barriers can be viewed from the perspective of particular types of barriers within a given category; from the perspective of the particular stages (e.g., the various barriers that can interfere with access and those that can interfere with patient–provider communication); or from the perspective of the interaction of barriers and stages. Third is the idea that barriers are modifiable. This is important, because it highlights that a shift in emphasis from descriptive to interventional studies is possible.

Barriers to Care

Barriers to care can have negative effects on access, navigation, the clinical encounter, and implementation of recommended interventions. Because parents or guardians have direct experience of barriers to care, and are thus well positioned to report on them, Seid and colleagues developed and validated the Barriers to Care Questionnaire (BCQ) as a measure of barriers to care from the parent's perspective (Seid, Sobo, Gelhard, & Varni, 2004). "Worse barriers," as measured by the BCQ, have been shown to be related to being uninsured, not having a regular doctor, not getting care when needed, worse primary care experiences, and lower HRQOL (Seid, 2008; Seid et al., 2004). Based on an extensive review of the literature on patient/family health care experiences and focus groups of parents of children with chronic health conditions, the barriers-to-care construct used in the BCQ (Seid et al., 2004; Sobo, Seid, & Reyes Gelhard, 2006) has been operationalized as consisting of (1) pragmatics, (2) health beliefs, (3) expectations related to quality of care available from the health care system, (4) skills and knowledge needed to navigate the health care system, and (5) marginalization.

- *Pragmatics* are practical considerations in obtaining necessary care, such as cost, financial resources, the availability of time off from work, child care, proximity to a health service institution, transportation options, and an institution's open hours. Research has shown that such factors are associated with late or no initiation of necessary preventive care (Byrd, Mullen, Selwyn, & Lorimor, 1996). They also seem to mitigate against receipt of proper curative procedures, hospitalizations, or prescriptions (Flores, Abreu, Olivar, & Kastner, 1998).
- *Health beliefs* (Good, 1994) are understandings about the cause, course, and cure of disease or illness, as well as ideas about the meaning and value of health and illness for the individual and the family. Health beliefs can affect medical care seeking. For instance, the understandings regarding *caida de mollera* or fallen fontanelle and the resulting health-care-seeking patterns in the U.S. Southwest have been documented (Trotter, Ortiz de Montellano, & Logan, 1989). Health beliefs or ethnomedical knowledge regarding many childhood ailments have been documented, as have the health beliefs that lead parents to resist procedures for their children, (Anderson, Toledo, & Hazam, 1982; Mosnaim et al., 2006; Robledo, Wilson, & Gray, 1999).

Importantly, health beliefs vary across individual members of a given cultural or social group (Foster, 1994; Weller, Pachter, Trotter, & Baer, 1993). Furthermore, they are not monolithic or immutable. Research has shown that they may shift according to context; they may be fairly fluid, depending on available resources and short-term outcomes. They may be altered to accommodate the particular illness episode in question; they may serve to validate rather than proscribe action, surfacing in *ex post facto* rationalizations (Foster, 1994). Furthermore, people are easily able to accommodate new information (e.g., health education messages) in terms of existing health beliefs (Sobo, 1995). This can sometimes mean that new information is applied in ways that might seem nonsensical to those imparting it. Despite the research that has been done on expectations and health beliefs, scientists are far from fully understanding the impacts of these factors. It is known that expectations can be altered and health beliefs can be negotiated (Kleinman, Eisenberg, & Good, 1978), perhaps most effectively through culturally and linguistically appropriate disease-specific education.

• *Expectations* of the health care system are often based on previous experiences. These have been explored, for example, among African Americans, whose historical experience of the health care system has included negative and exploitative encounters (Henry J. Kaiser Family Foundation, 2000; Sobo, 1995; Thomas & Quinn, 1991). Skepticism regarding medical care in general has also been examined (Fiscella, Franks, & Clancy, 1998), and low expectations (e.g., the perception that there will be barriers to care) have been shown to correlate with later initiation of care and nonuse of care (Byrd et al., 1996).

• The particular *skills and knowledge* necessary for negotiating the health care system have received much less scrutiny than the other dimensions of the barriers-to-care construct defined above. This dimension of barriers to care includes the learned strategies or behaviors necessary for accessing and obtaining care, for making best use of the clinical encounter, and for overcoming barriers to implementing recommended care. An empirical example entails guardians of children with asthma asking providers to prescribe more than one inhaler at one time, to obviate the need for multiple copayments (Sobo et al., 2006). These strategies and their actualization rest on such variables as literacy and organizational/planning skills (including the capacity to complete paperwork and follow through on health system communications), as well as on biomedical literacy and knowledge of the health system itself (Sobo & Seid, 2003). Possession of (or knowledge about where and how to find) information on care availability, eligibility requirements, and so on is key, as is facility with the culture of the formal health care system.

• *Marginalization* refers to an individual's interpretation of experiences within the health care system that lead to being less proactive, informed, and activated. The current health care system is fragmented, arbitrary, difficult to understand, laced with barriers, and inherently unbalanced with respect to power and control (Kreps, 1996). Marginalization results when these health care system characteristics are interpreted as being specific to the individual or his or her social, ethnic, religious, or other group memberships and are therefore internalized. Importantly, the same experience can be interpreted in many different ways—based in part on attributions for the cause of that experience, and in part on understandings regarding the broader context in which the experience is played out. Bad service that is not interpreted as being related to oneself or one's social identity does not marginalize, while a perceived personal affront may do so.

Children's and Parents' Experience of the Health Care System

Understanding the ways that children and their parents actually experience care is crucial if we are to understand how health care affects the psychological well-being of families and children. Their perceptions and experiences of barriers to care may differ in important ways from those of health care professionals. These differences signify, among other things, the sometimes vast social, cultural, and economic gaps that separate families and health care professionals. Professionals are acculturated to the world of health care, while parents experience this world (initially at least) as foreign and opaque—as a new and different culture (Sobo & Seid, 2003).

Accessing the System

To gain health care to begin with, a family must be aware of the presence of health and community resources. Awareness is not always the case, especially for immigrant families (Yu, Huang, Schwalberg, & Kogan, 2005), but also for isolated new parents of any origin. Once awareness is raised, and if family members have the financial means to do so, they must access a care site—for example, by phoning or coming in person to get an appointment or a place in the queue for care. This is often easier said than done.

Access depends, for example, upon whether a timely appointment can be secured and whether office hours are compatible with a family's schedule. Having to wait too many days or weeks can be a problem; so can scattered appointments for parents of more than one child or a child with multiple providers. Once a suitable appointment has been secured, getting to the care site can be difficult, as can arranging care for other dependents. Missed work and missed school are also often problematic (Crain, Kercsmar, Weiss, Mitchell, & Lynn, 1998; Mosnaim et al., 2006; Sobo et al., 2006).

Navigating the System

Some of the skills that parents need to master if they are to navigate the care system go beyond simply learning the system's language and layout. Due to the health care system's fragmentation, parents also must learn how to case-manage access to multiple providers and services. Research finds that parents are often shocked at how much of this work is left up to them; it is even more salient with more complex conditions, due to the variety of specialist care that needs to be organized and articulated (Sobo, 2007).

The idea that learning to navigate the health care system is like entering a foreign world is reflected in the discourses used by parents at the grassroots level (Sobo, in press). For instance, literature for parents of newly diagnosed children has likened the diagnosis to planning a vacation to Italy, only to be rerouted to the Netherlands. This idea was introduced into circulation by parent and peer educator Emily Perl Kingsley in a widely disseminated 1987 essay, "Welcome to Holland." The essay is included, for instance, as part of the National Down Syndrome Congress's "new parent package" (*www.ndsccenter.org/resources/package1.php*).

The Clinical Encounter

Once a family figures out where to go for what and makes it to a care site for a particular appointment, there are shared tasks within the clinical encounter that must be accomplished in order for the encounter to be productive (Von Korff, Gruman, Schaefer, Curry, & Wagner, 1997). Parents, children, and clinicians must collaborate in what has been termed a "treatment alliance" to exchange information, arrive at an understanding of the problem and potential solutions, and develop and communicate a plan. The degree to which these tasks are successfully accomplished influences patients' perceptions of the treatment alliance with their health care provider (Fuertes et al., 2007) and self-efficacy (Heisler et al., 2003). These in turn influence subsequent processes, such as adherence (Broers et al., 2005; Dimatteo, 2004; Maddigan, Majumdar, & Johnson, 2005; Maly, Bourque, & Engelhardt, 1999), and ultimately outcomes, such as HRQOL (Cote, Farris, & Feeny, 2003; Hays et al., 1994; Maddigan et al., 2005; Varni, Jacobs, & Seid, 2000). Continual development of the treatment alliance (Dimatteo, 2004; Fuertes et al., 2007; Gavin, Wamboldt, Sorokin, Levy, & Wamboldt, 1999; Roter, 2000) is key.

Here again, barriers can interfere. Systematic research has shown that in addition to their initial lack of familiarity with the health care system's world, parents have found it problematic that they are in a different social position in this world vis-à-vis professionals (Sobo & Seid, 2003). The way that physicians communicate may itself be a barrier. As early as 1968, Barbara Korsch's seminal work laid bare the gap in child–parent–physician communication (Korsch, Gozzi, & Francis, 1968). Her findings showed that physicians tended to use medical jargon and to interact with mothers in a paternalistic fashion, and that mothers were highly dissatisfied with the clinical interaction. Although awareness of these issues is now high, and physician education now includes consideration of the parent–physician relationship, research continues to document that clinicians are still not very good judges of parents' information needs and wants (Seid et al., 2004). As well, parents continue to experience social, cultural, and linguistic barriers in their interactions with physicians (Mosnaim et al., 2006).

In terms of the clinical encounter in particular, this means that parents must learn to understand biomedical jargon or to ask for clarification (i.e., they must have certain skills). It also means that if parents encounter such barriers, their expectations of future interactions are more likely to be negative. Moreover, it raises the possibility that some parents will view problems with communication as their own failing (i.e., marginalization may be a barrier), rather than a failing of the health care system.

In addition to barriers to good communication with a particular provider, families may also have to contend with coordinating communication among providers. Parents are frustrated by the lack of coordinated communication among doctors, residents, fellows, and interns, which is evidenced when they have to answer the same set of questions over and over, and when conflicting information is given by the various clinicians (Sobo et al., 2006). Furthermore, some parents feel the need to "push" information to providers, especially if a child sees more than one provider or if a condition is rare or complex (Sobo et al., 2006). Thus the knowledge management that parents must undertake entails not only amassing and digesting information on services, scientific advances, guidelines for care, and other options, but also pressing this information on providers as appropriate and advocating for its appropriate use, as well as advocating for providers to look for further information on their own (Sobo, 2007).

Implementing the Care Plan

Negative expectations of care, including not only the quality of the clinical encounter but also the reception patients and families receive from front office staff, can cause problems later when implementation of a care plan is at stake. When staff members seem uncaring or biased, and their responses to families are perceived as including socioeconomic, lifestyle, ethnic/racial, and/or linguistic prejudice, patients and families may feel marginalized; therefore, they may not want to come back or follow through (Sobo et al., 2006).

Even when children receive optimal treatment and care plans are made clear to parents, numerous barriers exist to implementing the prescribed care. These include financial shortfalls, a lack of knowledge or skills to navigate the bureaucracy in order to implement the care plan, or a refusal of advice. The latter can happen if clinical advice conflicts with a person's health knowledge and the conflict is not addressed. It can happen on a wider scale among groups with a history of negative experiences with the health system and a fear that clinicians will deliberately harm them or experiment on them (Snow, 1993).

Barriers to implementation (like those to access, etc.) exist across the dimensions of pragmatics, health beliefs, expectations, skills/knowledge, and marginalization. To reinforce this point, we review some of the barriers to implementation that have been well documented for families of children with asthma (Leickly et al., 1998). For example, Mansour, Lanphear, and DeWitt (2000) cite the inability to pay for medications (pragmatics), as well as health beliefs about the use, safety, and long-term complications of asthma medication use (health beliefs), as barriers to implementing optimal asthma care. Wade, Holden, Lynn, Mitchell, and Ewart (2000) have documented a link between parental expectations (expectations) and problem-solving skills (skills) on the one hand, and asthma functional status and symptoms on the other, and recommend that these variables deserve further investigation and possible intervention. Conn and colleagues (2005) found that 34% of surveyed parents had strong concerns about asthma medication side effects, and that these concerns were significantly related to nonadherence. Similarly, parents' understandings about the links among certain types of medication, prevention activities, and the overall health of the asthmatic child can render doctors' orders inappropriate (Mansour et al., 2000).

Cultural understandings about the health, etiology, and treatment of asthma, as well as other conditions, have been well described for groups that do not subscribe to the medical model (itself highly cultural, of course; see Lupton, 2003). For example, Robledo and colleagues (1999) used structured qualitative interviews to explore knowledge and care of respiratory illnesses in a small group of mothers of Mexican origin living in the United States. They reported that these mothers held strong nonbiomedical beliefs regarding the cause of and treatment of respiratory illnesses. Similarly, Bearison, Minian, and Granowetter (2002) interviewed mothers of Dominican children with moderate to severe asthma. They found that although most mothers' understanding of the causes of asthma were consistent with standard biomedical beliefs about asthma, this understanding was supplemented by popular Dominican beliefs about illness and treatment. As a result, mothers treated their children's asthma differently, depending on whether the treatment was for prevention or for controlling an asthma attack. Mothers were likely to *treat* an acute asthma attack by using medically prescribed regimens, but were likely to rely on indigenous medical beliefs, such as those regarding humoral balance or thermal regulation of the body, to *prevent* attacks. There was a general mistrust of biomedically prescribed preventive medications, with mothers citing the overuse of pharmaceuticals in the United States, fear of dependency, and physicians' apparent failure to disclose possible side effects.

Implications for Interventions

We have posited that (1) all families face at least some barriers to care in their interactions with the health care system; (2) a child's and parent's subjective experience of the health care system is important; (3) several different kinds of barriers can exist at different stages of the journey through the health care system; and (4) barriers are modifiable. Taken together, these suppositions can drive the development of interventions to improve families' and children's interactions with the health care system. To gain a fuller idea of future directions in interventions, we now consider those that have already been tested.

Accessing the System

Most interventions targeting access tend to be addressed at pragmatic barriers, such as cost and provider availability. These types of interventions are imperative, as they have the potential to affect large numbers of children. A key example is the federal government's State Children's Health Insurance Program (SCHIP), designed to provide access to publicly funded health care for children of the working poor (families earning too much to qualify for Medicaid but not enough to afford private health insurance, or not working for an employer that offers coverage). Many studies document the success of SCHIP in improving access to care (Dick et al., 2004; Kenney & Chang, 2004; Newacheck, Brindis, Cart, Marchi, & Irwin, 1999; Szilagyi et al., 2004), and many have linked the program to improved asthma care quality (Szilagyi et al., 2006) as well as improved HRQOL (Seid, Varni, Cummings, & Schonlau, 2006).

However, pragmatic barriers are not the only barriers to access. As other research on SCHIP has shown, knowledge and skills also play a part. As Yu and Seid (2006) describe, many parents of eligible but uninsured children were simply not aware of the SCHIP program, misunderstood the eligibility requirements or costs, or found the application process too difficult.

The effects of improved access on pediatric health outcomes have also been demonstrated on a smaller scale. For instance, scheduling a follow-up primary care appointment for pediatric patients following an emergency department visit for asthma was shown to significantly improve the likelihood of primary care follow-up (Baren et al., 2006). Similarly, among pediatric patients visiting the emergency department for asthma, providing a single follow-up appointment at an emergency department–based asthma clinic decreased unscheduled asthma care and improved asthma self-management over a 6-month period (Teach, Crain, Quint, Hylan, & Joseph, 2006). In sum, removing barriers to access can improve health outcomes.

Navigating the System

There is a small but growing literature regarding what are termed "patient navigator" interventions. Patient navigators are essentially liaisons: They are people who help patients overcome perceived barriers to care (Dohan & Schrag, 2005). The specific services offered by patient navigators are diverse, and depend on the barriers they identify and the strategies they adopt to eliminate or reduce those barriers (Dohan & Schrag,

2005). Often a navigator serves the function of brokering patient relationships with service providers. Most patient navigator programs focus on adults, and many concern services for cancer care.

There are few clinical trials of patient navigator interventions. Many examples measure outcomes, but do not explicitly determine whether changes in process (i.e., reduced barriers) are the mechanism by which the outcomes are produced. Notwithstanding, they have lent support to the idea that navigators can improve access to and navigation through the health care system.

Rahm, Sukhanova, Ellis, and Mouchawar (2007), for example, tested a navigator intervention to improve follow-up to genetic counseling for cancer. The navigator called patients who had had genetic testing, explained genetic counseling to them (knowledge), helped patients make appointments (logistics, skills), and called again to remind them prior to their appointment that they were expected in the clinic. Results showed that the intervention group had higher counseling rates and shorter times to counseling than the usual-care control group. Similarly, Jandorf, Gutierrez, Lopez, Christie, and Itzkowitz (2005) tested a patient navigator intervention in increasing colorectal cancer screening. The navigator in this case also educated the patients, helped them make appointments, and reminded them of their appointments prior to the scheduled time. In this randomized controlled trial, rates of screening were 16% in the navigator group and 5% in the usual-care control group. Given the complexity of the health care environment that children and families must often negotiate, interventions that aid with navigation merit investigation among the pediatric population.

The Clinical Encounter

Interventions at the level of the clinical encounter tend to focus on either the patient and family, or the provider. Studies focused on the patient and family mainly serve to stimulate the patient to take a more active role in the clinical visit via information giving and brief skills training, and most have focused on adult populations. For example, previsit questionnaires and leaflets have been used to focus patients and help them formulate questions in advance of their consultation. In one of the few pediatric studies in this area, Triggs and Perrin (1989) found that when parents completed a brief checklist of developmental concerns prior to seeing their pediatrician, psychosocial concerns were discussed more frequently during the visit. Similarly, adolescent girls who completed a computerized assessment of their health behaviors while waiting for their health care provider and then discussed the results with the provider demonstrated improved nutrition and physical activity levels (Patrick et al., 2001).

There are many more pediatric intervention studies that target the provider, with a general goal of improving providers' communication skills and knowledge base. Clark and colleagues have reported a randomized controlled trial examining the effects of an interactive seminar designed to improve physician support and problem-solving efforts undertaken with their patients with asthma and their families. This intervention was shown to improve asthma education, use of written medication management strategies, and parents' perception of asthma care; it also resulted in a decrease in nonemergency office visits (Clark et al., 1998). Many of the demonstrated gains in physician behavior were maintained at a 2-year follow-up, with patients in the intervention group also having fewer hospitalizations than controls (Clark et al., 2000). This same intervention has been shown to reduce emergency department use and hospitalization rates for asthma among children from low-income families (Brown, Bratton, Cabana, Kaciroti, & Clark, 2004).

In a follow-up to this initial work, Cabana and colleagues (2006) report on a randomized control trial examining the effects on health care utilization of an updated version of the intervention (termed Physician Asthma Care Education). In addition to improved provider communication, patients of physicians who received the intervention had a significant decrease in days limited by asthma symptoms and reduction in emergency department visits for asthma.

Similarly, Wissow and colleagues (2008) have recently reported the results of a randomized trial of brief provider training that incorporated communication skills training for pediatric primary care physicians and targeted mental health symptoms. Significant reductions in parent mental health symptoms and children's impairment across a range of behavioral and emotional problems were reported. Taken together, these findings suggest that reducing barriers that occur in the patient–provider encounter is an important avenue for improving children's health outcomes.

Implementing the Care Plan

As described earlier, there are clearly several barriers that come into play with regard to implementation of a prescribed treatment plan. Although many studies have focused on directly improving adherence to health care behaviors, it is important to make a distinction between these and studies that have attempted to improve adherence indirectly, by overcoming barriers to care. Much of the adherence intervention literature of the former type targets families or patients, usually in settings outside the health care system (i.e., where most adherence behavior takes place). However, consistent with the theme of understanding the effects of the family's interactions with the health care system, it is also important to consider interventions that target the health care system (i.e., families' experiences) and the potential these have for improving adherence. Unfortunately, the literature here is sparse.

Notwithstanding, studies in this area have examined strategies to increase the likelihood that treatment information delivered by providers will be retained. Often these strategies incorporate clinicians (within the clinical encounter, as described above), as well as strategies at the level of the clinic or broader health system, such as standardized instructions. For example, Isaacman, Purvis, Gyuro, Anderson, and Smith (1992) found that parents who received either standardized oral or oral and written instructions for their children's otitis media had improved recall with regard to disease information, signs and symptoms, medication administration and fewer repeat emergency department visits 3 days after discharge, in comparison to a control group. Beyond studies such as this, there have been few if any attempts to improve adherence by changing the patient or family's experience of the health care system.

Future Research

Research on families' interactions with the health care system, its effects, and ways to intervene to improve experiences and outcomes is still in its infancy. Accordingly, the literature cited above, framing the interaction between families and the health care system in terms of barriers to care, is largely descriptive. Much of it is formative and hypothesis-generating rather than summative or hypothesis-testing.

Precisely for this reason, the present literature's effect on the future course of research in this area should not be underestimated. For instance, the development of a validated measure of barriers to care (Seid, 2008; Seid et al., 2004) can serve to spur further research on correlates and consequences of barriers to care. This should lead to a fuller understanding of potential intervention targets, and to better interventions as well; knowing which barriers are related to which outcomes will facilitate this. But barriers themselves are only part of the picture.

Our analysis of barriers to care suggests that interventions may be thought of as targeting specific types of *processes* that *form* barriers. Amelioration of these, and thus of specific barriers, may have specific effects on outcomes, and these can be measured in rigorous implementation studies. Findings to date suggest that various intervention approaches show promise in improving patients' health outcomes (Baren et al., 2006; Dick et al., 2004; Kenney & Chang, 2004; Rahm et al., 2007; Seid et al., 2006; Wissow et al., 2008)—but promise is not the same as actual trial-tested results. Much work is needed in this area, particularly rigorous trials with well-specified interventions and objective measures of disease process as well as of HRQOL.

Beyond what has already been reported or is presently under study, other avenues might be explored. For example, another branch of intervention studies that may bear fruit derives from knowledge available in the marketing, design, and hospitality industries. These industries have developed methods for designing highly engineered environments that enhance both customers' experiences and profitability. Consider, as an example, the Starbucks phenomenon. Starbucks is extremely effective at selling expensive coffee. In part, this has to do with the attributes of the coffee itself. But part of what draws customers in and keeps them coming back has to do with the "Starbucks experience" (Michelli, 2007)—the lighting, the furnishings, the music, the baristas, the status conferred through a Starbucks cup in hand. Similarly, grocery stores are highly engineered. Where foods are placed in the store, how much shelf space is devoted to a product, whether that product is between hand and eye level (prime real estate for higher-priced/higher-profit items) or on the lowest shelf, and which items go on the coveted end-of-aisle display shelves are subject to highly detailed analyses.

In contrast, if the health care experience for the general public is engineered at all (with the exception of expensive boutique hospitals serving the elite classes), it is designed with the provider in mind. Certainly one set of research questions has to do with how to create a better experience. A far more difficult set of questions—and one, perhaps, with farther-reaching implications—asks what differences to health outcomes this would make. There is a cliché that patients don't care about a surgeon's bedside manner as long as the surgeon has good hands and technical proficiency. However, just as the retail and hospitality industries have realized that fulfilling experiences breed brand loyalty, so has the health care industry discovered that disappointing experiences can breed mistrust, lowered expectations of treatment efficacy, and outright avoidance or hostility. Research is needed to determine whether and how positive experiences with health care lead to improved adherence among families and children, and thus to better clinical and HRQOL outcomes for the children served.

Implications for the Pediatric Psychologist's Role

Although much research is still needed, particularly in the realm of intervention studies, some implications for clinical practice can be surmised from our review. Conceptualizing barriers to care as a multidimensional construct and as a process variable offers the practitioner numerous avenues for intervention.

Pediatric psychologists have the expertise, skill set, and position within health care delivery systems to uniquely influence such factors as access and navigation, the clinical encounter, and implementation of the care plan. Understanding that indicators of success for our patients, such as improved adherence and HRQOL, can be directly affected by experiences within the health care delivery system itself leads us to broaden our intervention targets beyond the patient, family, or even classroom to the actual system of care delivery. For instance, pediatric psychologists could work with providers individually or in teams to develop more effective ways of educating patients about what to expect during their visit to the health care setting, or to provide navigation support for patients at higher risk for experiencing barriers to care.

Within the clinical encounter itself, pediatric psychologists are well versed in the skills necessary to help patients and families identify their needs and perceptions, communicate these to the health care team, and empower parents in their role as care providers. It is important to recognize the value of such services and the role they play in decreasing barriers to care. Beyond the patient and family, pediatric psychologists can also help mitigate barriers in the clinical encounter via work with the health care team in such areas as communication skills, cultural differences, and strategies for empowering patients.

Finally, our analysis has shown that numerous problems may arise during attempts to implement a treatment plan. Pediatric psychologists have the skill set necessary for an appreciation of context that highlights process, and are therefore well positioned to understand the barriers interfering with implementation of treatment and to develop feasible interventions to ameliorate the problems based on this understanding. To do so, it is crucial to keep in view the interconnections between different types of barriers to care and the different domains in which they occur. Few families will experience a single barrier in a single domain. Having been trained already to appreciate contextual complexity, pediatric psychologists have a unique role to play. In doing so, they can have a significant impact on patients' and families' interactions with the health care system.

References

Aday, L. (1993). *At risk in America: The health and health care needs of vulnerable populations in the United States.* San Francisco: Jossey-Bass.

Anderson, B. G., Toledo, J. R., & Hazam, N. (1982). An approach to the resolution of Mexican-American resistance to diagnostic and remedial pediatric heart care. In N. J. Chrisman & T. W. Maretzki (Eds.), *Clinically applied anthropology* (pp. 325–350). Dordrecht, The Netherlands: Reidel.

Baren, J. M., Boudreaux, E. D., Brenner, B. E., Cydulka, R. K., Rowe, B. H., Clark, S., et al. (2006). Randomized controlled trial of emergency department interventions to improve primary care follow-up for patients with acute asthma. *Chest, 129,* 257–265.

Bearison, D., Minian, N., & Granowetter, L. (2002). Medical management of asthma and folk medicine in a hispanic community. *Journal of Pediatric Psychology, 27*, 385–392.

Broers, S., Smets, E., Bindels, P., Evertsz, F. B., Calff, M., & de Haes, H. (2005). Training general practitioners in behavior change counseling to improve asthma medication adherence. *Patient Education and Counseling, 58*, 279–287.

Brown, R., Bratton, S. L., Cabana, M. D., Kaciroti, N., & Clark, N. M. (2004). Physician asthma education program improves outcomes for children of low-income families. *Chest, 126*, 369–374.

Byrd, T., Mullen, P., Selwyn, B., & Lorimor, R. (1996). Initiation of prenatal care by low-income Hispanic women in Houston. *Public Health Reports, 111*, 536–540.

Cabana, M. D., Slish, K. K., Evans, D., Mellins, R. B., Brown, R. W., Lin, X., et al. (2006). Impact of physician asthma care education on patient outcomes. *Pediatrics, 117*, 2149–2157.

Clark, N. M., Gong, M., Schork, M. A., Evans, D., Roloff, D., Hurwitz, M., et al. (1998). Impact of education for physicians on patient outcomes. *Pediatrics, 101*, 831–836.

Clark, N. M., Gong, M., Schork, M. A., Kaciroti, N., Evans, D., Roloff, D., et al. (2000). Long-term effects of asthma education for physicians on patient satisfaction and use of health services. *European Respiratory Journal, 16*, 15–21.

Conn, K. M., Halterman, J. S., Fisher, S. G., Yoos, H. L., Chin, N. P., & Szilagyi, P. G. (2005). Parental beliefs about medications and medication adherence among urban children with asthma. *Ambulatory Pediatrics, 5*, 306–310.

Cote, I., Farris, K., & Feeny, D. (2003). Is adherence to drug treatment correlated with health-related quality of life? *Quality of Life Research, 12*, 621–633.

Crain, E. F., Kercsmar, C., Weiss, K. B., Mitchell, H., & Lynn, H. (1998). Reported difficulties in access to quality care for children with asthma in the inner city. *Archives of Pediatrics and Adolescent Medicine, 152*, 333–339.

Dick, A. W., Brach, C., Allison, R. A., Shenkman, E., Shone, L. P., Szilagyi, P. G., et al. (2004). SCHIP's impact in three states: How do the most vulnerable children fare? *Health Affairs, 23*, 63–75.

Dimatteo, M. R. (2004). The role of effective communication with children and their families in fostering adherence to pediatric regimens. *Patient Education and Counseling, 55*, 339–344.

Dohan, D., & Schrag, D. (2005). Using navigators to improve care of underserved patients. *Cancer, 104*, 848–855.

Donabedian, A. (1966). Evaluating the quality of medical care. *Milbank Memorial Fund Quarterly, 44*(Suppl.), 166–206.

Donabedian, A. (1988). The quality of health care: How can it be assessed? *Journal of the American Medical Association, 260*, 1743–1748.

Drotar, D. (1997). Relating parent and family functioning to the psychological adjustment of children with chronic health conditions: What have we learned? What do we need to know? *Journal of Pediatric Psychology, 22*, 149–165.

Fiscella, K., Franks, P., & Clancy, C. M. (1998). Skepticism toward medical care and health care utilization. *Medical Care, 36*, 180–189.

Flores, G., Abreu, M., Olivar, M. A., & Kastner, B. (1998). Access barriers to health care for Latino children. *Archives of Pediatrics and Adolescent Medicine, 152*, 1119–1125.

Foster, G. M. (1994). *Hippocrates' Latin American legacy: Humoral medicine in the New World*. Langhorne, PA: Gordon & Breach.

Fredericks, E., Lopez, M., Magee, J., Shieck, V., & Opipari-Arrigan, L. (2007). Psychological functioning, nonadherence and health outcomes after pediatric liver transplantation. *American Journal of Transplantation, 7*, 1974–1983.

Fuertes, J. N., Mislowack, A., Bennett, J., Paul, L., Gilbert, T. C., Fontan, G., et al. (2007). The physician–patient working alliance. *Patient Education and Counseling, 66,* 29–36.

Gavin, L. A., Wamboldt, M. Z., Sorokin, N., Levy, S. Y., & Wamboldt, F. S. (1999). Treatment alliance and its association with family functioning, adherence, and medical outcome in adolescents with severe, chronic asthma. *Journal of Pediatric Psychology, 24,* 355–365.

Good, B. J. (1994). *Medicine, rationality, and experience: An anthropological perspective.* Cambridge, UK: Cambridge University Press.

Hays, R. D., Kravitz, R. L., Mazel, R. M., Sherbourne, C. D., DiMatteo, M. R., Rogers, W. H., et al. (1994). The impact of patient adherence on health outcomes for patients with chronic disease in the Medical Outcomes Study. *Journal of Behavioral Medicine, 17,* 347–360.

Heisler, M., Vijan, S., Anderson, R. M., Ubel, P. A., Bernstein, S. J., & Hofer, T. P. (2003). When do patients and their physicians agree on diabetes treatment goals and strategies, and what difference does it make? *Journal of General Internal Medicine, 18,* 893–902.

Henry J. Kaiser Family Foundation. (2000). *Kaiser Commission on Key Facts: Medicaid and the uninsured.* Washington, DC: Author.

Isaacman, D. J., Purvis, K., Gyuro, J., Anderson, Y., & Smith, D. (1992). Standardized instructions: Do they improve communication of discharge information from the emergency department? *Pediatrics, 89,* 1204–1208.

Jandorf, L., Gutierrez, Y., Lopez, J., Christie, J., & Itzkowitz, S. H. (2005). Use of a patient navigator to increase colorectal cancer screening in an urban neighborhood health clinic. *Journal of Urban Health, 82,* 216–224.

Kenney, G., & Chang, D. I. (2004). The State Children's Health Insurance Program: Successes, shortcomings, and challenges. *Health Affairs, 23,* 51–62.

Kleinman, A., Eisenberg, L., & Good, B. (1978). Culture, illness, and care: Clinical lessons from anthropologic and cross-cultural research. *Annals of Internal Medicine, 88,* 251–258.

Korsch, B. M., Gozzi, E. K., & Francis, V. (1968). Gaps in doctor–patient communication: 1. Doctor–patient interaction and patient satisfaction. *Pediatrics, 42,* 855–871.

Kreps, G. L. (1996). Communicating to promote justice in the modern health care system. *Journal of Health Communication, 1*(1), 99–109.

La Greca, A. M., & Bearman, K. J. (2002). The Diabetes Social Support Questionnaire—Family Version: Evaluating adolescents' diabetes-specific support from family members. *Journal of Pediatric Psychology, 27,* 665–676.

La Greca, A. M., Bearman, K. J., & Moore, H. (2002). Peer relations of youth with pediatric conditions and health risks: Promoting social support and healthy lifestyles. *Journal of Developmental and Behavioral Pediatrics, 23,* 271–280.

Leickly, F. E., Wade, S. L., Crain, E., Kruszon-Moran, D., Wright, E. C., & Evans, R., III. (1998). Self-reported adherence, management behavior, and barriers to care after an emergency department visit by inner city children with asthma. *Pediatrics, 101,* e8.

Lewin, A. B., Heidgerken, A. D., Geffken, G. R., Williams, L. B., Storch, E. A., Gelfand, K. M., et al. (2006). The relation between family factors and metabolic control: The role of diabetes adherence. *Journal of Pediatric Psychology, 31,* 174–183.

Lupton, D. (2003). *Medicine as culture: Illness, disease, and the body in Western societies.* London: Sage.

Maddigan, S. L., Majumdar, S. R., & Johnson, J. A. (2005). Understanding the complex associations between patient–provider relationships, self-care behaviours, and health-related quality of life in Type 2 diabetes: A structural equation modeling approach. *Quality of Life Research, 14,* 1489–1500.

Maly, R. C., Bourque, L. B., & Engelhardt, R. F. (1999). A randomized controlled trial of facilitating information giving to patients with chronic medical conditions: Effects on outcomes of care. *Journal of Family Practice, 48,* 356–363.

Mansour, M. E., Lanphear, B. P., & DeWitt, T. G. (2000). Barriers to asthma care in urban children: Parent perspectives. *Pediatrics, 106,* 512–519.

Michelli, J. (2007). *The Starbucks experience: Five principles for turning ordinary into extraordinary.* New York: McGraw-Hill.

Mosnaim, G., Kohrman, C., Sharp, L. K., Wolf, M. E., Sadowski, L. S., Ramos, L., et al. (2006). Coping with asthma in immigrant Hispanic families: A focus group study. *Annals of Allergy, Asthma, and Immunology, 97,* 477–483.

Newacheck, P. W., Brindis, C. D., Cart, C. U., Marchi, K., & Irwin, C. E. (1999). Adolescent health insurance coverage: Recent changes and access to care. *Pediatrics, 104,* 195–202.

Patrick, K., Sallis, J. F., Prochaska, J. J., Lydston, D. D., Calfas, K. J., Zabinski, M. F., et al. (2001). A multicomponent program for nutrition and physical activity change in primary care: PACE+ for adolescents. *Archives of Pediatrics and Adolescent Medicine, 155,* 940–946.

Rahm, A. K., Sukhanova, A., Ellis, J., & Mouchawar, J. (2007). Increasing utilization of cancer genetic counseling services using a patient navigator model. *Journal of Genetic Counseling, 16,* 171–177.

Robledo, L., Wilson, A. H., & Gray, P. (1999). Hispanic mothers' knowledge and care of their children with respiratory illnesses: A pilot study. *Journal of Pediatric Nursing, 14,* 239–247.

Roter, D. (2000). The enduring and evolving nature of the patient–physician relationship. *Patient Education and Counseling, 39,* 5–15.

Sales, J., Fivush, R., & Teague, G. W. (2008). The role of parental coping in children with asthma's psychological well-being and asthma-related quality of life. *Journal of Pediatric Psychology, 33,* 208–219.

Seid, M. (2008). Barriers to care and primary care for vulnerable children with asthma. *Pediatrics, 122,* 994–1002.

Seid, M., Sobo, E. J., Gelhard, L. R., & Varni, J. W. (2004). Parents' reports of barriers to care for children with special health care needs: Development and validation of the barriers to care questionnaire. *Ambulatory Pediatrics, 4,* 323–331.

Seid, M., Sobo, E. J., Zivkovic, M., Nelson, M., & Davodi-Far, M. (2003). Conceptual models of quality of care and health-related quality of life for vulnerable children. In E. J. Sobo & P. S. Kurtin (Eds.), *Child health services research: Applications, innovation and insights* (pp. 243–274). San Francisco: Jossey-Bass.

Seid, M., Varni, J. W., Cummings, L., & Schonlau, M. (2006). The impact of realized access to care on health-related quality of life: A two-year prospective cohort study of children in the California State Children's Health Insurance Program. *Journal of Pediatrics, 149,* 354–361.

Seid, M., Varni, J. W., & Kurtin, P. S. (2000). Measuring quality of care for vulnerable children: Challenges and conceptualization of a pediatric outcome measure of quality. *American Journal of Medical Quality, 15,* 182–188.

Snow, L. F. (1993). *Walkin' over medicine.* Boulder, CO: Westview Press.

Sobo, E. J. (1995). *Choosing unsafe sex: AIDS-risk denial among disadvantaged women.* Philadelphia: University of Pennsylvania Press.

Sobo, E. J. (2007). Mastering the health care system for children with special health care needs. In E. Sobo & P. Kurtin (Eds.), *Optimizing care for young children with special health care needs: Knowledge and strategies for navigating the system* (pp. 209–234). Baltimore: Brookes.

Sobo, E. J. (in press). Caring for children with special healthcare needs: "Once we got there, it was fine." In L. Manderson & C. Smith-Morris (Eds.), *Chronic conditions, fluid states: Globalization and the anthropology of illness.* New Brunswick, NJ: Rutgers University Press.

Sobo, E. J., & Seid, M. (2003). Cultural issues in health services delivery: What kind of "competence" is needed, and from whom? *Annals of Behavioral Science and Medical Education*, *9*, 97–100.

Sobo, E. J., Seid, M., & Reyes Gelhard, L. (2006). Parent-identified barriers to pediatric health care: A process-oriented model. *Health Services Research*, *41*, 148–172.

Szilagyi, P. G., Dick, A. W., Klein, J. D., Shone, L. P., Zwanziger, J., Bajorska, A., et al. (2006). Improved asthma care after enrollment in the State Children's Health Insurance Program in New York. *Pediatrics*, *117*, 486–496.

Szilagyi, P. G., Dick, A. W., Klein, J. D., Shone, L. P., Zwanziger, J., & McInerny, T. (2004). Improved access and quality of care after enrollment in the New York State Children's Health Insurance Program (SCHIP). *Pediatrics*, *113*, e395–e404.

Teach, S. J., Crain, E. F., Quint, D. M., Hylan, M. L., & Joseph, J. G. (2006). Improved asthma outcomes in a high-morbidity pediatric population: Results of an emergency department-based randomized clinical trial. *Archives of Pediatrics and Adolescent Medicine*, *160*, 535–541.

Thomas, S., & Quinn, S. (1991). The Tuskegee syphilis study, 1932–1972: Implications for HIV education and AIDS risk education programs in the black community. *American Journal of Public Health*, *81*, 1498–1505.

Triggs, E. G., & Perrin, E. C. (1989). Listening carefully. Improving communication about behavior and development: Recognizing parental concerns. *Clinical Pediatrics*, *28*, 185–192.

Trotter, R. T., Ortiz de Montellano, B., & Logan, M. H. (1989). Fallen Fontanelle in the American Southwest: Its origin, epidemiology, and possible organic causes. *Medical Anthropology*, *10*, 211–221.

Varni, J. W., Jacobs, J. R., & Seid, M. (2000). Adherence to treatment as a predictor of health-related quality of life: An integrative conceptual model. In D. Drotar (Ed.), *Promoting adherence to medical treatment in childhood chronic illness: Concepts, methods, and interventions* (pp. 287–306). Mahwah, NJ: Erlbaum.

Von Korff, M., Gruman, J., Schaefer, J., Curry, S. J., & Wagner, E. H. (1997). Collaborative management of chronic illness. *Annals of Internal Medicine*, *127*, 1097–1102.

Wade, S. L., Holden, G., Lynn, H., Mitchell, H., & Ewart, C. (2000). Cognitive-behavioral predictors of asthma morbidity in inner-city children. *Journal of Developmental and Behavioral Pediatrics*, *21*, 340–346.

Weller, S. C., Pachter, L. M., Trotter, R. T., & Baer, R. D. (1993). *Empacho* in four Latino groups: A study of intra- and inter-cultural variation in beliefs. *Medical Anthropology*, *15*, 109–136.

Wissow, L. S., Gadomski, A., Roter, D., Larson, S., Brown, J., Zachary, C., et al. (2008). Improving child and parent mental health in primary care: A cluster-randomized trial of communication skills training. *Pediatrics*, *121*, 266–275.

Yu, H., & Seid, M. (2006). Uninsurance among children eligible for the State Children's Health Insurance Program: Results from a national survey. *Managed Care Interface*, *19*, 31–39.

Yu, S. M., Huang, Z. J., Schwalberg, R. H., & Kogan, M. D. (2005). Parental awareness of health and community resources among immigrant families. *Maternal and Child Health Journal*, *9*, 27–34.

PART VI

Emerging Issues

CHAPTER 48

Genetics and Genetic Testing

KENNETH P. TERCYAK

The completion of the sequencing of the human genome is expected to significantly alter our understanding of the hereditary basis of several common chronic diseases and related conditions, including diabetes, heart disease, high cholesterol, high blood pressure, osteoporosis, and some forms of cancer (Pang, Baum, & Lam, 2000). As a result, the ability to predict the onset of disease will be enhanced, and more advanced and effective disease prevention and control strategies are likely to result (Gottesman & Collins, 1994).

Predictive genetic tests are typically offered to asymptomatic persons to assist in determining their risks of developing given diseases later in life (Chung, 2007). Some of the more well-known predictive genetic tests are those for Huntington disease, breast cancer, and hemochromatosis. When partnered with information such as family history, environmental exposures, and lifestyle behavior, risk information learned through genetic testing can guide medical decision making—including informing decisions about prevention and treatment options that are likely to be effective for a given individual's risk profile (Beery & Williams, 2007).

Though there are many reasons to be optimistic about the benefits of genetic testing for individuals, their potentially at-risk family members, and segments of the general population, knowledge generated from genetic tests is not without hazard or debate. This includes a host of ethical, legal, social, and psychological issues surrounding genetic forecasting of future health states, including risks of social stigmatization; loss of privacy control over protected health information; educational, employment, and insurance discrimination; uncertainty, psychological distress, and regret; and fatalistic thoughts about genetic determinism of disease (Burke, Pinsky, & Press, 2001). Nowhere are these issues more pronounced than when genetic testing is raised in the context of children's health (Dinc & Terzioglu, 2006). Though many diagnostic and predictive genetic tests may be beneficially utilized with children (Twomey, 2006), predictive genetic testing in children is often limited to only those disease circumstances where known prevention and intervention options exist. Presently, this represents only a fraction of diseases—though the proportion is expected to grow over time (Chung, 2007).

As genetic testing proliferates, greater numbers of adults may participate. These adults are often parents of minor-age children who question whether their children could have inherited parental disease risk (Tercyak, Peshkin, Demarco, et al., 2007). Regardless of whether children directly participate in predictive genetic testing, they may become aware of their family's history of disease, their parents' genetic test results, and outcomes related to these circumstances, thereby generating questions and uncertainties about their own future health status (Wilfond & Ross, in press). These realities are propelling a reexamination of what is known about the risks and benefits of predictive and other forms of genetic testing in and affecting children, including testing for adult-onset diseases (Kopelman, 2007).

Predictive and Preventive Medicine in the Genomic Era

Among the leading causes of death in the United States are diabetes, heart disease, and cancer (Mokdad, Marks, Stroup, & Gerberding, 2004). However, among the actual causes of death, which are defined as modifiable behavioral risk factors, are tobacco use, poor diet and physical inactivity, alcohol consumption, and others. These behaviors are typically initiated during childhood and adolescence, and there is a need to more effectively prevent their onset and reform public health approaches to prevention (Mokdad et al., 2004; Tercyak, 2008). Consistent with this call for early prevention, the Healthy People 2010 initiative established behavioral objectives relevant to the health and well-being of young people. Park, Brindis, Chang, and Irwin (2008) recently published a midcourse review of national progress toward achieving Healthy People 2010's adolescent objectives. Two of these objectives—adult chronic disease prevention, and mental health and substance use prevention—hold special significance, given the active research taking place to uncover their hereditary origins (see Hirschhorn & Daly, 2005, for a review).

Implications for Child and Family Health

It is widely recognized that childhood is an optimal time in human development for preventing illness and promoting health (Tercyak, 2008). When viewed from a developmental perspective, changes may be facilitated by many agents and resources, including a child's family, school, health care system, and community.

Given the recent advances in studying the complex roles of genes, the environment, and lifestyle behaviors in the risk and progression of disease throughout the lifespan ("epigenetics"), and the structure and function of genes ("genomics"), it is becoming clear that increasing attention will be paid to children and their families (Kenner, Gallo, & Bryant, 2005). Children may someday benefit from these advances, including increased knowledge of the genetic determinants of disease, new methods to diagnose and treat presymptomatic diseases before full-blown onset, and perhaps gene therapies (Williams & Lessick, 1996).

Promoting predictive and preventive medicine requires the engagement of many stakeholders, including affected adults, their children, and health care providers. Children growing up in the genomic medicine era will face complex decisions about considering predictive genetic testing (Moore, Khoury, & Bradley, 2005). Children's emerging cognitive capacities will have an impact on their role in the decision-making process, and will affect the nature and type of questions they consider in these encounters (Chouinard, 2007). Adolescents, and adolescent girls in particular, may be early adopters of predictive genetic testing—possibly owing to their maturity, concern for family, and women's health issues (Harel, Abuelo, & Kazura, 2003). Thus there is a high burden placed upon parents and health care providers alike to assist children and families with genetic testing decisions (Jacobs & Deatrick, 1999).

Genetic Testing

A "gene" is a unit of inheritance passed from parent to offspring. More specifically, it is a sequence of chromosomal deoxyribonucleic acid (DNA) that usually contains the information necessary for making a specific protein in the body (see Nussbaum, McInnes, & Willard, 2007, for a review). Humans are believed to have about 20,000 genes, though the exact number has not been determined. These genes combine to form 23 pairs of "chromosomes" (packages of genes; 46 total). Each parent contributes one chromosome to each pair, so children inherit half of their chromosomes from their mothers and half from their fathers. One's full complement of DNA is called a "genotype," and each child of a parent who carries a disease-causing gene has a 50% chance of inheriting that same gene if the condition is "dominantly" inherited (i.e., almost always results in a specific characteristic or affected state). "Recessively" inherited conditions appear only if children have received two copies of a disease-causing gene, one from each parent.

The expression of genes in the form of an observable trait, characteristic, or presence–absence of a disease ("phenotype") cannot always be predicted in advance. Some medical diseases are caused by permanent structural alterations (mutations) in DNA, and these are called "single-gene diseases." In dominantly inherited single-gene diseases, there is usually a 1:1 genotype–phenotype correspondence, meaning that having the altered gene leads to disease nearly 100% of the time. An example of a dominantly inherited disease is hypochondroplasia (i.e., a form of short-limbed dwarfism), and an example of a recessively inherited disease is cystic fibrosis. Other diseases are caused by rearrangements to, duplications of, or omissions from the whole chromosome that invariably disrupt the genes residing on those chromosomes; still other diseases are caused by a complex interplay of one or more gene mutations interacting with the environment ("multifactorial diseases"). Chromosomal diseases include Down syndrome and trisomy 18; multifactorial diseases include some forms of cancer and diabetes.

Multifactorial diseases are of particular interest, because genotype–phenotype correspondence is more variable than in dominantly inherited single-gene diseases, and because not all at-risk individuals go on to become medically affected. In many cases, it may be important to identify (prior to the onset of symptoms) those who are at risk to develop the disease, so that appropriate steps may be taken to prevent or control the disease. These steps may include lifestyle modifications, such as diet, physical activity, and smoking behavior, along with medical management (e.g., targeted screening). However, more research is necessary to prove the long-term effectiveness of initiating such changes in childhood among those who are genetically susceptible, and clinical testing is not yet available to identify children at risk.

Guidelines for Use of Genetic Testing

Genetic testing is the clinical tool used to predict the likelihood of disease occurrence, to identify individuals who carry disease-causing mutations, and to establish prenatal and clinical diagnosis or prognosis (Ansell, Ackerman, Black, Roberts, & Tefferi, 2003). The predictive ability of genetic tests is best viewed as a continuum of predictive capability, from 100% predictive though tests that indicate very small risk elevations. Genetic testing is similar to other kinds of laboratory testing that may be recommended by a health care provider, though several features make it unique. For example, genetic testing may be used for diagnostic purposes, medical management, and personal decision making, and results usually apply both to the individual undergoing testing and to other biological family members (McPherson, 2006).

In the case of children and adolescents, several points have been raised about when it is appropriate to use genetic testing. The main points to consider prior to initiating testing are these: (1) Testing should produce timely medical benefits, which means that steps to prevent or treat the disease are presently known, or that testing provides medical knowledge to promote the patient's current health and well-being; (2) substantial psychosocial benefits to competent adolescents should be gained from testing (e.g., it should reduce anxiety and uncertainty or should influence reproductive, educational, vocational, insurance, or lifestyle decisions and behaviors); and (3) if the benefits of the test are not available until adulthood, then testing should be deferred.

These points were set forth jointly by the American Society of Human Genetics and the American College of Medical Genetics (1995), and affirmed by the American Academy of Pediatrics (Nelson et al., 2001); similar recommendations have been offered by several other national and foreign health organizations (Borry, Stultiens, Nys, Cassiman, & Dierickx, 2006). In the case of genetic testing for pediatric diseases that are typically diagnosed at about the time of birth, or during childhood or adolescence, the indications for testing are clear. Less clear is the rationale for predictive testing, where results estimate the likelihood that a child will experience the disease at some point during his or her lifetime (including adulthood).

Genetic Health Care

In families who have experienced chronic illness, especially those predisposed to hereditary diseases, the potential is high that children's psychosocial development will be affected by such events. Children and adolescents, especially those who have had affected relatives, are likely to have experienced multiple losses as a result of these conditions (Fanos, 1997). Behavioral research suggests that nearly 50% or more of children who grow up in families at increased cancer risk report worrying about their and their family members' chances of developing cancer (Tercyak, Peshkin, Streisand, & Lerman, 2001). Data from community samples suggest that children's thoughts about cancer are not infrequent, especially among those who may be at elevated risk (Chin et al., 1998). In a study of perceived vulnerability to common diseases, 34% of adolescents and their parents believed that they were more likely to develop cancer than were their peers, and 46% believed they were just as likely as others to be affected by cancer during their lifetimes (Ponder, Lee, Green, & Richards, 1996).

Genetic testing is usually performed in the context of a genetic counseling consultation. In traditional genetic counseling, the counselor's (consultant's) interaction with the patient (client/consultant) is characterized by a nondirective approach (Latimer, 2007), as individuals are encouraged to make decisions in accordance with their own preferences and values (e.g., with regard to reproductive choices or the decision about whether or not to undergo genetic testing). However, this approach may be modified when individuals are being counseled about diseases or conditions for which effective screening and risk reduction options are available, or when evidence-based guidelines recommend a certain course of action (Resta et al., 2006).

Decisions and Outcomes

Undergoing genetic testing may be a unique health care decision, as the implications of the results usually hold meaning not only for the individuals being tested but also for their family members, especially blood relatives. In the medical literature, this has been termed "genetic exceptionalism"—underscoring the potential implications of inherited disease risk information for individual families, and the potential for persons to be discriminated against on the basis of this information (Diergaarde et al., 2007). Recently, the notion of genetic exceptionalism has been challenged on the grounds that other (nongenetic) medical tests share these characteristics, and that genetics are but one element contributing to human health and well-being (Kakuk, 2008). Many do not endorse a view of genetic exceptionalism, but view genetic tests like other medical tests, in that the information is personal and should be protected (Diergaarde et al., 2007).

Diabetes

There is a burgeoning literature on the psychosocial, behavioral, and related impacts of predictive testing for diabetes, including Type 1 diabetes and maturity-onset diabetes of the young (MODY). With respect to Type 1 diabetes, Johnson and colleagues (Johnson, Riley, Hansen, & Nurick, 1990; Johnson & Tercyak, 1995) were among the first to examine stress and coping among children informed of their elevated risk of developing Type 1 diabetes years before the onset of clinical symptoms, by virtue of their positive result on an antibody screening test. School-age children reported a sharp rise in their anxiety states upon learning this news, as did their parents. These anxiety states lessened over time, suggesting an acute, transient emotional impact of at-risk notification, followed by a return to the normal psychological state.

Of particular interest for these studies were how children came to view their at-risk status, and ultimately how they coped with it (Johnson et al., 1990; Johnson & Tercyak, 1995). Children were less likely than parents to believe they would eventually develop Type 1 diabetes, and used a combination of avoidance, problem-focused coping, and social support–gathering strategies to accommodate this perception. Anxiety and fatalistic thinking about the likelihood of developing diabetes contributed to another inter-

esting finding—lifestyle behavior changes (e.g., diet, physical activity modifications) following at-risk notification. These changes were probably an effort to prevent or delay
the onset of Type 1 diabetes, though there are no proven methods to do so.

There has also been considerable work examining psychological reactions and
other outcomes among parents to genetic screening programs for Type 1 diabetes risk
among newborn infants. Learning about infant genetic risk does not produce significant
anxiety among parents (Simonen et al., 2006; Yu et al., 1999). The presence of some
psychological disruptions, particularly among mothers, has been noted (Lernmark et
al., 2004), though these results may be subtle and likely to occur among only a subset of women (Johnson, Baughcum, Carmichael, She, & Schatz, 2004). Interestingly,
maternal understanding of infants' Type 1 diabetes at-risk status appears to vary from
infants' actual risk estimates, with more than 20% of mothers tending to underestimate
infant/child risk over time (Hood, Johnson, Baughcum, She, & Schatz, 2006). As also
observed previously, a majority of mothers of tested infants reported engaging their
children in diabetes prevention behaviors as they grew up (Baughcum et al., 2005).
These findings underscore the importance of patient education, counseling, and family
support—particularly in light of the propensity for mothers to engage their children in
unproven preventive strategies.

Though far less is known about predictive genetic testing for MODY, recent advances
make it a strong candidate for social and behavioral studies of anticipated test uptake
and impact (Ellard, Bellanne-Chantelot, & Hattersley, 2008). The available literature
includes a single-case report of predictive genetic testing for MODY in a young child.
The desire to pursue such testing was due in part to the identified family's strong history
of diabetes and interest in reducing uncertainty about the child's future health (Shepherd
et al., 2001). Adults who participate in MODY-predictive genetic testing appear to do so
out of strong concern for their children's risks and the desire to reduce uncertainty about
the likelihood of developing diabetes (Liljestrom et al., 2005). Though most are satisfied
with testing, a majority believe that childhood is the time in the life course when such
testing should be offered (Liljestrom et al., 2005). MODY appears to be a model disease
in which to explore such issues to better inform clinicians, families, and those at risk.
Currently, the available literature is small, and more work in this area is needed.

Heart Disease

The genetic origins of heart disease, like those of most chronic diseases affecting humans,
are actively being explored. For children and families, recent advances in understanding inherited cardiac arrhythmias is expected to lead to the proliferation of a number
of diagnostic and predictive tests for such risks as long-QT syndrome (LQTS; fast, chaotic heartbeats recorded on an electrocardiogram's QT waveform interval, which can
result in fainting and sudden death) (Etheridge et al., 2007). The short-term psychological effects of testing children for inherited LQTS were recently investigated (Hendriks,
Grosfeld, Wilde, et al., 2005). Among parents of children who were determined to be
gene carriers (at risk for LQTS), 50% showed clinical elevations in their levels of distress, and parents who were more familiar with LQTS and who had more children at
risk for LQTS were the most distressed.

In a follow-up to this work, researchers examined long-term psychological distress
outcomes among parents over a year later (Hendriks, Grosfeld, van Tintelen, et al.,

2005). The results showed persistently elevated worry and distress among parents of children who were carriers, particularly among those who were distressed upon first learning the news that their children were at risk. Other work suggests that parents of LQTS-prone children live with a fear that their children may die suddenly, thereby placing a significant psychological burden upon the family system (Farnsworth, Fosyth, Haglund, & Ackerman, 2006).

Inherited forms of heart disease also include a focus on familial hypercholesterolemia (FH), which is a dominantly inherited genetic condition resulting in elevated low-density lipoprotein cholesterol levels at birth and heart attacks at an early age (Civeira, 2004). There is a small but growing literature on psychosocial aspects of this form of diagnostic genetic testing in children, concluding that psychological distress reactions are relatively uncommon (Tonstad, 2001). Works examining adults' quality of life following their notification of being at risk for FH suggest that they may be prone to experience anxiety, fear of heart disease onset, and decreased well-being (Andersen, Jensen, Juul, & Faergeman, 1997). However, a majority of individuals ultimately experience a good quality of life (Agard, Bolmsjo, Hermeren, & Wahlstom, 2005), remain in favor of family screening for FH, and respond favorably to such screening if approached (van Maarle, Stouthard, Marang-van de Mheen, Klazinga, & Bonsel, 2001). Unfortunately, there is also a strong likelihood that family members will not substantially alter their lifestyle behaviors in response to positive screening results (e.g., risk reduction via modifications in diet, physical activity, smoking behavior) (Marteau et al., 2004). Parents and children, however, are likely to show different responses (de Jongh et al., 2003).

Cancer

Cancer represents another important, complex set of diseases for which various predisposition tests currently exist. These include predictive genetic tests that forecast the onset of ataxia telangiectasia, familial adenomatous polyposis (FAP), Li–Fraumeni syndrome, the multiple endocrine neoplasias, the neurofibromatoses, retinoblastoma, Von Hippel–Lindau syndrome, and Wilms tumor syndromes. These are model syndromes for which genetic testing and tumor surveillance may be appropriate for children (see Rao, Rothman, & Nichols, 2008, for a review).

With respect to hereditary cancer genetic testing in children, numerous medical, psychological, and ethical issues have been raised (Strahm & Malkin, 2006). For example, the American Society of Clinical Oncology (2003) recommends that cancer genetic testing in children be predicated on the principles of informed consent prior to testing, and that it should be done only if the result will have an impact on medical management decision making. It is understood that genetic testing may bring psychological consequences to tested children and their families, including differences in parental attitudes toward at-risk children and their normal-risk siblings, the experience of survivor guilt among children who are tested but who turn out not to be gene carriers, and elevated anxiety among those who are carriers (Strahm & Malkin, 2006).

There are several reasons why children may be tested for cancer susceptibility, including (1) clarification of diagnostic information for children with cancer; (2) targeted screening, prevention, or early detection of childhood neoplasias among those determined to be gene carriers, or the elimination of aggressive screening among noncarriers; and (3) satisfaction of a parent's or child's desire to learn about the child's genetic risk

(Patenaude, 1996). Furthermore, many parents of children at risk express an interest in having their children tested for predisposing gene mutations for a variety of cancerous and noncancerous disorders (Tercyak, Peshkin, DeMarco, Brogan, & Lerman, 2002). Parental interest, however, is not sufficient grounds for offering such testing in clinical circumstances without a more complete understanding of the potential pros and cons of that decision (Borry, Stultiens, Nys, & Dierickx, 2007).

One procedure that has been relatively well utilized is predictive testing for FAP—a rare medical condition that, if left untreated, may lead to colon cancer. Inherited in an autosomal dominant fashion, each child of a parent with FAP has a 50% chance of acquiring the mutation, resulting in a greater than 90% lifetime risk of disease (Rustgi, 2007). Children are eligible for gene screening, because polyps may develop during childhood and are detectable by sigmoidoscopy (recommended annually). Removal of a portion of the affected colon is recommended to prevent colon cancer from developing. An advantage of FAP testing in childhood is to spare at least some children from continuing frequent and invasive cancer surveillance procedures.

Very little is known about the characteristics of families who choose to have their children undergo screening for FAP gene mutations. Data suggest that in the short term, the process of testing is agreeable to children and their parents (Codori, Petersen, Boyd, Brandt, & Giardiello, 1996). However, children with FAP gene mutations are more likely to experience features of depression if their mothers are affected with FAP; children of affected mothers are also more likely to report greater anxiety after testing. A recent report did not identify long-term psychosocial consequences (Michie, Bobrow, & Marteau, 2001), underscoring the relative safety of FAP gene testing for children (Codori et al., 2003).

Other Medical Conditions

Though psychosocial aspects of predictive and other forms of genetic testing in children for all diseases is beyond the scope of this chapter, some medical conditions pose unique challenges or serve as useful case examples to illustrate broader issues of concern. Two such conditions are diagnostic and carrier genetic testing for fragile X syndrome, and predictive genetic testing for multiple-disease profiling.

Research in fragile X syndrome—the commonest cause of inherited cognitive impairments, including learning disabilities and/or severe intellectual disabilities or mental retardation—has generated a wealth of information about the psychological and behavioral aspects of diagnostic and carrier genetic testing in children and their parents. One study explored the notion of when in the life course might be the most appropriate time to learn about a fragile X at-risk status and undergo genetic testing, and identified childhood as the most frequently cited period (McConkie-Rosell, Spiridigliozzi, Sullivan, Dawson, & Lachiewicz, 2002). Notifying younger children was believed to provide more time to adjust to the news, whereas notifying older children and adolescents was believed to coincide with children's cognitive maturity levels and their abilities to understand, adjust, and cope with the information and the need to engage in family planning. Other work suggests that knowing one's fragile X genetic status may affect adolescents' concepts of themselves—including adolescents who are obligate gene carriers (McConkie-Rosell, Spiridigliozzi, Melvin, Dawson, & Lachiewicz, 2008)—and that these experiences may persist into the long term and foster unique genetic identities among these individuals (McConkie-Rosell, Spiridigliozzi, Sullivan, Dawson, & Lachiewicz, 2001).

Multiple-disease risk profiling is accomplished when genetic testing for two or more different conditions is implemented simultaneously (i.e., multiplex genetic testing) (American Medical Association, 1998). A robust example of multiplex genetic testing is work carried out by the National Human Genome Research Institute (*www.genome. gov*) at the National Institutes of Health (NIH). Through the NIH Multiplex Initiative, genetic testing for eight common conditions (Type 2 diabetes, heart disease, high cholesterol, high blood pressure, osteoporosis, lung cancer, colorectal cancer, and malignant melanoma) is available to healthy young adults, based on the results of 15 different disease-related genes of interest. The initiative represents a convergence of evidence generated across several fields of study (e.g., genetics, biostatistics, clinical medicine, epidemiology) to improve disease prediction (McBride et al., 2008). However, there is skepticism as to whether or not the explanatory power of multiplex genetic testing can deliver adequately on its promise, largely owing to the facts that the effect of genes on disease may be relatively small, there are likely to be many more genes involved in disease than are currently understood, and genotype–phenotype correspondence is poor (Janssens, Pardo, Steyerberg, & van Duijn, 2004). In a related fashion, others have expressed concern about how to adequately educate and counsel potential participants of multiplex genetic testing about its risks and benefits, so as to permit them to make a fully informed choice about doing so (American Medical Association, 1998). This represents a core area of interest for the NIH Multiplex Initiative, and new data are expected to shed light on this issue (McBride et al., 2008). Again, given the implications of childhood environmental exposures and lifestyle behaviors on the onset of disease in adulthood (Tercyak & Tyc, 2006), multiplex genetic testing may hold the greatest promise for primary prevention among the young and healthy, especially children.

Tobacco Use

There is no doubt that tobacco use is a major public health problem, and that this problem often begins during adolescence (Mathers, Toumbourou, Catalano, Williams, & Patton, 2006). Recent studies have observed variations in several candidate genes, which, together with certain environmental characteristics, may lead to smoking uptake and nicotine dependence (Munafo & Johnstone, 2008). One such study found that earlier smoking onset (prior to age 19 years) was associated with a polymorphism in the dopamine transporter gene (SLC6A3), and that this relationship may be associated with susceptibility to nicotine dependence (Ling, Niu, Feng, Xing, & Xu, 2004). Comings and colleagues (1996) noted that the dopamine D2 receptor (DRD2) gene is associated with earlier smoking initiation. Others have noted an association of the A1 allele of the DRD2 dopamine receptor gene with cigarette smoking progression (Audrain-McGovern, Lerman, Wileyto, Rodriguez, & Shields, 2004).

The identification of genetic variants may permit individually tailored treatments for smoking prevention and cessation (i.e., pharmacogenetics), which may reduce smoking rates. A survey of physicians suggests that over 75% of them would be interested in adopting a test allowing them to tailor smoking cessation treatments for patients (Shields et al., 2005); a more recent survey among adolescent health care providers suggests greater caution among those professionals when considering genetic testing for nicotine addiction susceptibility among adolescent patients (O'Neill et al., in press; Tercyak, Peshkin, Abraham, Wine, & Walker, 2007), even though adolescents themselves are reasonably enthusiastic (Tercyak, Peshkin, Wine, & Walker, 2006).

Cross-Cutting Issues

Given the complexity of human health and well-being (i.e., they are multiply determined by a complicated interplay of biological, psychological, and social processes), it is not surprising that a "transdisciplinary" perspective has been advocated for study (Albrecht, Freeman, & Higginbotham, 1998). Transdisciplinary science is characterized by integrating the natural, social, and behavioral sciences in a context that transcends traditional disciplinary boundaries (Choi & Pak, 2006). Studying the ethical, legal, and psychosocial aspects of predictive and other forms of genetic testing affords an opportunity to conduct transdisciplinary research as it relies on basic discoveries in human molecular genetics and translates those discoveries into real-world settings, with an emphasis on how individuals and populations may interact with them.

The Ethical, Legal, and Social Implications Research Program of the National Human Genome Research Institute at NIH sponsors much of the transdisciplinary work in this area (*www.genome.gov*). Transdisciplinary challenges in genomic research that interface with this research program have been described elsewhere (Collins, Green, Guttmacher, & Guyer, 2003). Two are particularly worth highlighting, because they could serve as a more immediate focus of efforts within child health psychology: factors influencing the translation of genetic information, and implications of genetic bases of human traits and behaviors.

First, factors influencing the translation of genetic information include a focus on how family members view and communicate with one another about risk information. Family communication is a cornerstone of clinical genetics, and it is also a core area of psychological inquiry. This makes family communication, and communication with children, about genetic testing important to examine from a pediatric psychology perspective.

There is a rapidly growing literature on the prevalence, decisions, and outcomes of family communication about genetic information—often focusing on the communication of genetic test results to potentially affected relatives. Within child health psychology, my colleagues and I have examined the frequency with which parents who have participated in genetic counseling and testing for inherited breast/ovarian cancer risks (BRCA1 and BRCA2 gene alterations) inform their minor-age children about parental genetic test results. In one study, it was observed that 47% of parents shared the news of their BRCA1 or BRCA2 genetic status with their children (Tercyak, Hughes, et al., 2001). In another study (Tercyak et al., 2002), similarly high rates of disclosure to minor-age children were reported, as well as a significant influence of child age on parental decision making: Older children were more likely to be informed of their parents' genetic test results than were younger children. That work also noted that parental disclosure of genetic test results to children was more likely to occur in the presence of more open parent–child communication styles, suggesting that family behavioral interactions are predictive of whether or not parents choose to share genetic risk information with their children. Perhaps least well understood are the psychosocial responses of children to learning of the news of their familial risk of adult-onset cancer. A small case series has suggested psychological resilience in this setting (Tercyak, Peshkin, et al., 2001), but more work is needed to better identify the unique psychological needs and resources of this potentially vulnerable population.

Second, the implications of genetic bases of human traits and behaviors include a focus on how genes and the environment may interact to produce highly complex phenotypes, such as those that might be studied by behavioral geneticists who are interested in individual differences in human behavior (e.g., intelligence, personality, psychopathology, substance use). Pediatric, clinical child, and developmental psychologists have much to offer these pursuits, as they appreciate not only a longitudinal perspective in the development of health and well-being throughout the lifespan, but also the importance of well-defined behavioral phenotypes.

Conclusion

This chapter has reviewed recent progress in understanding the genomic basis of several complex diseases that affect the lives of many in the United States, including children and their families. This progress in no way diminishes the well-recognized and important roles of environment and lifestyle in the onset of disease as well. Rather, it reflects a transdisciplinary, biopsychosocial perspective on health and well-being, and an appreciation of the interplay among genes, behavior, and the environment in promoting or compromising health. Through these and other advances, it is anticipated that we will be poised to better understand, and therefore better prevent, leading causes of death and disease. Much of this knowledge and progress may ultimately be directly applied to the youngest members of our society, who are still in the process of forming stable lifestyle behaviors. In light of the increased recognition of hereditary predispositions to disease, owing to the results of predictive and other forms of genetic testing, the health outcomes of these individuals and their families could be beneficially altered. However, these advances are predicated on the offer of safe and effective genetic tests—an offer that is multifaceted and more complex when the focus is children. It remains to be seen how best to inform, educate, and counsel children and their parents about genetic testing; how to manage and reduce potential iatrogenic psychosocial effects of at-risk notification; and how to raise children in families and a society that are still adapting to the uncertainties of future forecasted health states.

For these reasons, it is critically important that pediatric psychologists become immersed in genetics and genetic testing. As researchers, providers of health care to children, and influencers of public policy, pediatric psychologists are very well poised to contribute to the transdisciplinary genome science, including science at the nexus of ethical, legal, and social issues in genetic testing. Doing so in a cogent manner is likely to require additional training in genetics on the part of those in the field (Patenaude, 2003); however, this is no different from the additional training required of other specialists who seek to continue to make meaningful contributions to their fields in light of genetic breakthroughs (Fields, Nickerson, Waterston, & Ramsey, 2006). Given that pediatric psychologists are already working within many research and clinical settings that focus on complex, multifactorial diseases, an expansion of biopsychosocial work to embrace genetic knowledge is likely to serve both the field's and the public health's interest well.

References

Agard, A., Bolmsjo, I. A., Hermeren, G., & Wahlstom, J. (2005). Familial hypercholesterolemia: Ethical, practical and psychological problems from the perspective of patients. *Patient Education and Counseling, 57,* 162–167.

Albrecht, G., Freeman, S., & Higginbotham, N. (1998). Complexity and human health: The case for a transdisciplinary paradigm. *Culture, Medicine and Psychiatry, 22,* 55–92.

American Medical Association. (1998). Multiplex genetic testing. The Council on Ethical and Judicial Affairs, American Medical Association. *The Hastings Center Report, 28,* 15–21.

American Society of Clinical Oncology. (2003). American Society of Clinical Oncology policy statement update: Genetic testing for cancer susceptibility. *Journal of Clinical Oncology, 21,* 2397–2406.

American Society of Human Genetics and American College of Medical Genetics. (1995). Points to consider: Ethical, legal, and psychosocial implications of genetic testing in children and adolescents. *American Journal of Human Genetics, 57,* 1233–1241.

Andersen, L. K., Jensen, H. K., Juul, S., & Faergeman, O. (1997). Patients' attitudes toward detection of heterozygous familial hypercholesterolemia. *Archives of Internal Medicine, 157,* 553–560.

Ansell, S. M., Ackerman, M. J., Black, J. L., Roberts, L. R., & Tefferi, A. (2003). Primer on medical genomics. Part VI: Genomics and molecular genetics in clinical practice. *Mayo Clinic Proceedings, 78,* 307–317.

Audrain-McGovern, J., Lerman, C., Wileyto, E. P., Rodriguez, D., & Shields, P. G. (2004). Interacting effects of genetic predisposition and depression on adolescent smoking progression. *American Journal of Psychiatry, 161,* 1224–1230.

Baughcum, A. E., Johnson, S. B., Carmichael, S. K., Lewin, A. B., She, J. X., & Schatz, D. A. (2005). Maternal efforts to prevent Type 1 diabetes in at-risk children. *Diabetes Care, 28,* 916–921.

Beery, T. A., & Williams, J. K. (2007). Risk reduction and health promotion behaviors following genetic testing for adult-onset disorders. *Genetic Testing, 11,* 111–123.

Borry, P., Stultiens, L., Nys, H., & Dierickx, K. (2007). Attitudes towards predictive genetic testing in minors for familial breast cancer: A systematic review. *Critical Reviews in Oncology/ Hematology, 64,* 173–181.

Borry, P., Stultiens, L., Nys, H., Cassiman, J. J., & Dierickx, K. (2006). Presymptomatic and predictive genetic testing in minors: A systematic review of guidelines and position papers. *Clinical Genetics, 70,* 374–381.

Burke, W., Pinsky, L. E., & Press, N. A. (2001). Categorizing genetic tests to identify their ethical, legal, and social implications. *American Journal of Medical Genetics, 106,* 233–240.

Chin, D. G., Schonfeld, D. J., O'Hare, L. L., Mayne, S. T., Salovey, P., Showalter, D. R., et al. (1998). Elementary school-age children's developmental understanding of the causes of cancer. *Journal of Developmental and Behavioral Pediatrics, 19,* 397–403.

Choi, B. C., & Pak, A. W. (2006). Multidisciplinarity, interdisciplinarity and transdisciplinarity in health research, services, education and policy: 1. Definitions, objectives, and evidence of effectiveness. *Clinical and Investigative Medicine, 29,* 351–364.

Chouinard, M. M. (2007). Children's questions: A mechanism for cognitive development. *Monographs of the Society for Research in Child Development, 72*(1), vii–112.

Chung, W. K. (2007). Implementation of genetics to personalize medicine. *Gender Medicine, 4,* 248–265.

Civeira, F. (2004). Guidelines for the diagnosis and management of heterozygous familial hypercholesterolemia. *Atherosclerosis, 173,* 55–68.

Codori, A. M., Petersen, G. M., Boyd, P. A., Brandt, J., & Giardiello, F. M. (1996). Genetic testing for cancer in children: Short-term psychological effect. *Archives of Pediatrics and Adolescent Medicine, 150,* 1131–1138.

Codori, A. M., Zawacki, K. L., Petersen, G. M., Miglioretti, D. L., Bacon, J. A., Trimbath, J. D., et al. (2003). Genetic testing for hereditary colorectal cancer in children: Long-term psychological effects. *American Journal of Medical Genetics: Part A, 116,* 117–128.

Collins, F. S., Green, E. D., Guttmacher, A. E., & Guyer, M. S. (2003). A vision for the future of genomics research. *Nature, 422,* 835–847.

Comings, D. E., Ferry, L., Bradshaw-Robinson, S., Burchette, R., Chiu, C., & Muhleman, D. (1996). The dopamine D2 receptor (DRD2) gene: A genetic risk factor in smoking. *Pharmacogenetics, 6,* 73–79.

de Jongh, S., Kerckhoffs, M. C., Grootenhuis, M. A., Bakker, H. D., Heymans, H. S., & Last, B. F. (2003). Quality of life, anxiety and concerns among statin-treated children with familial hypercholesterolaemia and their parents. *Acta Paediatrica, 92,* 1096–1101.

Diergaarde, B., Bowen, D. J., Ludman, E. J., Culver, J. O., Press, N., & Burke, W. (2007). Genetic information: Special or not? Responses from focus groups with members of a health maintenance organization. *American Journal of Medical Genetics: Part A, 143,* 564–569.

Dinc, L., & Terzioglu, F. (2006). The psychological impact of genetic testing on parents. *Journal of Clinical Nursing, 15,* 45–51.

Ellard, S., Bellanne-Chantelot, C., & Hattersley, A. T. (2008). Best practice guidelines for the molecular genetic diagnosis of maturity-onset diabetes of the young. *Diabetologia, 51,* 546–553.

Etheridge, S. P., Sanatani, S., Cohen, M. I., Albaro, C. A., Saarel, E. V., & Bradley, D. J. (2007). Long QT syndrome in children in the era of implantable defibrillators. *Journal of the American College of Cardiology, 50,* 1335–1340.

Fanos, J. H. (1997). Developmental tasks of childhood and adolescence: Implications for genetic testing. *American Journal of Medical Genetics, 71,* 22–28.

Farnsworth, M. M., Fosyth, D., Haglund, C., & Ackerman, M. J. (2006). When I go in to wake them … I wonder: Parental perceptions about congenital long QT syndrome. *Journal of the American Academy of Nurse Practitioners, 18,* 284–290.

Fields, S., Nickerson, D. A., Waterston, R. H., & Ramsey, P. G. (2006). Positioning a medical school for modern biomedical research: The Department of Genome Sciences at the University of Washington School of Medicine. *Academic Medicine, 81,* 882–885.

Gottesman, M. M., & Collins, F. S. (1994). The role of the Human Genome Project in disease prevention. *Preventive Medicine, 23,* 591–594.

Harel, A., Abuelo, D., & Kazura, A. (2003). Adolescents and genetic testing: What do they think about it? *Journal of Adolescent Health, 33,* 489–494.

Hendriks, K. S., Grosfeld, F. J., van Tintelen, J. P., van Langen, I. M., Wilde, A. A., van den Bout, J., et al. (2005). Can parents adjust to the idea that their child is at risk for a sudden death?: Psychological impact of risk for long QT syndrome. *American Journal of Medical Genetics: Part A, 138,* 107–112.

Hendriks, K. S., Grosfeld, F. J., Wilde, A. A., van den Bout, J., van Langen, I. M., van Tintelen, J. P., et al. (2005). High distress in parents whose children undergo predictive testing for long QT syndrome. *Community Genetics, 8,* 103–113.

Hirschhorn, J. N., & Daly, M. J. (2005). Genome-wide association studies for common diseases and complex traits. *Nature Reviews Genetics, 6,* 95–108.

Hood, K. K., Johnson, S. B., Baughcum, A. E., She, J. X., & Schatz, D. A. (2006). Maternal understanding of infant diabetes risk: Differential effects of maternal anxiety and depression. *Genetics in Medicine, 8,* 665–670.

Jacobs, L. A., & Deatrick, J. A. (1999). The individual, the family, and genetic testing. *Journal of Professional Nursing, 15,* 313–324.

Janssens, A. C., Pardo, M. C., Steyerberg, E. W., & van Duijn, C. M. (2004). Revisiting the clinical validity of multiplex genetic testing in complex diseases. *American Journal of Human Genetics, 74,* 585–588.

Johnson, S. B., Baughcum, A. E., Carmichael, S. K., She, J. X., & Schatz, D. A. (2004). Maternal anxiety associated with newborn genetic screening for Type 1 diabetes. *Diabetes Care, 27,* 392–397.

Johnson, S. B., Riley, W. J., Hansen, C. A., & Nurick, M. A. (1990). Psychological impact of islet cell-antibody screening. Preliminary results. *Diabetes Care, 13,* 93–97.

Johnson, S. B., & Tercyak, K. P. (1995). Psychological impact of islet cell antibody screening for IDDM on children, adults, and their family members. *Diabetes Care, 18,* 1370–1372.

Kakuk, P. (2008). Gene concepts and genethics: Beyond exceptionalism. *Science and Engineering Ethics, 14,* 357–375.

Kenner, C., Gallo, A. M., & Bryant, K. D. (2005). Promoting children's health through understanding of genetics and genomics. *Journal of Nursing Scholarship, 37,* 308–314.

Kopelman, L. M. (2007). Using the best interests standard to decide whether to test children for untreatable, late-onset genetic diseases. *Journal of Medicine and Philosophy, 32,* 375–394.

Latimer, J. (2007). Becoming in-formed: Genetic counselling, ambiguity and choice. *Health Care Analysis, 15,* 13–23.

Lernmark, B., Elding-Larsson, H., Hansson, G., Lindberg, B., Lynch, K., & Sjoblad, S. (2004). Parent responses to participation in genetic screening for diabetes risk. *Pediatric Diabetes, 5,* 174–181.

Liljestrom, B., Aktan-Collan, K., Isomaa, B., Sarelin, L., Uutela, A., Groop, L., et al. (2005). Genetic testing for maturity onset diabetes of the young: Uptake, attitudes and comparison with hereditary non-polyposis colorectal cancer. *Diabetologia, 48,* 242–250.

Ling, D., Niu, T., Feng, Y., Xing, H., & Xu, X. (2004). Association between polymorphism of the dopamine transporter gene and early smoking onset: An interaction risk on nicotine dependence. *Journal of Human Genetics, 49,* 35–39.

Marteau, T., Senior, V., Humphries, S. E., Bobrow, M., Cranston, T., Crook, M. A., et al. (2004). Psychological impact of genetic testing for familial hypercholesterolemia within a previously aware population: A randomized controlled trial. *American Journal of Medical Genetics: Part A, 128,* 285–293.

Mathers, M., Toumbourou, J. W., Catalano, R. F., Williams, J., & Patton, G. C. (2006). Consequences of youth tobacco use: A review of prospective behavioural studies. *Addiction, 101,* 948–958.

McBride, C. M., Alford, S. H., Reid, R. J., Larson, E. B., Baxevanis, A. D., & Brody, L. C. (2008). Putting science over supposition in the arena of personalized genomics. *Nature Genetics, 40,* 939–942.

McConkie-Rosell, A., Spiridigliozzi, G. A., Melvin, E., Dawson, D. V., & Lachiewicz, A. M. (2008). Living with genetic risk: Effect on adolescent self-concept. *American Journal of Medical Genetics: Part C, 148,* 56–69.

McConkie-Rosell, A., Spiridigliozzi, G. A., Sullivan, J. A., Dawson, D. V., & Lachiewicz, A. M. (2001). Longitudinal study of the carrier testing process for fragile X syndrome: Perceptions and coping. *American Journal of Medical Genetics, 98,* 37–45.

McConkie-Rosell, A., Spiridigliozzi, G. A., Sullivan, J. A., Dawson, D. V., & Lachiewicz, A. M. (2002). Carrier testing in fragile X syndrome: When to tell and test. *American Journal of Medical Genetics, 110,* 36–44.

McPherson, E. (2006). Genetic diagnosis and testing in clinical practice. *Clinical Medicine and Research, 4,* 123–129.

Michie, S., Bobrow, M., & Marteau, T. M. (2001). Predictive genetic testing in children and adults: A study of emotional impact. *Journal of Medical Genetics, 38,* 519–526.

Mokdad, A. H., Marks, J. S., Stroup, D. F., & Gerberding, J. L. (2004). Actual causes of death in the United States, 2000. *Journal of the American Medical Association, 291*, 1238–1245.

Moore, C. A., Khoury, M. J., & Bradley, L. A. (2005). From genetics to genomics: Using gene-based medicine to prevent disease and promote health in children. *Seminars in Perinatology, 29*, 135–143.

Munafo, M. R., & Johnstone, E. C. (2008). Genes and cigarette smoking. *Addiction, 103*, 893–904.

Nelson, R. M., Botkjin, J. R., Kodish, E. D., Levetown, M., Truman, J. T., Wilfond, B. S., et al. (2001). Ethical issues with genetic testing in pediatrics. *Pediatrics, 107*, 1451–1455.

Nussbaum, R. L., McInnes, R. R., & Willard, H. F. (2007). *Thompson & Thompson genetics in medicine* (7th ed.). Philadelphia: Saunders/Elsevier.

O'Neill, S. C., Luta, G., Peshkin, B. N., Abraham, A., Walker, L. R., & Tercyak, K. P. (in press). Adolescent medical providers' willingness to recommend genetic susceptibility testing for nicotine addiction and lung cancer risk to adolescents. *Journal of Pediatric Psychology.*

Pang, C. P., Baum, L., & Lam, D. S. (2000). Hunting for disease genes in multi-functional diseases. *Clinical Chemistry and Laboratory Medicine, 38*, 819–825.

Park, M. J., Brindis, C. D., Chang, F., & Irwin, C. E. (2008). A midcourse review of the Healthy People 2010: 21 critical health objectives for adolescents and young adults. *Journal of Adolescent Health, 42*, 329–334.

Patenaude, A. F. (1996). The genetic testing of children for cancer susceptibility: Ethical, legal, and social issues. *Behavioral Sciences and the Law, 14*, 393–410.

Patenaude, A. F. (2003). Pediatric psychology training and genetics: What will twenty-first-century pediatric psychologists need to know? *Journal of Pediatric Psychology, 28*, 135–145.

Ponder, M., Lee, J., Green, J., & Richards, M. (1996). Family history and perceived vulnerability to some common diseases: A study of young people and their parents. *Journal of Medical Genetics, 33*, 485–492.

Rao, A., Rothman, J., & Nichols, K. E. (2008). Genetic testing and tumor surveillance for children with cancer predisposition syndromes. *Current Opinion in Pediatrics, 20*, 1–7.

Resta, R., Biesecker, B. B., Bennett, R. L., Blum, S., Hahn, S. E., Strecker, M. N., et al. (2006). A new definition of genetic counseling: National Society of Genetic Counselors' Task Force report. *Journal of Genetic Counseling, 15*, 77–83.

Rustgi, A. K. (2007). The genetics of hereditary colon cancer. *Genes and Development, 21*, 2525–2538.

Shepherd, M., Ellis, I., Ahmad, A. M., Todd, P. J., Bowen-Jones, D., Mannion, G., et al. (2001). Predictive genetic testing in maturity-onset diabetes of the young (MODY). *Diabetic Medicine, 18*, 417–421.

Shields, A. E., Blumenthal, D., Weiss, K. B., Comstock, C. B., Currivan, D., & Lerman, C. (2005). Barriers to translating emerging genetic research on smoking into clinical practice: Perspectives of primary care physicians. *Journal of General Internal Medicine, 20*, 131–138.

Simonen, P., Korhonen, T., Simell, T., Keskinen, P., Karkkainen, M., Knip, M., et al. (2006). Parental reactions to information about increased genetic risk of Type 1 diabetes mellitus in infants. *Archives of Pediatrics and Adolescent Medicine, 160*, 1131–1136.

Strahm, B., & Malkin, D. (2006). Hereditary cancer predisposition in children: Genetic basis and clinical implications. *International Journal of Cancer, 119*, 2001–2006.

Tercyak, K. P. (2008). Editorial: Prevention in child health psychology and the *Journal of Pediatric Psychology. Journal of Pediatric Psychology, 33*, 31–34.

Tercyak, K. P., Hughes, C., Main, D., Snyder, C., Lynch, J. F., Lynch, H. T., et al. (2001). Parental communication of BRCA1/2 genetic test results to children. *Patient Education and Counseling, 42*, 213–224.

Tercyak, K. P., Peshkin, B. N., Abraham, A., Wine, L., & Walker, L. R. (2007). Interest in genetic counseling and testing for adolescent nicotine addiction susceptibility among a sample of adolescent medicine providers attending a scientific conference on adolescent health. *Journal of Adolescent Health, 41,* 42–50.

Tercyak, K. P., Peshkin, B. N., Demarco, T. A., Brogan, B. M., & Lerman, C. (2002). Parent–child factors and their effect on communicating BRCA1/2 test results to children. *Patient Education and Counseling, 47,* 145–153.

Tercyak, K. P., Peshkin, B. N., Demarco, T. A., Patenaude, A. F., Schneider, K. A., Garber, J. E., et al. (2007). Information needs of mothers regarding communicating BRCA1/2 cancer genetic test results to their children. *Genetic Testing, 11,* 249–255.

Tercyak, K. P., Peshkin, B. N., Streisand, R., & Lerman, C. (2001). Psychological issues among children of hereditary breast cancer gene (BRCA1/2) testing participants. *Psycho-Oncology, 10,* 336–346.

Tercyak, K. P., Peshkin, B. N., Wine, L. A., & Walker, L. R. (2006). Interest of adolescents in genetic testing for nicotine addiction susceptibility. *Preventive Medicine, 42,* 60–65.

Tercyak, K. P., & Tyc, V. L. (2006). Opportunities and challenges in the prevention and control of cancer and other chronic diseases: Children's diet and nutrition and weight and physical activity. *Journal of Pediatric Psychology, 31,* 750–763.

Tonstad, S. (2001). Stratification of risk in children with familial hypercholesterolemia with focus on psychosocial issues. *Nutrition, Metabolism, and Cardiovascular Diseases, 11*(Suppl. 5), 64–67.

Twomey, J. G. (2006). Issues in genetic testing of children. *American Journal of Maternal Child Nursing, 31,* 156–163.

van Maarle, M. C., Stouthard, M. E., Marang-van de Mheen, P. J., Klazinga, N. S., & Bonsel, G. J. (2001). How disturbing is it to be approached for a genetic cascade screening programme for familial hypercholesterolaemia?: Psychological impact and screenees' views. *Community Genetics, 4,* 244–252.

Wilfond, B., & Ross, L. F. (in press). From genetics to genomics: Ethics, policy, and parental decision-making. *Journal of Pediatric Psychology.*

Williams, J. K., & Lessick, M. (1996). Genome research: Implications for children. *Pediatric Nursing, 22,* 40–46.

Yu, M. S., Norris, J. M., Mitchell, C. M., Butler-Simon, N., Groshek, M., Follansbee, D., et al. (1999). Impact on maternal parenting stress of receipt of genetic information regarding risk of diabetes in newborn infants. *American Journal of Medical Genetics, 86,* 219–226.

CHAPTER 49

Translating Clinical Child Neuroscience to Practice

New Directions

MIKLE SOUTH
JULIE WOLF
LAUREN HERLIHY

The field of developmental cognitive neuroscience is growing extraordinarily fast. Complementary branches of research into genetics, neuroimaging, and animal models of human behavior are providing valuable insights into both typical and atypical development. "Translational science" is the term used to describe the "two-way street" on which there is an active exchange between basic scientists and practicing clinicians (National Institutes of Health, 2008). In this chapter, we consider how knowledge gained from neuroscience research can inform pediatric psychology practice.

We begin with a brief overview of techniques and general principles for the field. Although other pediatric psychology conditions are relevant, we focus in depth on the neurobiology of two specific conditions as examples of the kind of work that can be and is being done in this area: autism spectrum disorders (ASDs) and attention-deficit/ hyperactivity disorder (ADHD). Both conditions are seen frequently in pediatric psychology settings, and both have been subjects of substantial neuroscience research over the past decade. However, their specific inclusion here is intended only to provide examples of the potential for clinically informed neuroscience research. We have included a recommended reading list at the end of this chapter with information on other topics of interest to pediatric psychology.

Overview of Child Clinical Neuroscience

Diagnostic Categories and Dimensional Definitions

The conceptualization of psychopathology as discrete categories, such as in the *Diagnostic and Statistical Manual of Mental Disorders*, fourth edition, text revision (DSM-

IV-TR; American Psychiatric Association, 2000), is a tremendous challenge for clinical neuroscience research. Such categories do not readily account for overlap of symptoms across diagnostic boundaries, or for the heterogeneity of symptom expression across individuals within a particular diagnostic group (South, Ozonoff, & Schultz, 2008). Alternatively, proponents of a dimensional systems approach view typical and atypical behavior as variations in degree along one or more continuous dimensions of behavior or personality (Cuthbert, 2005; Reiger, 2007). Thus children with quite different categorical diagnoses may be conceptualized as falling at opposite extremes of the same construct of inhibition/constraint. For example, a child diagnosed with ADHD is likely to be impulsive and disinhibited, while a child diagnosed with an anxiety disorder is likely to be too cautious and overinhibited.

Such dimensional descriptions are frequently more productive for neuroscience research. For example, Todd and colleagues (2005) reanalyzed data from three studies of genetic associations in ADHD. The three studies had originally found no link between ADHD (as defined by the DSM-IV-TR) and variation in two genes that are related to dopamine function in the brain. There were likewise no genotype associations between genotype and the DSM-IV-TR subtypes of ADHD (i.e., predominantly inattentive, predominantly hyperactive–impulsive, and combined). However, there was significant linkage for both genes when the authors used a population-based, dimensional definition of ADHD as the dependent variable. Todd and colleagues suggest (1) that inconsistent results across many genetic studies may be the consequence of error that arises from diagnostic heterogeneity; and (2) that valid dimensional definitions will lead to better understanding of underlying disease processes. Neuroscience research using dimensional approaches often focuses on subclinical markers called "endophenotypes," as described in the next section.

Clinical Neuroscience and the Description of Endophenotypes

An important challenge for strictly dimensional classification systems is to demonstrate clinical utility (Cuthbert, 2005). One important avenue for doing so is the definition of intermediate "endophenotypes" (i.e., measurable characteristics that lie on the pathway between genes and observed symptom expression) (Gottesman & Gould, 2003). Endophenotypes are subclinical biomarkers that are related to categorical symptoms, but are one step closer to the genetic foundations for that behavior. For example, one frequent symptom of autism is impaired use of such nonverbal behaviors as eye-to-eye gaze. Yet there may be multiple underlying reasons for the limited use of eye contact that could be considered as separate endophenotypes. For instance, one child may be less motivated than usual to interact with other people, perhaps because of *hypoactivity* in the brain's emotion regulation systems, including the amygdala (Schultz, 2005); a different child may actively avoid eye contact because of social anxiety that arises due to *hyperactivity* of the amygdala (Dalton et al., 2005). The similar outward behavior of these two children—defined symptomatically as markedly impaired eye gaze—is based on different genetic makeups that would probably respond effectively to quite distinct interventions.

Neuroscience technology is well suited for research to identify such endophenotypes. For instance, functional magnetic resonance imaging (fMRI) is a noninvasive neuroimaging technique that can measure brain activity within the amygdala during experiments that track eye gaze (Dalton et al., 2005), thus helping to describe the neural processes that underlie outward behavior. Neuroimaging techniques can also measure changes in brain function in response to treatment (e.g., see McClure et al., 2007, for pediatric anxiety; Odegard, Ring, Smith, Biggan, & Black, 2008, for dyslexia; Plizska et al., 2006, for ADHD). As noted below, most neuroscience research is still limited to group comparisons and cannot yet draw reliable conclusions about individual cases. Theoretically, however, it is feasible that intermediate endophenotypes could inform treatment. Thus, if impaired eye gaze in autism is shown to stem from anxious avoidance, which results from poor comprehension of facial expressions (see Schultz, 2005), then teaching a young child diagnosed with autism to better comprehend facial expressions may lead to better eye gaze and improved social development.

Brief Overview of Techniques

Understanding genetic and neurobehavioral heterogeneity for any particular disorder will require multiple techniques and applications. Here we summarize evidence from three methods that are particularly rich in application to clinical practice: functional neuroimaging, especially fMRI; genetics research; and brain–behavior research using animal models.

Functional Magnetic Resonance Imaging

fMRI is the newest major neuroimaging modality, but now is among the most widely used in pediatric research.

Technique. fMRI measures levels of oxygen during blood flow in the brain, which is interpreted as a reflection of neural activity in response to specific stimuli or tasks. Functional imaging studies often utilize one of two major designs: Block designs explore the contrast in brain activity between two or more conditions (such as viewing a series of face photos vs. a series of house photos); event-related designs measure brain activity in response to specific stimuli or tasks.

Advantages. Unlike most other functional imaging techniques, fMRI does not involve any ionizing radiation. It is therefore safe for use with participants of any age, as well as for repeated/longitudinal studies. fMRI has excellent spatial resolution: Typical studies use 1-mm or 1.5-mm resolution, but newer studies routinely use even better resolutions that allow for the identification of precise regions associated with specific behavioral functions.

Limitations. Because of strict movement tolerances, fMRI is generally not practical for studying children below 10 or 11 years of age. Although there clearly exist specific structure-to-function associations in the brain, most behaviors arise from the interaction of multiple regions and systems, which are more difficult to capture and understand with a single technique; the development of analytic methods for tracing psychophysical interactions across the brain is encouraging (e.g., Marreiros, Kiebel, & Friston, 2008). To date, virtually all fMRI studies report findings from group comparisons; clinical utility for individual cases has yet to be demonstrated (Bush, 2008).

Other imaging technologies are also yielding promising results. Functional imaging techniques include evoked response potentials, which are especially useful for studies of very young children (e.g., Ackles, 2008), and single-photon emission computed tomography (SPECT). Structural imaging techniques, including quantitative MRI and diffusion tensor imaging (DTI), can also be used effectively with young children (e.g., Cleavinger et al., 2008).

Behavioral Genetics

Tercyak (Chapter 48, this volume) provides a thorough review of contributions from behavioral genetics, including the limitations that have accompanied candidate gene and linkage studies over the past two decades. This chapter reviews just a few genetics studies with functional implications for ASDs and ADHD.

Technique. Quantitative trait loci (QTL) analyses are used to identify regions of the genome that show likely associations with dimensional behavioral phenotypes. Another powerful method is the use of DNA microarray technologies to scan thousands of genetic markers at a time. This is helpful for identifying copy number variations (small changes in DNA) that may be important for the influence of gene expression on the development of atypical behavior.

Advantages. It is unlikely that there are any single-gene causes of psychiatric disorders. However, ascertainment of multiple genes that are associated with vulnerability for atypical behavior may be able to identify patterns of gene function that are related to causal pathways. For example, at least seven autism susceptibility genes appear to be important for neuronal regulation of synaptic development, suggesting that disordered synaptic development may be a vital precursor to ASDs (for a review, see Sutcliffe, 2008). Better understanding of the influence of environmental factors on gene expression is important for individual treatment, as well as for larger social policy discussions (Moffitt, Caspi, & Rutter, 2005). Recent advances into epigenetics may provide improved understanding of environmental influences, such as nutrition and stress, on the expression of genes that are relevant to psychological health.

Limitations. Genetic methods are limited by poor definitions of behavioral phenotypes, especially within the current category-based diagnostic system. Also, there remains little understanding of how multiple genes work together (and within varying environmental contexts) to influence clinical symptoms and syndromes (Anderson, 2008).

Animal Models

Research with many species has provided substantial knowledge about the brain mechanisms that contribute to emotion and cognition in humans.

Technique. Using a variety of techniques, researchers create animals with genetic "knockouts" (i.e., specific genes that have been rendered inoperative). Brain lesion techniques, often using neurotoxins (e.g., ibotenic acid), are also used to create animal models that mimic important dimensions of psychopathology, such as impulsivity, stereotyped behavior, anxiety, and reduced social behavior. Direct electrophysiological recording of brain activity is frequently used in animal research.

Advantages. The primary advantage of using animals is to take advantage of research paradigms that are not possible in humans due to ethical constraints. The shorter life cycles of many species allow for efficient investigation of developmental processes. In addition, gene knockout and brain lesion methods allow for the manipulation of very specific regions and behaviors.

Limitations. Qualitative and quantitative differences between humans and other animal species in brains and behavior make it imperative that translation from one model to the other be done with caution and care (Crawley, 2007). Although some specific behaviors (such as stereotypies) are good targets for animal research, it can be difficult to capture the complexity and richness of many human phenomena, including social interactions.

Autism Spectrum Disorders

The ASDs include autism, Asperger's disorder, and pervasive developmental disorder not otherwise specified (PDD-NOS). The hallmark features include impaired social interaction and communication, accompanied by restricted or repetitive behaviors and interests (see Campbell, Segall, & Dommestrup, Chapter 34, this volume, for a thorough description). Recent neuroscience research in ASDs has focused on deficits in social perception, which may be consequences of atypical social motivation. A second current research theme suggests that ASD symptoms arise from abnormal neural connectivity, marked by restricted long-range connections and overabundant short-range connections within the brain. We summarize both lines of research and then consider applications to treatment.

Social Perception and Motivation

fMRI Studies

In typical development, the fusiform face area (FFA) is actively involved specifically in face perception (Kanwisher, McDermott, & Chun, 1997), although it also appears to be engaged while individuals who are experts view stimuli in their area of expertise (e.g., birds for an ornithologist). In stark contrast to typical face perception, numerous studies of ASD samples have reported underactivation of the FFA during face perception tasks (for a review, see Schultz, 2005). The Schultz lab has also recently found significant and negative correlations between FFA activity and scores on standardized measures of social deficits, indicating that hypoactivation of the FFA is an endophenotype with strong clinical relevance (R. T. Schultz, personal communication, May 7, 2008). It is not yet known whether FFA dysfunction is a primary cause of ASD symptoms, or is secondary to problems in other neural systems, such as the limbic system (particularly the amygdala).

Together with evidence from structural imaging, human postmortem tissue research, and animal models, there is growing support for critical contributions of amygdala dysfunction to multiple symptoms of autism (see Bachevalier & Loveland, 2006). Schultz (2005) and others argue that underdevelopment of perceptual processing regions (such as the FFA) comes as a consequence of failure in the amygdala-based reward system. The logic is as follows: In early infancy in ASDs, the amygdala does not attach extra emotional salience to faces and other social stimuli, compared to other complex objects in the environment. Thus infants with ASDs do not pay special attention to social cues. Because perceptual processing regions depend on repeated experience (i.e., expertise) to develop properly, the failure to attach special importance to social stimuli leads to underdeveloped specialization of the FFA and other social-perceptual systems. Therefore, frequent findings of FFA hypoactivity in ASDs reflect a more fundamental deficit in social perception and motivation.

Genetic Studies

The first reported biomarker for autism was an increased level in blood platelets of the neurotransmitter serotonin, first noted in 1961 and since replicated many times (see Anderson, 2002). The amygdala and nearby brain regions are rich in serotonin receptors, consistent with strong theoretical and empirical grounds to suspect that abnormal serotonin function in the amygdala could contribute to multiple characteristics of autism, including core symptoms of social dysfunction (Skuse, 2006). Nonetheless, studies of the serotonin transporter gene SLC6A4 have yielded inconsistent results to date. This may be due to heterogeneity of samples or methods, or may arise because quite distinct genetic mechanisms (e.g., overtransmission of the short form vs. the long form of the allele) can lead to somewhat similar phenotypes. In any case, there remains great interest in research on the genetic basis for amygdala dysfunction in autism.

Animal Models

Social cognition has also been studied extensively in animals, especially in rodents and in nonhuman primates. In their review of the animal literature, Bachevalier and Loveland (2006) concluded that a circuit between the amygdala and orbito-frontal cortex (OFC) is essential for social bonding and self-regulation of emotional behavior. Variability in ASD symptom severity is probably due to the degree and the timing of disruption of this circuit. Importantly, symptom development is probably most dependent on problems within the connections among the amygdala, the OFC, the hippocampus, and other key structures. This implies that atypical social motivation in ASDs may arise from problems in connections between the amygdala and other key structures, rather than within the amygdala itself (see also South, Ozonoff, Suchy, et al., 2008). This notion provides an important unifying link between the two themes (social motivation and neural connectivity) that are discussed in this chapter.

Beyond studies specifically for social cognition, a number of mouse models for other autism symptoms have been developed (e.g., for stereotyped behavior). These usually have limited validity for autism as a complex developmental syndrome. However, Crawley and colleagues (McFarlane et al., 2008) have recently reported their work with a mouse strain (BTBR T+tf/j) that exhibits the whole ASD triad of social deficits, atypical communication, and repetitive (self-grooming) behaviors. The simultaneous presence of all core domains of ASD symptoms in this mouse model holds tremendous promise for future investigation of genetic and behavioral foundations to these disorders.

Neural Connectivity

fMRI Studies

Findings from structural and functional neuroimaging studies suggest that early brain overgrowth in ASDs may lead to overconnectivity in some localized brain regions, and that overall there is increased neural "noise," which leads to reduced efficiency of information processing (Haist, Adamo, Westerfield, Courchesne, & Townsend, 2005). This model posits that there are too few long-range neural connections to promote the integration of information across different brain networks. This is consistent with neuropsychological studies of ASDs that indicate a bias toward local, detail-oriented information processing, rather than the holistic or gestalt-oriented approach seen in typical development.

For example, an early fMRI study (Ring et al., 1999) using a version of the Embedded Figures Task demonstrated that their group with ASDs, compared to controls, showed increased activation in early visual processing areas (in occipito-temporal regions). The same group showed reduced activation in prefrontal cortex, almost as if the information from visual processing regions had become stuck in a neural "bottleneck" and did not ever arrive in the frontal lobes. More recent fMRI studies in ASDs have consistently demonstrated marked restriction in activation across extended brain networks, but especially for connections to the frontal lobes, for a number of different kinds of cognitive tasks (Just, Cherkassky, Keller, Kana, & Minshew, 2007). These findings fit well with the information bottleneck theory and may also partially explain known behavioral impairments in such executive function tasks as planning, organization, and inhibition. The Infant Brain Imaging Study Network (2008) is conducting a longitudinal investigation of neural connectivity in high-risk infants (siblings of older probands already diagnosed with autism), which should provide an important window into developmental processes in ASDs.

Genetic Studies

Morrow and colleagues (2008) have highlighted the involvement, for some families affected by ASDs, of several genes that are actively regulated by neuronal activity. That is, the function of those genes is dependent upon activity in the synapse, and is likely to play a critical role in learning. A recent review of autism-related genes shows that at least seven known susceptibility genes for ASDs are involved in the regulation of neuronal activity that is likely to guide synaptic development (Sutcliffe, 2008). The notion that dysregulation of these genes in very early development could inhibit the formation of synaptic connections in the brain also fits well with behavioral and neuroimaging results.

Animal Models

An intriguing recent mouse study by Tabuchi and colleagues (2007) explored the effects of a specific knockout of the neuroligin 3 gene—a mutation seen in a small percentage of individuals diagnosed with ASDs. In addition to poor social functioning, the animals surprisingly showed an increase in *inhibitory* synaptic transmission, with no effect on excitatory transmission. Theoretically, such increased inhibition of neural impulses in the developing brain could lead to underdevelopment of neural connectivity. In sum, neuropsychological findings of simultaneous overfocus on details and underfocus on integration of information are supported by neuroimaging, genetics, and animal models of brain development in ASDs.

Clinical Neuroscience Applications to Treatment of ASDs

In this section, we bring the social motivation and neural connectivity concepts together. Knowledge regarding atypical neural connectivity in autism not only helps to explain how existing treatments work, but emphatically underscores the need for intervention as early as possible. Hebb's law (Hebb, 1949) is oversimplistically summarized as "Neurons that fire together, wire together." Following this maxim, the requirement for therapeutic intervention in autism is to build artificially, through targeted and repeated practice, those neural networks that have not developed naturally. Because subsequent brain development greatly depends on what has come before, the creation of better functional networks earlier in life should lead to healthier later development.

Deficits in social motivation appear to be very early precursors to autism. For example, a recent eye-tracking study was able to define a cluster of 6-month-old infants who attended more to the mother's mouth than to her eyes during a still-face paradigm; 10 of the 11 infants in that cluster had an older sibling already diagnosed with autism (Merin, Young, Ozonoff, & Rogers, 2007). If the development of ASDs is known to be a meaningful risk, effective treatment should begin in infancy, focusing on building both the motivation to attend to social information and the explicit skills that are required to interact successfully with others. Social motivation is therefore a prime target for early intervention.

Behavioral Interventions

Traditional treatment models for ASDs have focused on teaching social skills in an explicit manner, as children with ASDs do not seem to pick up on these rules implicitly (Campbell et al., Chapter 34, this volume). Such paradigms involve didactic instruction, modeling, coaching, role playing, and reinforcement/feedback (Pierce & Schreibman, 1997). A number of approaches have also employed typically developing peers as tutors and peer models (e.g., Kamps et al., 1992). Outcome research has shown improvements in several areas: play skills, social initiation, eye contact, experience sharing, interest in peers, problem-solving skills, and emotional knowledge.

In line with a social motivation theory of autism, several recent models of social skill development have moved away from explicit teaching in favor of a more experiential approach. These interventions seek to increase the motivation that underlies social behavior, rather than simply to teach explicit skills with no attention to the underlying motivation. Relationship development intervention (RDI; see Gutstein, Burgess, & Montfort, 2007) uses fun and rewarding social activities in which social skills are necessary to accomplish a task, but very little explicit instruction of skills is involved. RDI is a lifespan model: Based on developmental stage, various treatment "levels" address specific aspects of socialization, such as attunement, referencing, coordination, collaboration, joint attention, perspective taking, sharing ideas, and forming friendships. Gutstein and colleagues (2007) have reported one demonstration of effectiveness for RDI. More research is needed to determine the effectiveness of RDI and other experiential models.

There are now several programs that seek to combine the benefits of both explicit and experiential models by teaching necessary skills while also addressing participants' motivation to engage with social stimuli. Let's Face It! (Tanaka, Lincoln, & Hegg, 2003; Wolf et al., 2008) is a computer-based intervention designed to provide intensive training in face-processing skills for children with ASDs. The software includes a number of arcade-like games that target such skills as face matching, emotion identification, facial identity recognition, face salience, immediate memory for faces, and eye gaze interpretation. Thus specific face-processing skills are taught while the computer game medium creates a motivating and fun platform for skill development. Other studies have also shown effectiveness for computer-based platforms used to teach face-processing skills to individuals with ASDs (e.g., Faja, Aylward, Bernier, & Dawson, 2008). Similarly, Gray's (1998) "social stories" and "comic strip conversations" help children to learn social information through a medium that may be more fun and motivating than traditional instructional techniques.

Pharmacotherapy

Consistent with neuroscience research regarding the role of serotonin in ASDs, selective serotonin reuptake inhibitors have shown some efficacy in treatment. Medication therapy is generally targeted toward comorbid symptoms (such as anxiety or aggressive behavior), as there is as yet no known pharmacological treatment for the core symptom domains in ASDs (Kolevzon, Mathewson, & Hollander, 2006). The dopamine antagonist risperidone has been approved by the U.S. Food and Drug Administration for cases of severe aggression and self-injury in autism, and considerable animal research on other neurotransmitter symptoms relevant to autism is in progress. Please see Scahill (2008) for a discussion of the risks and benefits of medication for ASDs, in general, and the use of risperidone in particular.

Attention-Deficit/Hyperactivity Disorder

ADHD is a set of conditions commonly seen by pediatric psychologists, affecting some 3–5% of the population. Primary symptoms include inattention, impulsivity, and hyperactivity (see Daly, Cohen, Carpenter, & Brown, Chapter 36, this volume, for a thorough description). As in children with ASDs, there is considerable heterogeneity in presentation and degree of symptoms in children diagnosed with ADHD. Clinical researchers have made compelling arguments for separating the primarily inattentive subtype of ADHD from the combined subtype (referring to inattention *and* hyperactivity–impulsivity). In this chapter, these subtypes are generally considered together, for two reasons. First, many neuroscience-based research studies either did not report subtype analyses or only included one subtype. Second, despite the different behavioral profiles, there is only mixed evidence supporting the existence of separate neuropsychological dimensions;

many recent studies have shown little or no difference in subtype cognitive profiles, despite differences in behavioral profiles (Geurts, Verté, Oosterlaan, Roeyers, & Sergeant, 2005). Future research on the neurocognitive correlates of ADHD clearly needs to pursue the validity of endophenotypes that might distinguish these subcategories.

This section follows two related themes: first, the role of impaired response inhibition, meaning the ability to utilize effortful control in order to suppress a prepotent or impulsive action (reviewed in Wodka et al., 2007); and second, the role of the dopamine system, including indicators of response to pharmacological treatment.

Response Inhibition

fMRI Studies

The most consistent executive function difficulty reported in behavioral studies of ADHD is response inhibition, including evidence for impaired inhibition (1) of motor responses, (2) during executive function/cognitive control tasks, and (3) of emotional behavior (see Barkley, 1997). fMRI research on both children and adults with ADHD has consistently shown hypoactivation of the dorsal anterior cingulate cortex (dACC) during response inhibition tasks (see Bush, Valera, & Seidman, 2005). The dACC subserves a number of relevant cognitive functions (such as evaluation of errors) and is tightly connected to the prefrontal cortex. Bush and colleagues (2005) conceptualized that *decreased* activation of the dACC in ADHD leads to inefficient decision making. This leads to increased errors, which lead to *increased* activation of other areas of the ACC that are involved in error monitoring. Evidence that neighboring brain regions—even different aspects of the same structure—can have quite different functions provides a set of vital problems for future neuroimaging investigations (see Bush et al., 2005; Durston, Mulder, Casey, Ziermans, & Van Engeland, 2006).

Neuroimaging studies of children with ADHD have also demonstrated atypical structure (reduced volume) and function (reduced activation) in a network involving the frontal cortex and the striatum (Rubia, Smith, Brammer, Toone, & Taylor, 2005). Casey, Durston, and Fossella (2001) have argued that the prefrontal cortex has a critical role in *interference control*, whereas the striatum is involved in *response inhibition*. Both functions are believed to be fundamentally impaired in ADHD. An elegant study of parent–child dyads (Casey et al., 2007) defined functional regions of interest by using MRI during a response inhibition task (a go/no-go task). The authors then examined the association of findings from DTI, used to map white matter fiber pathways, in these functional regions of interest. In dyads affected by ADHD, there were significant correlations between white matter measurements and functional activation in the inferior frontal gyrus and the caudate nucleus (part of the striatum). This study provides further evidence that disruptions in frontal and striatal systems contribute to the cognitive profile of ADHD; it also suggests that these disruptions may be highly heritable.

Genetic Studies

A recent review of possible cognitive endophenotypes for ADHD concluded that response inhibition demonstrates many qualities of an intermediate step between genes and cognitive function (Crosbie, Pérusse, Barr, & Schachar, 2007). Among important criteria for acceptance as an endophenotype, the influence of response inhibition on ADHD symptoms appears to be independent of conduct problems, anxiety, or learning disabilities. There is also some evidence of familiality of response inhibition—for instance, in some unaffected siblings of children with ADHD. However, twin and family studies of this trait are not well developed, and estimates of heritability are not reliable. Several studies have examined response inhibition in the context of the dopamine system (discussed below). A QTL study by Cornish and colleagues (2005) found a significant relationship between one variant of the dopamine transporter gene (DAT1) and extreme scores of response inhibition in a general population sample. In contrast, the D4 dopamine receptor has shown inconsistent associations with response inhibition.

Animal Models

Likewise in mice, knockout of the D4 receptor has not shown association with an analogue to response inhibition in humans (Helms, Gubner, Wilhelm, Mitchell, & Grandy, 2008). Studies of dopamine-related stimulant medications in rats have not reliably demonstrated effects on response inhibition. In contrast, several studies of the norepinephrine reuptake inhibitor atomoxetine have led to decreased impulsivity in rats, including improved behavioral inhibition (see Robinson et al., 2008).

In summary, response inhibition remains a pertinent behavioral correlate of ADHD. Neuroimaging research provides support for the atypical brain activity in ADHD during response inhibition tasks, particularly in frontal lobe networks. However, work to identify the genetic and neurotransmitter substrates of response inhibition has not consistently shown expected associations. The role of dopamine systems in some, but not all, ADHD symptoms is a rich area of study in neuroscience.

The Dopamine System and Response to Stimulants

The first-line pharmacological treatment for ADHD is methylphenidate (most commonly known by the brand name Ritalin), a stimulant that blocks presynaptic reuptake of dopamine and norepinephrine. Although current research is examining several neurotransmitter systems in ADHD, interest in the dopamine system in ADHD—including predictors of response to stimulant medication—remains a dominant theme.

fMRI Studies

The striatum (recall the neuroimaging findings regarding response inhibition noted above) is rich in dopamine receptors and is likely to be a primary site for stimulant activation during pharmacological treatment of ADHD. Neuroimaging studies using several modalities (e.g., fMRI, positron emission tomography, SPECT) have shown that methylphenidate affects regional blood flow in dorsolateral prefrontal cortex and the striatum, as well as in the thalamus (Bush, 2008). Methylphenidate appears to increase the efficiency of brain functioning over time, perhaps through stimulation of catecholamines (including dopamine and norepinephrine), which in turn enhances regulatory control of the prefrontal cortex (Brennan & Arnsten, 2008). Epstein and colleagues (2007) found important differences between youths and adults in the brain response to methylphenidate, highlighting the importance of developmental factors. There is also a clear need to expand research on other affected areas of the brain, particularly the parietal cortex and the cerebellum (see Bush, 2008).

Genetic Studies

Genes related to dopamine regulation have been a major target of ADHD research. Manor and colleagues (2004) reported a link between variation in the D5 receptor gene in ADHD and performance on a continuous performance task before, but not after, participants took methylphenidate; this suggests an association between gene configuration and performance style on behavioral inhibition tasks. Similar associations, including a link between genotype and dose response (see Joober et al., 2007), have been reported in other dopamine receptor genes (including genetic variants for D2 and D4 receptors), and also for the dopamine transporter gene DAT1. As for ASDs, however, it appears that there are no genes of "major effect"—that is, sufficient by themselves to cause ADHD. Rather, it is likely that multiple genes make small contributions to the overall brain and behavioral phenotypes.

Animal Models

Because of the frequency of ADHD diagnosis and subsequent stimulant prescription, there are many important public health questions regarding the use of methylphenidate and other stimulants (Furman, 2005). Although these drugs are generally considered safe for long-term use, there remain many concerns, including questions about interactions between long-term effects and age of treatment onset; use with comorbid conditions (including epilepsy and tic disorders); potential for abuse; and efficacy versus other potentially safer treatment courses. It is therefore critical to ask the question: Who will benefit most from stimulant interventions? Animal studies are particularly well suited for research in this area.

Studies with rats have confirmed the activation of methylphenidate in prefrontal cortex (e.g., Gray et al., 2007). One study of treatment response (Blondeau & Dellu-Hagedorn, 2006) characterized five groups of rats based on dimensional measures of attention, impulsivity, and hyperactivity. In the "combined" subgroup marked by both inattention and impulsivity, methylphenidate increased impulsivity during a five-choice serial reaction time test, whereas the nonstimulant atomoxetine decreased impulsivity. There was no effect of either drug on the nonaffected subgroup. Studies such as this one that aim to predict treatment response—whether the endophenotypes are behavioral, cognitive, or biological—are critical for the next generation of research.

Clinical Neuroscience Applications to Treatment of ADHD

Individualized Behavioral Treatment

As with all psychological conditions, treatment for ADHD needs to be fitted to each individual. There is strong evidence that impaired response inhibition is common in ADHD, but this is clearly not universal. A child diagnosed with primarily inattentive symptoms, for example, may show more deficits in working memory than in response inhibition (see Diamond, 2005); therefore, treatment should be targeted to the needs of each child. It is an important tenet of translational neuroscience to rely on the experienced judgment of the clinician. What applications can then be gained from neuroscience techniques?

Neuroimaging studies suggest that deficits in response inhibition may occur as a consequence of inefficient information processing in the prefrontal cortex and ACC. This indicates that for individuals with ADHD accompanied by difficulties in response inhibition, frontal regions may be slow to involve other, supporting neural networks in response to changing task demands (Fassbender & Schweitzer, 2006). This paradigm provides support for many existing treatment strategies, such as ensuring adequate time to complete tasks and providing adequate external support for decision-making situations (where a child with ADHD may not process information well enough to make the best choices).

Whereas typically developing individuals are able to utilize verbal strategies to deal with new or changing task requirements, individuals with limited response inhibition are forced to depend on lower-level sensory and motor processing approaches; they must make a greater cognitive effort to understand and to respond to new information. Nonverbal instructional strategies are therefore essential, especially for tasks that involve planning and error monitoring. Such strategies could include combinations of written and spoken instructions and feedback; explicit coaching and reminding about errors and problems that might otherwise be overlooked; and repeated practice to monitor and inhibit motor, cognitive, and behavioral impulsivity.

A frequent frustration with children who struggle with ADHD is the feeling that they could do many difficult tasks, if only they would try! Neuroscience cannot excuse motivational deficits, but there is evidence that the motivational system develops atypically in ADHD. In particular, there appear to be an intrinsic aversion to delays of any sort, which may easily lead to impulsivity. Although further research is needed to clarify the mechanisms that underlie atypical function of the dopamine-based reward system in ADHD, it is apparent that behavioral interventions will benefit from careful tracking of and response to both motivators and punishments for each individual. More work is especially needed to explain how dysfunction in the dopamine system is related to the high risk for substance use and abuse in ADHD, especially during the transition from adolescence to adulthood (Biederman, 2003). In the meantime, the potential for substance abuse should be consistently monitored for teenagers diagnosed with ADHD.

Summary

The guiding question for this chapter has been this: How can knowledge of neuroscience inform pediatric psychology practice? The translational "two-way street" between basic research and clinical practice is clearly in its early stages of development, but moving rapidly forward. We anticipate that the next edition of this *Handbook* may include translational findings within many of the specific chapters. In the meantime, it is important that practicing clinicians actively and regularly consider how findings from neuroscience research may be relevant to treatment of any developmental concern. For example, understanding that an important form of reading disability arises as a consequence of phonological processing difficulties has made a dramatic impact on the development of effective reading interventions (see Shaywitz, Lyon, & Shaywitz, 2006).

Conversely, investigators in clinically based neuroscience research must take care to account for the rich complexity of the behaviors and individuals seen in clinical settings, and to ensure that important findings from basic research are disseminated to practice settings in a timely and effective manner.

Recommended Readings

For more in-depth discussions of clinical neuroscience in other areas of interest to pediatric psychology, we recommend the following:

ADHD and Conduct Problems: Nigg, J. T., & Casey, B. J. (2005). An integrative theory of attention-deficit/hyperactivity disorder based on the cognitive and affective neurosciences. *Development and Psychopathology, 17,* 785–806.

Attachment/Bonding: Swain, J. E., Lorberbaum, J. P., Kose, S., & Strathearn, L. (2007). Brain basis of early parent–infant interactions: Psychology, physiology, and *in vivo* functional neuroimaging studies. *Journal of Child Psychology and Psychiatry, 48,* 262–287.

Autism Spectrum Disorders: South, M., Ozonoff, S., & Schultz, R. T. (2008). Neurocognitive development in autism. In C. A. Nelson & M. Luciana (Eds.), *Handbook of developmental cognitive neuroscience* (2nd ed., pp. 701–716). Cambridge, MA: MIT Press.

Childhood Anxiety: Pine, D. S. (2007). Research review: A neuroscience framework for pediatric anxiety disorders. *Journal of Child Psychology and Psychiatry, 48,* 631–648.

Childhood Depression: Miller, A. (2007). Social neuroscience of child and adolescent depression. *Brain and Cognition, 65,* 47–68.

Learning Disabilities: Fawcett, A. J., & Nicolson, R. I. (2007). Dyslexia, learning, and pedagogical neuroscience. *Developmental Medicine and Child Neurology, 49,* 306–311.

Acknowledgments

We would like to thank Michael Crowley and Bob Schultz for their conceptual input, and Annahir Cariello, Julianne Dana, Kandice Ellett, Cassie Niersel, and Carolyn Talley for their assistance in preparing the manuscript.

References

Ackles, P. (2008). Stimulus novelty and cognitive-related ERP components of the infant brain. *Perceptual and Motor Skills, 106,* 3–20.

American Psychiatric Association. (2000). *Diagnostic and statistical manual of mental disorders: DSM-IV-TR* (4th ed., text rev.). Washington, DC: Author.

Anderson, G. M. (2002). Genetics of childhood disorders: XLV. Autism, part 4: Serotonin in autism. *Journal of the American Academy of Child and Adolescent Psychiatry, 41,* 1513–1516.

Anderson, G. M. (2008). The potential role for emergence in autism. *Autism Research, 1,* 18–30.

Bachevalier, J., & Loveland, K. A. (2006). The orbitofrontal–amygdala circuit and self-regulation of social-emotional behavior in autism. *Neuroscience and Biobehavioral Reviews, 30,* 1–21.

Barkley, R. A. (1997). Behavioral inhibition, sustained attention, and executive functions: Constructing a unifying theory of AD/HD. *Psychological Bulletin, 121,* 65–94.

Biederman, J. (2003). Pharmacotherapy for attention-deficit/hyperactivity disorder (AD/HD) decreases the risk for substance abuse: Findings from a longitudinal follow-up of youths with and without AD/HD. *Journal of Clinical Psychiatry, 64,* 3–8.

Blondeau, C., & Dellu-Hagedorn, F. (2006). Dimensional analysis of AD/HD subtypes in rats. *Biological Psychiatry, 61,* 1340–1350.

Brennan, A., & Arnsten, A. (2008). Neuronal mechanisms underlying attention deficit hyperactivity disorder: The influence of arousal on prefrontal cortical function. *Annals of the New York Academy of Sciences, 1129,* 236–245.

Bush, G. (2008). Neuroimaging of attention deficit hyperactivity disorder: Can new imaging findings be integrated in clinical practice? *Child and Adolescent Psychiatric Clinics of North America, 17,* 385–404.

Bush, G., Valera, E. M., & Seidman, L. J. (2005). Functional neuroimaging of attention-deficit/hyperactivity disorder: A review and suggested future directions. *Biological Psychiatry, 57,* 1273–1284.

Casey, B. J., Durston, S., & Fossella, J. (2001). A mechanistic model of cognitive control: Clinical, neuroimaging, and lesion studies. *Clinical Neuroscience Research, 1,* 267–282.

Casey, B. J., Epstein, J. N., Buhle, J., Liston, C., Davidson, M. C., Tonev, S. T., et al. (2007). Frontostriatal connectivity and its role in cognitive control in parent–child dyads with AD/HD. *American Journal of Psychiatry, 164,* 1729–1736.

Cleavinger, H., Bigler, E., Johnson, J., Lu, J., McMahon, W., & Lainhart, J. (2008). Quantitative magnetic resonance image analysis of the cerebellum in macrocephalic and normocephalic children and adults with autism. *Journal of the International Neuropsychological Society, 14,* 401–413.

Cornish, K. M., Manly, T., Savage, R., Swanson, J., Morisano, D., Bulter, N., et al. (2005). Association of the dopamine transporter (DAT1) 10/10-repeat genotype with ADHD symptoms and response inhibition in a general population sample. *Molecular Psychiatry, 10,* 686–698.

Crawley, J. N. (2007). Mouse behavioral assays relevant to the symptoms of autism. *Brain Pathology, 17,* 448–459.

Crosbie, J., Pérusse, D., Barr, C. L., & Schachar, R. J. (2007). Validating psychiatric endophenotypes: Inhibitory control and attention deficit hyperactivity disorder. *Neuroscience and Biobehavioral Reviews, 32,* 40–55.

Cuthbert, B. N. (2005). Dimensional models of psychopathology: Research agenda and clinical utility. *Journal of Abnormal Psychology, 114,* 565–569.

Dalton, K. M., Nacewicz, B. M., Johnstone, T., Schaefer, H. S., Gernsbacher, M. A., Goldsmith, H. H., et al. (2005). Gaze fixation and the neural circuitry of face processing in autism. *Nature Neuroscience, 8,* 519–526.

Diamond, A. (2005). Attention-deficit disorder (attention-deficit/hyperactivity disorder without hyperactivity): A neurobiologically and behaviorally distinct disorder from attention-deficit/hyperactivity disorder (with hyperactivity). *Development and Psychopathology, 17,* 807–825.

Durston, S., Mulder, M., Casey, B. J., Ziermans, T., & Van Engeland, H. (2006). Activation in ventral prefrontal cortex is sensitive to genetic vulnerability for attention-deficit hyperactivity disorder. *Biological Psychiatry, 60,* 1062–1070.

Epstein, J. N., Casey, B. J., Tonev, S. T., Davidson, M. C., Reiss, A. L., Garrett, A., et al. (2007) AD/HD- and medication-related brain activation differences in concordantly affected parent–child dyads with AD/HD. *Journal of Child Psychology and Psychiatry, 48,* 899–913.

Faja, S., Aylward, E., Bernier, R., & Dawson, G. (2008). Becoming a face expert: A computerized face-training program for high-functioning individuals with autism spectrum disorders. *Developmental Neuropsychology, 33,* 1–24.

Fassbender, C., & Schweitzer, J. B. (2006). Is there evidence for neural compensation in attention deficit hyperactivity disorder?: A review of the functional neuroimaging literature. *Clinical Psychology Review*, 26, 445–465.

Furman, L. (2005). What is attention-deficit hyperactivity disorder (AD/HD)? *Journal of Child Neurology*, 20, 994–1002.

Geurts, H. M., Verté, S., Oosterlaan, J., Roeyers, H., & Sergeant, J. A. (2005). ADHD subtypes: Do they differ in their executive functioning profile? *Archives of Clinical Neuropsychology*, 20, 457–477.

Gottesman, I. I., & Gould, T. G. (2003). The endophenotype concept in psychiatry: Etymology and strategic intentions. *American Journal of Psychiatry*, 160, 636–645.

Gray, C. A. (1998). Social stories and comic strip conversations with students with Asperger syndrome and high-functioning autism. In E. Schopler, G. B. Mesibov, & L. J. Kunce (Eds.), *Asperger syndrome or high-functioning autism?* (pp. 167–198). New York: Plenum Press.

Gray, J. D., Punsoni, M., Tabori, N. E., Melton, J. T., Fanslow, V., Ward, M. J., et al. (2007). Methylphenidate administration to juvenile rats alters brain areas involved in cognition, motivated behaviors, appetite, and stress. *Journal of Neuroscience*, 27, 7196–7207.

Gutstein, S. E., Burgess, A. F., & Montfort, K. (2007). Evaluation of the Relationship Development Intervention program. *Autism*, 11, 397–411.

Haist, F., Adamo, M., Westerfield, M., Courchesne, E., & Townsend, J. (2005). The functional neuroanatomy of spatial attention in autism spectrum disorder. *Developmental Neuropsychology*, 27, 425– 458.

Hebb, D. O. (1949). *The organization of behavior.* New York: Wiley.

Helms, C. M., Gubner, N. R., Wilhelm, C. J., Mitchell, S. H., & Grandy, D. K. (2008). D4 receptor deficiency in mice has limited effects on impulsivity and novelty seeking. *Pharmacology, Biochemistry, and Behavior*, 90, 387–393.

Infant Brain Imaging Study Network. (2008). *Brain development in autism: Infant siblings.* Retrieved July 18, 2008, from *www.babysibsimaging.org*

Joober, R., Grizenko, N., Sengupta, S., Amor, L., Schmitz, N., Schwartz, G., et al. (2007). Dopamine transporter 3'-UTR VNTR genotype and AD/HD: A pharmaco-behavioural genetic study with methylphenidate. *Neuropsychopharmacology*, 32, 1370–1376.

Just, M., Cherkassky, V., Keller, T., Kana, R., & Minshew, N. (2007). Functional and anatomical cortical underconnectivity in autism: Evidence from an FMRI study of an executive function task and corpus callosum morphometry. *Cerebral Cortex*, 17, 951–961.

Kamps, D. M., Leonard, B. R., Vernon, S., Dugan, E. P., Delquadri, J. C., Gershon, B., et al. (1992). Teaching social skills to students with autism to increase peer interactions in an integrated first-grade classroom. *Journal of Applied Behavior Analysis*, 25, 281–288.

Kanwisher, N., McDermott, J., & Chun, M. M. (1997). The fusiform face area: A module in human extrastriate cortex specialized for face perception. *Journal of Neuroscience*, 17, 4302–4311.

Kolevzon, A., Mathewson, K., & Hollander, E. (2006). Selective serotonin reuptake inhibitors in autism: A review of efficacy and tolerability. *Journal of Clinical Psychiatry*, 67, 407–414.

Manor, I., Corbex, M., Eisenberg, J., Gritsenkso, I., Bachner-Melman, R., Tyano, S., et al. (2004). Association of the dopamine D5 receptor with attention deficit hyperactivity disorder (AD/HD) and scores on a continuous performance test (TOVA). *American Journal of Medical Genetics: Part B. Neuropsychiatric Genetics*, 127, 73–77.

Marreiros, A., Kiebel, S., & Friston, K. (2008). Dynamic causal modelling for fMRI: A two-state model. *NeuroImage*, 39, 269–278.

McClure, E. B., Adler, A., Monk, C. S., Cameron, J., Smith, S., Nelson, E. E., et al. (2007). fMRI predictors of treatment outcome in pediatric anxiety disorders. *Psychopharmacology*, 191, 97–105.

McFarlane, H. G., Kusek, G. K., Yang, M., Phoenix, J. L., Bolivar, V. J., & Crawley, J. N.

(2008). Autism-like behavioral phenotypes in BTBR T+tf/J mice. *Genes, Brain, and Behavior, 7,* 152–163.

Merin, N., Young, G. S., Ozonoff, S., & Rogers, S. J. (2007). Visual fixation patterns during reciprocal social interaction distinguish a subgroup of 6-month-old infants at-risk for autism from comparison infants. *Journal of Autism and Developmental Disorders, 37,* 108–121.

Moffitt, T. E., Caspi, A., & Rutter, M. (2005). Strategy for investigating interactions between measured genes and measured environments. *Archives of General Psychiatry, 62,* 473–481.

Morrow, E. M., Yoo, S., Flavell, S. W., Kim, T., Lin, Y., Hill, R. S., et al. (2008). Identifying autism loci and genes by tracing recent shared ancestry. *Science, 321,* 218–223.

National Institutes of Health. (2008). *NIH Roadmap for Medical Research.* Retrieved July 18, 2008, from *nihroadmap.nih.gov/clinicalresearch/overview-translational.asp*

Odegard, T., Ring, J., Smith, S., Biggan, J., & Black, J. (2008). Differentiating the neural response to intervention in children with developmental dyslexia. *Annals of Dyslexia, 58,* 1–14.

Pierce, K., & Schreibman, L. (1997). Multiple peer use of pivotal response training to increase social behaviors of classmates with autism: Results from trained and untrained peers. *Journal of Applied Behavior Analysis, 30,* 157–160.

Plizska, S. R., Glahn, D. C., Semrud-Clikeman, M., Franklin, C., Perez, R., III, Xiong, J., et al. (2006). Neuroimaging of inhibitory control areas in children with attention deficit hyperactivity disorder who were treatment naive or in long-term treatment. *American Journal of Psychiatry, 163,* 1052–1060.

Reiger, D. A. (2007). Dimensional approaches to psychiatric classification: Refining the research agenda for DSM-V: An introduction. *International Journal of Methods in Psychiatric Research, 16*(Suppl. 1), S1–S5.

Ring, H. A., Baron-Cohen, S., Wheelwright, S., Williams, S. C., Brammer, M., Andrew, C., et al. (1999). Cerebral correlates of preserved cognitive skills in autism: A functional MRI study of embedded figures task performance. *Brain, 122,* 1305–1315.

Robinson, E. S., Eagle, D. M., Mar, A. C., Bari, A., Banerjee, G., Jiang, X., et al. (2008). Similar effects of the selective noradrenaline reuptake inhibitor atomoxetine on three distinct forms of impulsivity in the rat. *Neuropsychopharmacology, 33,* 1028–1037.

Rubia, K., Smith, A. B., Brammer, M. J., Toone, B., & Taylor, E. (2005). Abnormal brain activation during inhibition and error detection in medication-naive adolescents with AD/HD. *American Journal of Psychiatry, 162,* 1067–1075.

Scahill, L. (2008). How do I decide whether or not to use medication for my child with autism? Should I try behavior therapy first? *Journal of Autism and Developmental Disorders, 38,* 1197–1198.

Schultz, R. T. (2005). Developmental deficits in social perception in autism: The role of the amygdala and fusiform face area. *International Journal of Developmental Neuroscience, 23,* 125–141.

Shaywitz, B. A., Lyon, G. R., & Shaywitz, S. E. (2006). The role of functional magnetic resonance imaging in understanding reading and dyslexia. *Developmental Neuropsychology, 30,* 613–632.

Skuse, D. (2006). Genetic influences on the neural basis of social cognition. *Philosophical Transactions of the Royal Society of London, Series B, 361,* 2129–2141.

South, M., Ozonoff, S., & Schultz, R. T. (2008). Neurocognitive development in autism. In C. A. Nelson & M. Luciana (Eds.), *Handbook of developmental cognitive neuroscience* (2nd ed., pp. 701–716). Cambridge, MA: MIT Press.

South, M., Ozonoff, S., Suchy, Y., Kesner, R. P., McMahon, W. M., & Lainhart, J. E. (2008). Intact emotion facilitation for nonsocial stimuli in autism: Is amygdala impairment in autism specific for social information? *Journal of the International Neuropsychological Society, 14,* 42–54.

Sutcliffe, J. S. (2008). Genetics. Insights into the pathogenesis of autism. *Science, 321,* 208–209.

Tabuchi, K., Blundell, J., Etherton, M. R., Hammer, R. E., Liu, X., Powell, C. M., et al. (2008). A neuroligin-3 mutation implicated in autism increases inhibitory synaptic transmission in mice. *Science, 318,* 71–76.

Tanaka, J., Lincoln, S., & Hegg, L. (2003). A framework for the study and treatment of face processing deficits in autism. In H. Leder & G. Swartzer (Eds.), *The development of face processing* (pp. 101–119). Berlin: Hogrefe.

Todd, R. D., Huang, H., Smalley, S. L., Nelson, S. F., Willcutt, E. G., Pennington, B. F., et al. (2005). Collaborative analysis of DRD4 and DAT genotypes in population-defined AD/HD subtypes. *Journal of Child Psychology and Psychiatry, 46,* 1067–1073.

Wodka, E. L., Mahone, E. M., Blankner, J. G., Larson, J. C. G., Fotedar, S., Denckla, M. B., et al. (2007). Evidence that response inhibition is a primary deficit in AD/HD. *Journal of Clinical and Experimental Neuropsychology, 29,* 345–356.

Wolf, J. M., Tanaka, J. W., Klaiman, C., Koenig, K., Cockburn, J., Herlihy, L., et al. (2008). *Let's Face It!: A computer-based intervention for strengthening face processing skills in individuals with autism spectrum disorders.* Paper presented at the 7th International Meeting for Autism Research, London.

CHAPTER 50

Allergic Reactions in Children
Implications for Pediatric Psychology

KIMBERLEE M. ROY
YELENA P. WU
MICHAEL C. ROBERTS

Allergies, or the body's immunological response to normally innocuous substances as toxins, affect millions of people in the United States. For children, population estimates range from 40% for hay fever (Academy of Allergy, Asthma, and Immunology, 2000) to 8% for food allergies (Wood, 2003) to 15% for atopic dermatitis (Leung, 2003). Allergic reactions can occur in response to a variety of substances, including pollen, dust, animals, foods, insect bites, latex, and medications. In the past several years, research into the effects of allergies has begun to find that children with allergies face many physical and psychosocial challenges and effects, akin to those confronted by children with other chronic illnesses. This chapter outlines the medical aspects of allergic disorders in children, reviews the relatively small literature on the psychological effects of allergies, and discusses the future of this expanding field of investigation and application.

Description of the Allergic Response

The body's allergic response takes place in three stages: sensitization, mast cell activation, and prolonged immune activation (Muth, 2002). In the first stage the allergen encounters the immune system; although no reaction is produced at this stage, the body is primed for future encounters with the allergen. Antibodies are created for that particular substance. These antibodies are then distributed to mast cells in the body. In the second stage, the allergen encounters the body again. The body recognizes the allergen as harmful, and histamines and leukotrienes are released. These chemicals cause the symptoms recognized as an allergy attack. In the third stage, prolonged immune activation, mast cells continue to release histamines and leukotrienes and attract other cells to the area. These other cells continue to release histamines and leukotrienes, and the increased production of chemicals can cause cell damage.

The effects of the allergic response often depend on the type of allergen encountered. The most common reaction involves hay fever symptoms, including sneezing, sinus congestion, watering eyes, and coughing. Allergens can also cause skin reactions (such as hives and atopic dermatitis) or gastrointestinal symptoms (such as stomach upset and diarrhea). If the reaction is severe, systemic anaphylaxis can occur. Early anaphylactic symptoms may include oral tingling, a sensation of tightening airways, abdominal pain, nausea, vomiting, and skin flushing. These symptoms can progress into greater respiratory difficulty, hypotension, and dysrhythmias if left untreated, as typically develop in fatal and near-fatal cases. To qualify as a true anaphylactic reaction, the reaction must be multisystemic (Foucard & Malmheden-Yman, 2001).

Diagnosis

The diagnosis of an allergy is often made by a careful assessment of the patient's medical history, including reactions to substances and family history of allergies. Allergies are often comorbid with one another and with asthma (McQuaid, Mitchell, & Esteban, 2006), so it is essential to ascertain which allergens are causing the allergic reaction. To increase diagnostic certainty, a skin prick test may be completed: The individual is exposed to a series of environmental allergens concentrated in liquid form, applied to pins, and scratched into the skin on the back and/or arms. If an allergy to a substance is present, a red wheal (hive) appears where the skin has been scratched. Allergists measure the size of the wheal to determine the level of reactivity to the substance. When the wheal is too small to be considered reactive but is still present, a larger amount of the allergen is injected into the skin, and a further reaction is awaited. Skin prick tests are painful and can cause itchiness and bruising. Another skin reaction method involves spreading the allergen on a patch placed on the skin. After a period of time, the patch is removed, and red wheals are looked for. This is useful for ascertaining contact reaction when pin pricks or injection are not feasible (chemicals).

Another method is radioallergosorbent testing (RAST), which looks for the blood concentration of immunoglobulin E, a type of protein in the blood plasma that acts as an antibody in allergic reactions (Zepf, 2002). Unfortunately, RAST can yield inconsistent results and cannot diagnose an allergy. Rather, RAST can only suggest the potential for an allergy. Oral challenges are often the only definitive way to make a diagnosis of food allergy. The "gold standard" of oral food challenges is the double-blind placebo-controlled challenge (Bahna, 2007). Because such challenges can lead to severe anaphylactic symptoms, they should only be conducted in a hospital setting by an experienced specialist (Sampson, 2002). The risk of severe anaphylactic symptoms in such a challenge, however, may lead some parents to eliminate potential allergens from their children's environment without confirmation of a diagnosis.

Treatment

Treatment of allergies varies, depending on the type of allergy. For example, atopic dermatitis (itchy, inflamed skin) is often treated with topical ointments and corticosteroids, whereas treatment for allergic rhinitis (hay fever symptoms in reaction to an environmental substance) includes over-the-counter or prescription medications such as antihistamines and decongestants (Muth, 2002). Traditional antihistamines are generally available over the counter and can relieve such symptoms as sneezing and watery eyes by blocking the release of histamines by immune cells. A side effect of traditional antihistamines is that they tend to cause drowsiness. For this reason, traditional antihistamines are sometimes combined with decongestants, which have stimulating side effects that counteract the drowsiness. However, decongestants can cause nervousness, restlessness, or insomnia. Newer forms of antihistamines perform the same tasks as traditional ones, but do so without any sedating effects. Although some of the newer antihistamines are available over the counter, many are still available by prescription and cost significantly more than traditional medications. Intranasal corticosteroids may be used and cause fewer side effects than traditional antihistamines, but are less effective at treating watery and itchy eyes. Oral corticosteroids may be used on a limited basis (3–7 days) for more severe and treatment-resistant allergy symptoms.

When children are being treated for allergic rhinitis, nonpharmacological approaches, such as removing the allergen from the environment, are preferred (Smith & McGhan, 2002). When this is not feasible, oral antihistamines and nonsteroid intranasal treatments are the next choice. The sedating effects of some antihistamines can be beneficial for children (e.g., allowing them to sleep comfortably), but may have daytime effects that interfere with educational functioning and social interactions. Intranasal corticosteroids are effective in children, but they may have a temporary stunting effect on growth, and dosages should be small and monitored (Smith & McGhan, 2002). Allergen immunotherapy, or "allergy shots," can be used in people who have yearly, recurrent, seasonal symptoms of long duration, or perennial symptoms. However, allergy shots are not recommended for preschool-age children, because anaphylaxis (although rare) can occur. Treatment is also not recommended for more than 3–5 years' duration (Muth, 2002).

For some allergies, including foods, latex, bee stings, and medications, avoidance of the allergen is the only treatment. For this reason, children with these types of allergies are recommended to have emergency kits available at all times (American Academy of Pediatrics, 2001), including diphenhydramine and a shot of autoinjectable epinephrine (Epipen or Epipen Jr.) to treat symptoms after an exposure.

Challenges for Children with Allergies and Their Families

Children with allergies face numerous challenges that may differ, depending on the severity and type of their allergies. These challenges range from living with uncomfortable allergy symptoms to constant vigilance for possible allergen exposure. Although many children and their families adjust well, children with allergies may exhibit a range of psychosocial problems. However, there is little evidence for a causal relationship between allergies and psychosocial problems (or vice versa). Allergies may affect several areas of functioning and development, including individuation from parents, socialization outside the family, and establishment of peer relations. This is similar to findings for children with asthma, an ailment that also can cause the sudden onset of life-threatening symptoms (see McQuaid & Abramson, Chapter 17, this volume).

Some research suggests that children with allergies may be more likely to be withdrawn and to exhibit internalizing disorders such as depression (e.g., Bell, 1992; Watten & Faleide, 1996), and that this tendency may be due to genetic causes (Wamboldt, Schmitz, & Mrazek, 1998). Conversely, other research suggests that children with internalizing disorders are more likely to have allergies (e.g., Infante, Slattery, Klein, & Essex, 2007). The few studies that have examined the relationship between internalizing disorders and allergies (not asthma) have focused on anxiety disorders. For example, children with panic disorder appear to be more likely to have allergies (Kovalenko et al., 2001). In addition, Slattery and colleagues (2002) reported that children with separation anxiety disorder had higher rates of atopic disorders (asthma, hives, hay fever, and eczema). However, there is considerably more research supporting the connection between anxiety disorders and allergies in adults (Teufel et al., 2007).

One explanation for the increased rate of internalizing problems is that children with allergies may be shy and have behaviorally inhibited temperaments (Bell, 1992; Kagan, Snidman, Julia-Sellers, & Johnson, 1991; Lilljeqvist, Smorvik, & Faleide, 2002). Another possible explanation is the isolation that children may feel or the teasing they may endure because of their allergies (Lewis-Jones, 2006).

Children with allergies may also exhibit a range of externalizing behaviors, such as aggression (Watten & Faleide, 1996) and hyperactivity (Roth, Beyreiss, Schlenzka, & Beyer, 1991). Roth and colleagues (1991) suggested that there might be a common biological mechanism underlying attention/hyperactivity problems and some allergies (e.g., eczema and food allergies). However, support for this hypothesis is mixed (Miller, 1995). Perhaps adding to the confusion is that children may present with inattention and hyperactivity due to allergy symptoms, and these symptoms can lead to a misdiagnosis of attention-deficit/hyperactivity disorder (ADHD) (McLeod, 2004). In addition, children with allergies such as hay fever may have more sleep and academic difficulties, and these may contribute to ADHD-type symptoms (Brawley et al., 2004).

Children with allergies may have difficulty sleeping (i.e., problems with falling asleep and interrupted sleep). Like hay fever, certain food allergies (e.g., an allergy to cow's milk) are especially likely to affect children's sleep (Kahn et al., 2001). Allergy-related scratching or diarrhea may awaken children and cause sleepiness and impaired functioning during the day (Lewis-Jones, 2006). In the case of atopic dermatitis, even children with controlled symptoms may experience sleep difficulties (Reuveni, Chapnick, Tal, & Tarasiuk, 1999).

Children with allergies may encounter a variety of challenges related to their allergies in the school setting. Children with food allergies need to be monitored closely for the foods they are exposed to, as well as for the classmates they are permitted to sit next to during meals and snacks. Children may also need to be monitored on field trips and on the playground (McIntyre, Sheetz, Carroll, & Young, 2005). It is recommended that schools institute protocols for how allergic events should be handled (McIntyre et al., 2005). Some parents choose to home-school their children with allergies, due to the unpredictability of allergen exposure in the school environment and perhaps due to the allergy severity (Bollinger et al., 2006). Few studies of academic achievement in children with allergies have been conducted, but one study conducted in Sweden has suggested that children with severe rhinitis are more likely to have poor grades (Sundberg, Toren, Hoglund, Aberg, & Brisman, 2007). In addition, children who have poor sleep can have academic difficulties that may lead to the development of learning disabilities (Reuveni et al., 1999).

Some allergies such as eczema may have obvious physical effects that impede children's social functioning (Lewis-Jones, 2006; McLeod, 2004; Miller, 1995). Furthermore, to prevent exposure to allergens, children may be restricted in the social events (e.g., birthday parties) they attend (Bollinger et al., 2006). Although minimizing children's exposure to allergens can be necessary for avoiding impairing or dangerous allergic responses, the impact on children's social development and functioning may be considerable.

The demands of caring for a child with allergies can greatly affect family functioning on a daily basis (Sicherer, Noone, & Munoz-Furlong, 2001). For example, food preparation in a family where a child has food allergies can be a daily challenge, and family members' activities may be restricted by such allergies (Bollinger et al., 2006). Caregivers may also experience stress (Bollinger et al., 2006), disturbed sleep, and higher levels of anxiety and depression (Moore, David, Murray, Child, & Arkwright, 2006). Conversely, characteristics of the family, such as a parent's encouragement of a child's independence, may affect the child's allergy symptoms (Dennis, Rostill, Reed, & Gill, 2006).

Role of Pediatric Psychologists in Treating Children with Allergies

Given the numerous challenges children with allergies and their families face, pediatric psychologists can play an important role in treating allergies and improving medical outcomes (Capoore, Rowland Payne, & Goldin, 1998). Although the intervention research is somewhat limited, the existing literature suggests that a biopsychosocial approach may be most useful in working with family members of a child with an allergy (Barankin & DeKoven, 2002). Anxiety related to the child's allergy is often an important target of intervention. Although some level of anxiety and vigilance is adaptive, a pediatric psychologist can help family members manage anxiety by providing education to the parents and child about the psychosocial impact of allergies, teaching the child relaxation techniques, working with the child's school to prevent exposure to allergens, minimizing the child's feelings of being singled out because of the allergy, and supporting parents in their coping with their child's allergy. In addition, interventions may include supporting children during anxiety-provoking and painful procedures such as allergy testing (Jeffs, 2007). The specific interventions used will depend on how a child's or family's anxiety is related to the allergy and how the allergy affects the child's and family's lives. Given the prevalence of allergies in children, pediatric psychologists may also consider using a support group format or group intervention (Monga & Manassis, 2006).

Because a child's allergy affects all members of the family (Lauritzen, 2004), interventions often address family members' concerns and adjustment. In some cases, supporting parents' psychological adjustment may have beneficial effects on children's adjustment to their allergy (Dennis et al., 2006; Monga & Manassis, 2006). A balance between easing parents' worries and helping them to encourage their children's developmentally appropriate independence on the one hand, and acknowledging needed levels of vigilance on the other, is very important to attain in these families. At other times, pediatric psychologists may need to work with families to improve adherence to allergy medications (Blaiss, 2004) or to help families minimize their children's exposure to allergens (Maloney, Chapman, & Sicherer, 2006). Pediatric psychologists can also help families understand the connections between their children's allergies and such outcomes as quality of life. There are several quality-of-life measures for specific allergic conditions that may be useful (e.g., Lewis-Jones, 2006; Meltzer, 2001; Roberts, Hurley, & Lack, 2003; Teufel et al., 2007).

Future Directions

Many challenges that children with allergies and their families face can be addressed through collaborative efforts among the children, the families, the medical team, school personnel, and pediatric psychologists. Although the research literature on the relationship between psychosocial functioning and childhood allergies is growing, substantial work remains to be done. Future research should continue to explore the psychosocial and quality of life outcomes associated with a range of childhood allergies. Also, studies should address the complex interplay among the biology underlying allergies (e.g., immune activation), children's and families' psychosocial functioning, and children's medical outcomes. Together, these studies will provide a strong basis for the interventions that pediatric psychologists can then design, implement, test, and disseminate, so that children with allergies and their families achieve the best possible medical and psychological outcomes.

References

Academy of Allergy, Asthma, and Immunology. (2000). *The allergy report: Science-based findings on the diagnosis and treatment of allergic children.* Milwaukee, WI: Author.

American Academy of Pediatrics. (2001). Guidelines for emergency medical care in school (RE9954). *Pediatrics, 107,* 435–436.

Bahna, S. L. (2007). Food challenges procedure: Optimal choice for clinical practice. *Asthma and Allergy Proceedings, 28,* 640–646.

Barankin, B., & DeKoven, J. (2002). Psychosocial effect of common skin diseases. *Canadian Family Physician, 48,* 712–716.

Bell, I. R. (1992). Allergens, physical irritants, depression, and shyness. *Journal of Applied Developmental Psychology, 13,* 125–133.

Blaiss, M. S. (2004). Allergic rhinitis and impairment issues in schoolchildren: A consensus report. *Current Medical Research and Opinion, 20,* 1937–1952.

Bollinger, M. E., Dahlquist, L. M., Mudd, K., Sonntag, C., Dillinger, L., & Mckenna, K. (2006). The impact of food allergy on the daily activities of children and their families. *Annals of Allergy, Asthma, and Immunology, 96,* 415–421.

Brawley, A., Silverman, B., Kearney, S., Guanzon, D., Owens, M., Bennett, H., et al. (2004). Allergic rhinitis in children with attention-deficit/hyperactivity disorder. *Annals of Allergy, Asthma, and Immunology, 92,* 663–667.

Capoore, H. S., Rowland Payne, C. M. E., & Goldin, D. (1998). Does psychological intervention help chronic skin conditions? *Postgraduate Medical Journal, 74,* 662–664.

Dennis, H., Rostill, H., Reed, J., & Gill, S. (2006). Factors promoting adjustment to childhood atopic eczema. *Journal of Child Health Care, 10,* 126–139.

Foucard, T., & Malmheden-Yman, I. (2001). Food-induced anaphylaxis. *Pediatric Allergy Immunology, 12*(Suppl. 14), 97–101.

Infante, M., Slattery, M. J., Klein, M. H., & Essex, M. J. (2007). Association of internalizing disorders and allergies in a child and adolescent psychiatry clinical sample. *Journal of Clinical Psychiatry, 68,* 1419–1425.

Jeffs, D. A. (2007). A pilot study of distraction for adolescents during allergy testing. *Journal for Specialists in Pediatric Nursing, 12,* 170–185.

Kagan, J., Snidman, N., Julia-Sellers, M., & Johnson, M. O. (1991). Temperament and allergic symptoms. *Psychosomatic Medicine, 53,* 332–340.

Kahn, A., Mozin, M. J., Groswasser, J., Sottiaux, M., Dan, B., Scaillet, S., et al. (2001). Sleep disorders and childhood allergy. In G. Stores & L. Wiggs (Eds.), *Sleep disturbance in children and adolescents with disorders of development* (pp. 137–139). London: Mac Keith Press.

Kovalenko, P. A., Hoven, C. W., Wu, P., Wicks, J., Mandell, D. J., & Tiet, Q. (2001). Associations between allergy and anxiety disorders in youth. *Australian and New Zealand Journal of Psychiatry, 35,* 815–821.

Lauritzen, S. O. (2004). Lay voices on allergic conditions in children: Parents' narratives and the negotiation of a diagnosis. *Social Science and Medicine, 58,* 1299–1308.

Leung, D. Y. M. (2003). Atopic dermatitis (atopic eczema). In M. Hill (Ed.), *Fitzpatrick's dermatology in general medicine* (6th ed., pp. 1180–1194). New York: McGraw-Hill.

Lewis-Jones, S. (2006). Quality of life and childhood atopic dermatitis: The misery of living with childhood eczema. *International Journal of Clinical Practice, 60,* 984–992.

Lilljeqvist, A. C., Smorvik, D., & Faleide, A. O. (2002). Temperamental differences between healthy, asthmatic, and allergic children before onset of illness: A longitudinal prospective study of asthma development. *Journal of Genetic Psychology, 163,* 219–227.

Maloney, J. M., Chapman, M. D., & Sicherer, S. H. (2006). Peanut allergen exposure through saliva: Assessment and interventions to reduce exposure. *Journal of Allergy and Clinical Immunology, 118,* 719–724.

McIntyre, C. L., Sheetz, A. H., Carroll, C. R., & Young, M. C. (2005). Administration of epinephrine for life-threatening allergic reactions in school settings. *Pediatrics, 116,* 1134–1140.

McLeod, R. P. (2004). Lumps, bumps, and things that go itch in your office! *Journal of School Nursing, 20,* 57–59.

McQuaid, E. L., Mitchell, D. K., & Esteban, C. A. (2006). Allergies and asthma. In G. G. Bear & K. M. Minke (Eds.), *Children's needs III: Development, prevention, and intervention* (pp. 909–924). Bethesda, MD: National Association of School Psychologists.

Meltzer, E. O. (2001). Quality of life in adults and children with allergic rhinitis. *Journal of Allergy and Clinical Immunology, 108,* S45–S53.

Miller, K. (1995). Psychoneurological aspects of food allergy. In B. E. Leonard & K. Miller (Eds.), *Stress, the immune system, and psychiatry* (pp. 185–206). New York: Wiley.

Monga, S., & Manassis, K. (2006). Treating anxiety in children with life-threatening anaphylactic conditions. *Journal of the American Academy of Child and Adolescent Psychiatry, 45,* 1007–1010.

Moore, K., David, T. J., Murray, C. S., Child, F., & Arkwright, P. D. (2006). Effect of childhood eczema and asthma on parental sleep and well-being: A prospective comparative study. *British Journal of Dermatology, 154,* 514–518.

Muth, A. S. (Ed.). (2002). *Allergies sourcebook* (2nd ed.). Detroit, MI: Omnigraphics.

Reuveni, H., Chapnick, G., Tal, A., & Tarasiuk, A. (1999). Sleep fragmentation in children with atopic dermatitis. *Archives of Pediatrics and Adolescent Medicine, 153,* 249–253.

Roberts, G., Hurley, C., & Lack, G. (2003). Development of a quality-of-life assessment for the allergic child or teenager with multisystem allergic disease. *Journal of Allergy and Clinical Immunology, 111,* 491–497.

Roth, N., Beyreiss, J., Schlenzka, K., & Beyer, H. (1991). Coincidence of attention deficit disorder and atopic disorders in children: Empirical findings and hypothetical background. *Journal of Abnormal Child Psychology, 19,* 1–13.

Sampson, H. A. (2002). Peanut allergy. *New England Journal of Medicine, 346,* 1294–1299.

Sicherer, S. H., Noone, S. A., & Munoz-Furlong, A. (2001). The impact of childhood food allergy on quality of life. *Annals of Allergy, Asthma, and Immunology, 87*, 461–464.

Slattery, M. J., Klein, D. F., Mannuzza, S., Moulton, J. L., Pine, D. S., & Klein, D. G. (2002). Relationship between separation anxiety disorder, parental panic disorder, and atopic disorders in children: A controlled high-risk study. *Journal of the American Academy of Child and Adolescent Psychiatry, 41*, 947–954.

Smith, M. D., & McGhan, W. F. (2002). Allergy's sting: It's partly economic. In A. S. Muth (Ed.), *Allergies sourcebook* (2nd ed., pp. 12–15). Detroit, MI: Omnigraphics.

Sundberg, R., Toren, K., Hoglund, D., Aberg, N., & Brisman, J. (2007). Nasal symptoms are associated with school performance in adolescents. *Journal of Adolescent Health, 40*, 581–583.

Teufel, M., Biedermann, T., Rapps, N., Hausteiner, C., Henningsen, P., Enck, P., et al. (2007). Psychological burden of food allergy. *World Journal of Gastroenterology, 13*, 3456–3465.

Wamboldt, M. Z., Schmitz, S., & Mrazek, D. (1998). Genetic association between atopy and behavioral symptoms in middle childhood. *Journal of Child Psychology and Psychiatry, 39*, 1007–1016.

Watten, R. G., & Faleide, A. O. (1996). Behavioural and mental health profiles in childhood hay fever. *British Journal of Health Psychology, 1*, 349–355.

Wood, R. A. (2003). The natural history of food allergy. *Pediatrics, 111*, 1631–1637.

Zepf, B. (2002). Guidelines, recommendations on peanut allergy. *American Family Physician*, 1–3. Retrieved February 7, 2003, from *www.aafp.org/afp/20020901/tips/12.html*

CHAPTER 51

Positive Psychology in Pediatric Psychology

LAMIA P. BARAKAT
ELIZABETH R. PULGARON
LAUREN C. DANIEL

With historical roots in literature, philosophy, and theology, and expressed in psychology's goals of enhancing the lives of individuals, the recently coined term "positive psychology" reflects a conceptual focus on and empirical study of virtue, positive emotion, and well-being (Linley, Joseph, Harrington, & Wood, 2006). Positive psychology has as its foundation both humanistic approaches emphasizing exploration of potentialities (e.g., Maslow, 1968) and efforts to understand adaptive coping, hardiness, and other characteristics of resilience in the face of stressful and traumatic experiences (Lazarus, 2003). Going a step further, Seligman and Csikszentmihalyi (2000) have stated that positive psychology "is about valued subjective experiences: well-being, contentment, and satisfaction (in the past); hope and optimism (for the future); and flow and happiness (in the present)" (p. 5). The core of this conceptualization is that an essential aim of psychology is to understand not only psychopathology and negative reactions to trauma, but adaptation, positive emotion, adaptive coping, and hope (Affleck & Tennen, 1996; Gable & Haidt, 2005; Linley et al., 2006). Research in this young field has expanded rapidly.

Pediatric psychology has a long tradition of understanding resilience (defined in terms of protective vs. risk factors) in the context of chronic conditions in childhood. And yet positive psychology as framed by its originators is just emerging in the pediatric psychology literature, with a noticeable shift toward emphasis on resilience (more broadly defined) and positive outcomes, as well as on protective factors. In contrast, there is a more comprehensive positive psychology literature in the areas of clinical child and adolescent psychology and of adult health psychology. Therefore, positive psychology research in these related specialty areas is presented first, to help frame the emerging work in the intersection of positive psychology with pediatric psychology.

Positive Psychology and Clinical Child and Adolescent Psychology

Clinical child and adolescent psychology has long endeavored to understand the resilience of children, informed by such seminal works as Emmy Werner's (1992) longitudinal study of factors promoting resilience for at-risk children on the Hawaiian island of Kauai. Garmezy and Rutter (1983) emphasized the central importance of identifying and promoting protective factors to improve long-term outcomes; they outlined protective factors that reduce risk or the consequences of risk, promote self-esteem and self-efficacy, and create new possibilities. More recently, Goldstein and Brooks (2006) noted that the study of resilience processes has evolved, due to increasing adversities faced by youths and efforts to apply findings on adaptive and maladaptive developmental trajectories to interventions promoting resilience. Current research, moving beyond resilience defined solely in terms of protective factors to evaluate more broadly defined positive developmental outcomes, has turned to understanding subjective aspects of quality of life (e.g., life satisfaction, social relations, emotions) (Huebner, 2004). Self-esteem, hope, and social responsibility have also been addressed in the clinical child and adolescent literature as representing positive aspects of functioning (Huebner & Gilman, 2003). Therefore, studies assessing positive outcomes (more broadly defined) and outlining factors that promote resilience (more specifically defined) are established aspects of the clinical child and adolescent literature.

Positive Psychology and Adult Health Psychology

Beginning almost three decades ago, adult health psychology applied concepts now encompassed by positive psychology to resilience in the face of illness. The exploration of factors linked to resilience was catalyzed by the work of Taylor (1983), who highlighted the importance of positive reinterpretation in helping adults cope with stressful life experiences, particularly life-threatening health conditions. More recent work specifying how positive emotions may result in better-maintained health and decreased likelihood of developing illness has documented the importance of two positive emotions—hope and curiosity—in possibly preventing hypertension and diabetes, independent of the role negative emotions may play in promoting these diseases (Richman et al., 2005). In addition, the realization that trauma may result in recovery and resilience as well as distress (Bonanno, 2004), and the emerging concept of "posttraumatic growth" (PTG), have found their way into the literature on life-threatening health conditions, particularly with cancer survivors (Helgeson, Reynolds, & Tomlin, 2006). To summarize, the health psychology literature reflects a solid base of research on positive appraisals, active coping, personality characteristics associated with health, and PTG. Although many of these studies predated the birth of positive psychology, the movement toward increased examination of hope, positive emotion, and well-being has informed future directions for investigation of health and disease management and outcomes.

Research on Positive Psychology within Pediatric Psychology

Research endeavors within pediatric psychology were initially framed by clinical work with children and families experiencing significant distress in the face of chronic illness. Identification of maladjustment, potential derailing of children from their developmental trajectories, and weakening of the family system were therefore frequent topics of empirical study. The effort to evaluate resilience as more broadly defined in the clinical child and adolescent psychology literature, in addition to the study of risk and protective factors, emerged with recognition of the norm of adaptive outcomes (Noll & Kupst, 2007). That is, despite psychological risk factors associated with childhood chronic illnesses (Lavigne & Faier-Routman, 1992), current research indicates that the majority of children with chronic conditions fare just as well as their healthy peers and sometimes even better (e.g., Barakat et al., 1997; Eiser, Hill, & Vance, 2000; Lee, Gortmaker, McIntosh, Hughes, & Oleske, 2006; Phipps, Larson, Long, & Rai, 2006; Trzepacz, Vannatta, Davies, Stehbens, & Noll, 2003). Noll and Kupst (2007) have proposed that hardiness explains how well children and adolescents who experience cancer do in the face of adversity; the same conclusions may be drawn for children with other chronic conditions. The process of defining adaptation (including resilience and more optimal outcomes) among children, adolescents, and their families remains incomplete (Ahern, Kiehl, Soel, & Byers, 2006). Yet research at the intersection of positive psychology and pediatric psychology includes investigations of resilience defined broadly in terms of positive outcomes (health-related quality of life [HRQOL] and PTG), as well as examinations of the protective factors associated with resilience.

Resilience in Children with Chronic Conditions

Health-Related Quality of Life

The study of HRQOL provides a unique opportunity for pediatric psychologists to identify adaptive outcomes for children with chronic conditions (Roberts, Brown, Johnson, & Reinke, 2005). Substantial effort has been committed to measurement of HRQOL, in part to identify the ways in which chronic conditions and their treatments may affect functioning across various domains. HRQOL may be differentiated from the concept of well-being (Spieth & Harris, 1996), in that it encompasses the domains of physical, psychological, and social functioning that are directly affected by chronic illness. Studies show a range of functioning, depending on the type of chronic illness and the intensity and duration of its treatments. For example, in an assessment of physical, psychological, spiritual, and social aspects of HRQOL, pediatric cancer survivors generally reported positive outcomes (Zebrack & Chesler, 2002). However, Sawyer and colleagues (2004) reported that children and adolescents with asthma, diabetes, or cystic fibrosis reported lower levels of HRQOL than those from a community sample. It should be noted that effect sizes for some of the findings were small, and that differences were identified among the three chronic illness groups.

HRQOL measurement entails either general or disease-specific approaches (Spieth & Harris, 1996), and much of this literature has been based on research using the Pediatric Quality of Life Inventory (Varni, Seid, & Rode, 1999) or the Child Health Questionnaire (Landgraf, Abetz, & Ware, 1996). Given that many studies have found a lack of concordance between child and parent reports, with children typically endorsing higher HRQOL levels, corresponding parent and child versions of these measures are of benefit (Sawyer et al., 2004). Capitalizing on well-developed HRQOL measurement to further define adaptive outcomes, pediatric psychologists may identify areas of functioning that are relatively immune from deleterious aspects of illness and treatment, in addition to targeting those domains of HRQOL for which there is increased risk.

Posttraumatic Growth

In one of the first studies to undertake evaluation of PTG in the context of chronic conditions in children, using the Perceptions of Changes in Self scale of the Impact of Traumatic Stressors Interview Schedule, both pediatric cancer survivors and their mothers reported more changes for the better (in self, relationships, and future plans) than changes for the worse as a result of having experienced cancer and its treatment (Kazak, Stuber, Barakat, & Meeske, 1996). In a replication, Barakat, Alderfer, and Kazak (2006) found that about 90% of mothers, 80% of fathers, and 85% of adolescent survivors of cancer reported at least one positive outcome of the cancer and its treatment, and that almost a third of the survivors reported four or more positive changes. Interestingly, for survivors (but not mothers or fathers), PTG and posttraumatic stress were positively correlated, suggesting an association of PTG with distress.

Additional measures of PTG have been described in the pediatric psychology literature. A new measure for potential use in future research is the Benefit Finding Scale for Children, which consists of items such as "Having had my illness has helped me become a stronger person." Although the scale is still in early stages of development, the authors have reported good internal reliability (Phipps, Long, & Ogden, 2007). Positive correlations of scores on this measure with optimism and self-esteem were noted, as was a negative correlation with anxiety. Another scale, the Child Attitude Toward Illness Scale (Austin & Huberty, 1993), has been used in previous research to determine children's positive or negative feelings about their chronic condition. Thus, although few studies to date have focused on PTG, promising measures of the concept are emerging in the literature. Findings based on a few selected samples are suggestive of positive changes and/or perspectives on the illness experience, but the positive association of PTG and distress must be further explored. When measures of PTG are taken together with HRQOL measures, resilience for children with chronic conditions may be identified, and a broader picture of positive (and negative) outcomes for these children may be drawn.

Protective Factors for Children with Chronic Conditions

As in both clinical child and adolescent psychology and adult health psychology, description of risk and protective or resistance factors in the context of pediatric psychology predates positive psychology (Wallander, Varni, Babani, Banis, & Wilcox, 1989). Risk and resistance models incorporate varied influences on psychosocial outcomes in pediatric populations. Resistance factors mediate or moderate the relationship between risk factors (illness-related and sociodemographic) with psychosocial outcomes, and are explored here as protective elements that may result in adaptation. Although various protective factors are outlined in these models, self-esteem, optimism, repressive adaptive style, active coping, social support, and family functioning are reviewed here, as these variables may indicate opportunities for preventive interventions for children with chronic conditions.

Self-Esteem

In line with studies from the clinical child and adolescent psychology literature, research comparing populations with chronic illnesses to normative values and to healthy controls suggests links between positive outcomes and self-esteem (or self-appraisal of worth). For example, survivors of childhood cancer rated their self-concept more positively than either norm populations or healthy children did (Anholt, Fritz, & Keener, 1993). In two studies of youths with sickle cell disease, children reported no difference from norms in self-perceptions and social competence (Lemanek, Horwitz, & Ohene-Frempong, 1994), and adolescents reported higher self-esteem than norms (Simon, Barakat, Patterson, & Dampier, 2009). Simon and colleagues (2009) also found that self-esteem was inversely correlated with internalizing symptoms and that inadequacy was positively correlated with internalizing symptoms. In another study of adolescents with sickle cell disease, teens with higher self-esteem reported significantly fewer symptoms of anxiety and depression (Burlew, Telfair, Colangelo, & Wright, 2000). Clearly, self-esteem appears to serve a protective function.

Hope/Optimism

A solid proportion of the research on the role of positive appraisals or expectations in promoting resilience in chronic illness has used the Children's Hope Scale (Snyder et al., 1997), which outlines components of agency and pathways in attaining desired goals. In a study of children with asthma, hope was a significant predictor of treatment adherence when disease variables were controlled for (Berg, Rapoff, Snyder, & Belmont, 2007). Families with high levels of hope and low levels of medical uncertainty were found to have greater adherence to treatment plans after organ transplants (Maikranz, Steele, Dreyer, Stratman, & Bovaird, 2007). In addition, adolescent burn survivors with higher levels of hope experienced lower levels of externalizing behavior problems, and in combination with social support, hope significantly predicted global self-worth (Bauman, Snyder, Rapoff, Mani, & Thompson, 1998). Studies of optimism (the expectation of positive outcomes) with children and adolescents with chronic conditions confirm it too as a protective factor. For adolescents with sickle cell disease, optimism moderated the relationship between pain and opioid use (Pence, Valrie, Gil, Redding-Lallinger, & Daeschner, 2007), and a significant inverse relationship between optimism and school absences was found for those with asthma (Vinson, 2002).

Repressive Adaptive Style

"Repressive adaptive style" (characterized by high defensiveness and low anxiety) represents the tendency to underreport distress in those who have faced significant adversity (Phipps & Srivastava, 1997) that has not been linked to adverse effects (Phipps, 2007). Phipps and colleagues (2006) described that repressive adaptive style emerges in response to diagnosis of a chronic condition and is maintained across time. And, although this adaptive style seems counterintuitive as a facilitator of PTG, research suggests that it may be associated with adaptation. In an initial study of repressive adaptive style in childhood cancer (Canning, Canning, & Boyce, 1992) and a replication (Phipps & Srivastava, 1997), when adolescents with cancer were compared to healthy controls, higher levels of repressive adaptive style accounted for group differences on depression. Extending these findings and comparing children with cancer to a group of children with other chronic illnesses and a healthy control group, Phipps, Steele, Hall, and Leigh (2001) found that the children with cancer or other chronic illnesses reported higher levels of repressive adaptive style than healthy children did. Moreover, repressive adaptive style in children with cancer and their parents has been related to lower levels of post-traumatic stress symptoms than other adaptive styles have been (Phipps et al., 2006).

Active Coping

Although repressive adaptive style may aid children in coping with inevitable and uncontrollable aspects of chronic illness, active coping (seeking to solve problems and obtain environmental supports) may be necessary in facing more controllable disease-related problems. Active coping has predicted social adjustment in teens with a variety of chronic illnesses (Meijer, Sinnema, Bijstra, Mellenbergh, & Wolters, 2002). Furthermore, active coping has been demonstrated as a moderator of the relationship between hope and anxiety in children with sickle cell disease, and those who used high levels of active coping, support coping, or distraction coping reported lower levels of anxiety (Lewis & Kliewer, 1996). Similarly, following a pain coping intervention, use of active coping strategies for sickle cell pain was related to fewer emergency room visits in a sample of children (Gil et al., 2001) and fewer physical limitations during pain episodes in teens (Gil, Williams, Thompson, & Kinney, 1991). In contrast to these supportive studies, other research demonstrated that coping strategies did not bolster adjustment in children with sickle cell disease (Lutz, Barakat, Smith-Whitley, & Ohene-Frempong, 2004). In addition, an intervention targeting self-care coping for children with cancer found no improvements in self-esteem, self-efficacy, hopefulness, or distress (Hinds et al., 2000). Thus more research is needed to clarify the aspects of active coping that are most adaptive for children with chronic conditions.

Social Support

Social support (or family, friend, and community networks that provide for various needs) has been hypothesized as central to adaptive outcomes for children with chronic health conditions and their caregivers. Although this hypothesis has substantial support among children with developmental and physical disabilities (Dunst, Trivette, & Cross, 1996), the findings are less consistent among samples with chronic illnesses (see Decker, 2007, for a review of findings in adolescents with cancer). Yet perceived social support has been linked to lower self-reports of anxiety and depression, and to lower parent reports of internalizing and externalizing symptoms, in children newly diagnosed with cancer (Varni, Katz, Colegrove, & Dolgin, 1994); it was also related to greater disease knowledge and self-management behaviors in teens with asthma (Sin, Kang, & Weaver, 2005). Moreover, interventions focused on increasing social support have resulted in positive effects (Chernoff et al., 2002; Funck-Brentano et al., 2005).

Family Functioning

Adaptive family functioning—generally defined as including higher family cohesion, organization, and expressiveness; lower family conflict and control; and lower parenting stress—has been solidly supported as a resistance factor associated with a number of positive medical and psychological outcomes, including increased HRQOL (Barakat, Lash, Lutz, & Nicolaou, 2006; Newby, Brown, Pawletko, Gold, & Whitt, 2000; Soliday, Kool, & Lande, 2001; Vinson, 2002; Wallander et al., 1989). For instance, the family environment variables of cohesion and expressiveness predicted lower psychological distress and greater adaptation in children newly diagnosed with cancer (Varni, Katz, Colegrove, & Dolgin, 1996), and family satisfaction, as reported by mothers of cancer survivors, was inversely related to reports of posttraumatic stress symptoms in their children (Kazak et al., 1997). Research on sickle cell disease provides further support for family functioning as a resilience factor: Family cohesion moderated the association of negative parental affect and externalizing behavior problems for children and adolescents (Ievers, Brown, Lambert, Hsu, & Eckman, 1998), and lower parenting stress predicted better health outcomes for adolescents 1 year later (Barakat et al., 2007).

Conclusions

As highlighted by this overview of positive psychology in pediatric psychology, future investigation of positive outcomes and factors associated with resilience in the context of childhood illness offers many avenues. Indeed, the foundation has been laid by research on HRQOL and PTG as adaptive outcomes, as well as investigation of protective factors that explain resilience. Yet further expansion of positive psychology within pediatric psychology will demand extension of these pediatric psychology literatures, as well as development of concepts and theories consistent with positive psychology but unique to pediatric psychology. The literature review for this chapter turned up many dissertations focusing on resilience for children with chronic conditions, but few of these studies have as yet made their way into the published literature. Clearly, it will be important to support investigators in translating this work into long-standing, well-developed research programs, with results disseminated to the pediatric psychology community.

As noted by others (Roberts et al., 2005), of primary importance in achieving aspirations envisioned by the field of positive psychology is a redefinition of adaptation from the absence of psychopathology to recovery and resilience, as defined in terms of optimal outcomes (such as PTG, HRQOL, life satisfaction, and well-being). Although showing that children with chronic conditions and their families fare well in comparison with norms/peers on measures of psychopathology is an encouraging first step, the time is ripe to turn attention to assessment of broadly defined positive outcomes. The field is just establishing a literature base for the advancement of developmentally appropriate measures of growth and resilience, as well as models of these concepts specific to children and their families within the context of pediatrics. Furthermore, because the studies reviewed here are primarily cross-sectional, providing only snapshots of functioning, demonstrations of the temporal stability of positive outcomes and their associations with distress are necessary (i.e., clarifications of responses initially, over time, and [when appropriate] after treatment).

Related to these goals, prospective research is needed to address protective factors associated with resilience, such as self-esteem, social support, and family functioning, instead of focusing on risk and/or relying on cross-sectional methodologies. Current research on resilience pointing to reciprocal associations of risk and resistance over time (Goldstein & Harris, 2006), and investigations of other concepts (e.g., well-being and life satisfaction) associated with positive psychology (Huebner, 2004), may inform these efforts and support advances in pediatric psychology.

Finally, intervention research will be important for considering how to maintain or improve functioning for the majority of children and their families who adapt well, while also informing interventions to improve outcomes for those at risk (Drotar, 2006). Although a number of interventions promoting protective factors have been shown to have favorable effects (e.g., Chernoff et al., 2002; Funck-Brentano et al., 2005; Gil et al., 2001), a key question for future research remains how to translate what we learn about adaptive processes to working with those in distress. Continued study of resilience, as well as determination of the clinical utility of other positive psychology concepts and methods for working with children who have chronic conditions, will be necessary to the development of clinical practices and interventions that promote adaptation.

References

Affleck, G., & Tennen, H. (1996). Construing benefits from adversity: Adaptational significance and dispositional underpinnings. *Journal of Personality, 64,* 899–922.

Ahern, N. R., Kiehl, E. M., Sole, M. L., & Byers, J. (2006). A review of instruments measuring resilience. *Issues in Comprehensive Pediatric Nursing, 29,* 103–125.

Anholt, U. V., Fritz, G. K., & Keener, M. (1993). Self-concept in survivors of childhood and adolescent cancer. *Journal of Psychosocial Oncology, 11,* 1–16.

Austin, J. K., & Huberty, T. J. (1993). Development of the Child Attitude toward Illness Scale. *Journal of Pediatric Psychology, 18,* 467–480.

Barakat, L. P., Alderfer, M. A., & Kazak, A. E. (2006). Posttraumatic growth in adolescent survivors of cancer and their mothers and fathers. *Journal of Pediatric Psychology, 31,* 413–419.

Barakat, L. P., Kazak, A. E., Meadows, A. T., Casey, R., Meeske, K., & Stuber, M. L. (1997). Families surviving childhood cancer: A comparison of posttraumatic stress symptoms with families of healthy children. *Journal of Pediatric Psychology, 22,* 843–859.

Barakat, L. P., Lash, L., Lutz, M. J., & Nicolaou, D. C. (2006). Psychosocial adaptation of children and adolescents with sickle cell disease. In R. T. Brown (Ed.), *Comprehensive handbook of childhood cancer and sickle cell disease: A biopsychosocial approach* (pp. 471–495). New York: Oxford University Press.

Barakat, L. P., Patterson, C. A., Weinberger, B. S., Simon, K., Gonzalez, E. R., & Dampier, C. (2007). A prospective study of the role of coping and family functioning in health outcomes for adolescents with sickle cell disease. *Journal of Pediatric Hematology/Oncology, 29*(11), 752–760.

Bauman, D. D., Snyder, C. R., Rapoff, M. A., Mani, M. M., & Thompson, R. (1998). Hope and social support in the psychological adjustment of children who have survived burn injuries and their matched controls. *Children's Health Care, 27,* 15–30.

Berg, C. J., Rapoff, M. A., Snyder, C. R., & Belmont, J. M. (2007). The relationship of children's hope to pediatric asthma treatment adherence. *Journal of Positive Psychology, 2,* 176–184.

Bonanno, G. A. (2004). Loss, trauma, and human resilience. *American Psychologist, 59*, 20–28.

Burlew, K., Telfair, J., Colangelo, L., & Wright, E. C. (2000). Factors that influence adolescent adaptation to sickle cell disease. *Journal of Pediatric Psychology, 25*, 287–299.

Canning, E. H., Canning, R. D., & Boyce, W. T. (1992). Depressive symptoms and adaptive style in children with cancer. *Journal of the American Academy of Child and Adolescent Psychiatry, 31*, 1120–1124.

Chernoff, R. G., Ireys, H. T., DeVet, K. A., Kim, Y. J., Chernoff, R. G., Ireys, H. T., et al. (2002). A randomized, controlled trial of a community-based support program for families of children with chronic illness: Pediatric outcomes. *Archives of Pediatrics and Adolescent Medicine, 156*, 533–539.

Decker, C. L. (2007). Social support and adolescent cancer survivors: A review of the literature. *Psycho-Oncology, 16*, 1–11.

Drotar, D. (2006). *Psychological interventions in childhood chronic illness.* Washington, DC: American Psychological Association.

Dunst, C. J., Trivette, C. M., & Cross, A. H. (1996). Mediating influences of social support: Personal, family and child outcomes. *American Journal of Mental Deficiency, 90*, 403–417.

Eiser, C., Hill, J. J., & Vance, Y. H. (2000). Examining the psychological consequences of surviving childhood cancer: Systematic review as a research method in pediatric psychology. *Journal of Pediatric Psychology, 25*, 449–460.

Funck-Brentano, I., Dalban, C., Veber, F., Quartier, P., Hefez, S., Costagliola, D., et al. (2005). Evaluation of a peer support group therapy for HIV-infected adolescents. *AIDS, 19*, 1501–1508.

Gable, S. L., & Haidt, J. (2005). What (and why) is positive psychology? *Review of General Psychology, 9*, 103–110.

Garmezy, N., & Rutter, M. (Eds.). (1983). *Stress, coping and development in children.* New York: McGraw-Hill.

Gil, K. M., Anthony, K. K., Carson, J. W., Redding-Lallinger, R., Daeschner, C. W., & Ware, R. E. (2001). Daily coping practice predicts treatment effects in children with sickle cell disease. *Journal of Pediatric Psychology, 26*, 163–173.

Gil, K. M., Williams, D. A., Thompson, R. J., & Kinney, T. R. (1991). Sickle cell disease in children and adolescents: The relation of child and parent pain coping strategies to adjustment. *Journal of Pediatric Psychology, 16*, 643–663.

Goldstein, S., & Brooks, R. B. (2006). Why study resilience? In S. Goldstein & R. B. Brooks (Eds.), *Handbook of resilience in children* (pp. 3–15). New York: Springer.

Helgeson, V., Reynolds, K. A., & Tomlin, P. L. (2006). A meta-analytic review of benefit finding and growth. *Journal of Consulting and Clinical Psychology, 74*, 797–816.

Hinds, P. S., Quargneti, A., Bush, A. J., Pratt, C., Fairclough, D., Rissmiller, G., et al. (2000). An evaluation of the impact of a self-care coping intervention on psychological and clinical outcomes in adolescents with newly diagnosed cancer. *European Journal of Oncology Nursing, 4*, 6–17.

Huebner, E. S. (2004). Research on assessment of life satisfaction of children and adolescents. *Social Indicators Research, 66*, 3–33.

Huebner, E. S., & Gilman, R. (2003). Toward a focus on positive psychology in school psychology. *School Psychology Quarterly, 18*, 99–102.

Ievers, C. E., Brown, R. T., Lambert, R. G., Hsu, L., & Eckman, J. R. (1998). Family functioning and social support in the adaptation of caregivers of children with sickle cell syndromes. *Journal of Pediatric Psychology, 23*, 377–388.

Kazak, A. E., Barakat, L. P., Meeske, K., Dimitri, C., Meadows, A. T., Casey, R., et al. (1997). Posttraumatic stress, family functioning, and social support in survivors of childhood leukemia and their mothers and fathers. *Journal of Consulting and Clinical Psychology, 65*, 120–129.

Kazak, A. E., Stuber, M. L., Barakat, L. P., & Meeske, K. (1996). Assessing posttraumatic stress related to medical illness and treatment: The Impact of Traumatic Stressors Interview Schedule (ITSIS). *Families, Systems and Health, 14,* 365–380.

Landgraf, J. M., Abetz, L., & Ware, J. E. (1996). *The CHQ user's manual.* Boston: The Health Institute, New England Medical Center.

Lavigne, J. V., & Faier-Routman, J. (1992). Psychological adjustment to pediatric physical disorder: A meta-analytic review. *Journal of Pediatric Psychology, 17,* 133–157.

Lazarus, R. S. (2003). Does the positive psychology movement have legs? *Psychological Inquiry, 13,* 93–109.

Lee, G. M., Gortmaker, S. L., McIntosh, K., Hughes, M. D., & Oleske, J. M. (2006). Quality of life for children and adolescents: Impact of HIV infection and antiretroviral treatment. *Pediatrics, 117,* 273–283.

Lemanek, K., Horwitz, W., & Ohene-Frempong, K. (1994). A multiperspective investigation of social competence in children with sickle cell disease. *Journal of Pediatric Psychology, 19,* 443–456.

Lewis, H. A., & Kliewer, W. (1996). Hope, coping and adjustment among children with sickle cell disease: Test of mediator and moderator models. *Journal of Pediatric Psychology, 21,* 25–41.

Linley, P. A., Joseph, S., Harrington, S., & Wood, A. M. (2006). Positive psychology: Past, present and (possible) future. *Journal of Positive Psychology, 1,* 3–16.

Lutz, M. J., Barakat, L. P., Smith-Whitley, K., & Ohene-Frempong, K. (2004). Psychological adjustment of children with sickle cell disease: Family functioning and coping. *Rehabilitation Psychology, 49,* 224–232.

Maikranz, J. M., Steele, R. G., Dreyer, M., Stratman, A., & Bovaird, J. A. (2007). The relationship of hope and illness-related uncertainty to emotional adjustment and adherence among pediatric renal and liver transplant recipients. *Journal of Pediatric Psychology, 32,* 571–581.

Maslow, A. H. (1968). *Toward a psychology of being* (2nd ed.). Princeton, NJ: Van Norstrand.

Meijer, S. A., Sinnema, G., Bijstra, J. O., Mellenbergh, G. J., & Wolters, W. H. G. (2002). Coping styles and locus of control as predictors for psychological adjustment of adolescents with a chronic illness. *Social Science and Medicine, 54,* 1453–1461.

Newby, W. L., Brown, R. T., Pawletko, T. M., Gold, S. H., & Whitt, J. K. (2000). Social skills and psychological adjustment of child and adolescent cancer survivors. *Psycho-Oncology, 9,* 113–126.

Noll, R. B., & Kupst, M. J. (2007). The psychological impact of pediatric cancer hardiness: The exception or the rule? *Journal of Pediatric Psychology, 32,* 1089–1098.

Pence, L., Valrie, C. R., Gil, K. M., Redding-Lallinger, R., & Daeschner, C. (2007). Optimism predicting daily pain medication use in adolescents with sickle cell disease. *Journal of Pain and Symptom Management, 33,* 302–309.

Phipps, S. (2007). Adaptive style in children with cancer: Implications for a positive psychology approach. *Journal of Pediatric Psychology, 32,* 1055–1066.

Phipps, S., Larson, S., Long, A., & Rai, S. N. (2006). Adaptive style and symptoms of posttraumatic stress in children with cancer and their parents. *Journal of Pediatric Psychology, 31,* 298–309.

Phipps, S., Long, A. M., & Ogden, J. (2007). Benefit Finding Scale for Children: Preliminary findings from a childhood cancer population. *Journal of Pediatric Psychology, 23,* 1264–1271.

Phipps, S., & Srivastava, D. K. (1997). Repressive adaptation in children with cancer. *Health Psychology, 16,* 521–528.

Phipps, S., Steele, R. G., Hall, K., & Leigh, L. (2001). Repressive adaptation in children with cancer: A replication and extension. *Health Psychology, 20,* 445–451.

Richman, L. S., Kubzansky, L., Maselko, J., Kawachi, I., Choo, P., & Bauer, M. (2005). Positive emotional and health: Going beyond the negative. *Health Psychology, 24,* 422–429.

Roberts, M. C., Brown, K. J., Johnson, R. J., & Reinke, J. (2005). Positive psychology for children: Development, prevention, and promotion. In C. R. Snyder (Ed.), *Handbook of positive psychology* (pp. 663–675). New York: Oxford University Press.

Sawyer, M. G., Reynolds, K. E., Couper, J. J., French, D. I., Kennedy, J. D., Martin, A. J., et al. (2004). Health-related quality of life of children and adolescents with chronic illness: A two year prospective study. *Quality of Life Research, 13,* 1309–1319.

Seligman, M. E. P., & Csikszentmihalyi, M. (2000). Positive psychology: An introduction. *American Psychologist, 56,* 216–217.

Simon, K., Barakat, L. P., Patterson, C. A., & Dampier, C. (2009). Symptoms of depression and anxiety in adolescents with sickle cell disease: The role of intrapersonal characteristics and stress processing variables. *Child Psychiatry and Human Development, 40*(2), 317–330.

Sin, M. K., Kang, D. H., & Weaver, M. (2005). Relationships of asthma knowledge, self-management, and social support in African American adolescents with asthma. *International Journal of Nursing Studies, 42,* 307–313.

Snyder, C. R., Hoza, B., Pelham, W. E., Rapoff, M., Ware, L., Danovsky, M., et al. (1997). The development and validation of the Children's Hope Scale. *Journal of Pediatric Psychology, 22,* 399–421.

Soliday, E., Kool, E., & Lande, M. B. (2001). Family environment, child behavior, and medical indicators in children with kidney disease. *Child Psychiatry and Human Development, 31,* 279–295.

Spieth, L. E., & Harris, C. V. (1996). Assessment of health-related quality of life in children and adolescents: An integrative review. *Journal of Pediatric Psychology, 21,* 175–193.

Taylor, S. (1983). Adjustment to threatening events: A theory of cognitive adaptation. *American Psychologist, 38,* 1161–1173.

Trzepacz, A. M., Vannatta, K., Davies, W. H., Stehbens, J. A., & Noll, R. B. (2003). Social, emotional and behavioral functioning of children with hemophilia. *Journal of Developmental and Behavioral Pediatrics, 24,* 225–232.

Varni, J. W., Katz, E. R., Colegrove, R., & Dolgin, M. (1994). Perceived social support and adjustment of children with newly diagnosed cancer. *Journal of Developmental and Behavioral Pediatrics, 15,* 20–26.

Varni, J. W., Katz, E. R., Colegrove, R., & Dolgin, M. (1996). Family functioning predictors of adjustment in children with newly diagnosed cancer: A prospective analysis. *Journal of Child Psychology and Psychiatry, 37,* 321–328.

Varni, J. W., Seid, M., & Rode, C. A. (1999). The PedsQL: Measurement model for the Pediatric Quality of Life Inventory. *Medical Care, 37,* 126–39.

Vinson, J. A. (2002). Children with asthma: Initial development of the child resilience model. *Pediatric Nursing, 28,* 149–158.

Wallander, J. L., Varni, J. W., Babani, L., Banis, H. T., & Wilcox, K. T. (1989). Family resources as resistance factors for psychological maladjustment in chronically ill and handicapped children. *Journal of Pediatric Psychology, 14,* 157–173.

Werner, E. E. (1992). The children of Kauai: Resiliency and recovery in adolescence and adulthood. *Journal of Adolescent Health, 13,* 262–268.

Zebrack, B. J., & Chesler, M. A. (2002). Quality of life in childhood cancer survivors. *Psycho-Oncology, 11,* 132–141.

CHAPTER 52

Individual and Organizational Collaborations

A Roadmap for Effective Advocacy

F. DANIEL ARMSTRONG

In the 1970s, the new field of pediatric psychology was faced with a single overriding task: establishing credibility as a specialty discipline that could be recognized for its unique contribution to the well-being of children with medical conditions. The need to create an identity that was part of psychology and pediatrics, yet at the same time distinct, forced the field to emphasize its unique aspects—often at the expense of meaningful integrated collaboration with other disciplines and organizations. Nearly 40 years later, pediatric psychology is firmly established as a defined discipline, respected by colleagues in the fields of psychology, pediatrics, dentistry, nursing, surgery, and the neurosciences. With this respect comes the expectation that pediatric psychologists will fully participate in the changing landscape that emphasizes interdisciplinary collaboration, thereby moving to transdisciplinary approaches to research and clinical care.

This expectation translates into opportunities for pediatric psychology that have not yet been realized. Interdisciplinary and transdisciplinary collaboration most commonly occurs between individuals in a collaborative office setting with pediatricians or as part of a collaborative research team (Kazak et al., 2007). Similarly, interdisciplinary and transdisciplinary collaboration may involve joint advocacy on behalf of groups of patients in a practice or a specific type of research initiative. Sometimes the issues of concern are much larger than individuals, and the actions needed for solution may require collaborations at a systems level, most frequently involving multiple organizations that share a mission or focus. These types of organizational collaborations represent an entirely different level of challenge, but also represent an opportunity for substantive and far-reaching impact on many individuals.

In this chapter, models for both individual and organizational collaboration are described, with special emphasis on how pediatric psychologists can acquire the skills to participate effectively in both types of collaboration. Many positive outcomes may result from this type of collaboration, including improved care delivery and advancement of scientific knowledge. Sometimes the outcome of collaboration is shared advocacy leading to changes in public policy, which subsequently results in improvements in the lives of many.

Disciplinary, Multidisciplinary, Interdisciplinary, and Transdisciplinary: What Is the Difference?

Psychologists, like professionals in other disciplines, have defined the boundaries of what constitutes psychological practice. State laws determine the knowledge areas and competencies necessary for practice, and training programs are accredited for teaching these core knowledge areas and competencies. Legally and professionally, all this defines what it means to be a psychologist. As members of a specialty, pediatric psychologists have historically defined their mission in terms of the types of patients seen, the types of problems addressed, and the types of research conducted (Society of Pediatric Psychology [SPP], 2008). Disciplinary identity ensures that all individuals providing service or conducting research will share a core knowledge and acquire a core set of similar skills.

As disciplines grow, new information and skills are acquired. The skills that previously defined the discipline often lose their traditional focus as new challenges are recognized. In these situations, collaborations develop with other disciplines to fulfill the prior need and allow progress. A classic example is the role that psychologists play in directly intervening with children experiencing pain and/or distress during invasive medical procedures. Early in the development of the field, its entrée into the medical world was the ability to teach children to relax, use modifications of systematic desensitization, and restructure environments so that the children would be less behaviorally disruptive when given shots, lumbar punctures, or other painful but necessary medical procedures (Tsao & Zeltzer, 2008; Uman, Chambers, McGrath, & Kisely, 2008). As knowledge was translated into models of clinical intervention and then into clinical practice, pediatric psychologists found that being directly involved in the treatment of every child undergoing medical procedures in a busy medical practice became unmanageable. At the same time, pediatricians and anesthesiologists, working independently, developed new, safe, and effective analgesic medications that substantially improved the experience of painful procedures. While this was happening, a new group of professionals in another discipline, child life, began to take on an increasingly important role in clinical settings, initially providing play opportunities and then providing interventions. In due time, the disciplines of pediatric psychology, pediatric oncology, pediatric anesthesiology, and child life began to work together from a multidisciplinary perspective to address pain during invasive medical procedures. Some children were treated with medication, while others received behavioral interventions, more frequently provided by child life specialists than by psychologists. Multidisciplinary clinics were born, with each discipline providing a specific component of a broader multidisciplinary intervention. The concept of several disciplines doing their own thing in the same place received the designation "multidisciplinary."

In time, the individuals working as part of multidisciplinary teams discovered that they often had overlapping and complementary skills. New types of interactions between professionals began to occur, with a focus on integration of knowledge as opposed to parallel presentation of discipline-specific knowledge. This new integration of disciplines became known as "interdisciplinary" (Guralnick, 2000). In the clinical setting (to continue the example from above), interdisciplinary collaborations involved combinations of pharmaceutical and behavioral interventions, with anesthesiologists and psychologists working as a team. As federal training programs, such as Leadership Education in Neurodevelopmental Disabilities (LEND; Maternal and Child Health Bureau, 2008), began to require training in interdisciplinary clinical applications, the concept of interdisciplinary collaborations began to spread to research programs. In fact, as part of the National Institutes of Health (NIH) Roadmap for Medical Research, research activities require demonstration of interdisciplinary scientific methodology for funding (NIH, 2008). For pediatric psychologists, the transition from multidisciplinary collaboration to interdisciplinary collaboration has emerged slowly but has proven to be a very effective model in the delivery of clinical care, particularly for children with such complex conditions as cancer, HIV, diabetes, and traumatic brain injury. It has also emerged into a research model that brings together several disciplines around problems of significant behavioral, biological, and genetic complexity (Armstrong, 2006).

As interdisciplinary models have proven successful and collaborations between professionals in clinical and research activities have matured, a new concept of "transdisciplinary" collaboration has emerged. "Transdisciplinary" implies a level of integration and synergy that blurs the lines between discipline-specific knowledge and methods in such a way that the resulting outcome is unique and not discernible from a single discipline's perspective (Armstrong & Reaman, 2005). Again, for example, in the clinical setting, psychologists and anesthesiologists determine the "best fit" between a child's style and pharmaceutical or behavioral intervention. Transdisciplinary collaboration does not occur easily. It is often the product of years of working together to the point where all involved have learned not only to think like their colleagues, but to think with their colleagues in entirely new ways.

Collaboration Applications

Pediatric psychologists have been on the cutting edge of multidisciplinary, interdisciplinary, and transdisciplinary collaboration, with evidence of success in the context of clinical care, research, and institutional and professional organization initiatives. The following sections provide an overview of the challenges and opportunities that have been encountered, as well as some of the strategies that have proven effective.

Clinical Collaboration

Because pediatric psychology has "grown up" in the hospital setting, clinical care has, of necessity, involved collaboration. Effective working relationships with pediatricians, pediatric subspecialists, nurses, therapists, and other children's health care providers are required for access to children with health concerns. For children with complex diseases or other conditions, such as cancer, diabetes, sickle cell disease, or those treated with organ transplantation, careful coordination of care combined with continuity of care has become the norm. In many medical centers, and particularly in children's hospitals, the clinical involvement of the pediatric psychologist has shifted from being one of several consultants (multidisciplinary) to being an integral member of ongoing clinical teams (interdisciplinary). Increasingly, specialized (by training or experience) pediatric psychologists are being hired as full-time members of pediatric specialty programs (e.g., cancer centers, sickle cell centers, HIV treatment programs, cystic fibrosis centers) to provide highly integrated transdisciplinary care (Grant, Economou, Ferrell, & Bhatia, 2007). One concrete indicator of this process is that psychological services are now starting to be included as part of a bundle of services in terms of reimbursement.

The skills necessary for success in a clinical (inpatient, outpatient, or community) environment include (1) expertise in the application of disciplinary knowledge; (2) significant shared knowledge and expertise in the areas where collaboration is required; and (3) the commitment and the personal social skills necessary to facilitate ongoing information exchange and shared learning among collaborators. One of the hallmarks of successful high-level interdisciplinary or transdisciplinary collaboration is that the conversations of all members of the team focus on children, and not on the information and skill set focus of individual team members. On these successful teams, each person talks as much if not more about what the others bring to the discussion than about their own area of expertise.

Research Collaboration

Pediatric psychologists have been involved in collaborative approaches to research since the field was established. Models of collaboration have typically involved (1) a psychologist assuming the principal investigator's role in a study primarily involving a behavioral question, with pediatricians or investigators from other disciplines contributing in a secondary role; (2) a pediatrician or an investigator from another discipline serving as the principal investigator in a study primarily focused on nonbehavioral issues, with the psychologist contributing measurement and methodology expertise; or (3) the psychologist and pediatrician serving as co–principal investigators on research questions that are integrally related and of equal importance. In each of these cases, access to a patient population may require collaboration. All of these models provide benefits that include increased collegiality, cross-disciplinary learning, increased respect for one another as investigators and as representatives of legitimate scientific study, and the development of collegial working relationships that may last for decades (Armstrong & Drotar, 2000; Armstrong & Reaman, 2005; Whitsett, Armstrong, & Pollock, 2006). Although these types of collaborations are primarily beneficial, there are some potential limitations. Disagreements among collaborators (e.g., decisions about what measures to use, authorship order) can escalate to a level of conflict that jeopardizes progress on important scientific investigations. If unresolved, these conflicts can jeopardize the careers of each of the investigators involved, as well as an institution's commitment to a particular line of research.

Because of the complexity of many child health research topics, as well as the relatively low prevalence of certain childhood diseases, collaboration may represent the only way that meaningful research can take place. Increasingly, interdisciplinary approaches are needed to understand the interrelationships among biological mechanisms, social and environmental factors, and psychological and behavioral factors that affect child health outcomes. Studies of neurocognitive functioning in children treated for cancer increasingly require collaborations between psychologists and neuroscientists in the fields of imaging, biochemistry, and genetics. Studies of pain in children require collaborations among psychologists, anesthesiologists, and pharmacologists. These are but two examples where collaborations are essential to define the scope of a problem and to design interventions that affect outcome. These collaborations require specialized expertise, access to state-of-the-art equipment and methodology, and access to patient populations that will permit adequately powered studies to be conducted.

Because most institutions do not have access to patient populations of sufficient size to carry out descriptive, epidemiological, or randomized intervention trials, collaboration in child health research has frequently expanded to include investigators from multiple disciplines at multiple centers. Recognizing the benefits of this type of collaboration, the NIH has established clinical trial groups to conduct multicenter, multi-investigator research. Most of the significant recent advances in the treatment of childhood cancer have been attributed to multicenter, multi-investigator clinical trials conducted by cooperative groups funded by the National Cancer Institute (Armstrong & Reaman, 2005). Similar kinds of advances have occurred because of collaborative research conducted by the Cooperative Study of Sickle Cell Disease (Farber, Koshy, & Kinney, 1985); the Pediatric AIDS Clinical Trials Group (Rosendorf et al., 1993), which has evolved into the Pediatric HIV/AIDS Cohort Study (Pediatric HIV/AIDS Cohort Study, 2008); and the Diabetes Control and Complications Trial (Diabetes Control and Complications Trial Research Group, 1993).

Multicenter, multi-investigator collaborative research has a number of benefits. These include (1) access to sufficient and representative patient populations; (2) access for patients to participation in clinical research; (3) accurate description of the extent of a particular observed finding in the disease population; (4) access to specialized core resources that might not be available in a single institution; (5) access to high-quality biostatistical and data management support; (6) infrastructure to support long-term management of a participant cohort; and (7) increased opportunities for research funding. The benefit of collaborative, multicenter research should not be underestimated, since this model may permit research questions to be asked and answered rapidly, leading to faster dissemination and translation into clinical and community practice. Finally, multicenter collaborations offer investigators employed by small institutions the opportunity to contribute innovative ideas that would be impossible to test outside the multicenter collaborative model (Armstrong & Reaman, 2005).

Multicenter, multi-investigator collaborative research is, however, not without its limitations. The process of bringing an idea to the level of a multicenter trial can be burdensome and extremely laborious. Most multicenter collaborative groups have extensive requirements for review at multiple levels. This, combined with the current regulatory requirements of institutional review boards and fiscal compliance, can produce profound delays in implementation of meaningful research. Similarly, prioritization of resources can undermine scientific questions that are not perceived as important within the context of the collaborative group, and competition between institutions for funding and attribution of grant awards represents a substantial barrier. Other challenges include (1) variability in measurement; (2) difficulty in maintaining standardized data collection and quality control; (3) difficulty in implementing interventions across multiple sites; (4) investigator attrition and turnover; and (5) the cost of conducting research at multiple sites (Armstrong & Drotar, 2000; Whitsett et al., 2006). Without adequate resources, the scientific quality of studies may be compromised or abandoned altogether.

Nevertheless, on balance, there are many reasons for pediatric psychologists to consider collaborative research endeavors. The development of cross-disciplinary and cross-institutional relationships has been a primary driver of progress in research on many child health conditions that involve a primary behavioral or psychological component. Were it not for these collaborations, much of the work in pain assessment and treatment, neurodevelopmental outcomes, behavioral adherence with medical regimens, health-related quality of life, and bioethics would not have taken place. Perhaps most importantly, the growing pains associated with multicenter and multi-investigator research are opening opportunities for transdisciplinary research that bring together investigators from multiple fields in psychology, biology, biochemistry, genetics, imaging, biomedical engineering, physics, ethics, and education. Collaboration in research on newborn screening for rare conditions for which there is no current treatment is an example of an effort that involves pediatricians, geneticists, biochemists (those developing the newborn screening tests), psychologists, ethicists, and educators (Bailey, Armstrong, Kemper, Skinner, & Warren, 2008). These transdisciplinary, collaborative research models are only beginning to be developed, but they offer opportunities for comprehensive views of disease and the development of innovative, multifocused approaches to intervention (Armstrong, 2006).

Organizational Collaboration

Collaborations on clinical and research programs typically occur because they contribute to a broad mission of improved child health and because they benefit the individuals involved. Collaborations between and among organizations occur for similar reasons. Mission alignment that leads to improved child health outcomes is one benefit of organizational collaboration. At a different level, organizational collaboration occurs because of direct benefits (e.g., financial; institutional research ranking) for the participating organizations. Despite these benefits, organizational collaborations are often difficult to bring about, for a number of reasons. These include (1) concerns by the potentially collaborating organizations that they will lose their unique identity; (2) difficulties in resolving organizational and structural differences that pose barriers to collaboration; (3) difficulties in obtaining consensus among individual members of the organizations that collaboration is desirable; (4) differences in culture and style; (5) concerns that the contributions and returns from the collaboration will be unequally distributed; and (6) difficulties with concretely defining a shared mission and the mechanism for carrying it out. These challenges are substantial, and are often sufficient to interfere with or completely block successful collaboration. However, organizations that successfully develop effective collaborations around a shared mission frequently find not only that the mission is advanced, but that the overall health of the individual organizations is improved. Although there have been a number of cross-disciplinary collaborations (e.g., the SPP and the Society of Developmental and Behavioral Pediatrics), the collaboration between the SPP and the American Academy of Pediatrics (AAP) is an illustrative example of effective collaboration on a shared mission, with mutual benefits.

The SPP–APP Collaboration

In 1995, the Executive Committee of the SPP initiated a strategic planning process. One of the initiatives that emerged was the creation of a task force to promote collaboration between the SPP and the AAP. The rationale behind this initiative was that collaboration would advance the SPP's mission more rapidly than continued isolated efforts would. The Pediatric Interface Task Force thus became the first organizational effort by pediatric psychologists to create interorganizational synergy to address global concerns of child health. The steps in this process involved exchanges of information, creation of opportunities for joint contribution to policy statements, reciprocal committee appointments, and joint advocacy on child health issues. These steps represent an effective model for other collaborations.

For the initial step, the SPP invited a pediatrician to moderate a symposium on developmental and behavioral pediatrics at the American Psychological Association (APA) convention. Second, after work with the leadership of APA, a SPP member was appointed to the AAP Committee on Psychosocial Aspects of Child and Family Health (COPACFH). At the same time, another SPP member was appointed to the AAP Media Committee at the request of the APA. Third, the SPP invited Robert Hahnemann, MD, then the president of the AAP, to give the keynote address for the SPP at the APA Convention. He left the membership with this memorable statement: "I wish that every child can be touched by a pediatrician and a pediatric psychologist" (Armstrong, 1998). Each of these exchanges diminished concerns about collaboration, and strengthened the working relationship around a common mission of improving child health.

The collaboration did not stop at the point of sharing speakers and committee appointments. Over the next 12 years, the SPP and AAP joined forces on a number of important advocacy and policy initiatives. The SPP was part of a multiorganizational consensus conference on insurance reimbursement and children's access to mental health services (AAP, 2000). SPP participation on AAP committees led to collaboration on more than 17 AAP policy statements and task force reports. These included a statement on parental discipline (AAP COPACFH, 1998); a statement on coping with terror and disaster (AAP COPACFH, 1999); the revision of the "new morbidity" statement (AAP COPACFH, 2001a); a joint statement on assessment and treatment of pain in children, featuring an additional collaboration between the AAP and the American Pain Society (AAP COPACFH & American Pain Society Task Force, 2001); and a much-publicized statement on coparent adoption (AAP COPACFH, 2002). Further evidence of the level of comfort with collaboration was the inclusion of the SPP representative on policy statements typically not associated with behavioral health, such as the prenatal visit (AAP COPACFH, 2001b).

Again, the steps taken by the SPP and the AAP serve as a model for organizational collaboration. Reciprocal relationships were established, and advocacy for children became a centerpiece of the collaborative effort. Clearly, the shared mission of the two organizations was enhanced by this collaboration. Pediatricians and psychologists became highly aware of the benefits of collaboration, not only on organization committees, but in hospitals and outpatient settings in the community. Collaborative practice models emerged in a number of communities (Foy & Earls, 2005). Pediatric psychologists also assumed leadership roles in traditionally physician-led training, research, and clinical programs in clinical pediatric departments, centers, and medical schools.

Clearly, the benefits to each organization have proved to be substantial and long-lasting. Most importantly, the benefit of a shared mission has led to stronger advocacy positions on behalf of children.

Advocacy Out of Collaboration

As a result of these collaborative efforts, pediatric psychologists began to be included in substantial advocacy initiatives alongside their pediatrician colleagues outside the structure of the AAP–SPP relationship. In February 1999, representatives from the SPP were invited to join the APA president, the AAP president, and the director of the National Institute of Mental Health (NIMH) for a planning initiative at NIMH on research to provide mental health services to young children in the pediatric medical home. The SPP was also asked to provide representation on the AAP's Task Force on the Family, which resulted in a seminal publication highlighting the diversity of families and their influence on children (AAP, 2003). In addition, the SPP participated in the American Cancer Society-sponsored summit to develop a national plan for the care of children with cancer (American Cancer Society, 2002), and was asked to provide commentary to the Institute of Medicine of the National Academy of Sciences (Armstrong, 2001) on death and dying issues for children (Field & Behrman, 2003). The outcomes of these collaborative advocacy efforts have included changes in state laws related to adoption by gay and lesbian parents, modifications in reimbursement for hospice care of children, and enactment of the Caroline Pryce Walker Conquer Childhood Cancer Act in 2008.

The organizational collaboration between the SPP and the AAP began in a conventional manner, with representation on one another's committees, reciprocal speaking engagements, and shared policy initiatives. Over time, strong relationships have permeated the leadership of departments of pediatrics in medical schools and hospitals; led to innovative programs of child health care in community settings; and resulted in integrated training programs for pediatricians and psychologists in residency, internship, and fellowship settings. Above all, the collaboration between the SPP and the AAP made it possible for the two organizations to speak in a combined voice on behalf of children, and in the process, to influence policy that affects children's lives.

Conclusions and Implications

Collaboration—whether among individuals involved in clinical, research, or educational activities, or among large organizations with different perspectives and memberships—represents a unique opportunity both to carry out a mission and to benefit the individuals or the organizations. Pediatric psychology has grown as a field, and the SPP has grown as an organization, because of the willingness of individuals and the organization to collaborate with other individuals and organizations in related fields. As a result, clinical care has improved; research not possible by individuals is successfully performed; and trainees learn to build integrated "medical homes" that benefit their communities. There are many pitfalls to collaboration, not the least of which is the possible loss of a professional's or professional organization's unique identity. However, there is evidence that loss of a unique identity within the context of a collaborative relationship can be transformative, with the resulting new identity being one that elevates the individual's and organization's contribution to the mission of improving the lives of children.

Health care in the United States is very likely to change in the coming decades. Advances in genetics and genomics, combined with new approaches to health care financing, reimbursement, and access, will change the way that most professions (not just psychology) are practiced. Multidisciplinary, interdisciplinary, and transdisciplinary clinical and translational models are being developed and tested, and are a predominant focus of research at the NIH. As these research models emphasize collaboration, clinical approaches are certain to do the same. The field's strong history of collaboration and development of clinical, research, and advocacy models positions pediatric psychologists to adapt and lead as new challenges and opportunities emerge.

Acknowledgments

Preparation of this chapter was supported in part by grants from the Maternal and Child Health Bureau (No. MCJ-129147-05-05), the Administration on Developmental Disabilities (No. 90DD0408), Children's Medical Services of the Florida Department of Health (No. C0Q03), and the National Heart, Lung, and Blood Institute (No. 1U54HL090569-01).

References

American Academy of Pediatrics (AAP). (2000). Policy statement: Insurance coverage of mental health and substance abuse services for children and adolescents: A consensus statement. *Pediatrics, 106,* 860–862.

American Academy of Pediatrics (AAP). (2003). Family pediatrics: Report of the Task Force on the Family. *Pediatrics, 111,* 1541–1571.

American Academy of Pediatrics (AAP), Committee on Psychosocial Aspects of Child and Family Health (COPACFH). (1998). Policy statement: Guidance for effective discipline. *Pediatrics, 101,* 723–728.

American Academy of Pediatrics (AAP), Committee on Psychosocial Aspects of Child and Family Health (COPACFH). (1999). Policy statement: How pediatricians can respond to the psychosocial implications of disasters. *Pediatrics, 103,* 521–523.

American Academy of Pediatrics (AAP), Committee on Psychosocial Aspects of Child and Family Health (COPACFH). (2001a). Policy statement: The new morbidity revisited: A renewed commitment to the psychosocial aspects of pediatric care. *Pediatrics, 108,* 1227–1230.

American Academy of Pediatrics (AAP), Committee on Psychosocial Aspects of Child and Family Health (COPACFH). (2001b). Policy statement: The prenatal visit. *Pediatrics, 107,* 1456–1458.

American Academy of Pediatrics (AAP), Committee on Psychosocial Aspects of Child and Family Health (COPACFH). (2002). Policy statement: Co-parent or second-parent adoption by same-sex parents. *Pediatrics, 109,* 339–340.

American Academy of Pediatrics (AAP), Committee on Psychosocial Aspects of Child and Family Health (COPACFH), & American Pain Society, Task Force on Pain in Infants, Children, and Adolescents. (2001). Policy statement: The assessment and management of acute pain in infants, children, and adolescents. *Pediatrics, 108,* 793–797.

American Cancer Society. (2002). *National action plan for childhood cancer: Report of the National Summit Meetings on Childhood Cancer.* Atlanta, GA: Author.

Armstrong, F. D. (1998). American Academy of Pediatrics president addresses SPP at APA. *SPP Progress Notes, 22*, 13, 21.

Armstrong, F. D. (2001). Invited statement, Society of Pediatric Psychology, Division 54, American Psychological Association to Institute of Medicine, National Academies of Sciences: Care of children who are dying, and their families. *SPP Progress Notes, 25*(3), 9–10.

Armstrong, F. D. (2006). Neurodevelopment and chronic illness: Mechanisms of disease and treatment. *Mental Retardation and Developmental Disabilities Research Reviews, 12*, 168–173.

Armstrong, F. D., & Drotar, D. (2000). Multi-institutional and multi-disciplinary research collaboration: Strategies and lessons from cooperative trials. In D. Drotar (Ed.), *Handbook of research in pediatric and clinical child psychology: Practical strategies and methods* (pp. 281–303). New York: Kluwer Academic/Plenum Press.

Armstrong, F. D., & Reaman, G. H. (2005). Psychological research in childhood cancer: The Children's Oncology Group perspective. *Journal of Pediatric Psychology, 30*, 89–97.

Bailey, D. B., Armstrong, F. D., Kemper, A. R., Skinner, D., & Warren, S. F. (2008). Supporting family adaptation to presymptomatic and "untreatable" conditions in an era of expanded newborn screening. *Journal of Pediatric Psychology*, DOI: 10.1093/jpepsy/jsn032.

Diabetes Control and Complications Trial Research Group. (1993). The effect of intensive treatment of diabetes on the development and progression of long-term complications in insulin-dependent diabetes mellitus. *New England Journal of Medicine, 329*, 977–986.

Farber, M. D., Koshy, M., & Kinney, T. R. (1985). Cooperative Study of Sickle Cell Disease: Demographic and socioeconomic characteristics of patients and families with sickle cell disease. *Journal of Chronic Diseases, 38*, 495–505.

Field, M. J., & Behrman, R. E. (Eds.). (2003). *When children die: Improving palliative and end-of-life care for children and their families.* Washington, DC: National Academy Press.

Foy, J. M., & Earls, M. E. (2005). A process for developing community consensus regarding the diagnosis and management of attention-deficit/hyperactivity disorder. *Pediatrics, 115*, e97–e104.

Grant, M., Economou, D., Ferrell, B., & Bhatia, S. (2007). Preparing professional staff to care for cancer survivors. *Journal of Cancer Survivorship, 1*, 98–106.

Guralnick, M. J. (2000). Interdisciplinary assessment for young children. In M. J. Gurlanick (Ed.), *Interdisciplinary clinical assessment of young children with developmental disabilities* (pp. 3–15). Baltimore: Brookes.

Kazak, A. E., Rourke, M. T., Alderfer, M. A., Pai, A., Reilly, A. F., & Meadows, A. T. (2007). Evidence-based assessment, intervention and psychosocial care in pediatric oncology: A blueprint for comprehensive services across treatment. *Journal of Pediatric Psychology, 32*, 1099–1110.

Maternal and Child Health Bureau. (2008). MCH training program: Our goals. Retrieved March 10, 2009, from *mchb.hrsa.gov/training/goals_interpractice.asp*

National Institutes of Health (NIH). (2008). NIH Roadmap for Medical Research: Interdisciplinary research. Retrieved March 9, 2009, from *nihroadmap.nih.gov/interdisciplinary*

Pediatric HIV/AIDS Cohort Study. (2008). Overview. Retrieved March 9, 2009, from *phacs. nichdclinicalstudies.org/overview.asp*

Rosendorf, L. L., Dafni, U., Amato, D. A., Lunghofer, B., Bartlett, J. G., Leedom, J. M., et al. (1993). Performance evaluation in multi-center clinical trials: Development of a model by the AIDS Clinical Trials Group. *Controlled Clinical Trials, 14*, 523–537.

Society of Pediatric Psychology (SPP). (2008). *Mission statement: Who we are.* Retrieved from *www.societyofpediatricpsychology.org/~division54/who/index.shtml*

Tsao, J. C., & Zeltzer, L. K. (2008). Commentary: Evidence-based assessment of pediatric pain. *Journal of Pediatric Psychology, 33*, 956–957.

Uman, L. S., Chambers, C. T., McGrath, P. J., & Kisely, S. (2008). A systematic review of randomized controlled trials examining psychological interventions for needle-related procedural pain and distress in children and adolescents. An abbreviated Cochrane review. *Journal of Pediatric Psychology, 33*, 842–854.

Whitsett, S. F., Armstrong, F. D., & Pollock, B. H. (2006). Research opportunities and collaborative multi-site studies in psychosocial hematology/oncology. In R. T. Brown (Ed.), *Pediatric hematology/oncology: A biopsychosocial approach* (pp. 547–556). New York: Oxford University Press.

Index